EIGHTH EDITION

Fitness Professional's Handbook

Barbara Bushman, PhD, FACSM

Editor

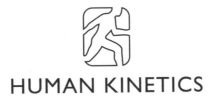

HUMAN KINETICS

Library of Congress Cataloging-in-Publication Data

Names: Bushman, Barbara, editor. | Howley, Edward T., 1943- Fitness professional's handbook.

Title: Fitness professional's handbook / Barbara Bushman, PhD, FACSM, editor.

Description: Eighth edition. | Champaign, IL : Human Kinetics, [2025] | Seventh edition published in 2017. | Includes bibliographical references and index.

Identifiers: LCCN 2023020116 (print) | LCCN 2023020117 (ebook) | ISBN 9781718217829 (print : alk. paper) | ISBN 9781718217836 (epub) | ISBN 9781718217843 (pdf)

Subjects: LCSH: Physical fitness--Handbooks, manuals, etc. | Physical fitness--Testing--Handbooks, manuals, etc. | Exercise--Physiological aspects--Handbooks, manuals, etc. | Health. | Health behavior. | Nutrition.

Classification: LCC GV481 .H734 2025 (print) | LCC GV481 (ebook) | DDC 613.7--dc23/eng/20230518

LC record available at https://lccn.loc.gov/2023020116

LC ebook record available at https://lccn.loc.gov/2023020117

ISBN: 978-1-7182-1782-9 (print)

Senior Acquisitions Editor: Michelle Earle; **Managing Editor:** Hannah Werner; **Copyeditor:** Marissa Wold Uhrina; **Proofreader:** Leigh Keylock; **Indexer:** Beth Nauman-Montana; **Permissions Manager:** Laurel Mitchell; **Graphic Designer:** Dawn Sills; **Cover Designer:** Keri Evans; **Cover Design Specialist:** Susan Rothermel Allen; **Cover Graphic:** DrPixel/Moment/Getty Images; **Photographs:** © Human Kinetics, unless otherwise noted; **Photo Asset Manager:** Laura Fitch; **Photo Production Specialist:** Amy M. Rose; **Photo Production Manager:** Jason Allen; **Senior Art Manager:** Kelly Hendren; **Illustrations:** © Human Kinetics, unless otherwise noted; **Printer:** Premier Print Group

Printed in the United States of America   10 9 8 7 6 5 4 3 2 1

Human Kinetics
1607 N. Market Street
Champaign, IL 61820
USA

United States and International
Website: **US.HumanKinetics.com**
Email: info@hkusa.com
Phone: 1-800-747-4457

Canada
Website: **Canada.HumanKinetics.com**
Email: info@hkcanada.com

E8928

To Tobin, for always encouraging me in all my adventures. Words cannot convey how much your love and support mean to me. Thankful to God for bringing us together over 30 years ago at the university natatorium when I was an injured runner doing deep water run training and you were a lifeguard at the pool. Forever and always, we are Team Bushman.

And to my family, by birth and through marriage, for being such a blessing in my life. A special dedication to my father-in-law, Ed, and my dad, Ken, who both passed away during the time span when I was working on this book. To Dad, for a lifetime of encouragement and for asking me so often how this project was coming along, I really wish you could have seen the completed book.

—*Barbara Bushman*

CONTENTS

PREFACE

You can make a difference. For many of us, an underlying goal when making career decisions is to have a positive impact on others. What area of life is more important than health? The term *healthspan* has been used to reflect the years of healthy living without being hampered by diseases. To promote good health, the value of moving more is firmly supported by research. The evidence that regular physical activity and structured exercise are good for health and fitness is overwhelming—and is a theme running throughout this book. Fitness professionals are uniquely qualified to help individuals, as well as whole communities, develop the habit of exercise in order to reap the benefits of improved physical fitness and prevention of (or treatment for) chronic diseases. Fitness professionals can make a real difference! In this role, being knowledgeable and current with information in the field is key, with the understanding that this will take an ongoing commitment as new research leads to updated recommendations and guidelines. This text will help you learn the foundational information that fitness professionals need. You will learn how to screen participants for exercise programs, evaluate the various components of fitness, and prescribe exercise to improve each fitness component. In addition, you will learn how to promote safe and effective exercise programs in various situations. Throughout the book you will become familiar with guidelines from governmental sources (e.g., *Physical Activity Guidelines for Americans*) as well as professional organizations (e.g., American College of Sports Medicine); organizations regularly release updates that will become resources in your ongoing quest to remain current. Rather than being daunting, the constant growth in knowledge is an exciting aspect of our field.

Updates to the Eighth Edition

At regular intervals, professional societies, such as the American College of Sports Medicine (ACSM) and the American Heart Association (AHA), and government agencies, such as the United States Department of Health and Human Services, update physical activity recommendations for the general public and for special segments of the population such as older adults and people with chronic diseases. This book reflects the latest information that will help you help others. Regardless of whether you pursue a career in the fitness industry or in an allied health field, you will find the information in this textbook valuable as you build your professional skill set.

In this edition of the text, some reorganization of topics has occurred to enhance the presentation of content, and each chapter has been updated based on available standards, guidelines, and research. Additional case studies, application points, and research insights have been added throughout the book to deepen your knowledge and understanding of the information. Two new chapters provide an overview of assessment and considerations for comprehensive program design. The pharmacology content previously found in various chapters has been pulled together in one extended feature that will serve as a helpful resource on the impact that various medications have on the body's responses to physical activity. Here is a snapshot of each chapter:

- Chapter 1, Health and Fitness Benefits of Physical Activity and Exercise, discusses the current physical activity guidelines within a framework of how recommendations have evolved over time. It updates the leading causes of death, introduces the concern with sedentary behavior even for those who meet physical activity guidelines, and explores the value of fitness for future health outcomes.

- Chapter 2, Preparticipation Screening, includes the revised Physical Activity Readiness Questionnaire for Everyone (PAR-Q+) and Pre-Activity Screening Questionnaire (PASQ) as well as an example of a health screening questionnaire (HSQ). ACSM's preparticipation health screening process is described in detail, including how to determine if medical clearance is recommended, and considerations for determining if a referral to a supervised program is necessary. A key new feature in this edition is a dedicated section on pharmacology that covers major drug categories, including how medications may affect heart rate, blood pressure, and the response to exercise.

- Chapter 3, Anatomy in Action: Functional Movement, includes information on bones and joints, muscle groups, and exercise tips by region of the body. In addition, muscle involvement in selected activities has been combined with common mechanical errors to emphasize interrelationships between them. A new case study demonstrates how knowledge of musculoskeletal anatomy, biomechanics, and joint torque come together to answer a practical question.

- Chapter 4, Physiology in Action: Exercise Physiology, presents information on aerobic and anaerobic energy production, factors affecting aerobic exercise and the responses to training, skeletal muscle structure and muscle contraction, adaptations within the neuromuscular system to improve muscular fitness, and impacts of environmental conditions.

- Chapter 5, Fueling for Activity: Dietary Considerations, provides updated information on the *2020-2025 Dietary Guidelines for Americans* and insights on evaluation of ergogenic aids. New content on scope of practice is provided to help fitness professionals understand when referral is needed.

- Chapter 6, Energy Costs of Physical Activity, includes background on how to estimate the energy cost of activities. Examples throughout the chapter provide step-by-step guidance so you can clearly see how to complete the calculations. Steps on how to use the Compendium of Physical Activities will allow for estimation of energy cost of a wide variety of activities. Information on wearable technology to track energy expenditure has been updated.

- Chapter 7, Overview of Assessment, is a new chapter to this edition and provides the foundation for the assessment chapters in this part of the book. This chapter explains how to maximize accuracy and develop a logical sequence for fitness testing. Key aspects of informed consent and procedures to maximize safety are included. Of particular importance is discussion of how to explain test results to clients in a way that is meaningful and relevant.

- Chapter 8, Cardiorespiratory Fitness Assessments, provides considerations related to the type of testing used to evaluate aerobic fitness as well as the mode of exercise used. Discussion of how to maximize accuracy in measurements of heart rate and blood pressure is provided. Examples of submaximal, maximal, and field tests are included. In addition, content related to tests for youth and older adults has been added.

- Chapter 9, Muscular Fitness Assessments, includes various methods of assessing muscular fitness (new to this edition are handgrip strength tests and vertical jump) and how to interpret test results. Content related to tests for youth and older adults, as well as considerations for clients with cardiovascular disease, is included.

- Chapter 10, Flexibility and Neuromotor Fitness Assessments, includes updated information related to flexibility and new content on neuromotor fitness. This chapter covers factors that influence flexibility and neuromotor fitness as well as assessments for each.

- Chapter 11, Body Composition Assessments, discusses potential concerns related to obesity and disease risk. Assessments ranging from simple measures such as waist circumference to more complex measures that might be used in research settings are discussed. Specific guidance on increasing accuracy of all measurements is included, particularly for skinfolds, which can provide insights on composition with careful site determination and techniques.

- Chapter 12, Electrocardiogram (ECG) Assessment, retains the valuable background, basic rhythms, and ECG changes with myocardial infarction from prior editions while expanding content related to angina pectoris.

- Chapter 13, Exercise Prescription for Aerobic Fitness, discusses the optimal exercise dose associated with health outcomes and the importance of progression and safety in an exercise prescription. A new section on how to use metabolic calculations within an exercise prescription has been added, expanding on content introduced in chapter 6. New content related to high-intensity interval training is included as well as updates to the section on environmental impacts on exercise prescription.

- Chapter 14, Exercise Prescription for Muscular Fitness, includes an expanded section on the health-related benefits of resistance training and several new research insights. Material throughout has been updated to reflect the most current guidelines and recommendations.

- Chapter 15, Exercise Prescription for Flexibility and Neuromotor Fitness, includes considerations for both flexibility and neuromotor fitness in relation to day-to-day function, safety when being physically active, and avoiding low-back pain. New to this edition is the coverage of neuromotor fitness, including examples of activities.

- Chapter 16, Putting Together a Comprehensive Program, is a new chapter that discusses how to pull all the various components into a complete exercise program for a client. Training principles are discussed, with a focus on providing appropriate programs for the client's status and goals. Expanded discussion on developing the optimal training stimulus and balancing activity level with nutritional requirements will help fitness professionals optimize outcomes *and* safety for clients.

- Chapter 17, Youth, has been extensively updated to reflect public health physical activity guidelines for youth, an area of importance given some trends in youth physical activity. Program design that integrates health- and skill-related physical fitness is discussed along with strategies to promote ongoing participation.

- Chapter 18, Older Adults, expands the discussion on the influence of exercise on changes in cardiorespiratory fitness and muscle mass with age. A complete exercise program is emphasized including aerobic and muscular fitness as well as flexibility and neuromotor fitness.

- Chapter 19, Pregnancy, is now a separate chapter, and thus content has been expanded, with discussion of the benefits of physical activity and exercise during pregnancy. With a focus on promoting safety, new screening tools, a discussion of contraindications for exercise, and signs and symptoms that warrant stopping exercise are included. General recommendations on physical activity for healthy women during pregnancy and postpartum are provided, along with new content on pelvic floor training.

• Chapter 20, Weight Management, is a newly organized chapter that includes a discussion of obesity and the role energy balance plays in weight management. Healthy guidelines for both losing weight and gaining weight are provided. Insights on eating disorders, including recognition of the signs, are discussed.

• Chapter 21, Chronic Diseases, is a new chapter that includes updated topic areas from the prior edition on cardiovascular disease, pulmonary disease, diabetes, and osteoporosis, as well as new content on cancer.

• Chapter 22, Behavior Modification, emphasizes both the transtheoretical model of behavior change and self-determination theory. Examples and strategies to facilitate behavior change and enhance motivation for physical activity will be beneficial in understanding how to apply the theories when interacting with clients. Additional insights on the impact of the environment are included.

• Chapter 23, Injury Prevention and Management, provides detailed information on the development of emergency action plans as well as providing acute care for injuries. Various conditions are discussed including delayed-onset muscle soreness, exertional rhabdomyolysis, community-associated methicillin-resistant *Staphylococcus aureus*, sickle cell trait, and traumatic brain injury. New content using the 50/30/20/10 rule for conditioning and the FIT rule for strength training is provided related to safe return to activity.

• Chapter 24, Legal Considerations, provides updates on injury data and a more detailed description of the professional standard of care and scope of practice. New case law examples on risk management have been included throughout the chapter.

Although many updates have been made throughout the book, former users of the text will be comfortable with this new edition. The text continues to reference *ACSM's Guidelines for Exercise Testing and Prescription* as a valuable source of standards and expectations for fitness professionals in addition to other position statements and stands as well as current research articles. The text is helpful for those interested in taking certification exams (e.g., ACSM) as well as serving as a reference for fitness professionals in the field. Study questions at the end of each chapter help with review of the content. This edition also includes interesting sidebars, useful key points, case study questions and answers, a glossary, and extensive references, making it a useful textbook for students as well as a valuable reference for practitioners.

Intended Audience

This text continues to be written for the upper-level undergraduate or beginning graduate student with a general background in anatomy and physiology. The purpose of the text is to provide information required in the areas of fitness testing and prescription to screen participants, carry out standardized fitness tests to evaluate the major components of fitness, and write appropriate exercise prescriptions. Many academic programs incorporate laboratory experiences to drive the mastery of skills needed to accomplish these tasks. In that way, the class is not simply an academic experience but one that allows a person to move into practicum or internship experiences with the requisite skills and abilities. This text will work seamlessly with most laboratory experiences associated with fitness assessment because of its attention to detail regarding the most common fitness tests, from pretest concerns to careful evaluation of results.

Text Organization

Part I, Physical Activity and Exercise: Realizing Benefits and Maximizing Safety, contains two chapters that provide an overview of the connections among health and fitness, general information to set up the remainder of the text, and a step-by-step approach to screening participants for fitness programs.

Part II, Foundations, covers basic anatomy, biomechanics, and exercise physiology, useful for a quick review. In addition, chapters are provided on nutrition assessment and how to evaluate the caloric cost of activity, both of which are central to energy balance.

Part III, Fitness Assessments, provides extensive detail on how to assess cardiorespiratory fitness, muscular fitness, flexibility and neuromotor fitness, and body composition. In addition, a chapter on ECG provides helpful background information on this valuable assessment of cardiac function.

Part IV, Exercise Prescription, provides a separate chapter on how to deal with the test results for each of the fitness components assessed in part III, and it describes how to formulate an exercise prescription consistent with a client's goals and abilities. A new chapter provides examples of progression for beginner, intermediate, and established exercisers.

Part V, Special Populations and Conditions, provides chapters on exercise testing and prescription for the following: youth; older adults; pregnant women; and people with cardiovascular disease, pulmonary disease, diabetes, cancer, and osteoporosis. In addition, a chapter devoted to weight management is included.

Part VI, Exercise Programming Considerations, includes chapters on scientific approaches to changing behavior, injury prevention and management, and legal considerations.

Special Features in the Eighth Edition

Many items in the textbook will help you identify and retain key information.

- *Objectives* quickly outline the main points of the chapter and highlight the learning goals for the topics covered.
- *Key Points* summarize important facts.
- *Glossary* definitions are provided at the end of the book for reference on key terms.
- *Research Insight* boxes cover important research topics for each chapter. Additional highlight boxes on special topics and tips can be found in each chapter as well.
- *Application Point* boxes provide connections between content and aspects of training.
- *Case Studies* within the chapters, written by experts in their fields, provide examples of application of content.
- *Procedures* for common fitness tests are highlighted so that they are easy to find and use.
- *Review Questions* covering important material are included at the end of every chapter.
- *Practice Case Studies* at the end of the chapters let readers apply the concepts covered in the chapter. Answers to these case studies are provided so that readers can quickly check their responses.
- *Video* icons let readers know when a demonstration is available on a topic.
- *References* are numbered and organized by chapter at the end of the book. These resources will help the reader discover additional sources of information.

HK*Propel* Online Content

A valuable feature of this text for students is HK*Propel*, which includes 25 video clips that correspond to key techniques covered in the book. (Note: You must have an Internet connection in order to view this streaming video content.) See the card at the front of the print book for your unique HK*Propel* access code. For ebook users, reference the HK*Propel* access code instructions on the page immediately following the book cover.

When a demonstration is available on a topic, you will see a video icon that looks like this:

To view the videos, log in to HK*Propel*. The video numbers along the right side of the video players correspond with video number cross-references in the book, and the title under the player corresponds with the exercise or procedure title in the book. Scroll through the list of clips until you find the video you want to watch. Select that clip and the full video will play.

Instructor Resources

In addition to the thoroughly updated content, this edition also offers several instructor resources to aid in teaching a class with this textbook:

- The updated *instructor guide* includes a syllabus; a course outline that details lecture topics and lab and classroom activities; practical exam checklists for students and instructors; and a lab assignment grading sheet for use by instructors.
- The *test package* includes 720 questions, including true-false, fill-in-the-blank, multiple-choice, multiple-response, and essay questions. The questions have been updated to reflect the new content added to the text. Instructors may also create their own customized quizzes or tests from the test bank questions to assign to students directly through HK*Propel*. Multiple-choice and true-false questions are automatically graded, and instructors can easily review student scores in the platform.
- The Microsoft PowerPoint *presentation package* contains over 800 slides that present the textbook material in a lecture-friendly format, including art, photos, and tables pulled from the text as well as tables and figures that are unique to the PowerPoint.
- The *image bank* contains most of the art, tables, and content photos. Instructors may use the art, tables, and photos to create class presentations.
- The ready-made *chapter quizzes* are learning management system (LMS) compatible and can be used to measure student learning of the most important concepts for each chapter. They include 240 questions in multiple-choice and true-false formats. Each quiz may also be downloaded or assigned to students within HK*Propel*. The chapter quizzes are automatically graded, with scores available for review in the platform.

ACKNOWLEDGMENTS

The founding editors, Dr. Ed Howley and Dr. Don Franks, along with editor Dr. Dixie Thompson, have developed this amazing textbook focused on encouraging the next generation of fitness professionals who are knowledgeable and effective. Since the first edition in 1986, this textbook has been updated and expanded as new developments and discoveries advance the field. I want to express my deep gratitude for their tireless efforts over the years and for their support in continuing the legacy of this book with the current edition.

Many wonderful authors have contributed to this textbook. Their passion for the content, along with their ability to organize and present crucial information in a user-friendly way to help fitness professionals move forward in their careers, is foundational to the ongoing success of this book. First, I would like to recognize and thank the following people for their contributions to previous editions:

David R. Bassett Jr., PhD
Sue Carver, ATC, MPT, CMT
Scott A. Conger, PhD
Laura Horvath Gagnon, PT, DPT, PhD, OCS, IMT
Ralph La Forge, MS
Jean Lewis, EdD (deceased)
Wendell Liemohn, PhD
Kyle McInnis, ScD
Michael Shipe, PhD, RCEP

Second, I want to express my deep gratitude to the individuals who have authored or revised chapters or developed case studies for this current edition. Their dedication to their respective specialty areas and willingness to contribute to this textbook have been pivotal in providing significant updates and new features throughout the book. I am so grateful for their involvement and encourage readers to review the About the Contributors and About the Case Study Contributors sections for background on these amazing professionals.

Physical Activity and Exercise: Realizing Benefits and Maximizing Safety

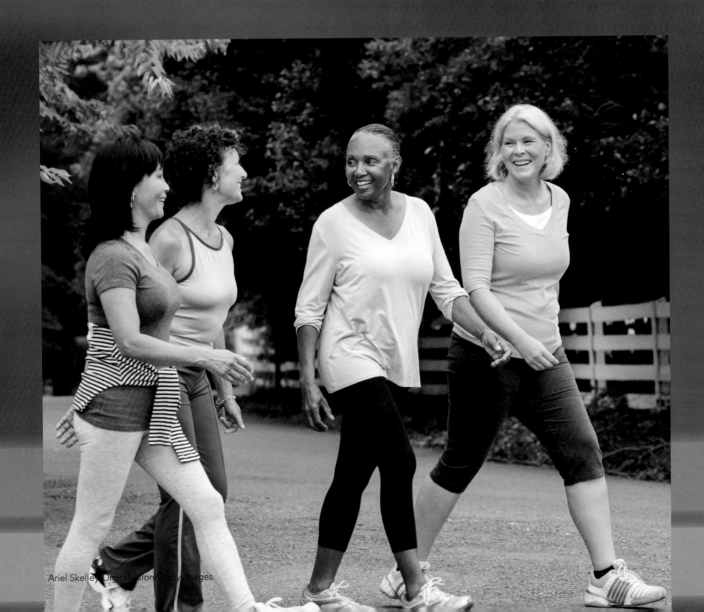

Physical activity is an essential element of health and well-being. With that in mind, this book is written for current and future fitness professionals who help individuals, communities, and groups gain the benefits of regular physical activity in a positive and safe environment.

The chapters of part I provide the background underlying the study of physical activity and its relevance to fitness. In chapter 1, the current evidence regarding physical activity and health is summarized, and insights are provided into the connections between health and fitness. In chapter 2, a process for screening potential fitness participants, criteria for medical referrals, and suggestions on the development of supervised and unsupervised programs are provided.

Health and Fitness Benefits of Physical Activity and Exercise

Barbara A. Bushman

OBJECTIVES

The reader will be able to do the following:

1. Contrast the physical activity requirements for achieving health benefits, fitness, and performance
2. Describe the difference between lifespan and healthspan
3. Compare the leading causes of death with the most common behavioral factors that lead to early death
4. Define common terms used in the field of exercise science, including physical activity, exercise, and physical fitness
5. Describe the difference between absolute and relative intensity for physical activity
6. Explain the difference between moderate-intensity and vigorous-intensity physical activity, and how volume of physical activity is calculated
7. List the health-related benefits gained through regular participation in physical activity and exercise, including activities that focus on aerobic and muscular fitness
8. Contrast the changes in physical activity guidelines over the past 50 years in terms of exercise volume, intensity, and outcomes
9. Describe the physical activity recommendations for realizing substantial health benefits provided in the *Physical Activity Guidelines for Americans*, 2nd edition
10. Describe recommendations related to physical activity to lose weight or to maintain weight loss
11. Define *adverse events*, and explain how the potential for such events affects the intensity of physical activity recommended for those who have been sedentary
12. Explain why lack of physical activity and low levels of fitness are more important to address than being overweight as far as the risk of chronic disease is concerned
13. Describe the difference between health-related fitness and performance-related fitness
14. Describe the continuum of physical activity recommendations for realizing health, fitness, and performance goals

Throughout this text the question of "How much exercise is enough?" is addressed. The answer requires an understanding of "Enough for what?" In other words, what is the client's goal? Is it fitness, performance, or avoidance of disease? Exercise recommendations usually describe the frequency (number of days per week), intensity (strenuousness of the activity), and duration (time) of activity in each session. As figure 1.1 shows, the frequency (F), intensity (I), time (T), and type (T) of activity vary depending on the goal. On the left side of the figure, avoidance of disease (e.g., lowering the risk of heart disease or type 2 diabetes) can be achieved with moderate-intensity activity done 30 minutes per day, 5 days per week. To achieve cardiorespiratory fitness (CRF), as well as the health benefits associated with moderate-intensity physical activity, vigorous (hard) exercise is done 3 to 4 days per week, 30 to 45 minutes per day, which is equivalent to running about 3 miles (5 kilometers) 3 to 4 days per week. What about those who want to be elite marathon runners? In contrast to the previous two examples, elite marathon runners work at the extreme end of the intensity scale (very hard) for hours every day.

This text focuses on the amount of physical activity and exercise needed for health and fitness rather than on the performance of elite athletes. However, the information on nutrition, CRF, body composition, strength, and flexibility forms the foundation for those who want to achieve performance-related goals, and will therefore be helpful for those training for performance as well. In this chapter the focus is on how physical activity is connected to health and fitness. Later chapters provide more extensive detail about how to help sedentary people become active and active people become more fit.

Health and Avoidance of Disease

What does being healthy mean? For some it is the simple avoidance of disease, but it is also more than that. Health has been defined as a "state of complete physical, mental, and social well-being and not merely the absence of disease or infirmity" (46). Positive health is associated with one's capacity to enjoy life and withstand challenges. Negative health is associated with morbidity (incidence of disease) and premature mortality (40). While *lifespan* simply reflects the number of days of one's life without consideration of quality of life, *healthspan* reflects positive health and has been defined as "the number of years an individual is healthy and free from debilitating disease" (7). Factors associated with healthspan include being physically active, consuming nutritious foods, not smoking, and maintaining a healthy body weight (7). The highest quality of life includes mental alertness and curiosity, positive emotional feelings, meaningful relationships with others, awareness and involvement in societal strivings, recognition of the broader forces of life, and the physical capacity to accomplish personal goals with vigor. Although physical activity plays a major role in the physical dimension, it also contributes to learning, relationships, and a sense of limitations when confronting environmental challenges. An optimal quality of life requires individuals to strive, grow, and develop, even if never reaching the highest level of positive health. So, what are the risks or challenges to health and well-being?

Factors Affecting Health and Disease

The leading causes of death describe the specific diseases and situations linked to dying. In 2019, the top seven

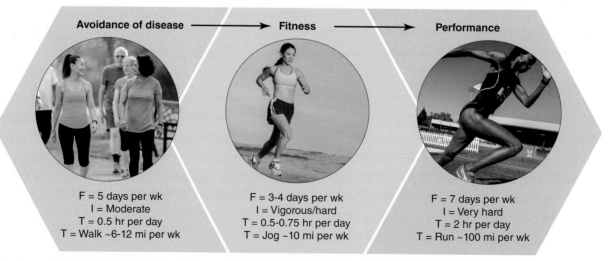

Avoidance of disease → Fitness → Performance

F = 5 days per wk
I = Moderate
T = 0.5 hr per day
T = Walk ~6-12 mi per wk

F = 3-4 days per wk
I = Vigorous/hard
T = 0.5-0.75 hr per day
T = Jog ~10 mi per wk

F = 7 days per wk
I = Very hard
T = 2 hr per day
T = Run ~100 mi per wk

FIGURE 1.1   How much physical activity is enough? FITT reflects frequency, intensity, time, and type.
Photo on far left: FatCamera/E+/Getty Images

leading causes of death were heart disease (23.1%), malignant neoplasms (cancers) (21.0%), accidents (unintentional injuries) (6.1%), chronic lower respiratory diseases (5.5%), cerebrovascular diseases (stroke) (5.3%), Alzheimer's disease (4.3%), and diabetes mellitus (3.1%) (22). In 2020, COVID-19 entered the list as the third leading cause of death following heart disease and cancer, and above accidents, stroke, chronic lower respiratory disease, Alzheimer's disease, and diabetes (28). Most of the top seven leading causes of death are chronic degenerative diseases whose onset can be delayed or prevented. Risk factors associated with chronic diseases can be divided into three categories (see figure 1.2) (45).

Inherited or Biological Factors

These factors include the following:

- *Age:* Older adults have more chronic diseases than younger people.
- *Sex:* Men develop cardiovascular disease (CVD) at an earlier age than women, but women experience more strokes than men (6).
- *Race:* African Americans develop about 30% more heart disease than non-Hispanic white Americans (42).
- *Susceptibility to disease:* Several diseases have a genetic component that increases the potential for having them.

People can achieve health and fitness goals up to their genetic potential, but it is not possible to establish the relative portion of a person's health that is determined by heredity. Although heredity influences physical activity, fitness, and health (33), most people can lead healthy or unhealthy lives regardless of their genetic makeup. Thus, genetic background neither dooms a person to poor health nor guarantees good health.

Environment

Individuals are born not only with fixed genetic potentials but also into environments that affect development. An environment includes physical factors (e.g., climate, water, altitude, pollution), socioeconomic factors (e.g., income, housing, education, workplace), and family (e.g., parental values, divorce, extended family, friends) that affect opportunities to be active, levels of fitness, and health statuses. Some elements, such as nutrition or air quality, have a direct effect. Other elements, such as the values and behaviors of role models, have an indirect influence. When working with clients, it is important to understand many aspects of their past and current circumstances in order to help them make lifestyle changes.

Behaviors

Whereas the leading causes of death describe the diseases that kill, the *actual causes* of death describe behaviors that are linked to those diseases (see the right side of figure 1.2). Top behaviors include smoking, poor diet, physical inactivity, and alcohol as well as microbial and toxic agents and illicit drug use (32). Smoking has been a top actual cause of death for a long time (26, 27). That smoking is on the list should be no surprise given its connection to both lung cancer and CVD. The existence of smoking-cessation programs and laws restricting areas where people can smoke speak to the seriousness with which society takes that risk to health. Poor diet and physical inactivity, along with alcohol consumption, are other behavior choices that affect health. The emphasis on healthy eating at work and school and on the creation of new parks and bike trails to enhance opportunities to be physically active are examples of responses to these actual causes of death. Healthy eating and physical activity affect many factors that influence health and disease. Clearly, the ability to help clients establish and reinforce the behaviors of healthy eating and physical activity will

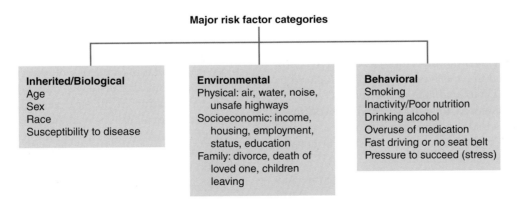

FIGURE 1.2 Major categories of risk factors with examples of each.

Adapted from "Healthy People," *The Surgeon General's Report on Health Promotion and Disease Prevention* (1979).

do much to improve their health and well-being. (See chapter 5 for information on nutrition and chapter 22 for steps to help clients change their behaviors.) This chapter introduces the role that physical activity and fitness play in a healthy lifestyle.

Important Definitions

The field of exercise science has many terms, so first it is helpful to establish a common framework for terminology to facilitate understanding of the various parts of an exercise prescription or physical activity recommendation (11, 39, 40, 41).

- *Physical activity* is defined as any bodily movement produced by skeletal muscle that results in energy expenditure. It is associated with occupation, leisure time, household chores, and sport.
- *Exercise* is a subset of physical activity that is planned, structured, and repetitive and has the objective of improving or maintaining physical fitness.
- *Physical fitness* refers to a set of health- or skill-related attributes that can be measured by specific tests.
- *Health-related fitness* refers to muscular strength and endurance, CRF, flexibility, and body composition.
- *Skill-related (performance-related) fitness* refers to agility, balance, coordination, speed, power, and reaction time.
- *Absolute intensity* describes the rate of work (i.e., how much energy is expended per minute) and can be expressed in a number of ways:
  - Kilocalories (kcal) of energy produced per minute ($kcal \cdot min^{-1}$)
  - Milliliters of oxygen consumed per kilogram of body weight per minute ($ml \cdot kg^{-1} \cdot min^{-1}$)
  - Metabolic equivalents (METs), where 1 MET is taken as resting metabolic rate (RMR) and is equal to $3.5 \ ml \cdot kg^{-1} \cdot min^{-1}$; exercise intensity is given as a multiple of the MET (e.g., 3 METs, 6 METs)
- *Relative intensity* describes the degree of effort required to expend energy and is influenced by CRF or maximal aerobic power ($\dot{V}O_2max$). A person with a CRF of 10 METs who is working at 6 METs is at a relative intensity of 60% $\dot{V}O_2max$ (6 METs ÷ 10 METs × 100). This will be covered in more detail in chapter 13.
- *Moderate intensity* refers to an absolute intensity of 3 to 5.9 METs and a relative intensity of 40% to 59% $\dot{V}O_2R$ or as a level 5 or 6 on a 10-point scale (with 10 being the highest level of activity).

- *Vigorous intensity* refers to an absolute intensity of 6 or more METs and a relative intensity of 60% to 89% $\dot{V}O_2R$ or as a level 7 or 8 on a 10-point scale (with 10 being the highest level of activity).
- *Frequency* refers to the number of days per week physical activity is done.
- *Duration* refers to the amount of time a physical activity is done.
- *Volume* refers to the total amount of energy expended, or work accomplished in an activity, and it is equal to the product of the absolute intensity, frequency, and time. For example, a person expending $5 \ kcal \cdot min^{-1}$ for 20 minutes on 3 days per week will have an exercise volume of $300 \ kcal \cdot wk^{-1}$ ($5 \ kcal \cdot min^{-1} \times 20$ minutes per day × 3 days per week). The volume can also be expressed using the MET scale: A 10 MET activity done 3 days per week for 20 minutes per day generates a volume of $600 \ MET\text{-}min \cdot wk^{-1}$ (10 METs × 3 days per week × 20 minutes per day).

Physical Activity and Health

From the beginning of recorded history, philosophers and health professionals have observed that regular physical activity is an essential part of a healthy life. Hippocrates wrote the following in *On Regimen in Acute Diseases*, in about 400 BC:

> . . . food and exercise, while possessing opposite qualities, yet . . . work together to produce health. . . . And it is necessary, as it appears, to discern the power of various exercises, both natural exercises and artificial, to know which of them tends to increase flesh and which to lessen it; and not only this, but also to proportion exercise to bulk of food, to the constitution of the patient, to the age of the individual . . . (24)

Over the past five decades, thousands of studies have examined the relationship between physical activity and the risk of various diseases and death. The overwhelming conclusion is that regular participation in physical activity results in a reduced risk of numerous diseases and of death from all causes. As shown in figure 1.3, regular participation in physical activity reduces the risk of death from all causes by about 40% (relative risk decreased from 1.0 to 0.6). Doing physical activity on a regular basis also has been shown to have a positive impact on the following (39, 41):

- *Cardiorespiratory health:* Physical activity reduces the risk of heart disease and stroke, lowers blood pressure (BP), improves the blood lipid profile, and increases CRF.

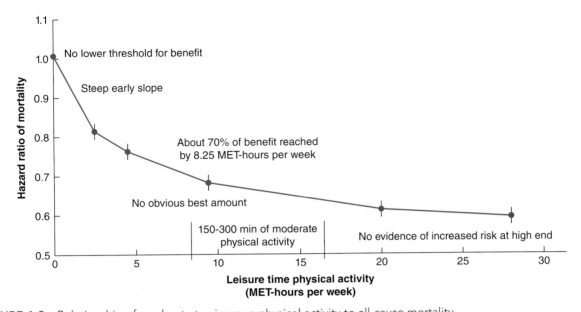

FIGURE 1.3 Relationship of moderate to vigorous physical activity to all-cause mortality.

Reprinted from U.S. Department of Health and Human Services, "Physical Activity Guidelines for Americans," 2nd ed. (Washington, DC: U.S. Department of Health and Human Services), 2018.

- *Metabolic health:* Physical activity reduces the risk of developing type 2 diabetes and helps control blood glucose in those who already have type 2 diabetes.
- *Musculoskeletal health:* Physical activity slows the loss of bone density that occurs with aging, and it lowers the risk of hip fractures. In addition, it improves pain management in people with arthritis. Finally, progressive muscle-strengthening activities increase or preserve muscle mass, strength, and power.
- *Cancer:* Physically active people have a lower risk of many cancers, including cancers of the bladder, breast, colon, endometrium, esophagus, kidney, lung, and stomach.
- *Brain health:* Physical activity lowers the risk of depression and age-related cognitive decline, reduces anxiety, and improves the quality of sleep. See figure 1.4 for insight on how physical activity is related to both acute and habitual (chronic) benefits on brain health.
- *Functional ability and fall prevention:* Physical activity reduces the risk of functional limitations (e.g., ability to do activities of daily living) and, for older adults, lowers the risk of falling and fall-related injuries.

Physical Activity Guidelines

Given the large number of benefits derived from participation in physical activity, it should be no surprise that professional societies such as the American College of Sports Medicine (ACSM), the American Heart Association (AHA), and various governmental agencies (e.g., Centers for Disease Control and Prevention [CDC]) have developed physical activity guidelines for the general public. The following paragraphs provide a brief overview of how the focus of these guidelines shifted from fitness to public health outcomes over the past 50 years.

Focus on Intensity

In the early and mid-1970s, three major organizations published guidelines or recommendations for improving fitness and health:

1. In 1972, the AHA published *Exercise Testing and Training of Apparently Healthy Individuals: A Handbook for Physicians* (5). The exercise prescription was to begin at a relative intensity of 60% $\dot{V}O_2$max for 15 to 20 minutes, 3 days per week.

2. In 1973, the YMCA published the first edition of *The Y's Way to Physical Fitness* (17). The exercise prescription was to exercise at 80% $\dot{V}O_2$max for 40 to 45 minutes, 3 days per week.

3. In 1975, ACSM published the first edition of *ACSM's Guidelines for Exercise Testing and Prescription* (1). The exercise prescription was to exercise at approximately 70% to 90% $\dot{V}O_2$max for 20 to 45 minutes, 3 to 5 days per week.

In each case the focus was on higher-intensity exercise, with both CRF and health outcomes being important.

Outcome	Population	Benefit	Acute	Habitual
Cognition	Children ages 6 to 13 years	Improved cognition (performance on academic achievement tests, executive function, processing speed, memory)	✔	✔
	Adults	Reduced risk of dementia (including Alzheimer's disease)		✔
	Adults older than age 50 years	Improved cognition (executive function, attention, memory, crystallized intelligence,* processing speed)		✔
Quality of life	Adults	Improved quality of life		✔
Depressed mood and depression	Children ages 6 to 17 years and adults	Reduced risk of depression Reduced depressed mood		✔
Anxiety	Adults	Reduced short-term feelings of anxiety (state anxiety)	✔	
	Adults	Reduced long-term feelings and signs of anxiety (trait anxiety) for people with and without anxiety disorders		✔
Sleep	Adults	Improved sleep outcomes (increased sleep efficiency, sleep quality, deep sleep; reduced daytime sleepiness, frequency of use of medication to aid sleep)		✔
	Adults	Improved sleep outcomes that increase with duration of acute episode	✔	

Note: The Advisory Committee rated the evidence of health benefits of physical activity as strong, moderate, limited, or grade not assignable. Only outcomes with strong or moderate evidence of effect are included in the table.

*Crystallized intelligence is the ability to retrieve and use information that has been acquired over time. It is different from fluid intelligence, which is the ability to store and manipulate new information.

FIGURE 1.4 Benefits of physical activity on brain health.

Reprinted from U.S. Department of Health and Human Services, "Physical Activity Guidelines for Americans," 2nd ed. (Washington, DC: U.S. Department of Health and Human Services), 2018.

Focus on Volume

In 1978, ACSM published its first position stand (2): "The Recommended Quantity and Quality of Exercise for Developing and Maintaining Fitness in Healthy Adults." The focus was on improving CRF as well as achieving health outcomes. The emphasis was again on higher-intensity exercise to achieve these goals. However, in that same year, a now classic study on Harvard alumni by Paffenbarger, Wing, and Hyde (29) showed a 36% lower risk of developing a heart attack in those who accumulated 2,000 kcal or more of leisure-time physical activity per week (that did not have to be done at a high intensity). This study and many that followed shifted the focus to three variables associated with physical activity guidelines:

1. Activity volume (e.g., kcal expended) rather than intensity

2. Health outcomes (e.g., reduced risk of heart attack) rather than CRF

3. Leisure-time activity rather than structured exercise programs

Throughout the 1980s the body of research showing a strong relationship between regular participation in physical activity and a lower risk of chronic disease grew. The idea that physical activity and exercise were linked to a reduced risk of chronic disease was explored (9, 10, 11). Dr. William Haskell took a leadership role in explaining potential links among physical activity, fitness, and health (19, 20). Figure 1.5 shows the following:

- Early understanding reflected that physical activity improved fitness, which, in turn, was linked to improved health outcomes (figure 1.5a).

- However, it was just as likely that physical activity could improve health and fitness separately and by different mechanisms (figure 1.5b).

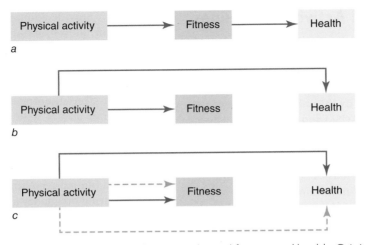

FIGURE 1.5 Possible causal relations among physical activity, physical fitness, and health. Original models (a) assumed that health gains due to physical activity were dependent on improved fitness, but a later model (b) proposed that physical activity can improve both health and fitness separately and probably by different mechanisms. Consistent with (b), the last model (c) suggests that some physical activity programs can improve one and not the other.

- Lastly, some physical activity programs could improve fitness and not health outcomes, and vice versa (figure 1.5c).

These distinctions helped shape the understanding of how physical activity is connected to fitness and health outcomes—that is, physical activity could achieve health outcomes independent of fitness.

One of the most important decisions that accelerated the drive to promote physical activity in a public health context occurred in 1992, when the AHA made physical inactivity a major risk factor for CVD, the same as smoking, high BP, and high serum cholesterol (15). Following up on that important decision, in 1995 the ACSM and CDC published their public health physical activity recommendation to reduce the risk of chronic disease (30): "Every U.S. adult should accumulate 30 minutes or more of moderate-intensity physical activity on most, preferably all, days of the week." The shift in focus was clearly spelled out, with exercise volume (total kcal expended) being crucial and somewhat independent of intensity (as long as it was equal to or higher than moderate intensity). It is important to remember that this was a minimum recommendation (*at least* 30 minutes, 5 times per week) for realizing health benefits. In the following year, the U.S. Surgeon General's report on physical activity and health was published (38). This document supported the 1995 ACSM and CDC statement and brought even more attention to the need for Americans to become physically active. The emphasis on physical activity from a public health perspective also was incorporated into subsequent editions of *ACSM's Guidelines for Exercise Testing and Prescription.*

Focus on Weight

The United States and many other industrialized countries have seen an incredible increase in the prevalence of overweight and obesity over the last 30 years. In the United States, 42.4% of adults are obese, and the combined overweight and obesity prevalence is 73.1% (16). The increase in obesity during the 1990s prompted the Institute of Medicine (IOM) to evaluate the research on how much physical activity was needed to prevent weight gain (23). The IOM recommended 60 minutes of moderate-intensity activity daily to prevent weight gain and achieve the full health benefits of physical activity, twice the amount that ACSM and the CDC recommended for reducing the risk of chronic diseases. This was supported by recommendations from the International Association for the Study of Obesity (IASO) to engage in 60 minutes per day of physical activity to prevent weight gain (35) and the International Obesity Task Force (IOTF) recommendation of 60 to 90 minutes of activity daily to prevent weight regain in those who have lost a great deal of weight (13). The 2020-2025 *Dietary Guidelines for Americans* recommends adults need at least 150 to 300 minutes of moderate-intensity activity per week (44). The *Physical Activity Guidelines for Americans* notes more activity than 150 minutes per week will be needed to lose weight or to keep weight off and that some will need to do 300 or more minutes per week to meet body-weight goals (41) (chapter 20 provides more information on weight management). The current *ACSM Guidelines* suggest an initial target of 150 minutes per week, with progression to at least 250 minutes per week of moderate to vigorous exercise spread out over 5 to 7 days per week to promote long-term weight loss maintenance (4).

Current Physical Activity Guidelines

As revisions to recommendations occurred, there was confusion among both fitness professionals and the general public about how much activity was enough. Which was it—30, 60, or 90 minutes per session? Was moderate-intensity activity the only way to achieve these various goals? In 2007, ACSM and the AHA published an updated position stand on physical activity and health that addressed some of these questions (21):

- *Moderate or vigorous:* The position stand supported the 1995 minimum recommendation of 30 minutes of moderate-intensity activity 5 days per week for reducing the risk of chronic disease. However, one could do 20 minutes of vigorous-intensity activity 3 days per week to achieve the same goal or do some combination of both.

- *More is better:* Doing more than the minimum (e.g., doing 60 minutes of moderate-intensity activity 5 days per week) increases health benefits.

This brief historical tour through physical activity recommendations shows how guidelines change as research reveals more about the effects of physical activity. The review also provides a jumping-off point for a comprehensive series of recommendations that affects much of what is presented in this text. In 2008, the U.S. Department of Health and Human Services (HHS) published the *Physical Activity Guidelines for Americans*—the first set of national physical activity recommendations related to health and fitness (39). This document was based on an extensive review of the literature that was carried out by an advisory committee (40). These guidelines provide physical activity recommendations for children and adolescents, adults, older adults (65 years and older), women during and following pregnancy, people with disabilities, and people with chronic medical conditions. The *Physical Activity Guidelines for Americans* was updated based on a new literature review (31); the second edition, released in 2018, expanded coverage to include guidance for preschool children (41). The following is a brief summary of the recommendations (41):

- Preschool children should be active throughout the day with a variety of activities.

- Children and adolescents should include 60 minutes or more of moderate to vigorous activity daily, including aerobic, muscle-strengthening, and bone-strengthening activities.

- Adults should move more and sit less. Aerobic activity should include at least 150 to 300 minutes of moderate-intensity activity or 75 to 150 minutes of vigorous activity, or an equivalent combination of moderate and vigorous activity on a weekly basis. Greater amounts of activity can provide additional health benefits. In addition, muscle-strengthening activities should be included on 2 or more days per week.

- Older adults should include multicomponent physical activity including aerobic, muscular-strengthening, and balance activities. For older adults who cannot reach 150 minutes per week of moderate-intensity activity, being as active as abilities and conditions allow is encouraged.

- Additional recommendations related to activity during pregnancy and the postpartum period, as well as for adults with chronic health conditions and disabilities, are included; individuals should consult with their health care provider to maximize safety.

- Realizing the overall safety of physical activity, gradual progression, selection of activities appropriate to a given fitness level and goals, adherence to safe practices, and consultation with a health care provider for those with chronic conditions or symptoms are also suggested.

Strength Training

A majority of studies examining the relationship between physical activity and chronic disease measured only aerobic activity. That said, ACSM has recommended exercises to enhance muscular strength and endurance since their 1990 position stand (3), and that has remained the case since then. The *2008 Physical Activity Guidelines for Americans* and the more recent 2018 second edition provides guidelines for improving muscular strength and endurance. Recommendations include the following (21, 39, 41):

- Do exercises for the all the major muscle groups: legs, hips, back, chest, abdomen, shoulders, and arms.

- To maximize strength development, use a resistance that allows 8 to 12 repetitions (number of times each lift is done in 1 set) of each exercise, at which point fatigue is experienced.

- One set of each exercise is sufficient, although more can be gained with 2 or 3 sets.

- Do resistance training on at least 2 days each week.

There is no question that muscular strength and endurance activities provide benefits, including improvements in muscle mass, strength, and bone health (39). But evidence also suggests that resistance training is associated with a lower risk of all-cause mortality, potentially linked to the role that increased muscle mass plays in glucose metabolism (21), as well as a lower risk of cancer mortality (34). Chapter 14 provides more details

RESEARCH INSIGHT

Focus on Physical Activity or Sedentary Behavior?

A great deal of time is spent sitting, whether at work, in a car, or in front of the TV or computer. In the United States children and adults spend about 7.7 hours per day during waking time being sedentary (41). Investigators have pointed to a link between sedentary behavior and increased risk of chronic diseases—even in people who meet the physical activity guidelines. Risk related to sedentary behavior is dependent on the amount of physical activity. The following visual from the current *Physical Activity Guidelines for Americans* depicts all-cause mortality risk as it relates to daily sitting time and engagement in physical activity.

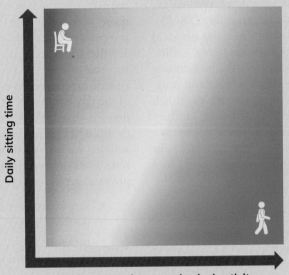

Moderate to vigorous physical activity
Risk of all-cause mortality decreases
as one moves from red to green.

Heat map.

Reprinted from U.S. Department of Health and Human Services, "Physical Activity Guidelines for Americans," 2nd ed. (Washington, DC: U.S. Department of Health and Human Services), 2018.

In this figure, the horizontal axis shows moderate to vigorous activity in minutes, and the vertical axis shows sitting time in hours. The colors reflect the risk of all-cause mortality, with red showing higher risk and green lower risk; the intermediate colors of orange and yellow show decreasing risk, from the higher risk associated with red to lower risk reflected by green. The greatest risk is for individuals who have low physical activity and high sitting time (upper corner in red). The lowest risk is for those who are very physically active and do not have much sitting time during the day (lower corner in green). Encouragingly, even for those who have a high number of hours sitting, notice across the top of the figure, the colors shift to orange, yellow, and even green as the amount of physical activity increases. Thus, including high volumes of moderate to vigorous activity (considered to be about 60 to 75 minutes per day of moderate activities or 30 to 40 minutes per day of vigorous physical activity) can help lower risk that is associated with high volumes of sitting. On the other hand, note that even low time spent sitting does not remove all risk resulting from a lack of moderate to vigorous physical activity (lower left corner is shaded in orange). From a broad perspective, promotion of physical activity along with a reduction in sedentary time is a winning combination.

about the importance of resistance training in an exercise program to improve health and reduce the risk of chronic diseases (8).

Individuals need adequate muscular strength and endurance to be able to carry out activities of daily living, do leisure activities (e.g., gardening, mowing, sport), and realize performance goals. An increase in muscle mass has implications beyond sport performance, because muscle mass contributes to the number of calories expended per day. This is tied to energy balance and the ability to maintain body weight with age. In addition, adequate endurance of the muscles in the trunk (core) is important to reduce the risk of low-back pain. As strength declines with aging, the ability of older adults to maintain an independent lifestyle is compromised. The evaluation of muscular fitness is discussed in chapter 9, and the design of programs to improve muscular strength and muscular endurance is presented in chapter 14.

Despite what is known about the effects of aerobic and resistance training on health and fitness, participation rates by adults over the age of 18 are not what they should be. However, results have been more encouraging for aerobic activity than for resistance training (18, 43). In 2020, 47.9% of American adults met the physical activity guidelines for aerobic activity described earlier. In contrast, 31.9% met the muscle-strengthening activity guidelines, and only 25.2% met both aerobic and muscle-strengthening activity guidelines (43), leaving much room for improvement. In the United States, Healthy People 2030 provides national objectives to improve health and well-being, promoting strategies to help people throughout the lifespan to be more physically active (43).

Adverse Events

In contrast to the many benefits of participating in physical activity, there is also the potential for an adverse outcome: an injury or medical complication (e.g., heart attack). Figure 1.6 captures factors that can increase the risk of injury associated with participation in physical activity. The risk is greater for older, less fit individuals who have little experience doing physical activity. The risk of musculoskeletal injuries increases with the amount of activity done (i.e., more risk for someone running 30 miles [48 kilometers] a week compared with 10 miles [16 kilometers] a week), as well as the amount of increase in physical activity, whether intensity or volume, when changing workouts. Participation in collision sports has a higher injury risk than participation in noncollision sports. Finally, both equipment and environmental factors can contribute to injury risk. Cardiac events such as a heart attack or sudden death are rare, but the risk is higher when someone becomes more active than usual, emphasizing the need for a progressive introduction to physical activity (4). Figure 1.7 illustrates that although the risk of a cardiac event increases for an active person during exercise, the overall risk of cardiac arrest is considerably lower for the rest of the day compared with a sedentary person. The good news is that healthy people have a low risk of adverse events when participating in moderate-intensity physical activity such as brisk walking (40, 41). To reduce the risks associated with exercise testing and participation in physical activity programs, fitness professionals should

- screen individuals using health-risk questionnaires (chapter 2 and chapter 24),
- measure important physiological variables at rest before taking exercise tests (chapters in part III), and
- gradually progress each individual through a physical activity program (chapters in part IV).

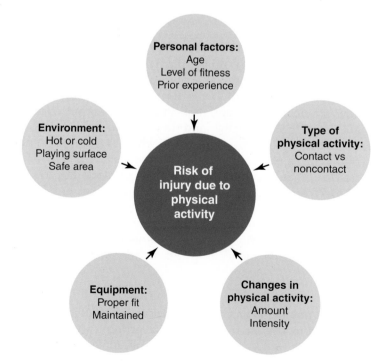

FIGURE 1.6   Factors affecting the risk of injury due to participation in physical activity.

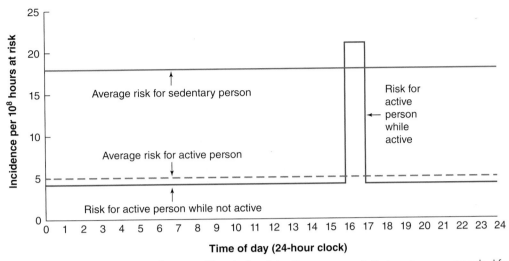

FIGURE 1.7   Risk of cardiac arrest based on usual level of activity. Strenuous activity is not recommended for a sedentary person and is not shown on this graph.

From U.S. Department of Health and Human Services (DHHS), *Physical Activity Guidelines Advisory Committee Report 2008*, Fig. G10.5, (2008), G10-22.

KEY POINT

Current physical activity guidelines recommend moderate-intensity or vigorous-intensity aerobic physical activity to realize substantial health benefits along with strengthening exercises to help maintain muscle mass and bone health. These recommendations have evolved as a result of a growing research base that shows the substantial health benefits that can be realized through regular physical activity.

Fitness

Figure 1.1 presented health (avoidance of disease), fitness, and performance as three distinct goals, with a physical activity recommendation tied to each. It should be clear at this point, however, that health and fitness goals are not so much distinct as connected. They are two sides of the same coin—a coin that represents an investment in achieving health outcomes through regular participation in physical activity. As previously stated, health outcomes are realized by doing a minimum of

- 150 minutes per week of moderate-intensity physical activity or
- 75 minutes per week of vigorous-intensity physical activity.

The vigorous-intensity recommendation is the traditional exercise prescription for increasing or maintaining CRF.

Intensity: Moderate Versus Vigorous

Are there any benefits to doing vigorous versus moderate physical activity? Swain and Franklin (37) addressed this question in a systematic review of the literature examining the relationship of physical activity to the incidence of CVD and risk factors for CVD. In their review, it was important to control for the total energy expenditure associated with the physical activity in order to accurately compare the difference between moderate-intensity and vigorous-intensity activity; for any duration of vigorous activity, more energy would be expended compared with moderate activity. Their findings follow.

- The vast majority of epidemiological studies found a greater reduction in the risk of CVD with vigorous-intensity (≥6 METs) than with moderate-intensity (3-5.9 METs) physical activity. In addition, more favorable risk-factor profiles were observed for people engaged in vigorous as opposed to moderate activity.

- Clinical intervention studies generally showed greater improvement in diastolic blood pressure, glucose control, and CRF after vigorous-intensity physical activity versus moderate-intensity activity. However, no intensity effect was observed on improvements in systolic blood pressure, blood lipid profile, or body-fat loss.

Thus, although moderate-intensity physical activity was good, vigorous-intensity activity was better. In addition, one can obtain faster and larger gains in CRF with vigorous-intensity exercise programs. However, as mentioned, fitness professionals must use good judgment when working with individual clients, recognizing that vigorous-intensity exercise is associated with more adverse events and that some clients may simply wish to stay with a successful moderate-intensity program that meets their needs rather than progress to a vigorous-intensity exercise program.

Fitness or Fatness: Which Is More Important?

Some investigators, notably Dr. Steven Blair and colleagues, have used CRF as an index of physical activity, reasoning that more-active people would have higher levels of CRF. Many of the classic studies linking physical activity to various health outcomes have used this approach and have both confirmed and expanded on research that uses questionnaires or objective measures of physical activity (e.g., pedometers or accelerometers) to obtain information on the activity levels of individuals. The advantage of using CRF as a measure of physical activity is that it can be objectively determined using treadmill or cycle ergometer tests (see chapter 8), and it is easily tracked over time. Having information on CRF as a measure of physical activity also elicits another question—Which is more important in terms of health status: having a higher level of physical activity or having a lower body fatness?

This is no small question given the attention to the obesity epidemic. Obesity is linked to a variety of chronic diseases. However, from a health-promotion perspective, should the focus be more on getting people to be physically active or on achieving a healthy body weight? Figure 1.8 is an example of the kind of data that allow one to separate the impact of fitness from fatness (12). In this study, investigators measured the CRF and body fatness of individuals with diabetes and then followed them over time to determine how many died from CVD. Those who had a high fitness score and were at a

normal body weight were used as the reference group to compare with the others; this group was assigned a risk value of 1.0. For the normal-weight group, those who had low fitness levels had about a fourfold greater risk of dying from CVD compared with those who had high fitness levels, indicating the importance of being fit. This was also true for the other weight classes. In contrast, looking across the figure, moving from normal weight to overweight and then to obese had little impact on the risk of dying from CVD in this group of subjects. Similar observations have been made for a wide variety of health outcomes (14, 25, 36). In addition, recent work shows that a change in fitness, not fatness, is the best predictor of future health outcomes.

The message is clear: Being physically active provides substantial health benefits independent of body weight. This is consistent with a central theme of the *Physical Activity Guidelines for Americans*: Health-related benefits of physical activity occur in people of all body weights and whether one is gaining or losing weight (41). The primary focus, then, should be on getting people physically active so they can realize the health benefits and then consider body weight as the physical activity program is being established. This is a powerful message to current and future fitness professionals.

Performance

The term *performance* means different things to different people. At its most basic level, it means being able to complete daily tasks efficiently; at a higher level, it speaks to an ability to engage successfully in sport-related performance.

Completing Daily Tasks

To get through the day efficiently, fundamental motor skills are required that allow individuals to accomplish various tasks. Tasks include being able to move from place to place and push, pull, pick up, carry, and perform other tasks requiring the hands and arms. Moderate levels of muscular strength and muscular endurance, flexibility, body composition or relative leanness, and CRF are essential for these routine tasks. Although successful daily living is important at all ages, it is a top priority for the elderly because it allows them to live independently. In addition, a person's lifestyle adds other needs. Contrast, for example, a computer programmer, a firefighter, and a parent staying at home with an infant. The computer programmer needs stretching and relaxation activities to prevent low-back and postural problems and can benefit from short activity breaks. The firefighter is sedentary for most of the time but must be able to respond quickly with near-maximal levels of anaerobic energy and muscular strength and endurance, all within an adverse environment with heavy equipment. Thus,

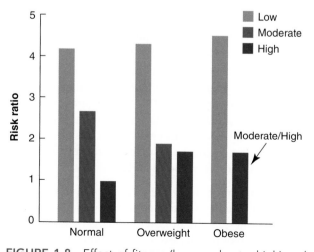

FIGURE 1.8 Effect of fitness (low, moderate, high) and fatness on the risk of death from CVD in men with diabetes.
Based on Church et al. (2005).

this person must engage in regular vigorous aerobic, anaerobic, and resistance exercise to maintain the conditioning necessary to respond to emergencies. The parent needs flexibility, strength, and endurance to lift and carry the infant and other items through an obstacle course of toys, clothes, and so on (in addition to learning to perform these tasks under sleep deprivation). The term *functional fitness* describes fitness programming that uses a variety of exercises to simulate routine tasks rather than using traditional aerobic or resistance training exercises.

Achieving Desired Sport Performance

Some clients may want to engage in selected sports such as tennis, basketball, and golf or in high-performance endurance competitions such as triathlons, 100K bike races, or 10K runs. In addition to requiring good physical fitness, most of these activities require specific motor abilities—agility, balance, coordination, power, and speed—as well as the particular skills of the sport.

Clearly, high fitness levels are desirable as an athletic base, but individuals also have specific needs depending on their sport. Compare, for example, 10K runners, basketball players, and golfers. The runners rely on aerobic power that comes from distance running, with careful stretching and attention to muscular fitness. Basketball players depend on aerobic and anaerobic energy; coordination; and specific passing, shooting, and defensive skills. Golfers require a moderate cardiorespiratory base, muscular power, and coordination of a complex

skill used in a variety of settings (e.g., fairway, sand traps, woods). Although it is beyond the scope of this textbook to discuss performance across all sports and competitions, reflect on the connection between fitness in all the areas (aerobic, muscular, flexibility) and what is needed for performance. The Human Kinetics website (US.HumanKinetics.com) is a resource for information on publications dealing with performance of a wide variety of sports.

KEY POINT

Being physically fit (achieving appropriate levels of CRF, body composition, strength, and flexibility) is linked to a low risk of health problems and an improved ability to engage in daily tasks with adequate energy. A higher level of these fitness components is associated with sport performance, along with attention to the unique skills related to each sport or game.

Pulling It All Together

As this chapter draws to an end, reconsider the initial question of how much exercise is enough. The goals of health, fitness, and performance represent a continuum of outcomes that result from regular participation in physical activity and exercise (see figure 1.9). Participa-

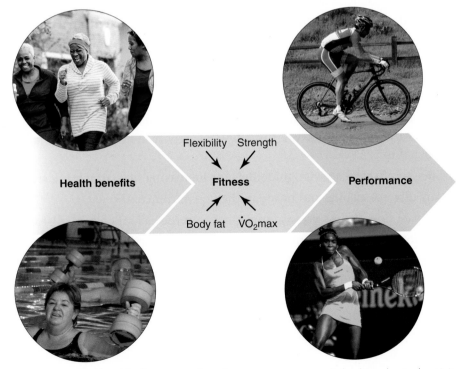

FIGURE 1.9 The continuum of health, fitness, and performance outcomes linked to physical activity.

Photo on top left: kali9/E+/Getty Images

15

tion in both moderate- and vigorous-intensity physical activity is associated with numerous substantial health benefits and improvement in the various fitness components of CRF, body composition, flexibility, and strength. Achieving a level of fitness is a first step in the quest to realizing performance-related goals. The progression from moderate physical activity to structured vigorous exercise programs and then sports and games reflects a logical pathway that minimizes risk and maximizes the chance of success along the way.

One of the most frustrating yet exciting aspects of dealing with health problems is that people can modify their health status and control major health risks. The frustrating side is that many people find it difficult to change an unhealthy lifestyle. The exciting element is that, with help, they can gain control of their health. The opportunity to help people change their unhealthy lifestyles carries the responsibility of making recommendations based on the best scientific evidence available. This text provides the background to evaluate health-related risk factors and behaviors, test the various fitness components, and prescribe exercise to improve each.

KEY POINT

Fitness professionals live in an exciting time because of the increasing evidence and recognition that regular physical activity is essential to a good life. It is a worthwhile challenge to motivate people to begin and continue an active lifestyle, especially when there is so much competition for everyone's time.

1

LEARNING AIDS

REVIEW QUESTIONS

1. What are the differences in the physical activity requirements for achieving health benefits, fitness, and performance?
2. List the top seven leading causes of death, and compare them with the behaviors linked to the top actual causes of death.
3. What is the difference between absolute and relative intensity?
4. What is moderate-intensity and vigorous-intensity physical activity in terms of METs?
5. Calculate the volume of physical activity done per week for someone exercising at 5 METs for 40 minutes per day, 3 days per week.
6. How does regular participation in physical activity affect the top two leading causes of death?
7. What does the *2018 Physical Activity Guidelines for Americans* recommend for moderate-intensity and vigorous-intensity physical activity in order to realize substantial health benefits?
8. Describe the physical activity guidelines for increasing or maintaining strength.
9. What are adverse events, and how can they be minimized?
10. What impact does fitness versus fatness have on the risk of chronic disease?
11. What performance-related fitness components are linked to sport?
12. Describe the continuum of physical activity recommendations for realizing health, fitness, and performance goals.

CASE STUDIES

1. A client complains that she has been deceived by all the physical activity recommendations you have given her over the past several years. She just read a government report indicating that a person only has to do moderate-intensity physical activity (walking) to achieve health benefits. She wants to know if she should continue her vigorous exercise program in which she exercises at her target heart rate for 30 minutes 3 to 4 days per week or whether she should switch to a walking program. How do you respond?

2. You have just presented a speech on physical fitness to a local service club. One of the members says that he knows of two men who died in incidents related to exercise during the past few years and that he has read of other exercise-related deaths. He has decided that it is safer to lead a quiet life and not take the risk of exercising. How do you respond?

3. You are working with an obese client who has been sedentary for several years. He indicates that he would like to lose weight before beginning a physical activity program. What information might you provide to encourage him to begin a moderate-intensity physical activity program as plans are developed to accomplish weight-loss goals?

Answers to Case Studies

1. You might state that the physical activity recommendations in the government report were aimed at people who are currently sedentary and not those who are habitually active and involved in vigorous exercise. In addition, you might indicate that participation in vigorous exercise is associated with other health-related benefits (increases in CRF, or $\dot{V}O_2max$) that are more difficult to achieve with moderate-intensity exercise.

2. You might respond by acknowledging that there are risks related to exercise, but the risk of death is very low for someone making a gradual transition from a sedentary lifestyle to one involving moderate-intensity physical activity. In addition, deterioration of the cardiovascular system through sedentary living causes a much higher risk of major health problems compared with being active. Finally, exercise-related risks can be minimized by starting slowly and gradually increasing the amount and intensity of exercise.

3. You might begin by telling him that the health-related benefits of physical activity occur in all people, independent of body weight or body fatness. Further, it is important to establish a pattern of physical activity as one of the new behaviors needed to help maintain the weight loss once the goal is achieved.

2

Preparticipation Screening

Barbara A. Bushman and Lauren R. Chaney

OBJECTIVES

The reader will be able to do the following:

1. Understand the purpose of evaluating the health status of potential participants in fitness programs and identify appropriate instruments for the preparticipation health screening process

2. Identify the presence of cardiovascular, metabolic, or renal disease, including signs and symptoms

3. Describe the categories of participants who should receive medical clearance before undergoing exercise testing or participation

4. Identify primary risk factors for cardiovascular disease and understand how they are used in providing educational counseling regarding disease prevention and management

5. Recommend an appropriate fitness program for participants based on their preparticipation health screening and fitness test results

6. Understand the impact of various medications on participants' responses to exercise

2

Despite the growing evidence of the benefits of physical activity and continued evolution of guidelines related to physical activity and health (35), fitness professionals in clinical, community, and commercial settings will encounter people with low cardiorespiratory fitness (CRF) and an array of health and medical conditions. The fitness professional is responsible for communicating clearly with participants regarding testing and programming and for properly screening prospective exercise participants to determine whether medical clearance is warranted before fitness testing or initiation of a regular physical activity program. This chapter provides background on screening recommendations; the fitness professional also must be aware of institutional or facility policies and legal requirements when tailoring interactions with individual clients.

Upon joining a fitness facility or program, an individual is likely given a protective legal document to read and sign such as a waiver (release of liability), an assumption of risk, or an informed consent. These documents can provide an effective defense (legal liability protection) for fitness facilities and professionals if they are ever named as defendants in a negligence lawsuit. The waiver and assumption of risk defenses are described in chapter 24. Prior to preparticipation health screening, the American College of Sports Medicine (ACSM) recommends an informed consent as the first step (8).

The informed consent document is intended to document clear communication with the participant of the purpose and procedures, risks and discomforts, potential benefits, responsibilities of the participant, how data collected will be handled, opportunity to ask questions, and option to withdraw at any time (7). An example of an informed consent document is included in chapter 7, and others are available elsewhere (7, 8); informed consent documents should be reviewed for acceptability by local authorities such as the legal counsel of a facility or the institutional review board (8).

After the informed consent is the preparticipation screening process. To screen an exercise participant, the fitness professional should begin with a preparticipation screening questionnaire, such as the Physical Activity Readiness Questionnaire for Everyone or the Pre-Activity Screening Questionnaire (8, 19, 22). These two questionnaires are discussed in detail later in this chapter. The Exercise Preparticipation Health Screening Questionnaire for Exercise Professionals is another potential screening questionnaire (41). Additionally, a more comprehensive health screening questionnaire (HSQ) (also referred to as a *health history questionnaire*, HHQ) will be of value in gathering pertinent information on health risks and medical history, as described later in this chapter.

In some instances, medical clearance or referral of the participant to a medically based supervised exercise program may be necessary before engaging in an exercise program. Agreement is not universal about when medical clearance is necessary before exercise participation or when supervised exercise in a clinical setting is warranted. To help the fitness professional make these decisions, this chapter includes recommendations of the American Heart Association (AHA) and ACSM. When in doubt, the fitness professional should rely on the participant's primary care physician and the fitness director (or medical director) of the facility to make the final decision regarding approval for exercise participation. Safety is always the top priority when working with clients, and each situation is unique.

A preparticipation screening and HSQ will contain a significant amount of personal health information, which must be kept in a way that is "private, confidential, and secure" (6). A participant's medical history and fitness test results should be shared only with authorized individuals, which may include other health care or fitness professionals who will be working with the participant, and should only be discussed in a private setting in which other staff or participants cannot overhear. In situations where medical clearance is required, the medical clearance form can include a release form section that requires the client's signature so that the health care professional can release pertinent medical information to the fitness professional, if warranted, in accordance with the Health Insurance Portability and Accountability Act of 1996 (HIPAA) (36). Written authorization is required from the client, according to HIPAA regulations (36), when a client's protected health information (PHI) is provided to a third party (e.g., when a medical clearance form containing PHI is returned directly to a fitness professional). It is best and most time efficient for individuals to deliver or send the medical clearance form to their health care provider and to return the completed form to the fitness professional. Additional legal concerns that may be involved in the exercise testing and prescription process are addressed in chapter 24. It is beyond the scope of this textbook to cover all potential legal requirements in each area; various resources are available (for example, 6, 21).

Aside from legal rights that protect personal health information, the fitness professional should consider that many participants may feel uncomfortable sharing their medical history. Using a professional yet conversational style to ask questions about medical diagnoses can help to alleviate the discomfort that clients may feel. For instance, when participants have checked the box for having a heart attack, relevant questions providing further insight into their medical history would include the following: "Are your heart symptoms present? If so, are they stable?" "Has your heart attack affected your activities of daily life?" "Have you been able to return to the activities you were doing before the event?" "Did you participate in cardiac rehabilitation?" "Were you given any restrictions?" The participant's responses should be documented on the HSQ. Reviewing the form conversationally allows the fitness professional to learn more about the participant's health status and to convey empathy, making participants more likely to perceive the fitness professional as being genuinely concerned with helping them improve their health.

If prospective exercise participants refuse to complete a preparticipation screening form, they cannot be properly screened. When participants object to preparticipation screening procedures, the fitness professional should inform them of the benefits of screening and the potential risks of not completing the screening, as well as reassure them that all information is kept private, confidential, and secure. If prospective participants still refuse, ACSM recommends that they be permitted to sign a release or waiver before exercising, as permitted by law (6). An example of a preparticipation screening refusal form that includes a waiver can be found elsewhere (20, 21). The release or waiver should entail the following: acknowledgment that a preparticipation screening was provided, that the participant has been informed of the risks inherent in fitness activities, that the participant has chosen not to be screened, that the participant assumes personal responsibility, and that the participant releases the facility from any claims or suits arising from exercise participation. If someone chooses not to sign the waiver or release, the facility has the option of denying participation to the extent permitted by law (6). It is strongly recommended that a facility consult with a competent lawyer to establish policies and procedures regarding refusal for participation and the use of a waiver or release.

Screening Forms

The AHA and ACSM recommend that exercise facilities provide their adult members with a preparticipation screening that is consistent with the exercise programs they plan to pursue. Although an exercise facility may not have a legal responsibility to conduct a preparticipation screening, this screening is in the best interest of exercise participants. The primary purpose is to identify both those individuals not known to be at risk as well as those with known risk of a cardiovascular event when active (9). The results of the preparticipation screening should be interpreted and documented by qualified staff (6, 7, 8, 9).

Regarding apparently healthy people, the risk of cardiovascular events during physical activity is remarkably low (adjusted risk of 1-3 per 1,000,000 participant hours), although increased age, greater physical activity level, and the presence of cardiovascular disease (CVD) risk factors are associated with greater risk (23, 24, 33). Light- to moderate-intensity physical activity appears to carry the same incidence of cardiovascular events as resting condition; vigorous physical activity does increase risk in susceptible individuals, especially when the activity is sudden or sporadic (54). A well-designed and properly evaluated preparticipation health screening serves several purposes, including identifying symptoms of chronic diseases that increase the risk of cardiovascular events during exercise participation, recognizing people with clinically significant diseases or conditions that warrant participation in medically supervised programs, and determining if people should seek medical clearance prior to fitness testing or exercise participation (9, 54). Preparticipation screening is the first step in the fitness professional's health risk appraisal of exercise participants and future testing and prescription as recommended by ACSM (8, 41, 47), including the following:

- Make a classification as to whether the individual currently exercises regularly.
- Review medical history for established cardiovascular, metabolic, or renal disease.
- Identify signs and symptoms of cardiovascular, metabolic, or renal disease.
- Determine the level of desired aerobic exercise intensity.
- Establish if medical clearance is necessary.
- Administer fitness tests and evaluate results.
- Develop an individualized exercise prescription.
- Evaluate progress with follow-up tests.

Preparticipation screening questionnaires can be self-guided or can be administered by fitness professionals. This section will describe the PAR-Q+ and PASQ, two potential screening tools. The focus of the preparticipation screening is to provide a means by which the level of risk can be determined that indicates the need to consult with a health care provider prior to physical activity (6). In addition, an HSQ should be included to gather additional information reflecting a broader medical history (7).

Physical Activity Readiness Questionnaire for Everyone

The Physical Activity Readiness Questionnaire for Everyone (PAR-Q+; see form 2.1 or access www.eparmedx.com

for a current online version) was designed to replace the Physical Activity Readiness Questionnaire (PAR-Q) (45). The PAR-Q+ is a preparticipation screening questionnaire for people who want to pursue moderate (i.e., 40%-59% $\dot{V}O_2R$) to vigorous (i.e., ≥60% $\dot{V}O_2R$) physical activity. The PAR-Q+ is designed (and has been validated) to reduce the barriers to physical activity participation for people with and without established chronic disease. The original PAR-Q produced an inordinate number of false positives with older adults (60 years of age and older), especially among those with orthopedic problems. This resulted in almost 20% of participants being referred to medical personnel before being cleared for physical activity versus only 1% for the present version (58). If participants answer *no* to all seven questions in the self-administered questionnaire (form 2.1), they are cleared for physical activity participation (58, 59).

If participants answer *yes* to any of the seven questions on the PAR-Q+, they are directed to complete additional questions about whether they have signs or symptoms of chronic disease or established chronic disease (i.e., orthopedic, cancer, cardiovascular, metabolic, or pulmonary disease). If each response is *no* to the additional questions, the participant is cleared for physical activity participation. If participants answer *yes* to any of the additional questions, they are directed to contact a qualified exercise professional (i.e., individuals with university training in exercise sciences with current valid certification) or complete an online questionnaire, the ePARmed-X+ (http://eparmedx.com), to further clarify the risk associated with exercise participation (14, 45, 58, 59).

The ePARmed-X+ is an interactive online tool that provides a more extensive questionnaire about the presence of specific medical conditions (e.g., diabetes, low-back pain, arrhythmias), whether a physician is actively managing the conditions, and how severe the conditions are. Based on their answers, participants are recommended to either visit their physician or a qualified exercise professional for further information regarding appropriate exercise participation (14, 58, 59).

Pre-Activity Screening Questionnaire

The Pre-Activity Screening Questionnaire (PASQ; see form 2.2) is a preparticipation screening that classifies a client's current physical activity level and desired future level of physical activity along with reviewing medical conditions related to cardiovascular, metabolic, or renal disease and their major signs and symptoms. The PASQ provided in this text is based on recommendations for preparticipation screening proposed by the ACSM (8), and also is discussed in chapter 24. The goals of the screening process are to identify individuals (8, 47)

1. who warrant medical clearance before beginning an exercise program or increasing the frequency, intensity, or volume of their current program;

2. who have clinically significant disease(s) that could benefit from participating in a medically supervised program; and

3. who have medical conditions that preclude them from exercise participation until these conditions subside or are more effectively controlled.

Screening is used along with good clinical judgment, with referrals to a health care provider or changes in an exercise program to more vigorous activity to be individualized (8).

Health Screening Questionnaire

In addition to the use of a preparticipation screening such as the PAR-Q+ or PASQ, an HSQ will provide needed information to assess risk and develop an appropriate plan for a given participant. A general example of an HSQ is provided in form 2.3. The HSQ should provide information to assess risk factors, past history of CVD, present status of signs or symptoms of CVD, medical history (related to other chronic diseases, illnesses, surgeries, musculoskeletal or joint injuries), past and present health habits (e.g., physical activity and diet), and medications (prescribed or over the counter) (7).

No questionnaire can address all possible medical conditions that might warrant physician clearance or might affect exercise testing or exercise programs. Thus, the fitness professional should ask additional questions relevant to the participant's medical history while reviewing the HSQ with the participant. The line of questioning should be directed by any condition that is checked as being present. In doing so, medical diagnoses or symptoms that may place the participant at additional cardiovascular risk during exercise are more likely to be addressed. The HSQ should be tailored so that it is applicable to the participant population (i.e., form 2.3 is a general example; forms should be customized as needed).

Assessing the presence of a client's primary risk factors for CVD (e.g., hypertension) to determine their CVD risk classification (i.e., low, moderate, or high) as part of the decision-making process for medical clearance prior to exercise participation is no longer recommended. However, fitness professionals are encouraged to evaluate the CVD risk factor assessment as part of the health risk appraisal because this information can be used in decisions related to exercise testing and prescription (8). The information from a review of risk factors along with the HSQ should be evaluated *before* conducting any fitness testing or recommending exercise prescriptions.

2023 PAR-Q+

The Physical Activity Readiness Questionnaire for Everyone

The health benefits of regular physical activity are clear; more people should engage in physical activity every day of the week. Participating in physical activity is very safe for MOST people. This questionnaire will tell you whether it is necessary for you to seek further advice from your doctor OR a qualified exercise professional before becoming more physically active.

GENERAL HEALTH QUESTIONS

Please read the 7 questions below carefully and answer each one honestly: check YES or NO.	YES	NO
1) Has your doctor ever said that you have a heart condition ☐ OR high blood pressure ☐?	☐	☐
2) Do you feel pain in your chest at rest, during your daily activities of living, OR when you do physical activity?	☐	☐
3) Do you lose balance because of dizziness OR have you lost consciousness in the last 12 months? Please answer NO if your dizziness was associated with over-breathing (including during vigorous exercise).	☐	☐
4) Have you ever been diagnosed with another chronic medical condition (other than heart disease or high blood pressure)? PLEASE LIST CONDITION(S) HERE: _____	☐	☐
5) Are you currently taking prescribed medications for a chronic medical condition? PLEASE LIST CONDITION(S) AND MEDICATIONS HERE: _____	☐	☐
6) Do you currently have (or have had within the past 12 months) a bone, joint, or soft tissue (muscle, ligament, or tendon) problem that could be made worse by becoming more physically active? Please answer NO if you had a problem in the past, but it does not limit your current ability to be physically active. PLEASE LIST CONDITION(S) HERE: _____	☐	☐
7) Has your doctor ever said that you should only do medically supervised physical activity?	☐	☐

☑ **If you answered NO to all of the questions above, you are cleared for physical activity.**
Please sign the PARTICIPANT DECLARATION. You do not need to complete Pages 2 and 3.

- ▶ Start becoming much more physically active – start slowly and build up gradually.
- ▶ Follow Global Physical Activity Guidelines for your age (https://www.who.int/publications/i/item/9789240015128).
- ▶ You may take part in a health and fitness appraisal.
- ▶ If you are over the age of 45 yr and NOT accustomed to regular vigorous to maximal effort exercise, consult a qualified exercise professional before engaging in this intensity of exercise.
- ▶ If you have any further questions, contact a qualified exercise professional.

PARTICIPANT DECLARATION

If you are less than the legal age required for consent or require the assent of a care provider, your parent, guardian or care provider must also sign this form.

I, the undersigned, have read, understood to my full satisfaction and completed this questionnaire. I acknowledge that this physical activity clearance is valid for a maximum of 12 months from the date it is completed and becomes invalid if my condition changes. I also acknowledge that the community/fitness center may retain a copy of this form for its records. In these instances, it will maintain the confidentiality of the same, complying with applicable law.

NAME _____ DATE _____

SIGNATURE _____ WITNESS _____

SIGNATURE OF PARENT/GUARDIAN/CARE PROVIDER _____

⬭ **If you answered YES to one or more of the questions above, COMPLETE PAGES 2 AND 3.**

⚠ **Delay becoming more active if:**

- ✓ You have a temporary illness such as a cold or fever; it is best to wait until you feel better.
- ✓ You are pregnant - talk to your health care practitioner, your physician, a qualified exercise professional, and/or complete the ePARmed-X+ at www.eparmedx.com before becoming more physically active.
- ✓ Your health changes - answer the questions on Pages 2 and 3 of this document and/or talk to your doctor or a qualified exercise professional before continuing with any physical activity program.

(continued)

FORM 2.1 *(continued)*

2023 PAR-Q+
FOLLOW-UP QUESTIONS ABOUT YOUR MEDICAL CONDITION(S)

1. Do you have Arthritis, Osteoporosis, or Back Problems?

If the above condition(s) is/are present, answer questions 1a-1c.   If **NO** ☐ go to question 2

1a.	Do you have difficulty controlling your condition with medications or other physician-prescribed therapies? (Answer **NO** if you are not currently taking medications or other treatments)	YES ☐ NO ☐
1b.	Do you have joint problems causing pain, a recent fracture or fracture caused by osteoporosis or cancer, displaced vertebra (e.g., spondylolisthesis), and/or spondylolysis/pars defect (a crack in the bony ring on the back of the spinal column)?	YES ☐ NO ☐
1c.	Have you had steroid injections or taken steroid tablets regularly for more than 3 months?	YES ☐ NO ☐

2. Do you currently have Cancer of any kind?

If the above condition(s) is/are present, answer questions 2a-2b   If **NO** ☐ go to question 3

2a.	Does your cancer diagnosis include any of the following types: lung/bronchogenic, multiple myeloma (cancer of plasma cells), head, and/or neck?	YES ☐ NO ☐
2b.	Are you currently receiving cancer therapy (such as chemotheraphy or radiotherapy)?	YES ☐ NO ☐

3. Do you have a Heart or Cardiovascular Condition? This includes Coronary Artery Disease, Heart Failure, Diagnosed Abnormality of Heart Rhythm

If the above condition(s) is/are present, answer questions 3a-3d   If **NO** ☐ go to question 4

3a.	Do you have difficulty controlling your condition with medications or other physician-prescribed therapies? (Answer **NO** if you are not currently taking medications or other treatments)	YES ☐ NO ☐
3b.	Do you have an irregular heart beat that requires medical management? (e.g., atrial fibrillation, premature ventricular contraction)	YES ☐ NO ☐
3c.	Do you have chronic heart failure?	YES ☐ NO ☐
3d.	Do you have diagnosed coronary artery (cardiovascular) disease and have not participated in regular physical activity in the last 2 months?	YES ☐ NO ☐

4. Do you currently have High Blood Pressure?

If the above condition(s) is/are present, answer questions 4a-4b   If **NO** ☐ go to question 5

4a.	Do you have difficulty controlling your condition with medications or other physician-prescribed therapies? (Answer **NO** if you are not currently taking medications or other treatments)	YES ☐ NO ☐
4b.	Do you have a resting blood pressure equal to or greater than 160/90 mmHg with or without medication? (Answer **YES** if you do not know your resting blood pressure)	YES ☐ NO ☐

5. Do you have any Metabolic Conditions? This includes Type 1 Diabetes, Type 2 Diabetes, Pre-Diabetes

If the above condition(s) is/are present, answer questions 5a-5e   If **NO** ☐ go to question 6

5a.	Do you often have difficulty controlling your blood sugar levels with foods, medications, or other physician-prescribed therapies?	YES ☐ NO ☐
5b.	Do you often suffer from signs and symptoms of low blood sugar (hypoglycemia) following exercise and/or during activities of daily living? Signs of hypoglycemia may include shakiness, nervousness, unusual irritability, abnormal sweating, dizziness or light-headedness, mental confusion, difficulty speaking, weakness, or sleepiness.	YES ☐ NO ☐
5c.	Do you have any signs or symptoms of diabetes complications such as heart or vascular disease and/or complications affecting your eyes, kidneys, **OR** the sensation in your toes and feet?	YES ☐ NO ☐
5d.	Do you have other metabolic conditions (such as current pregnancy-related diabetes, chronic kidney disease, or liver problems)?	YES ☐ NO ☐
5e.	Are you planning to engage in what for you is unusually high (or vigorous) intensity exercise in the near future?	YES ☐ NO ☐

2023 PAR-Q+

6. **Do you have any Mental Health Problems or Learning Difficulties?** This includes Alzheimer's, Dementia, Depression, Anxiety Disorder, Eating Disorder, Psychotic Disorder, Intellectual Disability, Down Syndrome

If the above condition(s) is/are present, answer questions 6a-6b   If **NO** ☐ go to question 7

6a.	Do you have difficulty controlling your condition with medications or other physician-prescribed therapies? (Answer **NO** if you are not currently taking medications or other treatments)	YES ☐ NO ☐
6b.	Do you have Down Syndrome **AND** back problems affecting nerves or muscles?	YES ☐ NO ☐

7. **Do you have a Respiratory Disease?** This includes Chronic Obstructive Pulmonary Disease, Asthma, Pulmonary High Blood Pressure

If the above condition(s) is/are present, answer questions 7a-7d   If **NO** ☐ go to question 8

7a.	Do you have difficulty controlling your condition with medications or other physician-prescribed therapies? (Answer **NO** if you are not currently taking medications or other treatments)	YES ☐ NO ☐
7b.	Has your doctor ever said your blood oxygen level is low at rest or during exercise and/or that you require supplemental oxygen therapy?	YES ☐ NO ☐
7c.	If asthmatic, do you currently have symptoms of chest tightness, wheezing, laboured breathing, consistent cough (more than 2 days/week), or have you used your rescue medication more than twice in the last week?	YES ☐ NO ☐
7d.	Has your doctor ever said you have high blood pressure in the blood vessels of your lungs?	YES ☐ NO ☐

8. **Do you have a Spinal Cord Injury?** This includes Tetraplegia and Paraplegia

If the above condition(s) is/are present, answer questions 8a-8c   If **NO** ☐ go to question 9

8a.	Do you have difficulty controlling your condition with medications or other physician-prescribed therapies? (Answer **NO** if you are not currently taking medications or other treatments)	YES ☐ NO ☐
8b.	Do you commonly exhibit low resting blood pressure significant enough to cause dizziness, light-headedness, and/or fainting?	YES ☐ NO ☐
8c.	Has your physician indicated that you exhibit sudden bouts of high blood pressure (known as Autonomic Dysreflexia)?	YES ☐ NO ☐

9. **Have you had a Stroke?** This includes Transient Ischemic Attack (TIA) or Cerebrovascular Event

If the above condition(s) is/are present, answer questions 9a-9c   If **NO** ☐ go to question 10

9a.	Do you have difficulty controlling your condition with medications or other physician-prescribed therapies? (Answer **NO** if you are not currently taking medications or other treatments)	YES ☐ NO ☐
9b.	Do you have any impairment in walking or mobility?	YES ☐ NO ☐
9c.	Have you experienced a stroke or impairment in nerves or muscles in the past 6 months?	YES ☐ NO ☐

10. **Do you have any other medical condition not listed above or do you have two or more medical conditions?**

If you have other medical conditions, answer questions 10a-10c   If **NO** ☐ read the Page 4 recommendations

10a.	Have you experienced a blackout, fainted, or lost consciousness as a result of a head injury within the last 12 months **OR** have you had a diagnosed concussion within the last 12 months?	YES ☐ NO ☐
10b.	Do you have a medical condition that is not listed (such as epilepsy, neurological conditions, kidney problems)?	YES ☐ NO ☐
10c.	Do you currently live with two or more medical conditions?	YES ☐ NO ☐

PLEASE LIST YOUR MEDICAL CONDITION(S) AND ANY RELATED MEDICATIONS HERE: _____

_____

GO to Page 4 for recommendations about your current medical condition(s) and sign the PARTICIPANT DECLARATION.

2023 PAR-Q+

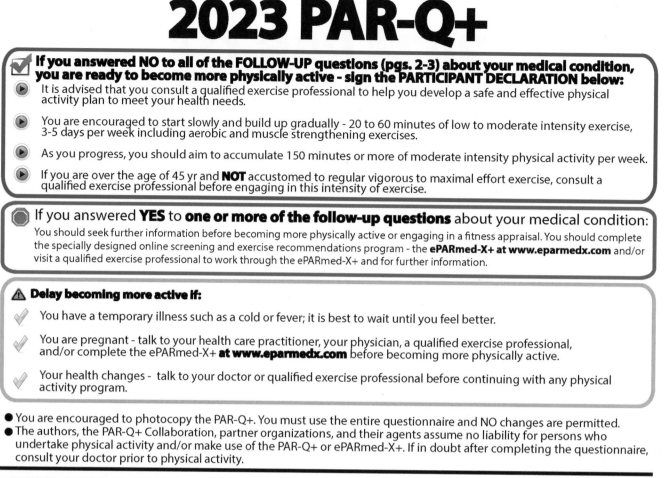

☑ **If you answered NO to all of the FOLLOW-UP questions (pgs. 2-3) about your medical condition, you are ready to become more physically active - sign the PARTICIPANT DECLARATION below:**

▶ It is advised that you consult a qualified exercise professional to help you develop a safe and effective physical activity plan to meet your health needs.

▶ You are encouraged to start slowly and build up gradually - 20 to 60 minutes of low to moderate intensity exercise, 3-5 days per week including aerobic and muscle strengthening exercises.

▶ As you progress, you should aim to accumulate 150 minutes or more of moderate intensity physical activity per week.

▶ If you are over the age of 45 yr and **NOT** accustomed to regular vigorous to maximal effort exercise, consult a qualified exercise professional before engaging in this intensity of exercise.

🛑 **If you answered YES to one or more of the follow-up questions about your medical condition:**

You should seek further information before becoming more physically active or engaging in a fitness appraisal. You should complete the specially designed online screening and exercise recommendations program - the **ePARmed-X+ at www.eparmedx.com** and/or visit a qualified exercise professional to work through the ePARmed-X+ and for further information.

⚠ **Delay becoming more active if:**

✔ You have a temporary illness such as a cold or fever; it is best to wait until you feel better.

✔ You are pregnant - talk to your health care practitioner, your physician, a qualified exercise professional, and/or complete the ePARmed-X+ **at www.eparmedx.com** before becoming more physically active.

✔ Your health changes - talk to your doctor or qualified exercise professional before continuing with any physical activity program.

● You are encouraged to photocopy the PAR-Q+. You must use the entire questionnaire and NO changes are permitted.
● The authors, the PAR-Q+ Collaboration, partner organizations, and their agents assume no liability for persons who undertake physical activity and/or make use of the PAR-Q+ or ePARmed-X+. If in doubt after completing the questionnaire, consult your doctor prior to physical activity.

PARTICIPANT DECLARATION

● All persons who have completed the PAR-Q+ please read and sign the declaration below.

● If you are less than the legal age required for consent or require the assent of a care provider, your parent, guardian or care provider must also sign this form.

I, the undersigned, have read, understood to my full satisfaction and completed this questionnaire. I acknowledge that this physical activity clearance is valid for a maximum of 12 months from the date it is completed and becomes invalid if my condition changes. I also acknowledge that the community/fitness center may retain a copy of this form for records. In these instances, it will maintain the confidentiality of the same, complying with applicable law.

NAME _____ DATE _____

SIGNATURE _____ WITNESS _____

SIGNATURE OF PARENT/GUARDIAN/CARE PROVIDER _____

––––––– For more information, please contact –––––––
www.eparmedx.com
Email: eparmedx@gmail.com

Citation for PAR-Q+
Warburton DER, Jamnik VK, Bredin SSD, and Gledhill N on behalf of the PAR-Q+ Collaboration.
The Physical Activity Readiness Questionnaire for Everyone (PAR-Q+) and Electronic Physical Activity
Readiness Medical Examination (ePARmed-X+). Health & Fitness Journal of Canada 4(2):3-23, 2011.

The PAR-Q+ was created using the evidence-based AGREE process (1) by the PAR-Q+ Collaboration chaired by Dr. Darren E. R. Warburton with Dr. Norman Gledhill, Dr. Veronica Jamnik, and Dr. Donald C. McKenzie (2). Production of this document has been made possible through financial contributions from the Public Health Agency of Canada and the BC Ministry of Health Services. The views expressed herein do not necessarily represent the views of the Public Health Agency of Canada or the BC Ministry of Health Services.

Key References
1. Jamnik VK, Warburton DER, Makarski J, McKenzie DC, Shephard RJ, Stone J, and Gledhill N. Enhancing the effectiveness of clearance for physical activity participation; background and overall process. APNM 36(S1):S3-S13, 2011.
2. Warburton DER, Gledhill N, Jamnik VK, Bredin SSD, McKenzie DC, Stone J, Charlesworth S, and Shephard RJ. Evidence-based risk assessment and recommendations for physical activity clearance; Consensus Document. APNM 36(S1):S266-s298, 2011.
3. Chisholm DM, Collis ML, Kulak LL, Davenport W, and Gruber N. Physical activity readiness. British Columbia Medical Journal. 1975;17:375-378.
4. Thomas S, Reading J, and Shephard RJ. Revision of the Physical Activity Readiness Questionnaire (PAR-Q). Canadian Journal of Sport Science 1992;17:4 338-345.

Reprinted by permission from the PAR-Q+ Collaboration and the authors of the PAR-Q+ (Dr. Darren Warburton, Dr. Norman Gledhill, Dr. Veronica Jamnik, and Dr. Shannon Bredin).

FORM 2.2   PASQ (Pre-Activity Screening Questionnaire)

INSTRUCTIONS

Please complete all four sections of this form. A staff member who is an exercise professional in our facility will review it and inform you if medical clearance is needed prior to engaging in physical activity.

SECTION 1—CURRENT PHYSICAL ACTIVITY

When answering the questions in this section, please note the following definitions:

Moderate Intensity: An activity that causes noticeable increases in heart rate and breathing (e.g., brisk walking)

Vigorous Intensity: An activity that causes substantial increases in heart rate and breathing (e.g., jogging)

Over the last three months, have you regularly performed physical activity for at least 30 minutes, three days/week at a moderate intensity level?   ○Yes   ○No

If yes, which of the following best describes any vigorous-intensity activity in your regular routine the last 3 months?

_____I participate in some or all vigorous-intensity activity

_____None, but I want to begin some vigorous-intensity activity

_____None, and I want to continue moderate-intensity activity

SECTION 2—MEDICAL CONDITIONS

Please check (✔) any of the following medical conditions that you currently have or have had.

_____Heart attack

_____Heart surgery

_____Cardiac catheterization

_____Coronary angioplasty (PTCA)

_____Heart valve disease

_____Heart failure

_____Heart transplantation

_____Congenital heart disease

_____Abnormal heart rhythm

_____Pacemaker/implantable cardiac defibrillator

_____Peripheral vascular disease (PVD or PAD): disease affecting blood vessels in arms, hands, legs, and feet

_____Cerebrovascular disease—stroke or TIA (transient ischemic attack)

_____Type 1 or Type 2 diabetes

_____Renal (kidney) disease

(continued)

FORM 2.2 *(continued)*

SECTION 3—SIGNS OR SYMPTOMS

Please check (✔) any of the signs or symptoms that you have *recently* experienced.

_____Pain, discomfort in the chest, neck, jaw, or arms at rest *or* upon exertion

_____Shortness of breath at rest *or* with mild exertion

_____Dizziness or loss of consciousness during *or* shortly after exercise

_____Shortness of breath occurring at rest *or* 2-5 hours after the onset of sleep

_____Edema (swelling) in both ankles that is most evident at night *or* swelling in a limb

_____An unpleasant awareness of forceful *or* rapid beating of the heart

_____Pain in the legs *or* elsewhere while walking; often more severe when walking upstairs or uphill

_____Known heart murmur

_____Unusual fatigue *or* shortness of breath with usual activities

SECTION 4—ACKNOWLEDGMENT, FOLLOW-UP, AND SIGNATURE

I acknowledge that I have read this questionnaire in its entirety and have responded accurately, completely, and to the best of my knowledge. Any questions regarding the items on this questionnaire were answered to my satisfaction. Also, if my health status changes at any time, I understand that I am responsible to inform a staff member at this facility of any such changes. I also understand that the PASQ is not a substitution for a medical examination.

Please note: The authors of the PASQ assume no liability for individuals who participate in physical activity and/or complete the PASQ. If questions arise after completing the PASQ, seek the advice of your health care provider prior to physical activity.

Participant's Name—Please Print _____

Participant's Signature _____

Date _____

FORM 2.3 Example Health Status Questionnaire (HSQ)

SECTION 1—PERSONAL AND EMERGENCY CONTACT INFORMATION

Name: _____ Date of birth: _____

Address: _____

Phone: _____ (OK to text message to this number: Yes or No)

Physician's name: _____

Height: _____ Weight: _____

Person to contact in case of emergency: _____

Emergency contact phone: _____

SECTION 2—CURRENT AND PLANNED PHYSICAL ACTIVITY LEVEL

Have you been performing planned, structured physical activity for at least 30 minutes a day at a moderate intensity on at least 3 days per week for at least the last 3 months?
○ Yes   ○ No
If yes, please list typical weekly activities in which you currently engage *and* note if any changes in your exercise program are desired.

_____

_____

If no, please note the frequency, intensity, time, and type of exercise you plan to perform.

_____

_____

Please check all true statements for sections 3-4.

SECTION 3—MEDICAL CONDITIONS

Have you had or do you currently have any of the following?

_____ A heart attack

_____ Heart surgery, cardiac catheterization, or coronary angioplasty

_____ Pacemaker, implantable cardiac defibrillator/rhythm disturbance

_____ Heart valve disease   _____ High cholesterol

_____ Heart failure   _____ Diabetes

_____ Heart transplantation   _____ Renal disease

_____ Congenital heart disease   _____ Asthma

_____ High blood pressure   _____ Cancer

_____ Other medical condition (please specify: _____)

SECTION 4—SYMPTOMS

Do you currently experience any of the following?

_____ Chest discomfort with exertion   _____ Unreasonable breathlessness

_____ Dizziness, fainting, or blackouts   _____ Ankle swelling

_____ Unpleasant awareness of a forceful, rapid, or irregular heart rate

_____ Burning or cramping sensations in your lower legs when walking a short distance

The fitness professional should be informed immediately of any changes that occur in your health status.

(continued)

FORM 2.3 *(continued)*

SECTION 5—CIGARETTE SMOKING

Are you a current smoker? ○ Yes   ○ No
If no, select one of the following:
_____ Never smoked
_____ Quit (list approximate date when quit smoking)
Are you exposed to environmental tobacco smoke? ○ Yes   ○ No

SECTION 6—HISTORY OF SURGERIES OR HOSPITALIZATION

Please list any surgeries or hospitalizations, including the date of the occurrence.

_____

_____

_____

SECTION 7—HISTORY OF MUSCULOSKELETAL OR JOINT INJURIES

Please list any injuries that have affected your ability to be physically active, including the date of injury and the duration of impact.

_____

_____

_____

SECTION 8—FAMILY HISTORY

Do you have any immediate family members with the following? If so, list relationship.

_____ Heart attack   _____ Diabetes

_____ Heart surgery (e.g., bypass, stent)   _____ Cancer

_____ Sudden death

SECTION 9—PRESCRIBED OR OVER-THE-COUNTER MEDICATIONS

Are you currently taking any medication? ○ Yes   ○ No
If yes, please list all of your prescribed and over-the-counter medications and how often you take them, whether daily (D) or as needed (PRN).

_____

_____

Of the medications you have listed, are there any you do not take as prescribed?

_____

_____

To be completed by fitness professional:
Medical clearance required   ○ Yes   ○ No
If *yes*, note date it was received: _____

PATIENT INFORMATION RELEASE FORM

If it is recommended that you receive medical clearance prior to exercise participation, you agree that it is permissible to seek this approval from your physician in compliance with the Health Insurance Portability and Accountability Act of 1996 (HIPAA).

Participant signature: _____ Date: _____

Fitness professional signature: _____ Date: _____

Adapted from ACSM (2022); ACSM (2022).

Evaluation of Screening Forms

Initially, the participant's preparticipation screening should be evaluated to ascertain if medical clearance is necessary prior to beginning an exercise program based on the following:

1. The individual's current physical activity level
2. Known cardiovascular, metabolic, or renal disease or signs and symptoms of these diseases
3. Desired exercise intensity

Addressing these three factors will help the fitness professional identify those individuals who should not pursue unaccustomed vigorous-intensity exercise that may expose them to an unnecessary increased risk for sudden cardiac death or acute myocardial infarction (8, 47). Participants who do not require medical clearance can undergo fitness testing, and the results should be evaluated relative to norms or be used to track progress. With this information, the fitness professional can develop an appropriate exercise prescription for improving the participant's health and fitness in relation to present health status and physical activity level. To maintain up-to-date records of the participant's health status, ask participants to promptly report any significant change in health status and readminister the HSQ annually (6).

Make a Classification on Exercise Status

The first step in evaluating health status entails determining whether the individual currently participates in regular exercise. Participants should be classified as a current exerciser if they have been performing planned, structured physical activity of at least moderate intensity (i.e., 40%-59% $\dot{V}O_2R$) for at least 30 minutes a day on 3 or more days a week during the past 3 months. This classification helps identify those individuals unaccustomed to regular physical activity and for whom exercise may place unwarranted demands on the cardiovascular system and increase the risk of complications (e.g., myocardial infarction) (8, 47).

Review Medical History

The next step involves identifying if the participant has been previously diagnosed with CVD including heart disease, peripheral vascular disease, and cerebrovascular disease (i.e., stroke); metabolic disease including diabetes mellitus (type 1 or 2 diabetes); or renal disease.

The fitness professional should ask the participant if a physician or other qualified health care provider has ever diagnosed them with any of these diseases. Prior diagnosis of one of these diseases alone does not warrant medical clearance; the fitness professional also should consider whether the participant is a regular exerciser, the participant's medical history, and the participant's desired aerobic exercise intensity (8, 47).

Identify Signs and Symptoms

Table 2.1 provides information to assist with identifying major signs and symptoms indicative of undiagnosed cardiovascular, metabolic, or renal disease. To acknowledge any of these signs or symptoms would mean the individual is symptomatic and should receive medical clearance from an appropriate health care provider before pursuing a regular exercise program, even if they are currently participating in regular exercise (i.e., discontinue exercise if these are reported) (8, 47). Conversely, participants who do not present with the conditions in table 2.1 would be considered to be asymptomatic. Note that just because participants have one of these signs or symptoms, it does not mean that they have cardiovascular, metabolic, or renal disease. The fitness professional should evaluate the signs and symptoms within the context of the participant's recent medical history and seek additional information to further qualify the participant's responses. For instance, a participant may present with a resting heart rate (RHR) greater than 100 bpm but have no other symptoms suggestive of CVD. Upon further inquiry, the fitness professional finds that the participant has rushed to make the appointment and recently consumed a large dose of caffeine. Thus, the elevated heart rate (HR) may be the result of these recent events rather than an indication of possible CVD; rechecking RHR would be appropriate. This scenario demonstrates the importance of the fitness professional asking additional questions to interpret the preparticipation screening properly (8, 47).

KEY POINT

Evaluation of the preparticipation screening helps the fitness professional determine whether a participant

1. is a current, regular exerciser;
2. has established cardiovascular, metabolic, or renal disease; and
3. shows signs or symptoms suggestive of these diseases.

These criteria help determine whether it is appropriate for the participant to undergo fitness testing or begin regular physical activity or if medical clearance is recommended before doing so (8). All health screening information should be kept private, confidential, and secure.

Table 2.1 Major Signs or Symptoms of Cardiovascular, Metabolic, and Renal Diseases

Sign or symptom	Clarification and significance
Angina (i.e., heart pain) in the chest, neck, jaw, arms, or other areas; women may also present with unusual nausea	Angina is a hallmark of heart disease and indicates the blood supply to the heart is insufficient (i.e., ischemia). Key features of angina include a constricting or heavy feeling in the middle of the chest, shoulders, back, or arms, or in the neck, cheeks, or teeth. These sensations may be provoked by exercise or exertion and other forms of stress, cold temperature, or after meals.
Palpitations or tachycardia (i.e., RHR >100 bpm)	A palpitation is the unpleasant awareness of a forceful or rapid heartbeat, which may indicate an irregular heartbeat. The fitness professional may be able to sense the palpitation by taking the HR manually at the carotid or radial artery. Palpitations can originate from unusual stress, fever, anemia, or a high cardiac output. Tachycardia is a common palpitation, and it can be due to recent actions (e.g., caffeine ingestion) or a sign of other cardiovascular problems.
Shortness of breath at rest or with mild exertion	Dyspnea is an abnormally uncomfortable awareness of breathing and is a principal symptom of cardiac and pulmonary disease. It occurs naturally during heavy exertion in individuals with high CRF and during mild exertion in untrained individuals. Dyspnea may be considered abnormal when it occurs at an atypical (e.g., low-intensity) level of exertion for an individual.
Dizziness or syncope	Syncope is the loss of consciousness and occurs most often due to lack of blood flow to the brain. Dizziness and especially syncope during exercise can be the product of cardiac disorders that prevent the normal increase or decrease in cardiac output. These cardiac output disorders are potentially life threatening. Dizziness or syncope can occur in healthy individuals after completing an exercise bout and should be addressed. These symptoms may occur because of reduced blood flow back to the heart.
Ankle edema	Ankle edema is an unnatural accumulation of fluid surrounding the ankles and is characteristic of congestive heart failure (CHF), a common form of CVD. Individuals with CHF may exhibit generalized edema, whereas swelling in one limb may result from a venous thrombosis or blockage in the lymphatic system.
Intermittent claudication	Intermittent claudication is a burning or cramping pain in the lower extremities that is exacerbated by exertion. It occurs in a muscle with inadequate blood supply secondary to localized atherosclerosis. The pain should be consistent at a given exertion level and should resolve within 1-2 minutes after exercise cessation. Intermittent claudication is more prevalent in individuals with CHD and type 1 or 2 diabetes.
Orthopnea or paroxysmal nocturnal dyspnea	Orthopnea is dyspnea that occurs when lying at rest, with relief occurring by sitting upright or standing. Paroxysmal nocturnal dyspnea occurs during sleep, with relief by sitting up or standing. Both conditions reflect left ventricular dysfunction; nocturnal dyspnea also may be seen in individuals with chronic obstructive pulmonary disease.
Known heart murmur	Heart murmurs may be of no concern or may indicate cardiovascular disease. Realize that common causes of exertion-related sudden cardiac death, including hypertrophic cardiomyopathy and aortic stenosis, must be ruled out.
Unusual fatigue or shortness of breath with usual activities	This may be benign or may be a sign of the onset or change in status of cardiovascular or metabolic diseases.

Adapted by permission from American College of Sports Medicine, *ACSM's Guidelines for Exercise Testing and Prescription*, 11th ed. (Philadelphia, PA: Wolters Kluwer, 2022).

Determine Desired Level of Activity

Determining the desired aerobic exercise intensity level is also included in the preparticipation screening process. The fitness professional should consider the individual's proposed exercise intensity, properly classify it (i.e., light, moderate, or vigorous), and compare it to the individual's current exercise level. Aerobic exercise intensity is commonly classified as follows: light (i.e., ≤40% $\dot{V}O_2R$), moderate (i.e., 40%-59% $\dot{V}O_2R$), and vigorous (i.e., ≥60% $\dot{V}O_2R$) (8, 47). Thus, the fitness professional can readily discern if the participant plans to make changes to the exercise volume or to the aerobic exercise intensity that will be performed. Compared to light- to moderate-intensity aerobic exercise, vigorous-intensity aerobic exercise is more likely to initiate acute cardiovascular events in selected individuals (29, 53). Thus, the desired level of aerobic exercise intensity should be considered before recommending medical clearance prior to exercise participation.

KEY POINT

Analyzing current and desired exercise intensity, disease status, and presence of signs or symptoms are considered when determining whether a participant requires medical clearance before exercising, undergoing fitness testing, or progressing the intensity or volume of their exercise regimen.

Establish If Medical Clearance Is Recommended

At this juncture, the fitness professional should consider the individual's current exercise status; the presence of diagnosed cardiovascular, metabolic, or renal disease; signs or symptoms indicative of these diseases; and the participant's desired aerobic intensity level. The ACSM has provided a preparticipation screening algorithm (see figure 2.1) to help fitness professionals make this decision. Each determination must be made on a case-by-case basis. The starting point of the logic model is based on the subject's participation in regular exercise, then decisions are made based on disease and symptom status. It may help the fitness professional to consider these three caveats to determine if medical clearance is recommended.

1. Individuals who have not been diagnosed with cardiovascular, metabolic, or renal disease and who do not demonstrate signs or symptoms of these diseases do not require medical clearance, whether they are current, regular exercisers or not.

2. Individuals with signs and symptoms indicative of cardiovascular, metabolic, or renal disease are always recommended to receive medical clearance, regardless of their disease status or whether they are current, regular exercisers.

3. Individuals with established cardiovascular, metabolic, or renal disease who are asymptomatic need medical clearance prior to aerobic exercise participation if they are not regular exercisers. In contrast, participants with these same characteristics who are regular exercisers only need medical clearance if they plan to pursue vigorous-intensity aerobic exercise.

These guidelines, combined with the fitness professional's sound judgment, help determine whether a participant requires medical clearance prior to exercise participation (8, 7, 47). It is important to note that the last portion of the algorithm addresses aerobic exercise progression.

When medical clearance before exercise participation is recommended, a referral to the individual's health care provider should be made. The type of medical clearance (e.g., verbal communications, electrocardiogram monitoring during a graded exercise test, or more advanced testing) should be determined by the health care provider to whom the participant is referred, because no universally recommended screening test has been established (8). A written clearance along with any instruction or restrictions can be requested by the fitness professional, and continued communication between the health care provider and fitness professional is encouraged (8).

Steps Following the Screening Process

With the information gathered within the preparticipation and health screenings, and assuming medical clearance is either not required or has been obtained, the fitness professional can move forward working with the client.

Administer Fitness Tests and Evaluate Results

The next step of the health appraisal involves administering and evaluating fitness tests. When combined with the HSQ, the test results provide greater insight into an individual's current level of physical fitness. Common measurements obtained before fitness testing are HR and blood pressure (BP), percent body fat, waist circumference, and flexibility. Next, a submaximal graded exercise test can be conducted to determine how the participant's HR, BP, and rating of perceived exertion (RPE) respond to gradually increasing exercise workloads. Additional

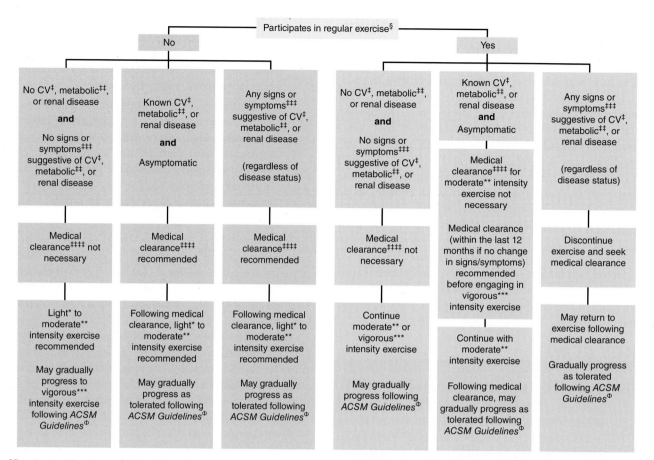

§Exercise participation, performing planned, structured physical activity at least 30 minutes at moderate intensity on at least 3 d ·wk⁻¹ for at least the last 3 months.

*Light-intensity exercise, 30% to <40% HRR or V̇O₂R, 2 to <3 METs, 9–11 RPE, an intensity that causes slight increases in HR and breathing.

**Moderate-intensity exercise, 40% to <60% HRR or V̇O₂R, 3 to <6 METs, 12–13 RPE, an intensity that causes noticeable increases in HR and breathing.

***Vigorous-intensity exercise, ≥60% HRR or V̇O₂R, ≥6 METs, ≥14 RPE, an intensity that causes substantial increases in HR and breathing.

‡CVD, cardiac, peripheral vascular, or cerebrovascular disease.

‡‡Metabolic disease, type 1 and 2 diabetes mellitus.

‡‡‡Signs and symptoms, at rest or during activity; includes pain, discomfort in the chest, neck, jaw, arms, or other areas that may result from ischemia; shortness of breath at rest or with mild exertion; dizziness or syncope; orthopnea or paroxysmal nocturnal dyspnea; ankle edema; palpitations or tachycardia; intermittent claudication; known heart murmur; or unusual fatigue or shortness of breath with usual activities.

‡‡‡‡Medical clearance, approval from a health care professional to engage in exercise.

ΦSee the most current edition of *ACSM's Guidelines for Exercise Testing and Prescription*.

FIGURE 2.1 ACSM preparticipation screening algorithm for aerobic exercise participation.

Reprinted by permission from D. Riebe, B. Franklin, P. Thompson, et al., "Updating ACSM's Recommendations for Exercise Preparticipation Health Screening," *Medicine in Science in Sports and Exercise* 47 (2015): 2473-79.

fitness tests may be used to determine muscular strength and endurance, flexibility, and functional fitness. Chapter 7 includes an overview of testing, and other chapters in part III include fitness testing procedures. Indications for stopping an exercise test are discussed in detail in chapter 8 and include the participant complaining of chest pain, inappropriate BP or HR responses, pronounced shortness of breath at low exercise intensities, signs of poor perfusion, or severe fatigue (8). If symptoms suggestive of CVD occur during fitness testing, the fit-

ness professional should stop the test and seek medical assistance if needed. Medical clearance would be recommended before conducting additional exercise testing or permitting the client to begin exercising in the facility. The results of the fitness tests can be compared with normative data based on the participant's age and sex (8) or can simply be tracked over time to chart progress. The fitness test values, combined with the participant's medical history and exercise goals, should serve as the framework for the exercise prescription.

Develop an Individualized Exercise Prescription

At this point, the fitness professional should be prepared to address the next step in the health appraisal process: setting up the exercise prescription by following current guidelines (8). An appropriate exercise prescription considers a person's health status, personal goals, and fitness test results. Chapters in part IV of this textbook address exercise prescriptions for aerobic fitness, muscular fitness, flexibility, and neuromotor function for generally healthy adults. In addition, chapters in part V provide background on exercise prescription for special populations.

Evaluate Progress With Follow-Up Tests

The participant's exercise goals and health status are certain to change over time, which necessitates the last step in the health appraisal: evaluating progress with follow-up tests. Fitness tests should be repeated periodically and a health screening readministered. Follow-ups involving fitness tests and updates to the participant's health status serve several purposes: documenting the participant's health and fitness progress, identifying any changes in health status or response to activity, and indicating whether changes in the exercise prescription or level of supervision are necessary (8). No specific guidance exists on the timing of follow-up testing. Follow-up fitness tests may be conducted 2 to 3 months after the participant has been exercising regularly, with biannual testing thereafter. For established exercisers, annual testing may be sufficient to provide feedback on training status.

Fitness Program Decisions

This chapter has addressed the guidelines supported by the ACSM concerning when medical clearance is necessary before a participant undergoes fitness testing or begins an exercise program. The following section discusses additional criteria to consider as the fitness professional decides which of the following actions to pursue:

- Immediate referral for medical clearance
- Admission to one of the following fitness programs:
  - Clinic-based supervised exercise program
  - Appropriately prescribed exercise under the supervision of a fitness professional
  - Vigorous-intensity exercise program
  - Any unsupervised physical activity

- Educational information, seminars, or referral to other health professionals

Fitness professionals will encounter people who are on the verge of meeting the criteria for medical clearance. Do they require medical clearance? Should they possibly exercise in a clinical supervised program? The following section provides considerations to help resolve these dilemmas, realizing that each case will be unique.

Determining If Referral to a Supervised Program Is Necessary

The fitness professional should consider the participant's health status and desired activity level to determine whether referral to a supervised exercise program is necessary. A clinical supervised program has a medical director (or committee), who provides oversight of the program, and professionally qualified staff, who have academic training in and clinical knowledge of monitoring special populations who are at a significantly higher risk for cardiac complications during exercise (e.g., people diagnosed with cardiovascular, metabolic, or renal disease) (8). These types of programs are also better suited for people with special conditions (e.g., emphysema, chronic bronchitis, cancer, epilepsy) that warrant additional supervision by medically qualified personnel (e.g., nurses or clinical exercise physiologists) who have experience with special populations.

For example, consider a 65-year-old male who experiences unreasonable breathlessness at rest, and upon further inquiry it is noted that he has chronic bronchitis and typically requires supplemental oxygen when exercising. The participant has been walking regularly and independently but never monitors his blood oxygen levels (i.e., oxygen saturation levels). In this case, the pulmonary condition dictates that the participant's oxygen levels should be monitored before, during, and after exercise participation to ensure that oxygen saturation levels are maintained. This individual would benefit from initially exercising in a clinic-based supervised exercise program, such as a supervised pulmonary rehabilitation or cardiac rehabilitation program. As with medical clearance, no universal guidelines exist for referring an individual to supervised programs. Each exercise facility should have standards regarding the health conditions it considers itself qualified to supervise, and these standards should be based on the qualifications of its fitness professionals, the availability of medical equipment (e.g., supplemental oxygen, automatic external defibrillator [AED]), and its emergency preparedness (9). The safety of the participant is a priority in each of these decisions; when unsure, fitness professionals should consult with a supervisor or physician to determine whether referral to a supervised program is necessary.

Obtaining Medical Clearance

Obtaining medical clearance is recommended in professionally staffed fitness facilities and programs, based on predetermined screening criteria. After determining that a person requires medical clearance, the fitness professional should immediately inform the participant of this requirement. The appropriate health care personnel, typically the participant's primary care physician, should provide the medical clearance and will determine how the medical clearance will be granted (6, 8). A sample medical clearance form is presented in form 2.4. Another option, specific to the use of the PASQ, can be accessed from the Fitness Law Academy (https://www.fitness lawacademy.com/forms-and-documents). Both forms provide the health care professional with the option to refer the patient to a clinic-based supervised exercise facility. When the health care professional makes this recommendation, the fitness professional should contact the participant promptly and place the participant in contact with the nearest clinic-based supervised exercise facility. In accordance with HIPAA regulations, the request for medical clearance must be accompanied by a written notation indicating that the participant understands that personal health information will be shared with appropriate health care professionals (i.e., medical release form) (36).

Medical clearance can be sought in one of two ways. First, the participant can be given the paperwork to be signed by an appropriate health care professional. Afterward, the participant can return the paperwork to the fitness professional for verification. This has been suggested to be the most expedient method given the established relationship between the participant and the medical provider (19). Second, if a written authorization to release medical records has been signed by the participant (i.e., the medical release form), fitness professionals can contact the appropriate health care professional and provide the medical release form to the physician's administrative office along with the medical clearance form. If the fitness professional sends the medical clearance form directly to the participant's physician, the physician may require that the patient sign the clinic's HIPAA authorized medical release form before returning it to the fitness professional, if the completed clearance form contains the patient's PHI. The workload of many health care professionals does not allow them to respond quickly to each medical request they receive. Thus, it is recommended to wait 3 business days before sending a second medical clearance request. Thereafter, participants should be encouraged to contact the health care professional personally to expedite the return of the medical clearance form. Participants requiring medical clearance should be informed of the facility's preparticipation screening protocol so they understand that their clearance to begin exercising may take time. Although they may have to wait to exercise, participants should be assured that the steps taken in accordance with established protocols are serving their health interests.

To prevent the delay of fitness tests for individuals requiring medical clearance, the preparticipation screening procedures could be completed and submitted to the appropriate fitness professional for review 2 to 3 business days before a fitness test is scheduled. This will provide time to secure medical clearance and ensure that the appropriate paperwork is completed before the fitness test, allowing the participant to begin an exercise program shortly thereafter.

KEY POINT

The fitness professional should consider the participant's health status and desired activity level, as well as the facility's preparticipation screening standards and emergency preparedness, to determine whether referral to a clinical supervised exercise program is necessary. If necessary, medical clearance should be obtained or appropriate medical personnel contacted prior to exercise testing and participation.

Education Regarding CVD Risk Factors

A thorough health risk appraisal includes a medical history and CVD risk factor assessment. Identifying and effectively controlling CVD risk factors is an important objective of overall CVD prevention and management even though it is no longer a part of the preparticipation screening process (8). Fitness professionals are encouraged to review CVD risk factors with participants to ascertain if they meet the requirements for positive CVD risk factors (see table 2.2). Fitness professionals are encouraged to be conservative when identifying CVD risk factors. When a specific risk factor is unknown or unavailable, it is designated as a risk factor. It is common practice to sum the number of positive CVD risk factors. It is important to note that elevated high-density lipoprotein cholesterol (HDL-C) levels $\geq$HDL 60 mg $\cdot$ dl^{-1} (1.55 mmol $\cdot$ L^{-1}) are considered to be a negative CVD risk factor, which provides a cardioprotective benefit. Participants with HDL-C levels $\geq$HDL 60 mg $\cdot$ dl^{-1} (1.55 mmol $\cdot$ L^{-1}) should have one positive CVD risk factor subtracted from the sum of the positive CVD risk factors (8, 5).

FORM 2.4   Sample Medical Clearance Form*

Dear _____:

Your patient _____ would like to begin an exercise program at our fitness facility, _____. We would appreciate your medical opinion and recommendations concerning participation in regular exercise at our facility. The exercise program may include aerobic training, strength training, flexibility exercises, and neuromotor activities (e.g., balance, agility), which will be appropriately increased in duration and intensity over time. Please provide the following information and return this form to the fitness professional working with your patient.

Name: _____

Address: _____

AUTHORIZATION

I consent to and authorize my health care professional to release health information, specifically concerning my ability to participate in an exercise program and fitness assessment, to _____. By completing this form, the health care professional is not assuming any responsibility for the exercise and assessment program.

Participant's signature _____ Date _____

Fitness professional's signature _____ Date _____

HEALTH CARE PROFESSIONAL RECOMMENDATIONS

Please identify any recommendations or restrictions for your patient regarding the following:

○ I believe no contraindications to exercise exist and the client can begin an exercise program.

○ I believe some contraindications to exercise may exist and the client can begin an exercise program with the following cautions: _____.

○ I believe contraindications to exercise exist and the following activities should be avoided: _____.

○ I believe contraindications to exercise exist and the client should *not* begin an exercise program.

If this client has completed a graded exercise test, please provide a copy of the final exercise test report and interpretation.

Health care professional's signature _____

Health care professional's name _____

Address _____

Thank you for your consideration.

_____

(Signature of fitness professional)

*Must be accompanied by a medical release form in accordance with HIPAA regulations.

Table 2.2 Atherosclerotic Cardiovascular Disease Risk-Factor Thresholds

Positive risk factors[a]	Defining criteria
Age	Men ≥45 years; women ≥55 years
Family history	Myocardial infarction, coronary revascularization, or sudden death before age 55 in father or other male first-degree relative or before age 65 in mother or other female first-degree relative
Cigarette smoking	Current cigarette smoker, quit within previous 6 months, or exposure to environmental tobacco smoke
Physical inactivity	Not meeting minimum threshold of 500-1,000 MET-min of moderate to vigorous physical activity or 150 minutes of moderate-intensity or 75 minutes of vigorous-intensity physical activity
Body mass index (BMI)/waist circumference	BMI ≥30 kg · m^{-2} or waist girth >40 inches (102 centimeters) for men and >35 inches (88 centimeters) for women
Blood pressure	SBP ≥130 mmHg and/or DBP ≥80 mmHg based on an average of 2 or more occasions or on antihypertensive medication
Lipids	LDL-C ≥130 mg · dl^{-1} (3.37 mmol · L^{-1}) or HDL-C <40 mg · dl^{-1} (1.04 mmol · L^{-1}) in men and <50 mg · dl^{-1} (1.30 mmol · L^{-1}) in women or non-HDL-C ≥160 (4.14 mmol · L^{-1}) or on lipid-lowering medication. If total serum cholesterol is all that is available, use ≥200 mg · dl^{-1} (5.18 mmol · L^{-1})
Blood glucose	Fasting plasma glucose ≥100 mg · dl^{-1} (5.55 mmol · L^{-1}); or 2-hour plasma glucose values in oral glucose tolerance test ≥140 mg · dl^{-1} (7.77 mmol · L^{-1}); or HbA1C ≥5.7%

Negative risk factor	Defining criteria
HDL-C[b]	≥60 mg · dl^{-1} (1.55 mmol · L^{-1})

SBP = systolic blood pressure, DBP = diastolic blood pressure, HDL = high-density lipoprotein, LDL = low-density lipoprotein, non-HDL-C = total cholesterol minus HDL-C, HbA1C = glycated hemoglobin, MET = metabolic equivalent

[a]If the presence of or absence of a CVD risk factor is not disclosed or unavailable, that CVD risk factor should be counted as a risk factor.

[b]It is common to sum risk factors in making clinical judgments. If HDL-C is high, subtract one risk factor from the sum of positive risk factors because high HDL-C decreases CVD risk.

Adapted by permission from American College of Sports Medicine, *ACSM's Guidelines for Exercise Testing and Prescription*, 11th ed. (Philadelphia, PA: Wolters Kluwer, 2022), 47.

Fitness professionals should inform participants about their risk factors for CVD and the significance of those factors. Initially, they should explain the meaning of a risk factor (i.e., a clinical diagnosis or lifestyle behavior that increases the chances of developing heart disease). The fitness professional should then address which risk factors can be modified, which include all of the factors except family history and age. The participant should be informed that regular physical activity can have a positive influence on most risk factors for CVD and decrease the risk of developing new ones (8, 10). The reality that regular physical activity can help manage and prevent these risk factors can serve as powerful motivation for long-term exercise adherence.

The clinical significance of a given risk factor is predicated on its severity, and thus a risk-factor continuum should be considered (27, 28). Risk factors can be determined simply by noting the thresholds in table 2.2. A person who has a resting BP of ≥130/80 mmHg or is taking antihypertensive medication would be classified as hypertensive. Beginning at 115/75 mmHg, however, CVD risk doubles with each increment of 20/10 mmHg—the higher the BP, the higher the CVD risk (30). Considerable research evidence shows that increasing levels of abdominal obesity, blood glucose, smoking, and low-density lipoprotein cholesterol (LDL-C) are associated with additional CVD risk (17, 25, 32, 51, 52). Therefore, the presence and magnitude of the risk factor should be considered in order to quantify the CVD risk. Furthermore, risk factors exert an independent effect on CVD risk and also interact with one another to further increase CVD risk. For instance, the presence of obesity alone increases CVD risk 15% to 25%, but when it is present with high cholesterol and elevated fasting blood glucose, CVD risk increases approximately 65% to 85% (38, 39, 62). The degree of increased risk for multiple risk factors is determined by their combination and severity. To do this, various tools are available. In the past, the

Framingham algorithm was used, which quantified the severity of a participant's individual risk factors and overall relative risk for developing CVD (34, 60). Currently, the Framingham Heart Study recommends a CVD Risk Calculator, which considers age, sex, race, total cholesterol, HDL-C, systolic BP, BP-lowering medication use, diabetes status, and smoking status; a link to an online calculator is provided at this reference (26).

In addition, the fitness professional should discuss sensible lifestyle changes participants can pursue to control their CVD risk factors. However, information alone is unlikely to lead participants to make significant changes. Chapter 22 provides several approaches to supporting positive behavior change that fitness professionals can use to help the participant. In addition, the fitness professional can inform the participant of support groups and upcoming educational seminars, and may recommend other health professionals (e.g., dietitians) who can assist with healthy lifestyle choices.

Changing Health or Fitness Status

People who regularly participate in physical activity are likely to experience positive changes in their fitness level (e.g., greater CRF) and more effectively manage their risk factors (e.g., lower resting BP). These changes can be readily observed by noting changes in participants' exercise duration or intensity and in resting BP measurements. Changes such as these improve quality of life and reduce the risk for chronic disease.

However, new medical conditions may develop and not be readily apparent after a participant completes a preparticipation screening and fitness tests. Unless specifically asked about new conditions, participants may not report this information. For instance, a participant may begin to experience chest pain during exercise but may keep this information private. The preparticipation screening directs participants to contact the fitness director to report when they experience significant changes in their health status, but not all clients will understand the importance of this communication. Although some people will notify staff members when health changes occur, others will not. Open communication with clients is important. Also, semiannual fitness retesting and annual re-administration of the HSQ are advisable to determine whether participants who are experiencing changes in health status should seek medical clearance or be assigned to a clinic-based supervised program (6).

If participants develop symptoms such as significant chest pain during exercise or other signs or symptoms suggestive of undiagnosed cardiovascular, metabolic, or renal disease, they should stop exercising and be required to obtain medical clearance (8). Additional situations in which moderate- and vigorous-intensity exercise should be discontinued include musculoskeletal problems exac-

erbated with activity and severe psychological, medical, or drug or alcohol problems that are not responding to therapy (5). In addition, exercise should be deferred with major changes in resting BP (8). It is the responsibility of the fitness professional to determine the length of time between follow-up fitness tests or health screening administrations to ensure participants are pursuing an appropriate exercise program.

KEY POINT

Fitness professionals should be aware of temporary or chronic conditions that alter a participant's health status and warrant medical clearance, additional supervision, or changes in exercise recommendations. These conditions can be identified with periodic re-administration of the HSQ and follow-up fitness tests.

Understanding Common Medications

Within the HSQ, the participant should be asked to document prescribed and over-the-counter medications. Although knowledge of all aspects of pharmacology is beyond the scope of the fitness professional, awareness of common medications and their effects is valuable. Information on medications provides additional insight into the medical history and diagnosed CVD risk factors. Some participants may indicate that they do not have a given medical condition because they are taking medication to treat the condition. However, taking a prescription medication to manage a chronic disease does not mean that the condition is absent, just that it is more likely to be controlled. For example, a participant may indicate that they do not have high cholesterol but lists Lipitor as one of their medications. Lipitor is in a class of drugs known as *statins* and is prescribed to treat high cholesterol. Thus, the participant still has the CVD risk factor related to lipids, and the fitness professional should note this accordingly.

In addition, the fitness professional should be able to determine whether a prescribed medication will alter the typical physiological responses to physical activity. For example, if a participant is taking a medication from the class of drugs known as *beta-blockers*, the fitness professional should be aware that the participant's HR will be substantially reduced (e.g., may not exceed 120 bpm) even though the participant is exercising vigorously. This response should not be considered abnormal; instead, it indicates the effectiveness of the medication and necessitates the use of other ways to monitor exercise intensity such as use of a perceived exertion scale. The following section provides background on common medication categories, including how various medications may affect physiological responses to exercise (i.e., HR and BP responses).

The medications in this section are listed with both generic and brand names. Generic drugs can look physically different than their brand-name counterparts; however, the Food and Drug Administration (FDA) requires generic drugs (and their brand-name counterparts) to have the same active ingredient, strength, uses, form, route of administration, and labeling. Additionally, many medications have multiple indications, which may not be included in this chapter. Further, notable side effects are listed in the following section and may be of interest to the fitness professional when working with a client; however, the list is not all encompassing. For more details about medications, several sources are available and should be consulted, including https://medlineplus.gov/druginformation.html and https://dailymed.nlm.nih.gov/dailymed/index.cfm.

Hypertension

Eight different antihypertensive drug classes will be discussed, each with a different mechanism of action:

1. Diuretics, which increase excretion of electrolytes and water
2. Calcium channel blockers (CCBs), which interfere with calcium movement during polarization of the heart
3. Angiotensin-converting enzyme (ACE) inhibitors, which decrease production of the powerful vasoconstrictor angiotensin II
4. Angiotensin II receptor blockers (ARBs), which block the action of angiotensin II
5. Beta-blockers, which compete with epinephrine and norepinephrine on target organs
6. Aldosterone receptor antagonists, which compete with aldosterone receptors in the kidney
7. Central alpha-2 agonists, which reduce the effects of norepinephrine in the central nervous system (CNS)
8. Direct vasodilators, which dilate arterioles

See table 2.3 for examples of these medications; their notable side effects; and their impacts on HR, BP, and exercise response.

Thiazide-type diuretics, calcium channel blockers, ACE inhibitors, and ARBs are considered first-line medications for treatment of hypertension. These agents are used to treat the majority of patients with hypertension. Many of these medications can be used for other indications in addition to blood pressure management. To review FDA-approved indications, refer to medication package inserts or sources discussed previously.

Thiazide-Type Diuretics and Loop Diuretics

Diuretics act by increasing the excretion of electrolytes (e.g., sodium, potassium, chloride) and water; the different classes of diuretics work on different parts of the kidney (12, 40, 42, 48, 56). By decreasing the fluid volume in the body, blood pressure is lowered. A potential concern is low blood levels of potassium (hypokalemia), which could induce arrythmias (43). To avoid this, consumption of potassium-rich foods is recommended. Some may use a potassium supplement or potassium-sparing diuretics (2).

Calcium Channel Blockers (CCBs)

These drugs interfere with the slow calcium currents that occur during depolarization in cardiac and vascular smooth muscle (40, 42, 56). By inhibiting calcium entry into vascular smooth muscle and myocardial cells, blood vessels dilate (40, 42, 56). Dilation of blood vessels will help lower BP (40, 42, 56). The dihydropyridine (DHP) CCBs are more selective for the vasculature when compared to the non-dihydropyridines (NON-DHP), which are more selective for the heart and tend to reduce HR in addition to some BP lowering effects (44).

The effects of CCBs on exercise prescription and training have been studied. The regression equations relating percent HR max (%HRmax) and percent $\dot{V}O_2$max (%$\dot{V}O_2$max) have been found to be the same in patients taking diltiazem and in unmedicated patients (11). Verapamil (Calan) and nifedipine (Procardia) are assumed not to alter the relationship between %HRmax and %$\dot{V}O_2$max. CCBs are not thought to adversely affect endurance training in healthy subjects or in patients with coronary artery disease (37).

MacGowan and colleagues showed that verapamil does not diminish training responses in healthy, young subjects (40). The public perception of a calcium blocker may be that it blocks the absorption of dietary and supplemental calcium, thus leading to increased risk of osteoporosis. This is not true because the CCBs work at the cellular level.

Renin-Angiotensin Aldosterone System Inhibitors

These medications act at different points within the renin-angiotensin system to decrease vasoconstriction (42, 56). Two main classes are the angiotensin-converting enzyme (ACE) inhibitors and angiotensin II receptor blockers (ARBs).

Angiotensin-converting enzyme inhibitors (generic names end in -pril) lower BP by inhibiting ACE, an enzyme that converts angiotensin I to angiotensin II, which is a powerful vasoconstrictor (42, 56). These medications are also associated with increased brady-kinin, which can produce a cough, a well-known side effect of ACE inhibitors (42, 56). Of note, this class of medications has been shown to be protective of kidney function (2, 3, 56).

ARBs (generic names end in -sartan) are medications that also work through the renin-angiotensin system (2). These agents block the effects of angiotensin II without affecting ACE (2). Because of this, they do not produce a cough; they also exhibit kidney-protective effects (2).

Beta-Blockers

Knowledge of the location of beta-receptors is helpful in understanding the impact of these medications. Beta-1 receptors are found in the heart. Beta-2 receptors are found in the lungs. This can be easily remembered because humans have one heart and two lungs.

Beta-blockers (generic names end in -olol) work by blocking the effects of catecholamines (especially nor-epinephrine) at beta-1, beta-2, and/or alpha-1 adrenergic receptors (42, 56). When the beta-blocker antagonizes beta-1 and beta-2 receptors, it causes a decrease in HR (42, 56). Some beta-blockers are able to inhibit alpha-1 receptors (along with beta receptors) (42, 56). The block-ade of alpha-1 receptors relaxes blood vessels and adds another mechanism of lowering BP (42, 56). Overall, beta-blockers decrease vasoconstriction and improve heart function (42, 56).

Patients who are on beta-blockers require special consideration related to the use of HR in an exercise pre-scription. Heart rate max must be measured (rather than estimated) to calculate an appropriate target HR (THR) for anyone taking beta-blockers, and this measurement should be repeated after any change in beta-blocking medicines. The commonly used formula (i.e., 220 – age) for estimating maximal HR is invalid if the client was on beta-blockers at the time of testing and cannot be used to calculate THR. For these patients, a THR is some-times computed by adding 20 to 30 bpm to the client's resting HR while standing. However, in view of the wide differences in physiological responses to beta blockade, another approach is to use RPE ratings, with patients targeting exercise intensity between 11 and 14 on the Borg RPE scale (i.e., light to somewhat hard effort) (4).

All beta-blockers can mask the majority of symptoms associated with low blood sugar (hypoglycemia), such as shakiness, increased HR, and nervousness—except one: sweating. It's important to remind patients on beta-blockers to check their blood sugar if unexpected sweating occurs (61).

Propranolol can reduce airway flow by blocking beta-2 receptors, thus making it difficult to breathe (42). This effect is small in most individuals (42). However, in patients with asthma or other lung diseases, this effect is potentially dangerous, and thus non-selective beta-blockers (i.e., block both beta-1 and beta-2 recep-tors) are best avoided in individuals with lung disease, such as asthma (42).

Aldosterone Receptor Antagonists

Aldosterone receptor antagonists (ARAs) compete with aldosterone at receptor sites in the kidney; ARAs cause increased amounts of sodium and water to be excreted, while potassium is retained (42, 56). Spironolactone is non-selective, so it blocks aldosterone and androgen. Because it blocks androgen, it is associated with hor-monal side effects (42, 56). Eplerenone is selective, so it only blocks aldosterone and does not exhibit hormonal side effects (42, 56).

Centrally Acting Alpha-2 Adrenergic Agonists

The impact on the sympathetic nervous system will help lower BP as well as HR (15). Thus, bradycardia is a potential side effect of note for the fitness professional (2, 42, 56).

Direct Vasodilators

Vasodilators decrease BP by relaxing vascular smooth muscle (2, 42). This class of medications has a varia-ble effect on HR (2, 42). For example, hydralazine is associated with an increase in HR, whereas minoxidil is not (2, 42).

Angina

Angina is chest pain or discomfort due to a reduced blood flow. Nitrates are used to prevent or stop attacks of angina pectoris (chest pain) (2). Nitrates exist in several forms, including patches, ointments, long-acting tablets, and sublingual tablets (2, 42). They are produced from amyl nitrate (a volatile agent), which is rendered nonexplosive by adding an inert chemical such as lactose (2). Nitrates relax most smooth muscle, including arteries and veins (2, 42). This helps reduce the workload and oxygen requirement of the heart (2, 42). Patients may take longer-acting tablet forms of nitrates such as isosorbide dinitrate and isosorbide mononitrate to prevent anginal attacks, whereas sublingual nitroglycerin tablets are used to treat acute anginal episodes (2). See table 2.4 for examples of these medications; their notable side effects; and their impacts on HR, BP, and exercise response.

Table 2.3 Hypertension Medications

Examples of drugs in class	Notable side effects	Impact on HR, BP, and exercise response
THIAZIDE-TYPE DIURETICS		
• Hydrochlorothiazide (Hydrodiuril) • Chlorthalidone (Thalitone)	• ↓ K, Mg, Na, H • ↑ Ca, UA, LDL, TG, blood glucose • Orthostatic hypotension • Photosensitivity • Dehydration	• ↓ BP • ↓ cardiac output • ↓ plasma volume • ↓ peripheral vascular resistance
LOOP DIURETICS		
• Furosemide (Lasix) • Bumetanide (Bumex) • Torsemide (Demadex)	• ↓ K, Mg, Na, Cl, Ca (different from thiazides, which ↑ Ca) • ↑ HCO_3, UA, blood glucose, triglycerides, total cholesterol • Hearing impairment • Dehydration	• ↓ BP
DHP—CALCIUM CHANNEL BLOCKERS		
• Nifedipine (Adalat CC, Procardia XL) • Amlodipine (Norvasc)	• Peripheral edema • Headache • Flushing • Palpitations	• ↓ BP • Reflex tachycardia • ↑ oxygen delivery to the heart muscle • ↓ peripheral vascular resistance • ↓ oxygen consumption and requirements of the heart
NON-DHP—CALCIUM CHANNEL BLOCKERS		
• Diltiazem (Cardizem) • Verapamil (Calan SR)	• Peripheral edema • Constipation • Headache	• ↓ BP • ↓ HR • ↓ oxygen demand of the heart • ↓ total systemic resistance
ACE INHIBITORS AND ARBS		
ACE inhibitors: • Lisinopril (Prinivil) • Quinapril (Accupril) • Ramipril (Altace) ARBs: • Losartan (Cozaar) • Valsartan (Diovan) • Olmesartan (Benicar)	• ↑ K • ↑ sCr • Dizziness • Headache • Cough (only with ACE inhibitors) • Avoid in women who are planning to become pregnant or who are pregnant • Avoid concomitant use of ACE inhibitor with an ARB or direct renin inhibitor due to increased risk of hypotension, syncope, increased K, and changes in kidney function	• ↓ BP • ↓ systemic vascular resistance • ↑ cardiac output • ↓ peripheral arterial resistance
BETA-1 (SELECTIVE) BETA-BLOCKERS		
• Metoprolol succinate (Toprol XL) • Metoprolol tartrate (Lopressor) • Atenolol (Tenormin)	• Fatigue • Dizziness • Cold extremities	• ↓ BP • ↓ HR • ↓ cardiac output
BETA-1 AND BETA-2 (NON-SELECTIVE) BETA-BLOCKERS		
• Propranolol (Inderal LA/XL)	• Fatigue • Dizziness • Cold extremities	• ↓ BP • ↓ HR • ↓ cardiac output
NON-SELECTIVE BETA-BLOCKERS AND ALPHA-1 BLOCKER		
• Carvedilol (Coreg) • Labetalol (Trandate)	• Peripheral edema • Fatigue • Dizziness • Cold extremities	• ↓ BP • ↓ HR • ↓ cardiac output • ↓ peripheral vascular resistance

Examples of drugs in class	Notable side effects	Impact on HR, BP, and exercise response
BETA-1 SELECTIVE BLOCKER WITH NITRIC OXIDE–DEPENDENT VASODILATION		
• Nebivolol (Bystolic)	• Fatigue • Nausea • ↑ TG • ↓ HDL • Dizziness • Cold extremities	• ↓ BP • ↓ HR • ↓ myocardial contractility • ↓ peripheral vascular resistance
ALDOSTERONE RECEPTOR ANTAGONISTS		
• Spironolactone (Aldactone) • Eplerenone (Inspra)	• ↑ K, blood glucose • ↓ Na, Mg, Ca • Dizziness • Dehydration • Spironolactone: gynecomastia, breast tenderness, impotence, irregular menses	• ↓ BP • May cause changes in HR
CENTRALLY ACTING ALPHA-2 ADRENERGIC AGONISTS		
• Clonidine (Catapres) • Guanfacine (Tenex)	• Sedation • Dizziness • Dry mouth • Avoid sudden discontinuation, which could lead to withdrawal syndrome (e.g., rebound hypertension, headache, tremors, sweating)	• ↓ BP • ↓ HR • ↓ peripheral resistance • ↓ kidney vascular resistance
DIRECT VASODILATORS		
• Hydralazine (Alpresoline) • Minoxidil*	• Edema • Headache • Flushing • Palpitations • Nausea • Vomiting • Hydralazine: drug-induced lupus syndrome • Minoxidil: monitor for abnormal amount of hair growth on face, back, arms, and legs	• ↓ BP • HR (variable response) • ↓ peripheral vascular resistance • ↑ stroke volume • ↑ cardiac output

*When used as a topical agent (versus a tablet for BP) this medication is commonly known as Rogaine.

Ca = calcium; Cl = chlorine; CK = creatine kinase; H = hydrogen; HCO_3 = bicarbonate; K = potassium; Mg = magnesium; Na = sodium; sCr = serum creatinine; TG = triglycerides; UA = uric acid

Source: National Library of Medicine.

Table 2.4   Angina Medications

Examples of drugs in class	Notable side effects	Impact on HR, BP, and exercise response
NITRATES		
• Isosorbide dinitrate* (Isordil) • Isosorbide mononitrate* (Imdur) • Nitroglycerin (Nitrostat, Nitrobid)	• Headache • Dizziness • Flushing • Syncope	• ↓ BP • ↓ systemic vascular resistance • ↓ systolic arterial pressure • ↓ afterload • ↓ preload

For nitroglycerin tablets, take at the onset of chest pain. *Do not take* more than 3 doses within 15 minutes. Call 911 if chest pain persists or worsens 3 to 5 minutes after the first dose.

*Long-acting agents, taken daily to prevent chest pain.

Source: National Library of Medicine.

Hyperlipidemia

Several types of medications are used by people who are unable to adequately control lipids through diet and exercise. The first group is the bile acid sequestering agents, including cholestyramine (Questran) and colesevelam (Welchol), which bind to bile acids and reduce reabsorption. This mechanism is associated with reduced LDL plasma levels and decrease in serum cholesterol levels. Ezetimibe (Zetia) is an azetidione-based cholesterol inhibitor that prevents intestinal absorption of lipids (2). Niacin (Niaspan) has many different mechanisms that result in reduced cholesterol. It is associated with significant flushing, which could interfere with exercise (2). Fibrates are used primarily for elevated triglycerides and include gemfibrozil (Lopid), fenofibrate (Tricor), and fenofibric acid (Trilipix) (2).

Statins (generics end in -statin) are some of the most effective and best-tolerated agents for treating high cholesterol (2, 42). Statins work by inhibiting HMG-CoA reductase, an enzyme involved in production of cholesterol (2, 42). A notable side effect is that they can cause a significant degree of muscle problems (e.g., myalgia, myositis, and even rhabdomyolysis) that could negatively affect exercise (2, 42). Additionally, they are teratogenic, and use should be avoided in women who are planning to become pregnant or who are pregnant (42). See table 2.5 for examples of these medications; their notable side effects; and their impacts on HR, BP, and exercise response.

Anticoagulants and Antiplatelets ("Blood Thinners")

The term *blood thinners* is often used, although rather than thinning the blood, these medications lower the risk of blood clots (42). Clots that form in the arteries, veins, and heart can lead to heart attacks, strokes, and blockages that can cause other health problems. Two general categories of blood thinners are anticoagulants, which affect various proteins (factors) involved with the coagulation process, and antiplatelet drugs, which prevent platelets from binding together, thus preventing blood clots from forming (2).

Two categories of oral anticoagulants include direct oral anticoagulants (DOACs) and vitamin K antagonists. DOACs inhibit specific clotting factors, which reduces clotting activity (42). A vitamin K antagonist blocks vitamin K, which is required for the activation of certain clotting factors (2, 42). Without adequate vitamin K, the liver still produces clotting factors, but they do not have clotting activity (42). One consideration with the use of vitamin K antagonists (i.e., warfarin) is the need for careful

Table 2.5 Hyperlipidemia Medications

Examples of drugs in class	Notable side effects	Impact on HR, BP, and exercise response
STATINS		
• Atorvastatin (Lipitor) • Rosuvastatin[a] (Crestor) • Simvastatin (Zocor) • Pravastatin[a] (Pravachol)	Muscle pain: Presents as muscle soreness, tiredness, or weakness; symmetrical in large adjacent muscle groups in the legs, back, arms. Symptoms usually occur within 6 weeks of starting treatment but can develop at any time. Severity presentation varies: • *Myopathy*: General term for disease of muscle • *Myalgia*: Muscle soreness and tenderness without CK[b] elevations • *Myositis*: Muscle symptoms with ↑ CK • *Rhabdomyolysis*: Muscle symptoms with very high CK (>10,000) + muscle protein in the urine (myoglobinuria), which can lead to acute renal failure Risk factors include sporadic heavy exercise, being elderly or female, low BMI	Data are inconsistent
BILE ACID SEQUESTERING AGENTS, AZETIDIONE-BASED CHOLESTEROL INHIBITORS, NIACIN, FIBRATES		
• Cholestyramine (Questran), colesevelam (Welchol) • Ezetimibe (Zetia) • Niacin (Niaspan) • Gemfibrozil (Lopid), fenofibrate (Tricor), fenofibrate acid (Trilipix)	• Indigestion (colesevelam, gemfibrozil) • Constipation (colesevelam) • Joint pain (ezetimibe) • Flushing (niacin)	• Unlikely to affect exercise • Flushing (niacin) may impact exercise

[a]Pravastatin and rosuvastatin are the most hydrophilic (water-loving) statins. Hydrophilic statins are less likely to enter non-liver cells such as myocytes (muscle cells) and thus might have less risk of myopathy.

[b]CK = creatine kinase

Sources: National Library of Medicine; Abd and Jacobson (2011).

monitoring using the international normalized ratio (INR) (42). In many cases, the therapeutic INR range is 2-3 but this may vary depending on the patient and their diagnosis. The higher the INR, the more likely bleeding will occur; the lower the INR, the more likely clots will form. Foods high in vitamin K will decrease the INR, which will increase the risk of clotting, so awareness of dietary sources is important. Example of foods high in vitamin K include broccoli, cabbage, cauliflower, coriander, spinach, brussels sprouts, canola oil, chickpeas, collard greens, green kale, and tea (green or black). Anticoagulants are often used to treat deep vein thromboses (DVT) and pulmonary embolisms (PE) (42). Additionally, patients with atrial fibrillation are at a higher risk for stroke when compared to the general population; therefore, depending on the patient's risk factors, it is recommended to use anticoagulants to prevent a stroke in this patient population (42). Antiplatelet drugs, P2Y12 inhibitors, block platelet activation and aggregation (42). They are commonly used in patients with acute coronary syndrome to prevent clotting after placement of a coronary stent (42). Neither anticoagulants nor antiplatelets are likely to directly affect exercise testing or training, but they do increase the risk of bruising and can lead to serious, potentially life-threatening bleeding. See table 2.6 for examples of these medications; their notable side effects; and their impacts on HR, BP, and exercise response.

Diabetes

A substantial number of participants in fitness programs may have hyperglycemia, or elevated levels of blood glucose, which can be due to type 2 diabetes mellitus. In this condition, the pancreas can produce insulin, but it is unable to produce enough to maintain normal blood glucose control or the body has become resistant to the insulin that is produced (50, 55). Treatment consists of oral antiglycemic agents or insulin, and some of these agents can cause hypoglycemia or low blood sugar (50, 55). Hypoglycemia is potentially dangerous, and the fitness professional should be cognizant of any changes in alertness and orientation in clients taking any medication that can lower plasma glucose concentrations (50). Additional background and considerations when working with individuals with diabetes are found in chapter 21. See table 2.7 for examples of these medications; their notable side effects; and their impacts on HR, BP, and exercise response.

Oral Antiglycemic Agents

Several categories of oral antiglycemic agents exist with differing mechanisms of action, with the common goal of maintaining normal blood glucose. Depending on the patient's comorbidities (e.g., heart failure, chronic kidney disease) and treatment goals, the American Diabetes Association (ADA) recommends the following for initial medication interventions of type 2 diabetes mellitus: metformin, glucagon-like peptide-1 receptor agonists (GLP-1 RA), or sodium glucose co-transporter 2 (SGLT2) inhibitors (50). Metformin reduces glucose production in the liver, increases insulin sensitivity (which means glucose is being absorbed into the body tissues versus circulating in the blood and causing high blood glucose levels), and decreases absorption of glucose in the intestines, which lowers overall blood glucose (50, 55). GLP-1 RA (generics end in -utide or -atide) activate glucagon-like peptide-1 receptors, which reduces glucagon, increases insulin secretion, slows gastric emptying, and increases satiety (42, 55). Because of this, they are associated with weight loss. Interestingly, some drugs in

Table 2.6 Anticoagulant and Antiplatelet Medications

Examples of drugs in class	Notable side effects	Impact on HR, BP, and exercise response
VITAMIN K ANTAGONIST		
• Warfarin (Coumadin)	• Bleeding • Bruising • Skin necrosis • Purple toe syndrome • Avoid in women who are planning to become pregnant or who are pregnant	Exercise may affect INR (increase or decrease)
DOACS		
• Dabigatran (Pradaxa) • Apixaban (Eliquis) • Rivaroxaban (Xarelto)	• Bleeding • Bruising • Anemia	Unlikely to affect exercise
P2Y$_{12}$ INHIBITORS		
• Clopidogrel (Plavix) • Prasugrel (Effient) • Ticagrelor (Brillinta)	• Bleeding • Bruising • Shortness of breath (ticagrelor) • ↑ sCr, UA (ticagrelor)	Unlikely to affect exercise

INR = international normalized ratio; sCr = serum creatinine; UA = uric acid

Source: National Library of Medicine.

this class, such as semaglutide, have been approved for use in chronic weight management. SGLT2 inhibitors reduce reabsorption of filtered glucose in the kidneys, which increases glucose excretion in the urine (42, 55). Through this mechanism, they can also decrease blood pressure (42, 55). Some of the beneficial effects of SGLT2 inhibitors for individuals with heart failure have been suggested to be related to this effect on blood pressure (42). The thiazolidinediones decrease insulin resistance and increase glucose uptake into muscle and fat tissue (2, 42, 50, 55). Dipeptidyl-peptidase-4 (DPP-4) inhibitors (generics end in -gliptin) block the breakdown of GLP-1 (42). This reduces glucagon and increases insulin secretion, which lowers blood glucose (55). Sulfonylureas stimulate insulin release from the beta cells in the pancreas (2, 42, 55).

Insulin

Insulin is required for individuals with type 1 diabetes, and, in some cases, insulin is recommended for treatment of type 2 diabetes mellitus (2, 42, 55). It activates insulin receptors, which decreases glucose production in the liver and increases glucose uptake by fat and skeletal muscle tissue (42, 55). Insulin exists in many different forms.

1. Long-acting (e.g., insulin glargine) and ultra-long-acting insulin (e.g., insulin degludec) have a longer duration of action (approximately 24 hours or more) with flatter, more constant plasma concentrations (42, 55). Onset of action is a couple hours after administration (42).

2. Intermediate-acting insulin, insulin neutral protamine hagedorn (NPH), has an onset of action 2 to 4 hours after administration, and the duration of treatment is 12 to 18 hours (42, 55).

3. Short-acting (e.g., insulin regular) and rapid-acting (e.g., insulin aspart) insulin have a quick onset (approximately 15-30 minutes) and short duration of action (2-6 hours) (42).

4. Insulin mixes are a combination of intermediate-acting and short-acting insulin (42, 55). An example of this is Humalog 75/25, which is made up of 75% intermediate-acting insulin and 25% short-acting insulin (42, 55).

Depression and Anxiety

Depending on the severity and pattern of depressive episodes over time, health care providers may offer psychotherapy or antidepressant medications, or both. Antidepressant medications are most commonly used to help relieve the distress of depression or anxiety. They are also used to help with other conditions such as obsessive-compulsive disorder, eating disorders, post-traumatic stress disorder, and pain (42).

Antidepressants can take up to several weeks—typically 4 to 6—to be fully effective (16, 42). Early signs that the medication is working include improved sleep, appetite, and energy. Improvement in mood usually comes later. It should be noted that antidepressants have a boxed warning for increased risk of suicidal thoughts and behaviors in children, adolescents, and young adults. Patients, of all ages, should be monitored closely for worsening and/or emergence of suicidal thoughts and behaviors when starting an antidepressant (42).

Antidepressants come in many different classes; some of the most common are selective serotonin reuptake inhibitors (SSRIs) and serotonin and norepinephrine reuptake inhibitors (SNRIs). SSRIs increase serotonin by blocking its reuptake in the neuronal synapse (18, 42, 49). SNRIs have a similar mechanism to SSRIs, in which they increase serotonin and norepinephrine by blocking reuptake (18, 42, 49). Besides depression and anxiety, duloxetine, a SNRI, is FDA approved for treatment of neuropathic pain associated with diabetes mellitus and chronic, musculoskeletal pain (42, 49). See table 2.8 for

Table 2.7 Diabetes Medications

Examples of drugs in class	Notable side effects	Impact on HR, BP, and exercise response
BIGUANIDE		
• Metformin (Glucophage)	• Diarrhea • Nausea • Vomiting • Flatulence • Heartburn • Risk of lactic acidosis	• Data are inconsistent • *Hypoglycemia:* None • *Weight change:* Neutral (potential for modest loss)
THIAZOLIDINES		
• Pioglitazone (Actos)	• Edema • Bone fractures	• *Hypoglycemia:* Not alone, but increases the effect of insulin when used in combination • *Weight change:* Gain

Examples of drugs in class	Notable side effects	Impact on HR, BP, and exercise response
SGLT2 INHIBITORS		
• Empagliflozin (Jardiance) • Dapagliflozin (Farxiga)	• Urinary tract infection • Genital fungal infection • Increased urination • Ketoacidosis • Volume depletion	• *Hypoglycemia:* Not alone, but increases the effect of insulin when used in combination • *Weight change:* Loss • ↓ BP • ↓ preload • ↓ afterload
DPP-4 INHIBITORS		
• Sitagliptin (Januvia) • Alogliptin (Nesina)	• Headache • Joint pain • Common cold	• *Hypoglycemia:* Not alone, but increases the effect of insulin when used in combination • *Weight change:* Neutral
SULFONYLUREAS		
• Glipizide (Glucotrol) • Glimepiride (Amaryl) • Glyburide (Glynase)	• Hypoglycemia • Nausea • Diarrhea	• *Hypoglycemia:* Yes; ensure patients check their blood sugar prior to exercise • *Weight change:* Gain
GLP-1 RA		
• Dulaglutide (Trulicity [injection]) • Semaglutide (Ozempic [injection], Rybelsus [oral]) • Tirzepatide (Mounjaro [injection])	• Nausea • Vomiting • Diarrhea • ↓ appetite • Heartburn • Injection site reactions	• *Hypoglycemia:* Not alone, but increases the effect of insulin when used in combination • *Weight change:* Loss
INSULIN		
• Insulin (injection)	• Injection site reactions • ↓ K • Lipodystrophy	• *Hypoglycemia:* Yes; ensure patients check their blood sugar prior to exercise • *Weight change:* Gain

K = potassium

Sources: National Library of Medicine; Standards of Care in Diabetes—2023: Pharmacologic Approaches to Glycemic Treatment.

Table 2.8   Depression and Anxiety Medications

Examples of drugs in class	Notable side effects	Impact on HR, BP, and exercise response
SSRIS		
• Citalopram (Celexa) • Escitalopram (Lexapro) • Fluoxetine (Prozac) • Paroxetine (Paxil) • Sertraline (Zoloft)	• Nausea • Diarrhea • Dry mouth • Headache • ↓ Na (usually associated with syndrome of inappropriate antidiuretic hormone secretion [SIADH]) • Discontinuation syndrome (avoid abruptly stopping [e.g., dizziness, headache, irritability]) • Serotonin syndrome (when used in common with other serotonergic drugs) • Sexual side effects (↓ sex drive, erectile dysfunction)	
SNRIS		
• Venlafaxine (Effexor) • Duloxetine (Cymbalta)	Similar to SSRIs	• ↑ BP (due to norepinephrine activity) • ↑ HR (due to norepinephrine activity)

Source: National Library of Medicine.

examples of these medications; their notable side effects; and their impacts on HR, BP, and exercise response.

Pain

Pain medication is defined broadly as any medication that relieves pain. Many different pain medicines exist, and certain pains respond better to some medicines than others. Each person may have a slightly different response to each pain reliever. See table 2.9 for examples of these medications; their notable side effects; and their impacts on HR, BP, and exercise response.

Nonsteroidal Anti-Inflammatory Drugs (NSAIDs)

NSAIDs decrease the formation of prostaglandins, which results in decreased inflammation, alleviation of pain, and reduced fever (42). There are two types of NSAIDs: nonselective NSAIDs (ibuprofen) and selective NSAIDs (celecoxib). Of note, NSAIDs have three boxed warnings:

1. *CV risk*: can cause an increased risk of serious cardiovascular thrombotic events, myocardial infarction, and stroke, which can be fatal (42)

2. *Gastrointestinal (GI) risk*: can increase the risk of serious GI events, such as bleeding, ulceration, and perforation of the stomach or intestines, which can be fatal (42)

3. *Coronary artery bypass graft (CABG) surgery*: NSAID use is contraindicated after CABG surgery (42)

Opioids

Opioids can be used for acute and chronic pain. These medications activate opioid receptors in the CNS (42). This process produces pain relief and also can cause euphoria and reduced breathing (also known as *respiratory depression*) (42). Most opioids are considered schedule II controlled substances, which means they have a potential for abuse and misuse can lead to death (42).

Chronic Obstructive Pulmonary Disease (COPD) and Asthma

Bronchodilators relax smooth muscle or decrease inflammation surrounding airways in the lungs and relieve the symptoms of asthma, COPD, and related lung disorders. These medications are used in the form of an inhaler; however, some can be taken orally. Bronchodilators tend to reduce dynamic hyperinflation at rest and during exercise and improve exercise performance (13, 16, 31).

The long-acting inhalers are used for maintenance therapy to *prevent* breathing issues (31, 42). They are usually dosed once or twice daily, and their effect can last up to 12 to 24 hours (42). The short-acting inhalers, also referred to as *rescue therapy*, are used as needed to *treat* asthma attacks or breathing issues (31), and are usually

Table 2.9 Pain Medications

Examples of drugs in class	Notable side effects	Impact on HR, BP, and exercise response
NONSELECTIVE NSAIDS		
• Ibuprofen (Advil) • Naproxen (Aleve)	• Heartburn • Nausea • Stomach bleeding • Stomach ulcers • Acute kidney injury	• ↑ BP
SELECTIVE NSAIDS		
• Celecoxib (Celebrex) • Meloxicam (Mobic) • Diclofenac (Voltaren)	• Severe skin reactions (celecoxib) • Stomach bleeding • Stomach ulcers • Heartburn • Acute kidney injury	• ↑ BP
OPIOIDS		
• Fentanyl (Duragesic) • Hydrocodone (Hycodan) • Oxycodone (OxyContin) • Morphine (MS Contin) • Tramadol (Ultram)*	• Constipation • Nausea • Vomiting • Sedation • Dizziness • Reduced breathing • Misuse can lead to death	Data are inconsistent

*Also increases norepinephrine and serotonin.

Source: National Library of Medicine.

dosed every 4 to 6 hours as their effect is much shorter than long-acting inhalers (42). Unlike long-acting inhalers (or inhaled corticosteroids), short-acting inhalers are only to be used as needed (31).

This chapter will review three different classes of inhalers:

1. Beta-2 agonists
2. Muscarinic antagonists
3. Inhaled corticosteroids

In addition to inhalers, oral steroids will be reviewed. Beta-2 agonists activate the beta-2 receptors (2, 31, 42). They work by relaxing bronchial smooth muscle and increasing the airway lumen (2, 31, 42). Because they activate beta-2 receptors, they can increase HR and BP, although most of their effect is on the smooth muscle found in airways (2, 31, 42). There are two different forms: long acting and short acting (2, 31, 42). Muscarinic antagonists work by blocking the effect of acetylcholine, a neurotransmitter, which results in relaxation of bronchial smooth muscle (31, 42). They are also available as long acting and short acting (2, 31, 42). Inhaled corticosteroids (ICS) and oral steroids act as anti-inflammatory agents and thus have a major role

in the treatment and prevention of asthma and COPD (2, 31, 42). They work by decreasing inflammation in the airway, which improves lung function (2, 31, 42). Inhaled corticosteroids are specifically long acting. Oral steroids can be used for COPD exacerbations or chronically for severe, persistent asthma, but they cause several systemic side effects when used chronically (31, 42). See table 2.10 for examples of these medications; their notable side effects; and their impacts on HR, BP, and exercise response.

Attention Deficit/Hyperactivity Disorder (ADHD)

ADHD is characterized by symptoms of inattention, hyperactivity, and impulsivity (49). Defects in the dopamine pathways can play a role in ADHD, so the primary treatment is stimulant medications, which increase dopamine and norepinephrine levels in the brain. This is thought to enhance behavioral activity (42, 49). Like opioids, stimulants are considered schedule II controlled substances, which means that they have a potential for abuse and misuse can lead to death (42, 49). In addition to stimulants, non-stimulant products are also used for the treatment of ADHD. These include medications

Table 2.10   COPD and Asthma Medications

Examples of drugs in class	Notable side effects	Impact on HR, BP, and exercise response
INHALED CORTICOSTEROIDS (ICS)		
Long acting: • Beclomethasone (Qvar) • Budesonide (Pulmicort) • Fluticasone propionate (Flovent)	• Hoarseness and weakness of voice • Fungal infection of the mouth	• *Weight change:* Gain (less likely with inhaled than with oral)
ORAL STEROIDS		
• Prednisone (Deltasone) • Budesonide (Uceris)	• Osteoporosis • Growth suppression • ↑ blood glucose • Impaired mental status	• ↑ BP • *Weight change:* Gain (more likely with oral)
BETA-2 AGONISTS		
Long acting: • Salmeterol (Severent) • Formoterol (Foradil) Short acting: • Albuterol (Proair HFA)	• Muscle tremor • ↓ K • Restlessness	• ↑ BP • ↑ HR
MUSCARINIC ANTAGONISTS		
Long acting: • Tiotropium (Spiriva, Handihaler/Respimat) • Glycopyrrolate (Seebri Neohaler) Short acting: • Ipratropium (Atrovent HFA)	• Dry mouth • Cough • Bitter taste	Data are inconsistent

K = potassium

Source: National Library of Medicine.

such as viloxazine (Qelbree), atomoxetine (Strattera), clonidine (Kapvay), and guanfacine (Intuniv). Clonidine and guanfacine are commonly used to treat ADHD in children and adolescents and can decrease HR and BP. Besides ADHD, clonidine and guanfacine are FDA approved for the treatment of hypertension (see Hypertension section). In contrast, viloxazine and atomoxetine can be used to treat ADHD in children, adolescents, and adults, and, like stimulants, can increase HR and BP (42). See table 2.11 for examples of these medications; their notable side effects; and their impacts on HR, BP, and exercise response.

Tobacco Cessation

Nicotine gums, nasal sprays, and patches are used as smoking substitutes for people who are trying to stop smoking (2, 42, 46). They work by stimulating the CNS and peripheral nervous system, which reduces the symptoms of nicotine withdrawal and provides a safer alternative to using tobacco products (2, 42, 46). They also may cause dopamine release, which creates a pleasurable and relaxing effect (42). With nicotine gum and lozenges, the nicotine is absorbed through the oral mucosa, providing sufficient plasma nicotine concentrations to curb the craving to smoke (2, 42, 46). Nicotine nasal spray allows nicotine to be rapidly absorbed through blood vessels in the nose (2, 42, 46). With transdermal nicotine patches, the nicotine is absorbed slowly through the skin; it should be placed on the upper body or upper outer arm, particularly on nonhairy, clean, dry skin (42). It may be recommended to take the patch off at night to avoid vivid dreams (42). The inhaler should be used with caution in patients with a history of lung disease such as asthma (42). Nicotine can affect the exercise response, particularly if a person uses nicotine replacement therapy but also continues to smoke (42). In particular, the fitness professional should note that HR and BP will be increased (42). Medical contraindications to nicotine replacement therapy include recent myocardial infarction or stroke (57). See table 2.12 for examples of these medications; their notable side effects; and their impacts on HR, BP, and exercise response.

Table 2.11   ADHD Medications

Examples of drugs in class	Notable side effects	Impact on HR, BP, and exercise response
STIMULANTS		
• Methylphenidate (Ritalin, Concerta) • Dexmethylphenidate (Focalin) • Dextroamphetamine/amphetamine (Adderall) • Lisdexamfetamine (Vyvanse)[a]	• Insomnia • ↓ appetite • Headache • Irritability • Nausea • Misuse can lead to death	• ↑ BP • ↑ HR • *Weight change:* Loss
NON-STIMULANTS—NOREPINEPHRINE REUPTAKE INHIBITORS		
• Viloxazine (Qelbree) • Atomoxetine (Straterra)	• Sedation • ↓ appetite • Headache • Abdominal pain • Nausea	• ↑ BP • ↑ HR • *Weight change:* Loss
NON-STIMULANTS—CENTRALLY ACTING ALPHA-2 ADRENERGIC AGONISTS[b]		
• Clonidine (Kapvay) • Guanfacine (Intuniv)	• Sedation • Dizziness • Dry mouth • Avoid sudden discontinuation, which could lead to withdrawal syndrome (e.g., rebound hypertension, headache, tremors, sweating)	• ↓ BP • ↓ HR • *Weight change:* Gain

[a]Besides ADHD, lisdexamfetamine is FDA approved for the treatment of binge eating disorder.

[b]Note that different brand names are used for different indications.

Source: National Library of Medicine.

Table 2.12 Tobacco Cessation Medications

Examples of drugs in class	Notable side effects	Impact on HR, BP, and exercise response
NICOTINE REPLACEMENT THERAPY		
• Nicotine patch (NicoDerm CQ) • Nicotine polacrilex gum (Nicorette) • Nicotine lozenge (Nicorette) • Nicotine inhaler (Nicotrol Inhaler) • Nicotine nasal spray (Nicotrol NS)	• Headache • Dizziness • Nervousness • Insomnia • Heartburn • *Patch:* Vivid dreams, skin irritation • *Inhaler:* Mouth and throat irritation • *Nasal spray:* Nasal irritation, watery eyes, sneezing, transient changes in taste and smell	• ↑ BP • ↑ HR

Source: National Library of Medicine.

2

LEARNING AIDS

REVIEW QUESTIONS

1. What is the first step in the preparticipation screening process, and what is its main objective?

2. What is the purpose of using the PAR-Q+ or PASQ?

3. If a prospective exercise participant chooses not to complete a PAR-Q+ or PASQ, what is the next course of action?

4. Explain a sign or symptom that may indicate a participant has cardiovascular, metabolic, or renal disease.

5. Patient education involves the identification of primary risk factors for CVD. Explain what a primary risk is, and provide three examples, including the threshold for each.

6. Consider a 35-year-old female who is 5 feet 6 inches (168 centimeters) and weighs 160 pounds (72.7 kilograms), smokes occasionally on the weekends, and walks 3 days per week for 35 minutes. Her health screening indicates that she does not have high BP or cholesterol or type 2 diabetes. Her resting BP is 118/60 mmHg, and her RHR is 85 bpm. What are her primary risk factors, and why did you designate them as such?

7. Why is it important to consider participants' HDL-C levels when determining the number of risk factors?

8. What is an example of a chronic disease that puts an individual at high risk for cardiovascular complications during exercise participation?

9. Provide an example of a medical condition that would require medical clearance prior to exercise testing or participation.

10. Why is it important to determine if a prospective exercise participant is a current, regular exerciser?

11. After obtaining fitness test results, with what standards should the fitness professional compare them?

12. Explain two scenarios in which a participant may be referred to a clinic-based supervised exercise program.

13. How can HR and BP change due to various medications prescribed for hypertension?

14. What is a notable side effect of statins that could affect exercise?

15. Describe the mechanism of action of oral antiglycemic agents compared to various types of insulin.

16. What are potential changes in HR and BP for pulmonary patients taking beta-2 agonists?

17. How might nicotine replacement therapy affect the usefulness of HR measures taken during submaximal exercise testing to estimate aerobic capacity?

CASE STUDIES

1. A 46-year-old male, employed as a computer programmer, has not exercised regularly for 5 years. He has not been diagnosed with cardiovascular, metabolic, or renal disease, nor does he report any major signs or symptoms suggestive of these diseases. He wants to begin a walking program. His height is 178 centimeters, weight is 88.7 kilograms, and thus he has a BMI of 28.0 kg · m^{-2}. His father suffered a heart attack (myocardial infarction [MI]) at 52 years of age. Additionally, his resting HR is 74 bpm, with a BP of 122/78 mmHg. His LDL-C is 115 mg · dl^{-1}, HDL-C is 47 mg · dl^{-1}, and fasting blood glucose level is 88 mg · dl^{-1}. He does not smoke, and he takes medication (a diuretic) for hypertension.

   a. Does he warrant medical clearance prior to exercise participation? Why or why not?

   b. Identify his primary risk factors for CVD, including the clinical basis for each one.

2. A 61-year-old female, a retired accountant, has been physically inactive for 15 years and wants to lose weight. She was diagnosed with type 2 diabetes 12 years ago, and her last fasting blood glucose level was 145 mg · dl^{-1}. She does not smoke, nor does she report any major signs or symptoms suggestive of CVD or renal disease. She is 5 feet 4 inches and weighs 178 pounds. Her waist circumference is 37 inches. Her resting blood pressure is 124/74 mmHg, with a total cholesterol of 225 mg · dl^{-1} and an LDL-C level of 147 mg · dl^{-1}.

   a. Does she warrant medical clearance prior to exercise participation? Why or why not?

   b. Identify her primary risk factors for CVD, including the clinical basis for each one.

3. A 23-year-old graduate student who has been running 5 miles (8 kilometers) 4 to 5 days per week for the past 3 years is interested in performing high-intensity interval training in order to improve her running speed. She does not report any major signs or symptoms suggestive of cardiovascular, metabolic, or renal disease. She is 5 feet 5 inches (165 centimeters) and weighs 125 pounds (56.8 kilograms). She has a resting HR of 56 bpm, resting BP of 114/64 mmHg, and total cholesterol of 175 mg · dl^{-1} with an LDL-C level of 95 mg · dl^{-1} and an HDL-C level of 64 mg · dl^{-1}. Her mother was diagnosed with heart disease at 53 years of age but underwent successful heart surgery.

   a. Does she warrant medical clearance prior to exercise participation? Why or why not?

   b. Identify her primary risk factors for CVD, including the clinical basis for each one.

4. A 57-year-old sales representative who walks 3 days per week for 30 minutes per day wants to begin running 2 to 3 days per week. He had a heart attack at age 51 and has been exercising regularly ever since. He reports no major signs or symptoms suggestive of cardiovascular, metabolic, or renal disease but has not seen a physician

in 2 years. He is 6 feet (183 centimeters), weighs 205 pounds (93.2 kilograms), and has a waist circumference of 38 inches (97 centimeters). His resting BP is 124/78 mmHg, and he is a nonsmoker, takes atenolol to manage his blood pressure, and does not know his cholesterol levels. His father died from a heart attack at 66 years of age, and his brother had heart surgery (coronary artery bypass graft) at 59 years of age.

a. Does he warrant medical clearance prior to exercise participation? Why or why not?

b. Identify his primary risk factors for CVD, including the clinical basis for each one.

Answers to Case Studies

1. For case study #1 consider the following:

   a. He is not a regular exerciser but does not report established cardiovascular, metabolic, or renal disease, nor signs or symptoms suggestive of these diseases. He wants to pursue a light- to moderate-intensity aerobic exercise regimen, and thus medical clearance is not required prior to exercise participation.

   b. He demonstrates four CVD risk factors: age (≥45 years of age), family history (first-degree male relative ≤55 years of age with an MI), blood pressure (on antihypertensive medication), and physical inactivity (currently not engaging in physical activity).

2. For case study #2 consider the following:

   a. She reports no signs and symptoms of CVD or renal disease, but she is not a regular exerciser and has been diagnosed with a metabolic disease (type 2 diabetes). Thus medical clearance is recommended prior to exercise participation. Following medical clearance, she should start with light- to moderate-intensity exercise.

   b. She exhibits a series of CVD risk factors, including age (≥55 years of age), BMI/waist circumference (BMI ≥30 kg · m^{-2}, waist >35 inches), physical inactivity (currently physically inactive), lipids (total cholesterol ≥200 mg · dl^{-1}; LDL-C ≥130 mg · dl^{-1}), and blood glucose (fasting BG ≥100 mg · dl^{-1}), as expected with her diagnosis of type 2 diabetes, a metabolic disease.

3. For case study #3 consider the following:

   a. She is a current, regular exerciser with no history of cardiovascular, metabolic, or renal disease, nor signs and symptoms of these diseases. She is interested in performing higher-intensity aerobic exercise, and medical clearance is not necessary prior to doing so.

   b. Although she does report one risk factor (family history—mother was diagnosed with heart disease ≤55 years of age), she also demonstrates a negative risk factor (HDL ≥60 mg · dl^{-1}), which negates her positive risk factor. This results in a net of no primary risk factors.

4. For case study #4 consider the following:

   a. Although he is a current, regular exerciser, he has known CVD (i.e., heart attack) and wants to pursue vigorous-intensity aerobic exercise (i.e., running). Furthermore, he has not visited his physician in 2 years and thus needs to obtain medical clearance prior to his pursuit of a vigorous-intensity aerobic exercise program.

   b. He presents with several CVD risk factors, including age (≥55 years of age), lipids (because his cholesterol levels are unknown), and blood pressure (takes antihypertensive medication).

Foundations

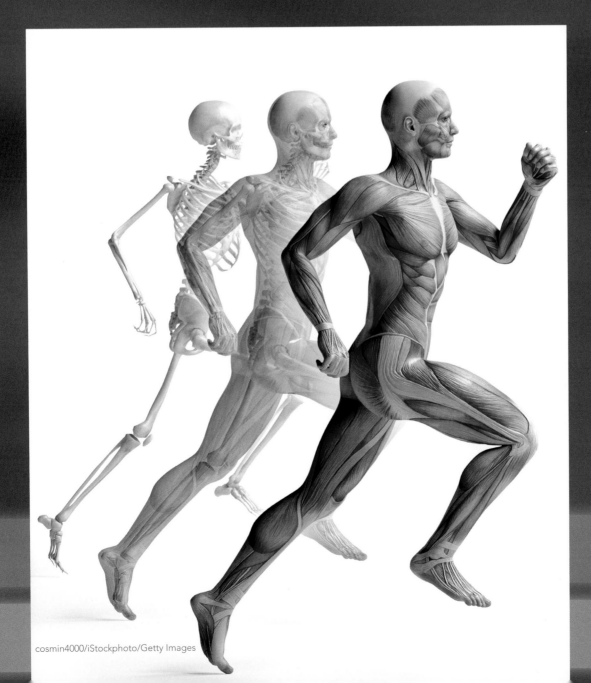

Part II provides the basic scientific foundation for understanding the structure and function of the human body, nutrition, and energy expenditure. In chapter 3 the bones, joints, and muscles of the body and their biomechanical functions during common physical activities are reviewed. In chapter 4 the concepts of energy production, muscle function, and the physiological response to acute and chronic exercise are examined. In chapter 5 nutrition and the impact of diet are discussed. In chapter 6 the energy cost of physical activity and exercise is addressed.

Anatomy in Action: Functional Movement

Clare E. Milner

OBJECTIVES

The reader will be able to do the following:

1. Identify the major bones of the skeletal system and classify them by shape
2. Name each synovial joint and demonstrate the movements possible
3. Explain how concentric, eccentric, and isometric muscle actions differ
4. List the major muscles in each muscle group, and identify the major actions at the joints involved (shoulder girdle, shoulder joint, elbow joint, radioulnar joint, wrist joint, lumbosacral joint, vertebral column, hip joint, knee joint, ankle joint, and subtalar joint)
5. Cite common exercises involving the major muscle groups and point out potential errors in their execution
6. Describe the three factors that determine stability and describe the relationships among them during physical activity
7. Explain how contracting muscles produce torque at a joint
8. Describe how a person can change positions of body segments to alter the resistance torque when exercising
9. Define the mechanical principles of *rotational inertia* and *angular momentum* as applied to human movement
10. Describe the key muscle groups involved in locomotion, throwing, cycling, jumping, swimming, and carrying objects
11. Discuss common errors seen in locomotion, throwing, and striking

3

The fitness professional must have knowledge of the bones, joints, and muscles; must understand muscle forces and other forces (e.g., gravity); and must be able to apply biomechanical principles to human movement. With this knowledge, the fitness professional is better equipped to direct safe physical activity for participants seeking the health-related benefits of exercise. This knowledge also helps earn the respect of clients, who will view the instructor as a professional in the field rather than a technician who may know what to do but not why. This chapter is a summary; for greater detail on anatomy and biomechanics, see the reference list (1-7).

Skeletal Anatomy

Most of the 200 distinct bones in the human skeleton are involved in movement. Their high mineral component gives them rigidity, while their protein component reduces their brittleness. The two types of bone tissue are cortical and trabecular bone. Cortical, or compact, bone is the dense, hard outer layer of a bone. Trabecular bone, also known as spongy or cancellous bone, has a lattice-like structure to provide greater internal strength along the lines of stress within a bone but with less overall weight than solid bone. Bones are living tissue and are constantly being remodeled in adaptation to the loading demands placed on them. Bones are divided into four classifications according to their shape: long, short, flat, and irregular.

Long Bones

The long bones, found in the limbs and the fingers and toes, serve primarily as levers for movement. Each long bone has several distinct features. The diaphysis, or shaft, is made up of thick, compact bone surrounding the hollow medullary cavity. It is characteristic of long bones where the shaft is longer than it is wide. The epiphyses, or expanded ends, are composed of spongy bone with a thin outer layer of compact bone. The articular cartilage is a thin layer of hyaline cartilage covering the articulating surfaces (the surfaces of a bone that come into contact with another bone to form a joint) that provides a smooth, low-friction surface and helps absorb shock. The periosteum is a fibrous membrane covering the entire bone (except where the articular cartilage is present) to serve as an attachment site for muscles (see figure 3.1). Examples of long bones include the femur in the thigh, the ulna in the forearm, and the phalanges in the digits.

Short, Flat, and Irregular Bones

In addition to long bones, the skeleton is made up of short bones, flat bones, and irregularly shaped bones (see figure 3.2). The tarsals (in the ankle) and carpals (in the

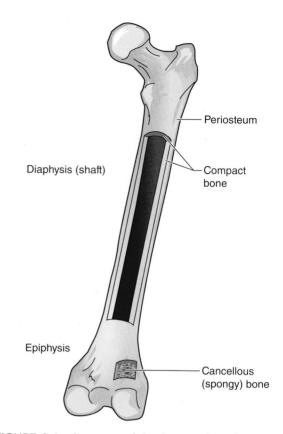

FIGURE 3.1 Structure of the femur, a long bone in the thigh.

wrist) are the short bones, and they are approximately as wide as they are long. Their composition (internal trabecular bone covered with a thin outside layer of cortical bone) provides light weight and strength. Their roughly cubic shape decreases the potential for movement between adjacent bones. The flat bones, such as the ribs, ilia (wings of the pelvis), and scapulae (shoulder blades), serve primarily as broad sites for muscle attachments and, in the case of the ribs and ilia, to enclose cavities and protect internal organs. These bones have a broad, flattened structure. They are composed of trabecular bone covered with a thin layer of cortical bone. The ischium (inferior part of the pelvis), pubis (anterior part of the pelvis), and vertebrae are irregularly shaped bones that protect internal parts and support the body in addition

KEY POINT

Bones are living tissues that are light in weight but strong and stiff. The combination of solid cortical bone on the outside and a lightweight scaffold of trabecular bone inside provides strength with less weight than solid bone.

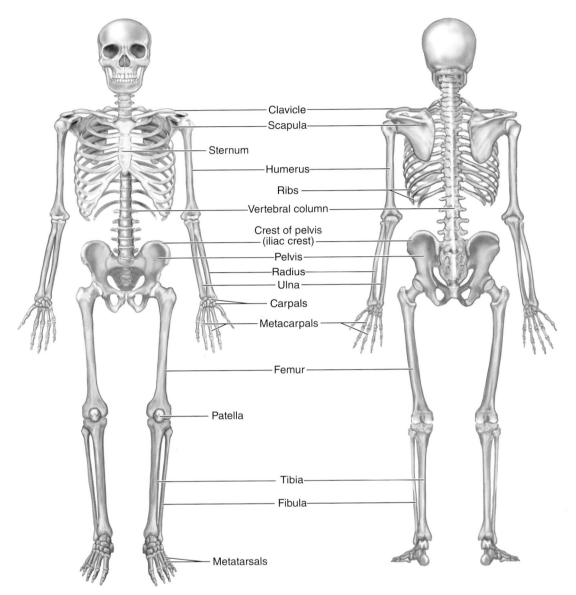

FIGURE 3.2 Anterior (front) and posterior (back) views of the human skeleton in the anatomical position.

to being sites for muscle attachments. An additional category of bone, sesamoid, is reserved for those few bones in the body that are embedded within a tendon. The role of these bones is to modify the way a tendon crosses a joint. The patella (kneecap) is a sesamoid bone embedded in the quadriceps tendon at the knee.

Ossification of Bones

The skeleton begins as a cartilaginous structure that is gradually replaced by bone during growth and maturation in a process known as *ossification*. This process begins at the diaphysis of long bones (in centers of ossification) and spreads toward the epiphyses. The epiphyseal plates between the diaphysis and epiphyses are the growth areas where the cartilage is replaced by bone;

bone growth continues in length and width until the epiphyseal plates are completely ossified. During growth, cartilage is added first and then eventually replaced by bone. When no further cartilage is produced and the cartilage has been replaced by bone, growth ceases. Secondary centers of ossification develop in the epiphyses and in some bony protuberances, such as the tibial tuberosity and the articular condyles of the humerus;

KEY POINT

Ossification is the replacement of cartilage with bone during growth. Generally, bone growth is completed by the late teens.

Planes and Axes of Movement

Anatomical terminology enables the accurate description of position and movement of the human body. To describe joint movements, reference is made to rotation around one or more of three axes and to movement in one of three cardinal planes. These planes are perpendicular to each other and represent a side view (sagittal plane), front or back view (frontal or coronal plane), and top view, looking down from above (transverse plane). Movement observed in each plane is a rotation around an axis that is perpendicular to the plane. The reference position for describing movement is the anatomical position (standing erect, arms hanging at sides, palms facing forward, feet shoulder-width apart; see figure 3.3). The mediolateral axis is perpendicular to the sagittal plane, and joint rotations about this axis are flexion and extension. The anteroposterior axis is perpendicular to the frontal plane, and joint rotations about this axis are abduction and adduction. The longitudinal or vertical axis is perpendicular to the transverse plane, and rotations about this axis are internal and external rotation. Joint rotations are described according to how the distal segment (body part just below the joint) moves relative to the proximal segment (body part just above the joint).

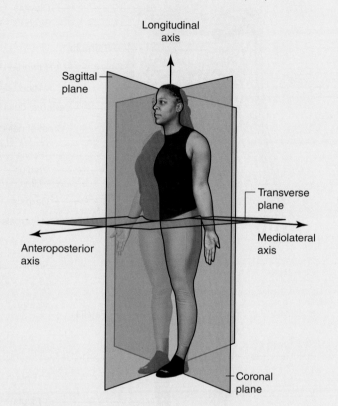

FIGURE 3.3   The anatomical position and the cardinal planes and axes of movement.

however, short bones have one center of ossification. The age when growth plates close varies among individuals. Although bone fusion at some centers of ossification may occur by puberty or earlier, most of the long bones do not completely ossify until the late teens. Premature closing, which results in a shorter bone length, can be caused by trauma, abnormal stresses, or malnutrition.

Structure and Function of Joints

Joints, which are the places where two or more bones meet, or articulate, are often classified according to the amount of movement that can take place at those sites. Ligaments, which are tough, fibrous bands of connective tissue, connect bones to each other across all joints. Joints are classified as synarthrodial, amphiarthrodial, or synovial based on how much they can move. Synar-

throdial joints are immovable joints. The bones merge into each other and are bound together by fibrous tissue that is continuous with the periosteum. The sutures, or lines of junction, of the cranial (skull) bones are prime examples of this type of joint. Amphiarthrodial joints, or cartilaginous joints, allow only slight movement between bones. Usually a fibrocartilage disc separates the bones, and movement can occur only by deformation of the disc. Examples of these joints are the tibiofibular and sacroiliac joints and the joints between the bodies of the vertebrae in the spine.

Diarthrodial joints, more commonly known as synovial joints, are freely movable joints that allow greater movement direction and range; most of the joint movements during physical activity occur at these joints. The synovial joints are the most common type and include most joints of the extremities. Strong, inelastic ligaments, along with connective and muscle tissue crossing the joint, maintain their stability. Synovial joints have several distinguishing characteristics. The articulating surfaces of the bones are covered by articular cartilage, a type of hyaline cartilage that reduces friction and contributes to shock absorption between the bones. Each joint is completely enclosed by an articular capsule, whose thickness varies from thin and loose to thick and tight. The synovial membrane lines the inner surface of the capsule. It secretes synovial fluid into the joint cavity, the space enclosed by the articular capsule. Synovial fluid bathes the joint to nourish the articular cartilage and reduce friction when bones move. Normally, the joint cavity is small and therefore contains little synovial fluid, but an injury to the joint can increase the secretion of synovial fluid and cause swelling.

Some synovial joints, such as the sternoclavicular and knee joints, also have a partial or complete fibrocartilage disc between the bones to aid shock absorption and, in the case of the knee, to give greater stability to the joint. The partial, C-shaped discs between the femur and the tibia at the knee are called *menisci*. To reduce friction or rubbing as tendons move during muscle contraction, tendons often are surrounded by tendon sheaths—cylindrical, tunnel-like sacs lined with synovial membrane. For example, the two proximal tendons of the biceps brachii pass through these tunnels in the bicipital groove of the humerus. Bursae, or sacs of synovial fluid that lie between muscles, tendons, and bones, also reduce friction between the tissues and act as shock absorbers. Many bursae are found around the shoulder, elbow, hip, and knee. Bursitis, or the inflammation of a bursa, can result from repeated friction or mechanical irritation.

The primary movement at a joint is rotation about one or more axes. Some joints may exhibit a small amount of sliding (translation) between the bones. The limits to direction and range of motion at a joint are determined primarily by the shape of the bones at their articulating ends. Depending on the bone shape, joints may rotate about one, two, or three axes.

The type of joint determines the movements that occur within that joint:

- Ball-and-socket joints, which are found at the hip and shoulder, allow a wide range of movement in all directions as the ball rotates within the socket.
- Hinge joints, such as the elbow and ankle joints, have only one axis of rotation due to the structure of the interlocking bones.
- Other types of joints include ellipsoidal joints, such as the wrist, and saddle joints, such as the sternoclavicular joint, whose shapes permit rotation about two axes.
- Pivot joints, such as the proximal radioulnar joint, permit rotation about one axis only: the longitudinal axis.

- Gliding joints, such as between the tarsal bones in the foot, have minimal sliding movement between the bones.

The length of the ligaments and to a lesser extent their elasticity, or ability to stretch passively and return to their normal length, also limit range of motion. For example, the iliofemoral ligament at the anterior hip joint is a strong but short ligament that limits hip extension.

KEY POINT

The moveable joints in the body are diarthrodial (synovial) joints. The bony surfaces are covered in smooth articular cartilage, and the joint cavity is filled with synovial fluid, which lubricates the joint. The limits to range and direction of motion at a joint are determined by the shape of the articulating bones and the length of ligaments crossing the joint.

Joint Movements

Specific terminology is used to describe the direction of movement at the various joints. This ensures that movements are described accurately and can be immediately understood. The anatomical position (see figure 3.3) serves as a point of reference. Terminology generally relates to movements within planes and about axes. Flexion and extension are movements in the sagittal plane about a mediolateral axis. Flexion is moving the distal segment forward and upward from the anatomical position to bring two body segments closer together. Extension is the return from flexion, moving the segment in the opposite direction. Abduction and adduction are movements in the frontal plane about an anteroposterior axis. Abduction is moving the distal segment out to the side and away from the body from the anatomical position, whereas adduction is the return toward the anatomical position from abduction, moving the segment in the opposite direction. Internal and external rotation are movements in the transverse plane about a longitudinal axis. Internal rotation is turning a segment toward the midline of the body from the anatomical position. External rotation is the return toward the anatomical position, turning the segment in the opposite direction. Exceptions to these general descriptions are noted where they occur for specific joints.

The body can be divided into two regions: the axial skeleton and the appendicular skeleton. The axial skeleton forms the main axis of the body and consists of the bones and joints of the vertebral column. The appendicular skeleton consists of all four extremities, which are appended (attached) to the axial skeleton. The appendicular skeleton can be further subdivided into the upper extremities and lower extremities.

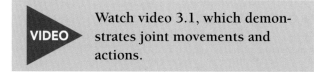

Watch video 3.1, which demonstrates joint movements and actions.

KEY POINT

Synovial joints rotate about one or more of the three primary axes of movement in the body, with some joints having additional movements (table 3.1). Anatomical terminology enables these movements to be described accurately and concisely.

Table 3.1 Movements at Main Synovial Joints

Joint	Movements
AXIAL SKELETON	
Vertebral column	Flexion, extension; lateral flexion; rotation
Lumbosacral joint	Anterior pelvic tilt, posterior pelvic tilt
APPENDICULAR SKELETON: UPPER EXTREMITY	
Shoulder girdle (scapulothoracic joint)	Elevation, depression; protraction (abduction), retraction (adduction); upward rotation, downward rotation
Shoulder joint (glenohumeral joint)	Flexion, extension; abduction, adduction; internal rotation, external rotation; horizontal adduction, horizontal abduction
Elbow joint	Flexion, extension
Radioulnar joint	Pronation, supination
Wrist joint	Flexion, extension; abduction (radial flexion), adduction (ulnar flexion)
Metacarpophalangeal joints	Flexion, extension; abduction, adduction
APPENDICULAR SKELETON: LOWER EXTREMITY	
Hip joint	Flexion, extension; abduction, adduction; internal rotation, external rotation
Knee joint	Flexion, extension
Ankle joint	Plantarflexion, dorsiflexion
Subtalar joint	Eversion, inversion

Skeletal Muscle

Skeletal, or voluntary, muscles consist of thousands of muscle fibers (e.g., the brachioradialis has approximately 130,000 fibers; the gastrocnemius has more than 1 million) plus connective tissue. Each fiber is enclosed by the endomysium, a type of connective tissue. The fascicles, or bundles of fibers grouped together, are surrounded by the perimysium, and the entire muscle is enclosed by the epimysium. The tendon is the passive part of the muscle and is made up of elastic connective tissue. Each muscle attaches to bone at the periosteum or alternatively to deep, thick fascial tissue via tendons and the perimysium and epimysium connective tissues. The size and shape of tendons depend on the functions and shape of the muscles. Some tendons can be easily seen and palpated just under the surface of the skin,

such as the hamstring muscle tendons at the sides of the posterior aspect of the knee and the Achilles tendon inserting into the posterior heel. Other muscles, such as the supraspinatus and infraspinatus (muscles of the rotator cuff in the shoulder), are attached directly to the bone with no observable tendon. Broad and flat tendons, such as the proximal tendinous sheath of the latissimus dorsi, are aponeuroses. Refer to figure 3.4 for anterior and posterior views of surface muscles. Other muscles lie underneath the surface muscles.

Forces That Cause Movement

Joint movement is caused primarily by either the shortening of a muscle or the action of gravity, although other forces, such as another person pushing or pulling on a body part, may cause joint movement. Whether a muscle contraction causes movement depends on the combined

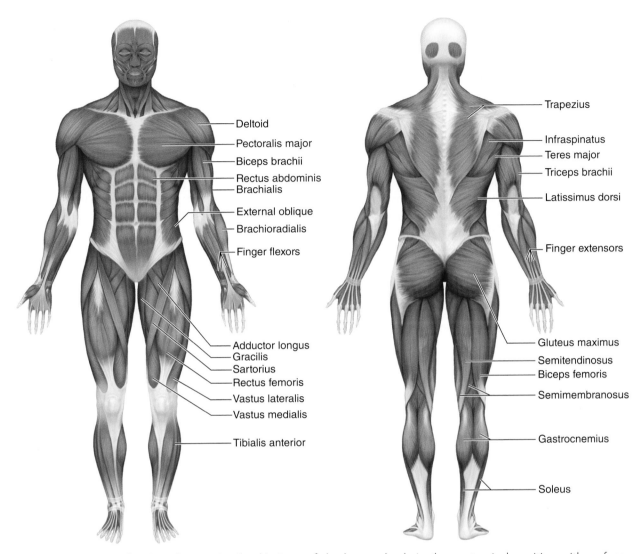

FIGURE 3.4 Anterior (front) and posterior (back) views of the human body in the anatomical position with surface muscles illustrated.

effect of the force developed and the amount of resistance from other forces.

Forces That Resist or Prevent Movement

The same forces that can cause movement may also resist or prevent movement. Joint movement caused by gravity can be resisted or decelerated by eccentric muscle action (which lengthens the muscle; see the section on eccentric action later in the chapter). Gravity always resists movement occurring in a direction away from the earth. Other forces that can resist movement include internal soft-tissue restriction by ligaments and tendons. Outside the body, exercise bands, hydraulic or air-pressure devices on resistance training equipment, and the drag provided by water against bodies moving through it can resist movement.

Muscle Action

Each muscle fiber is innervated, or receives stimuli, by a branch of a motor neuron. A motor unit consists of a single motor neuron, its branches, and all the muscle fibers that it innervates. With a sufficiently strong stimulus, each muscle fiber within that motor unit responds maximally; muscular tension increases as a result of the stimulation of more motor units (recruitment) or an increased rate of stimulation (summation). A muscle whose primary purpose is a strength or power movement (e.g., the gastrocnemius) rather than a delicate movement (e.g., the finger muscles) has a large number of muscle fibers and many muscle fibers per motor unit. When a muscle develops tension, it tends to shorten toward the middle, pulling on all of its bony attachments. Whether the attached bones move as a result of that muscle action depends on the amount of muscle force and the resistance to that movement from other forces. The three major muscle actions are concentric, eccentric, and isometric.

Concentric Action

Concentric action occurs when a muscle shortens under tension. This shortening pulls the points of attachment on each bone closer to each other, causing movement at the joint. Figure 3.5 illustrates elbow flexion moving a dumbbell against gravity as a result of a concentric action. The muscles responsible for flexion act with sufficient force to shorten, which pulls the forearm toward the humerus. Although the pull is on all the bones of attachment, usually only the bone farthest from the trunk (i.e., more distal) moves during a concentric action. To stand up from a semisquat position, the body must extend at the hip joints and knee joints, but gravity resists that extension. The muscles must develop sufficient force to overcome the force of gravity as the muscle shortens in a concentric action, pulling on the bones to cause extension. Resistance training with free weights uses gravity as the resistance. The use of pulleys in resistance training machines changes the direction of the force needed to overcome gravity acting on the weight stack, offering resistance to movement in other directions. Water resists the movement of submerged body parts in all directions.

To exercise muscles by using gravity as the resisting force, the movements must be done in the direction opposite the pull of gravity (i.e., away from the earth). Shoulder abduction from a standing position occurs opposite the pull of gravity, so a concentric action is required by the muscles that will pull the humerus into the abducted position. Movements such as shoulder horizontal abduction and adduction executed from a standing position occur parallel to the ground and therefore are not resisted by gravity. During these movements, gravity is still trying to draw the upper limb toward the earth (requiring concentric action of the shoulder abductors to overcome it). To perform horizontal abduction and adduction against the resistance of gravity, the performer must get into a position in which these movements are away from the pull of gravity. To horizontally abduct the shoulder against gravity, the performer can lie prone on a bench or stand with the trunk flexed 90° at the hip. Horizontal adduction against gravity can be done from a supine position on a bench.

A concentric action is also necessary for a rapid movement, regardless of the direction of other forces. When an external force could cause the desired movement without any muscular action but would be too slow, concentric actions produce the desired speed. An example of this is seen in the upper-limb movements during the second count of a jumping jack, when the arms adduct from their abducted position. Gravity would adduct the arms, but concentrically acting muscles speed up the adduction.

A muscle that is very effective in causing a certain joint movement is a prime mover, or agonist. Assistant movers are smaller muscles that make a smaller contribution to the same movement. For example, the peroneus longus and brevis are prime movers for eversion of the foot, but they assist plantar flexion of the ankle joint only a little. During a concentric action, muscles that act opposite to the muscles causing the concentric action, the antagonist muscles, are mostly passive and lengthen as the agonists shorten. For example, for the elbow to flex against gravity, the muscles responsible for elbow flexion act concentrically, while the antagonists, or the muscles responsible for elbow extension, relax and lengthen passively.

Watch video 3.2, which shows concentric and eccentric muscle actions as demonstrated in the biceps curl.

Eccentric Action

An eccentric action occurs when a muscle generates tension that is not great enough to cause movement but instead slows the speed of movement in the opposite direction caused by another force (see figure 3.5). The muscle exerts force, but its length increases while it is

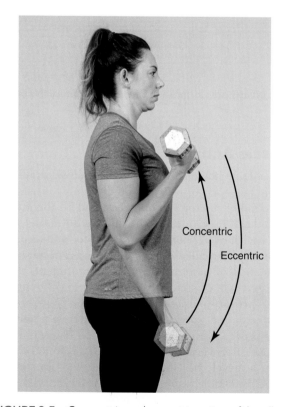

FIGURE 3.5 Concentric and eccentric action of the elbow flexors during a biceps curl.

under tension. Shoulder abduction requires concentric action, but gravity will adduct the upper limb back to the side of the body. To adduct the upper limb more slowly than gravity does, the same muscles that acted concentrically to abduct the upper limb now act eccentrically to control the speed of the upper limb. Eccentric actions also may occur when the maximum effort of a muscle is not great enough to overcome the opposing force. Movement due to the opposing force will still occur despite the maximally activated muscle, which is lengthening under tension. An example of this may occur when a person with the elbow joint flexed to 90° is handed a heavy weight. The exerciser tries to flex the elbow joint or even maintain the 90° position but lacks the strength to do so. The elbow joint extends despite the efforts to flex it. Muscles that are antagonists to the eccentrically acting muscles will passively shorten during the movement.

Ballistic Movement

A ballistic movement is a fast movement that occurs when resistance is minimal, as in throwing a ball, and requires a burst of concentric action to initiate it. Once movement has begun, these initial muscles relax because any further action would slow the movement. Other muscles actively guide the movement in the appropriate direction. At the end of the movement, eccentric action of muscles that are antagonist to the initial muscles decelerates and stops the movement. For example, one of the most important movements in throwing is internal rotation of the shoulder joint. The muscles responsible for internal rotation act quickly and concentrically to begin the throwing motion. After the ball is released, the muscles responsible for external rotation act eccentrically to slow and stop the movement during the follow-through. The reverse is true for the windup, or preparation for the actual throw.

Jumping jacks require repeated ballistic movements in which opposing muscles come into play. The upper-limb movements require concentric action by the agonist muscles to initiate the rapid movement. Once the movement is initiated, these muscles relax. To stop the abduction movement and initiate the upper-limb movement in the opposite direction, muscles antagonistic to those that acted concentrically act eccentrically to decelerate the movement and then act concentrically to initiate the next movement (adduction).

Isometric Action

During an isometric action, or static action, the muscle exerts a force that is equal in magnitude to an opposing force. The muscle length does not change and the joint position is maintained: The contractile part of the muscle is active, but there is no overall change in the entire muscle length. Holding the upper limb in an abducted position or maintaining a semisquat position requires isometric action, producing just enough muscle force to counteract the pull of gravity and result in no movement. The effort involved in trying to move an immovable object (e.g., pushing against a wall) is another example of an isometric action; although the amount of muscular force can be maximal, the joint does not move (see figure 3.6).

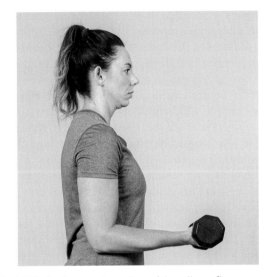

FIGURE 3.6 Isometric action of the elbow flexor muscles holding a dumbbell.

The posterior pelvic tilt desired during some exercises is maintained by isometric action of the anterior trunk muscles after they have acted concentrically to tilt the pelvis backward. During all resistance exercises that involve the arms or legs, the trunk muscles should act isometrically to stabilize the trunk and help prevent injury.

KEY POINT

During concentric muscle action, the muscle shortens and the joint moves in the direction the muscle is pulling. During eccentric muscle action, the muscle lengthens and the joint moves in the opposite direction than the muscle is pulling. During isometric muscle contraction, the muscle length does not change and the joint does not move.

Role of Muscles

Skeletal muscles can act in several ways and have a variety of effects on joint movement. They can cause movement via concentric action or decelerate movement caused by another force via eccentric action. Muscles also may act isometrically to stabilize or prevent undesirable movement. For example, during a push-up, gravity tends to cause the lumbar spine to hyperextend. Isometric action of the trunk muscles prevents this sagging and stabilizes the lumbar region in a neutral position.

Another function of muscle is to counteract an undesirable action caused by the concentric action of another muscle. The concentric action of many muscles causes more than one movement at the same joint or causes movement at more than one joint. If only one of those movements is intended, another muscle must act to prevent the undesirable movement. For example, concentric action of fibers in the upper trapezius both elevates and adducts the scapula. If only adduction is desired, fibers in the lower trapezius, which cause depression and adduction, neutralize the undesirable scapula elevation. In this example, different fibers of the same large trapezius muscle neutralize the unwanted action. As another example, the biceps brachii causes both elbow flexion and radioulnar supination, so for only flexion to occur, the pronator teres counteracts the supination movement.

Muscles can also guide movements caused by other muscles. During activities against a great resistance, such as lifting free weights, additional muscles help maintain balance and proper direction of the movement. After the force of a prime mover has initiated a ballistic movement, other muscles guide the movement in the proper direction.

KEY POINT

The major roles of the muscles are to cause movement (concentric action) regardless of an opposing force, decelerate or control the speed of movement (eccentric action) caused by another force, and prevent movement (isometric action). Other muscle functions include counteracting an undesirable action caused by the concentric action of another muscle and guiding movements caused by another muscle.

Muscle Groups

A muscle group includes all of the muscles that cause the same movement at the same joint. The group is named for the joint where the movement takes place and for the movement commonly caused by the concentric action of those muscles. The elbow flexors, for example, are a muscle group composed of the muscles responsible for flexion at the elbow joint when the muscles act concentrically. Table 3.2 lists the prime and assistant movers at each joint. A muscle group also may act eccentrically to control the opposite motion at the joint. For example, the elbow flexor muscle group flexes the elbow joint during

Table 3.2 Muscle Groups at Each Joint

Joint	Prime movers (assistant movers in parentheses)
AXIAL SKELETON	
Vertebral column (thoracic and lumbar areas)	Flexors—rectus abdominis, external oblique, internal oblique
	Extensors—erector spinae group
	Rotators—internal oblique, external oblique, erector spinae, rotatores, multifidus
	Lateral flexors—internal oblique, external oblique, quadratus lumborum, multifidus, rotatores (erector spinae group)
Lumbosacral joint	Anterior pelvic tilters—iliopsoas (rectus femoris)
	Posterior pelvic tilters—rectus abdominis, internal oblique (external oblique, gluteus maximus)
APPENDICULAR SKELETON: UPPER EXTREMITY	
Shoulder girdle (scapulothoracic joint)	Protractors—serratus anterior, pectoralis minor
	Retractors—middle fibers of trapezius, rhomboids (upper and lower fibers of trapezius)
	Upward rotators—upper and lower fibers of trapezius, serratus anterior
	Downward rotators—rhomboids, pectoralis minor
	Elevators—levator scapulae, upper fibers of trapezius, rhomboids
	Depressors—lower fibers of trapezius, pectoralis minor
Shoulder joint (glenohumeral joint)	Flexors—anterior deltoid, clavicular portion of pectoralis major (short head of biceps brachii)
	Extensors—sternal portion of pectoralis major, latissimus dorsi, teres major (posterior deltoid, long head of triceps brachii, infraspinatus, teres minor)

Joint	Prime movers (assistant movers in parentheses)
APPENDICULAR SKELETON: UPPER EXTREMITY	
Shoulder joint (glenohumeral joint)	Abductors—middle deltoid, supraspinatus (anterior deltoid, long head of biceps brachii)
	Adductors—latissimus dorsi, teres major, sternal portion of pectoralis major (short head of biceps brachii, long head of triceps brachii)
	External rotators—infraspinatus*, teres minor* (posterior deltoid)
	Internal rotators—pectoralis major, subscapularis*, latissimus dorsi, teres major (anterior deltoid, supraspinatus*)
	Horizontal adductors—both portions of pectoralis major, anterior deltoid
	Horizontal abductors—latissimus dorsi, teres major, infraspinatus, teres minor, posterior deltoid
Elbow joint	Flexors—brachialis, biceps brachii, brachioradialis (pronator teres, flexor carpi ulnaris and radialis)
	Extensors—triceps brachii (anconeus, extensor carpi ulnaris and radialis)
Radioulnar joint	Pronators—pronator quadratus, pronator teres, brachioradialis
	Supinators—supinator, biceps brachii, brachioradialis
Wrist joint	Flexors—flexor carpi ulnaris, flexor carpi radialis (flexor digitorum superficialis and profundus)
	Extensors—extensor carpi ulnaris, extensor carpi radialis longus and brevis (extensor digitorum)
	Abductors (radial flexors)—flexor carpi radialis, extensor carpi radialis longus and brevis (extensor pollicis)
	Adductors (ulnar flexors)—flexor carpi ulnaris, extensor carpi ulnaris
Metacarpophalangeal joint	Flexors—flexor digitorum superficialis, flexor digitorum profundus, flexor pollicis longus, flexor pollicis brevis, flexor digiti minimi, interossei, lumbricals
	Extensors—extensor digitorum, extensor indicis, extensor digiti minimi, extensor pollicis longus, extensor pollicis brevis, interossei
	Abductors—interossei
	Adductors—interossei
APPENDICULAR SKELETON: LOWER EXTREMITY	
Hip joint	Flexors—iliopsoas, pectineus, rectus femoris (sartorius, tensor fasciae latae, gracilis, adductor longus and brevis)
	Extensors—gluteus maximus, biceps femoris, semitendinosus, semimembranosus
	Abductors—gluteus medius (tensor fasciae latae, iliopsoas, sartorius)
	Internal rotators—gluteus maximus, the six deep external rotator muscles (iliopsoas, sartorius)
	External rotators—gluteus minimus, gluteus medius (tensor fasciae latae, pectineus)
Knee joint	Flexors—biceps femoris, semimembranosus, semitendinosus (sartorius, gracilis, gastrocnemius, plantaris)
	Extensors—rectus femoris, vastus medialis, vastus lateralis, vastus intermedius
Ankle joint	Plantar flexors—gastrocnemius, soleus (peroneus longus, peroneus brevis, tibialis posterior, flexor digitorum, flexor hallucis longus)
	Dorsiflexors—tibialis anterior, extensor digitorum longus, peroneus tertius (extensor hallucis longus)
Subtalar joint	Invertors—tibialis anterior, tibialis posterior (extensor and flexor hallucis longus, flexor digitorum longus)
	Evertors—extensor digitorum longus, peroneus brevis, peroneus longus, peroneus tertius

*Rotator cuff muscles

an elbow curl. To return to the starting position, the pull of gravity extends the joint to the original position, but the elbow flexor muscle group is still exerting force to eccentrically control the speed of that movement (see figure 3.5). Maintaining the elbow in a flexed position requires an isometric action by those same elbow flexors (see figure 3.6). Specific muscles that cause more than one action at a joint or cause movement at more than one joint belong to more than one muscle group. For example, the flexor carpi ulnaris belongs in both the wrist flexor and wrist adductor muscle groups, and the biceps brachii is part of the elbow flexor and radioulnar supinator muscle groups.

KEY POINT

A muscle group includes all the muscles that act concentrically to cause a specific movement at a given joint.

Many errors that occur during exercise and movement activities result from a lack of knowledge of musculoskeletal anatomy rather than a lack of muscular strength or coordination. Applying basic knowledge allows exercisers to perform better and more safely. The following sections, from the axial through the appendicular skeleton, offer tips for exercising each major muscle group and avoiding common exercise mistakes.

Joints and Muscles of the Axial Skeleton

The axial skeleton forms the midline of the body. It consists of the skull, the vertebral column, and the rib cage, which attaches to the vertebral column.

Vertebral Column

The vertebral column contains 24 individual vertebrae and the sacrum. Although movement between adjacent vertebrae is just a few degrees, when combined over the whole vertebral column, the range of motion of the trunk is substantial. Movements of the trunk occur in all three planes: flexion and extension, lateral flexion to the left and right, and rotation to the left and right (see figure 3.7).

Lumbosacral Joint

The pelvis (see figure 3.8) tilts mainly at the joint formed by the fifth lumbar vertebra and the sacrum. A reference for the direction of pelvic tilt is a line between

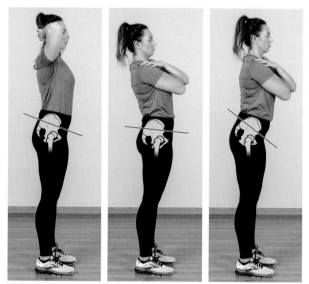

Normal   Posterior pelvic tilt   Anterior pelvic tilt

FIGURE 3.8   Movements of the lumbosacral joint and pelvis.

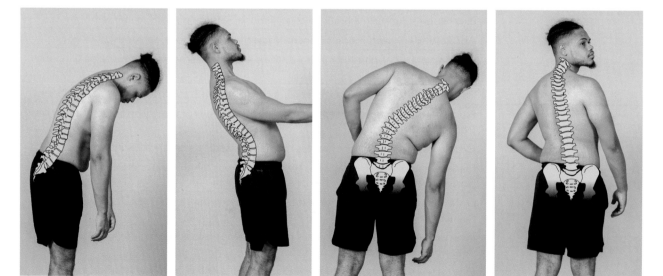

Flexion   Extension   Lateral flexion to right   Rotation to right

FIGURE 3.7   Movements of the vertebral column and trunk.

APPLICATION POINT

Exercise Tips

In general, neither neck hyperextension nor hyperflexion is desirable. The same pairs of muscles that act concentrically to cause flexion and extension can be strengthened or stretched, one side at a time, by cervical lateral flexion and rotation. Participants should tilt or turn the head from side to side rather than bend the neck forward or backward.

Many exercises require appropriate positioning of the lumbosacral joint and lumbar vertebrae and actions by the trunk muscles for either movement or stabilization. An abdominal curl-up or crunch should begin with a backward pelvic tilt that is maintained throughout the curl-up and return movement. If the backward pelvic tilt cannot be maintained or the exerciser feels tightness or an ache in the lumbar area, the exerciser should stop. If the problem is inadequate strength to maintain the backward tilt, the exercise should be modified to one that the exerciser has sufficient abdominal strength to perform correctly.

A full curl-up, in which the exerciser comes up to a sitting position, requires hip flexion by the hip flexor muscles during the last stages of the exercise. Initially, the abdominal muscles concentrically tilt the pelvis backward and then flex the vertebral column. Once flexion is achieved, these muscles act isometrically to keep the pelvis tilted backward and the trunk in a flexed position. During a full curl-up, the exerciser can feel a sticking point that occurs when the trunk flexion is complete and the hip flexors begin to bring the trunk to an upright position. Doing partial curl-ups or crunches helps eliminate the role of the hip flexors and maintain focus solely on strengthening the abdominal muscles.

The leg lift is considered an abdominal exercise, but often it is not taught correctly. From a supine position on the floor, the legs are lifted and held up by concentric and then isometric action of the hip flexors. Some of the hip flexors also pull the lumbosacral joint into a forward-tilted position. The abdominal muscles must prevent that forward tilt and maintain a flattened lumbar spine and posterior pelvic tilt. The backward pelvic tilt should precede the hip flexion, and, as in the case of the curl-up, if the proper tilt cannot be maintained, the exercise should not be done in that fashion.

The pelvis also tends to tilt forward during overhead upper-limb movements from a standing position. This can be prevented by keeping the arms in front of the ears and flexing the knees slightly.

When weights are lifted from a supine position, as in the bench press, there is a tendency to hyperextend the lumbar spine and tilt the pelvis forward. Although this tendency can allow the exerciser to lift a somewhat heavier weight, it does not increase the work of the upper-limb and chest muscles, and it puts the low back into a compromising position. Bench presses are best done with the hips and knees in a flexed position and the feet on the bench or a bench extension to maintain a posterior pelvic tilt. Upright presses are best done seated with the back supported.

the anterior and posterior superior iliac spines in the sagittal plane. When the pelvis tilts anteriorly, the angle between the horizontal and the line between the iliac spines increases. With posterior pelvic tilt, the angle of the line between the iliac spines becomes closer to the horizontal. Anterior pelvic tilt is accompanied by extension of the lumbar spine, whereas a backward tilt results in a flattening out of the lumbar spine.

Joints and Muscles of the Appendicular Skeleton: Upper Extremity

The upper extremity begins at the shoulder girdle. It continues through the arm, elbow, forearm (including radioulnar joints), and wrist to the hand.

Shoulder Girdle

The primary articulation between the scapula (shoulder blade) and the thoracic cage (ribs) is not a traditional joint because there is no direct contact between the bones, which have several muscles between them. However, there is a large range of motion of the scapula on the thoracic cage that has its own terminology. Vertical movements are *elevation* (upward movement) and *depression* (downward movement). Horizontal movements are *protraction* or *abduction* (out to the side) and *retraction* or *adduction* (in toward the spine). Rotational movements are *upward* and *downward rotation* (see figure 3.9). Movements of the shoulder girdle combine with movements of the shoulder joint to provide the large range of motion found at the shoulder. The shoulder girdle also includes the sternoclavicular joint, between

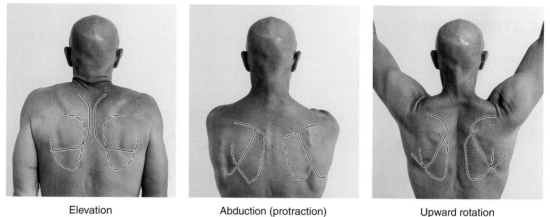

Elevation
Depression

Abduction (protraction)
Adduction (retraction)

Upward rotation
Downward rotation

FIGURE 3.9 Movements of the scapulae (scapulothoracic joint).

the sternum (breastbone) and clavicle (collarbone), and the acromioclavicular joint, between the scapula and clavicle. These joints move when the scapulothoracic joint moves.

Shoulder Joint

The glenohumeral joint is a ball-and-socket joint, so it can move in all directions—flexion, extension, abduc-

tion, adduction, internal and external rotation, and circumduction (tips of the fingers trace a circle in the sagittal plane). Horizontal adduction and horizontal abduction are additional movements of the upper limb toward and away from the midline when it is positioned in the transverse plane, or parallel to the ground (see figure 3.10).

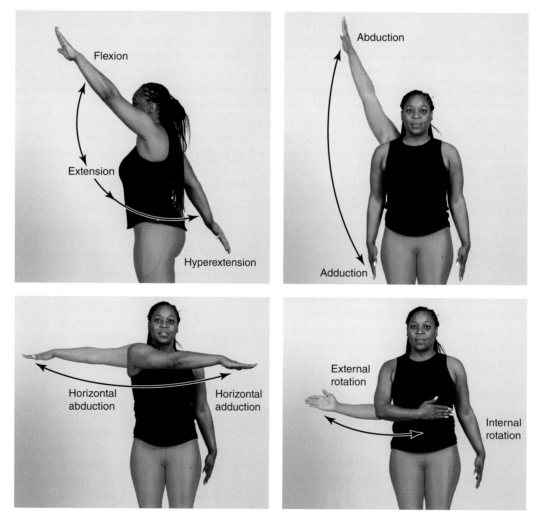

FIGURE 3.10 Movements of the shoulder (glenohumeral) joint.

The relationship between the scapulothoracic and shoulder joints is called *scapulohumeral rhythm*. The glenohumeral joint alone cannot reach the full range of motion seen at the shoulder because it is restricted by the bone structure at the joint. However, the glenoid fossa that makes up part of the glenohumeral joint is part of the scapula, so if the scapula also moves, greater range of motion can occur.

Elbow Joint

The elbow joint is the articulation between the humerus and the two forearm bones, the radius and ulna. The ulnohumeral joint is the primary joint, and as a hinge joint, it limits movements to flexion and extension (see figure 3.11). The radiohumeral joint is also part of the elbow joint, but it does not provide much bony stability. The ability of some people to hyperextend the elbow joint is due to differences in the shape of their articulating surfaces.

Radioulnar Joints

The radius and ulna articulate with each other both proximally and distally in the forearm. The joint movements are pronation and supination (see figure 3.12). Although the wrist is not involved in these movements, the position of the radioulnar joints can be identified by the direction the palms face. When the arms hang down alongside the trunk, the palms face forward in the supinated position and toward the back in the pronated position. In the supinated position, the radius and ulna are parallel with each other; in the pronated position, the radius lies across and on top of the ulna.

Wrist Joint

The wrist joint consists of the radiocarpal and ulnocarpal articulations between the forearm bones and the carpal bones of the wrist. Movements at the wrist include joint flexion, extension, abduction (radial flexion), and adduction (ulnar flexion) (see figure 3.13).

Metacarpophalangeal Joints of the Hand

The metacarpophalangeal joints are the knuckles of the hand. The second through the fifth joints move in flexion and extension as well as abduction and adduction of the fingers. The metacarpophalangeal joint of the thumb allows only flexion and extension. The ability of the opposable thumb to touch the tips of all the other digits comes from movement at the carpometacarpal joint. The interphalangeal joints of the fingers and thumb are hinge joints that flex and extend.

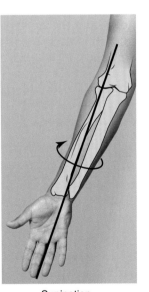
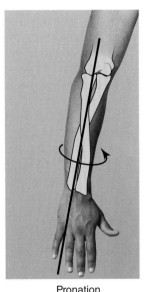
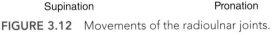

FIGURE 3.12 Movements of the radioulnar joints.

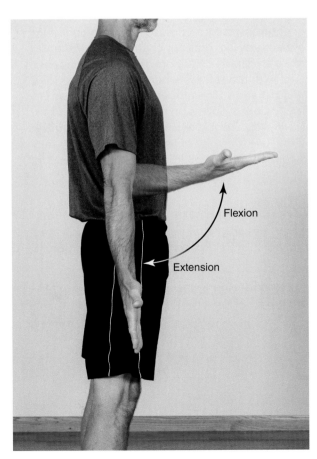

FIGURE 3.11 Movements of the elbow joint.

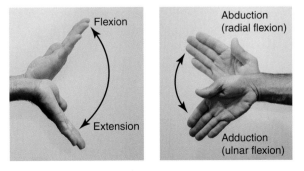

FIGURE 3.13 Movements of the wrist joint.

APPLICATION POINT

Exercise Tips for the Upper Extremity

This section offers tips for exercising muscles of the upper extremity. Functional movements as well as exercises with weights are suggested.

Shoulder Girdle and Shoulder Joint Muscles

Movement can be enhanced and more muscles involved if shoulder girdle movements are deliberately incorporated with shoulder joint movements. These muscles can be optimally involved in the following exercises and movements:

- *Forward reaching:* Glenohumeral joint flexion can be accompanied by scapular elevation and upward rotation if the exerciser reaches the fingertips as far forward as possible.
- *Push-up:* At the completion of a push-up, the scapulae can be protracted to raise the chest a bit more off the floor.
- *Overhead reaching:* Normally, some scapular elevation is involved when the upper limb is overhead. A conscious effort to reach as high as possible will involve the scapula elevators more. Conversely, a deliberate attempt to keep the shoulders down and the neck long requires concentric action by the scapula depressors.
- *Sideward reaching:* During horizontal abduction at the shoulder joint, the upper limb can be moved farther back with scapular retraction.

Elbow and Radioulnar Joint Muscles

Flexion against resistance requires concentric action of the flexor muscles at the elbow joint. The degree to which these muscles are strengthened, however, is affected by supination and pronation—a good point to remember when instructing participants on how to perform curls. The biceps brachii attaches to the radius, and this bone rotates when the forearm pronates, stretching out the biceps and reducing its contribution to elbow flexion. Thus, elbow flexion with the radioulnar joint in a pronated position (a reverse curl) is a weaker movement than a traditional curl with the forearm in a supinated position. The brachialis muscle is not affected by the position of the radioulnar joint because it is attached to the ulna, so its relationship to the humerus does not change with pronation and supination of the radius. Thus, a reverse curl puts more emphasis on the brachialis at the expense of the biceps. Further, the brachioradialis muscle can act with more force when the radioulnar joint is in a neutral position midway between pronation and supination. The elbow extensor muscles are not affected by the position of the radioulnar joint. Triceps push-downs, in which elbow extension occurs with the radioulnar joints in the pronated position, require the wrist flexors to stabilize the wrist joint, whereas triceps pull-downs (supinated position) use the wrist extensors, which are usually much weaker than the flexors. Exercisers who want to concentrate on building the elbow extensors should perform triceps push-downs.

Wrist Joint Muscles

During wrist flexion and extension curls, the wrist muscles are affected by the position of the radioulnar joints. Gravity acts as resistance for wrist flexion when the radioulnar joints are in the supinated position and as resistance for extension when the radioulnar joints are in the pronated position.

Metacarpophalangeal Joint Muscles

These gripping muscles can be strengthened in flexion by squeezing a small rubber ball. The extensor, adductor, and abductor muscles can be strengthened by placing a rubber band over the fingers and moving various combinations of fingers in adduction and abduction against the resistance of the band.

Joints and Muscles of the Appendicular Skeleton: Lower Extremity

The lower extremity begins at the pelvic girdle. It continues through the hip, thigh, knee, leg, and ankle to the foot.

Hip Joint

The hip joint is a ball-and-socket joint similar to the shoulder (glenohumeral joint), but the bony socket at the hip is much deeper compared with the shoulder. The deep socket makes the hip more stable than the shoulder at the expense of total range of motion (see figure 3.14). For example, there is less extension at the hip than at the shoulder. Movements at the hip joint are flexion, extension, abduction, adduction, internal and external rotation, and circumduction (a movement combining flexion, extension, abduction, and adduction that results in the foot moving in a circular motion).

Knee Joint

The tibiofemoral joint is the primary knee joint. The knee does not have good bony stability in flexion due to the flattened surface of the tibial plateau; therefore, it relies on ligaments to provide stability, making it vulnerable to injury. Flexion and extension are the major movements at the knee (see figure 3.15). When the knee is in a flexed position, limited rotation, abduction, and adduction are possible.

Ankle Joint

Also called the *talocrural joint*, the ankle joint is limited to movement in one plane only. Plantar flexion is pointing the foot downward and dorsiflexion is pulling the foot up toward the shin (see figure 3.16).

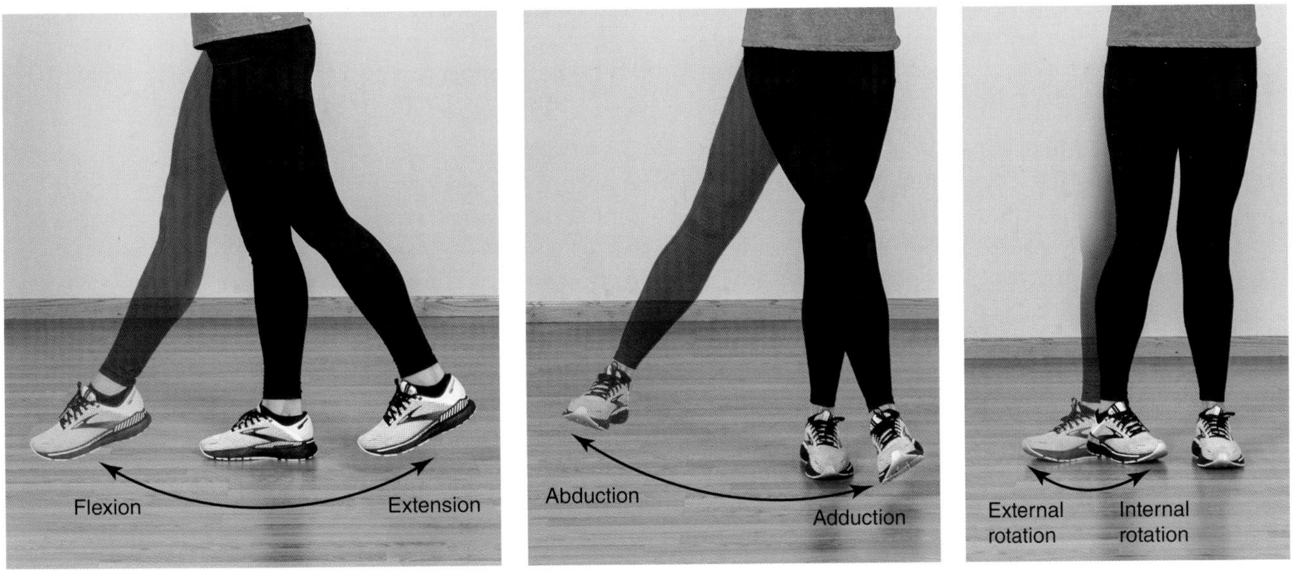

FIGURE 3.14 Movements of the hip joint.

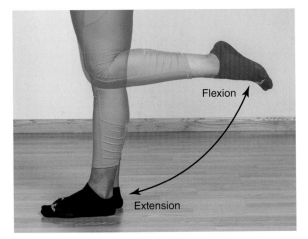

FIGURE 3.15 Movements of the knee joint.

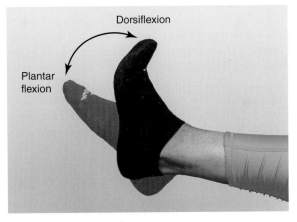

FIGURE 3.16 Movements of the ankle joint.

Subtalar Joint

The subtalar joint contributes to pronation and supination movements of the foot. In the frontal plane, these movements are eversion and inversion (see figure 3.17). In combination with other foot joints, the subtalar joint lowers the medial longitudinal arch (pronation) via a combination of eversion, dorsiflexion, and abduction. The opposite movement is supination, and it raises the arch via a combination of inversion, plantar flexion, and adduction.

APPLICATION POINT

Exercise Tips for the Lower Extremity

This section offers tips for exercising muscles of the lower extremity. Functional movements as well as exercises with weights are suggested.

Hip Joint Muscles

A common error during side-lying leg raises for the hip abductors is the attempt to move the foot as high as possible. Because the range of motion for true abduction is limited (about 45°), the exerciser will externally rotate the top limb, which turns the foot out and allows it to go higher. However, this rotation changes the muscle involvement more to the hip flexors. To exercise the primary abductor muscles, the limb should not be rotated and the toes should face forward, not upward.

In backward lower-limb movements for strengthening the gluteus muscles, hip extension is limited primarily by the tightness of the hip ligaments. A limb can appear to be more extended if it is accompanied by a forward pelvic tilt. The exerciser should be cautioned to keep the pelvis in its neutral position in order to focus on the gluteal muscles, even though some apparent hip extension is lost.

Knee Joint Muscles

Hyperflexion can strain and stretch knee ligaments and put pressure on the menisci. Therefore, a maximum squat depth to a 90° angle at the knee joint is recommended. During any lunging movements or forward–back stride positions in which the front knee is flexed, the knee should be over or in back of the foot and not in front. Any knee position that puts a twisting pressure on the knee joint should also be avoided. The hurdler position, with one limb out to the back and side with a flexed knee, should be avoided; instead, both legs should be out in front.

A common exercise position is standing with feet shoulder-width apart. The exerciser should have the feet turned slightly outward (7°-10°). The appropriate toe-out position is one that positions the kneecaps facing forward. During any squatting or standing movement, the knee should be in line directly above the foot (not moving to the outside or inside of the foot) to avoid straining the lateral and medial knee ligaments and to develop good lower-extremity positioning habits. Performing the exercise in front of a mirror is recommended to enable the exerciser to monitor the position of the knee relative to the foot.

Ankle Joint Muscles

If the squat exercise is performed with the heels of the feet resting on a low block, the soleus muscles are exercised more than they would be if the feet were flat. This position with the heels up shortens the gastrocnemius muscles even more (they are already shortened by the flexed knee), limiting their ability to generate force. The soleus muscles, which do not cross the knees, are not shortened to the same extent. To increase the force production of the gastrocnemius muscles, the squat could be done with the balls of the feet on the block. The mountain climber especially would benefit from this modification because it mimics the knee and ankle positions in climbing. Individual limits to range of motion at the ankle joint should also be taken into consideration during the squat. Exercisers with limited dorsiflexion benefit from placing the heels on a low block to prevent them from going onto tiptoes at the bottom of the squat. This ensures they maintain a stable base and can perform the exercise safely.

Subtalar Joint Muscles

The subtalar joint plays a role in adapting to uneven surfaces. One way of exercising the invertors and evertors is to walk across, instead of up and down, a ramp or hill.

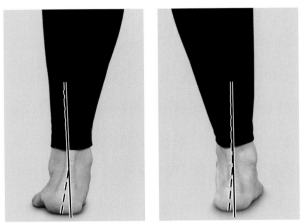

Eversion   Inversion

FIGURE 3.17 Movements of the subtalar joint. Left foot is everted and right foot is inverted.

KEY POINT

During exercises involving the vertebral column and lumbosacral joints, participants should remember to achieve a posterior (backward) pelvic tilt before initiating the exercise and should maintain the tilt throughout the exercise to protect the lumbar spine. For exercises involving the knee, participants should remember to keep the knee in line above the foot when observing themselves in a mirror. The knee should also stay behind or above the foot when observed from the side.

Basic Biomechanical Concepts for Human Movement

Biomechanics is the study of how the joints of the human body move and the forces that contribute to or hinder those movements. Understanding key principles of biomechanics is necessary to fully understand human movement. Some of these concepts are described next.

Stability

Stability is a feature of the whole body and is influenced by the position of all parts of the body. It is the ability to maintain a stable, balanced position following a disruption such as being touched by an opposing player. In order to maintain balance, an individual's center of gravity must fall within the area of the base of support. In the simple case of standing on two feet with arms at the sides, a roughly rectangular base of support is formed from the toes of each foot to the heels of each foot. With weight evenly distributed on both feet, the center of gravity is in the middle of the base of support (see figure 3.18). Changing the foot position will change the shape and area of the base of support. Changing the position of the body or holding an object will alter the location of the center of gravity within the base of support.

Stability is proportional to the distance from the center of gravity to the edge of the base of support in the direction that an external force would propel the person. Figure 3.19 compares more and less stable positions relative to a force applied in a mediolateral direction. With the feet apart, if one leans so that the line of gravity falls directly over one foot and a pushing force is applied in

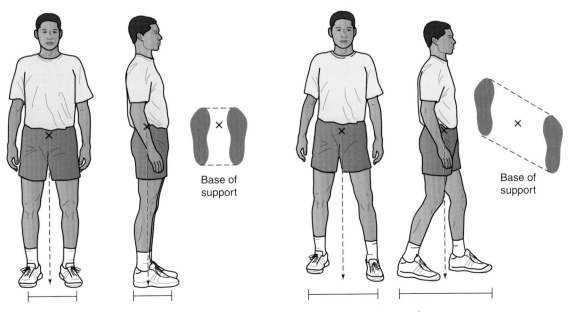

Base of support

Base of support

FIGURE 3.18 The relationships among center of gravity, body position, and base of support.

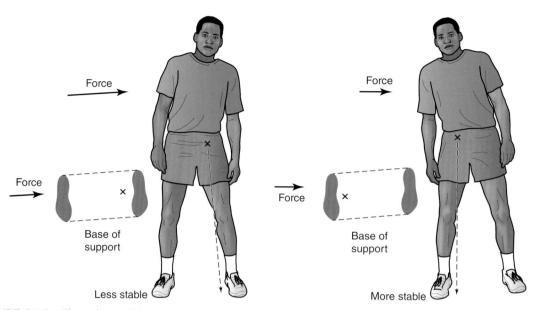

FIGURE 3.19 The relationships among the direction of a perturbing force, center of gravity, and base of support in more and less stable positions.

the same direction of the lean, the result is less stability than if the feet were together but with the line of gravity along the edge of the foot closer to the applied force. A wide base of support in the anticipated direction of perturbation typically provides greater stability. A lower body position and the accompanying lower center of gravity also contribute to a more stable position. For example, a football lineman may have a triangular base of support between one hand in contact with the ground and both feet. He will squat to lower his center of gravity and lean forward so that his center of gravity is as far as possible from the edge of the base of support in the direction he anticipates an opponent will try to move him (backward). Stability is also directly proportional to body weight. With all other factors being equal, a heavy person is more stable than a lighter one. Thus, a 300-pound (136-kilogram) lineman in a three-point squat is more stable than a 200-pound (91-kilogram) lineman in the same position.

Stability may be increased by moving the feet apart to widen the base of support and by flexing the knees and hips to lower the center of gravity. A wide base of support compromises the ability to respond quickly due to the large change in position required to initiate movement. During standing exercises that require balance, stability can also be aided by holding or pushing against a nearby object such as a wall or chair. Many exercises can be executed from a sitting position, which increases the base of support and lowers the center of gravity. To help maintain stability against a potentially perturbing force, the weight should be shifted toward that force. Just before walking begins, a position close to instability is attained by shifting the center of gravity in the direction of the intended movement, closer to the anterior limits of the base of support. During walking, as the line of gravity moves outside the base of support, a new base of support is established when the other foot makes contact and stability is restored. In basketball, a guard who takes a charge from a forward will fall more quickly and easily if the guard is in an unstable position—standing erect with feet closer together and weight on the heels at the moment of the collision.

KEY POINT

Stability is directly proportional to the distance of the center of gravity from the edge of the base of support. It is inversely proportional to the height of the center of gravity above the base of support, and it is directly proportional to the weight of the body. For greater stability during standing, the knees should be flexed, the feet spread apart in the direction of an oncoming force, and body weight shifted toward the force.

Torque

A force is any push or pull that is applied to a person or object. In the body, when a force is applied at a distance from a joint, it produces a torque (T), which will typically rotate the joint. Torque is the product of the magnitude of the force (F) and the force arm (FA), which is the perpendicular distance from the axis of rotation to the direction of application of that force. Torque is also referred to as *moment*, and the torque arm is also called the *moment arm*. Torque can be expressed as follows:

$$T = F \times FA$$

When two opposing forces act to produce rotation in opposite directions, one of the forces is typically designated as the resistance force (R), and its force arm is called the *resistance arm* (RA), producing a resistance torque (T_R) as follows:

$$T_R = R \times RA$$

In considering torque produced by a muscle to cause movement against gravity or some other external force, F and FA are designated for the muscle and R and RA are designated for gravity or other opposing forces.

Applying Torque to Muscle Action

Muscle action is a force. The force arm is the perpendicular distance from the axis of rotation of the joint to the line of action of the force from its point of application (where the muscle attaches to the bone being moved). Figure 3.20 illustrates the direction of pull of the biceps brachii on the radius with the elbow flexed to 90°. The force arm is the perpendicular distance from the elbow joint to this line of force. If the muscle insertion were closer to the joint, the force arm would be smaller, and the same force would produce less torque, or more muscle force would be required to produce the same torque. Joint position also affects torque. Figure 3.21 shows the direction of pull of the biceps brachii with the elbow in a more extended position. Note that the force arm is not always parallel to the bone. The more extended elbow position shortens the force arm, so the same muscle force produces less torque at that joint angle, or more muscle force is required to generate the same torque. This is why a dumbbell biceps curl feels harder at the start of the flexion movement compared with the middle of the flexion movement. It is crucial to remember that the force arm is the perpendicular distance from the line of action of the force to the axis of rotation, not the distance along the bone from the point of attachment of the muscle tendon on the bone to the joint axis.

Torque Resulting From Other Forces

The force of gravity directed vertically downward is treated as a resistance force. The resistance produced by gravity acting on a body part is the weight of the object. The resistance arm is the perpendicular distance from the axis of rotation to the point within the object that represents its center of gravity. The torque is the product of the resistance force and the resistance arm. Figure 3.22 illustrates the torque produced by gravity acting on the forearm and hand, which acts to extend the elbow. This torque can be increased by adding mass such as a dumbbell to increase both the magnitude of force (total weight of forearm and hand plus the added mass) and the length of the resistance arm if the mass is added farther from the axis of rotation. The resistance arm of a force

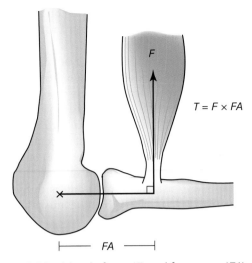

FIGURE 3.20   Muscle force (*F*) and force arm (*FA*) of the biceps brachii with the elbow joint flexed to 90°.

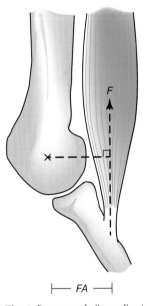

FIGURE 3.21   The influence of elbow flexion less than 90° at the elbow joint on the force arm (*FA*) of the biceps brachii. Note that *FA* is perpendicular to the muscle force (*F*).

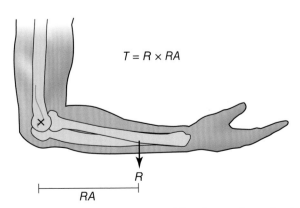

FIGURE 3.22   Extensor torque (*T*) is the product of resistance force (*R*), located at the center of gravity of the forearm and hand, and the resistance arm (*RA*).

applied by someone pushing or pulling on a limb is the perpendicular distance from the axis of rotation to the point of application of the push or pull.

For muscle contraction to move a bone, the muscle force generated must produce a torque greater than the opposing or resistance torque. In this case, the muscle action is concentric and the joint moves in the direction of the muscle torque. If the resistance torque is greater than the muscle torque, the muscle acts eccentrically and lengthens under tension. In this case, the joint moves in the opposite direction of the muscle torque (in the direction of the resistance torque) and is only slowed down by the muscle torque. When the muscular torque equals the resistance torque, no movement occurs and the muscle acts isometrically.

KEY POINT

Torque at a joint is the product of the force and the perpendicular distance to the axis of rotation, known as the *force arm*. Torque due to muscle force is often resisted by a resistance torque due to gravity or another external force. The direction of joint movement depends on whether muscle torque or resistance torque is greater.

APPLICATION POINT

Applying Torque to Exercise

Knowledge of torque can be used to modify exercises for individuals. The amount of muscle force required by the exercise can be tailored to a person's needs by altering the amount of resistance force, the resistance arm, or both in order to change the resistance torque. For example, resistance torque can be increased by adding external weight so that greater muscle force is required to overcome it (figure 3.23a). The resistance torque also can be changed by altering the position of the body parts. Figure 3.23b shows an exerciser reducing the required muscle force by not holding added weight, thus decreasing both the resistance force and the resistance arm, and then by flexing the elbow to further shorten the resistance arm and the resistance force (figure 3.23c).

During an abdominal crunch, the position of the arms determines the length of the resistance arm and therefore the amount of resistance torque against which the abdominal muscles have to work to flex the trunk and lift the shoulders off the floor. The arms may be held at the sides of the body to bring the upper-body mass closer to the axis of rotation and reduce the required muscle force. To increase the challenge of this exercise, the arms can be raised with the hands on the back of the head. The resistance arm can be increased by holding a weight with the arms straight out overhead, which increases the resistance torque and therefore increases the muscle force required to perform the exercise.

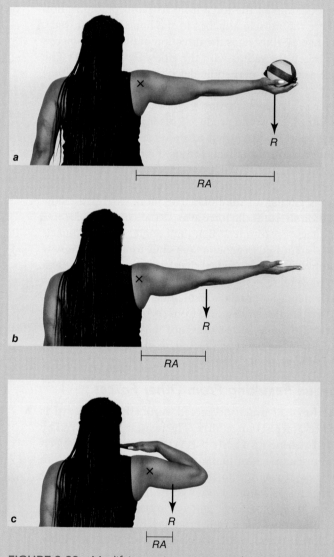

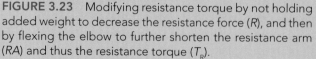

FIGURE 3.23 Modifying resistance torque by not holding added weight to decrease the resistance force (*R*), and then by flexing the elbow to further shorten the resistance arm (*RA*) and thus the resistance torque (T_R).

CASE STUDY

Carrying Bag Options: Musculoskeletal Anatomy and Biomechanics of Carrying Objects

Case Study Contributor: Clare Milner

Kendra has a new job and will be walking between the transit station and her workplace each day. She is looking forward to getting more steps to help achieve her fitness goals, but she has some questions about the best option for carrying her laptop and personal items during the walk. Kendra is considering a few different bag options, including a laptop bag that has a long cross-body strap or a backpack with a laptop pocket. She has heard that backpacks are recommended for students carrying schoolbooks and is wondering if the backpack would be the better choice for her and why it is preferred. Using your knowledge of musculoskeletal anatomy, the biomechanics of carrying objects, and joint torque, how would you explain to Kendra the effect each bag option will have on her body so that she can make an informed decision?

The different bag styles will affect Kendra's body and place demands on the joints and muscles in different ways. Using the cross-body strap on the laptop bag is a better option than a bag with a short carry handle. With the cross-body strap, the trunk supports the weight of the bag and its contents instead of the smaller muscles of the upper limb and hand. However, since the bag is positioned on one side of the body, the trunk muscles will need to generate a force in the frontal plane and create a torque to counteract the resistance torque created by the weight of the bag and its resistance arm. The resistance arm is the distance between the center of gravity of the bag and the axis of rotation of the vertebral column. The weight of the bag acts to laterally flex the vertebral column and trunk and must be counteracted by muscle force to maintain an upright trunk. The muscles of the axial skeleton, primarily the obliques and quadratus lumborum, will generate an isometric force on the opposite side of the body to the bag to counteract its resistance torque.

Carrying her laptop in a backpack will provide Kendra with the most comfort during her daily walks. The backpack positions the weight closer to the vertebral column, which creates a shorter resistance arm for the resistance force created by the weight of the backpack. In this case, the resistance torque of the backpack acts to extend the trunk and vertebral column in the sagittal plane. This action must be counteracted by generating an isometric flexion torque using the anterior trunk muscles, primarily rectus abdominis. Importantly, the shorter resistance arm means that the weight of the bag carried on the back compared to the side of the body will generate a smaller resistance torque and so require less muscle force to maintain an upright trunk position.

KEY POINT

> The torque that resists limb movements can be altered by modifying the amount of the resistance force and by changing the length of the resistance arm.

Rotational Inertia

Rotational inertia, or the resistance to change in the rotation of a body segment around a joint axis, depends on the mass of the segment and its distribution around the joint. Rotational inertia is also referred to as the *moment of inertia*. A lower limb, for example, has more rotational inertia than an upper limb not only because it is heavier but also because its mass is concentrated a greater distance away from its axis of rotation. A swinging softball bat held by its striking end has less rotational inertia than when held at the handle. When holding the bat by the striking end, most of its mass is close to the axis of rotation, which reduces its rotational inertia and makes it easier to swing. However, with less mass at the striking end, the bat will not move the ball very far. Optimal weight and weight distribution of the bat is a trade-off against how quickly the bat can be swung.

The rotational inertia of body segments before or during movement depends on the mass of the segments, which cannot be changed, and on the distribution of the mass around the joints, which can be manipulated. For example, an upper limb with the elbow extended has a greater rotational inertia than with the elbow flexed. Similarly, a lower limb with an extended knee has more rotational inertia than with the knee flexed. The amount of muscle force necessary to cause rapid limb movement is proportional to the rotational inertia of the limb to be moved. During jogging, the knee of the recovery limb is partially flexed to reduce the rotational inertia around

APPLICATION POINT

Applying Angular Momentum to Exercise

The concept of angular momentum can be applied to ballistic limb movements during exercise. A fast-moving body segment is decelerated by eccentric muscle actions; a faster movement, a greater mass, or a greater desired deceleration requires greater muscle force to decelerate the body segment. Care must be taken when performing rapid ballistic limb movements, especially when using added weight. The movements may generate great momentum, and considerable muscle strength may be required to decelerate and eventually stop them. This may result in damage to the muscle or the rotating joint if the momentum cannot be controlled.

Transfer of angular momentum from one body segment to another can be achieved by stabilizing the initial moving body part at a joint, which causes angular movement of another body part. For example, when an exerciser performs an abdominal crunch to exercise the trunk flexors, flinging the arms forward from an overhead position transfers their momentum to the trunk. This decreases the amount of muscular force needed from the trunk flexors and makes the exercise easier. In another example, a jump with a turn in the air can be better achieved if, just before takeoff, the arms are swung forcibly across the body in the intended direction of the spin.

the hip joint. Less muscular force is then needed to swing the recovery leg forward compared with a more extended knee, which reduces local fatigue of the hip flexors. In sprinting, on the other hand, the quicker the recovery limb is brought forward, the faster the running speed. Powerful actions of the hip flexors, along with maximal knee flexion, result in the recovery limb coming forward sooner and thus an increase in overall speed. Another example of rapid movement to which this principle can be applied is jumping jacks. Keeping the elbow flexed reduces the rotational inertia of the upper limb. This may reduce the amount of muscle force required from the shoulder abductor and adductor muscle groups to maintain a certain cadence, or, if greater muscle force is applied, it may result in faster movements.

Angular Momentum

Angular momentum, or the quantity of angular motion, is expressed as the product of angular velocity and rotational inertia. A moving body part possesses angular momentum; the faster it moves and the greater its rota-

KEY POINT

Rotational inertia can be decreased by moving the mass of the limb closer to the joint axis and vice versa. The amount of eccentric force necessary to decelerate a moving body segment is proportional to its angular momentum (rotational inertia × angular velocity). Angular momentum can be transferred from one body segment to another.

tional inertia, the greater the angular momentum. The amount of force necessary to change angular momentum is proportional to the amount of the momentum.

Muscle Groups and the Mechanics of Physical Activity

Human movement is caused or controlled by muscle forces. The following sections briefly review the involvement of muscle groups in some common physical activities (see table 3.3). Success in physical activities depends in part on properly executing movement. Some of the more common errors are also discussed in the following sections.

Walking and Running

The phases and muscle groups involved in walking and running are similar. However, more forceful muscle actions are needed during running as speed increases and greater joint ranges of motion are observed (see figures 3.24 and 3.25).

Muscle Groups

The two phases of gait are the stance phase and the swing phase. The swing phase ends and the stance phase begins at foot contact; the stance phase ends at toe-off, when the swing phase begins. The key difference between walking and running is that during walking either one or both feet are on the ground at all times, but during running only one foot is on the ground at a time. In between foot contacts during running there is a flight phase when neither foot is in contact with the ground.

Table 3.3 Movements and Muscles Involved in Locomotion, Throwing, Cycling, Jumping, and Swimming

Major muscle group	Movement task
Hip extensors	Locomotion—push-off; cycling; jumping; swimming—front crawl, back crawl, sidestroke
Hip flexors	Locomotion—recovery; swimming—front crawl, back crawl, sidestroke
Hip abductors	Swimming—breaststroke; throwing
Hip adductors	Swimming—breaststroke
Hip external and internal rotators	Throwing
Knee extensors	Locomotion—landing; cycling; jumping
Knee flexors	Locomotion—recovery
Ankle plantar flexors	Locomotion—push-off, landing; jumping
Ankle dorsiflexors	Locomotion—recovery
Shoulder joint flexors	Underhand throwing
Shoulder joint extensors	Swimming—front crawl
Shoulder joint internal and external rotators	Throwing
Anterior shoulder joint muscles	Swimming—back crawl, sidestroke lead arm; throwing
Posterior shoulder joint muscles	Swimming—sidestroke trail arm, breaststroke; throwing—windup
Shoulder girdle upward and downward rotators	Swimming—breaststroke, sidestroke lead arm, front crawl, back crawl
Shoulder girdle protractors	Swimming—back crawl; throwing
Shoulder girdle retractors	Swimming—front crawl, breaststroke; throwing—windup
Shoulder girdle elevators	Swimming—front crawl, back crawl, sidestroke lead arm, breaststroke
Elbow flexors	Throwing
Elbow extensors	Throwing
Trunk flexors	Throwing
Trunk rotators	Throwing

Gait cycle

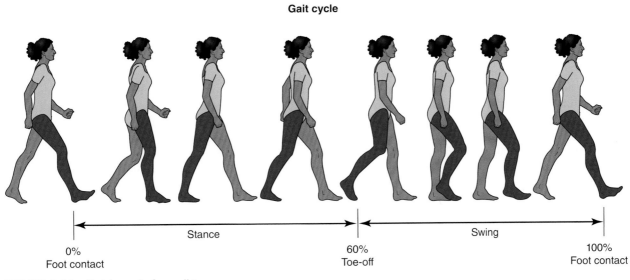

FIGURE 3.24 Stride cycle for walking.

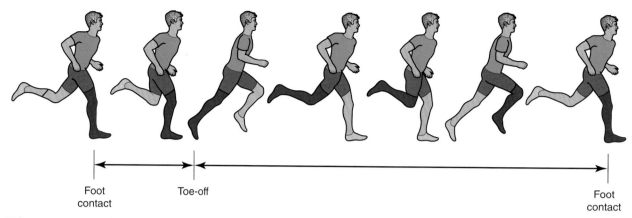

Foot contact   Toe-off   Foot contact

FIGURE 3.25 Stride cycle for running.

Just before foot contact, the hip extensors act eccentrically to decelerate the swinging forward limb. At foot contact with the ground, the knee extensors act eccentrically to control knee flexion against gravity and cushion the impact. The heel touches the ground first during walking and distance running. Following heel contact, the ankle dorsiflexors act eccentrically to lower the ball of the foot onto the ground. As running speed increases, the pattern of contact changes and the flat foot or the ball of the foot makes contact with the ground first. A small proportion of runners contact the ground with the flat foot or the ball of the foot at all speeds.

During the stance phase, the body moves forward over the stationary foot as the hip extends and the ankle dorsiflexes. Before push-off, the hip continues to extend as the knee extends and the ankle plantar flexes. At this point the swinging limb has moved forward in front of the body in preparation for the next foot contact. The push-off is accomplished by the concentric action of the hip extensors and ankle plantar flexors. The gluteus maximus assumes a greater role in hip extension as speed increases.

At the beginning of the swing phase, the hip flexors act concentrically to begin the forward limb swing. This is a ballistic movement, so the momentum initiated by the hip flexors continues the motion passively. Hip flexion is accompanied by pelvic rotation to bring the swinging limb in front of the body. The knee flexes at the beginning of the swing to reduce the rotational inertia of the swing limb. The knee extensors then initiate knee extension prior to foot contact, and the knee flexors work eccentrically to control knee extension at the end of the swing phase. The ankle joint is dorsiflexed to clear the foot from the ground and prepare for foot contact. Speed is a product of stride length and stride frequency; thus, one or both factors can be increased to increase speed. Greater hip range of motion contributes to greater stride length. Rapid recovery of the swing leg via rapid hip flexion during the swing phase is vital to prepare for foot contact at the start of the next stance phase.

In the upper body, arm swing requires shoulder flexion and extension. As speed increases, the swing becomes more vigorous, and there is more elbow flexion. For the greatest efficiency, the arms should move in the sagittal plane. To increase the involvement of the upper limbs for exercise, a walker can exaggerate the shoulder flexion and extension movements.

Walking or running up an incline elicits greater action from the gluteus maximus muscle at the hip and from the knee extensors to raise the body against gravity. The ankle dorsiflexors are more active immediately before landing in order to match the position of the ankle joint to the angle of the incline. Because the ankle is in a more dorsiflexed position, the plantar flexors begin acting during push-off from a more stretched position. For these reasons, hill climbing requires greater flexibility in the plantar flexors, especially the soleus muscle, and greater strength in the dorsiflexors. During downhill running, there is more eccentric action by the knee extensors at foot contact compared with uphill running. As a result, these muscle groups are more apt to become fatigued and to be sore afterward.

Running in place requires the ankle plantar flexors to propel the body upward against gravity; thus, they work more than any of the other lower-extremity muscle groups in this activity. The knee extensors are primarily involved in eccentric action to cushion the landing at foot contact. During running in place, the ball of the foot touches the ground first. Therefore, the plantar flexors are active during the landing, acting eccentrically to control the speed and amount of ankle dorsiflexion. Additional muscles are involved in moving the limb immediately after push-off and before the foot lands again, including hip flexion and extension and knee flexion that brings the foot up to the front.

Common Mechanical Errors

Some novice runners have a tendency to run with stiff legs or with insufficient knee flexion of the recovery limb. This results in a greater rotational inertia of the limb, which means the hip flexors must exert greater force than they would if the knee were more flexed. Keeping the knees stiff during foot contact can also expose the stance limb to greater forces and increase the potential for bone or soft-tissue injury.

Another potential error is the direction of upper- and lower-limb movements. All movements should be executed in the anterior and posterior directions. Excessively swinging the hands across the trunk rotates the upper trunk; in reaction, the lower trunk rotates in the opposite direction. This excess transverse-plane rotation does not contribute to forward motion of the runner. Excessive movements that do not contribute to forward motion are energetically wasteful.

Some runners propel themselves too high off the ground during the airborne phase. Again, excessive movement, this time in the vertical direction, does not contribute to forward motion of the runner. Typically, this bouncing style of running also shortens stride length. The runner must now increase stride frequency to maintain running speed.

Slapping the feet onto the ground in a noisy running style can increase the impact forces that the limbs are exposed to every time they strike the ground. The tactile and aural cues of running softly and quietly may enable runners to reduce their impact forces.

Cycling

Cycling is a predominantly lower-body activity. The upper body provides stable support for the lower limbs to generate force and transfer it to the pedal.

Muscle Groups

The main force in cycling comes from concentric contraction of the hip and knee extensors during the downward part of the pedal stroke. Ankle plantar flexors are also involved in maintaining the foot in a stable position to allow the transfer of forces to the pedal. With toe clips or clip-in shoes, riders can use the hip and knee flexors and ankle dorsiflexors on the upward part of the pedal stroke to help return the pedal to the top position. However, this technique requires conscious effort to develop.

Common Mechanical Errors

Good alignment of the lower limb in the frontal plane is important in reducing the risk of knee pain in cyclists. Allowing the knee to move into a varus or valgus position may change how forces are transmitted across the knee joint, potentially overloading tissues. Correct fit of the rider on the bicycle is essential in reducing such errors. Seat height and fore–aft position, as well as handlebar height and distance from the seat, have a large effect on body segment alignment and joint motions during cycling. Toe clips can help to maintain the ball of the foot over the pedal axle, creating a stable platform to push against on the downstroke.

Jumping and Landing

Jumping and landing are common in many team sports, such as basketball, volleyball, and soccer. Several individual sports also have jumping and landing components, including gymnastics and tennis.

Muscle Groups

The hip and knee extensors, followed by the ankle plantar flexors, forcibly propel the body upward against gravity. The amount of trunk flexion primarily determines the angle of takeoff. The trunk extends, and the arms flex from an extended position just before the lower-limb joints extend. If the reach height of the arms is important, as in a jump ball in basketball or in a tennis smash, the scapulae elevate. During the landing, the hip and knee extensors and the ankle plantar flexors act eccentrically to control the rate of flexion of the lower-body joints and absorb the impact forces.

Common Mechanical Errors

Landing with an upright body position and stiff knees fails to take advantage of the shock-absorbing capabilities of the lower-extremity joints and results in high impact forces, which increase the risk of injury. In particular, landing from a jump in this extended position is a risk factor for knee ligament injury. Conversely, using a deep knee flexion reduces performance because the time taken to reverse the joint motions in preparation for takeoff is extended, and explosiveness is lost. In the frontal plane, landing from a jump with a valgus collapse of the knees has been associated with increased risk of noncontact knee injury, particularly in female athletes participating in sports with a jumping component, such as basketball.

Overarm Throwing

Overarm throwing is a component of many team sports. Examples include American football, baseball, softball, and cricket.

Muscle Groups

Throwing is performed in three phases: the windup, or preparation; the execution, or actual throw; and the follow-through, or recovery. Figure 3.26 illustrates the sequence of the execution phase.

In preparation for throwing, the weight shifts to the back foot, the back hip internally rotates (because the foot is fixed on the ground, rotation is seen at the pelvis), and the trunk rotates with some lateral flexion and extension. In the upper limb, the shoulder externally rotates, and there is some horizontal abduction of the throwing arm accompanied by retraction of the scapula, flexion of the elbow, and extension of the wrist. The movements of the throwing arm are ballistic. The external rotation at the shoulder is fast and powerful. Toward the end of the windup, the internal rotators begin to act eccentrically

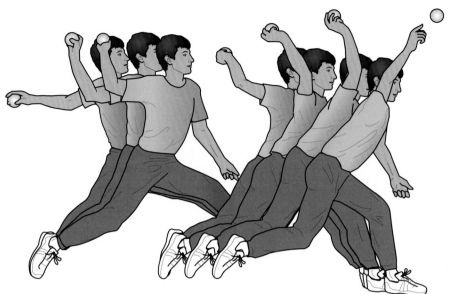

FIGURE 3.26 The execution phase of an overarm throw.

to decelerate the external rotation in preparation for the actual throw.

The weight shift forward is the initial movement in the execution of the throw. This is accomplished by the hip abductors, extensors, and external rotators; the ankle plantar flexors; and the subtalar evertors of the back limb. The front hip rotates internally. The trunk then flexes laterally in the direction opposite to that of the windup, rotates, and flexes. There is a forcible internal rotation of the shoulder, along with scapular protraction. Although some horizontal adduction occurs, the contribution of the shoulder in an overhand throw mostly comes from this internal rotation. The elbow extends, and the wrist moves toward flexion. Depending on the desired spin on the ball, the forearm pronators and the wrist abductors or adductors also may be involved.

Because the actions at the shoulder and elbow joints are vigorous ballistic movements, the shoulder external rotators and horizontal abductors act eccentrically to decelerate the movements during the follow-through. The elbow flexors act eccentrically to prevent elbow hyperextension.

Common Mechanical Errors

The speed of the ball in the hand just before release is the speed of the ball immediately after it leaves the hand. The more joints involved in the throwing motion, the greater the ball speed when it is released. Most throwing problems that result in low velocity, such as pushing the ball rather than throwing it, stem from a lack of trunk rotation or from poor timing of this rotation with the movements of the shoulder joint. The thrower should rotate the trunk and hips during the windup so the pelvis is sideways to the intended direction of the throw and the shoulders are rotated even more to the back. As the hips and then

the trunk rotate forward to begin the throw, the upper limb lags behind. This sets up a whipping action of the upper limb and allows adequate time for the important shoulder internal rotation. Without the trunk rotation, the resulting inadequate shoulder rotation produces a pushing motion during the throw.

KEY POINT

Common mechanical errors in locomotion include running with stiff legs, swinging the arms across the trunk, lifting too high off the ground, and slapping the feet. Common errors in cycling and jumping relate to alignment of the lower extremities in the frontal plane. The most common mechanical errors in throwing are insufficient trunk rotation and poor timing among the trunk, hip, and upper-limb movements.

Lifting and Carrying Objects

The object to be lifted from the ground should be located close to the lifter's spread feet or even between them. The lifter squats, keeping the trunk as erect as possible. The lift should be accomplished by the powerful lower limbs rather than the spine or arms.

Muscle Groups

Lifting begins by keeping the trunk in an upright position and then tilting the pelvis backward and keeping the abdominal muscles activated; the knee extensors along with the hip extensors then act concentrically. The lift should be slow and smooth, not jerky (see figure 3.27).

The weight should be carried close to the body, with the trunk assuming a position that allows the center of gravity to fall within the area of the base of support. The trunk lateral flexors are more active when the weight is carried on one side, the extensors are more active when the weight is in front, and the abdominal muscles are more active when the weight is carried across the top of the back, as in backpacking.

Common Mechanical Errors

Insufficient lower-limb strength can result in poor lifting technique. In particular, emphasis shifts to the lumbar spine and trunk extensors to lift the object. The high forces generated at the lumbar spine can result in injury. Protect the lower back during lifting by using a wide lifting belt or activating the trunk musculature to provide support.

KEY POINT

The steps of proper lifting are to place the feet close to the object, keep the trunk upright, tilt the pelvis backward, and slowly extend the hips and knees while continuing to activate the abdominal muscles.

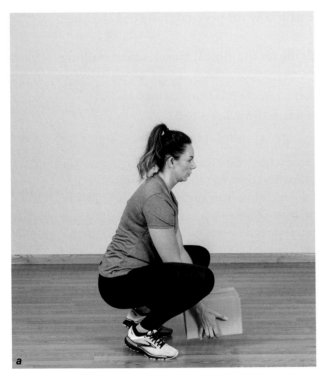 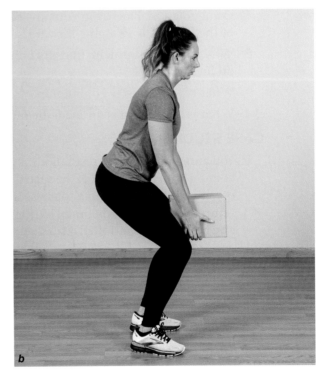

FIGURE 3.27   Lifting technique.

LEARNING AIDS

REVIEW QUESTIONS

1. Name the three cardinal planes and their associated axes.

2. Using the shoulder (glenohumeral) joint as an example, explain why a ball-and-socket joint is so mobile.

3. Explain how the trunk has such a large range of motion even though each intervertebral joint within it has only a few degrees of motion.

4. Explain from an anatomical viewpoint why the knee is vulnerable to injury.

5. Identify the phase of a squat exercise in which the quadriceps femoris is acting (a) concentrically and (b) eccentrically.

6. Explain in terms of torque how an abdominal crunch is more difficult when the arms are extended overhead compared with folded across the chest.

7. Using rotational inertia in your answer, explain why runners naturally flex the knee of the leg that is swinging forward.

8. Why is walking up an incline more challenging for the gluteal muscles than walking on level ground?

9. What type of muscle contractions are involved in exercises performed in water?

10. What is a common error made by novices when throwing a ball?

CASE STUDIES

1. You are supervising the resistance training area when you hear a lot of clanging noises coming from the vicinity of the seated leg press. You discover that the exerciser at that machine is not controlling the descent of the weights. You suggest that they slowly return the weights rather than letting them drop. They ask you why—they don't see any benefit in a controlled return other than reduced noise. What do you tell them?

2. Alice wants to know why she can move a heavier weight when she does wrist curls with her palms up than with her palms down and why she can do more pull-ups with her palms facing her than with her palms facing away. How do you answer her?

3. José complains that his lower back aches somewhat when he reaches overhead while standing in place during the cool-down portion of an aerobics class. What should he do during this movement to prevent the aching?

Answers to Case Studies

1. Explain to the exerciser that the hip and knee extensors that are used to push against the weights are also working to control the descent. The press requires concentric contraction; the return requires eccentric contraction. Both kinds of contractions lead to increased strength.

2. When she is doing the wrist curls with her palms down (radioulnar pronated position), the wrist extensors are the contracting muscles; when her palms are up (supinated position), the wrist flexors are the working muscles. The wrist flexors are usually stronger than the wrist extensors.

   The explanation is different for the pull-ups. The elbow flexor muscles are working regardless of the position of the radioulnar joint. However, when the palms are facing away (pronation), the distal tendon of the biceps brachii is wrapped around the radius bone, and therefore this muscle cannot exert as much force as when the palms are facing toward the body (supinated position).

3. He should make a conscious effort to maintain a backward pelvic tilt. He should also keep his arms in front of his head instead of by his ears and his knees slightly flexed to help maintain the backward tilt.

4

Physiology in Action: Exercise Physiology

Brian Parr and Barbara A. Bushman

OBJECTIVES

The reader will be able to do the following:

1. Explain how muscle produces energy aerobically and anaerobically, and evaluate the importance of aerobic and anaerobic energy production in physical activity and exercise
2. Describe the various fuels for muscle work and how exercise intensity and duration affect the respiratory exchange ratio
3. Describe how exercise tests, training, heredity, sex, age, altitude, and cardiovascular and pulmonary diseases influence maximal oxygen uptake ($\dot{V}O_2max$)
4. Describe how ventilatory threshold and lactate threshold indicate fitness as well as predict performance in endurance events
5. Describe how heart rate, stroke volume, cardiac output, oxygen extraction, and blood pressure change during a graded exercise test and the effect of endurance training on those responses
6. Describe the structure of skeletal muscle and the sliding-filament theory of muscle contraction
7. Describe the power, speed, endurance, and metabolism of the types of muscle fibers
8. Summarize the impact of genetics, sex, and training on muscle fiber types
9. Describe the impact of sensory receptors on flexibility and strength
10. Summarize the effects of training on adaptations within the neuromuscular system to improve muscular strength and endurance
11. Summarize the effects of endurance training on muscular, metabolic, and cardiorespiratory responses to submaximal work and on $\dot{V}O_2max$, and describe how reducing or ceasing training affects $\dot{V}O_2max$
12. Contrast the importance of the various mechanisms for heat loss during heavy exercise and during submaximal exercise in a hot environment

4

Fitness professionals need to know basic exercise physiology when working with clients—for example, to prescribe appropriate activities, understand weight-loss concerns, and explain to participants what happens when training in a hot and humid environment. A single chapter cannot cover the extensive detail found in texts devoted to exercise physiology; instead, select topics will be summarized and, where possible, application will be made to exercise testing and prescription. For additional background and details, several texts on exercise physiology are listed in the references (23, 55, 56, 61, 71, 85).

Energy and Work

Energy is essential for all bodily functions. Several kinds of energy exist in biological systems, including

- electrical energy in the nerves and muscles,
- chemical energy in the synthesis of molecules,
- mechanical energy in the contraction of muscle, and
- thermal energy, derived from all of these processes, which helps maintain body temperature.

The ultimate source of the energy found in biological systems is the sun. The radiant energy from the sun is captured by plants and used to convert simple atoms and molecules into carbohydrate, fat, and protein. The sun's energy is trapped within the chemical bonds of these food molecules.

For the cells to use this energy, they must break down the foodstuffs in a manner that conserves most of the energy contained in the bonds of the carbohydrate, fat, and protein. In addition, the final product of the breakdown must be a molecule the cell can use—adenosine triphosphate (ATP). Cells use ATP as the primary energy source for biological work, whether this work is electrical, mechanical, or chemical.

During muscular activity, ATP is constantly converted to adenosine diphosphate (ADP) and inorganic phosphate (Pi) in order to provide the energy needed for the work. The ATP must be replaced as quickly as it is used if the muscle is to continue to generate force. Muscles have multiple systems for replacing ATP for both short- and long-duration activities such as when running at high speeds for short periods of time (e.g., 100-meter dash) or at slower speeds for longer distances (e.g., marathon). Two broad types of reactions that are available to regenerate the ATP are anaerobic reactions for anaerobic energy, which can regenerate ATP rapidly and do not require oxygen, and aerobic reactions for aerobic energy, which are slower to activate but can sustain ATP regeneration for long periods of time and require oxygen.

Anaerobic Energy Sources

One-enzyme reactions and one multiple-enzyme pathway can replace ATP at a fast rate. These energy systems allow muscle to continue to generate force during strenuous activities or help make the transition from rest to exercise as the slower aerobic system comes up to speed. In the most important of the one-enzyme reactions, phosphocreatine (PC) reacts with ADP to form ATP. The PC concentration in muscle is limited and along with the ATP stores can provide for energy needs for only about 3 to 15 seconds during all-out activity (55).

$$PC + ADP \rightarrow ATP + C$$

In the multiple-enzyme pathway called *glycolysis*, glucose is metabolized at a high rate and ATP is generated without requiring oxygen. Lactic acid is produced in the process and may lead to lactate and hydrogen ion (H^+) accumulation in the muscle and blood; the H^+ produced may interfere with the mechanism involved in muscle contraction, leading to fatigue (55). Glycolysis provides ATP at a higher rate and is a substantial contributor to the ATP needed in all-out activities lasting less than 2 minutes. In contrast, when glucose is metabolized aerobically, it represents a long-lasting source of ATP, producing about 16 times more ATP per glucose molecule than when metabolized anaerobically (55).

Aerobic Energy Production

The oxidative metabolism of carbohydrate (muscle glycogen and blood glucose) and fat (from both adipose tissue and intramuscular sources) provides the long-term sources of ATP for physical activities and exercise that typically are associated with health-related outcomes. The complete oxidation of these fuels takes place in the mitochondria of the cell, which increase in number with endurance training. The larger number of mitochondria increases the capacity of the muscle to use fat as a fuel because fat can only be metabolized via aerobic pathways.

$$\text{Carbohydrate or fat} + O_2 \rightarrow ATP$$

ATP production via aerobic mechanisms is slower than ATP production from anaerobic sources, and during lower-intensity submaximal work it may take 2 or 3 minutes before aerobic processes fully meet the ATP needs of the cell. One reason for this lag is the time required for the heart to increase the delivery of oxygen-enriched blood to the muscles at the rate needed to meet the ATP demands of the muscle. Another is the time required for the mitochondria to increase the rate of ATP production from resting levels to that needed to meet the exercise demand. Aerobic production of ATP is the primary means of supplying energy to the muscle in heavy exercise lasting more than 2 to 3 minutes and in longer-duration submaximal work.

Interaction of Exercise Intensity, Exercise Duration, and Energy Production

The proportion of energy coming from anaerobic sources is influenced by the intensity and duration of the activity. Figure 4.1 shows that during an all-out activity lasting less than 1 minute (e.g., a 400-meter dash), the muscles obtain most of their ATP from anaerobic sources. In a 2- to 3-minute maximal effort, approximately 50% of the energy comes from anaerobic sources and 50% comes from aerobic sources. In a 10-minute maximal effort, the anaerobic component drops to 15%. For a 30-minute all-out effort, the anaerobic component is about 5%, and it is even smaller in a submaximal 30-minute training session.

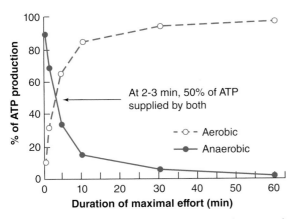

FIGURE 4.1 Percent of aerobic and anaerobic contributions to total energy supply during maximal work of various durations (71).

KEY POINT

ATP is supplied at a high rate by the anaerobic processes of PC breakdown and glycolysis. Anaerobic energy is important in short, explosive events and in physical activities requiring maximal effort for less than 2 minutes. ATP is supplied during prolonged exercise by the aerobic metabolism of carbohydrate and fat in the mitochondria of the muscle. This is the primary means of supplying energy to the muscle in maximal work lasting more than 2 minutes and in submaximal work.

Metabolic, Cardiovascular, and Respiratory Responses to Exercise

Within a complete exercise program, two main types of activities for a fitness professional to recommend are those that increase or maintain cardiorespiratory function and those that improve or maintain muscular fitness. Activities that demand aerobic energy production automatically cause the circulatory and respiratory systems to deliver oxygen to the muscle to meet the demand. The selected aerobic activities must be strenuous enough to challenge and thus improve the cardiorespiratory system. This crucial link between aerobic activities and cardiorespiratory function provides the basis for much of exercise programming. Muscular fitness requires activities that stress the muscle beyond normal levels to achieve improvements in muscular strength and endurance. The following sections summarize selected physiologic responses to aerobic and muscular-strengthening activities.

Measuring Oxygen Uptake

How does oxygen get to the mitochondria? First, oxygen enters the lungs during inhalation; it then diffuses from the alveoli of the lungs into the blood. Oxygen traveling in the blood is primarily bound to hemoglobin in the red blood cells, and the heart delivers the oxygen-enriched blood to the muscles. Oxygen then diffuses into the muscle cells and reaches the mitochondria, where it can be used (consumed) in the production of ATP.

Oxygen consumption ($\dot{V}O_2$) during exercise is measured by subtracting the volume of oxygen exhaled from the volume of oxygen inhaled.

$$\dot{V}O_2 = \text{volume } O_2 \text{ inhaled} - \text{volume } O_2 \text{ exhaled}$$

Additional information on measuring $\dot{V}O_2$ is provided in chapter 8. In general, the percentage of oxygen in room air is known, and the percentage of oxygen in the exhaled air and the total volume of air exhaled in liters per minute (i.e., the pulmonary ventilation) can be measured with specialized equipment. Thus, the oxygen consumption can be determined. The carbon dioxide produced in the mitochondria of the muscle diffuses into the blood by which it is carried back to the lungs. In the lungs, the carbon dioxide diffuses into the alveoli and is exhaled. Similar to the calculation for oxygen consumption, the carbon dioxide production can be calculated by examining the difference between the percentage of carbon dioxide in the room air and exhaled air.

The ratio of CO_2 production ($\dot{V}CO_2$) to oxygen consumption ($\dot{V}O_2$) in the mitochondria of the cell is called the respiratory quotient (*RQ*). However, because $\dot{V}CO_2$ and $\dot{V}O_2$ are measured at the mouth rather than at the tissue, this ratio is called the *respiratory exchange ratio* (*R*). This ratio can help us identify the type of fuel used during exercise as described in the next section.

$$R = \dot{V}CO_2 \div \dot{V}O_2$$

For example, for a $\dot{V}CO_2$ of 1.8 L · min^{-1} and a $\dot{V}O_2$ of 2.4 L · min^{-1}, the *R* would be calculated as follows:

$$R = 1.8 \text{ L} \cdot \text{min}^{-1} \div 2.4 \text{ L} \cdot \text{min}^{-1} = 0.75$$

Fuel Utilization During Exercise

In general, protein contributes little (less than 10%) to total energy production at rest and during exercise under normal circumstances, and for the purpose of this discussion it will be ignored (55). Ignoring protein leaves carbohydrate (muscle glycogen and blood glucose) and fat (adipose tissue and intramuscular fat) as the primary fuels for exercise. The ability of *R* to provide good information about the metabolism of fat and carbohydrate during exercise stems from the following observations about the metabolism of fat and glucose during steady-state exercise. Steady-state exercise reflects when the supply of oxygen and nutrients meets the body's demands for a given level of exercise.

When *R* = 1.0, 100% of the energy is derived from carbohydrate and 0% from fat; when *R* = 0.7, the reverse is true. When *R* = 0.85, approximately 50% of the energy comes from carbohydrate and 50% comes from fat (see the *Respiratory Quotients for Carbohydrate and Fat* sidebar). For the *R* measurement to be correct, the subject must be in a steady state. If lactate and hydrogen ions (H$^+$) are increasing in the blood, the plasma bicarbonate (HCO$_3^-$) buffer store reacts with the acid (H$^+$) and produces CO_2. The exerciser is stimulated to hyperventilate and "blow off" the CO_2, and thus the reaction occurs as follows:

$$H^+ + HCO_{3-} \rightarrow H_2CO_3 \rightarrow H_2O + CO_2$$

This CO_2 does not come from the aerobic metabolism of carbohydrate and fat, so when it is exhaled it results in an overestimation of the true value of *R*. During strenuous work, H$^+$ are produced in great amounts, and *R* can exceed 1.0.

Effect of Exercise Intensity on Fuel Utilization

R changes during increasing exercise intensity. The *R* increases at about 40% to 50% $\dot{V}O_2$max, indicating that carbohydrate is becoming a more dominant fuel source. Fat may provide more energy per gram, but it requires more oxygen to do so; in contrast, carbohydrate yields 6.3 ATP per molecule of oxygen compared to 5.6 ATP

Respiratory Quotients for Carbohydrate and Fat

For glucose (C$_6$H$_{12}$O$_6$),

$$C_6H_{12}O_6 + 6\ O_2 \rightarrow 6\ CO_2 + 6\ H_2O + \text{energy}$$

$$R = \frac{6\ CO_2}{6\ O_2} = 1.0$$

For palmitate (C$_{16}$H$_{32}$O$_2$, a fatty acid),

$$C_{16}H_{32}O_2 + 23\ O_2 \rightarrow 16\ CO_2 + 16\ H_2O + \text{energy}$$

$$R = \frac{16\ CO_2}{23\ O_2} = 0.7$$

per molecule of oxygen for fat (55). When using carbohydrate, muscle obtains about 6% more energy from each liter of oxygen (O$_2$) when carbohydrate is used (5 kcal · L^{-1}) compared with when fat is used (4.7 kcal · L^{-1}).

Carbohydrate fuels for muscular exercise include muscle glycogen and liver glycogen, with the latter used for maintaining the blood glucose concentration. Muscle glycogen is the primary carbohydrate fuel for heavy aerobic exercise lasting less than 2 hours, and inadequate muscle glycogen results in premature fatigue (13). As muscle glycogen is depleted during prolonged heavy exercise, blood glucose becomes more important in supplying the carbohydrate fuel. Toward the end of heavy exercise lasting 3 hours or more, blood glucose provides almost all the carbohydrate used by the muscles. Therefore, heavy exercise is limited by the availability of carbohydrate fuels, which must be either stored in abundance before exercise (muscle glycogen) or replaced through the ingestion of carbohydrate during exercise (blood glucose) (12).

Effect of Exercise Duration on Fuel Utilization

Figure 4.2 shows how *R* changes during a 90-minute test performed at 65% of the subject's $\dot{V}O_2$max (72). *R* decreases over time, indicating a greater reliance on fat as a fuel. The fat is derived from both intramuscular fat stores and adipose tissue, which releases free fatty acids into the blood to be carried to the muscle. Using more fat spares the remaining carbohydrate stores and extends the time to exhaustion.

Effect of Intensity on Fuel Utilization

A common question by people who are using exercise to promote weight loss relates to the best type of exercise to burn fat. The previous section explained that the percent

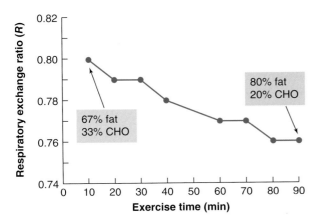

FIGURE 4.2 Changes in *R* (respiratory exchange ratio) during prolonged steady-state exercise (72). CHO = carbohydrates.

of energy derived from fat can be estimated using the *R*, where a value closer to 0.70 suggests greater fat use. Given that the *R* is lower during relatively lower-intensity exercise and during longer-duration exercise is the basis for the belief that "low and slow" exercise is most effective for burning fat and is the basis for many exercise weight-loss programs. However, if the goal is to use the greatest amount of fat (in grams) as a fuel during exercise, low intensity may not be optimal. This is because at a low intensity the total energy expenditure is relatively low, so the total amount of fat used may be low too, even though a high percentage of energy is coming from fat.

The maximal rate of fat metabolism during exercise is called FATmax (50) and occurs at the same intensity as the lactate threshold (1). At this intensity, the calculation based on the *R* and the total energy expenditure predicts the greatest rate of fat oxidation in g · min⁻¹.

Effect of Diet and Training on Fuel Utilization

The type of fuel used during exercise is affected by diet. A diet high in carbohydrate (versus an average diet) increases the muscle glycogen content and extends the time to exhaustion (48). Further, the muscle gains a greater capacity to increase its glycogen store if a person performs strenuous exercise before eating high-carbohydrate meals (48, 84). Finally, during prolonged heavy exercise, carbohydrate beverages help maintain the blood glucose concentration and extend the time to fatigue (12).

Endurance training increases the number of mitochondria in the muscles involved in the training program. Having more mitochondria increases the ability of the muscle to use fat as a fuel and to process the available carbohydrate aerobically. This ability spares the carbohydrate store and reduces lactate and H⁺ production, both of which favorably influence performance (43).

The respiratory exchange ratio (*R*) tracks fuel use during steady-state exercise. When *R* = 1.0, 100% of the energy is derived from carbohydrate; when *R* = 0.7, 100% of the energy is derived from fat. When hydrogen ions increase in the blood during heavy exercise, they are buffered by plasma bicarbonate. This buffering produces CO_2 and invalidates using *R* as an indicator of fuel use during exercise. As exercise intensity increases, *R* increases, indicating that carbohydrate plays a bigger role in generating ATP. During prolonged moderately strenuous exercise, *R* decreases over time, indicating that fat is being used more and carbohydrate is being spared.

Transition From Rest to Steady-State Aerobic Work

Anaerobic and aerobic sources of energy (ATP) are not distinct activities, but rather work together to allow the body to make the transition from rest to exercise. When a person steps onto a treadmill belt moving at a velocity of 200 m · min⁻¹ (7.5 mph), the ATP requirement increases from the low level needed to stand alongside the treadmill to the new level required to run at 200 m · min⁻¹. This change in the ATP supply to the muscle must take place in the first step on the treadmill. If this change fails to occur, the person will drift off the back of the treadmill. Many factors contribute to the body's ability to supply the needed ATP, as will be described in the following section.

Oxygen Uptake

The cardiovascular and respiratory systems cannot instantaneously increase the delivery of oxygen to the muscles to completely meet the ATP demands via aerobic processes. In the interval between the time a person steps onto the treadmill and the time the cardiovascular and respiratory systems deliver the required oxygen, anaerobic sources of energy supply the needed ATP. The volume of oxygen missing in the first few minutes of work is the oxygen deficit (figure 4.3). PC supplies some of the needed ATP, and the anaerobic breakdown of carbohydrate provides the rest until the oxidative mechanisms meet the ATP requirement. When the uptake of oxygen levels off during submaximal work, the oxygen uptake value represents the steady-state oxygen requirement for the activity. At this point, the ATP need of the cell is being met by the aerobic production of ATP in the mitochondria of the muscle.

RESEARCH INSIGHT

Effect of Diet on Fuel Utilization During Exercise

The intensity and duration of exercise are important determinants of the fuel used to produce ATP. In general, lower-intensity exercise relies more on fat as a fuel, primarily plasma free fatty acids (FFA), and higher-intensity exercise uses more carbohydrate as a fuel. The specific source of the carbohydrate depends on the duration of exercise. In the first 1 to 2 hours of exercise, muscle glycogen provides the majority of the carbohydrate for the working muscle. In longer bouts of exercise, blood glucose becomes the most important carbohydrate source.

Carbohydrate intake, either in the diet or during exercise, can influence the availability of carbohydrates, especially muscle glycogen. This is because carbohydrate stores in the body are relatively limited. A diet high in carbohydrates is associated with elevated muscle glycogen levels and improved endurance exercise performance. During prolonged exercise, the consumption of carbohydrates can maintain blood glucose levels and sustain exercise intensity by providing carbohydrates to the working muscle and preventing hypoglycemia. Therefore, the carbohydrate content of the diet before exercise and intake during exercise can enhance carbohydrate use as a fuel, especially during high-intensity exercise, because carbohydrate stores in the body are somewhat limited.

Plasma FFA is the major fat source for exercise and a primary fuel during light- to moderate-intensity exercise. It is generally thought that body stores of fat are sufficient for most types of exercise, even when consuming a relatively low-fat diet. But some research suggests that eating a high-fat diet can increase fat use during exercise (36). This has the effect of sparing carbohydrate use by the muscle, maintaining muscle glycogen and blood glucose levels for longer. However, this seems to be true with light- to moderate-intensity exercise but not high-intensity exercise, when carbohydrate is a primary fuel source and depletion of muscle glycogen and blood glucose is of most concern. A high-fat, low-carbohydrate diet is also associated with low muscle glycogen levels, which could impair performance in some types of exercise. For this reason, high-fat, low-carbohydrate diets are not recommended for athletes competing in events that rely on muscle glycogen and blood glucose as fuels for sustained muscular activity.

The carbohydrate content of the diet and intake during exercise is also important for minimizing the use of protein as a fuel. Recall that protein generally provides little energy during exercise. This is true as long as carbohydrate availability is sufficient. Consuming adequate carbohydrates in the diet prior to exercise and during exercise reduces the reliance on protein as a fuel and allows more accurate use of R to estimate the relative contribution of carbohydrate and fat to energy production. More about the effects of diet and exercise intensity and duration on fuel use during exercise can be found in the following sources (34, 36, 66, 86, 87).

When the participant stops running and steps off the treadmill, the ATP need of the muscles that were involved in the activity suddenly drops toward the resting value. However, the oxygen uptake remains above the pre-exercise resting level for several minutes, which suggests that ATP production is above the resting requirement. The oxygen uptake decreases quickly at first and then more gradually approaches the resting value. The time frame of this depends on the intensity and duration of the exercise; that is, the oxygen consumption returns quickly to pre-exercise resting level following light exercise but remains elevated longer after prolonged, high-intensity exercise.

This elevated oxygen uptake during recovery from exercise is the excess postexercise oxygen consumption (EPOC). Many factors affect EPOC, including replenish-

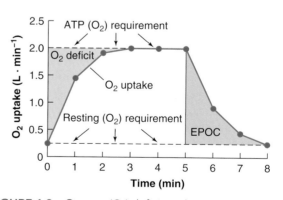

FIGURE 4.3 Oxygen (O_2) deficit and excess postexercise oxygen consumption (EPOC) during a 5-minute run on a treadmill.

ing oxygen borrowed from hemoglobin and myoglobin at the start of exercise and restoring ATP and PC of the muscle back to normal. (Remember that it was depleted somewhat at the onset of work.) This is why in the past EPOC has also been called the *oxygen debt* and *oxygen repayment*. However, the elevated oxygen consumption in recovery is also used to meet the ATP requirement for the higher heart rate (HR) and breathing during recovery (compared with rest), the increased body temperature (which increases metabolism and respiration), and elevated norepinephrine and epinephrine (55). The liver uses a small part of the elevated oxygen consumption to convert some of the lactate produced at the onset of work into glucose (71). Additionally, some of the lactate is converted to ATP in the mitochondria, which requires oxygen. This ATP can be used for muscular contraction during active recovery instead of simply stopping exercise completely. Active recovery results in a faster rate of lactate clearance from the muscle and blood (64) and is one reason why cooling down after exercise is recommended.

If an individual reaches the steady-state oxygen requirement earlier during the first minutes of work, a smaller oxygen deficit is incurred. The body depletes less PC and produces less lactate and H+. Endurance training speeds up the kinetics of oxygen transport; that is, it decreases the time needed to reach a steady state of oxygen uptake. People in poor condition, as well as people with cardiovascular or pulmonary disease, take longer to reach the steady-state oxygen requirement. They incur a larger oxygen deficit and must produce more ATP from the immediate and short-term sources of energy when beginning work or transitioning from one intensity to the next (38, 73).

Heart Rate and Pulmonary Ventilation

The link between the cardiorespiratory responses to work and the time it takes to reach the steady-state oxygen requirement should be no surprise. Figure 4.4 shows

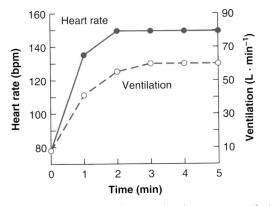

FIGURE 4.4 Response of HR and pulmonary ventilation during a 5-minute run on a treadmill.

how HR and pulmonary ventilation typically respond to a submaximal run test. The shape of the curve in each case resembles the curve for oxygen uptake described earlier.

In addition, the muscle contributes to the lag in oxygen uptake at the onset of work. An untrained muscle has relatively few mitochondria available to produce ATP aerobically and relatively few capillaries per muscle fiber to bring the oxygen-enriched arterial blood to those mitochondria. Following endurance training, both of these factors increase so that the muscle can produce more ATP aerobically at the onset of work. In addition, less lactate and H+ are produced at the onset of work, and the blood lactate and H+ concentrations are lower for a fixed submaximal work rate (38, 43, 73).

KEY POINT

At the onset of submaximal exercise, $\dot{V}O_2$ does not increase immediately (oxygen deficit), and some of the ATP must be supplied anaerobically by PC and glycolysis. At the end of exercise, $\dot{V}O_2$ remains elevated for some time (EPOC) to replenish PC stores, support the energy cost of the elevated HR and breathing, and synthesize glucose from lactate. Training reduces the oxygen deficit because $\dot{V}O_2$ increases more rapidly at the onset of work, allowing the steady-state oxygen requirement to be reached more quickly.

Physiology of Warm-Up and Cool-Down

The importance of a warm-up and cool-down as part of the training session is discussed in chapter 13. Given the current discussion of the metabolic events that occur at the onset and end of exercise, an exploration of the physiology of warming up and cooling down is relevant here.

The purpose of a warm-up is to prepare the body for activity. This includes increasing muscle temperature to increase enzyme activity. It also increases blood flow to bring oxygen and fuels to muscle. Together, this allows for increases in ATP production in the muscle at the onset of exercise, leading to improved performance (28). A warm-up should prepare the muscles for the movements used in the exercise session.

Cooling down provides a transition to recover from the exercise session to resting conditions. An active cool-down promotes blood flow from the extremities to maintain venous return, cardiac output, and blood pressure (BP) (9). This is especially important with upright exercise involving the legs. An active cool-down also clears metabolic wastes such as CO_2, lactate, and H^+ from the muscle more quickly.

For athletes, a warm-up and cool-down can improve performance at the onset of exercise and speed recovery after exercise. For fitness clients, it eases the transition into exercise and reduces the risk of dizziness or fainting after exercise, especially intense exercise.

Graded Exercise Test

Oxygen consumption and cardiorespiratory fitness (CRF) are clearly linked because oxygen delivery to tissue depends on lung and heart function. One of the most common tests used to evaluate cardiorespiratory function is a graded exercise test (GXT), in which participants exercise at progressively increasing work rates. During the test the participant may be monitored for cardiovascular variables (HR and BP), respiratory variables (pulmonary ventilation and respiratory frequency), and metabolic variables (oxygen uptake and blood lactate level). Chapter 8 provides details on GXT testing procedures. The manner in which a person responds to the GXT provides important information about cardiorespiratory function and the capacity for prolonged work.

Oxygen uptake is typically expressed per kilogram of body weight to facilitate comparisons between people or between tests for the same person over time. The $\dot{V}O_2$ value in liters per minute is simply multiplied by 1,000 to convert $\dot{V}O_2$ to $ml \cdot min^{-1}$, and that value is divided by the subject's body weight in kilograms to yield a value expressed in milliliters per kilogram per minute ($ml \cdot kg^{-1} \cdot min^{-1}$).

$$\dot{V}O_2 = 2.4\ L \cdot min^{-1} \cdot 1,000\ ml \cdot L^{-1} = 2,400\ ml \cdot min^{-1}$$

For a 60-kilogram person, this would be expressed as follows:

$$\dot{V}O_2 = 2,400\ ml \cdot min^{-1} \div 60\ kg = 40\ ml \cdot kg^{-1} \cdot min^{-1}$$

Figure 4.5 shows a GXT conducted on a treadmill in which the speed is constant at 3 mph (4.8 $km \cdot hr^{-1}$) and the grade changes 3% every 3 minutes. With each stage of the GXT, oxygen uptake increases to meet the ATP demand of the work rate. Also, the participant incurs a small oxygen deficit at each stage as the cardiovascular system tries to adjust to the new demand of the increased work rate.

Healthy individuals reach the steady-state oxygen requirement by 1.5 minutes or so of each GXT stage up to moderately heavy work (65, 67). People who have low CRF or who have cardiovascular and pulmonary diseases may not be able to reach the expected values in the same amount of time and might incur larger oxygen deficits with each stage of the test. Because these individuals do

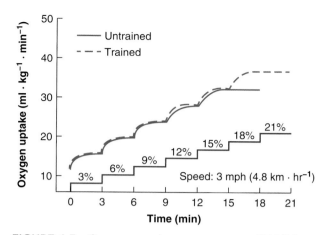

FIGURE 4.5 Oxygen uptake responses to a GXT (54).

not reach the expected steady-state demands of the test at each stage, the oxygen uptake measured at various stages of the test is lower than expected.

Toward the end of a GXT, a point is reached at which the work rate changes (e.g., the grade on the treadmill increases) but the oxygen uptake does not. In effect, the cardiovascular system has reached its limits for transporting oxygen to the muscle. This point is called *maximal aerobic power*, or *maximal oxygen uptake* ($\dot{V}O_2max$). A complete leveling off in oxygen consumption is not seen in many cases because the subject must work one stage past the actual point at which $\dot{V}O_2max$ is reached, requiring high motivation. Over the years, a variety of approaches have been used to obtain evidence that the subject has achieved $\dot{V}O_2max$ on the GXT (see the *Criteria for $\dot{V}O_2max$* Research Insight). Participation in a 10- to 20-week endurance training program typically increases $\dot{V}O_2max$. When trained people retake the GXT, they often reach the steady state sooner at light to moderate work rates and progress further into the test, at which time the greater $\dot{V}O_2max$ is measured.

Maximal aerobic power describes the greatest rate at which the body (primarily muscle) can produce ATP aerobically during dynamic exercise involving a large muscle mass (e.g., running, cycling). It is also the upper limit at which the cardiovascular system can deliver oxygen-enriched blood to the muscles. Thus, maximal aerobic power is not only a good index of CRF, but also a good predictor of performance capability in aerobic events such as distance running, cycling, cross-country skiing, and swimming (5, 6). In the apparently healthy person, maximal aerobic power is the quantitative limit at which the cardiovascular system can deliver oxygen to tissues. This usual interpretation must be tempered by the mode of exercise (test type) used to impose the work rate on the subject.

RESEARCH INSIGHT

Criteria for $\dot{V}O_2$max

When a plateau in $\dot{V}O_2$ did not occur in a GXT, several investigators used an approach in which they observed how much the $\dot{V}O_2$ increased in the last stage of the GXT. If the increase was small, well below the expected increase in $\dot{V}O_2$ for the final stage, it was taken as evidence of a plateau and that $\dot{V}O_2$max was achieved. A classic plateau criterion established by Taylor and colleagues (88) used an increase in $\dot{V}O_2$ in the last stage that was <2.1 ml · kg^{-1} · min^{-1} higher than the previous stage of the GXT, half the expected increase in $\dot{V}O_2$. In addition, other investigators identified a variety of secondary criteria (the plateau being the primary criterion) that could be used as evidence that the individual was working maximally when the highest $\dot{V}O_2$ was measured:

- An R greater than 1.10 (49). This indicated that lactate and H$^+$ levels were elevated and CO_2 was blown off in great amounts to help buffer the change in pH.
- A blood lactate concentration greater than 8 mmol · L^{-1}, about eight times the resting value (2). This also indicated that the individual was doing extreme work involving a sizable anaerobic component.
- An HR near that of the individual's age-predicted maximal HR. Given the error in estimating maximal HR, this approach has limitations as a criterion (see chapter 8).

These and other criteria have been used alone and in combination to establish whether or not the subject has achieved $\dot{V}O_2$max (46), but problems remain with this approach. The most recent approaches to confirming that a true $\dot{V}O_2$max has been reached in a GXT include doing a follow-up supramaximal test at an intensity higher than that achieved in the GXT. These follow-up tests have been used on the same day as the GXT (after a brief rest, the follow-up test begins) (21, 27), and on a different day (35, 75). These approaches have been very effective in confirming the $\dot{V}O_2$max value achieved on the GXT.

Test Type

For the average person, the highest value for maximal aerobic power is measured when the subject completes a GXT involving uphill running. A GXT conducted at a walking speed usually results in a $\dot{V}O_2$max value 4% to 6% below the graded running value, and a test on a cycle ergometer may yield a value 10% to 12% lower than the graded running value (25, 62, 63). If an individual works to exhaustion using an arm ergometer, the highest oxygen uptake value is less than 70% of that measured with the legs (29). Knowing these variations in maximal aerobic power is helpful in making recommendations about the intensity of various exercises needed to achieve the target or training HR. At any given submaximal work rate, most physiological responses (HR, BP, and blood lactate) are greater for arm work than for leg work (29, 83).

Training and Heredity

Endurance training increases $\dot{V}O_2$max by 5% to 25%, with the magnitude of the change depending, in part, on the initial level of fitness. A person with a low $\dot{V}O_2$max sees the largest change, but there is consider-

able individual variation in response (see chapter 13). Eventually, a point is reached where further training does not increase $\dot{V}O_2$max. Approximately 40% of the extremely high values of maximal aerobic power found in elite cross-country skiers and distance runners relates to a genetic predisposition to a superior cardiovascular system (7). Because typical endurance programs may increase $\dot{V}O_2$max by only 20% or so, it is unrealistic to expect a person with a $\dot{V}O_2$max of 40 ml · kg^{-1} · min^{-1} to increase to 80 ml · kg^{-1} · min^{-1}, a value measured in some elite cross-country skiers and distance runners (79). On the other hand, some who do intense interval training can achieve gains of 44% in $\dot{V}O_2$max (37).

Sex and Age

Women's $\dot{V}O_2$max values (ml · kg^{-1} · min^{-1}) are about 15% lower than men's, a difference that exists from ages 20 to 60, primarily because of differences in percent body fat and in hemoglobin levels. This 15% variation between men and women is an average value, and $\dot{V}O_2$max values overlap considerably in these populations (3). The average female has less hemoglobin and a smaller heart volume compared with the average male. To deliver the same volume of oxygen to the muscles, the woman must have a higher HR to compensate for the smaller stroke volume and a slightly higher cardiac output to compensate for the slightly lower hemoglobin concentration (3). In addition, the average woman typically has a smaller muscle mass with which to accomplish the work, which increases the HR response. These differences between women's and men's cardiovascular responses to cycle ergometry are shown in figure 4.6. Table 4.1 summarizes the differences in cardiovascular responses between men and women in response to exercise.

In most people, aging gradually but systematically reduces $\dot{V}O_2max$ by about 1% each year. $\dot{V}O_2max$ is influenced by physical activity and percent body fat, so people who remain active and maintain a healthy body weight (which is not the usual case) have higher $\dot{V}O_2max$ values across the age span. Endurance training by middle-aged people has the potential benefit of maintaining or elevating $\dot{V}O_2max$ to a level consistent with that of a younger, sedentary person (51, 52, 53).

Altitude

$\dot{V}O_2max$ decreases with increasing altitude. At 7,400 feet (2,300 meters), $\dot{V}O_2max$ is only 88% of the sea-level value. This decrease in $\dot{V}O_2max$ is attributable primarily to the reduction in arterial oxygen content that occurs as the oxygen pressure in the air decreases with increasing altitude. When the arterial oxygen content is lower, the heart must pump more blood per minute to meet the oxygen needs of any task. As a result, the HR response is higher at submaximal intensities performed at greater altitudes (45). Additional considerations for aerobic activity when at higher elevations are found in chapter 13.

Cardiovascular and Pulmonary Diseases

Cardiovascular and pulmonary diseases decrease $\dot{V}O_2max$ by diminishing the delivery of oxygen from the air to the blood and reducing the capacity of the heart to deliver blood to the muscles. Patients with cardiovascular disease (CVD) have some of the lowest $\dot{V}O_2max$ (functional capacity) values, but they also experience the largest changes in $\dot{V}O_2max$ from endurance training. Table 4.2 shows common values for $\dot{V}O_2max$ in a variety of populations (55, 71).

Blood Lactate and Pulmonary Ventilation

Muscle produces lactate and H^+, which are released into the blood. Figure 4.7 shows that during a GXT, blood lactate concentration changes little or not at all at the lower work rates; lactate is metabolized as fast as it is produced (8). As the GXT increases in intensity, a work rate is reached at which the blood lactate concentration suddenly increases. This work rate is referred to as the

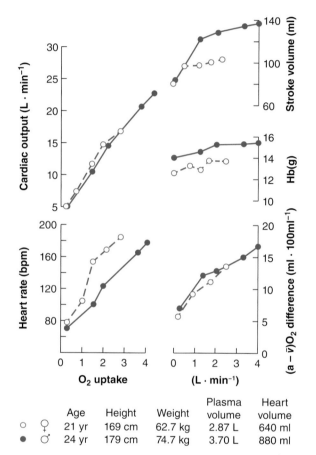

		Age	Height	Weight	Plasma volume	Heart volume
○	♀	21 yr	169 cm	62.7 kg	2.87 L	640 ml
●	♂	24 yr	179 cm	74.7 kg	3.70 L	880 ml

FIGURE 4.6 The cardiovascular responses of well-trained men and women to cycle ergometry. Hb = hemoglobin.

Reprinted by permission from P.-O. Åstrand and K. Rodahl, *Textbook of Work Physiology*, 4th ed. (Champaign, IL: Human Kinetics, 2003), 176.

Table 4.1   Cardiovascular Responses of Women Compared With Men

Variable	Rest	At same absolute $\dot{V}O_2$ (L · min⁻¹)	At same relative $\dot{V}O_2$ (ml · kg⁻¹ · min⁻¹)	At maximal work
Cardiac output	Same	Slightly higher	Same	Lower
Stroke volume	Lower	Lower	Lower	Lower
HR	Higher	Higher	Higher	Same

Table 4.2 Maximal Aerobic Power in Healthy and Diseased Populations

Population	$\dot{V}O_2MAX$ (ml · kg^{-1} · min^{-1})	
	Men	Women
Endurance athletes	65-94	60-75
Nonathletes		
Young adult (20-29 years)	43-52	33-42
Middle-aged adult (40-49 years)	36-44	26-35
Older adult (60-69 years)	31-38	22-30
Post-myocardial infarction patients	Approximately 22	Approximately 18
Severe pulmonary disease patients	Approximately 13	Approximately 13

Adapted from Kenney et al. (2021); Powers et al. (2024).

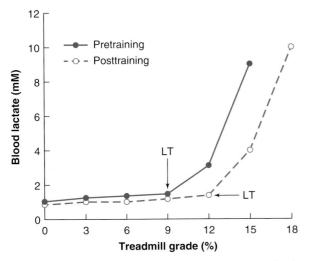

FIGURE 4.7 Training causes the LT to occur at a higher exercise intensity (24).

KEY POINT

Maximal oxygen uptake, $\dot{V}O_2max$, is the greatest rate at which oxygen can be delivered to working muscles during dynamic exercise. $\dot{V}O_2max$ is influenced by heredity and training, decreases about 1% per year with age, and is about 15% lower in women compared with men. $\dot{V}O_2max$ is lower at high altitudes. Cardiovascular and pulmonary diseases lower $\dot{V}O_2max$; however, people with CVD can potentially attain improvements in $\dot{V}O_2max$ through endurance training.

lactate threshold (LT), and it typically occurs between 50% and 80% $\dot{V}O_2max$. This sudden increase in the blood lactate concentration is sometimes called the *anaerobic threshold*, but because several conditions other than a lack of oxygen (hypoxia) at the muscle cell can result in lactate being produced and released into the blood, *lactate threshold* is the preferred term. Endurance training increases the number of mitochondria in the trained muscles, facilitating the aerobic metabolism of carbohydrate and the use of more fat as fuel. As a result, when the subject retakes the GXT following training, less lactate is produced and the LT occurs at a later stage of the test. LT is a good indicator of endurance performance and has been used to predict performance in endurance races (5, 6).

Pulmonary ventilation is the volume of air inhaled or exhaled per minute and is calculated by multiplying the frequency (*f*) of breathing by the tidal volume (*TV*), the volume of air moved in one breath.

$$\text{Ventilation (L · min}^{-1})$$
$$= TV \text{ (L · breath}^{-1}) \times f \text{ (breaths · min}^{-1})$$

An example of this follows:

$$30 \text{ L · min}^{-1} = 1.5 \text{ L · breath}^{-1} \times 20 \text{ breaths · min}^{-1}$$

Pulmonary ventilation increases linearly with work rate until 50% to 80% of $\dot{V}O_2max$, at which point a relative hyperventilation results (see figure 4.8). The inflection point in the pulmonary ventilation response is the ventilatory threshold (VT). The VT has been used as a noninvasive indicator of the LT and as a predictor of performance (20, 70). The increase in pulmonary ventilation is mediated by changes in the frequency of breathing (from about 10-12 breaths · min^{-1} at rest to 40-50 breaths · min^{-1} during maximal work) and in the TV (from 0.5 L · breath^{-1} at rest to 2-3 L · breath^{-1} in maximal work). Endurance training lowers pulmonary ventilation during submaximal work, so the VT occurs later in the GXT. The maximal value for pulmonary ventilation tends to change in the direction of $\dot{V}O_2max$.

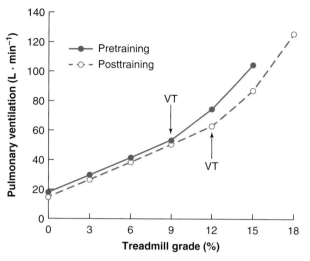

FIGURE 4.8 Following training, the VT occurs later in the GXT.

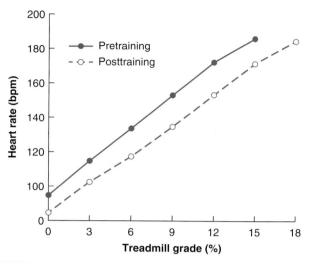

FIGURE 4.9 Training reduces the HR response to sub-maximal exercise (24).

KEY POINT

The points at which the blood lactate concentration and the pulmonary ventilation increase suddenly during a GXT are called the *lactate* and *ventilatory thresholds*, respectively. These typically occur between 50% and 80% $\dot{V}O_2$max. The LT and VT are good predictors of performance in endurance events (e.g., 10K runs, marathons).

Heart Rate

Once the HR reaches about 110 bpm, it increases linearly with work rate during a GXT until near-maximal efforts. Figure 4.9 shows how training influences the subject's HR response at the same work rates. The lower HR at submaximal work rates is a beneficial effect because it decreases the oxygen needed by the heart muscle. Maximal HR shows no change or is slightly reduced as a result of endurance training.

Stroke Volume

The volume of blood pumped by the heart per beat (ml · beat^{-1}) is the stroke volume (SV). For the typical person doing work in the upright position (e.g., cycling, walking), SV increases in the early stages of the GXT until about 40% $\dot{V}O_2$max is reached, and then it levels off (see figure 4.10) (3). Consequently, when $\dot{V}O_2$ is greater than 40% $\dot{V}O_2$max, HR is the sole factor responsible for the increased flow of blood from the heart to the working muscles. This is what makes HR a good indicator of the metabolic rate during exercise—it is linearly related to intensity from light exercise to heavy exercise. One of the

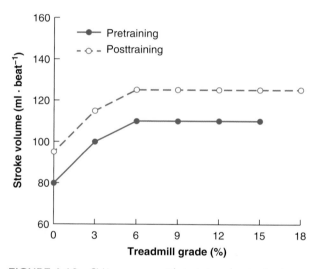

FIGURE 4.10 SV increases with training due to the larger volume of the ventricle (24).

primary effects of endurance training is an increase in SV at rest and during work; this increase is due to a larger volume of the ventricle that is linked, in part, to a larger blood volume (24). This allows a greater end-diastolic volume (EDV), the volume of blood in the heart just before contraction. Following endurance training, even if the same fraction of blood in the ventricle is pumped per beat (ejection fraction), the heart pumps more blood per minute at the same HR.

Cardiac Output

Cardiac output ($\dot{Q}$) is the volume of blood pumped by the heart per minute and is calculated by multiplying the HR (bpm) by the SV (ml · beat^{-1}).

RESEARCH INSIGHT

Stroke Volume in Elite Athletes

For most people, SV levels off at about 40% $\dot{V}O_2$max, making HR the sole factor increasing blood flow to the muscles at higher exercise intensities. However, there is clear evidence that this is not the case for highly trained endurance athletes. Interestingly, in these athletes, SV increases systematically with exercise intensity up to $\dot{V}O_2$max. This appears to be due to both enhanced filling of the ventricle before contraction (EDV) and greater emptying of the ventricle during contraction (ejection fraction), in contrast to what is observed in people of average fitness (31, 90).

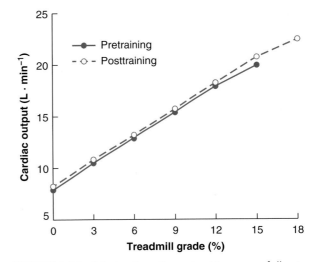

FIGURE 4.11 Maximal cardiac output increases following training (24).

$$\text{Cardiac output} = \text{HR} \times \text{SV}$$

$$\text{Cardiac output} = 60 \text{ bpm} \times 80 \text{ ml} \cdot \text{beat}^{-1}$$

$$\text{Cardiac output} = 4,800 \text{ ml} \cdot \text{min}^{-1}, \text{ or } 4.8 \text{ L} \cdot \text{min}^{-1}$$

Cardiac output increases linearly with work rate. Generally, the cardiac output response to light and moderate work is not affected by endurance training. What changes is how the cardiac output is achieved: with a lower HR and higher SV.

Maximal cardiac output (highest value reached in a GXT) is the most important cardiovascular variable determining maximal aerobic power because the oxygen-enriched blood (carrying about 0.2 L of O_2 per liter of blood) must be delivered to the muscle for the mitochondria to use. If a person's maximal cardiac output is 10 L · min^{-1}, only 2 L of O_2 would leave the heart each minute (i.e., 0.2 L of O_2 per liter of blood times a cardiac output of 10 L · min^{-1} = 2 L of O_2 · min^{-1}). A person with a maximal cardiac output of 30 L · min^{-1} would deliver 6 L of O_2 · min^{-1} to the tissues. Endurance training increases the maximal cardiac output and thus the delivery of oxygen to the muscles (see figure 4.11). This increase in maximal cardiac output is matched by greater capillary numbers in the muscle to allow the blood to move slowly enough through the muscle to maintain the time needed for oxygen to diffuse from the blood to the mitochondria (80). The increase in maximal cardiac output accounts for 50% of the increase in maximal oxygen uptake that occurs in previously sedentary people who engage in endurance training (77).

Oxygen Extraction

Two factors determine oxygen uptake at any time: the volume of blood delivered to the tissues per minute (cardiac output) and the volume of oxygen extracted from each liter of blood. Oxygen extraction is calculated by subtracting the oxygen content of mixed venous blood (as it returns to the heart) from the oxygen content of the arterial blood. This is the arteriovenous oxygen difference, or the $(a - \bar{v})O_2$ *difference.*

$$\dot{V}O_2 = \text{cardiac output} \times (a - \bar{v})O_2 \text{ difference}$$

For example, use the following values at rest to calculate the $(a - \bar{v})O_2$ difference:

$$\text{Cardiac output} = 5 \text{ L} \cdot \text{min}^{-1}$$

$$\text{Arterial oxygen content} = 200 \text{ ml of } O_2 \cdot \text{L}^{-1}$$

$$\text{Mixed venous oxygen content} = 150 \text{ ml of } O_2 \cdot \text{L}^{-1}$$

$$\dot{V}O_2 = 5 \text{ L} \cdot \text{min}^{-1} \times (200 - 150 \text{ ml of } O_2 \cdot \text{L}^{-1})$$

$$\dot{V}O_2 = 5 \text{ L} \cdot \text{min}^{-1} \times 50 \text{ ml of } O_2 \cdot \text{L}^{-1}$$

$$\dot{V}O_2 = 250 \text{ ml} \cdot \text{min}^{-1}$$

The $(a - \bar{v})O_2$ difference reflects the ability of the muscle to extract oxygen, and it increases with exercise intensity (see figure 4.12). The ability of tissue to extract oxygen is a function of the capillary-to-muscle-fiber ratio and the number of mitochondria in the muscle fiber. Endurance training increases both of these factors, thus increasing the maximal capacity to extract oxygen in the last stage of the GXT (75). This increase in the $(a - \bar{v})O_2$ difference accounts for about 50% of the increase in $\dot{V}O_2$max that occurs with endurance training in previously sedentary individuals (77).

In the general population, SV is the major variable influencing maximal cardiac output. Differences in maximal cardiac output and maximal aerobic power that exist between females and males, between trained

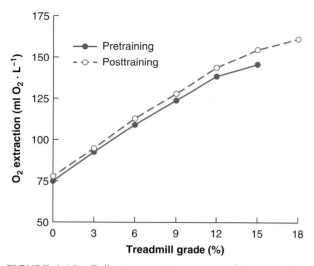

FIGURE 4.12 Following training, maximal O_2 extraction increases due to greater capillary and mitochondrial density in the trained muscles (24).

and untrained individuals, and between world-class endurance athletes and average fit individuals can be explained largely by differences in maximal SV. For example, in three groups of people who differed greatly in $\dot{V}O_2$max (5.2 versus 3.2 versus 1.6 L · min⁻¹), little difference was observed in maximal HR (range 190-200 bpm) and oxygen extraction (range 160-170 ml of O_2 · L⁻¹). In contrast, SV differed greatly between the groups (160 versus 100 versus 50 ml · beat⁻¹) (76). Clearly, maximal SV is the primary factor related to the differences in $\dot{V}O_2$max that exist from person to person.

Blood Pressure

BP is dependent on the balance between cardiac output and the resistance that blood vessels offer to blood flow (total peripheral resistance). The resistance to blood flow is altered by the constriction or dilation of arterioles, which are blood vessels located between the artery and the capillary.

$$BP = cardiac\ output \times total\ peripheral\ resistance$$

BP is sensed by baroreceptors in the arch of the aorta and in the carotid arteries. When BP changes, the baroreceptors send signals to the cardiovascular control center in the brain, which in turn alters cardiac output or the diameter of arterioles. For example, if a person who has been lying supine suddenly stands, blood pools in the lower extremities, SV decreases, and BP drops. If BP is not restored quickly, less blood flows to the brain and the person might faint. The baroreceptors monitor this decrease in BP, and the cardiovascular control center simultaneously increases the HR and reduces the diameter of the arterioles (to increase total peripheral resistance) to try to return BP to normal. During exer-

cise, the arterioles dilate in the active muscle to increase blood flow and meet metabolic demands. This dilation is matched with a constriction of arterioles in the liver, kidneys, and gastrointestinal tract and an increase in HR and SV, as already mentioned. These coordinated changes maintain BP and direct most of the cardiac output to the working muscles.

BP is monitored at each stage of a GXT. Figure 4.13 shows how systolic blood pressure (SBP) increases with each stage until maximum work tolerance is reached. Diastolic blood pressure (DBP) tends to remain the same or decrease during a GXT. See chapter 8 for criteria for terminating a GXT. Endurance training reduces the BP responses at fixed submaximal work rates.

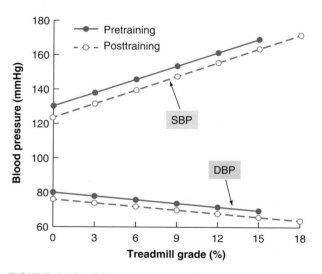

FIGURE 4.13 SBP increases until maximum work tolerance is reached. DBP remains steady or decreases.

KEY POINT

In people of average fitness, SV increases until about 40% $\dot{V}O_2$max, but both HR and cardiac output (HR × SV) increase linearly with work rate. Endurance training reduces HR and increases SV at rest and during exercise. In addition, maximal cardiac output is greater because maximal HR is generally unchanged. Variations in $\dot{V}O_2$max are primarily due to differences in maximal SV. Half of the increase in $\dot{V}O_2$max from endurance training is the result of an increase in maximal SV; the other half is due to an increase in oxygen extraction.

Two factors that determine the oxygen demand (work) of the heart during aerobic exercise are the HR and the SBP. The product of these two variables is called the *rate–pressure product*, or the *double product*, and is proportional to the myocardial oxygen demand (i.e., the volume of oxygen the heart muscle needs each minute to function properly). Factors that decrease the HR and BP responses to work increase the chance that the coronary blood supply to the heart muscle will adequately meet the oxygen demands of the heart. Endurance training decreases the HR and BP responses to fixed submaximal work and protects against any diminished blood supply (ischemia) to the myocardium. Drugs are also used to lower HR and BP to reduce the work of the heart (see chapter 2).

When a person does the same rate of work with the arms as with the legs, the HR and BP responses are considerably higher during the arm work. Given that the load on the heart and the potential for fatigue are greater for arm work, fitness professionals should choose activities that use the large muscle groups of the legs when possible. Such activities result in lower HR, BP, and perception of fatigue at the same work rate (29, 83), which allow one

KEY POINT

SBP increases with each stage of a GXT, whereas DBP remains the same or decreases. The work of the heart is proportional to the product of the HR and the SBP. Training lowers both, making it easier for the coronary arteries to meet the oxygen demand of the heart. HR and BP are higher during arm work compared with leg work at the same work rate.

to accomplish more work in a fixed time period than with arm exercise. That said, if participants need to increase their capacity for arm work related to employment or sport, structured progressive exercise programs should be implemented for that purpose.

Cardiovascular Responses to Isometric Exercise and Weightlifting

Most endurance exercise programs use dynamic activities involving large muscle masses to place loads on the cardiorespiratory system. The previous summary of the physiological responses to a GXT indicates that cardiovascular load is proportional to exercise intensity. But this is not necessarily the case for resistance training, in which a person can have a disproportionately high cardiovascular load relative to the exercise intensity. In a now classic study, a subject performed an isometric exercise test (sustained handgrip) at only 30% maximum voluntary contraction (MVC) strength while BP was monitored. In contrast to dynamic exercise, both the SBP and DBP increased over time, and SBP exceeded 220 mmHg. This kind of exercise puts a disproportionate load on the heart and is not recommended for older adults or people with heart disease (57). See chapter 14 for information on resistance training programs for patients with CVD.

Dynamic, heavy-resistance exercises can also cause extreme BP responses. Figure 4.14 shows the peak BP response achieved during exercise at 95% to 100% of the maximum weight that could be lifted one time (1RM). Both DBP and SBP are elevated, with average values exceeding 300/200 mmHg for the two-leg leg press done to fatigue. The elevation in pressure was believed to be caused by the compression of the arteries by the muscles,

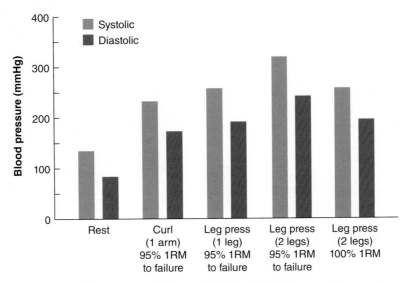

FIGURE 4.14 BP responses during weightlifting (59). RM = repetition maximum.

a reflex response attributable to the static component associated with near-maximal dynamic lifts, and by the Valsalva maneuver (trying to exhale forcefully against a closed airway), which can independently elevate BP (59). Another study reported peak values of about 190/140 mmHg for exercises of 50%, 70%, and 80% of 1RM done to fatigue in untrained lifters. Bodybuilders responded with lower BPs, indicating a cardiovascular adaptation to resistance training (26).

KEY POINT

> Isometric exercise and heavy-resistance exercise elicit high BP responses compared with dynamic endurance exercise. Both SBP and DBP increase with isometric and dynamic resistance training.

Understanding Muscle Structure and Function

Exercise means movement, and movement requires muscle action. Skeletal muscle must convert the chemical energy of ATP to mechanical work. How does a muscle do this?

Skeletal muscle is a complex structure composed of a variety of tissues, including nerve, muscle, and connective tissue. Figure 4.15 shows the basic structure of muscle. The epimysium is the connective tissue that surrounds the whole muscle; the perimysium surrounds bundles of muscle fibers called *fasciculi*; and each muscle fiber is surrounded by the endomysium, which overlies the muscle fiber's membrane, the sarcolemma. The connective tissue transmits the force, generated by the muscle, to the bone so that movement can occur. Each muscle fiber is composed of a large number of myofibrils, which run the full length of the muscle and give skeletal muscle its striated appearance. A myofibril is composed of a series of sarcomeres, the fundamental units of muscle contraction (figure 4.16). The sarcomere contains the thick filament myosin and the thin filament actin and is bounded by connective tissue called the *Z line* (55, 71, 89).

According to the sliding-filament theory of muscle contraction, the thin actin filaments slide over the thick myosin filaments, pulling the Z lines toward the center of the sarcomere. In this way the entire muscle shortens, but the contractile proteins do not change size.

For muscle to release the energy in ATP for shortening, an enzyme, ATPase, exists in muscle to split ATP and release the potential energy contained within its bonds. ATPase is found in an extension of the thick myosin filament, the myosin head, which also can bind to actin. The myosin head and its connection to the thick filament is called the *crossbridge*. ATP, the crossbridge, and actin interact to shorten the sarcomere (55) through these steps:

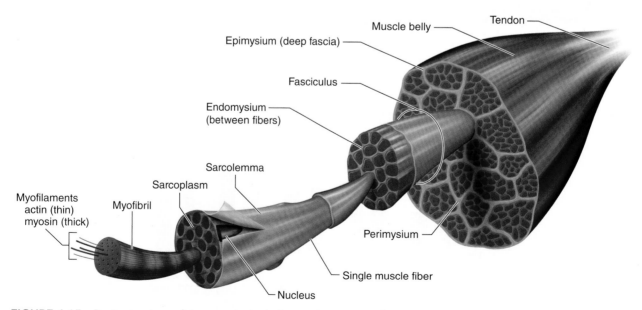

FIGURE 4.15 Basic structure of the muscle, including various types of connective tissue.

1. At the end of a contraction cycle the myosin crossbridge is tightly bound to actin.

2. ATP binds to the myosin, allowing its release from actin.

3. ATP is broken down (hydrolyzed) to ADP and Pi (which remain bound to myosin), and the myosin head moves away from the actin.

4. The energized crossbridge binds to a new actin molecule.

5. It then releases Pi to initiate movement referred to as the *power stroke* and pulls the thin filament (actin) toward the center of the sarcomere.

6. ADP is released from the myosin head, and ATP must be available to initiate the event in step 1.

The crossbridges are not always moving and the muscles are not always in contraction because at rest, two proteins that are associated with actin block the interaction of myosin with actin: troponin, which has the capacity to bind calcium, and tropomyosin. For a muscle contraction to occur, the first step is for the motor neuron associated with the muscle fiber to depolarize. When a motor neuron is depolarized, acetylcholine (ACh) is released and binds to receptors on the muscle fiber (figure 4.17). This will result in depolarization (excitation) of the muscle fiber. The wave of depolarization, or action potential, moves over the surface of the muscle fiber and deep into the muscle cell on communication channels called *T-tubules*. As the action potential moves down the T-tubules, calcium (Ca^{2+}) is released from

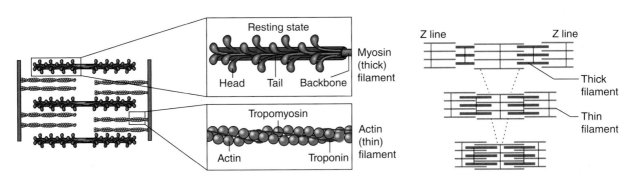

FIGURE 4.16 Detailed view of the myosin and actin filaments in a sarcomere, and changes in filament alignment in a myofibril during shortening.

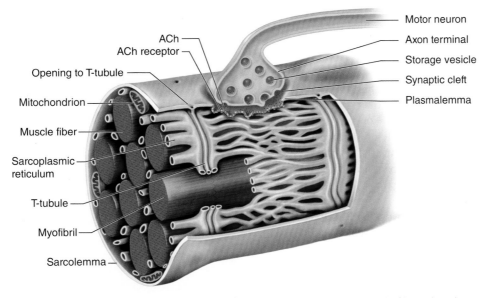

FIGURE 4.17 Myofibrils are surrounded by the sarcoplasmic reticulum within a muscle fiber; depolarization of a motor neuron allows for acetylcholine to be released and to bind with receptors to initiate depolarization of the muscle.

APPLICATION POINT

How Is an Understanding of the Sliding-Filament Theory Applicable to the Fitness Professional?

Consider how the relationship of actin and myosin relates to various types of contractions. An isometric contraction is one in which tension is developed without the muscle shortening. The myosin head binds to the actin and energy is released, but the sarcomere does not shorten because the myosin head will connect and disconnect to the actin in the same location repeatedly. Thus, an isometric contraction is still an active process, requiring ATP with the potential for improvement in muscular function and increase in muscle mass. In rehabilitative settings, isometric contractions allow for controlled force development at pain-free joint positions (68). Given that isometric contractions offer the ability to focus on weak points in a range of motion, this feature could be applied in various sport settings (68). Perhaps improvement in force production at a given joint position within a movement could overcome a biomechanical disadvantage (58). Limitations related to strength development at the trained angle and questions on how this transfers to dynamic movements are considerations (68). One recommendation is to incorporate isometric resistance training along with dynamic strength training (58).

In contrast to the lack of shortening of the sarcomere with isometric contractions, isotonic contractions involve a change in the length of the muscle. The sarcomere shortens during the concentric phase of the isotonic contraction, as when lifting a dumbbell. This is also referred to as *positive work* (42). Within an isotonic contraction is the lengthening phase (e.g., controlled lowering of a weight), which results in the forced separation of the myosin heads from the actin, lengthening the sarcomere while under tension. This is referred to as an *eccentric contraction*, or *negative work* (42). Eccentric contractions are part of supporting the body against gravity and to absorb shock, as with downhill running. Delayed-onset muscle soreness (DOMS; i.e., soreness that begins within a day and peaks 2-3 days after an activity rather than acute soreness during or immediately after an activity) is observed following eccentric muscle contractions or other novel activities (44). Although the exact mechanism behind the cause of DOMS is unknown, damage of muscle due to active lengthening during eccentric contractions or overstressing of single muscle fibers due to insufficient muscle recruitment coordination with unfamiliar activities may be involved (44).

storage areas in the muscle fibers called the *terminal cisternae* of the sarcoplasmic reticulum (SR). This calcium binds to troponin, which moves the tropomyosin off the binding sites on actin and allows the myosin head to attach to the actin filament. When the myosin head binds to actin, energy is released, the crossbridge moves, and the sarcomere shortens. This sequence of crossbridge cycling continues as long as calcium is present and the muscle can replace the ATP it uses. The muscle relaxes when the calcium is pumped back into the SR and troponin and tropomyosin can again block the interaction of actin and myosin (55). The two principal needs for ATP during exercise are crossbridge cycling and pumping the calcium back to the SR, both of which increase with exercise intensity.

Muscle Fiber Types and Performance

Muscle fibers vary in their abilities to produce ATP by the aerobic and anaerobic mechanisms described earlier in the chapter. Muscle fibers can be classified based on their biochemical properties, how they produce and use ATP to

KEY POINT

A muscle contraction cycle begins when ATP binds to myosin, allowing it to be released from actin. After the ATP is split to form a high-energy myosin crossbridge, the myosin head binds to another actin and releases energy; the crossbridge moves and pulls actin toward the center of the sarcomere. ATP must bind to and release the crossbridge from actin to start the process again. Calcium from the SR blocks inhibitory proteins (troponin and tropomyosin) and allows the myosin head to bind to actin to begin moving the crossbridge. Relaxation occurs when calcium is pumped back into the SR.

generate muscle contraction, and contractile properties such as the speed and force of contraction. Based on these properties, muscle fibers are organized into three types:

Table 4.3 Contractile and Biochemical Characteristics of Skeletal Muscle Fiber Types

	Type IIx Fast glycolytic (FG)	Type IIa Fast oxidative-glycolytic (FOG)	Type I Slow oxidative (SO)
Contraction speed	Very fast	Fast	Slow
Myosin ATPase activity	Very high	High	Low
Force production	Very high	High	Low
Fiber diameter	Large	Large	Small
Maximal power	Very high	High	Low
ATP production	Glycolytic	Glycolytic and oxidative	Oxidative
Primary fuel used	PC, glucose/glycogen	Glucose/glycogen, fat	Fat
Capillary, myoglobin, mitochondria content	Low	High	Very high
Fatigue resistance	Low	High	Very high

Data from McArdle et al. (2023); Powers et al. (2024).

fast glycolytic (IIx), fast oxidative-glycolytic (IIa), and slow oxidative (I). The biochemical and contractile properties of these fiber types are shown in table 4.3 (61, 71).

Oxidative fibers (type I) have an abundance of mitochondria, myoglobin, and capillaries, components that are involved in the delivery, uptake, and use of oxygen to produce ATP. These fibers have a high capacity to make ATP aerobically using fats as a fuel. By contrast, glycolytic fibers (type IIx) have a lower content of capillaries, myoglobin, and mitochondria, so they produce ATP anaerobically, primarily using phosphocreatine and muscle glycogen or glucose. This results in the production of lactate and H^+, which can lead to fatigue. Type IIa fibers have biochemical characteristics that are similar to type I fibers and contractile properties that are similar to type IIx fibers. For this reason, they are sometimes called *intermediate fibers*.

The speed of contraction is determined by myosin ATPase activity, the rate at which ATP is broken down by the myosin head. This myosin ATPase activity is based on different isoforms of the enzyme, which differ in the speed of ATP breakdown, so a muscle fiber with a low ATPase activity (type I) will contract more slowly, and a fiber with a high ATPase activity (type IIx) will contract more rapidly, which accounts for the difference in maximal contraction speed between fiber types. Type IIa fibers are considered intermediate fibers and have biochemical characteristics that are similar to type I fibers (oxidative, fatigue resistant) and contractile properties that are similar to IIx fibers (fast, high force).

The maximal force production of a muscle fiber is related to muscle fiber size. The diameter of a muscle fiber is an indication of the content of contractile proteins, actin and myosin. A larger diameter fiber has more actin and myosin, so it can form more crossbridges and generate more force than a smaller fiber. This accounts for much of the difference in force production between fiber types. Together, maximal force production and maximal contraction speed determine the maximal power output of a muscle fiber.

KEY POINT

Muscle fibers differ in speed of contraction, force, and resistance to fatigue. Type I fibers are slow, generate low force, and resist fatigue. Type IIa fibers are fast, generate high force, and resist fatigue. Type IIx fibers are fast, generate high force, and easily fatigue.

Muscle Fiber Types: Genetics, Sex, and Training

In the average male and female, about 52% of the muscle fibers are type I, with the fast-twitch fibers divided into approximately 33% type IIa and 13% type IIx (80, 81). However, the distribution of fiber types in the overall population is quite variable. Studies comparing identical and fraternal twins suggest that the distribution of fast and slow fibers is genetic. In addition, fast-twitch fibers cannot be converted to slow-twitch fibers, or vice versa, with endurance training (4). In contrast, the capacity of the muscle fiber to produce ATP aerobically (its oxidative capacity) seems to be easily altered by endurance training. This is seen as a conversion of IIx to IIa fiber types. Type IIx fibers are not found in some elite endurance athletes because these fibers have been converted to the oxidative version, type IIa (80). The increase in mitochondria and capillaries in endurance-trained muscles allows a person to meet ATP demands aerobically, with less glycogen depletion and lactate formation (43).

The tension, or force, generated by a muscle depends on more than the fiber type. Tension increases with the frequency of stimulation, from a single twitch to a complete tetanic contraction, with the latter being the typical type of muscle fiber contraction. In addition, the force of contraction depends on the degree to which the muscle fibers contract simultaneously (synchronous firing) and the number of muscle fibers recruited for the contraction. The latter factor, muscle fiber recruitment, is the most important.

During exercise, muscle fibers are recruited in groups called *motor units*, which include the motor neuron and all the muscle fibers it innervates, to produce the force necessary for the exercise task. When a motor unit is recruited, all muscle fibers contract maximally to generate force. The force produced by the muscle is dependent on the number of motor units recruited; more motor units recruited means more force is generated. It also depends on the muscle fiber type in the motor unit. Motor units with type IIx fibers will produce a very high force very quickly but will fatigue rapidly. A motor unit with type I fibers will produce less force but will not fatigue nearly as rapidly.

Figure 4.18 shows the order in which the various muscle fiber types are recruited as the intensity of exercise increases. The order is from the most to the least oxidative, from the slowest to the fastest fiber (type I to type IIa to type IIx) (78). This means that activities or events that require a high level of force to be generated quickly, such as sprinting and weightlifting, would require more

type IIx fibers than exercise at a lower relative intensity, such as distance running, which would use more type I fibers. This explains why the high force generated in sprinting or weightlifting cannot be sustained for long. The recruitment of fast glycolytic fibers during intense exercise (above 70% $\dot{V}O_2$max) results in the accumulation of lactate and H^+ in the muscle, which interferes with force production and contributes to muscle fatigue.

Since the type I and IIa motor units recruited are primarily oxidative, a submaximal intensity (<70% $\dot{V}O_2$max) can be sustained for longer. This means that lactate and H^+ production is lower and the muscle does not fatigue as rapidly. The muscle fiber recruitment pattern also has implications for training adaptations in the muscle. Although chronic light exercise (<40% $\dot{V}O_2$max) only recruits and causes a training effect in type I fibers, exercise beyond 70% $\dot{V}O_2$max involves all fiber types and will promote the conversion of type IIx to IIa fibers during endurance training (33). This response has important implications in the specificity of training and the potential for transferring training effects from one activity to another. If a muscle fiber is not used, it cannot become trained.

KEY POINT

Muscle tension depends on the frequency of the stimulation leading to a tetanus contraction, the synchronous firing of muscle fibers, and the recruitment of muscle fibers, with the latter being the most important. The order of recruitment of muscle fibers is from the most to the least oxidative. Light to moderate exercise uses type I muscle fibers, whereas moderate to vigorous exercise requires type IIa fibers in addition to the type I fibers already involved. Both of these fibers favor the aerobic metabolism of carbohydrate and fat. Heavy exercise requires type IIx fibers that favor anaerobic glycolysis, which increases the likelihood of lactate and hydrogen ion production.

Exercise-Induced Muscle Changes

When muscles work at high intensities for an extended period, especially early in a training program, a condition called *rhabdomyolysis* (often called *rhabdo*) can develop. Such exercise causes the breakdown of muscle, resulting in severe muscle soreness, edema (swelling), and the release of large proteins into the circulation that can cause kidney damage and death (55). Rhabdomyolysis is relatively rare and typically occurs following prolonged, intense exercise to which a person is unaccustomed. In contrast, progressively increasing the difficulty of a work-

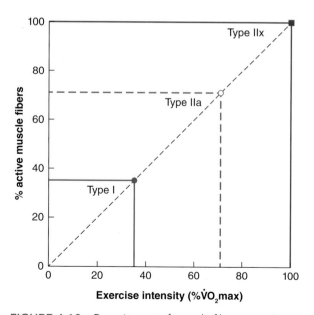

FIGURE 4.18 Recruitment of muscle fiber types in exercise of increasing intensity.

out from light to moderate to heavy over a long period of time minimizes the potential for such a problem. Appropriate progression is the foundation of the training recommendations highlighted throughout this book.

A more common and less severe consequence of high-intensity or prolonged exercise is delayed-onset muscle soreness (DOMS). Typically occurring 24 to 48 hours after exercise, DOMS is caused by microscopic damage to muscle fibers due to overloading, especially during the eccentric phase of contraction. This damage causes inflammation, edema, and soreness. Many people believe that DOMS is caused by lactic acid in the muscle. However, any lactic acid produced is cleared from the muscle shortly after exercise and would not be present days later to cause soreness. Interestingly, the inflammation in DOMS is an important part of the process that repairs damage and promotes protein synthesis and muscle growth. More information about the causes of DOMS and prevention and treatment techniques are found in the reviews by Cheung (10) and Dupuy (22).

Another common muscle issue during exercise is muscle cramps, which are involuntary and painful contractions. The exact cause of muscle cramps is a source of much research and debate, but two theories prevail. One suggests that muscle cramps are caused by water and electrolyte imbalances brought on by exercise-induced water and sodium losses in sweat. Since many muscle cramps occur after prolonged exercise in the heat, this makes intuitive sense. The other theory is that abnormal activity of the muscle spindle results in uncontrolled contraction. This is supported by the fact that passive stretching, which stimulates the Golgi tendon organ (GTO) and promotes muscle relaxation, often relieves cramps. It is possible that muscle cramps are caused by a combination of these mechanisms under different conditions, something that should become clearer with future research. The review by Maughan and Shirreffs (60) provides more information about the causes, potential treatments, and limitations of research involving muscle cramps.

Impact of Muscle Sensory Receptors on Flexibility and Strength

Muscle force production is regulated by the way the muscle fibers are stimulated and by the number and type of fibers recruited. This is typically thought of as a top-down process in which the conscious control of movement begins in the brain and is propagated along the spinal cord and motor neuron to activate the muscle. However, feedback from muscle sensory receptors called *proprioceptors* is important in regulating muscle contraction, affecting force production, flexibility, and adaptations to training. These muscle proprioceptors include the muscle spindle and GTO.

The muscle spindle is a grouping of sensory and motor neurons and specialized muscle fibers located in line with the muscle that are sensitive to and respond to changes in muscle length. A sudden change in muscle length stimulates the muscle spindle, resulting in contraction of the muscle. A classic example of this is the patellar tendon reflex in which tapping the patellar tendon leads to contraction of the quadriceps muscle. This same response also occurs during active stretching. A quick stretch can stimulate the muscle spindle and cause the muscle being stretched to contract. This is one reason why slow, static stretching traditionally has been recommended to improve flexibility while reducing the risk of injury (14).

The GTO is a sensory receptor located in the tendon that is sensitive to changes in muscle tension. When stimulated by increased tension (e.g., while lifting a heavy weight), the GTO inhibits the stimulation of the muscle and causes relaxation. For this reason, the GTO is thought of as a mechanism to protect against muscle damage from excessive loads. The GTO is also stimulated by passive stretching and results in the relaxation of the muscle, the basis for stretching techniques including proprioceptive neuromuscular facilitation (PNF) stretching.

Given the role of the muscle spindle and GTO in regulating muscle contraction, the improvement in muscular strength and flexibility as a result of training may include adaptations in these proprioceptors. It is thought that in response to resistance training the GTO stimulation and inhibition of muscle contraction is diminished, leading to increased strength (32). While the improvement in flexibility from stretching could be due to a change in feedback from the muscle spindle or other muscle sensory receptors, the research suggests that it is mostly due to an increase in stretch tolerance (69).

Muscular Adaptations to Endurance and Resistance Training

Skeletal muscle changes in response to exercise training to promote an improved capacity to participate in exercise. These adaptations are specific to the type of training (endurance or resistance), muscle groups used, and fiber types recruited. A historical look (33) and recent review (47) of training adaptations are recommended to learn more about this interesting topic.

The major muscle adaptation to endurance training is an increase in the oxidative capacity of the muscle due to an increase in capillaries, myoglobin, and mitochondria. This adaptation is brought about by changes in Ca^{+2}, ATP, and free radical levels in the muscle that occur during exercise that promote mitochondrial synthesis. This allows the muscle to produce more ATP aerobically using fat as a fuel, resulting in reduced lactate and H^+ production and improved fatigue resistance. This is consistent with a shift in fast fiber type from IIx to IIa, described previously in this chapter. The enhanced oxidative capacity increases the oxygen extraction by the muscle, part of the improvement in $\dot{V}O_2$max that occurs from endurance training. Together, endurance training allows an individual to exercise at a higher intensity for a longer time without fatigue.

The primary adaptation to resistance training is increased force production, or strength, by the muscle. This is commonly attributed to protein synthesis leading to a larger muscle size within which more contractile proteins can generate greater force. This could be due to an increase in muscle fiber size (hypertrophy) or the number of muscle fibers (hyperplasia). Most research suggests that muscle fiber hypertrophy is responsible for the majority of the increase in muscle size. Similar to the adaptations to endurance training, changes within the muscle during exercise stimulate protein synthesis, so hypertrophy only occurs in the muscle groups being trained.

However, hypertrophy is not the only adaptation that results in increased strength. Resistance training also leads to improvements in muscle activation including synchronous firing of motor units and reduced inhibitory mechanisms that result in greater force production. In most training studies, these neural adaptations are responsible for most of the strength gains in the initial several weeks of training, with hypertrophy occurring later.

Effects of Endurance Training and Detraining on Physiological Responses

Many observations have been made about the effects of endurance training on various physiological responses to exercise. In this section, the connection between effects will be discussed.

• Endurance training increases the number of mitochondria and capillaries in muscle, causing all active fibers to become more oxidative. This effect is manifested by the increase in type IIa fibers and decrease in type IIx fibers. These changes boost the endurance capacity of the muscle by allowing fat to be used for a greater percentage of energy production, sparing the muscle glycogen store and reducing lactate production. The LT shifts to the right, and performance times in endurance events improve.

• Endurance training decreases the time it takes to achieve a steady state in submaximal exercise. This reduces the oxygen deficit and reliance on PC and anaerobic glycolysis for energy.

• Endurance training enlarges the volume of the ventricle. This accommodates an increase in the EDV such that more blood is pumped out per beat. The increased SV is accompanied by a decrease in HR during submaximal work, so the cardiac output remains the same. The heart works less to meet the oxygen needs of the tissues at the same work rate. Table 4.4 summarizes these changes that result from endurance training.

• Maximal aerobic power increases with endurance training, the increase being inversely related to the initial $\dot{V}O_2$max. In formerly sedentary people, about 50% of the increase in $\dot{V}O_2$max results from greater maximal cardiac output, a change brought about by an increase in maximal SV, given that maximal HR either remains the same or decreases slightly. The other 50% of the increase in $\dot{V}O_2$max is attributable to an increase in oxygen extraction at the muscle, shown by an increase in the $(a - \bar{v})$ O_2 difference. This occurs as a result of higher numbers of capillaries and mitochondria in the trained muscles.

Transfer of Training

The training effects that have been discussed are observed only when the trained muscles are the muscles used in the exercise test. Although this may appear obvious for the decrease in blood lactate that is attributable to, in part, the greater numbers of mitochondria in the trained muscles, it is also linked to the changes that occur in the HR response to submaximal work following the training program. Figure 4.19 shows the results of repeated submaximal exercise tests conducted on subjects who trained only one leg on a cycle ergometer for 13 days. The HR response to a fixed submaximal work rate performed by the trained leg decreased as expected. At the end of the 13 days of training, the untrained leg was subjected to the same exercise test. The HR responded as if a training

Table 4.4   Effects of Endurance Training on Cardiovascular Response to a Graded Exercise Test

Variable	Rest	At same relative $\dot{V}O_2$ (ml · kg^{-1} · min^{-1})	At maximal work
Cardiac output	Same	Same	Higher
SV	Higher	Higher	Higher
HR	Lower	Lower	No change or slightly lower

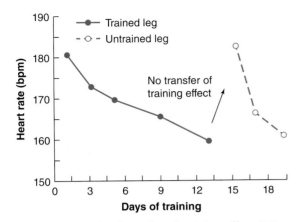

FIGURE 4.19 Lack of transfer of training effect (11).

effect had not occurred. This indicates that part of the reason the HR response to submaximal exercise decreases following training is because of feedback from the trained muscles to the cardiovascular control center, which, in turn, reduces sympathetic stimulation to the heart (11, 77). This finding has important implications for evaluating the effects of training programs. The expected training responses (lower lactate production, lower HR, greater fat use) are linked to testing the same muscle groups that were involved in the training. The probability of the training effect carrying over to another activity depends on the degree to which the new activity uses the muscles that were involved in the training program.

Detraining

How fast is a training effect lost? A number of investigations have explored this question by having subjects either reduce or completely cease training. Maximal

oxygen uptake is typically used as the principal measure to evaluate physiological changes due to detraining, but an individual's response to a submaximal work rate also has been used to track these changes over time.

Ceasing Training

The following study used subjects who had trained for 10 ± 3 years and agreed to cease training for 84 days (18). They were tested on days 12, 21, 56, and 84 of detraining. Figure 4.20 shows how their $\dot{V}O_2max$ decreased 7% within the first 12 days. Remember that $\dot{V}O_2max =$ cardiac output $\times$ $(a - \bar{v})O_2$ difference. The decrease in $\dot{V}O_2max$ was attributable entirely to a drop in maximal cardiac output because the maximal oxygen extraction, or $(a - \bar{v})O_2$ difference, was unchanged.

In turn, the lower maximal cardiac output was attributable entirely to a decrease in maximal SV because maximal HR actually increased during detraining. A subsequent study showed that the reduced SV was caused by a reduction in plasma volume that occurred in the first 12 days of no training (16). In contrast, the drop in $\dot{V}O_2max$ between days 21 and 84 was attributable to a decrease in the $(a - \bar{v})O_2$ difference because maximal cardiac output was unchanged (see figure 4.20). This lower oxygen extraction appeared to result from smaller numbers of mitochondria in the muscle, given that the number of capillaries surrounding each muscle fiber was unchanged (15).

The same subjects also completed a standard (fixed work rate) submaximal exercise test during the 84 days of no training (17). Figure 4.21 shows that HR and blood lactate responses to this work test increased throughout detraining. The higher responses relate to the fact that the same work rate required a greater percentage of

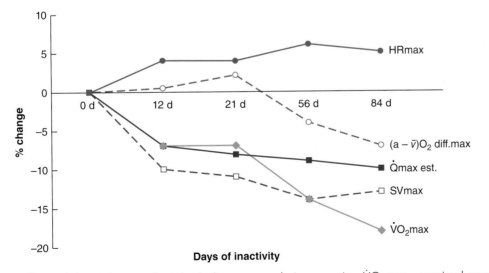

FIGURE 4.20 Effects of detraining on physiological responses during exercise. $\dot{V}O_2max$ = maximal oxygen uptake; $\dot{Q}$ max est. = estimated maximal cardiac output; $(a - \bar{v})O_2$ diff. max = maximal arteriovenous oxygen difference; HRmax = maximal heart rate; SVmax = maximal stroke volume.

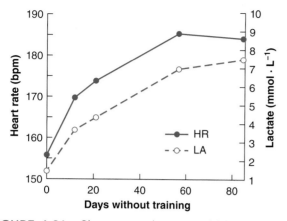

FIGURE 4.21 Changes in the HR and blood lactate responses to a standard exercise test taken during 84 days of detraining (17).

$\dot{V}O_2$max because the latter variable decreased throughout the detraining. The magnitude of change in HR and blood lactate responses to this submaximal work, however, makes them sensitive indicators of a person's training state.

Reduced Training

To evaluate the effect of reduced training, Hickson and colleagues (39, 40, 41) trained subjects for 10 weeks to increase $\dot{V}O_2$max. The training program was conducted 40 minutes per day, 6 days per week. Three days involved running at near-maximum intensity for 40 minutes; the other 3 days required six 5-minute bouts at near-maximum intensity on a cycle ergometer, with a 2-minute rest between work bouts. Subjects expended about 600 kcal on each day of exercise, or 3,600 kcal each week. At the end of this 10-week program, the subjects were divided into groups that trained at either a one-third or two-thirds reduction in the previous frequency (4 and 2 days per week, respectively), duration (26 and 13 minutes per day, respectively), or intensity (a one-third or two-thirds reduction in work done or distance run per 40-minute session).

Data collected on the maximal treadmill tests showed that cutting duration from 40 to 26 or 13 minutes or frequency from 6 to 4 or 2 days did not affect $\dot{V}O_2$max. In contrast, $\dot{V}O_2$max clearly fell when the intensity of training was reduced by either one-third or two-thirds. The subjects were able to maintain $\dot{V}O_2$max when the total exercise per week was cut from 3,600 to 1,200 kcal in the group whose exercise frequency and duration were reduced by two-thirds, but they were not able to maintain $\dot{V}O_2$max when the intensity was reduced, even though the subjects were still expending about 1,200 kcal · wk^{-1}. This shows that exercise intensity is critical in maintaining $\dot{V}O_2$max and that it takes less exercise to maintain than to achieve a specific level of $\dot{V}O_2$max.

KEY POINT

Endurance training increases the ability of a muscle to use fat as a fuel and to spare carbohydrate, decreases the time it takes to achieve a steady state during submaximal work, increases the size of the ventricle, and increases $\dot{V}O_2$max by increasing SV and oxygen extraction. Endurance training effects (lower HR, lower blood lactate) do not transfer when untrained muscles are used to perform the work. Maximal oxygen uptake decreases when training stops. The initial decrease is caused by a decrease in SV and, later, in oxygen extraction. Maximal oxygen uptake can be maintained by doing intense exercise, even when cutting exercise duration and frequency.

Regulating Body Temperature

Under resting conditions, the body's core temperature is 37 °C, and heat production and heat loss are balanced. Mechanisms of heat production include the basal metabolic rate, shivering, work, and exercise. During exercise, mechanical efficiency is about 20% or less, which means that 80% or more of energy production ($\dot{V}O_2$) is converted to heat. For example, if a client is working on a cycle ergometer at a rate requiring a $\dot{V}O_2$ of 2.0 L · min^{-1}, the energy production is about 10 kcal · min^{-1}. At 20% efficiency, 2 kcal · min^{-1} are used to do work and 8 kcal · min^{-1} are converted to heat. If most of this added heat is not lost, core temperature might quickly rise to dangerous levels. How does the body lose excess heat?

Heat-Loss Mechanisms

The body loses heat by four processes: radiation, conduction, convection, and evaporation. In radiation, heat transfers from the surface of one object to the surface of another, with no physical contact between the objects. Heat loss depends on the temperature gradient—that is, the temperature difference between the surfaces of the objects. When a person is seated at rest in a comfortable environment (21-22 °C), about 60% of body heat is lost through radiation to cooler objects. Conduction is the transfer of heat from one object to another by direct contact, and, like radiation, it depends on a temperature gradient. A person sitting on a cold marble bench loses body heat by conduction. Convection is a special case of conduction in which heat is transferred to air (or water) molecules, which become lighter and rise away from the body to be replaced by cold air (or water). Heat loss can be enhanced by increasing the movement of the air (or water) over the surface of the body. For example, a fan stimulates heat loss by placing more cold air molecules into contact with the skin.

All of these heat-loss mechanisms can be heat-gain mechanisms as well. Heat is gained from the sun by radiation across 93 million miles (150 million kilometers) of space, and heat can be gained by conduction as when sitting on hot sand at the beach. Similarly, if a fan were to place more hot air (warmer than skin temperature) into contact with the skin, heat would be gained. Heat gained from the environment adds to that generated by exercise and puts an additional strain on heat-loss mechanisms.

The fourth heat-loss mechanism is the evaporation of sweat. Sweating is the process of producing a watery solution over the surface of the body, and evaporation is a process in which liquid water converts to a gas. This conversion requires about 580 kcal of heat per liter of sweat evaporated. The heat for this comes from the body, and thus the body is cooled. At rest, about 25% of heat loss is caused by evaporation, but during exercise evaporation becomes the primary mechanism for heat loss.

Evaporation depends on the water vapor pressure gradient between the skin and air and does not directly depend on temperature. The water vapor pressure of the air relates to the relative humidity and the saturation pressure at that air temperature. For example, the relative humidity can be 90% in winter, but because the saturation pressure of cold air is low, the water vapor pressure of the air is also low, and water vapor can be seen rising from the body following exercise. In warm temperatures, however, the relative humidity is a good indicator of the water vapor pressure of the air. If the water vapor pressure of the air is too high, sweat will not evaporate, and sweat that does not evaporate does not cool the body (55).

Body Temperature Response to Exercise

Figure 4.22 shows that during exercise in a comfortable environment, the core temperature increases proportionally to the relative intensity (%$\dot{V}O_2$max) of the exercise and then levels off (82). The gain in body heat that occurs early in exercise triggers the heat-loss mechanisms discussed in the preceding section. After 10 to 20 minutes, heat loss equals heat production, and the core temperature remains steady (30). The most important heat-loss mechanisms during exercise are discussed in the next section.

Heat Loss During Exercise

Exercise intensity and environmental temperature influence which heat-loss mechanism is primarily responsible for maintaining a steady core temperature during exercise. When a person participates in progressively difficult exercise tests in an environment that allows heat loss by all four mechanisms, the contribution that convection and radiation make to overall heat loss is modest. Because the temperature gradient between the skin and the room does not change much during exercise, the rate of heat loss is relatively constant. To compensate for this, evaporation picks up when heat losses by convection and radiation plateau, and evaporation is responsible for most of the heat loss in heavy exercise (figure 4.23).

When a person performs steady-state exercise in a warmer environment, the role that evaporation plays becomes even more important. Figure 4.24 shows that as environmental temperature increases, the gradient for heat loss by convection and radiation decreases, and the rate of heat loss by these processes also decreases. As a result, evaporation must compensate to maintain core temperature.

In strenuous exercise or hot environments, evaporation is the most important process for losing heat and maintaining body temperature in a safe range. It should be no surprise, then, that factors affecting sweat production (such as dehydration) or sweat evaporation (such as impermeable clothing) are causes for concern.

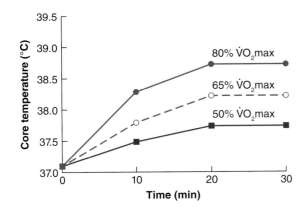

FIGURE 4.22 Core temperature increases over time as exercise intensity increases (3).

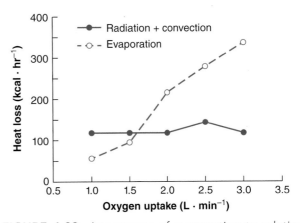

FIGURE 4.23 Importance of evaporation to relative work rate (82). Evaporation is more important at higher work rates.

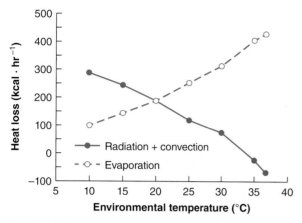

FIGURE 4.24 Importance of evaporation as a heat-loss mechanism during exercise as environmental temperature increases (3). At higher environmental temperatures, evaporation becomes more important.

Chapter 23 discusses how to prevent and treat heat-related disorders.

Training in a hot and humid environment for as few as 7 to 12 days results in specific adaptations that improve heat tolerance and, as a result, lower the trained person's body temperature during submaximal exercise (30). Adaptations that improve heat tolerance include the following:

- Increased plasma volume
- Earlier onset of sweating
- Higher sweat rate
- Reduced salt loss through sweat
- Reduced blood flow to the skin

KEY POINT

Heat can be lost from the body by radiation and convection when a temperature gradient exists between the skin and the environment; however, evaporation is the primary mechanism of heat loss during high-intensity exercise or during exercise in a hot environment. Body temperature increases in proportion to the relative work rate (%$\dot{V}O_2$max) during submaximal exercise. Acclimatization to heat can be achieved in 7 to 12 days of training in a hot, humid environment and improves one's ability to exercise safely.

LEARNING AIDS

REVIEW QUESTIONS

1. What are the two anaerobic sources of energy?

2. In an all-out run lasting 10 minutes, which energy system provides the greatest amount of energy?

3. Name the three fiber types, and indicate the order in which they are recruited as exercise intensity increases.

4. As exercise intensity increases, which substrate provides more energy—carbohydrate or fat?

5. Following an endurance training program, what changes in muscle allow more fat to be used as fuel during exercise?

6. Why is the HR response of women higher at the same work rate compared with men?

7. Draw a graph showing how oxygen uptake increases at the beginning of a submaximal exercise bout, and label the oxygen deficit.

8. Define or describe (graphically) the lactate threshold (LT). What happens to the LT as a result of an endurance training program?

9. Draw a graph of the HR response to a GXT, and show the effect of an endurance training program on the response.

10. For the average person, SV levels off at about 40% $\dot{V}O_2$max in a GXT. What causes the increase in cardiac output at higher exercise intensities?

11. Which cardiovascular variable—maximal HR, SV, or oxygen extraction—explains the large differences in $\dot{V}O_2$max observed across the population?

12. What happens to BP when the arms perform the same work rate as the legs?

13. What accounts for the decrease in $\dot{V}O_2$max with detraining?

14. Which is the most important training variable—intensity, frequency, or duration—linked to maintaining $\dot{V}O_2$max when training level is reduced?

15. What is the most important mechanism of heat loss during exercise?

CASE STUDIES

1. A female competitive distance runner took a GXT on a motor-driven treadmill in which the speed of the run increased 0.5 mph (0.8 km · hr^{-1}) each minute, with the test starting at 5 mph (8 km · hr^{-1}). Blood samples for lactate determination were obtained each minute, and the LT was found to occur at the 8 mph (13 km · hr^{-1}) stage of the test. Following an injury and a period of detraining, she repeated the test and found that the LT occurred at 6.5 mph (10.4 km · hr^{-1}). She wants to know what happened. What do you tell her?

2. A client with whom you have been working retakes a maximal GXT following 10 weeks of endurance training and finds that his HR is lower at each stage of the test. He is bothered by this because he thought his heart would be stronger and beat more times per minute. How do you help him understand what happened?

3. A female client is bothered by the fact that elite female runners who train as hard as elite male runners do not achieve the same performance times in distance races, and she wants to know why this is the case. How do you respond?

Answers to Case Studies

1. The LT is the point during a GXT when the blood lactate concentration suddenly increases. Following a period of detraining, there are fewer mitochondria in muscle and a reduced capacity to use fat as a fuel. As a result, more carbohydrate is used as fuel in glycolysis, and the usual breakdown products begin to accumulate in the cytoplasm of the muscle rather than going to the mitochondria. This results in increased lactate formation, and the LT occurs at a lower running speed. As she increases her training, the number of mitochondria in muscle will increase and the LT will again occur later in the GXT.

2. You need to confirm your client's feeling that the heart is stronger after training and can pump more blood per beat (increased SV). As a result, the heart does not have to beat as many times to deliver the same amount of oxygen to the tissues. This is a more efficient way for the heart to pump blood, and the heart does not have to work as hard at this lower rate.

3. You might begin by briefly stating that running speed in distance races relates to the amount of oxygen the runner can deliver to the muscles. When more oxygen can be delivered, the running speed is faster. The elite female distance runner differs from the elite male distance runner in three ways that have a bearing on this issue: Her heart size is smaller and she cannot pump as much oxygen-rich blood to the muscles per minute; the oxygen content of her blood is lower due to the lower hemoglobin concentration; and she is carrying relatively more body fat, which negatively affects sustained running speed even at the same level of fitness.

Fueling for Activity: Dietary Considerations

Laura J. Kruskall

OBJECTIVES

The reader will be able to do the following:

1. List the six classes of essential nutrients and describe their role in the proper functioning of the body
2. List the recommended percentage of calories from carbohydrate, fat, and protein
3. Understand the importance of vitamins and minerals and how to optimize them in a typical diet
4. Understand the role of the *Dietary Guidelines for Americans* in making healthy nutritional choices
5. Explain the relationship between blood lipid profile and cardiovascular disease, and explain the role of diet and exercise in modifying blood lipids
6. Know how to maintain hydration during exercise
7. Discuss the nutrient needs of a physically active person
8. Understand how dietary supplements are regulated and how to evaluate supplement claims
9. Understand the basic principles behind increasing glycogen storage before competition
10. List the importance and physiological consequences of suboptimal energy availability
11. Understand scope of practice as a fitness professional

Good nutrition results from eating a variety of foods in the proper quantities and with the appropriate distribution of nutrients for health promotion and disease prevention. Malnutrition, on the other hand, is the outcome of a diet in which underconsumption, overconsumption, or unbalanced consumption of nutrients leads to disease or increased susceptibility to disease. These definitions implicitly state that proper nutrition is essential to good health. A history of poor nutritional choices eventually may lead to health consequences such as increased risk of developing chronic conditions including cardiovascular disease (CVD), diabetes, obesity, and cancer (35).

With current media technologies, the public is bombarded with messages about nutrition, and it is often difficult for the layperson to distinguish sound nutrition information from misinformation. Fitness professionals can play an important role in conveying general, non-medical nutrition information. However, a Registered Dietitian Nutritionist (RDN) is a person who has had extensive education and supervised practice in nutrition and dietetics and is therefore the appropriate health care professional to perform a detailed nutrition assessment, complete a nutrition diagnosis, and provide a nutrition intervention specific to meet nutritional needs and personal goals. More on scope of practice is discussed later in the chapter (1, 2, 10).

Essential Nutrients

The body requires many nutrients for the maintenance, growth, and repair of tissues. Nutrients can be divided into six classes: carbohydrate, fat, protein, vitamins, minerals, and water (35). The Institute of Medicine (IOM) Food and Nutrition Board has established dietary reference intakes (DRI) to help people achieve a healthy intake of nutrients (13, 14, 22). The DRIs consist of recommended intakes for nutrients based on age and sex, including the recommended dietary allowances (RDA), or the amounts found to be adequate for approximately 97% of the population; adequate intakes (AI), or the amounts considered adequate although insufficient data exist to establish the appropriate RDA; and tolerable upper intake levels (UL), or the highest intakes believed to pose no health risk. Additionally, acceptable macronutrient distribution ranges (AMDR) have been established for fat, carbohydrate, and protein (14, 22).

Carbohydrate

Carbohydrate is a nutrient composed of carbon, hydrogen, and oxygen and is an essential source of energy in the body. Carbohydrates are categorized as monosaccharides, disaccharides, and polysaccharides. Examples of monosaccharides are glucose and fructose. Lactose and sucrose are two of the disaccharides, which are carbohydrate that forms when two monosaccharides combine.

The monosaccharides and disaccharides are sometimes called *simple sugars*. Simple sugars contribute significantly to the caloric content of foods such as fruit juices, soft drinks, and candy. The most important simple sugar in the human body is glucose. The molecular formula for glucose is $C_6H_{12}O_6$. Polysaccharides are complex carbohydrate formed by combining three or more sugar molecules. Starches and fiber are polysaccharides found in plants. Starches provide a source of dietary carbohydrate that the body can use for energy, while fiber is not digested and contributes to stool bulk. Rice, pasta, and whole-grain breads are just a few examples of foods that are high in complex carbohydrate. When carbohydrate is stored in the body, glucose molecules join together to form large molecules called *glycogen*. Glycogen is stored in the liver and skeletal muscle (35). Table 5.1 provides the approximate glucose and glycogen in the human body.

Grains, vegetables, and fruits are excellent sources of carbohydrate. The AMDR for carbohydrate is 45% to 65% of a person's total daily kcal (14, 22) (see figure 5.1). The minimum amount of carbohydrate intake for normal bodily functioning is $130 \text{ g} \cdot \text{day}^{-1}$, but the average carbohydrate intake of Americans is well beyond this RDA (14, 22, 35). The majority of carbohydrate calories

Table 5.1 Body Stores of Glucose and Glycogen

Source	Amount (grams)	Kcal
Blood glucose	5-25	20-100
Liver glycogen	70-110	280-440
Muscle glycogen	120-500	480-2,000

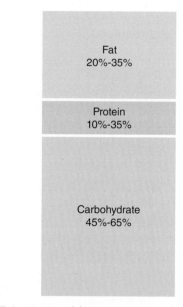

FIGURE 5.1 Acceptable macronutrient distribution range (AMDR) for carbohydrate, fat, and protein.

Based on Food and Nutrition Board (2005); National Institutes of Health (n.d.).

should come from high-quality, complex carbohydrate sources; foods with added sugar should be limited (31, 35). The reason for eating quality complex rather than simple carbohydrate is the higher nutrient density and dietary fiber of these foods. *Nutrient density* refers to the amount of essential nutrients in a food compared with the calories it contains (35). For example, a candy bar (containing simple sugars) has a low nutrient density, whereas a whole-grain muffin (containing complex carbohydrate and other essential nutrients) has a high nutrient density. Complex carbohydrate food choices can vary in quality and nutrients. For example, both a slice of highly processed white bread and a slice of whole-grain bread are classified as a complex carbohydrate food source, and both contain similar amounts of carbohydrate. However, the whole-grain bread contains other vitamins, minerals, and fiber important for health.

One of the benefits of consuming foods that are high in complex carbohydrate is that they also typically contain dietary fiber, a nonstarch polysaccharide that is found in plants and cannot be broken down by the human digestive system. Although fiber cannot be digested, it may help prevent hemorrhoids, constipation, and cancers of the digestive system because it helps food move quickly and easily through the digestive system. In addition, consuming water-soluble fiber has been shown to lower cholesterol levels (35). Unfortunately, more than 90% of women and 97% of men do not meet recommended intakes for dietary fiber of 38 g · day⁻¹ and 25 g · day⁻¹ for men and women aged 50 and younger, respectively (14, 22). For older men and women with lower energy requirements, the daily recommended levels are 30 grams and 21 grams, respectively (14, 22). *Dietary Guidelines for Americans, 2020-2025*, recommends that adults consume approximately 14 grams of fiber for every 1,000 kcal consumed. Excellent sources of dietary fiber are whole grains, vegetables, legumes, and fruits (31).

As mentioned earlier, carbohydrate is a vital source of energy in the human body. During high-intensity exercise, carbohydrate is the primary fuel source for energy production in the form of ATP. When carbohydrate is broken down in the human body, it yields approximately 4 kcal of energy per gram. This means that a person who eats 10 grams of carbohydrate gains approximately 40 kcal of energy to use or store as glycogen (35).

KEY POINT

The six classes of nutrients are carbohydrate, fat, protein, vitamins, minerals, and water. Carbohydrate contains 4 kcal per gram. Carbohydrate should contribute 45% to 65% of one's total daily energy intake, with limited energy intake coming from simple sugars.

Focus on Glycemic Index and Glycemic Load

When carbohydrate is ingested, blood glucose rises and subsequently insulin is released from the pancreas. The rapidity with which blood glucose rises after food intake is represented by the glycemic index (GI). Foods with a high GI cause a rapid spike in blood glucose, whereas foods with a low GI do not. A number of factors (e.g., biochemical composition, method of food preparation, fiber content) affect GI. Examples of foods with a high GI are grape juice, white rice, and soft drinks. Foods with a lower GI include apples, kidney beans, and milk. However, the change in blood glucose that occurs after eating a food depends both on the GI and on the quantity of carbohydrate in food. The glycemic load (GL) is a value that reflects the quality (i.e., the GI) and quantity of carbohydrate in a given food. To calculate GL, the GI of the food is multiplied by the grams of carbohydrate in the food, and the value is divided by 100. For example, a banana with a GI of 52 and 25 grams of carbohydrate would produce a GL of 13 (52 × 25 ÷ 100 = 13). A food with a large GL will dramatically increase blood glucose levels. The University of Sydney maintains a website where the GI and GL of various foods can be determined (28).

Controversy remains about the health impact of eating a diet rich in low-GI foods. Though some argue that a low-GI diet offers cardiovascular and metabolic benefits, the evidence is not strong. The Academy of Nutrition and Dietetics (1), the professional organization representing experts in food and nutrition, places only a minor emphasis on using the GI in making food choices and emphasizes that the total amount of carbohydrate is more important than GI. However, certain circumstances may arise where knowledge of GI is helpful. For example, someone with diabetes may be better able to control blood glucose with a balance of high- and low-GI foods. On the other hand, an endurance athlete needing to replenish glycogen stores quickly can choose high-GI foods to do so.

Fat

Fat is essential to a healthy diet and contributes to vital functions in the human body. Among the functions performed by the body's fat stores are temperature regulation, protection of vital organs, distribution of some vitamins, hormone regulation, energy production, and formation of cell membranes. Similar to carbohydrate, fat is composed of carbon, hydrogen, and oxygen; however, the chemical structure is different. Triglycerides are the primary storage form of fat in the body. These large molecules are composed of three fatty acid chains connected to a glycerol backbone. The majority of triglycerides are stored in adipose cells (i.e., fat cells), but these stored fats also can be found in other tissues like skeletal muscle as intramyocellular and extramyocellular lipid. The aerobic metabolism of triglycerides provides much of the energy needed during rest and low-intensity exercise. When metabolized, 1 gram of fat yields 9 kcal of energy. Phospholipids are another type of fat found in the body. As the name implies, these fats have phosphate groups attached to them. Phospholipids are important constituents of cell membranes. Lipoproteins are large molecules that allow fat to travel through the bloodstream. Cholesterol is a sterol, or a fatty substance in which carbon, hydrogen, and oxygen atoms are arranged in rings. In addition to the cholesterol consumed in the diet, the body constantly produces cholesterol, which is used in forming cell membranes and making steroidal hormones. Meat and eggs are the major sources of cholesterol in the typical American diet, but blood levels of cholesterol are influenced by factors other than consumption of dietary cholesterol. Thus, the *Dietary Guidelines for Americans* no longer emphasize cholesterol intake; instead the focus is on limiting dietary intake of saturated fat and trans fat (3, 31, 35).

Both animals and plants are sources of dietary fat. The AMDR for fat is 20% to 35% of total daily energy intake (14, 22) (figure 5.1). Saturated fat comes primarily from animal sources and is typically solid at room temperature. Plant sources of saturated fat include palm oil, coconut oil, and cocoa butter. The chemical structure of saturated fat contains no double bonds between carbon atoms; in other words, the fat is saturated with hydrogen atoms. A high intake of saturated fat directly relates to increased CVD. Therefore, one should limit consumption of saturated fat to less than 10% of total kcal (31). Unsaturated fat contains fewer hydrogen atoms because some double bonds exist between the carbon atoms. This type of fat is typically liquid at room temperature. Corn, peanut, canola, and soybean oil are sources of unsaturated fat. Trans fat is unsaturated fat that is common in many processed baked goods such as cookies and cakes. The intake of these fatty acids should be as low as possible because they are linked with negative health outcomes; the Food and Drug Administration (FDA) has mandated that food manufacturers phase out the use of trans fat, and amounts in a product are required to be displayed on the food label (31). The effects of various kinds of fat on health risk are discussed later in the chapter (see the section Diet, Exercise, and the Blood Lipid Profile).

Monounsaturated fatty acids, found in olive and canola oil, have a single double bond between carbon atoms in the fatty acid chain. Polyunsaturated fatty acids (e.g., fish, corn, soybean, and peanut oils) have two or more double bonds between carbon atoms. Two polyunsaturated fatty acids, alpha-linolenic acid (a type of omega-3 fatty acid) and linoleic acid (an omega-6 fatty acid), cannot be made by the body and must be consumed in the diet. The AI for alpha-linolenic acid is $1.6 \text{ g} \cdot \text{day}^{-1}$ for men and $1.1 \text{ g} \cdot \text{day}^{-1}$ for women (14, 22). Fish, walnuts, and canola oil are sources of this fatty acid. The AI for linoleic acid is $17 \text{ g} \cdot \text{day}^{-1}$ and $12 \text{ g} \cdot \text{day}^{-1}$ for men and women, respectively (14, 22). Sources include vegetable oils, nuts, avocados, and soybeans.

KEY POINT

The AMDR for fat is 20% to 35% of total daily energy intake, and less than 10% of total kcal should come from saturated fat. Intake of trans fat should be as low as possible. The breakdown of 1 gram of fat yields 9 kcal of energy.

Protein

Protein is a substance composed of carbon, hydrogen, oxygen, and nitrogen. All forms of protein are combinations of amino acids. Amino acids are molecules composed of an amino group (NH_3), a carboxyl group (COO), a hydrogen atom, a central carbon atom, and a side chain. The differences in the side chains give unique characteristics to each amino acid. Amino acids can combine in innumerable ways to form proteins, and it is estimated that tens of thousands of protein types exist in the body. The order of the linked amino acids provides the unique structure and function of protein that allow it to serve many functions in the body. Some of the most common functions are the following (35):

- Carry oxygen (hemoglobin)
- Fight disease (antibodies)
- Catalyze reactions (enzymes)
- Allow muscle contraction (actin, myosin, and troponin)
- Act as connective tissue (collagen)
- Clot blood (prothrombin)
- Act as a messenger (protein hormones such as growth hormone)

Of the 20 amino acids required by the human body, most can be constructed from other substances in the body; however, there are nine essential amino acids that the body cannot synthesize and so must be a part of one's regular diet. Eating a variety of protein-containing foods typically meets this need. Protein is found in both meat and plant products. Animal sources of protein such as meat, milk, and eggs contain the essential amino acids. Individual plant sources of protein such as beans, starchy vegetables, nuts, and grains do not always contain all essential amino acids when eaten in isolation. Because of this, vegetarian and vegan diets must contain a variety of protein-containing foods, and with careful planning protein needs can be met. Examples of foods that contain complementary proteins are legumes and grains, vegetables and nuts, and legumes and seeds. Foods that are incomplete protein sources do not have to be eaten in the same meal to gain the benefits. Eating a variety of these foods over days to a week is sufficient (35). In addition to protein, the nutrients that are of potential concern in vegetarian and vegan diets include fat, calcium, vitamin D, iron, zinc, iodine, riboflavin, and vitamin B_{12}. More information on the benefits and limitations of vegetarian diets can be found in the Position of the Academy of Nutrition and Dietetics, Dietitians of Canada, and the American College of Sports Medicine: Nutrition and Athletic Performance (24).

The AMDR for protein is 10% to 35% of total daily energy intake (figure 5.1) (14, 22). This amount ensures adequate protein for the growth, maintenance, and repair of cells. The adult RDA is 0.8 grams of protein for each kilogram of body weight (14, 22). As discussed later in this chapter, people who are training intensely have a higher protein requirement. Additionally, children need more protein to support their continually growing bodies.

In addition to the functions listed previously, protein can be metabolized for energy production. The breakdown of 1 gram of protein yields approximately 4 kcal of energy for the body. The contribution of protein to energy needs during exercise is usually quite small (<5%) in well-nourished individuals. However, during long bouts of exercise or when a person is not well nourished, protein may supply up to 15% of the body's energy needs (3).

KEY POINT

Protein is made of amino acids and serves numerous functions. To ensure that all needed amino acids are adequately available, people should eat a variety of protein-containing foods each day. The AMDR for protein is 10% to 35% of total daily energy intake. The breakdown of 1 gram of protein yields 4 kcal of energy.

Vitamins

Vitamins are organic substances that are essential to the normal functioning of the human body. Although vitamins do not contain energy for the body, they are essential in the metabolism of fat, carbohydrate, and protein. The body needs 14 vitamins for numerous processes, including blood clotting, protein synthesis, and bone formation. Because of the critical role vitamins play, they need to exist in proper quantities in the body. Major functions, important dietary sources, and recommended intakes of vitamins are listed in table 5.2. There are two major classifications of vitamins: fat soluble and water soluble (35).

The chemical structure of fat-soluble vitamins causes them to be transported and stored with lipids. The four fat-soluble vitamins are A, D, E, and K. Because these vitamins are stored in the body, it is not necessary to ingest large amounts daily; however, recommended amounts are required for physiological function (35). The DRI for vitamins are readily available and list individual vitamin requirements for men and women by age group. These DRI are intended for use in healthy individuals (22). The DRI may not be appropriate for people with a disease or certain health conditions.

The B vitamins and vitamin C are water-soluble vitamins. These vitamins are not stored in large quantities in the body and therefore must be consumed daily. Deficiencies related to water-soluble vitamins such as scurvy (vitamin C deficiency) and beriberi (thiamin deficiency) may occur rather quickly. Overconsuming either fat-soluble or water-soluble vitamins can lead to toxic effects; however, because fat-soluble vitamins are stored in the body, the potential for overdose with these substances is greater. Tolerable UL exist for many vitamins and minerals and are the highest level of daily intake that will likely not result in an adverse health outcome. These UL values are readily available for reference (22).

Minerals

Minerals are inorganic elements that serve a variety of functions in the human body. The minerals that appear in the largest quantities (calcium, phosphorus, potassium, sulfur, sodium, chloride, and magnesium) are often called *macrominerals* or *major minerals*. Other minerals are also essential to normal functioning of the body, but because they exist in smaller quantities, they are called *microminerals* or *trace elements* (35). Functions, dietary sources, and recommended intakes of minerals are listed in table 5.3.

Calcium is often inadequately consumed by Americans. It is important in the mineralization of bone, in muscle contraction, and in transmission of nervous impulses. Osteoporosis is a disease characterized by a decrease in the total amount of bone mineral in the body and in the strength of the remaining bone. This condi-

Table 5.2   Vitamins: Functions, Sources, and Dietary Reference Intakes for Adults Ages 19 to 50

Vitamin	Function	Sources	Adult RDA[a]		UL[b]
			Men	Women	
Thiamin (B$_1$)	Functions as part of a coenzyme to aid use of energy	Whole grains, nuts, lean pork	1.2 mg	1.1 mg	ND
Riboflavin (B$_2$)	Involved in energy metabolism as part of a coenzyme	Milk, yogurt, cheese	1.3 mg	1.1 mg	ND
Niacin	Facilitates energy production in cells	Lean meat, fish, poultry, grains	16 mg	14 mg	35 mg
B$_6$	Absorbs and metabolizes protein, aids in red blood cell formation	Lean meat, vegetables, whole grains	1.3 mg	1.3 mg	100 mg
Pantothenic acid	Aids in metabolism of carbohydrate, fat, and protein	Whole-grain cereals, bread, dark green vegetables	5 mg*	5 mg*	ND
Folic acid	Functions as coenzyme in synthesis of nucleic acids and protein	Green vegetables, beans, whole-wheat products	400 mcg	400 mcg	1,000 mcg
B$_{12}$	Involved in synthesis of nucleic acids, red blood cell formation	Only in animal foods, not plant foods	2.4 mcg	2.4 mcg	ND
Biotin	Functions as coenzyme in synthesis of fatty acids and glycogen	Egg yolk, dark green vegetables	30 mcg*	30 mcg*	ND
Choline	Important in cell membrane integrity and signaling, nerve transmission	Beef liver, chicken, codfish, wheat germ, cauliflower	550 mg*	425 mg*	3.5 g
C	Aids intracellular maintenance of bone, capillaries, and teeth	Citrus fruits, green peppers, tomatoes	90 mg	75 mg	2,000 mg
A	Aids vision, formation and maintenance of skin and mucous membranes	Carrots, sweet potatoes, butter, liver	900 mcg	700 mcg	3,000 mcg
D	Aids growth and formation of bones and teeth, aids calcium absorption	Eggs, tuna, liver, fortified milk	15 mcg	15 mcg	100 mcg
E	Protects polyunsaturated fat, prevents damage to cell membrane	Whole-grain cereals and breads, green leafy vegetables	15 mg	15 mg	1,000 mg
K	Important in blood clotting	Green leafy vegetables, peas, potatoes	120 mcg*	90 mcg*	ND

[a]Values are recommended daily allowance (RDA) for adults ages 19 to 50, unless marked with an asterisk. The requirements may vary for children, older adults, and pregnant or lactating women.

[b]Tolerable UL for adults aged 19 to 50. Intakes above the UL may lead to negative health consequences.

*Values are AI, indicating that sufficient data to set the RDA are unavailable.

ND = not yet determined

Adapted from Franks and Howley (1998); National Institutes of Health (n.d.).

tion is most common in the elderly but also may exist in younger people who have inadequate energy, calcium, or vitamin D intake or who suffer from menstrual dysfunction. Maximal bone density is achieved during the early adult years, and during older adult years, bone density declines in everyone. Those who achieve the highest bone density and maintain adequate intakes of calcium and vitamin D are most protected from osteoporosis. The DRIs for vitamin D are contained in table 5.2. The calcium RDA for adults aged 19 to 50 is 1,000 mg · day^{-1},

Table 5.3 Minerals: Functions, Sources, and Dietary Reference Intakes for Adults Ages 19 to 50

Mineral	Functions	Sources	Adult RDA[a]		UL[b]
			Men	Women	
Calcium	Bones, teeth, blood clotting, nerve and muscle function	Milk, sardines, dark green vegetables, nuts	1,000 mg	1,000 mg	2,500 mg
Chloride	Nerve and muscle function, water balance (with sodium)	Salt	2.3 g*	2.3 g*	3.6 g
Magnesium	Bone growth; nerve, muscle, enzyme function	Nuts, seafood, whole grains, leafy green vegetables	420 mg	320 mg	350 mg[c]
Phosphorus	Bones, teeth, energy transfer	Meats, poultry, seafood, eggs, milk, beans	700 mg	700 mg	4,000 mg
Potassium	Nerve and muscle function	Fresh vegetables, bananas, citrus fruits, milk, meats, fish	3,400 mg*	2,600 mg*	ND
Sodium	Nerve and muscle function, water balance	Salt	1.5 g*	1.5 g*	ND
Chromium	Glucose metabolism	Meats, liver, whole grains, dried beans	35 mcg*	25 mcg*	ND
Copper	Enzyme function, energy production	Meats, seafood, nuts, grains	900 mcg	900 mcg	10,000 mcg
Fluoride	Bone and teeth growth	Fluoridated drinking water, fish, milk	4 mg*	3 mg*	10 mg
Iodine	Thyroid hormone formation	Iodized salt, seafood	150 mcg	150 mcg	1,100 mcg
Iron	O_2 transport in red blood cells, enzyme function	Red meat, liver, eggs, beans, leafy vegetables, shellfish	8 mg	18 mg	45 mg
Manganese	Enzyme function	Whole grains, nuts, fruits, vegetables	2.3 mg*	1.8 mg*	11 mg
Molybdenum	Energy metabolism	Whole grains, organ meats, peas, beans	45 mcg	45 mcg	2,000 mcg
Selenium	Works with vitamin E	Meat, fish, whole grains, eggs	55 mcg	55 mcg	400 mcg
Zinc	Enzyme function, growth	Meat, shellfish, yeast, whole grains	11 mg	8 mg	40 mg

[a]Values are recommended daily allowance (RDA) for adults ages 19 to 50, unless marked with an asterisk. The requirements may vary for children, older adults, and pregnant or lactating women.

[b]Tolerable UL for adults aged 19 to 50. Intakes above the UL may lead to negative health consequences.

[c]Refers to pharmacological agents only and not to amounts contained in food and water. No evidence of ill effects from ingesting naturally occurring amounts in food and water.

*Values are AIs, indicating that sufficient data to set the RDA are unavailable.

ND = not yet determined

Adapted from Franks and Howley (1998); National Institutes of Health (n.d.).

with higher values for older adults and adolescents. Milk, dark green vegetables, and nuts are excellent sources of calcium. One cup (8 fluid ounces or 237 milliliters) of 1% milk has approximately 300 milligrams of calcium, which is almost one-third of the daily recommendation for a young adult (22, 35). See table 5.4 for daily calcium intake guidelines. Additional information on osteoporosis is found in chapter 21.

Iron is another mineral that is often underconsumed by Americans, and is a common nutrient deficiency in

the United States (35). In addition, getting adequate dietary iron is a concern in child and vegetarian or vegan athletes (3). In addition to being a critical component of hemoglobin and myoglobin, iron is necessary for the functioning of the immune system, the formation of brain neurotransmitters, and the functioning of the electron transport chain. The oxygen-carrying properties of hemoglobin depend on iron. There is a continual turnover of red blood cells in the body, and much of the iron used to form new hemoglobin comes from old red

Table 5.4 Guidelines for Daily Calcium Intake

Age	RDA (mg)
0-6 months	200*
7-12 months	260*
1-3 years	700
4-8 years	1,000
9-18 years	1,300
19-50 years	1,000
51-70 years men	1,000
51-70 years women	1,200
71 years and older	1,200
Pregnant or lactating 18 years or younger	1,300
Pregnant or lactating 19 years or older	1,000

*These values are AIs because insufficient evidence exists to clearly establish RDA for infants.

Data from National Institutes of Health (n.d.).

blood cells. However, iron is needed daily, and if iron reserves (liver, spleen, bone marrow) and intake are inadequate, hemoglobin cannot be formed and iron-deficiency anemia results. In this condition, the amount of hemoglobin in red blood cells falls, which decreases the capacity of the blood to transport oxygen (3, 35). The recommended intake of iron for males and postmenopausal women is 8 mg · day^{-1} (22). For females during the childbearing years, the recommended daily intake is 18 mg · day^{-1} (22). Red meat and eggs are excellent sources of heme iron. Additionally, spinach, lima and navy beans, and prune juice are excellent vegetarian sources of nonheme iron. Consuming vitamin C with meals increases the ability to absorb nonheme iron (3, 35).

Sodium, on the other hand, is a mineral that many Americans overconsume. High sodium intake has been linked with hypertension. The adult AI for sodium is 1,500 mg · day^{-1} (22). Adults should limit their daily sodium intake to no more than 2,300 mg · day^{-1} (13, 22, 31). People can reduce their sodium intake substantially by consuming fewer processed foods and adding less salt to foods when cooking.

Water

Water is considered an essential nutrient because of its vital role in the normal functioning of the body. It constitutes approximately 60% of the total body weight (13, 22, 35) and is essential in creating the environment in which all metabolic processes occur. Water is necessary to regulate temperature and transport substances throughout the body.

AI for total water is 3.7 L · day^{-1} for men and 2.7 L · day^{-1} for women (13, 22). Approximately 80% of this amount comes from beverages. As discussed later in this chapter, the amount needed for good health may be higher for individuals exercising intensely. Environmental conditions also can increase the need for water.

KEY POINT

Vitamins, minerals, and water do not provide energy but are essential to healthy functioning of the body. In general, most Americans would benefit from limiting sodium consumption (to decrease blood pressure) and getting recommended levels of calcium intake (to improve bone strength) and iron intake (to prevent anemia).

Focus on Antioxidant Vitamins

During metabolic processes, molecules or fragments of molecules form that can damage the body's tissues. These free radicals have at least one unpaired electron in their outer shells, and thus they are very chemically reactive. Lipid-rich cell membranes and DNA are highly susceptible to free radicals, and cell damage can occur when free radicals accumulate; for example, atherosclerosis is linked with free radicals. Some vitamins can react with free radicals and diminish the damage they cause. These antioxidant vitamins were hypothesized to counteract the effects of aging and decrease the likelihood of developing CVD and cancer. However, the scientific evidence finds that ingesting supplemental antioxidant vitamins does not play a prominent role in disease prevention, and in some cases negative side effects occur (20). For example, evidence suggests that high doses of beta-carotene (a precursor of vitamin A) may increase the risk of lung cancer in smokers, and high doses of vitamin E increase the risk of stroke and prostate cancer. However, studies continue to explore the potential health benefits and risks of these vitamins. Because of the toxic effects from an overdose of antioxidants, it is wise to avoid overconsuming these substances and stay within the established tolerable UL (22) (see table 5.2).

Examining Dietary Intake

The *Dietary Guidelines for Americans* (31) suggest engaging in regular physical activity and eating a balanced diet that contains the energy needed to achieve and sustain a healthy body weight. Keeping a food log (i.e., food diary or diet record) can help people reflect on their energy intake and eating habits. For this activity to yield valid results, the client should record everything that is consumed over a certain period of time. These records typically are kept for 3 to 4 days (with at least 1 day being a weekend day) and provide a general idea of a person's nutritional habits (3). Once the records are completed, several software packages are available to analyze the diet. A free USDA resource for analyzing one's diet, MyPlate, can be found at www.choosemyplate.gov (27). MyPlate provides dietary guidance based on factors such as age, sex, and level of activity. This guide is designed to help people choose foods that promote health and assist with achieving and maintaining a healthy weight. The MyPlate website allows the user to enter foods eaten and receive an analysis that compares them with recommended intake levels (26). This useful tool can help people determine whether they are in energy balance and consuming various foods and nutrients in healthy amounts.

Although food diaries provide important information, they come with limitations (2, 3, 35):

- People tend to underreport what they eat, whether intentional or due to lack of understanding of portion sizes.
- People do not keep records that are specific enough to provide quality information.
- People often temporarily change how they eat when they record their food intake.

The fitness professional can take steps to minimize these problems. First, make sure that clients understand the importance of completely and honestly recording what they eat. Emphasize to clients that the accuracy and usefulness of the food diary depend on the information provided. One of the most important results of completing a food record is that clients begin to become accountable for their food intake. By documenting the types and amounts of foods they eat, the clients begin to see for themselves opportunities to make healthier food choices. Additionally, provide clients with models or descriptions of how to accurately report food consumption. Providing explicit instructions will allow the client to create a more useful and accurate record. Additionally, the food diary should be user friendly and include cues to elicit complete responses. A sample food log with instructions is provided in form 5.1.

It also can be useful to examine the food diary for emotional or social cues to eating behaviors. For example, some people eat when depressed or only eat when alone. Such information can be helpful in making behavior

changes needed for weight loss and maintenance. More information on weight management is covered in chapter 20. It should be noted that analyzing a food record with general nutritional guidelines such as MyPlate or the *Dietary Guidelines for Americans* is acceptable in healthy clients. A more detailed nutrition assessment is the role of an RDN and requires a license to do so in many states. Similarly, a person trained and licensed in behavioral therapy or mental health may be required to be part of the care process if a significant relationship between mental challenges and food is observed. More on scope of practice is provided later in this chapter and in chapter 24.

KEY POINT

Accurate, detailed food diaries can be a useful tool in helping clients develop healthy dietary practices.

Recommendations for Dietary Intake

Dietary Guidelines for Americans, 2020-2025 (31) is a joint effort of the U.S. Department of Health and Human Services (HHS) and the U.S. Department of Agriculture (USDA). These recommendations can help people make healthy food choices, and they focus on lowering the risk of chronic disease and promoting health. The guidelines acknowledge the complex interaction of factors (personal, social, and environmental) that influence food consumption and identify a variety of healthy eating patterns that may be adopted. They point out common nutritional inadequacies and suggest ways to improve health outcomes through nutritional changes. For example, most Americans are too sedentary and weigh too much; thus, the guidelines suggest increasing physical activity and reducing calorie intake to a level that will lead to a healthy weight. The guidelines provide both general and specific recommendations. For instance, general recommendations include limiting consumption of added sugars and saturated fat. An example of a specific recommendation is to limit sodium consumption to <2,300 milligrams per day. A complete copy of *Dietary Guidelines for Americans* can be found using a simple Internet search engine. The 2020-2025 edition contains over 150 pages of nutrient recommendations and includes descriptive text of each nutrient recommendation, hyperlinks throughout the document that connect to related resources, and extensive appendices that are available for practical use (31).

These guidelines highlight nutrient recommendations for health promotion and disease prevention. Commonly, Americans underconsume some foods (i.e., fruits, veg-

FORM 5.1   Sample Food Log

INSTRUCTIONS

1. Record everything you eat, including foods and beverages eaten at meals and snacks.

2. Record carefully how the food was prepared. Be as descriptive as possible (e.g., "fried in corn oil" or "broiled in 1 tablespoon of margarine").

3. Be sure to indicate the amount of food eaten. Use typical household measures when possible (tsp = teaspoon; tbsp = tablespoon; c = cup; oz = ounce; g = gram).

4. Provide brand names and labels for packaged foods.

5. For composite foods such as sandwiches, casseroles, and soups, indicate the ingredients contained in the food. For example, a turkey sandwich might be described as "2 slices of whole-wheat bread, 1 oz of baked turkey breast without skin, 1 slice of tomato, 2 leaves of iceberg lettuce, and 1 tbsp light mayonnaise."

6. Indicate where and with whom you were when you ate. Describe your feelings at the time—were you worried, content, lonely, stressed, hungry? (Be honest.)

7. Carry this form with you so that you can write down foods as you eat them. Do not wait until the end of the day to record your food intake.

Food and drink	Description (e.g., amount, cooking method, brand name)	Location (e.g., place, with people or alone)	Feelings (e.g., hunger, anger, joy)	Time

etables, whole grains, calcium-containing foods) while overconsuming others (i.e., solid fat, added sugar, sodium-containing foods). See *Key Components of the Dietary Guidelines for Americans, 2020-2025*, which provides a summary of the four guidelines (31).

People can choose a variety of eating patterns to help achieve the goals set forward in the *Dietary Guidelines for Americans*. Table 5.5 outlines three viable approaches

to healthy eating: the Healthy U.S.-Style Eating Pattern, the Healthy Mediterranean-Style Eating Pattern, and the Healthy Vegetarian-Style Eating Pattern. The Healthy U.S.-Style Eating Pattern is based on the previously used USDA Food Patterns and the Dietary Approaches to Stop Hypertension (DASH) diet (21). This approach suggests daily amounts that people should consume from five major food groups (vegetables, fruits, grains,

Key Components of the Dietary Guidelines for Americans, 2020-2025

1. *Guideline 1.* Follow a Healthy Dietary Pattern at Every Life Stage
   - All food and beverage choices matter, and healthy eating can begin at any age.
   - Infants until about 6 months of age need to be fed human milk or iron-fortified infant formula if human milk is not available. Infants also need supplemental vitamin D as directed by their health care provider.
   - At the age of about 6 months, infants can be introduced to nutrient-dense foods. Introduce and encourage infants to consume a variety of foods from all food groups. Include foods rich in iron and zinc, particularly for infants who are fed human milk. Introduce potentially allergenic foods (one at a time) along with other complementary foods.
   - From 12 months through older adulthood, choose a healthy eating pattern at an appropriate energy level to help achieve and maintain a healthy body weight, support nutrient adequacy, and reduce the risk of chronic disease.

2. *Guideline 2.* Customize and Enjoy Food and Beverage Choices to Reflect Personal Preferences, Cultural Traditions, and Budgetary Considerations

   Individuals from all races, ages, and ethnicities can benefit from a healthy dietary intake. Consideration of cultural and personal preferences make these healthier dietary patterns easier to accomplish and maintain. The *Dietary Guidelines for Americans* includes some customization to address individual and diverse cultural needs and preferences in the United States.

3. *Guideline 3.* Focus on Meeting Food Group Needs With Nutrient-Dense Foods and Beverages, and Stay Within Calorie Limits

   Nutrient-dense foods provide energy nutrients, vitamins, minerals, and other health-promoting components and are limited in added sugars, saturated fat, and sodium. A healthy dietary pattern contains a variety of nutrient-dense foods from all or most food groups in proper amounts to meet nutrient needs while not exceeding energy requirements.

   A healthy dietary pattern includes these in the regular diet:
   - Vegetables of all types—dark green, red and orange, starchy, and other vegetables; beans, peas, and lentils
   - Fruits, especially whole fruit
   - Grains, at least half of which are whole grain
   - Dairy, including fat-free or low-fat milk, yogurt, and cheese, and/or lactose-free versions and fortified soy beverages and yogurt as alternatives
   - Protein foods, including lean meats, poultry, and eggs; seafood; beans, peas, and lentils; and nuts, seeds, and soy products
   - Oils, including vegetable oils and oils in food, such as seafood and nuts

4. *Guideline 4.* Limit Foods and Beverages Higher in Added Sugars, Saturated Fat, and Sodium, and Limit Alcoholic Beverages

   At most stages of life, it's a challenge to only meet nutrient needs with healthy foods and not consume an excess of foods that may taste good and are energy-dense. In order to maintain energy balance, there is not much room in the health dietary pattern for extra added sugars, saturated fat, sodium, or alcoholic beverages. A small amount of these can be included in the healthy dietary pattern, but larger quantities or regular consumption of these foods and beverages should be limited. The guidelines follow:
   - *Added sugars:* Less than 10% of calories per day starting at age 2. Avoid foods and beverages with added sugars for those younger than age 2.

(continued)

Key Components of the *Dietary Guidelines for Americans, 2020-2025* (continued)

- *Saturated fat:* Less than 10% of calories per day starting at age 2.
- *Sodium:* Less than 2,300 milligrams per day—and even less for children younger than age 14.
- *Alcoholic beverages:* Adults of legal drinking age can choose not to drink or to drink in moderation by limiting intake to 2 drinks or less in a day for men and 1 drink or less in a day for women, when alcohol is consumed. Drinking less is better for health than drinking more. Some adults should not drink alcohol, such as women who are pregnant.

Adapted from U.S. Department of Health and Human Services and U.S. Department of Agriculture (2020).

Table 5.5 Comparison of Healthy Eating Patterns*

Food group	Healthy U.S.-Style Eating Pattern	Healthy Vegetarian-Style Eating Pattern	Healthy Mediterranean-Style Eating Pattern
Fruits (cup)	2/day	2/day	2.5/day
Vegetables (cup)	2.5/day	2.5/day	2.5/day
Dark green	1.5/week	1.5/week	1.5/week
Red and orange	5.5/week	5.5/week	5.5/week
Starchy	5/week	5/week	5/week
Legumes	1.5/week	1.5/week	3-5/week
Other	4/week	4/week	4/week
Grains (oz)	6/day	6.5/day	6/day
Whole	≥3/day	3.5/day	3/day
Refined	≤3/day	3/day	3/day
Dairy (cup)	3/day	3/day	2/day
Protein (oz)	5.5/day	3.5/day	6.5/day
Meats (oz), poultry (oz), eggs (each)	26/week	3/week (eggs)	26/week
Seafood (oz)	8/week	—	15/week
Nuts, seeds (oz)	5/week or soy	7/week	5/week or soy
Soy products	5/week or nuts, seeds	8/week	5/week or nuts, seeds
Oils (g)	27/day	27/day	27/day
Limit on calories from other sources	240/day	250/day	240/day

*Average daily intake at or adjusted to a 2,000-calorie level.

From U.S. Department of Health and Human Services and U.S. Department of Agriculture (2020).

dairy products, and protein). These correspond with the five elements found in the MyPlate materials mentioned previously. Suggested limits on intake of certain products (e.g., solid fat) are also included. This plan is based on the established DRIs for nutrients and the *Dietary Guidelines for Americans*. It allows a great deal of flexibility in choosing foods and is adaptable to a vegetarian lifestyle.

The DASH diet was originally designed to help people control their blood pressure. This diet is characterized by sodium restriction; an emphasis on vegetables, fruits, low-fat milk products, whole grains, and lean proteins; and elimination or minimization of added sugars and processed meats and other foods. Scientific evidence strongly supports this dietary approach in reducing blood pressure and weight (21).

The Healthy Mediterranean-Style Eating Pattern has become popular in the United States in recent years. The pattern varies somewhat based on region but generally emphasizes grains (particularly whole grains), fruits, vegetables, olive oil, fish, and nuts. More monounsaturated fatty acids than saturated fatty acids are consumed in this pattern. Wine consumption with meals is also common. This eating pattern has been linked with a lower prevalence of CVD (31).

The FDA requires that most foods be labeled with nutrition information. These labels, titled Nutrition Facts (see figure 5.2), list the serving size, total calories, fat (including saturated and trans fat), cholesterol, sodium, carbohydrate (including dietary fiber and added sugar), protein, and vitamins and minerals contained in the food. Daily values (DV) are an important part of the label; they indicate the percentage of daily recommended levels of nutrients that are contained in a food. The DV inform the public about the nutritional content of food and are based on a daily intake of 2,000 kcal. The nutrition label contains the percentage of the recommended DV provided by nutrients found in the food. Nutrients listed as less than 5% of the DV would be a low source of the nutrient, while nutrients listed greater than 20% is a high source. For example, the suggested DV for potassium is 4.7 grams (4,700 milligrams); therefore, if a food contains 470 milligrams of potassium, it will constitute 10% of the recommended daily intake of potassium and be a good source of the nutrient. Additional information on food labels, including resources for health professionals, can be found by visiting the FDA website (33, 34).

KEY POINT

The *Dietary Guidelines for Americans* (31) encourage most people to eat fewer calories, be more active, and make wiser food choices. The Healthy U.S.-Style Eating Pattern, Healthy Mediterranean-Style Eating Pattern, and Healthy Vegetarian-Style Eating Pattern are approaches to healthy food consumption. Food labeling regulation allows consumers to evaluate the nutritional content of foods.

Diet, Exercise, and the Blood Lipid Profile

CVD is the leading cause of death in the United States. One of the primary risk factors for CVD is a poor blood lipid profile. Both diet and exercise can have a positive effect on this crucial risk factor.

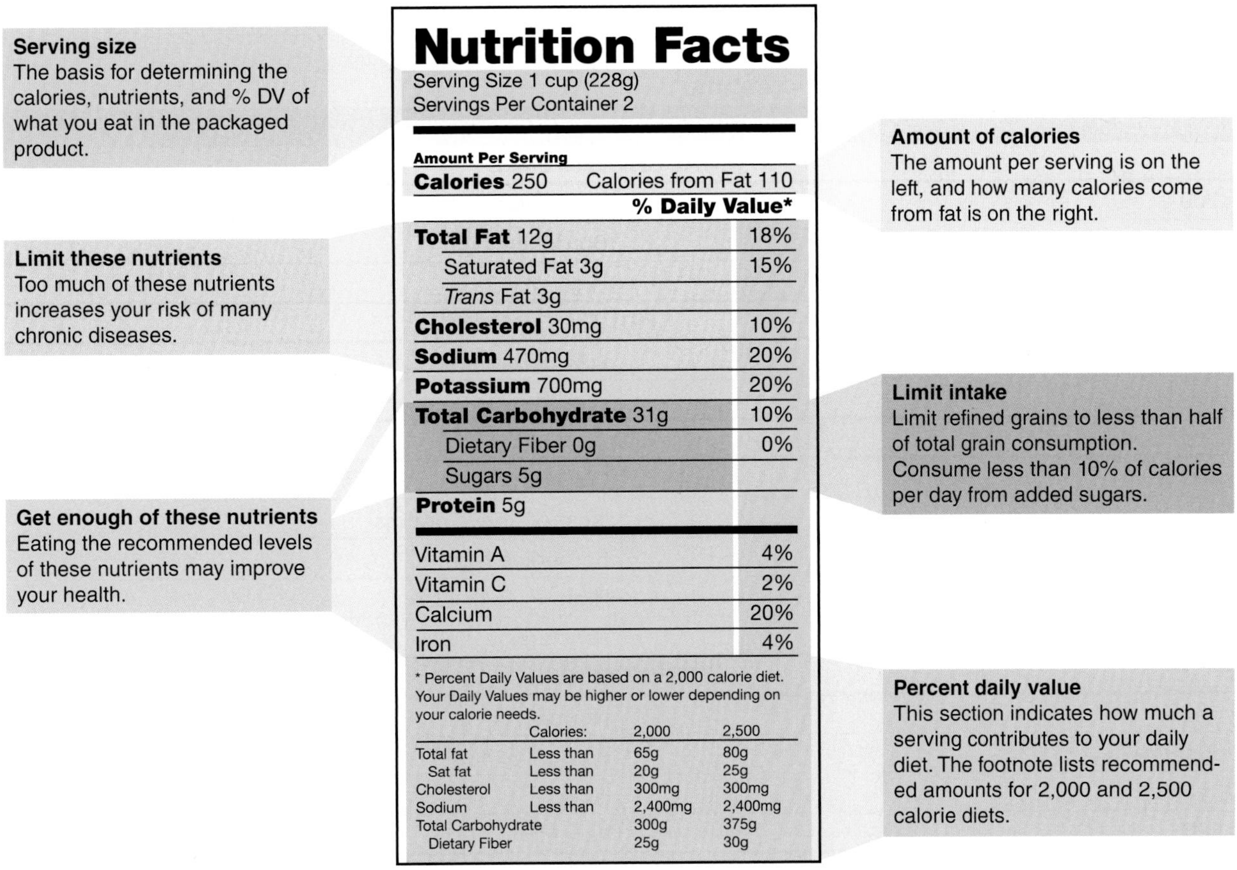

Serving size
The basis for determining the calories, nutrients, and % DV of what you eat in the packaged product.

Limit these nutrients
Too much of these nutrients increases your risk of many chronic diseases.

Get enough of these nutrients
Eating the recommended levels of these nutrients may improve your health.

Nutrition Facts

Serving Size 1 cup (228g)
Servings Per Container 2

Amount Per Serving	
Calories 250	Calories from Fat 110
	% Daily Value*
Total Fat 12g	18%
Saturated Fat 3g	15%
Trans Fat 3g	
Cholesterol 30mg	10%
Sodium 470mg	20%
Potassium 700mg	20%
Total Carbohydrate 31g	10%
Dietary Fiber 0g	0%
Sugars 5g	
Protein 5g	
Vitamin A	4%
Vitamin C	2%
Calcium	20%
Iron	4%

* Percent Daily Values are based on a 2,000 calorie diet. Your Daily Values may be higher or lower depending on your calorie needs.

	Calories:	2,000	2,500
Total fat	Less than	65g	80g
Sat fat	Less than	20g	25g
Cholesterol	Less than	300mg	300mg
Sodium	Less than	2,400mg	2,400mg
Total Carbohydrate		300g	375g
Dietary Fiber		25g	30g

Amount of calories
The amount per serving is on the left, and how many calories come from fat is on the right.

Limit intake
Limit refined grains to less than half of total grain consumption. Consume less than 10% of calories per day from added sugars.

Percent daily value
This section indicates how much a serving contributes to your daily diet. The footnote lists recommended amounts for 2,000 and 2,500 calorie diets.

FIGURE 5.2 Nutrition Facts label.

Based on Federal Food and Drug Administration.

Lipoproteins and Risk of Cardiovascular Disease

Because lipids are hydrophobic (i.e., not water soluble), they need to bind with some other substance to be transported in the blood. Lipoproteins are macromolecules composed of cholesterol, triglycerides, protein, and phospholipids. Classifications for these molecules are based on their size and makeup. The two classes of lipoproteins most closely linked with CVD are low-density lipoprotein (LDL) and high-density lipoprotein (HDL). LDL transports cholesterol and triglycerides from the liver to be used in various cellular processes. HDL retrieves cholesterol from the cells and returns it to the liver to be metabolized (5).

Elevated levels of total cholesterol (the sum of all forms of cholesterol) and low-density lipoprotein cholesterol (LDL-C) are linked with the development of atherosclerotic plaque in the arteries. Increased levels of high-density lipoprotein cholesterol (HDL-C) help prevent the atherosclerotic process. Heart-healthy guidelines for blood lipid values are total cholesterol levels below 200 mg · dl^{-1}, LDL-C values below 100 mg · dl^{-1}, and HDL values greater than 60 mg · dl^{-1}. Total cholesterol levels of 240 mg · dl^{-1} or higher, LDL-C values of 160 mg · dl^{-1} or higher, and HDL levels less than 40 mg · dl^{-1} in males and 50 mg · dl^{-1} in females are associated with greater risk of CVD (see table 5.6) (5).

Effects of Diet and Exercise on the Blood Lipid Profile

Consuming a diet low in saturated fat and cholesterol, losing weight, and participating in regular aerobic exercise all have been linked to positive changes in the blood lipid profile. The *2021 Dietary Guidance to Improve Cardiovascular Health: A Scientific Statement from the American Heart Association* (17) provides evidence-based dietary pattern guidance to promote cardiovascular health. The key recommendations include the following:

- Achieve and maintain a healthy body weight by adjusting energy intake and expenditure.
- Eat several servings and a variety of fruits and vegetables each day.
- Choose whole-grain foods and products over those that are processed.
- Choose healthy protein sources primarily from plants, fish, and seafood; low-fat or fat-free dairy products; and lean, unprocessed cuts of meat or poultry, if desired.
- Choose liquid plant oils instead of tropical oils and partially hydrogenated fats.
- Choose minimally processed foods instead of ultra-processed foods.

Table 5.6   Blood Lipid Classifications

Lipid level	Level rating
TOTAL CHOLESTEROL	
<200	Desirable
200-239	Borderline high
≥240	High
HDL-C	
<40 for males and <50 for females	Low/undesirable
≥60	High/desirable
LDL-C	
<100	Optimal
100-129	Near or above optimal
130-159	Borderline high
160-189	High
≥190	Very high
TRIGLYCERIDES	
<150	Normal
150-199	Borderline high
200-499	High
≥500	Very high

All values are mg · dl^{-1}.

Adapted from Johns Hopkins Medicine Lipid Panel (2022). Available: https://www.hopkinsmedicine.org/health/treatment-tests-and-therapies/lipid-panel#:~:text=Normal%3A%20Less%20than%20200%20mg,or%20above%20240%20mg%2FdL.

- Minimize the intake of foods and beverages containing added sugars.
- Choose prepared foods and cook with little or no salt.
- For those who drink alcohol, limit intake, and for those who do not drink alcohol, do not start.
- Apply these guidelines regularly wherever food is consumed.

Getting clients to adhere to these guidelines is a challenge because many factors contribute to dietary choices. More specific dietary guidelines for intake of saturated fat, trans fat, and cholesterol include the following:

- Limit total fat intake to 25% to 35% of total daily energy intake; if at the higher end of the range, care should be taken to ensure that most of the fat consumed comes from monounsaturated sources.
- Limit saturated fat intake to less than 10% of total kcal; this may be lower for someone with existing cardiovascular disease.
- Consume as little trans fat and dietary cholesterol as possible.

Consuming certain types of fat, such as omega-3 fatty acids, appears to benefit health. Omega-3 fatty acids are not abundant in the diet but are found in canola oil as well as in fish such as salmon and tuna. Omega-3 fatty acids are a polyunsaturated fat that get their name from the site of the first double bond in the fatty acid chain. American diets are typically low in omega-3 fatty acids and higher in omega-6 fatty acids (e.g., peanut, corn, and soybean oils), which are abundant in the diet. Bringing the intake of these two types of fat into better balance appears to improve the lipoprotein profile and lower the risk of CVD (25).

The Centers for Disease Control and Prevention recommends regular physical activity because it can help maintain a healthy weight and lower blood pressure, blood cholesterol, and blood glucose levels. The Surgeon General recommends 2 hours and 30 minutes of moderate-intensity exercise weekly for adults. Examples of moderate-intensity activity include brisk walking or bicycling. Children and adolescents should achieve a daily physical activity level of 1 hour (9).

KEY POINT

Elevated total cholesterol and LDL-C and depressed HDL-C are risk factors for CVD. Aerobic exercise; weight loss; and low intake of saturated fat, trans fat, and cholesterol improve the blood lipid profile. A balanced diet containing adequate amounts of omega-3 fatty acids also may have cardio-protective benefits.

Nutrition for Physically Active Individuals

Nutrition plays an important role in health, and it is also essential for optimal performance during physical activity. The *Position of the Academy of Nutrition and Dietetics, Dietitians of Canada, and the American College of Sports Medicine: Nutrition and Athletic Performance* (24) is a valuable resource on this topic coupled with the *ACSM Position Stand on Exercise and Fluid Replacement* (23). Fitness professionals should be familiar with these guidelines when working with athletes and active individuals. Remember that these are general guidelines and do not replace the individualized approach used by RDNs and, more importantly, those nutrition professionals who hold the Certified Specialist in Sports Dietetics (CSSD) advanced practice credential (10).

Hydration Before, During, and After Exercise

Sweating is the primary mechanism for heat dissipation during exercise. The amount of sweat lost during exer-

Focus on Trans Fat

Recent attention has focused on the health risks of trans-fatty acids (i.e., trans fat). Although small amounts of trans fat are found in animal products, the majority of this hydrogenated fat is found in processed foods produced from fat in plants. The hydrogenation process chemically transforms the spatial orientation of hydrogen atoms in the fat. This hardens the liquid plant oil and leads to a more stable product that is better suited for cooking. Consequently, many processed foods (e.g., cookies, chips, doughnuts, fries) can be prepared with trans fat. Foods high in trans fat have partially hydrogenated vegetable oils as a primary ingredient on their food label. The problem with trans fat is that, as saturated fat, it elevates LDL-C and lowers HDL-C; therefore, it should be avoided in order to improve the lipid profile (17, 31). When choosing a food containing a Nutrition Facts label, the amount of trans fat is required to be listed (32, 34).

cise depends on environmental heat and humidity, the type and intensity of exercise, and the characteristics of the exerciser. Dehydration reduces the capacity for sweating and can impair performance by decreasing strength, endurance, and coordination. As little as 2% to 3% of body weight loss due to fluid losses can impair performance. In addition, dehydration increases the risk of heat cramps, heat exhaustion, and heatstroke (see chapter 23).

Athletes and active individuals should consume 5 to 7 ml · kg^{-1} body weight of water or a sport beverage at least 4 hours prior to competition or activity (3, 23, 24). If this fluid consumption does not yield urine output (or urine is dark), additional water (3-5 ml · kg^{-1}) should be consumed 2 hours before the event (23). Fluid replacement during exercise is essential in activities that last an hour or longer, especially if they take place in hot, humid environments. Preventing excessive dehydration (>2% of body weight) should be the goal during exercise (practice or competition). Sweat rates vary dramatically based on environmental conditions, intensity of exercise, and individual characteristics; thus, fluid consumption must be based on each specific case. Consuming 400 to 800 milliliters of water during endurance exercise is adequate for many people (23, 24).

In activities whereby large amounts of sweat are lost, fluid should be fully replaced. Weighing before and after these types of activities is recommended. The participant should drink approximately 16 to 24 fluid ounces (approximately 450-675 milliliters) of water for each pound (0.5 kilogram) of weight lost (23, 24). If body weight has not returned to normal in the following days, additional water should be consumed before resuming exercise.

Protein Intake for Active Individuals

Athletes and individuals who are training intensely may benefit from increasing their protein intake above the level recommended for a sedentary person (i.e., 0.8 g · kg^{-1}). An individual training intensively in primarily endurance activities may benefit from consuming 1.2 to 1.4 grams of protein per kilogram of body weight (g · kg^{-1}). For those engaging in high-intensity, high-volume resistance training, a protein intake of 1.6 to 2.0 g · kg^{-1} may be needed (24). To this point, most of the studies in this area have focused on male athletes, so less is known about the protein needs of female athletes.

Additional protein requirements should be met through food choices, not through supplements. An upper limit to the rate at which muscle mass can be increased exists; therefore, excessive protein intake (i.e., above the recommendations) does not enhance performance or increase muscle mass (24). Because intensively training individuals have a higher energy intake, a diet with the normal distribution of macronutrients typically contains adequate amounts of protein, so purposefully consuming additional protein is usually not necessary (24). However, timing and spacing of dietary protein is important to maximize skeletal muscle protein synthesis with resistance training. Spacing daily protein needs throughout the day is recommended over consuming all or most daily protein in one meal. After exercise it is recommended to consume 15 to 25 grams of high-quality protein to provide amino acids for exercise-induced protein synthesis (24).

Another issue that sometimes arises is the adequacy of protein intake for individuals consuming vegetarian and vegan diets. Because plant protein is not digested as well as animal protein, it is suggested that people who are vegetarian and vegan need 10% more protein than omnivores. Because of the unique nutritional needs and potential for deficiency in certain vitamins and minerals, the vegetarian or vegan should receive consultation from an RDN or CSSD (24).

Ergogenic Aids

The search for nutritional and pharmacological agents that improve performance has led to the marketing of numerous products as ergogenic aids. Some ergogenic aids are sold as dietary supplements, while others are categorized as legal or illegal drugs. Some of these products (e.g., bee pollen, brewer's yeast) provide no scientifically proven physiological advantage. Other products, such as caffeine, may improve performance in some instances (3, 8, 15, 24) and have been regulated by various sporting agencies such as the International Olympic Committee (IOC). Some ergogenic aids must be strictly avoided, such as anabolic steroids, because of severe and sometimes fatal side effects (3, 8, 15, 24). For more information on rules regarding the use of ergogenic aids during competition, the following organizations can provide up-to-date resources:

United States Anti-Doping Agency (www.usada.org) (30)

World Anti-Doping Agency (www.wada-ama.org) (36)

Supplements 411 (29)

Banned Substances Control Group (7)

Informed Choice (12)

When it comes to learning about the scientific efficacy and safety of a dietary supplement, it is critical to use reliable sources. A good starting point is to review the information in the *Position of the Academy of Nutrition and Dietetics, Dietitians of Canada, and the American College of Sports Medicine: Nutrition and Athletic Performance* (24) and the *IOC Consensus Statement: Dietary Supplements and the High-Performance Athlete* (18). These resources provide a summary of those sports supplements that have scientific support for use versus those lacking evidence or that are banned or unsafe for use.

The Australian Institute of Sport (AIS) created and published some guiding principles that are used in their

Sports Supplements Framework (6). They created an ABCD classification system that ranks sport foods and supplement ingredients into four groups. The scientific evidence is carefully evaluated and reviewed, and then sport foods and supplements are categorized by efficacy, safety, and other practical considerations for use of the product. The AIS emphasizes the importance of asking the following questions before considering using a sport supplement (6):

- Is it safe? Lack of scientific evidence of harm does not mean the product is safe. It might mean only that no research is available.
- Is it permitted in sport?
- Is there evidence that it works?

It is important to understand the answers to these questions before deciding to use a supplement. The resources mentioned previously can be searched to determine if a product or substance is permissible for use. In addition to the position papers referenced, it is important for the fitness professional to be able to complete a thorough peer-reviewed literature search and understand the available scientific evidence regarding safety and efficacy.

There is often confusion as to whether the DRIs for vitamins and minerals apply to athletes and highly active individuals. They often consume vitamins and minerals in amounts higher than the DRI in an attempt to improve performance. Unless an actual nutrient deficiency is occurring, no evidence exists that this practice enhances performance. However, individuals who regularly restrict energy intake, eliminate whole food groups, or consume a poor diet may need additional attention or supplementation in order to prevent adverse health and performance outcomes. While athletes do not necessarily need more

if the diet is adequate, iron, calcium, vitamin D, and antioxidants are the most common micronutrients of concern that should be assessed in this population (24).

KEY POINT

Adequate hydration is essential to performance. Water should be consumed before, during, and after extended bouts of exercise. The typical protein RDA for adults (0.8 $g \cdot kg^{-1}$) is likely inadequate for athletes or those who train intensely. People who are training intensely should consume 1.2 to 2.0 $g \cdot kg^{-1}$ body weight. Ergogenic aids are pharmacological or nutritional agents thought to improve performance. Although some products may enhance performance, many highly touted products have no proven results. In healthy, well-nourished people, extra vitamins and minerals (i.e., above the RDA) do not improve performance.

Daily Carbohydrate Recommendations and Carbohydrate Loading

Adequate intake of carbohydrate is necessary for optimal performance in endurance events. Glucose is the major source of energy during moderate- to higher-intensity exercise; when blood glucose levels decline, the ability to continue exercise is limited. A physically active person should routinely consume daily carbohydrate in the range of 3.0 to 12.0 $g \cdot kg^{-1}$ body weight. This range of carbohydrate intake is broad and can be categorized as follows (24):

APPLICATION POINT

Practical Questions to Consider When Thinking About Taking a Dietary or Sport Supplement

Does the product contain proprietary ingredients? If the name of the compound is unknown, it cannot be evaluated.

How are words used? *Natural* does not always mean the product is safe.

Is the purpose to correct a diagnosed nutrient deficiency? A supplement may or may not be the answer. Sometimes a nutrient deficiency can be corrected through medical nutrition therapy by a qualified RDN.

Do a product's claims sound too good to be true, exaggerated, or unrealistic? Searching and understanding the peer-reviewed science is important.

Are a product's claims only from testimonials? This is not scientific evidence.

Is the data lacking regarding a product's safety? No news is not always good news; maybe research has not been done.

- 3 to 5 g · kg^{-1} for low-intensity activities or skill-based athletes
- 5 to 7 g · kg^{-1} for moderate-intensity activity for about an hour per day
- 6 to 10 g · kg^{-1} for moderate- to high-intensity activity lasting 1 to 3 hours per day
- 8 to 12 g · kg^{-1} for moderate- to high-intensity activity lasting over 4 to 5 hours per day

Carbohydrate loading is used to maximize glycogen storage before competition. This practice is most beneficial for athletes who compete in events requiring continuous activity lasting longer than 90 minutes, such as marathon running, and should be implemented a few days before the event. The current recommendation and protocol for carbohydrate loading includes the following (24):

- *Day 1:* No training, with diet containing 10 to 12 g · kg^{-1} body weight
- *Day 2:* No training, with diet containing 10 to 12 g · kg^{-1} body weight
- *Day 3:* Event or competition day. Use existing carbohydrate intake guidelines for before, during, and after exercise.

Carbohydrate Recommendations Before, During, and After Exercise

In addition to the total daily carbohydrate intake goals, it is important to space out carbohydrate intake before, during, and after endurance exercise. These guidelines are most important in longer-duration activities of an hour or more. The more time before an event or activity, the more time to ingest a greater quantity of carbohydrate and allow for that meal to be digested. If only a short time is available to eat before an event (i.e., an early morning race), lower amounts of carbohydrate need to be consumed to optimize digestion and absorption. Immediately before exercise, the guidelines for carbohydrate intake are as follows:

- *1 hour before:* 1 g · kg^{-1} body weight
- *2 hours before:* 2 g · kg^{-1} body weight
- *3 hours before:* 3 g · kg^{-1} body weight
- *4 hours before:* 4 g · kg^{-1} body weight

During events that involve continuous vigorous activity, it is beneficial to consume easily absorbed forms of carbohydrate such as sport drinks, gels, or gummies. Note that if carbohydrate is consumed in the gel or gummy form, an adequate amount of water must be consumed to meet hydration needs. Carbohydrate beverage solutions or sport drinks are composed of a 6% to 8% carbohydrate solution, which is optimal for absorption. In addition, sport drinks have multiple forms of sugars for optimal digestion and absorption and contain electrolytes lost in sweat. The guidelines for carbohydrate ingestion during exercise include the following (24):

- *Exercise less than 45 minutes:* Generally, no carbohydrate intake is needed.
- *Endurance exercise lasting 1 to 2.5 hours:* Consume 30 to 60 grams per hour.
- *Endurance exercise lasting greater than 2.5 to 3 hours:* Consume up to 90 grams per hour. *Note:* At this level of carbohydrate intake, multiple forms of sugar/carbohydrate, as commonly found in sport drinks, must be used.

For endurance activities in which glycogen depletion occurs, it is important to restore those levels before competing or exercising again. For optimal glycogen resynthesis, the recommendation is to consume 1.0 to 1.2 g · kg^{-1} body weight for the first 4 hours after activity, then to resume eating to meet daily carbohydrate intake goals (24).

KEY POINT

Intake of adequate carbohydrate is necessary for optimal performance. Carbohydrate loading benefits extended bouts of exercise. Carbohydrate intake during vigorous-intensity exercise can be beneficial, especially when exercise lasts 60 minutes or more. Recovery carbohydrate intake guidelines are recommended if glycogen stores need to be replenished quickly for another exercise bout or event.

Suboptimal Energy Availability

The Female Athlete Triad is a condition characterized by disordered eating, menstrual dysfunction, and low bone mineral density (11). This concept has since evolved into a broader spectrum of complications associated with optimal energy availability for sport and exercise, menstrual status, and bone health (24). Energy availability (EA) is defined as total energy intake minus exercise energy expenditure normalized to fat-free mass (FFM). In addition to complications with bone health, additional endocrine, gastrointestinal, cardiovascular, musculoskeletal, hematological, immunological, renal, psychological, and neuropsychiatric consequences associated with low EA have been identified. Relative Energy Deficiency in Sport (RED-S) is a condition that includes all of these physiological consequences of low EA and extends to male and female athletes with or without disordered eating or eating disorders. The optimal EA is 45 kcal · kg^{-1} FFM per day. Individuals with an EA lower than this may suffer from physiological and psychological consequences that translate into impaired performance and poor health (19, 24). For additional information on RED-S as well as the Female and Male Athlete Triad, see chapter 16.

KEY POINT

Low EA can lead to serious health consequences. Individuals who exhibit signs of the Triad or RED-S should be referred to a medical team, including a CSSD, for evaluation and intervention.

Scope of Practice

The Academy of Nutrition and Dietetics (known simply as the Academy) (1) oversees the practice credential Registered Dietitian Nutritionist (RD or RDN). RD and RDN are interchangeable; RDN is used in this chapter. This credential is granted and governed by the Commission on Dietetic Registration (CDR) of the Academy (1) and requires education and supervised practice accredited by the Accreditation Council for Education in Nutrition and Dietetics of the Academy. For those interested in working with athletes and active individuals, an additional board certification beyond the RDN credential is available, the CSSD (10). The person holding the CSSD credential has specialized experience in sport dietetics, conducts an appropriate nutrition assessment, and uses the data to provide safe and effective nutrition interventions aimed at promoting health and optimizing performance (10).

Currently, 48 states, the District of Columbia, and Puerto Rico have enacted statutory provisions regulating the practice of nutrition and dietetics either through state licensure or statutory certification. Because nutrition and dietetics are regulated at the level of the state and state statutes can change with time, fitness professionals must understand the regulations in their area. The Academy provides current information for each state and territory, so it is important to check for updates regularly (1).

State licensure supersedes both registration and certification. Thus, in states with licensure, only those with a license can practice nutrition and dietetics. Fitness professionals must understand the local laws and understand their level of nutrition knowledge and skills before communicating information to the public (16). This does not mean that only RDNs can provide nutrition education. Other health professionals may provide nutrition education to the public as long as it is general, nonmedical nutrition information. Education should be limited to healthy individuals and based on sound scientific nutrition principles. Conducting a nutrition assessment and providing a nutrition intervention is considered dietetics, and licensure is required for this in certain states. Further, if working with a person with a disease or health-related condition, the assessment of nutrition status and nutrition intervention is considered medical nutrition therapy and should be reserved for the RDN.

It is important to consider what information fitness professionals can provide to clients who seek nutritional advice while staying within their scope of practice (16). The *Dietary Guidelines for Americans* (31) contain general nutrition information that can be shared with clients. Additionally, it is within the scope of practice for fitness professionals to suggest healthy recipes, provide information about nutrients and their role in good health, and provide general, nonmedical nutrition information based on established guidelines such as those found in the *Dietary Guidelines for Americans* (31) and interactive systems such as MyPlate (27). Kruskall and colleagues (16) provide an overview of the scope of practice for fitness professionals and RDNs. Fitness professionals can serve an important role in helping clients think critically about what and how much they eat, with an ultimate goal of encouraging clients to make healthier food choices. Clients with special metabolic conditions such as diabetes mellitus should always be referred to an RDN for a nutrition assessment and subsequent intervention plan.

LEARNING AIDS

REVIEW QUESTIONS

1. What three nutrients provide energy for the body? How many calories result from the breakdown of each gram of these nutrients?

2. What is the AMDR for carbohydrate, protein, and fat?

3. What is the DRI for dietary fiber? How does this compare to the typical American intake?

4. What are trans-fatty acids? Why should they be avoided?

5. What is the RDA for iron for women of childbearing age? For men?

6. What nutrients do Americans typically overconsume? Underconsume?

7. What are desirable values of HDL-C, LDL-C, and total cholesterol?

8. What are general recommendations regarding fluid intake during exercise?

9. What is the amount of protein needed for intense endurance training? For strength training?

10. What are general recommendations to ensure adequate glycogen storage before competition?

11. What is RED-S?

12. Why is scope of practice important?

CASE STUDIES

1. A male college basketball player who weighs 190 pounds (86.4 kilograms) with a protein intake of 190 grams per day is considering additional protein supplements. Is his protein intake adequate? Would you recommend that he increase his protein intake?

2. Mr. Flanagan, a healthy 35-year-old male, recently became your client for fitness training. He is gradually improving his fitness and is becoming more interested in his overall wellness. He is beginning to ask questions about how he should eat. What advice do you provide to Mr. Flanagan?

3. Mrs. Ortez is an obese 55-year-old female with type 2 diabetes. She recently received physician clearance to join your fitness center. Her goals are to become regularly active, lose weight, and manage her diabetes with as little medication as possible. What dietary advice, if any, do you provide to Mrs. Ortez?

Answers to Case Studies

1. This athlete weighs 86.4 kilograms. The *Position of the Academy of Nutrition and Dietetics, Dietitians of Canada, and the American College of Sports Medicine: Nutrition and Athletic Performance* (24) recommends a maximum of 2.0 grams of protein for each kilogram of body weight. This athlete is consuming approximately 2.2 $g \cdot kg^{-1}$ (190 ÷ 86.4). Additional protein intake appears unwarranted. If the athlete is unable to maintain weight, endurance, or strength with his current eating habits, an RDN or CSSD should be consulted.

2. Mr. Flanagan is asking important questions about his overall wellness, and as a fitness professional, you are positioned to help him in several ways. First, point out to Mr. Flanagan the general recommendations contained in the *Dietary Guidelines for Americans* (31), which outline healthy eating practices that Americans should incorporate into their daily lives. Second, encourage Mr. Flanagan to begin tracking his dietary habits (see form 5.1). Tell him about the MyPlate website (27), and encourage him to examine how his food intake matches recommended levels. Third, provide Mr. Flanagan with recipes for healthy and easy-to-cook meals.

3. Because Mrs. Ortez has a metabolic disease, type 2 diabetes, it is important that she seek out advice from a number of medical professionals, including her physician and an RDN. However, as a fitness professional, you are a critical member of her overall wellness team. Here are things that you should do:

   • Encourage Mrs. Ortez to carefully follow the instructions of her physician regarding medications, weight loss, and any exercise limitations.

   • Encourage Mrs. Ortez to consult an RDN for a nutrition assessment and individualized nutrition intervention to help manage her diabetes.

   • Provide general recommendations from the *Dietary Guidelines for Americans* about healthy eating habits, but emphasize that these guidelines are not the medical nutrition therapy needed to manage her diabetes.

   • Provide examples of easy, low-calorie recipes.

   • Help her track her progress with exercise goals and weight loss, and monitor her response to exercise for any unhealthy signs.

6

Energy Costs of Physical Activity

Barbara A. Bushman

OBJECTIVES

The reader will be able to do the following:

1. Describe how measurements of oxygen consumption ($\dot{V}O_2$) can be used to estimate energy production, and list the number of calories derived per liter of oxygen (O_2) and per gram of carbohydrate, fat, and protein

2. Express energy expenditure as $L \cdot min^{-1}$, $kcal \cdot min^{-1}$, $ml \cdot kg^{-1} \cdot min^{-1}$, METs, and $kcal \cdot kg^{-1} \cdot hr^{-1}$

3. Estimate the oxygen cost of walking and running, including the cost of walking and running 1 mile (1.6 kilometers)

4. Estimate the oxygen cost of cycle ergometry for both arm and leg work

5. Estimate the oxygen cost of bench stepping

6. Identify the approximate energy cost of recreational activities, sport, and other activities, and describe the effect of environmental factors on the heart rate response to a fixed work rate

6

False promises about high energy expenditure often are used to lure people into joining a fitness program or buying a piece of exercise equipment. How can fitness professionals provide accurate insights for clients on what is real and what is not regarding energy expenditure? This chapter provides the background and examples to help answer those questions.

Measuring Energy Expenditure

The most common way to measure energy expenditure is indirect calorimetry. In this procedure, oxygen consumption ($\dot{V}O_2$), also referred to as oxygen uptake, is measured and energy expenditure is calculated using conversion factors. These factors (constants) are derived in a two-step process:

1. First, bomb calorimeter measurements reveal that the heat given off from the combustion of carbohydrate, fat, and protein yields approximately 4.0, 9.0, and 5.6 kcal of heat per gram, respectively. Because the nitrogen in protein cannot be completely oxidized in the body and is excreted as urea, the physiological value for protein is actually 4.0 kcal · g^{-1}.

2. Knowing how much oxygen is required to oxidize 1 gram of carbohydrate, fat, and protein allows one to calculate the number of calories of energy produced per liter of O_2 consumed. This is the caloric equivalent of oxygen. Values for carbohydrate, fat, and protein are listed in table 6.1.

Table 6.1 Measurements Associated With Oxidation of Carbohydrate, Fat, and Protein

Measurement	Carbohydrate	Fat	Protein*
Caloric density (kcal · g^{-1})	4.0	9.0	4.0
Caloric equivalent of 1 L of O_2 (kcal · L^{-1})	5.0	4.7	4.5
Respiratory quotient	1.0	0.7	0.8

*Does not include energy derived from the oxidation of nitrogen in the amino acids because the body excretes this as urea.

Based on Koebel (1984).

As shown in the table, carbohydrate gives about 6% more energy per liter of O_2 than fat gives (5.0 versus 4.7 kcal · L^{-1}), whereas fat gives more than twice as much energy per gram than carbohydrate gives (9 versus 4 kcal · g^{-1}). If a person is deriving energy from a 50–50 mixture of carbohydrate and fat during exercise, the caloric equivalent is approximately 4.85 kcal · L^{-1}, halfway between the value of 4.7 for fat and 5.0 for carbohydrate (22). The ratio of carbon dioxide produced to oxygen consumed at the cell is called the *respiratory quotient* (*RQ*). The same ratio, when measured by conventional gas exchange procedures, is called the *respiratory exchange ratio* (*R*) and is used to indicate fuel use (carbohydrate versus fat) during steady-state exercise (see chapter 4).

▶ **VIDEO** Watch video 6.1, which demonstrates measuring oxygen consumption.

KEY POINT

Oxygen consumption ($\dot{V}O_2$) can provide a measure of how much energy (calories) is produced by the body. The bomb calorimeter provides the number of calories gained per gram of food: 4 kcal · g^{-1} for carbohydrate, 9 kcal · g^{-1} for fat, and 4 kcal · g^{-1} for protein. Knowing how much oxygen is used to metabolize the food, 4.7 kcal · L^{-1} is obtained when fat is oxidized and 5.0 kcal · L^{-1} is obtained when carbohydrate is oxidized. When a 50–50 mixture of carbohydrate and fat is used for energy, 4.85 kcal · L^{-1} is obtained. However, for simplicity, a value of 5.0 kcal · L^{-1} may be used to convert oxygen uptake to kcal, with little loss of accuracy.

RESEARCH INSIGHT

Accuracy of Wearable Fitness Trackers

Pedometers use simple technology to track the number of steps taken and the total distance moved throughout the day. Accelerometer-based devices are used in research as well as in consumer-based activity trackers, also referred to as *wearable technology*. These devices track both steps and the intensity of activities to generate an estimate of energy expenditure, and they have a myriad of other features related to measuring heart rate (HR), monitoring sleep patterns, and estimating oxygen consumption. Questions remain on accuracy of information gathered by consumer-based activity trackers (23, 30). HR measures have been found to be both reliable and accurate, although wrist-worn devices may present challenges given the need to ensure the sensor is clean and is adequately secured. Accuracy of wearable devices to determine step count has been studied with both overestimation and underestimation found in activities of daily living. Estimation of energy expenditure via wearable technology has been found to be reliable but with poor validity. Several factors may affect validity, including difficulty in accounting for type and intensity of exercise and individual variation (e.g., body size and composition, energy balance, activity status). Thus, care should be taken in relying on individual values generated for fitness training; examining data trends over time may hold value (30). Research will continue in this area, and the fitness professional will benefit from remaining current with the continually unfolding technology.

Expressing Energy Expenditure

The energy requirement for an activity is calculated from the participant's steady-state oxygen uptake measured during an activity. Once the individual reaches steady-state oxygen uptake, the energy (ATP) supplied to the muscles is derived from aerobic metabolism. (See chapter 4 for more information on steady-state oxygen uptake.) The measured oxygen uptake then can be used to express energy expenditure in several ways. The five most common expressions follow.

1. $\dot{V}O_2$ *(L $\cdot$ min^{-1})*. The calculation of oxygen uptake yields a value expressed in liters of O_2 used per minute, sometimes called the *absolute* $\dot{V}O_2$. For example, the following data were collected for a man with a body weight of 80 kilograms performing a submaximal run on a treadmill. (*Note:* STPD refers to standardizing temperature, barometric pressure, and water vapor pressure: "standard temperature and pressure, dry.")

$$\text{Ventilation (STPD)} = 60 \text{ L} \cdot \text{min}^{-1}, \text{ inspired } O_2 = 20.93\%, \text{ and expired } O_2 = 16.93\%;$$
$$\text{and } \dot{V}O_2 (\text{L} \cdot \text{min}^{-1}) = 60 \text{ L} \cdot \text{min}^{-1} \times (20.93\% \text{ } O_2 - 16.93\% \text{ } O_2) = 2.4 \text{ L} \cdot \text{min}^{-1}$$

2. *Kilocalories per minute (kcal $\cdot$ min^{-1})*. Oxygen uptake can be expressed in kcal used per minute. The caloric equivalent of 1 liter of O_2 ranges from 4.7 kcal $\cdot$ L^{-1} for fat to 5.0 kcal $\cdot$ L^{-1} for carbohydrate. For practical purposes, 5.0 kcal per liter of O_2 is used to convert the oxygen uptake to kcal per minute. Energy expenditure is calculated by multiplying the kcal expended per minute (kcal $\cdot$ min^{-1}) by the duration of the activity in minutes. For example, if the 80-kilogram man mentioned previously ran on the treadmill for 30 minutes at a $\dot{V}O_2$ of 2.4 L $\cdot$ min^{-1}, the total energy expenditure can be calculated as follows:

$$\frac{2.4 \text{ L } O_2}{\text{min}} \times \frac{5 \text{ kcal}}{\text{L } O_2} = \frac{12 \text{ kcal}}{\text{min}}$$

$$\frac{12 \text{ kcal}}{\text{min}} \times 30 \text{ min} = 360 \text{ kcal}$$

3. $\dot{V}O_2$ *(ml $\cdot$ kg^{-1} $\cdot$ min^{-1})*. If the measured oxygen uptake, expressed in liters per minute, is multiplied by 1,000 to yield milliliters per minute and then divided by the individual's body weight in kilograms, the value is expressed in milliliters of O_2 per kilogram of body weight per

minute, or ml · kg^{-1} · min^{-1}. This expression, sometimes called the *relative* $\dot{V}O_2$, helps in comparing values for people of varying body sizes. See the following example for the 80-kilogram man with a $\dot{V}O_2$ of 2.4 L · min^{-1}:

$$\frac{2.4\,\text{L}}{\text{min}} \times \frac{1{,}000\,\text{ml}}{\text{L}} \div 80\,\text{kg} = 30\,\text{ml} \cdot \text{kg}^{-1} \cdot \text{min}^{-1}$$

4. *METs. MET* is a term used to describe a standard or reference resting metabolic rate. Actual resting metabolic rate varies and is less in females than in males and decreases with age (22). MET is taken, by convention, to be 3.5 ml · kg^{-1} · min^{-1}. This is called *1 MET*. Activities are expressed in terms of multiples of the MET unit, which is simply an alternative way of expressing oxygen uptake in ml · kg^{-1} · min^{-1}. For example, using the $\dot{V}O_2$ values presented previously in number 3, METs are calculated as follows:

$$30\,\text{ml} \cdot \text{kg}^{-1} \cdot \text{min}^{-1} \div 3.5\,\text{ml} \cdot \text{kg}^{-1} \cdot \text{min}^{-1} = 8.6\,\text{METs}$$

5. *Kilocalories per kilogram per hour (kcal · kg^{-1} · hr^{-1}).* The MET expression of energy expenditure carries a special bonus: It also indicates the number of calories the individual uses per kilogram of body weight per hour. In the example mentioned previously, the individual is working at 8.6 METs, or about 30 ml · kg^{-1} · min^{-1}. When this value is multiplied by 60 min · hr^{-1}, it equals 1,800 ml · kg^{-1} · hr^{-1}, or 1.8 L · kg^{-1} · hr^{-1}. Using the relationship described previously of 4.85 kcal per liter of O_2 (value assuming a 50–50 mix of carbohydrate and fat), the 1.8 is multiplied by 4.85 to give 8.7 kcal · kg^{-1} · hr^{-1}. The following steps show the details of this calculation. Given that the more general relationship of 5.0 kcal per liter of O_2 is often used, slight differences will occur (i.e., in this example if multiplying by 5.0 rather than 4.85, the result is 9.0 kcal · kg^{-1} · hr^{-1}).

$$8.6\,\text{METs} \times \frac{3.5\,\text{ml} \cdot \text{kg}^{-1} \cdot \text{min}^{-1}}{\text{MET}} = 30\,\text{ml} \cdot \text{kg}^{-1} \cdot \text{min}^{-1}$$

$$30\,\text{ml} \cdot \text{kg}^{-1} \cdot \text{min}^{-1} \times 60\,\text{min} \cdot \text{hr}^{-1} = 1{,}800\,\text{ml} \cdot \text{kg}^{-1} \cdot \text{hr}^{-1} = 1.8\,\text{L} \cdot \text{kg}^{-1} \cdot \text{hr}^{-1}$$

$$1.8\,\text{L} \cdot \text{kg}^{-1} \cdot \text{hr}^{-1} \times 4.85\,\text{kcal} \cdot \text{L}\,O_2^{-1} = 8.7\,\text{kcal} \cdot \text{kg}^{-1} \cdot \text{hr}^{-1}$$

As indicated in chapter 1, the volume of physical activity is linked to numerous health outcomes. The volume or amount of physical activity is easily calculated from the rate of energy expenditure and the duration of the activity. For example, if someone is exercising at an energy expenditure of 10 kcal · min^{-1} for 30 minutes, 300 kcal of energy are expended (10 × 30 = 300). The MET scale can also be used to calculate the volume of energy expenditure. If a person is exercising at 7 METs for 30 minutes, 210 MET-min of energy expenditure is accomplished (7 × 30 = 210). The *Physical Activity Guidelines for Americans* indicate that when people regularly accomplish 500 to 1,000 MET-min of physical activity per week, they realize substantial health benefits (32). In the case of the person working at 7 METs for 30-minute sessions, only three sessions a week would be needed to meet the low end of that physical activity range (3 × 210 = 630 MET-min), and five sessions (5 × 210 = 1,050 MET-min) would allow the person to reach the top end of the range. MET-min is helpful in examining total amount of activity over the course of a week that may be of varying types or intensity.

KEY POINT

Energy expenditure can be expressed in L · min^{-1}, kcal · min^{-1}, ml · kg^{-1} · min^{-1}, METs, and kcal · kg^{-1} · hr^{-1}:

- To convert L · min^{-1} to kcal · min^{-1}, multiply by 5.0 kcal · L^{-1}.
- To convert L · min^{-1} to ml · kg^{-1} · min^{-1}, multiply by 1,000 and divide by body weight in kilograms.
- To convert ml · kg^{-1} · min^{-1} to METs, divide by 3.5 ml · kg^{-1} · min^{-1}.
- To convert ml · kg^{-1} · min^{-1} to kcal · kg^{-1} · hr^{-1}, multiply by 60, divide by 1,000, and then multiply by 5.

Equations for Estimating
the Energy Cost of Activities

In the mid-1970s, the American College of Sports Medicine (ACSM) identified equations to estimate the steady-state energy requirement associated with common modes of activities, including walking, stepping, running, and cycle ergometry (3). Over the years, the equations have been modified to reflect the best information available, and this chapter discusses the current thinking in estimating energy costs (5). The oxygen uptake calculated from these equations is an estimate, and a typical standard deviation (SD) associated with the actual measured average value is about 10% (5, 12). Remember this normal variation in the energy costs of activities when using these equations in prescribing exercise.

The ACSM equations have been applied to graded exercise tests (GXTs) to estimate maximal aerobic power. This application gives reasonable estimates when the participants are healthy, and the rate at which the GXT progresses is slow enough to allow the individual to achieve steady-state oxygen uptake at each stage (27, 28). When the increments between the stages of the GXT are large or the person is somewhat unfit, oxygen uptake will not keep pace with each stage of the test. In these cases, the equations overestimate the actual measured oxygen uptake (20) because the equations are designed to estimate steady-state energy requirements. Thus, the recommendation is to not use these equations to calculate oxygen consumption during maximal tests, which by their nature are progressive and non-steady-state (5). For other available options, see the *Specialized Equations for Graded Exercise Tests* Research Insight.

When the ACSM equations were developed, an attempt was made to use a true physiological oxygen cost for each type of work. Each activity is broken down into the energy components. For example, in estimating the total oxygen cost of walking up a grade, the net oxygen cost of the horizontal walk (one component) is added to the net oxygen cost of the vertical (grade) walk (another component) and to the resting metabolic rate (final component), which is taken to be 1 MET ($3.5 \text{ ml} \cdot \text{kg}^{-1} \cdot \text{min}^{-1}$).

$$\text{Total O}_2 \text{ cost} = \text{net oxygen cost of activity} + 3.5 \text{ ml} \cdot \text{kg}^{-1} \cdot \text{min}^{-1}$$

For the equations to properly estimate the oxygen cost of the activity, the participant must follow instructions carefully (e.g., not hold on to the treadmill railing when walking or running, maintain the pedal cadence with leg or arm ergometry), and the work instruments (i.e., treadmill, cycle ergometer) must be calibrated so the settings are correct (see chapter 8).

RESEARCH INSIGHT

Specialized Equations for Graded Exercise Tests

All of the equations presented in this chapter estimate the energy cost of activities based on steady-state considerations. However, when a person completes a maximal GXT to volitional exhaustion (see chapter 8), they clearly are *not* in a steady state in the last stage of the test. When $\dot{V}O_2$max is estimated based on the steady-state equations, it is systematically higher than what is actually measured. To deal with this, investigators have developed unique equations for predicting $\dot{V}O_2$max for the treadmill (18) and cycle (31). Additionally, if the patient or client holds on to the treadmill railing during the test, the overestimation is even greater (17) because the patient is off-loading some of the work and can complete more stages of the test. Thus, investigators have developed specialized equations to account for holding on to the railing (26). An interesting approach was taken by Foster and colleagues (17) in which they used the steady-state equations (presented in this chapter) to predict the oxygen cost of the last stage of the treadmill test and then developed a prediction equation to estimate $\dot{V}O_2$max. It worked both for patients who held on to the treadmill railing and those who did not. Another example, specific to the standard Bruce treadmill protocol, requires only knowledge of the duration a client was able to continue before fatigue (18). This time (in minutes) is entered into the following equation to estimate $\dot{V}O_2$max:

$$\text{Estimated } \dot{V}O_2\text{max} = 14.8 - (1.379 \times \text{time}) + (0.451 \times \text{time}^2) - (0.012 \times \text{time}^3)$$

Energy Requirements of Walking, Running, Cycle Ergometry, and Stepping

The following sections provide equations to estimate the energy cost of walking, running, cycle ergometry, and stepping. These activities are common in adult fitness programs. Examples are provided to show how the equations are used in designing exercise programs.

Oxygen Cost of Walking

One of the most common activities in exercise programs and GXTs is walking. The oxygen cost of walking is determined by walking speed and whether the walker is on a horizontal or a graded surface. Prediction equations address these factors.

Walking Up a Grade

The following equation can be used to estimate the energy requirement between the walking speeds of 50 and 100 m · min^{-1}, or 1.9 and 3.7 mph. (Multiply miles per hour by 26.8 to obtain meters per minute. Divide meters per minute by 26.8 to obtain miles per hour.) The oxygen cost of walking up a grade is the sum of the oxygen cost of horizontal walking, the oxygen cost of the vertical component of walking on a grade, and the resting metabolic rate of 3.5 ml · kg^{-1} · min^{-1}. Dill (16) showed that the net cost of walking 1 m · min^{-1} on a horizontal surface is about 0.1 ml · kg^{-1} · min^{-1}. Studies have shown that the oxygen cost of moving (walking or stepping) 1 m · min^{-1} vertically is 1.8 ml · kg^{-1} · min^{-1} (9, 29). The vertical component (vertical velocity) is calculated by multiplying the grade (expressed as a fraction) times the speed in meters per minute. The equation for calculating the oxygen cost (ml · kg^{-1} · min^{-1}) of walking on a grade is as follows, with the 0.1 for the horizontal component and the 1.8 for the vertical component being constants (set values):

$$\dot{V}O_2 = (0.1 \text{ ml} \cdot \text{kg}^{-1} \cdot \text{min}^{-1} \times \text{horizontal velocity})$$
$$+ (1.8 \text{ ml} \cdot \text{kg}^{-1} \cdot \text{min}^{-1} \times \text{vertical velocity}) + 3.5 \text{ ml} \cdot \text{kg}^{-1} \cdot \text{min}^{-1}$$

QUESTION:

What is the total oxygen cost of walking 90 m · min^{-1} up a 12% grade?

ANSWER:

The horizontal component is calculated by multiplying the constant of 0.1 by the speed in m · min^{-1}. The vertical component is calculated by multiplying the constant of 1.8 by speed in m · min^{-1} by the grade expressed as a fraction. The following equations show how to calculate the total oxygen cost for walking 90 m · min^{-1} up a 12% grade. The first step is to write down the equation (simplified version without units of measure is shown), followed by filling in the information provided in the question, ensuring appropriate units of measure (speed must be in m · min^{-1} and grade expressed as a fraction):

$$\dot{V}O_2 = (0.1 \times \text{speed}) + (1.8 \times \text{speed} \times \text{grade}) + 3.5$$
$$\dot{V}O_2 = (0.1 \times 90) + (1.8 \times 90 \times 0.12) + 3.5 \text{ [multiply values within parentheses]}$$
$$\dot{V}O_2 = 9.0 + 19.44 + 3.5 \text{ [then add the three components]}$$
$$\dot{V}O_2 = 31.94 \text{ ml} \cdot \text{kg}^{-1} \cdot \text{min}^{-1}$$

By dividing by 3.5, the MET value can also be determined: 31.94 ÷ 3.5 = 9.1 METs.

The equations can be used to estimate the treadmill settings needed to elicit a specific oxygen uptake.

QUESTION:

How would the treadmill grade be set to achieve an energy requirement of 6 METs (21.0 ml · kg^{-1} · min^{-1}) when walking at 60 m · min^{-1}?

ANSWER:

The first step will be to write down the equation, and then fill in the information that is known.

$$\dot{V}O_2 = (0.1 \times \text{speed}) + (1.8 \times \text{speed} \times \text{grade}) + 3.5$$

Fill in the values that are known, including the oxygen cost ($\dot{V}O_2 = 21.0$ ml · kg⁻¹ · min⁻¹) and speed (60 m · min⁻¹):

$$21.0 = (0.1 \times 60) + (1.8 \times 60 \times \text{grade}) + 3.5$$

Then solve for grade by multiplying the values within the parentheses:

$$21.0 = (6.0) + (108 \times \text{grade}) + 3.5 \text{ [subtract 6 and 3.5 from both sides of the equation]}$$

$$11.5 = 108 \times \text{grade [divide both sides by 108]}$$

$$0.11 = \text{grade}$$

This fraction must be multiplied by 100 to convert to a percentage: $0.11 \times 100 = 11\%$.

Walking on a Level Surface

The equation for calculating the oxygen cost (ml · kg⁻¹ · min⁻¹) of walking on a flat surface is the same as for walking on a grade with the exception that no vertical component is included (as with a grade of 0%, the vertical component will calculate to be 0):

$$\dot{V}O_2 = (0.1 \text{ ml} \cdot \text{kg}^{-1} \cdot \text{min}^{-1} \times \text{horizontal velocity}) + 3.5 \text{ ml} \cdot \text{kg}^{-1} \cdot \text{min}^{-1}$$

QUESTION:

What are the estimated steady-state $\dot{V}O_2$ and METs for a walking speed of 90 m · min⁻¹ (3.4 mph)?

ANSWER:

The first step will be to write down the equation, and then fill in the information that is known, ensuring correct units of measure are used.

$$\dot{V}O_2 = (0.1 \times \text{speed}) + (1.8 \times \text{speed} \times \text{grade}) + 3.5$$

$$\dot{V}O_2 = (0.1 \times 90) + (1.8 \times 90 \times 0) + 3.5 \text{ [multiply values within parentheses,}$$
noting that the level treadmill is a grade of 0 and thus the vertical component is not a factor]

$$\dot{V}O_2 = (9.0) + (0) + 3.5 \text{ [add the values]}$$

$$\dot{V}O_2 = 12.5 \text{ ml} \cdot \text{kg}^{-1} \cdot \text{min}^{-1}$$

To determine METs, divide the 12.5 ml · kg⁻¹ · min⁻¹ by 3.5 to yield 3.6 METs.

The equations also can be used to predict the level of activity required to elicit a specific energy expenditure.

QUESTION:

A participant who is beginning an exercise program is told to exercise at 11.5 ml · kg⁻¹ · min⁻¹ to achieve the proper exercise intensity. What walking speed would be recommended with a level treadmill (no grade)?

ANSWER:

First write down the equation and insert the known values, ensuring correct units of measure.

$$\dot{V}O_2 = (0.1 \times \text{speed}) + (1.8 \times \text{speed} \times \text{grade}) + 3.5$$

$$11.5 = (0.1 \times \text{speed}) + (1.8 \times \text{speed} \times 0) + 3.5 \text{ [multiplying by 0 for the grade}$$
results in a value of 0 for the vertical component so it is no longer included]

$$11.5 = (0.1 \times \text{speed}) + 3.5 \text{ [subtract 3.5 from both sides of the equation]}$$

$$8 = (0.1 \times \text{speed}) \text{ [divide both sides by 0.1]}$$

$$80 = \text{speed}$$

The speed is in m · min⁻¹ and needs to be converted to miles per hour by dividing by 26.8. This results in a speed of 3.0 mph.

Walking at Various Speeds

The preceding equations are useful for walking speeds of 50 to 100 m · min⁻¹ (1.9-3.7 mph); beyond that, the oxygen requirement for walking has been found to increase in a curvilinear fashion (12). Other researchers have found the addition of height (measured in meters) to be important in predicting the oxygen consumption of walking on a level surface using the following equation (24). (Note that in this study $\dot{V}O_2$rest was assumed to be 3.3 ml · kg⁻¹ · min⁻¹; V is in m · s⁻¹, and Ht is in meters.)

$$\dot{V}O_2 \text{ in ml} \cdot \text{kg}^{-1} \cdot \text{min}^{-1} = \dot{V}O_2\text{rest} + 3.85 + (5.97 \times V^2 \div Ht)$$

One of the most common and useful ways to express the energy cost of walking is in kcal per minute. To determine the kcal · min⁻¹, convert the $\dot{V}O_2$ (in units of measure ml · kg⁻¹ · min⁻¹) to L · min⁻¹ by dividing by 1,000 and multiplying by body weight in kilograms. Then the relationship noted previously of 5.0 kcal per L O_2 can be used. For example, in the prior scenario of walking at 90 m · min⁻¹ (3.4 mph), the oxygen consumption was determined to be 12.5 ml · kg⁻¹ · min⁻¹, so for a 70-kilogram individual, this would be calculated as follows:

$$12.5 \div 1,000 \times 70 = 0.88 \text{ L} \cdot \text{min}^{-1}$$

$$0.88 \times 5.0 = 4.4 \text{ kcal} \cdot \text{min}^{-1}$$

Another method to determine kcal · min⁻¹ is to use METs. This is described in the sidebar *Using METs to Calculate Energy Costs.*

Oxygen Cost of Running

Running is common in fitness programs for apparently healthy people. It is possible to use the ACSM equations to estimate the oxygen cost of these activities for a broad range of speeds, generally from 130 to 350 m · min⁻¹ (equation is considered most accurate at speeds >134 m · min⁻¹ or 5 mph). The equations are also useful at speeds below 130 m · min⁻¹ as long as the person is actually running. The reality that a person can walk or run at speeds below 130 m · min⁻¹ complicates the issue. The oxygen cost of walking is less than that of running at slow speeds; however, at approximately 140 m · min⁻¹ (5.2 mph), the oxygen costs of running and walking are about the same. Above this speed, the oxygen cost of walking exceeds that of running (7).

Using METs to Calculate Energy Costs

MET values for activities can be used to estimate energy costs using the following simple equation (4):

$$\text{kcal} \cdot \text{min}^{-1} = (\text{METs} \times 3.5 \times \text{body weight in kg}) \div 200$$

For example, in the prior scenario of walking at 90 m · min⁻¹ (3.4 mph), the oxygen consumption was determined to be 12.5 ml · kg⁻¹ · min⁻¹, which equates to 3.6 METs. For a 70-kilogram individual, this would be calculated as follows. (Note that the 3.5 and 200 are constants in the equation.)

$$\text{kcal} \cdot \text{min}^{-1} = (3.6 \times 3.5 \times 70) \div 200$$

$$\text{kcal} \cdot \text{min}^{-1} = 4.4$$

If this individual walked at this speed for 30 minutes, the total caloric expenditure would be 132 kcal · min⁻¹.

How Body Weight Affects Energy Expenditure

Body weight is important when calculating how much energy a client may expend during exercise. A person weighing 220 pounds (100 kilograms) expends twice as many kcal per minute as a person weighing only 110 pounds (50 kilograms) when walking at the same speed. To reference the scenario of walking at 90 m · min^{-1} (3.4 mph), which was shown to require 3.6 METs, the kcal · min^{-1} for the two individuals would be calculated as follows:

For the individual weighing 100 kilograms:

$$\text{kcal} \cdot \text{min}^{-1} = (\text{METs} \times 3.5 \times \text{body weight in kg}) \div 200$$

$$\text{kcal} \cdot \text{min}^{-1} = (3.6 \times 3.5 \times 100) \div 200$$

$$\text{kcal} \cdot \text{min}^{-1} = 6.3$$

For the individual weighing 50 kilograms:

$$\text{kcal} \cdot \text{min}^{-1} = (\text{METs} \times 3.5 \times \text{body weight in kg}) \div 200$$

$$\text{kcal} \cdot \text{min}^{-1} = (3.6 \times 3.5 \times 50) \div 200$$

$$\text{kcal} \cdot \text{min}^{-1} = 3.15$$

Consequently, energy expenditure goals for clients in kcal will require a lighter person to exercise for a longer time compared with a heavier person. Consistent with that, as a client loses weight, the energy cost of walking at a given speed decreases because the energy cost depends on body weight. The participant can compensate for the lower energy cost by walking for a longer duration at that speed or by walking for the same duration at a higher speed.

Running Up a Grade

The net oxygen cost of running 1 m · min^{-1} on a horizontal surface is about twice that of walking, 0.2 ml · kg^{-1} · min^{-1} per m · min^{-1} (8, 11, 25). The equation gives reasonable estimates of the oxygen cost of running for the average person. However, it is well known that trained runners are more economical in terms of energy expenditure than the average person and that running economy varies within any group, trained or untrained (11, 15, 28). The oxygen cost of running up a grade is about half that of walking up a grade (10, 25). Some of the vertical lift associated with running on a flat surface is used to accomplish the grade work during inclined running, lowering the net oxygen requirement for the vertical work. The oxygen cost of running 1 m · min^{-1} vertically is about 0.9 ml · kg^{-1} · min^{-1}. As in the calculations for uphill walking, the vertical velocity is calculated by multiplying the fractional grade times the horizontal velocity. The following equation is used for calculating the oxygen cost of running up a grade.

$$\dot{V}O_2 = (0.2 \text{ ml} \cdot \text{kg}^{-1} \cdot \text{min}^{-1} \times \text{horizontal velocity})$$
$$+ (0.9 \text{ ml} \cdot \text{kg}^{-1} \cdot \text{min}^{-1} \times \text{vertical velocity}) + 3.5 \text{ ml} \cdot \text{kg}^{-1} \cdot \text{min}^{-1}$$

QUESTION:

What is the oxygen cost of running 150 m · min^{-1} (5.6 mph) up a 10% grade?

ANSWER:

The first step is to write down the equation. (A simplified version of the equation without units of measure is shown.)

$$\dot{V}O_2 = (0.2 \times \text{speed}) + (0.9 \times \text{speed} \times \text{grade}) + 3.5$$

Then fill in the information that is given in the question on speed and grade. Speed must be expressed in m · min^{-1} and the grade as a fraction (10% = 10 ÷ 100 = 0.10).

$$\dot{V}O_2 = (0.2 \times 150) + (0.9 \times 150 \times 0.10) + 3.5 \text{ [multiply values within parentheses]}$$

$$\dot{V}O_2 = (30) + (13.5) + 3.5 \text{ [add the three components together]}$$

$$\dot{V}O_2 = 47.0 \text{ ml} \cdot \text{kg}^{-1} \cdot \text{min}^{-1}$$

To determine METs, divide the 47.0 ml · kg^{-1} · min^{-1} by 3.5 to yield 13.4 METs.

QUESTION:

The oxygen cost of running 250 m · min^{-1} on a flat surface is about 53.5 ml · kg^{-1} · min^{-1}. What grade should be set on a treadmill for a speed of 200 m · min^{-1} to achieve the same $\dot{V}O_2$?

ANSWER:

First write down the equation for running:

$$\dot{V}O_2 = (0.2 \times \text{speed}) + (0.9 \times \text{speed} \times \text{grade}) + 3.5$$

Then, fill in the information provided in the question: $\dot{V}O_2$ is 53.5 ml · kg^{-1} · min^{-1}, and the speed selected is 200 m · min^{-1}.

$$53.5 = (0.2 \times 200) + (0.9 \times 200 \times \text{grade}) + 3.5 \text{ [multiply values within the parentheses]}$$

$$53.5 = (40) + (180 \times \text{grade}) + 3.5 \text{ [subtract the 40 and 3.5 from both sides of the equation]}$$

$$10 = (180 \times \text{grade}) \text{ [divide both sides of the equation by 180]}$$

$$0.06 = \text{grade}$$

This fraction must be multiplied by 100 to convert to a percentage: 0.06 × 100 = 6%. Thus a 6% grade will allow for a similar $\dot{V}O_2$.

Running on a Level Surface

As with walking, the equation for calculating the oxygen cost (ml · kg^{-1} · min^{-1}) of running on a flat surface is the same as when on a grade with the exception that no vertical component is included (as with a grade of 0%, the vertical component will calculate to be 0).

QUESTION:

A client with a body weight of 65 kilograms is running at a speed of 8 mph on a level treadmill. What is the estimated steady-state $\dot{V}O_2$ and METs? How many kcal would be expended if engaging in this activity for 45 minutes?

ANSWER:

First write down the equation:

$$\dot{V}O_2 = (0.2 \times \text{speed}) + (0.9 \times \text{speed} \times \text{grade}) + 3.5$$

Then fill in the information given in the question, taking care to ensure that the appropriate units of measure are used (speed in m · min^{-1}). Given that 1 mph is equal to 26.8 m · min^{-1}, the speed can be converted to m · min^{-1} (8 × 26.8 = 214.4). For a level treadmill, the grade is 0.

$$\dot{V}O_2 = (0.2 \times 214.4) + (0.9 \times 214.4 \times 0) + 3.5$$

$$\dot{V}O_2 = (42.9) + (0) + 3.5$$

$$\dot{V}O_2 = 46.4 \text{ ml} \cdot \text{kg}^{-1} \cdot \text{min}^{-1}$$

To determine METs, divide the 46.4 ml · kg^{-1} · min^{-1} by 3.5 to yield 13.3 METs.

Energy expenditure can be calculated in one of two ways:

1. *Option A:* To determine kcal · min^{-1}, divide the $\dot{V}O_2$ (in units of measure ml · kg^{-1} · min^{-1}) by 1,000 and multiply by body weight in kilograms to convert the units of measure to L · min^{-1}. Then the relationship noted previously of 5.0 kcal per liter of O_2 can be used. For this example, the runner's weight is 65 kilograms, so the calculations are as follows:

$$46.4 \div 1,000 \times 65 = 3.02 \text{ L} \cdot \text{min}^{-1}$$

$$3.02 \times 5.0 = 15.1 \text{ kcal} \cdot \text{min}^{-1}$$

2. *Option B:* Another method to determine kcal · min^{-1} is to use METs along with the person's body weight in kilograms. This is described in the sidebar *Using METs to Calculate Energy Costs.*

$$\text{kcal} \cdot \text{min}^{-1} = (\text{METs} \times 3.5 \times \text{body weight in kg}) \div 200$$

$$\text{kcal} \cdot \text{min}^{-1} = (13.3 \times 3.5 \times 65) \div 200$$

$$\text{kcal} \cdot \text{min}^{-1} = 15.1$$

Thus, either option will allow for determination of kcal · min^{-1} of 15.1. If the client runs for 45 minutes, this calculates to approximately 680 kcal ($15.1 \times 45 = 679.5$).

Running at Various Speeds

In contrast to the energy cost of walking, the energy cost of running increases linearly with increasing speed. As with walking, the energy cost is higher if body weight is greater.

Oxygen Cost of Walking and Running a Mile

Despite the vast amount of information regarding the costs of walking and running, a good deal of misunderstanding still exists. The energy cost of walking 1 mile (1.6 kilometers) is often suggested to be equal to that of running the same distance. In general, this is not the case (21). The equations for estimating the energy cost of walking and running can be used to estimate the caloric cost of walking and running 1 mile (1.6 kilometers)—information that is useful in achieving energy expenditure goals.

If a person (body weight 70 kilograms) walks at 3 mph (80 m · min^{-1}), this results in 1 mile (1.6 kilometers) completed in 20 minutes. The caloric cost for walking 1 mile (1.6 kilometers) for a 70-kilogram person is calculated as follows:

$$\dot{V}O_2 = (0.1 \times \text{speed}) + (1.8 \times \text{speed} \times \text{grade}) + 3.5$$

$$\dot{V}O_2 = (0.1 \times 80) + (1.8 \times 80 \times 0) + 3.5$$

$$\dot{V}O_2 = 11.5 \text{ ml} \cdot \text{kg}^{-1} \cdot \text{min}^{-1}$$

$$\dot{V}O_2 \text{ (ml} \cdot \text{mile}^{-1}) = 11.5 \text{ ml} \cdot \text{kg}^{-1} \cdot \text{min}^{-1} \times 70 \text{ kg} \times 20 \text{ min} \cdot \text{mi}^{-1} = 16,100 \text{ ml} \cdot \text{mi}^{-1}$$

and so

$$\dot{V}O_2 \text{ (L} \cdot \text{min}^{-1}) = 16,100 \text{ ml} \cdot \text{mi}^{-1} \div 1,000 \text{ ml} \cdot \text{L}^{-1} = 16.1 \text{ L} \cdot \text{mi}^{-1}$$

At about 5.0 kcal per liter of O$_2$, the gross caloric cost per mile of walking is 80.5 kcal (5 kcal · L^{-1} $\times$ 16.1 L · mi^{-1}). The net caloric cost for the mile walk can be calculated by subtracting the oxygen cost of 20 minutes of rest from the gross cost of the 3 mph walk. For this person,

- resting oxygen uptake = 3.5 ml · kg^{-1} · min^{-1} $\times$ 70 kg equals 245 ml · min^{-1};
- 20 minutes of rest (20 min $\times$ 245 ml · min^{-1}) equals 4,900 ml, or 4.9 L O$_2$;
- at 5.0 kcal · L^{-1}, 4.9 L O$_2$ equals 24.5 kcal for 20 minutes of rest (4.9 L O$_2$ $\times$ 5 kcal · L^{-1}); and
- the net cost of the mile walk is 80.5 kcal minus 24.5 kcal, or 56 kcal for each mile.

If the same person (body weight 70 kilograms) ran the mile at 6 mph (161 m · min^{-1}), the oxygen cost could be calculated by the following method.

$$\dot{V}O_2 = (0.2 \times \text{speed}) + (0.9 \times \text{speed} \times \text{grade}) + 3.5$$

$$\dot{V}O_2 = (0.2 \times 161) + (0.9 \times 161 \times 0) + 3.5$$

$$\dot{V}O_2 = (32.2) + (0) + 3.5$$

$$\dot{V}O_2 = 35.7 \text{ ml} \cdot \text{kg}^{-1} \cdot \text{min}^{-1}$$

$$\dot{V}O_2 \text{ (ml} \cdot \text{mi}^{-1}) = 35.7 \text{ ml} \cdot \text{kg}^{-1} \cdot \text{min}^{-1} \times 70 \text{ kg} \times 10 \text{ min} \cdot \text{mi}^{-1} = 25,000 \text{ ml} \cdot \text{mi}^{-1}$$

and so

$$\dot{V}O_2 \text{ (L} \cdot \text{min}^{-1}) = 25,000 \text{ ml} \cdot \text{mi}^{-1} \div 1,000 \text{ ml} \cdot \text{L}^{-1} = 25 \text{ L} \cdot \text{mi}^{-1}$$

At about 5.0 kcal per liter of O_2, 125 kcal are used to run 1 mile ($5 \text{ kcal} \cdot L^{-1} \times 25 \text{ L} \cdot mi^{-1}$). The gross caloric cost per 1 mile (or per 1.6 kilometers) is about 50% higher for running than for walking (125 versus 80 kcal). The net caloric cost of jogging or running 1 mile or 1.6 kilometers (calories used above resting), however, is about twice that of walking. For example, when we subtract the caloric cost for 10 minutes of rest (12 kcal) from the gross caloric cost of the run (125 kcal), the net cost is 113 kcal, or twice that for the walk (56 kcal). This follows from the net cost of running versus walking: $0.2 \text{ ml} \cdot kg^{-1} \cdot min^{-1}$ per $m \cdot min^{-1}$ versus $0.1 \text{ ml} \cdot kg^{-1} \cdot min^{-1}$ per $m \cdot min^{-1}$.

For weight control, the net cost of the activity is more applicable because it measures the energy used above that for rest or sitting. When a person walks at slow to moderate speeds (2-3.5 mph, or $54\text{-}94 \text{ m} \cdot min^{-1}$), the net cost of walking a mile (1.6 kilometers) is about half that of running the mile. This means that a person who runs a mile at 3 mph ($80 \text{ m} \cdot min^{-1}$) expends twice as many calories as someone who walks at the same speed. Because many people walk rather than run at these slower speeds, it is important to remember that the net energy cost of the mile is half that of running. For high walking speeds such as 5 mph ($134 \text{ m} \cdot min^{-1}$), or 1 mile in 12 minutes, however, the net energy cost of walking 1 mile is similar to that of running.

The net cost of running a mile (1.6 kilometers) is independent of speed. It does not matter whether participants run at 3 mph ($80 \text{ m} \cdot min^{-1}$) or run at 6 mph ($161 \text{ m} \cdot min^{-1}$)—the net caloric cost for running a mile is the same. At 6 mph, the participant expends energy at about twice the rate measured at 3 mph ($161 \text{ m} \cdot min^{-1}$), but because the mile is finished in half the time, the net energy expenditure is about the same. HR will, of course, be higher in the 6 mph ($161 \text{ m} \cdot min^{-1}$) run in order to deliver oxygen to the muscles at the higher rate.

KEY POINT

The oxygen cost of walking increases linearly between the speeds of 50 and 100 $m \cdot min^{-1}$; it increases faster at higher walking speeds. The oxygen cost of running increases linearly with speed from slow running (3 mph, or $80 \text{ m} \cdot min^{-1}$) to fast running. The net caloric cost of running a mile (1.6 kilometers) is twice that of walking a mile at a moderate pace.

Oxygen Cost of Cycle Ergometry

Cycle ergometry is a popular exercise done at a fitness center, at home, or as part of a rehabilitation program. Generally, cycle ergometry expends energy while causing less trauma to the ankle, knee, and hip joints compared with running. Cycle ergometers are used for conventional leg-exercise programs, but they are also available or adapted for arm exercise. The following sections describe how to estimate the energy costs of leg and arm cycle ergometry.

Leg Ergometry

In the previous activities the participants were carrying their body weight, and the oxygen requirement therefore was proportional to body weight ($ml \cdot kg^{-1} \cdot min^{-1}$). This is not the case in cycle ergometry, in which body weight is supported by the cycle seat and the work rate is determined primarily by the pedal rate and the resistance on the wheel. The oxygen requirement, in liters per minute, is approximately the same for people of all sizes for the same work rate. Thus, when a light person is doing the same work rate as a heavy person, the relative $\dot{V}O_2$ ($ml \cdot kg^{-1} \cdot min^{-1}$), or MET level, is higher for the lighter person.

The work rate is set on the simple, mechanically braked cycle ergometers by varying the force (weight, or load) on the wheel and the number of pedal revolutions per minute (rpm). On the Monark leg ergometer, the wheel travels 6 meters per pedal revolution. At a pedal rate of 50 rpm, the wheel moves a distance of 300 meters ($6 \text{ m} \times 50 \text{ rpm}$). If a 1-kilogram weight (force) is applied to the wheel, the work rate is $300 \text{ kgm} \cdot min^{-1}$ (kilogram-meters per minute = $m \cdot rev^{-1} \times rpm \times kg$). Work rates also are expressed in watts (W), where approximately $6 \text{ kgm} \cdot min^{-1}$ equals 1 W; the $300 \text{ kgm} \cdot min^{-1}$ work rate would be expressed as 50 watts (W). The work rate can be doubled by changing the force from 1 to 2 kilograms or by changing the pedal rate from 50 to 100 rpm. In contrast, some cycle ergometers are electronically controlled to deliver a specific work rate somewhat independent of pedal rate; as the pedal rate decreases, the load on the wheel increases proportionally to maintain the work rate (6).

The total oxygen cost of leg cycle ergometry is the sum of the resting oxygen uptake, the cost of unloaded cycling (movement of the legs against no resistance), and the cost of the work itself. The oxygen cost of doing 1 kilogram-meter of work is 1.8 milliliters. The energy required to move the pedals against no resistance has been estimated to be 1 MET, or 3.5 ml $\cdot$ kg^{-1} $\cdot$ min^{-1}. As with the other equations, resting oxygen uptake is 3.5 ml $\cdot$ kg^{-1} $\cdot$ min^{-1} (5). The estimates from the following equations are reasonable for work rates between approximately 150 and 1,200 kgm $\cdot$ min^{-1}. The equations for work rates expressed in kgm $\cdot$ min^{-1} follow.

$$\dot{V}O_2 \text{ (ml} \cdot \text{kg}^{-1} \cdot \text{min}^{-1}) = (1.8 \text{ ml O}_2 \cdot \text{kgm}^{-1} \times \text{work rate in kgm} \cdot \text{min}^{-1} \div \text{body weight in kg})$$
$$+ 3.5 \text{ ml} \cdot \text{kg}^{-1} \cdot \text{min}^{-1} + 3.5 \text{ ml} \cdot \text{kg}^{-1} \cdot \text{min}^{-1}$$

QUESTION:
What is the oxygen cost of doing 600 kgm $\cdot$ min^{-1} on a cycle ergometer for clients who weigh 50 kilograms and 100 kilograms?

ANSWER:
First consider the basic equation with the constants in place. (Note that the units of measure for $\dot{V}O_2$ is ml $\cdot$ kg^{-1} $\cdot$ min^{-1}.)

$$\dot{V}O_2 = (1.8 \times \text{work rate in kgm} \cdot \text{min}^{-1} \div \text{body weight in kg}) + 3.5 + 3.5$$

For the client who weighs 50 kilograms:

$$\dot{V}O_2 = (1.8 \times 600 \div 50) + 3.5 + 3.5 \text{ [multiply values within parentheses]}$$
$$\dot{V}O_2 = (21.6) + 3.5 + 3.5 \text{ [add the three components together]}$$
$$\dot{V}O_2 \text{ (ml} \cdot \text{kg}^{-1} \cdot \text{min}^{-1}) = 28.6 \text{ ml} \cdot \text{kg}^{-1} \cdot \text{min}^{-1}, \text{ or 8.2 METs}$$

For the client who weighs 100 kilograms:

$$\dot{V}O_2 = (1.8 \times 600 \div 100) + 3.5 + 3.5 \text{ [multiply values within parentheses]}$$
$$\dot{V}O_2 = (10.8) + 3.5 + 3.5 \text{ [add the three components together]}$$
$$\dot{V}O_2 \text{ (ml} \cdot \text{kg}^{-1} \cdot \text{min}^{-1}) = 17.8 \text{ ml} \cdot \text{kg}^{-1} \cdot \text{min}^{-1}, \text{ or 5.1 METs}$$

In some exercise programs, a participant might use a variety of exercise equipment to achieve a training effect and might want to set about the same intensity on each machine. The equation for the cycle ergometer can be used to set the load to achieve a particular MET value on the cycle ergometer and bring it in line with what is done during walking or running.

QUESTION:
A participant (body weight 70 kilograms) desires to work at 6 METs (21 ml $\cdot$ kg^{-1} $\cdot$ min^{-1}) to match the intensity of their walking program. What force (load) should be set on a Monark cycle ergometer at a pedal rate of 50 rpm?

ANSWER:
First write down the equation:

$$\dot{V}O_2 = (1.8 \times \text{work rate in kgm} \cdot \text{min}^{-1} \div \text{body weight in kg}) + 3.5 + 3.5$$

Then fill in the values that are given in the question, ensuring appropriate units of measure (use ml $\cdot$ kg^{-1} $\cdot$ min^{-1} for $\dot{V}O_2$):

$$21 = (1.8 \times \text{work rate} \div 70) + 3.5 + 3.5 \text{ [subtract 7 (3.5 + 3.5) from both sides of the equation]}$$
$$14 = (1.8 \times \text{work rate} \div 70) \text{ [multiply both sides by 70 and then divide both sides by 1.8]}$$
$$544 = \text{work rate (in kgm} \cdot \text{min}^{-1})$$

Considering the three components of work rate (m · rev^{-1} × rpm × kg), solve for kilograms (weight applied to the wheel) for the client who prefers a cadence of 50 rpm. (Recall for a Monark leg ergometer, the distance per revolution is 6 meters.)

$$544 \text{ kgm} \cdot \text{min}^{-1} = 6 \text{ m} \times 50 \text{ rpm} \times \text{kg [divide both sides by 6} \times 50, \text{ or } 300]$$

$$1.8 = \text{kg}$$

Arm Ergometry

A cycle ergometer can be used to exercise the muscles of the arms and shoulder girdle by modifying the pedals and placing the cycle on a table or by using equipment specifically designed for arm ergometry. Arm ergometry is used on a limited basis as a GXT to evaluate cardiovascular function. It is used more generally as a routine exercise in rehabilitation programs (19). Keep in mind a variety of factors when considering arm ergometry:

- $\dot{V}O_2$max for the arms is only 70% of that measured with the legs in a normal healthy population and is less in individuals who are unfit or elderly or in those with chronic diseases.
- The natural endurance of the muscles used in this work is less than that of the legs.
- The HR and blood pressure (BP) responses are higher for arm work compared with leg work at the same $\dot{V}O_2$.
- There is no need to account for unloaded arm cycling, but the oxygen cost of doing 1 kilogram-meter is about 3 ml $O_2 \cdot$ kgm^{-1} for arm work because of the inefficiency of the action (5).

The equation for estimating the oxygen cost of arm work for work rates expressed in kgm · min^{-1} is as follows:

$$\dot{V}O_2 \text{ (ml} \cdot \text{kg}^{-1} \cdot \text{min}^{-1}) = (3 \text{ ml } O_2 \cdot \text{kgm}^{-1} \times \text{work rate in kgm} \cdot \text{min}^{-1}$$
$$\div \text{ body weight in kg)} + 3.5 \text{ ml} \cdot \text{kg}^{-1} \cdot \text{min}^{-1}$$

QUESTION:

What is the oxygen requirement for a client (body weight 70 kilograms) doing 150 kgm · min^{-1} on an arm ergometer?

ANSWER:

First consider the basic equation with the constants in place. (Note that the units of measure for $\dot{V}O_2$ is ml · kg^{-1} · min^{-1}.)

$$\dot{V}O_2 = (3 \times \text{work rate in kgm} \cdot \text{min}^{-1} \div \text{body weight in kg)} + 3.5$$

Next, fill in the values provided within the question:

$$\dot{V}O_2 = (3 \times 150 \div 70) + 3.5 \text{ [complete the calculations within the parentheses and then add 3.5]}$$

$$\dot{V}O_2 = 9.93 \text{ ml} \cdot \text{kg}^{-1} \cdot \text{min}^{-1}, \text{ or } 2.8 \text{ METs}$$

In some situations, a participant may need guidance on the force (load) to set on the arm ergometer to achieve a target intensity. The equation for arm ergometry can be used to determine the load (weight) to achieve a particular MET value.

QUESTION:

A participant (body weight 70 kilograms) desires to work at 3 METs (10.5 ml · kg^{-1} · min^{-1}). What force (load) should be set on a Monark arm ergometer at a pedal rate of 50 rpm?

ANSWER:

First write down the equation:

$$\dot{V}O_2 = (3 \times \text{work rate in kgm} \cdot \text{min}^{-1} \div \text{body weight in kg)} + 3.5$$

Then fill in the values that are given in the question, ensuring appropriate units of measure (use ml · kg^{-1} · min^{-1} for $\dot{V}O_2$):

$$10.5 = (3 \times \text{work rate} \div 70) + 3.5 \text{ [subtract 3.5 from both sides of the equation]}$$

$$7 = (3 \times \text{work rate} \div 70) \text{ [multiply both sides by 70 and then divide both sides by 3]}$$

$$163 = \text{work rate (in kgm} \cdot \text{min}^{-1})$$

Considering the three components of work rate (m · rev^{-1} × rpm × kg), solve for kilograms (the load or weight applied to the wheel) for the client who prefers a cadence of 50 rpm. (Note that for a Monark arm ergometer, the distance per revolution is 2.4 meters.)

$$163 \text{ kgm} \cdot \text{min}^{-1} = 2.4 \text{ m} \times 50 \text{ rpm} \times \text{kg [divide both sides by 2.4} \times 50, \text{ or 120]}$$

$$1.4 = \text{kg}$$

KEY POINT

> The oxygen cost of cycle ergometry primarily depends on the work rate because body weight is supported. The net oxygen cost of leg ergometry is 1.8 ml · kgm^{-1} versus 3 ml · kgm^{-1} for arm ergometry. Physiological responses (e.g., HR and BP) are exaggerated for arm work compared with leg work at the same work rate because the oxygen cost is higher and represents a higher percentage of the arm $\dot{V}O_2$max.

Oxygen Cost of Bench Stepping

One of the most useful and inexpensive forms of exercise is bench stepping; it can be done at home and requires little or no equipment. The work rate is easily adjusted by simply increasing step height or cadence (number of lifts per minute). The total oxygen cost of this exercise is the sum of the costs of (a) stepping up with each foot, (b) stepping down with each foot, (c) moving back and forth on a level surface at the specified cadence, and (d) resting oxygen uptake (3.5 ml · kg^{-1} · min^{-1}). The oxygen cost of stepping up is 1.8 ml · kg^{-1} · min^{-1} per m · min^{-1}, as in walking (29). The oxygen cost of stepping down is a third of the cost of stepping up; therefore, the oxygen cost of stepping up and down is 1.33 times the cost of stepping up. The oxygen cost of stepping back and forth on a flat surface is equal to 0.2 ml O$_2$ per kilogram of body mass for each four-cycle step (5). A four-cycle step refers to stepping up with each foot and then back down with each foot. To determine step height, multiply inches by 0.0254 to obtain meters, or if step height is given in centimeters, divide by 100 to obtain meters. The equation for estimating the energy requirement for stepping follows:

$$\dot{V}O_2 \text{ (ml} \cdot \text{kg}^{-1} \cdot \text{min}^{-1}) = (0.2 \times \text{step rate})$$
$$+ (1.8 \times 1.33 \times \text{step rate} \times \text{step height in meters}) + 3.5 \text{ ml} \cdot \text{kg}^{-1} \cdot \text{min}^{-1}$$

QUESTION:
What is the oxygen requirement for stepping at a rate of 20 steps · min^{-1} on a 10-inch bench?

ANSWER:
First consider the basic equation with the constants in place (note that the units of measure for $\dot{V}O_2$ is ml · kg^{-1} · min^{-1}):

$$\dot{V}O_2 = (0.2 \times \text{step rate}) + (1.8 \times 1.33 \times \text{step rate} \times \text{step height in meters}) + 3.5$$

Next, fill in the values provided within the question (note that step height must be in meters, so to convert from inches to meters, multiply by 0.0254: 10 inches × 0.0254 = 0.25 meters).

$$\dot{V}O_2 = (0.2 \times 20) + (1.8 \times 1.33 \times 20 \times 0.25) + 3.5 \text{ [multiply values within parentheses]}$$

$$\dot{V}O_2 = (4) + (11.97) + 3.5 \text{ [add the three components together]}$$

$$\dot{V}O_2 = 19.47 \text{ ml} \cdot \text{kg}^{-1} \cdot \text{min}^{-1}, \text{ or 5.6 METs}$$

KEY POINT

The oxygen cost of bench stepping includes the cost of stepping up and down, moving horizontally back and forth, and resting oxygen uptake. The oxygen cost of stepping up is the same as in walking. The oxygen cost of stepping up and down is 1.33 times the cost of stepping up. The oxygen cost of stepping back and forth is 0.2 ml · kg^{-1} · min^{-1} times the step rate.

Energy Requirements of Other Activities

Clients have a wide variety of interests and range of options when it comes to the physical activities they use to achieve health and fitness goals. Fitness professionals can help clients understand the energy cost associated with physical activities using the calculated $\dot{V}O_2$ for steady-state activities of walking, running, leg and arm ergometry, and stepping, or by using MET values provided in the Compendium of Physical Activities (1, 2, 13, 14).

Using Calculated Oxygen Consumption

The determination of $\dot{V}O_2$ for walking, running, leg and arm ergometry, and stepping as described in this chapter assumes steady-state conditions. This allows for use of the relationship of 5.0 kcal per liter of O_2 to be used to calculate kcal · min^{-1}. Total kcal for a given workout can be determined as shown previously by multiplying the kcal · min^{-1} by the number of minutes engaged in that activity. Target duration to achieve a given target energy expenditure also can be calculated as shown in the following example.

The target energy expenditure for a client (body weight 85 kilograms) is set at 1,000 kcal · wk^{-1}. The client is comfortable walking on the treadmill at 3.5 mph with a 2% grade. The first step will be to calculate the $\dot{V}O_2$ by writing down the equation for walking, ensuring the values are in the correct units of measure. For speed, mph must be converted to m · min^{-1} by multiplying by 26.8 (3.5 × 26.8 = 93.8), and for grade, divide 2 by 100 to express as a fraction (2 ÷ 100 = 0.02).

$$\dot{V}O_2 = (0.1 \times \text{speed}) + (1.8 \times \text{speed} \times \text{grade}) + 3.5$$

$$\dot{V}O_2 = (0.1 \times 93.8) + (1.8 \times 93.8 \times 0.02) + 3.5 \text{ [multiply values within parentheses]}$$

$$\dot{V}O_2 = 9.38 + 3.38 + 3.5 \text{ [add the three components]}$$

$$\dot{V}O_2 = 16.26 \text{ ml · kg}^{-1} \cdot \text{min}^{-1}$$

The next step is to determine the kcal · min^{-1}. For this example, the $\dot{V}O_2$ (in units of measure ml · kg^{-1} · min^{-1}) will be converted to L · min^{-1}. (Recall, body weight of the client is 85 kilograms.) To determine kcal · min^{-1}, the L · min^{-1} is then multiplied by 5 (given 5.0 kcal per liter of O_2) as follows:

$$16.26 \div 1,000 \times 85 = 1.38 \text{ L · min}^{-1}$$

$$1.38 \times 5.0 = 6.9 \text{ kcal · min}^{-1}$$

Given the total target expenditure is 1,000 kcal, then

$$1,000 \text{ kcal · wk}^{-1} \div 6.9 \text{ kcal · min}^{-1} = 145 \text{ min · wk}^{-1}$$

Thus, approximately 30 minutes of walking on five days per week would achieve this target expenditure.

Using the Compendium of Physical Activities

The Compendium of Physical Activities is an excellent source of information about the energy cost of many physical activities, including leisure and occupational activities (1, 2). Dr. Bill Haskell of Stanford University conceptualized the compendium and developed a prototype that was used in studies examining physical activity, exercise, and fitness patterns in populations. In this way, investigators could link the energy expenditure of physical activity to various health outcomes and determine, for example, the relationship of physical activity to the risk of type 2 diabetes. In 1993, the first complete version of the compendium was published, followed by an update in 2000. Both articles offered a long list of activities that included specific codes to identify the activity and energy cost values expressed in METs, where 1 MET is equal to $3.5 \text{ ml} \cdot \text{kg}^{-1} \cdot \text{min}^{-1}$. A MET is also defined as $1 \text{ kcal} \cdot \text{kg}^{-1} \cdot \text{hr}^{-1}$. In 2011, an update of the compendium was published, but this time the list of activities, codes, and MET values were published on a website (2). A research team, led by Dr. Barbara Ainsworth, continues this work; the 2024 compendium provides a third update that expands on the 2011 compendium, such as introducing new content for older adults and for wheelchair activities (see https://pacompendium.com for the most current information).

The following example shows how to use the information on MET level as found on the Compendium of Physical Activities website to estimate the energy cost of activities. Keep in mind that the energy cost values in the compendium are measured or estimated values of a group; large interindividual variation in energy cost may exist for some activities. Other calculations that consider a person's characteristics (including age, sex, height, and body weight) have been proposed to reflect an individual's energy cost of activity by adjusting for differences in resting metabolic rate (2).

EXAMPLE

A client, who weighs 60 kilograms, bicycles to and from work each day (1 hour round trip, Monday through Friday) and wants to know how much energy is used each day in this activity and the weekly total (reflecting 5 days per week of biking to and from work).

1. For "bicycling to and from work, self-selected pace," the MET value is 6.8.

2. Using the equation provided earlier and information provided, determine the $\text{kcal} \cdot \text{min}^{-1}$:

$$\text{kcal} \cdot \text{min}^{-1} = (\text{METs} \times 3.5 \times \text{body weight in kg}) \div 200$$

$$\text{kcal} \cdot \text{min}^{-1} = (6.8 \times 3.5 \times 60) \div 200$$

$$\text{kcal} \cdot \text{min}^{-1} = 7.1$$

3. Thus, for the 1 hour (or 60 minutes) of biking to and from work, the energy expenditure per day is approximately 426 kcal ($7.1 \times 60 = 426$). For the week (reflecting 60 minutes per day on 5 days per week: $60 \times 5 = 300$ minutes), the energy expenditure would be 2,130 kcal ($7.1 \times 300 = 2,130$).

4. Another option in estimating energy cost would reflect the definition provided for 1 MET being equal to $1 \text{ kcal} \cdot \text{kg}^{-1} \cdot \text{hr}^{-1}$. For example, to calculate the weekly total for the client (body weight of 60 kilograms) who is exercising at this level (6.8 METs) for 5 hours per week (1 hour each day, Monday through Friday):

$$6.8 \text{ kcal} \cdot \text{kg}^{-1} \cdot \text{hr}^{-1} \times 60 \text{ kg} \times 5 \text{ hr} = 2,040 \text{ kcal}$$

5. There is a slight difference in the estimated total kcal for the week depending on the method used (2,130 kcal compared to 2,040 kcal). This is related to the value used for the number of kcal per liter of O_2 (see the Key Point earlier in the chapter that describes the use of 5.0 for ease of calculation rather than 4.85, which reflects using approximately a 50–50 mixture of carbohydrate and fat). The first method of calculating reflects use of the 5.0 kcal per liter of O_2 and the second is closer to 4.85 kcal per liter of O_2. This underscores that both of these indirect determinations of energy expenditure are approximations.

KEY POINT

The Compendium of Physical Activities is an excellent source of information about the energy cost of many physical activities, including leisure and occupational activities. Environmental factors such as heat, humidity, altitude, and pollution can increase the HR response to work while not affecting the energy cost. HR should be monitored more frequently in these settings to adjust the intensity of the activity downward to keep the person in the appropriate HR range (see chapter 13).

Environmental Concerns

Although changes in temperature, relative humidity, pollution, and altitude do not change the energy requirements for submaximal exercise, they do change the participant's response to the exercise. Remember that a person's HR response is the best indicator of the relative stress experienced due to the interaction of exercise intensity, exercise duration, and environmental factors. The participant should cut back on the intensity of the activity when environmental factors increase the HR response. The duration of the activity can be increased to accommodate any energy expenditure goal.

6

LEARNING AIDS

REVIEW QUESTIONS

1. What can an accelerometer measure that a pedometer cannot when monitoring physical activity?
2. How do you convert oxygen uptake in $L \cdot min^{-1}$ to $kcal \cdot min^{-1}$?
3. What is a MET equal to in $ml \cdot kg^{-1} \cdot min^{-1}$?
4. How much greater is the net oxygen cost of running $1 \, m \cdot min^{-1}$ on a flat surface compared with walking?
5. When a 50-kilogram person and an 80-kilogram person exercise at $600 \, kgm \cdot min^{-1}$ on a cycle ergometer, how do the oxygen uptakes compare in $L \cdot min^{-1}$ and $ml \cdot kg^{-1} \cdot min^{-1}$?

CASE STUDIES

1. A man (body weight 75 kilograms) walks at 3.5 mph for 30 minutes. How many calories does he expend?
2. A woman (body weight 60 kilograms) rides a cycle ergometer at a work rate of 100 watts. What is her oxygen uptake?
3. A college student (body weight 70 kilograms) runs 3 miles (4.8 kilometers) in 24 minutes. How many calories do they expend?
4. If a client (body weight 80 kilograms) is exercising at 8 METs for 30 minutes on 4 days per week, what is the caloric cost per week?
5. A client mentions they read that the same number of calories can be expended per mile whether they walk at 3 mph ($4.8 \, km \cdot hr^{-1}$) or run at 6 mph ($9.7 \, km \cdot hr^{-1}$). How do you respond?

Answers to Case Studies

1. The first step is to write down the walking equation:

$$\dot{V}O_2 = (0.1 \times speed) + (1.8 \times speed \times grade) + 3.5$$

Next, the speed must be converted to the correct units of measure ($m \cdot min^{-1}$) by multiplying 3.5 by 26.8 ($3.5 \times 26.8 = 93.8$) and inserted into the equation:

$$\dot{V}O_2 = (0.1 \times 93.8) + (1.8 \times 93.8 \times 0) + 3.5$$

$$\dot{V}O_2 = 12.9 \, ml \cdot kg^{-1} \cdot min^{-1} \text{ or 3.7 METs (calculated by } 12.9 \div 3.5 = 3.7)$$

Energy expenditure can be calculated in one of two ways:

Option A: To determine kcal · min^{-1}, multiply the $\dot{V}O_2$ (in units of measure ml · kg^{-1} · min^{-1}) by body weight and divide by 1,000 to convert the units of measure to L · min^{-1}. Then the relationship of 5.0 kcal per liter of O_2 can be used. For this case, the client's weight is 75 kilograms, so the calculations are as follows:

$$12.9 \div 1,000 \times 75 = 0.97 \text{ L} \cdot \text{min}^{-1}$$

$$0.97 \times 5.0 = 4.85 \text{ kcal} \cdot \text{min}^{-1}$$

Option B: Another method to determine kcal · min^{-1} is to use METs with the following equation:

$$\text{kcal} \cdot \text{min}^{-1} = (\text{METs} \times 3.5 \times \text{body weight in kg}) \div 200$$

$$\text{kcal} \cdot \text{min}^{-1} = (3.7 \times 3.5 \times 75) \div 200$$

$$\text{kcal} \cdot \text{min}^{-1} = 4.86$$

Thus, either option will allow for an estimation of approximately 4.9 kcal · min^{-1}. If he walks for 30 minutes, this calculates to 147 kcal ($4.9 \times 30 = 147$).

2. First consider the basic equation for leg ergometry:

$$\dot{V}O_2 = (1.8 \times \text{work rate in kgm} \cdot \text{min}^{-1} \div \text{body weight in kg}) + 3.5 + 3.5$$

Note that the work rate will need to be converted from watts to kgm · min^{-1} by multiplying by 6 in order to match the unit of measure required in the equation:

$$100 \text{ W} \times 6 = 600 \text{ kgm} \cdot \text{min}^{-1}$$

Now insert the known information into the equation:

$$\dot{V}O_2 = (1.8 \times 600 \div 60) + 3.5 + 3.5$$

$$\dot{V}O_2 = 25.0 \text{ ml} \cdot \text{kg}^{-1} \cdot \text{min}^{-1} \text{ or 7.1 METs (calculated by } 25.0 \div 3.5 = 7.1)$$

3. The first step is to write down the running equation:

$$\dot{V}O_2 = (0.2 \times \text{speed}) + (0.9 \times \text{speed} \times \text{grade}) + 3.5$$

Next, the speed must be determined in the correct units of measure (m · min^{-1}). Given that 1 mile is equal to 1,609 meters the distance of 3 miles is equal to 4,827 meters. This distance was run in 24 minutes, so determine m · min^{-1} by dividing 4,827 by 24 ($4,827 \div 24 = 201.1$ m · min^{-1}).

Now return to the running equation and enter in the known values:

$$\dot{V}O_2 = (0.2 \times 201.1) + (0.9 \times 201.1 \times 0) + 3.5$$

$$\dot{V}O_2 = (40.2) + (0) + 3.5$$

$$\dot{V}O_2 = 43.7 \text{ ml} \cdot \text{kg}^{-1} \cdot \text{min}^{-1} \text{ or 12.5 METs (calculated by } 43.7 \div 3.5 = 12.5)$$

Energy expenditure can be calculated in one of two ways:

Option A: Starting with $\dot{V}O_2$ (in units of measure ml · kg^{-1} · min^{-1}), convert to L · min^{-1}, and then use the relationship of 5.0 kcal per L O_2. For this case, the client's weight is 70 kilograms, so the calculations are:

$$43.7 \div 1,000 \times 70 = 3.06 \text{ L} \cdot \text{min}^{-1}$$

$$3.06 \times 5.0 = 15.3 \text{ kcal} \cdot \text{min}^{-1}$$

Option B: Another method to determine kcal · min^{-1} is to use METs with the following equation:

$$\text{kcal} \cdot \text{min}^{-1} = (\text{METs} \times 3.5 \times \text{body weight in kg}) \div 200$$

$$\text{kcal} \cdot \text{min}^{-1} = (12.5 \times 3.5 \times 70) \div 200$$

$$\text{kcal} \cdot \text{min}^{-1} = 15.3$$

Thus, either option will allow for determination of kcal · min^{-1} of 15.3. If they run for 24 min, this calculates to approximately 367 kcal ($15.3 \times 24 = 367.2$).

4. Knowing the MET value of the activity allows for estimation of energy expenditure using this equation:

$$\text{kcal} \cdot \text{min}^{-1} = (\text{METs} \times 3.5 \times \text{body weight in kg}) \div 200$$

$$\text{kcal} \cdot \text{min}^{-1} = (8 \times 3.5 \times 80) \div 200$$

$$\text{kcal} \cdot \text{min}^{-1} = 11.2$$

For a total of 2 hours per week (30 minutes $\times$ 4 days = 120 min $\cdot$ wk^{-1}), the energy cost is 1,344 kcal $\cdot$ wk^{-1} (120 $\times$ 11.2 = 1,344).

Another option for this calculation is using the relationship between MET and kcal $\cdot$ kg^{-1} $\cdot$ hr^{-1} provided in the Compendium of Physical Activities (2). Using this approach, 8 METs reflects approximately 8 kcal $\cdot$ kg^{-1} $\cdot$ hr^{-1}, so for an 80-kilogram client who exercises at this level for 2 hours per week, the calculations would be as follows:

$$8 \text{ kcal} \cdot \text{kg}^{-1} \cdot \text{hr}^{-1} \times 80 \text{ kg} \times 2 \text{ hr} = 1{,}280 \text{ kcal}$$

There is a difference in the two values given the use of 5.0 kcal per L O$_2$ assumed for the first option, whereas the second option reflects the 4.85 kcal per L O$_2$ as described earlier in the chapter. This difference underscores that these calculations are estimations rather than direct measures of energy expenditure.

5. You might indicate that the cost of running 1 m $\cdot$ min^{-1} (0.2 ml $\cdot$ kg^{-1} $\cdot$ min^{-1}) is about twice that for walking (0.1 ml $\cdot$ kg^{-1} $\cdot$ min^{-1}) due to the extra energy needed to propel the body off the ground and absorb the force of impact on each step. The net cost of running is thus higher than for walking.

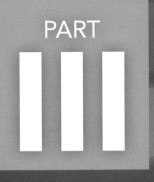

PART III

Fitness Assessments

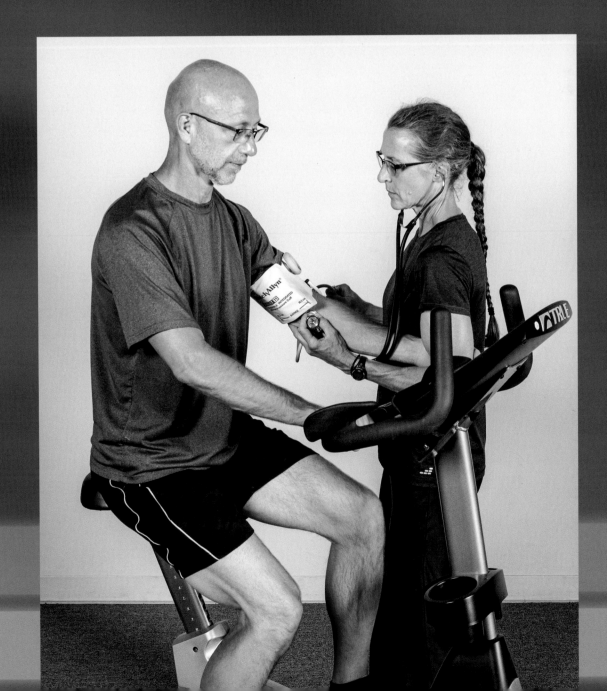

Fitness professionals must know how to measure the components of fitness and interpret the scores for clients. Chapter 7 provides an overview of assessment that includes important steps that must be taken prior to testing (e.g., informed consent, preparticipation and health screenings), selection of appropriate tests, how to obtain accurate results, and ways to explain results in a way that is meaningful to clients. The other chapters in part III cover the assessment of cardiorespiratory fitness (chapter 8), muscular fitness (chapter 9), flexibility and neuromotor fitness (chapter 10), body composition (chapter 11), and the heart's electrical activity or electrocardiogram (ECG) (chapter 12).

Overview of Assessment

Barbara A. Bushman

OBJECTIVES

The reader will be able to do the following:

1. Describe what is meant by reliability, objectivity, and validity
2. Explain ways to maximize accuracy (minimizing error) when conducting fitness testing
3. Explain the use of percentiles in evaluating test scores, including potential limitations
4. Discuss how fitness test results may need to be individualized to make them meaningful
5. List principles to enhance participation for people with disabilities
6. Describe a logical sequence for fitness testing
7. Identify key components of the informed consent document
8. Identify absolute and relative contraindications to exercise testing as noted by the American Heart Association
9. Identify common errors in the measurement of blood pressure and how to avoid those errors
10. Describe testing for aerobic fitness, muscular fitness, flexibility, and functional fitness
11. Discuss the need to use fitness testing, along with the client's activity, to develop an individualized exercise program

This chapter introduces considerations when selecting fitness tests and areas of fitness to be assessed as well as how fitness test results should be explained to clients and how to use results to develop individualized exercise programs. Assessment areas include cardiorespiratory fitness (CRF), body composition, muscular fitness, flexibility, and functional fitness (neuromotor function).

The first step in fitness testing is choosing fitness tests wisely. Consider the following factors when making a selection:

- *Reliability:* Does the test produce consistent results? Tests should give repeatable results.

- *Objectivity:* Do different test administrators get the same results from this test? Tests should give the same result regardless of the person administering the assessment.

- *Validity:* Does the test measure the characteristic of interest? Test results should reflect what is intended by the assessment.

Although a test can be reliable and objective and still not be valid, tests that are unreliable or lack objectivity cannot be valid. Once the consistency of the test is ensured, there are ways to determine whether the test measures what it is supposed to measure. For example, do experts agree that the test is valid? Does the test compare favorably with an established test (a standard) in the same area? This book includes fitness tests that reflect these characteristics.

Fitness professionals can do several things to maximize accuracy (i.e., minimize error) in testing:

- Properly prepare the person being tested so they are coming into the fitness test with needed rest and appropriate clothing and footwear.

- Organize the testing session so that all equipment is calibrated and in working order, the testing environment is controlled (e.g., room temperature is appropriate), and all participant files and forms are available and organized. Data scoring sheets should be available to record both resting measures and fitness testing data or scores as they are obtained (5).

- Ensure the client understands the purpose of the test and their responsibilities. For example, when conducting a submaximal bike test, maintenance of a particular pedal frequency is key to setting the work rate stipulated by the test protocol. Simply telling the client to "pedal at 50 rpm" is less effective than explaining the importance of the pedal frequency on work rate for accurately predicting their aerobic fitness. With the explanation, clients will understand their role in the test situation.

- Verify that correct form and techniques are used. Take time to clearly explain the test prior to beginning,

demonstrating body position or techniques if appropriate. Pay attention to the little details, and ensure the client understands what is being asked of them. Fitness professionals must provide sufficient supervision during all assessments to maximize the client's safety (5).

- Attend to details of the assessment, ensuring standardized procedures and protocols are carefully followed. If care is not taken to consistently administer the test, differences in results cannot be attributed to the training program. Thus, all tests must follow consistent and established implementation to be meaningful.

Fitness testing has many uses in a fitness setting, from prescribing exercise to refining programs (1). Fitness professionals must know how to interpret test scores and provide feedback to all program participants. The fitness professional can help participants evaluate their fitness test scores by doing the following:

- Explain the fitness test results in terminology that can be understood by the participant. See *Explaining Test Results* for more on this important aspect.

- Emphasize tracking status from their current level of fitness rather than only comparing with normative values.

- Provide recommendations based on the test data and on the participant's characteristics and goals.

One common approach to evaluating test scores is to compare the fitness participant with people of the same sex and similar age (i.e., use percentiles). *ACSM's Guidelines for Exercise Testing and Prescription* includes several normative tables related to physical fitness testing (1). Much of an individual's performance compared to others' is based on heredity and early experience, so there are limits to how much people can change even with great effort. Also, if differences exist in the comparison group (on whom the normative values have been established) and the fitness participant (e.g., differing racial or ethnic groups), normative values can be less meaningful or unsuitable to use. If appropriate normative values are not available, tracking scores over time can be of value. The emphasis should be individualized to help all people understand, achieve, and maintain CRF, healthy body composition, muscular fitness, flexibility, and functional fitness.

Although percentiles are included in some of the upcoming chapters, criteria to reach health standards would be more meaningful. Ideally, fitness standards should be based on what is needed for good health. Such standards are included for youth in the Healthy Fitness Zone standards within the FitnessGram (4). These are called *criterion-referenced standards*, with achievement of a given fitness score indicating a low risk of health problems (4). More research is needed to provide such fitness standards across the lifespan in various aspects

Explaining Test Results

For greatest effectiveness, fitness professionals must translate test results into meaningful application for clients. Over years of education, the fitness professional will have become comfortable with scientific terminology and the language of exercise. Too often this can result in overly technical explanations or involve wording that is unclear or even confusing to clients without a similar background. On the opposite extreme is overly simplifying concepts, which will also leave the client lacking in understanding. For example, how can maximal oxygen consumption ($\dot{V}O_2$max) be explained? An overly simple explanation might be that a relatively high $\dot{V}O_2$max means the heart is working well. Although not incorrect, the explanation is lacking. To say $\dot{V}O_2$max is a marker of aerobic fitness with no further explanation of what that means also leaves the client potentially confused. It is better to further explain that cardiorespiratory fitness is a reflection of the body's ability to take in and use oxygen; the greater one's ability to use oxygen at maximal levels of activity, the better the individual is able to engage in continuous activities that require repetitive large–muscle group movement such as running, cycling, or swimming. At lower levels of exertion that can be continued for a period of time, the client will be at a lower percentage of their $\dot{V}O_2$max as their cardiorespiratory fitness improves. Although the fitness professional understands advanced concepts (e.g., arteriovenous oxygen difference, calculation steps for $\dot{V}O_2$max), this level of detail typically is not appropriate, and inclusion within an explanation likely will result in greater confusion than clarity for the client. Thus, for each assessment component, the fitness professional should be able to explain what the tests mean regarding fitness without being too simplistic or too technical.

of fitness; as knowledge of the relationship between test scores and positive health is expanded, some standards may need to be modified and others defined.

Perhaps the more important question for fitness participants is what their health status will be 6 months, 2 years, or 20 years from now, as opposed to at this moment in life. In this way, individuals are encouraged to reflect on their current status (compared with health standards) in order to set reasonable, desirable, and achievable goals for the next testing time.

Test results can help people work toward and eventually achieve specific goals, but in some situations a particular fitness standard is not appropriate or reasonable for an individual. For example, the standards for running the mile cannot be used for people who swim for their fitness workouts or for people who use wheelchairs. However, individual goals for covering a certain distance in the water or in a wheelchair can be established. The fitness professional may set intermediary goals for a person who is very unfit. For example, a person who can only walk a quarter of a mile without stopping would be discouraged by discussing the standards for running 1 mile (1.6 kilometers). The initial goal for that person may be to work up to walking 1 mile without stopping. As indicated in chapter 22, it is important to set goals to help people begin and continue healthy behaviors.

Fitness and lifestyle behaviors (e.g., getting adequate exercise, nutrition, and rest; avoiding substance abuse; coping with stress) and fitness test scores are interrelated. The fitness professional should emphasize fitness behaviors that can be carried forward throughout life. It is more important for people to begin and continue regular physical activity than to reach a certain level or score on an exercise test. Likewise, it is more important for people to develop healthy eating habits than to have a certain percentage of body fat. By emphasizing healthy behaviors, fitness professionals can recognize people for their effort, and in the long run, living a consistent, healthy lifestyle is the best way for a client to improve fitness and overall health.

Many people have one or more chronic disease or disability, resulting in mild to severe limitations regarding physical activity. It is beyond the scope of this book to recommend specific activities and tests for all possible situations and conditions; however, evidence clearly shows that regular physical activity provides important health benefits for people with chronic health conditions and people with disabilities (8). The fitness professional can apply the following principles to enhance participation in physical activity for people with disabilities (7):

- *Access:* Participants with disabilities must have access to equipment and facilities they can use. This includes community (e.g., playgrounds, parks), schools, and fitness facilities.
- *Participation:* Fitness professionals should provide instruction and guidance in the use of exercise equipment and facilities.
- *Modifications:* Fitness tests and physical activities may have to be modified.

- *Adherence:* This is enhanced by offering multiple locations and socially engaging activities.
- *Regularity:* Regular participation is the key to health-related benefits for any population.

The fitness professional should involve experts in adapted physical education, therapeutic recreation, and special education for additional assistance as needed.

In addition to looking at test scores for individual clients, fitness professionals are challenged with determining whether programming is meeting clients' needs, asking themselves, for example, "Is my spin class improving the fitness of my attendees?" Analyzing test scores from various fitness classes can help the fitness professional decide what revisions to make in the overall fitness program. How many people drop out of various classes? What kinds of changes in CRF, body fatness, and muscular fitness are being made? How many injuries relate to the various classes? The answers to such questions help the fitness professional evaluate, revise, and improve fitness programs. Consider how programs are improving steadily rather than trying to reach perfection. This improvement can result from program evaluation.

Testing Sequence

The overall sequence of testing and activity prescription is shown in the sidebar *Sequence of Testing and Activity Prescription,* and the steps are described in this section. Following the informed consent process and a thorough review of preparticipation and health screenings (with medical clearance if required), the fitness professional will complete fitness testing and develop an individualized program for the participant. Opportunities for periodic retesting and revision of the program will follow as fitness gains are made. Although an optimal order of fitness testing has not been identified, a consistent testing sequence is recommended in which heart rate (HR) and blood pressure (BP) return to baseline levels and the same muscle group is not targeted in sequential tests or activities (1). A logical sequence for fitness testing can be followed that includes resting measures (HR, BP, body composition) and then assessment of CRF, muscular fitness, flexibility, and functional fitness.

Informed Consent

Fitness participants should be informed of all aspects of the testing process in terminology they can understand (1). An informed consent form is a document that outlines the pertinent information; verbal explanation of the informed consent is recommended (1). The informed consent form should clearly describe all the procedures and potential risks and benefits. The informed consent should include the responsibilities of the participant and clearly provide an opportunity for participants

---

Sequence of Testing and Activity Prescription

1. Informed consent
2. Preparticipation and health screenings
3. Resting cardiovascular tests and body composition assessment
4. Assessment for CRF
5. Assessment for muscular fitness
6. Assessment for flexibility and functional fitness
7. Development and implementation of an individualized exercise program
8. Periodic retest and activity revision

---

to ask questions. Questions and responses should be documented. Participants should understand that their data are confidential and that they can terminate any test or activity at any time should they feel uncomfortable. They should sign a written informed consent form after reading a description of the program and having all questions answered. A sample informed consent form is included in form 7.1. Any informed consent to be used should be reviewed by whatever authoritative body has oversight of that program (e.g., legal counsel of a facility, hospital risk management, university institution review board) to ensure that the informed consent and the planned process for gathering informed consent is acceptable (1). As noted within the informed consent, the client's information and data cannot be disclosed to any third party (e.g., client's physician) without a signed medical release. A sample medical release is provided to document the client's authorization to disclose personal information to another party (e.g., fitness testing data to the client's physician) (form 7.2).

Preparticipation and Health Screening

Chapter 2 describes procedures for conducting the preparticipation and health screenings prior to participation in exercise and exercise testing. On the basis of the information collected from the client, decisions can be made regarding participation in physical activity and exercise testing or the need for referral. The need for medical clearance is based on the individual's current level of physical activity; existence of signs or symptoms of known cardiovascular, metabolic, or renal disease; and the desired exercise intensity (1). Becoming familiar

FORM 7.1 Sample Informed Consent Form

The following is an example of a general consent form for exercise testing. The consent form should be developed and approved by administrative personnel associated with the setting where the testing and programming will occur, with review by legal counsel as needed (see chapter 24).

Testing purpose and explanation: In order to more safely participate in an exercise program, I hereby consent, voluntarily, to a series of exercise tests. Each test will assist in the determination of my overall physical fitness and will assess the following: cardiorespiratory fitness, body composition, muscular fitness, and flexibility. I shall perform a graded exercise test (GXT) by walking on a treadmill or riding a cycle ergometer. The GXT will begin at a low level and gradually increase in difficulty until my target heart rate is achieved. The test may be stopped at any time because of feelings of significant fatigue or for any other personal reason. Body composition will be determined using a skinfold test during which measures of a fold of skin and underlying tissue will be measured at various body locations. Muscular fitness will be assessed with a hand-grip test in which I will be asked to exert maximal grip force while holding the testing device and with a push-up test in which I will be asked to complete as many push-ups as possible without stopping to rest. A sit-and-reach test to assess my overall flexibility will require me to lean forward while seated on the floor to reach out as far as possible to touch a tape measure.

Risks and discomforts: I understand that the risks of the GXT or other test procedures may include abnormal heart rhythms, abnormal blood pressure response, fainting, and very rarely a heart attack or even death. In addition, there may be muscle soreness or strains, bruising, or other discomforts during or following testing. Every professional effort will be made to minimize these risks through proper administration of a completed health screening questionnaire (HSQ) as well as assessment of relevant health questions, supervision during the tests, and administration of tests using standardized procedures.

Responsibilities of the participant: I acknowledge that I have completed the HSQ and answered any health questions accurately. During the GXT or other tests, I will report any heart-related symptom (i.e., pain, pressure, tightness, or heaviness in the chest, neck, jaw, back, or arms) immediately. I have reported all medications (including nonprescription medications) taken on a regular basis, including today, to the appropriate staff member.

Benefits to be expected: I desire to pursue a GXT and additional fitness tests so that I may obtain better advice regarding my present level of cardiorespiratory and muscular fitness, flexibility, and body composition. This information will be used to prescribe an appropriate individualized exercise program. I understand that this test does not entirely eliminate risks in the proposed exercise program.

Inquiries: I understand that I can withdraw my consent or discontinue participation in any aspect of the fitness testing at any time without penalty or prejudice toward me. I have read the above statements and have had all of my questions answered to my satisfaction as indicated here: _____

_____

Use of health and fitness data: I have been informed that the information obtained from the HSQ and the fitness tests will be kept private and secure as required by the Health Insurance Portability and Accountability Act of 1996 (HIPAA) and/or other data privacy and security laws. However, I understand that these data may be shared with those who have a need to know (i.e., other fitness professionals employed at this facility who will be directly involved in the design/delivery of my exercise program). I also understand that these data will not be disclosed to any third parties (e.g., my physician or other health care providers) without my express written permission via a medical release.

_____	_____
Signature of participant	Date
_____	_____
Signature of witness	Date

FORM 7.2   Sample Medical Release Form

1. I _____ (*name of fitness participant*) hereby authorize the disclosure of the following personal information to a third party _____ (*name of third party such as the participant's physician*):

    _____ HSQ (health history data)

    _____ Fitness testing data

    _____ Other, please specify_____

    Third party's address and phone: _____

    _____

2. Purpose of the disclosure information: _____

3. I request that this release become invalid 90 days from the date I signed it.

4. I understand that this release can be revoked any time except to the extent that disclosure made in good faith has already occurred in release of this authorization.

5. Participant's signature:_____ Date: _____

6. Witness: _____ (please print)

Witness signature _____ Date: _____

*This form as well as all related forms should be developed in consultation with the facility's legal and medical advisors.

Adapted from Balady et al. (1998).

---

with the methods of obtaining this information from clients is essential in making appropriate judgments (see chapter 2). In addition, understanding potential impacts of medications is key to safe and accurate fitness test administration and exercise program development; medication impacts and additional resources to consult related to various medications are discussed in chapter 2.

The emphasis in the screening process is on the client's safety. The sidebar *American Heart Association's Contraindications to Exercise Testing* outlines situations and conditions that have been identified in which the risk of testing outweighs the possible benefits; these are considered absolute contraindications (i.e., reasons not to conduct the exercise test). Other conditions, referred to as *relative contraindications*, may increase the risk of exercise testing; people with these conditions only should be tested if a doctor determines that the need for the test outweighs the potential risk. Note that the American College of Sports Medicine (ACSM) interprets these contraindications as being for symptom-limited maximal exercise testing (1).

Resting Cardiovascular Tests and Body Composition Assessment

The first assessments typically include measurement of resting HR and BP. It is ideal to provide an environment without distractions (i.e., separate from activities within the facility) along with allowing the participant to use the restroom, because a full bladder, among other factors, can affect BP, as shown in *Avoiding Error in Resting Measures of Blood Pressure* (2). Additional details on how to assess BP are discussed more fully in chapter 8.

Body composition measures typically are made prior to other activities. Simple measures of weight in relation to height (i.e., body mass index) and circumference (e.g., waist, waist-to-hip ratio) can be easily tracked over time. Assessments that estimate body fat (e.g., skinfold measures) can also be included. Details on these assessments are found in chapter 11.

Tests for Cardiorespiratory Fitness

Although resting measures (HR, BP) provide baseline information, the fitness professional will also want to determine how the client's cardiorespiratory system responds to aerobic activity. Various levels of assessment can be made, including maximal exercise tests, submaximal exercise tests that can be used to estimate maximal aerobic capacity, and field tests that provide insights on CRF without requiring laboratory equipment (1). All these tests allow for evaluation of physiologic responses when the body is at work, and those responses are used in the assessment of CRF. Selection of the level of testing depends on several factors including the purpose of the test (e.g., diagnostic clinical assessment or submaximal test to estimate aerobic capacity for establishing a general CRF baseline), level of supervision and equipment (e.g., a field test requiring a measured course and a

American Heart Association's Contraindications to Exercise Testing

Absolute Contraindications

- Acute myocardial infarction (MI) within 2 days
- Ongoing unstable angina
- Uncontrolled cardiac arrhythmia with hemodynamic compromise
- Active endocarditis
- Symptomatic severe aortic stenosis
- Decompensated heart failure
- Acute pulmonary embolism, pulmonary infarction, or deep vein thrombosis
- Acute myocarditis or pericarditis
- Acute aortic dissection
- Physical disability that precludes safe and adequate testing

Relative Contraindications

- Known obstructive left main coronary artery stenosis
- Moderate to severe aortic stenosis with uncertain relation to symptoms
- Tachyarrhythmias with uncontrolled ventricular rates
- Acquired advanced or complete heart block
- Hypertrophic obstructive cardiomyopathy with severe resting gradient
- Recent stroke or transient ischemic attack
- Mental impairment with limited ability to cooperate
- Resting hypertension with systolic or diastolic blood pressures >200/110 mmHg
- Uncorrected medical conditions such as significant anemia, important electrolyte imbalance, and hyperthyroidism

Reprinted by permission from G.F. Fletcher et al., "Exercise Standards for Testing and Training: A Scientific Statement from the American Heart Association," *Circulation* 128, no. 8 (2013): 873-934.

stopwatch compared with a clinical maximal test that uses a treadmill and metabolic analysis system under the supervision of a physician), age of the participant (e.g., some tests are designed specifically for children, older adults, or those with physical limitations), and level of fitness (e.g., a field test that involves running would not be used for someone who is currently inactive). Details on maximal and submaximal tests, along with various field tests, are discussed in chapter 8.

Tests for Muscular Fitness

Muscular fitness is an umbrella term that encompasses muscular strength, muscular endurance, and muscular power. Muscular strength reflects the ability of the muscle or muscle group to generate maximal force (e.g., 1-repetition max, which is the maximal weight that can be lifted once but not multiple times). Muscular endurance reflects the ability of a muscle or muscle group to make repeated contractions or to sustain a contraction. Muscular power reflects the work done per unit of time. Muscular fitness has been described as being "an integral

portion of total health-related fitness" and "an integral part of performance-related fitness" (1). These descriptions reflect the importance of muscular fitness within activities of daily living (ADL) as well as in exercise, sport, and active recreation. Details on tests to assess the various aspects of muscular fitness are discussed in chapter 9. As with CRF testing, the participant's age, fitness level, and health status are considerations when selecting muscular fitness assessments.

Assessment for Flexibility and Functional Fitness

Flexibility is one of the components of fitness that may be overlooked given the relative lack of impact on health or mortality (8). Flexibility reflects the capacity to move joints freely throughout their normal range of motion; thus flexibility affects not only exercise performance and sport but also the ability to move within daily activities. Assessments for flexibility are discussed in chapter 10.

Functional fitness reflects various motor skills such as balance, coordination, gait, and agility (6). Training

Avoiding Error in Resting Measures of Blood Pressure

When taking BP measurements, the details matter, as shown in the following table (2). (*Note:* The values for potential error are not cumulative.)

Error	Correction	Potential increase in BP
Sitting with legs crossed	Feet should be flat on the floor with legs uncrossed	2-8 mmHg
Placing cuff over the top of clothing	Place cuff directly on the skin of the arm	5-50 mmHg
Using a cuff that is too small	Ensure the correct length and width of cuff is used (note marking on cuff that will show appropriate range)	2-10 mmHg
Taking a measurement when the client has a full bladder	Have client void the bladder prior to taking resting measures	10 mmHg
Talking by the client or talking to the client	No one should be talking during measurement of BP	10 mmHg
Having client hold out their arm for measurement	Support the arm during measurement	10 mmHg
Having client sit where the back and feet are not supported	Provide a seat with back support and at an appropriate height to allow feet to be flat on the floor	6 mmHg

Source: American Heart Association and American Medical Association. n.d. Target: BP, Measure Accurately. Accessed: February 2023. https://targetbp.org/blood-pressure-improvement-program/control-bp/measure-accurately/.

APPLICATION POINT

Identifying Errors in Blood Pressure Assessment

Examine the following picture to find five errors in BP measurement that could increase BP.

Answer: Errors in measurement can cause an increase in BP, including placing the cuff over clothing, having the client hold out their arm for measurement, having the client sit with the back and feet not supported, allowing the client's legs to be crossed, and talking with the client during the measurement.

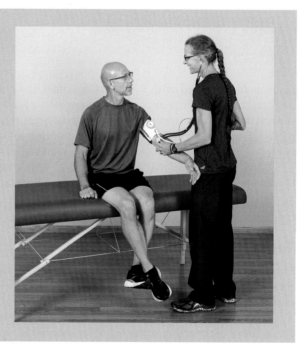

these aspects has been referred to as *neuromotor exercise training* and can be done along with resistance training and flexibility exercises in activities such as tai ji (tai chi), qigong, and yoga (6). Although research evidence has focused mainly on the benefits of neuromotor exercise training for the reduction of fall risk in older adults (1), consider the value of the motor skills enlisted in typical ADL. Assessments of the various components of functional fitness are found in chapter 10.

Development of and Participation in an Individualized Exercise Program

Equipped with the information gathered from resting measures and fitness tests, the fitness professional can develop an individualized exercise program. There is no one-size-fits-all exercise program because each person has a unique health status and goals. Additionally, fitness varies widely among individuals. A given individual may even differ in the various fitness components. Perhaps their level of aerobic fitness is low but muscular fitness is high, or they may have excellent flexibility but very poor balance. The fitness professional must review the various exercise test results to identify which areas of fitness need more (or less) attention (e.g., low level of aerobic fitness warrants more time devoted to this component of fitness) along with a careful discussion of client goals. (See chapter 22 for more on goal setting and encouraging adherence to life-long exercise.) Part III of this book focuses on aspects of exercise prescription to promote CRF, muscular fitness, flexibility, and functional (neuromotor) fitness. Chapter 16 includes sample programs that include the various components for beginners to established exercisers.

Periodic Retest and Activity Revision

To conduct an assessment only once may be helpful in setting up an exercise program but lacks the greater value that periodic testing can offer. A single assessment provides a snapshot of status at one point in time. This baseline information is used to develop an exercise program for the client. Repeating the assessment after 2 or 3 months of engaging in physical activity provides insight into the effectiveness of the exercise program for those starting out. For more established exercisers, biannual or annual assessments may be sufficient because large changes will be less likely. Progress can be celebrated, and lack of progress can be addressed with revisions of the exercise program.

LEARNING AIDS

REVIEW QUESTIONS

1. What is the difference between reliability and objectivity? Why are these two characteristics key to the validity of a test?

2. Describe and give examples of ways a fitness professional can increase accuracy of fitness testing.

3. How can a fitness professional help their client understand the meaning of fitness test scores?

4. What is the difference between percentile rankings and criterion-referenced standards?

5. List principles that can enhance participation in physical activity by people with disabilities.

6. Describe the content found in the informed consent document and why this communication tool is so important.

7. What is the difference between absolute and relative contraindications to exercise testing?

8. What are the five main areas that are assessed with fitness testing?

9. When interpreting fitness testing scores, what client characteristics should be considered when developing an exercise program for the client?

CASE STUDIES

1. You will be meeting with a new client to conduct fitness testing. What steps should you take to prepare for the session?

2. A new health club has contacted you to develop procedures for fitness testing that will be conducted by several fitness professionals. What areas of testing would you recommend and what factors would you consider when selecting specific assessments?

Answers to Case Studies

1. For exercise testing, all paperwork should be available and organized (i.e., informed consent, preparticipation and health screenings), the test environment should be prepared (i.e., as private of a location as possible and at an appropriate room temperature), and equipment should be ready (i.e., calibrated as needed and in working order). The client's file, including the data sheets to record resting and fitness test data, should be available to record measurements and scores immediately. The fitness professional should know the test protocols and be ready to explain the tests and test outcomes in a manner that is easily understood.

2. You will need to discuss with the health club owner what age and fitness level is anticipated for the clients as well as what equipment is available. Having a separate, private space for testing is optimal. Fitness assessments should include tests for CRF, muscular fitness, body composition, and flexibility, as well as potentially functional fitness. When selecting specific assessments, ensure that each is reliable, objective, and, to the extent possible, valid. Tests selected should be appropriate for the facility and background of employees (i.e., tests that do not require physician supervision if at a nonmedical facility). All employees who will be conducting fitness assessments should receive training to ensure consistent administration of the tests and appropriate knowledge of safety procedures.

Cardiorespiratory Fitness Assessments

Barbara A. Bushman

OBJECTIVES

The reader will be able to do the following:

1. Describe how cardiorespiratory fitness (CRF) relates to health and list reasons for and risks associated with testing CRF
2. List variables measured during a graded exercise test
3. Describe procedures used before, during, and after testing
4. Contrast the treadmill, cycle ergometer, and bench step as instruments for exercise testing
5. Contrast submaximal and maximal exercise tests
6. Describe the heart rate extrapolation procedures to estimate $\dot{V}O_2$max using submaximal treadmill, cycle, and bench-step exercise tests
7. Describe procedures for walking and running field tests to estimate CRF
8. Describe how to calibrate a treadmill and a Monark cycle ergometer

Higher levels of physical activity and cardiorespiratory fitness (CRF) are associated with reduced risks of chronic diseases and death. Consequently, it is important to focus on a healthy level of CRF as a lifelong goal that makes life more enjoyable and healthy. Those benefits alone merit the inclusion of CRF in any discussion about positive health (30). CRF, also called *cardiovascular* or *aerobic fitness*, is a good measure of the heart's ability to pump oxygen-rich blood to the muscles. Although the terms *cardio* (heart), *vascular* (blood vessels), *respiratory* (lungs and ventilation), and *aerobic* (working with oxygen) differ technically, they all reflect aspects of CRF. A person with a healthy heart that can pump great volumes of blood with each beat has a high level of CRF. CRF values are expressed in the following ways (as discussed in more detail in chapter 6):

- Liters of oxygen used by the body per minute ($L \cdot min^{-1}$)
- Milliliters of oxygen used per kilogram of body weight per minute ($ml \cdot kg^{-1} \cdot min^{-1}$)
- METs, multiples of resting metabolic rate, where $1\ MET = 3.5\ ml \cdot kg^{-1} \cdot min^{-1}$

A person with the ability to use $35\ ml \cdot kg^{-1} \cdot min^{-1}$ during maximal exercise is said to have a CRF equal to 10 METs ($35 \div 3.5 = 10$). Aerobic training programs increase the heart's ability to pump blood, so it is no surprise that such programs improve CRF.

Resting measures do not reveal how the cardiorespiratory system responds to activity, although lower resting HR is typically observed in individuals with higher CRF. Submaximal exercise tests can be used to estimate maximal aerobic capacity while not requiring maximal effort on the part of the participant. Maximal exercise tests, typically used in clinical, research, and athletic settings with appropriate supervision, also can be used to measure CRF. Field tests can provide insights on CRF without requiring laboratory equipment. All of these exercise tests can be used to evaluate various physiologic responses when the body is at work, and those responses are used in the assessment of CRF.

Results from CRF tests are used to write exercise recommendations, and they allow the fitness professional or physician to evaluate positive or negative changes in CRF resulting from physical conditioning, aging, illness, or inactivity. Given the current increase in obesity and inactivity in people of all ages, it makes sense to evaluate CRF throughout life, from early childhood to old age. This information indicates an individual's stand on cardiorespiratory health and alerts them to subtle lifestyle changes that may compromise positive health. The nature of the tests and the level of monitoring should vary across age groups to reflect the required information.

CRF testing depends on the purposes of the test, the type of person to be evaluated, and the work tasks available. Reasons for testing include the following:

- Determining physiological responses at rest and during submaximal or maximal work
- Providing a basis for exercise programming
- Evaluating the effectiveness of a training program
- Screening for coronary heart disease (CHD)
- Determining a person's ability to perform a specific work task

CRF can be measured or estimated with maximal graded exercise tests, submaximal tests, or even field tests. Choosing an appropriate test depends on several factors including age, fitness level, known health problems, and risks of CHD. The American College of Sports Medicine (ACSM) notes that the decision on whether a maximal or submaximal test is used depends on the reasons for the test, the individual's risk level, and the availability of needed equipment and qualified personnel (3). In health and fitness settings, CRF is typically assessed with submaximal exercise tests (3). Given that maximal tests require exercise to fatigue, these tests may not be appropriate in some situations (e.g., fitness facilities) and may require availability of emergency equipment (3). The American Heart Association has provided guidance on supervision of clinical exercise tests in a scientific statement, *Supervision of Exercise Testing by Nonphysicians: A Scientific Statement from the American Heart Association* (49). This statement focuses on clinical exercise testing and provides guidance on screening and recommended levels of supervision. Key factors for non-physician supervision include properly trained professionals who meet competency requirements, are trained in cardiopulmonary resuscitation, and are supported by a physician who is available for pretest assessments or any complications that arise (49).

Graded exercise tests (GXT) are exercise tests that have progressive stages (e.g., increasing speed and/or grade on a treadmill or increasing resistance or pedal cadence on a cycle ergometer). Exercise is thus used to place a load on the heart to determine the cardiovascular response and to see if the electrocardiogram (ECG) measurements change (24). Although submaximal exercise tests are not as effective as maximal tests in identifying disease, they are appropriate for making activity recommendations and determining functional responses to exercise (3). Any GXT protocol can be used for submaximal or maximal testing; the only difference is the criteria for stopping the test. Either type of test is stopped if any of the abnormal responses listed in the sidebar *ACSM's General Indications for Stopping an Exercise Test* occur (3). In the absence of abnormal responses, the submaximal test usually is terminated when the person reaches a certain HR (often 85% of maximum HR), and the maximal test is stopped when the person reaches voluntary exhaustion.

ACSM's General Indications for Stopping an Exercise Test*

- Onset of angina or angina-like symptoms
- Drop in systolic blood pressure (SBP) of ≥10 mmHg with an increase in work rate or if SBP decreases below the value obtained in the same position prior to testing
- Excessive rise in BP: systolic pressure of >250 mmHg and/or diastolic pressure of >115 mmHg
- Shortness of breath, wheezing, leg cramps, or claudication
- Signs of poor perfusion: light-headedness, confusion, ataxia, pallor, cyanosis, nausea, or cold and clammy skin
- Failure of HR to increase with increased exercise intensity
- Noticeable change in heart rhythm by palpation or auscultation
- Individual requests to stop
- Physical or verbal manifestations of severe fatigue
- Failure of the testing equipment

*Assumes that testing is nondiagnostic and is being performed without ECG monitoring.

Note that additional criteria for clinical testing can be found elsewhere (3).

Reprinted by permission from American College of Sports Medicine, *ACSM's Guidelines for Exercise Testing and Prescription*, 11th ed. (Philadelphia, PA: Wolters Kluwer, 2022), 78.

Field tests that require little equipment are covered at the end of the chapter. Field tests rely on the observation that for a person to walk or run at high speeds over long distances, the heart must pump great volumes of oxygen to the muscles. In this way, the average speed maintained in these tests gives an estimate of CRF. A higher average speed indicates a greater capacity to transport oxygen, resulting in a higher CRF score. An endurance run of a set distance for a given time or of a set time for a given distance provides information about a person's cardiorespiratory endurance as long as the run is 1 mile (1.6 kilometers) or longer. The advantages of an endurance run test include its moderately high correlation to maximum oxygen consumption, the use of a natural activity, and the large numbers of participants who can be tested in a short time. The disadvantages of endurance run tests are that it is difficult to monitor physiological responses and other factors may influence the outcome (e.g., motivation, environment). As such, field tests may not be appropriate for all populations.

As indicated in chapters 1 and 2, the risks associated with exercising are low compared with the benefits of being physically active. The risk of cardiac events with exercise testing varies depending on the prevalence of cardiovascular diseases in the group being tested (3). ACSM points out that the risk of exercise testing is low, as evidenced by research studies conducted for several decades that included a range of populations. Data from these studies show approximately 6 cardiac events per 10,000; given most studies involved maximal symptom limited tests, the risk of submaximal testing would be expected to be lower (3). Fitness professionals should emphasize that the overall CHD risk is greater for those who remain sedentary than for those who take an exercise test and then embark on a regular exercise program (3). This is consistent with evidence showing that low CRF directly relates to a higher risk of heart disease and death (12). The fitness professional should review the individual's health history and complete appropriate screenings to maximize safety. With some conditions the risk of exercise testing outweighs potential benefit; these are referred to as *absolute contraindications* to exercise testing. Other situations require an individualized assessment of the risk in relationship to benefit and are referred to as *relative contraindications* to exercise testing. The absolute and relative contraindications to exercise testing as described by the American Heart Association (26) are discussed in chapter 7.

KEY POINT

CRF is an important aspect of quality of life as well as a risk factor for CHD. The ability to use oxygen during exercise is the basis for CRF and can be expressed in $L \cdot min^{-1}$, $ml \cdot kg^{-1} \cdot min^{-1}$, and METs. CRF testing is used for programming exercise, screening for heart disease, and determining a person's ability to do a specific task. The risk of death attributable to exercise testing is very low.

Common Measures to Examine CRF

Various measurements can be taken, and repeated over time, that reflect CRF. Two of these measures are HR and BP, both of which can be done at rest and during submaximal or maximal exercise testing. Ensuring accurate and consistent measurement technique is key when measuring HR and BP. In addition, during exercise, the rating of perceived exertion (RPE) is typically recorded to gain insight on the subjective level of effort. Measurement or estimation of $\dot{V}O_2$max is also used to track CRF.

Heart Rate

HR is the number of times the heart contracts and is expressed in beats per minute (bpm). HR often is used as a fitness indicator at rest and during a standard submaximal exercise bout. Maximal HR is useful for guiding a client to exercise at a recommended intensity. This is referred to as a target heart rate range (THR) (see chapter 13). Although helpful within an exercise prescription, maximal HR is not a good fitness indicator because it changes little with training. Measured maximal HR is valuable when determining target or training HR, because age-based predictions are only estimates (i.e., actual HRmax may vary from the estimation based on equations such as 220 − age; HRmax estimations are discussed in chapter 13). Table 8.1 summarizes how endurance training affects HR in various situations.

When an ECG is recorded, the HR can be taken from the ECG recording (see chapter 12). Without an ECG, HR can be measured with a HR monitor (chest strap and receiver or watch), a stethoscope, or manual palpation of an artery (e.g., radial artery at the wrist). HR monitors are quite accurate and easy to use because HR is displayed in real time. Heart beats can be counted via auscultation, placing a stethoscope on the chest. More commonly, palpation of the pulse is used. When palpating, fingers (not the thumb) should be used, preferably at the wrist (radial artery). See *Palpating Pulse* for more details on manual palpation to determine HR. The pulse count at rest is typically taken for a full minute, or for 30 seconds and multiplied by 2 to determine the bpm (3). During exercise, the pulse count can be taken for 10 seconds, 15 seconds, or 30 seconds (2); longer durations are more accurate. The 10-, 15-, or 30-second count is multiplied

by 6, 4, or 2, respectively, to calculate bpm. When taken after exercise, measurement should begin soon after exercise ends (e.g., within 5 seconds) and should be taken for 10 or 15 seconds because the HR changes rapidly. For example, if a 10-second postexercise pulse count is 20, the HR is 120 bpm (6 × 20 = 120). When counting, start the timer on a beat that is counted as 0 (2).

Blood Pressure

Systolic (SBP) and diastolic (DBP) blood pressures can be measured at rest, during exercise, and after exercise. At rest, BP is classified as normal when SBP is less than 120 mmHg and DBP is less than 80 mmHg (62). With aerobic exercise, SBP is expected to increase with increasing exercise workload, while DBP tends to stay the same or even decrease. BP typically is measured during each stage of a GXT. If BP does not respond as predicted, an exercise test would need to be terminated (see sidebar *ACSM's General Indications for Stopping an Exercise Test*). BP should be taken upon completion of an exercise test and every 2 minutes for 6 to 8 minutes or longer if the BP has not returned to near baseline (pretest) levels (56). Given the valuable insights BP provides, the ability to measure BP accurately is vital for a fitness professional. Details to consider are provided in *Maximizing Accuracy of Blood Pressure*.

Rating of Perceived Exertion

Borg introduced rating of perceived exertion (RPE)—that is, how hard a person perceives exercise to be—using a scale from 6 to 20 (roughly based on resting to maximal HR, i.e., 60-200 bpm) (13). The Borg RPE scale has been used to judge the degree of effort experienced during an exercise test or an exercise session. For example, using the classic scale of 6 to 20, level of effort can be classified in the following way:

- Very light <10
- Light 10-11
- Moderate 12-13
- Vigorous 14-16
- Very hard 17-19
- Maximal 20

Relative level of effort for moderate and vigorous intensity can also be communicated with a scale of 0 to

Table 8.1 Effects of Endurance Training on Heart Rate

Condition	Effects of fitness on HR
Rest	↓
Standard submaximal work (same external work rate)	↓
Maximal work	No change
Set % of maximal	No change

Palpating Pulse

Palpating the pulse at a peripheral site allows the fitness professional to easily determine HR. Accessible sites include the radial artery and carotid artery. The radial pulse can be palpated at the proximal aspect of the wrist, just lateral to the flexor carpi radialis tendon (47). The carotid pulse can be found between the larynx and the anterior border of the sternocleidomastoid muscle on the right or left side of the neck (40). Although both radial and carotid pulses are easily accessible, the radial pulse is the typical site for determination of HR (40). Other reasons to select the radial pulse rather than the carotid pulse include the following:

- The carotid sinus is a baroreceptor or stretch receptor that can respond to mechanical stretch. If baroreceptors of the carotid sinus are activated (i.e., by applying too much pressure over the carotid sinus), HR would be decreased (4).

- The carotid pulse requires the fitness professional to be within the client's personal space (i.e., hand placed on the neck) to a greater extent than when accessing the radial pulse.

- The carotid pulse is impractical for use during exercise because the participant's movement would make stabilizing the area for measurement impossible.

Thus, the use of the radial pulse for rest as well as subsequent measurements during exercise is recommended.

When taking the radial pulse during exercise, ensure the participant's arm is supported, relaxed, and not in contact with the exercise equipment. This will aid in feeling the pulses rather than misinterpreting vibration of the equipment or movement of the arm or flexor tendons of the hand as a pulse (see the photo for positioning). The participant's hand on the nonmeasurement side can remain in contact with the equipment to help steady the person while the measurement is taken.

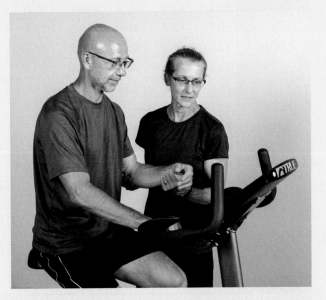

The fitness professional's arms are adducted (held tightly against the sides of the body), supporting the participant's lower arm at the elbow with one hand while palpating the radial pulse with the other hand in order to stabilize and support the client's arm to promote accurate HR measurement at the radial artery.

10, where a level 0 is sitting at rest and 10 is maximal effort. Using this scale, moderate-intensity activity is an effort level of 5 or 6 and vigorous-intensity activity begins at an effort level of 7 or 8 (59).

The relative effort concept can be used with a GXT to provide useful information during the test on the client's response and to serve as a reference for exercise prescription. The RPE scale can also be used in exercise prescriptions. When administering the RPE scale during a GXT, fitness professionals should provide the following instructions to the participant (1):

- During the exercise test pay close attention to how hard you feel the exercise work rate is.

- This feeling should reflect your total amount of exertion and fatigue, combining all sensations and feelings of physical stress, effort, and fatigue.

- Do not concern yourself with any one factor such as leg pain, shortness of breath, or exercise intensity, but try to concentrate on your total, inner feeling of exertion.

- Try not to underestimate or overestimate your feelings of exertion; be as accurate as you can.

Maximal Oxygen Consumption

Various methods will be discussed in this chapter to assess or estimate $\dot{V}O_2$max. These results can be helpful in developing and revising cardiorespiratory activity programs. The percentile values in table 8.2 provide opportunity for comparison with members of a group, based on age and sex. These percentile rankings are best used as reference points for participation progress, given the lack of a health criteria standard for CRF (as discussed in chapter 7).

Table 8.2 Percentile Values for Maximal Oxygen Uptake

Rating (percentile)	Age 20-29 M	Age 20-29 W	Age 30-39 M	Age 30-39 W	Age 40-49 M	Age 40-49 W	Age 50-59 M	Age 50-59 W	Age 60-69 M	Age 60-69 W	Age 70-79 M	Age 70-79 W
95	66.3	56.0	59.8	45.8	55.6	41.7	50.7	35.9	43.0	29.4	39.7	24.1
90	61.8	51.3	56.5	41.4	52.1	38.4	45.6	32.0	40.3	27.0	36.6	23.1
85	59.3	48.3	54.2	39.3	49.3	36.0	43.2	30.2	38.2	25.6	35.5	22.2
80	57.1	46.5	51.6	37.5	46.7	34.0	41.2	28.6	36.1	24.6	31.4	21.3
75	55.2	44.7	49.2	36.1	45.0	32.4	39.7	27.6	34.5	23.8	30.4	20.8
70	53.7	43.2	48.0	34.6	43.9	31.1	38.2	26.8	32.9	23.1	28.4	20.5
65	52.1	41.6	46.6	33.5	42.1	30.0	36.3	26.0	31.6	22.0	27.6	19.9
60	50.2	40.6	45.2	32.2	40.3	28.7	35.1	25.2	30.5	21.2	26.9	19.4
55	49.0	38.9	43.8	31.2	38.9	27.7	33.8	24.4	29.1	20.5	25.6	19.2
50	48.0	37.6	42.4	30.2	37.8	26.7	32.6	23.4	28.2	20.0	24.4	18.3
45	46.5	35.9	41.3	29.3	36.7	25.9	31.6	22.7	27.2	19.6	24.0	17.8
40	44.9	34.6	39.6	28.2	35.7	24.9	30.7	21.8	26.6	18.9	22.8	17.0
35	43.5	33.6	38.5	27.4	34.6	24.1	29.5	21.2	25.7	18.4	22.4	16.8
30	41.9	32.0	37.4	26.4	33.3	23.3	28.4	20.6	24.6	17.9	21.2	15.9
25	40.1	30.5	35.9	25.3	31.9	22.1	27.1	19.9	23.7	17.2	20.4	15.6
20	38.1	28.6	34.1	24.1	30.5	21.3	26.1	19.1	22.4	16.5	19.2	15.1
15	35.4	26.2	32.7	22.5	29.0	20.0	24.4	18.3	21.2	15.6	18.2	14.6
10	32.1	23.9	30.2	20.9	26.8	18.8	22.8	17.3	19.8	14.6	17.1	13.6
5	29.0	21.7	27.2	19.0	24.2	17.0	20.9	16.0	17.4	13.4	16.3	13.1

Values are in ml · kg^{-1} · min^{-1}; M = men; W = women; age in years. Fitness categories (percentile): Superior = 95; Excellent = 80-90; Good = 60-75; Fair = 40-55; Poor = 20-35; Very Poor = 5-15.

CRF Registry Advisory Board.

Maximizing Accuracy of Blood Pressure

To accurately measure BP, care must be taken to follow standard technique and avoid measurement errors. The setup is the first step, including the following (48):

- Select the proper cuff size. The bladder length should be 75% or greater of the patient's arm circumference and the length-to-width ratio of 2:1. Note that cuffs typically are labeled for ranges of arm circumference with lines to show whether the cuff size is correct when wrapped in place on the arm. Too large of a cuff will result in an erroneous lower reading, and too small of a cuff will result in a higher reading.

- The cuff should be on bare skin, not over clothing and not with sleeves rolled up (due to potential constriction or tourniquet effect).

- The cuff should be placed securely on the arm with space to allow for one finger to fit under the top and bottom edges of the cuff easily and for two fingers to fit very snugly.

For measurement at rest, attention must be taken to the following positioning and environment for the participant (48):

- When seated, the arm should be at the level of the heart, back should be supported, feet flat on the floor, and legs should not be crossed.

- The arm should be supported on a table or by the person taking the measurement to avoid elevated BP if the arm is held up by the participant; isometric contraction will elevate BP.

- Neither the participant nor the person taking the measurement should talk during the measurement.

Placement of the cuff should allow for the diaphragm or bell of the stethoscope to be placed over the brachial artery, which is located on the medial aspect of the antecubital fossa. The lower edge of the cuff should be approximately 2 centimeters above the antecubital fossa (48). The stethoscope earpieces should be oriented forward (i.e., toward the nose, so a memory cue is "you knows [nose] which way it goes"). Inflating the bladder of the cuff increases pressure around the arm, allowing for blood flow to be temporarily occluded through the brachial artery. The cuff should be inflated to at least 30 mmHg above the point the radial pulse disappears (48). No sound will be heard through the stethoscope at this point. Pressure is released from the bladder of the cuff at a rate of 2 mmHg per second or per heartbeat if HR is very slow (48). As pressure is released from the bladder of the cuff, blood is able to move back through the brachial artery at the highest pressure point (i.e., SBP); this will be a detectable sound, often described as a sharp tapping. The tapping will continue until blood flow is at the lowest point (DBP), at which point no audible sound will be heard. BP is recorded to the nearest even number at the onset of sound (SBP) and then the last audible sound (DBP).

BP measures during exercise are more challenging given the movement of the participant and noises related to exercise (e.g., foot strike on the treadmill). In addition to appropriate cuff size and placement, recommendations for exercise BP measures include the following (56):

- Place the BP monitor such that it is within 1 meter and can be viewed directly.
- Ensure the participant's shoulder and arm are relaxed; supporting the arm is key.
- Place the stethoscope bell or diaphragm over the brachial artery, avoiding excessive pressure, which can result in sounds heard below the DBP due to distortion of the artery.
- No talking should occur during measurement.

Although all these considerations may seem overwhelming, with practice and careful attention to technique, BP measures will become easier over time. Given the importance of assessing BP at rest and determining changes during exercise, accurate measures are vital.

In addition to technique, ensuring calibration of the sphygmomanometer is important. The manometer may be a mercury or an aneroid type. The mercury type is simple in design and was considered to be the standard for many decades, but it is not used in many clinical settings due to environmental concerns related to mercury toxicity (48). As a replacement to mercury devices, aneroid sphygmomanometers are commonly used, relying on metal bellows that expand and contract with changes in pressure. Aneroid units can experience a loss of calibration and thus should be monitored and calibrated regularly to ensure accuracy (48). A quick check to determine if an aneroid unit is out of calibration is to look at the calibration mark or zero point (25) (see the photos). If the indicator needle is outside of the oval when the cuff is fully deflated, the unit is out of calibration and should not be used. If the indicator needle falls within the oval, calibration issues still could exist because mechanical aspects of the gauge (e.g., springs, bellows) may wear, causing errors when pressure is applied (i.e., nonlinear errors may be present). Regular checks against a calibrated reference standard are recommended (25).

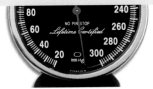

With needle outside the oval, you can be 100% sure the unit is OUT of calibration.

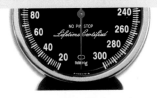

With needle inside the oval, you cannot be 100% sure the unit is in calibration. Periodically check against a calibrated reference standard.

Aneroid unit calibration mark: When the needle is outside the oval, the unit is out of calibration; when the needle is inside the oval, this does not guarantee the unit is in calibration, and the unit must be periodically checked against a calibrated reference standard.
©American Diagnostic Corporation 2023

KEY POINT

Common variables measured during a GXT include HR, BP, and RPE. Oxygen consumption can be measured at each stage of a test and at maximal exertion; $\dot{V}O_2$max can be estimated from the final stage achieved during a maximal GXT.

Graded Exercise Tests

This section explains how to administer a GXT and includes examples of various testing protocols. Because HR, BP, and RPE responses are influenced by several factors, variation in each factor from test to test should be carefully minimized. Some of these factors include

- temperature and relative humidity of the room;
- number of hours of sleep before testing;
- emotional state;
- hydration state;
- medication;
- time of day;
- time since last meal, cigarette smoking, caffeine intake, and exercise; and
- psychological environment of the test (i.e., the participant's comfort level with the surroundings during testing).

Attention to these factors increases the likelihood that changes in HR, BP, or RPE from one test to the next actually reflect changes in physical fitness and physical activity habits. A form such as the Sample Pretest Instructions for a Fitness Test (see form 8.1) helps ensure that the client is ready for testing.

Typical procedures to follow during GXTs are shown in *Steps to Administering a Graded Exercise Text*. A series of end points should be used to stop a GXT (3). These guidelines are for nondiagnostic testing performed without direct physician involvement or ECG monitoring. The assumption is that informed consent as well as preactivity screening and health history were completed, and the participant has been cleared, if necessary, for exercise testing and physical activity.

Modes of Exercise for Use in GXTs

An exercise test can be conducted using various modes of activity, given the ability to increase the workload systematically. When selecting the mode of exercise, the fitness professional must consider availability of equipment, participant experience and comfort, and testing aspects such as reproducibility and cost.

Bench Step

Bench stepping is economical and can be used for maximal testing as well as submaximal testing. The disadvantages include the limited number of stages for any one bench height, individual fitness level, and the difficulty of taking certain measurements during the test (e.g., BP).

Cycle Ergometer

Cycle ergometers are portable, moderately priced work instruments that allow easy measurement of HR and BP because the participant's upper body is essentially stationary. Their disadvantages, however, are that the exercise load is self-paced and that fatigued leg muscles may be a limiting factor. On mechanically braked cycle ergometers such as the Monark models, altering the pedal rate or the resistance on the flywheel changes the work rate. Generally, the pedal rate is constant during a GXT at a rate appropriate to the person being tested: 50 to 60 rpm for those of low to average fitness and 70 to 100 rpm

---

FORM 8.1   Sample Pretest Instructions for a Fitness Test

Name: _____ Test date: _____

Time: _____ Report to: _____

INSTRUCTIONS

Please observe the following:

1. Wear athletic shoes, shorts, and a loose-fitting shirt.
2. No food, drink (except water), tobacco, or caffeine for 3 hours before the test.
3. Do minimal physical activity on the day of the test.

CANCELLATION

If you cannot keep this appointment, please call _____ or _____.

Steps to Administering a Graded Exercise Test

Before Test Day

1. Ensure that testing personnel have been trained to implement the emergency action plan (see chapters 23 and 24).
2. Calibrate the exercise equipment (e.g., treadmill, cycle ergometer).
3. Make sure a scale, stadiometer, HR monitor, and sphygmomanometer are available.
4. Check supplies and data forms and that the RPE chart is clearly visible.
5. Select the appropriate test protocol for the participant.

Test Day

1. Ensure that the testing room is clean, quiet, and comfortable (e.g., temperature between 68 and 72 °F [20 and 22 °C], adequate ventilation).
2. Greet participant and verify that pretest instructions were followed.
3. Verify completion of informed consent (oral and written) and ensure all preparticipation and health screenings are complete.
4. Record age and measure height and weight. Calculate and record estimated HRmax and 70% and 85% HRmax.
5. Obtain resting HR and BP.
6a. Demonstrate how to do the step test and ask if the participant has any questions.
   - Have the participant practice the test protocol.
   - Make sure the participant can keep pace with the metronome or recording of step cadence.

OR

6b. Teach the participant how to use the cycle ergometer.
   - Adjust the seat height so the participant's knee is slightly flexed when the foot is at the bottom of the pedal swing and parallel to the floor.
   - Instruct the participant to keep pace (e.g., 50 rpm) with the metronome, speedometer, or digital display of pedal rate.
   - Tell the participant to lightly hold on to the handlebars and to release their hold when BP is taken.

OR

6c. Demonstrate how to get on and off and how to walk on the treadmill.
   - Have the participant hold on to the railing while getting a feel for belt speed by putting one foot on the belt to practice keeping up with the belt.
   - Have the participant step onto the belt, keeping eyes ahead and back straight, and walk in a relaxed manner with first one arm and then both arms swinging.
   - To maintain balance, the participant can touch the railing lightly with open hands, without grasping the railing.
7. Follow test protocol exactly.
   - Ask how the participant feels during the test.
   - Follow the criteria for terminating the test (e.g., %HRmax for a submaximal test).
   - HR, BP, and RPE are the usual variables recorded at each stage of the test.

Based on American College of Sports Medicine, *ACSM's Guidelines for Exercise Testing and Prescription,* 11th ed. (Philadelphia, PA: Wolters Kluwer, 2022).

for highly fit and competitive cyclists (31). A metronome or some other source of feedback such as a speedometer helps the person maintain the pedal rate. The resistance (load) on the wheel is increased sequentially to systematically overload the cardiovascular system. The starting work rate and the increment from one stage to the next depend on the fitness of the person being tested and the purpose of the test.

The cycle ergometer differs from the treadmill in that the seat supports the body weight, and the work rate depends primarily on pedal rate and the load on the wheel. This means that the relative $\dot{V}O_2$ at any work rate is higher for a smaller person than for a bigger person. In addition, the increments in the work rate demand a fixed increase in the $\dot{V}O_2$ (e.g., an increment of 150 kgm · min^{-1} equals a $\dot{V}O_2$ change of 270 ml · min^{-1}), forcing the small or unfit subject to make cardiovascular adjustments greater than those of a large or highly fit subject. Table 8.3 summarizes how differences in body weight affect the metabolic responses to weight-supported (e.g., cycle ergometry) and weight-carrying (e.g., bench stepping, walking, running) work tasks. Thus, for tasks in which body weight provides the resistance (weight-carrying tasks), a larger person achieves a greater absolute $\dot{V}O_2$ (L · min^{-1}) than a smaller person achieves, but both work at the same MET level. In cycling (a weight-supported task), the two people achieve a similar absolute $\dot{V}O_2$, but the larger person has a lower MET level.

Treadmill

Treadmill protocols are very reproducible because they set the pace for the subject, whereas the subject may go too slow or too fast on the bench step or the cycle ergometer. Treadmill tests can accommodate people of any fitness level and use the natural activities of walking and running, with the running tests placing the greatest potential load on the cardiovascular system. Treadmills, however, are expensive, are not portable, and make some measurements (e.g., BP) difficult. The type of treadmill test influences the measured $\dot{V}O_2$max, with the graded running test giving the highest value, the running test at 0% grade giving the next highest value, and the walking test giving the lowest value in comparison (9, 43).

To estimate $\dot{V}O_2$ by varying grade and speed, the grade and speed settings on the treadmill must be calibrated correctly (see details on how to calibrate a treadmill at the end of this chapter). Further, the subject cannot hold the treadmill railing during the test if the estimated $\dot{V}O_2$ values are going to be correct. For example, it was observed that HR decreased 17 bpm when a subject who was walking on a treadmill at 3.4 mph (5.5 km · hr^{-1}) and at a 14% grade held on to the treadmill railing (7). Holding on to the railing results in an overestimation of the $\dot{V}O_2$max because the HR is lower at any stage of the test and so the test lasts longer. With the treadmill test, there is no need to adjust the $\dot{V}O_2$ calculation for differences in body weight because the person being tested carries their own weight; therefore, the $\dot{V}O_2$ (ml · kg^{-1} · min^{-1}) is independent of body weight (45).

KEY POINT

CRF can be determined with bench stepping, cycle ergometers, or treadmills. The oxygen consumption values (expressed in ml · kg^{-1} · min^{-1}) are similar for most adults at specific stages of a treadmill or step test because the energy cost is proportional to body weight, which is carried by the test participant. In contrast, the absolute oxygen consumption (expressed in L · min^{-1}) is similar for most adults at each stage of a cycle ergometer test; however, the relative oxygen cost (ml · kg^{-1} · min^{-1}) is higher for lighter participants.

Testing Protocols

The following testing protocols are examples of tests used for various populations. These protocols can be used for submaximal or maximal testing, though it is important to remember that the criteria for stopping the test will not be the same. The first protocol, shown in table 8.4, could be used with deconditioned subjects

Table 8.3 Effect of Body Weight on Metabolic Responses to Various Work Tasks

| Work task | $\dot{V}O_2$MAX | | | | |
	L · min^{-1}	ml · kg^{-1} · min^{-1}	Energy production (kcal)	METs
Bench	↑	=	↑	=
Walk	↑	=	↑	=
Run	↑	=	↑	=
Body weight–supported cycle	=	↓	=	↓

MET = metabolic equivalent. Symbols (↑ or ↓ or =) indicate how a heavier person responds compared with a lighter person.

Table 8.4 Treadmill Protocols for Various Categories

Stage	METs	Speed (km · hr^{-1})	Grade (%)	Time (min)
		DECONDITIONED INDIVIDUALS[a]		
1	2.5	3.2	0.0	3
2	3.5	3.2	3.5	3
3	4.5	3.2	7.0	3
4	5.4	3.2	10.5	3
5	6.4	3.2	14.0	3
6	7.3	3.2	17.5	3
7	8.5	4.8	12.5	3
8	9.5	4.8	15.0	3
9	10.5	4.8	17.5	3
		NORMAL INACTIVE INDIVIDUALS[b]		
1	4.3	4.8	2.5	2
2	5.4	4.8	5.0	2
3	6.4	4.8	7.5	2
4	7.4	4.8	10.0	2
5	8.5	4.8	12.5	2
6	9.5	4.8	15.0	2
7	10.5	4.8	17.5	2
8	11.6	4.8	20.0	2
9	12.6	4.8	22.5	2
10	13.6	4.8	25.0	2
		YOUNG ACTIVE INDIVIDUALS[c]		
1	5.0	2.7	10.0	3
2	7.0	4.0	12.0	3
3	9.5	5.4	14.0	3
4	13.0	6.7	16.0	3
5	16.0	8.0	18.0	3

MET = metabolic equivalent.

[a]From Naughton and Haider (1973). [b]From Balke (1970). [c]From Bruce (1972).

who would start at a low MET level, walk slowly, and increase 1 MET per 3-minute stage (50). The Balke standard protocol (11) could be used for inactive adults by having them start at a higher MET level and progress 1 MET per 2-minute stage. More active or younger people could be tested on the Bruce protocol (15), which starts at a moderate MET level and goes up 2 or 3 METs per 3-minute stage. Unfortunately, some testing centers use the same testing protocol for all people, with the result that the initial stage is often too high or too low and the work increments for each stage are too small or too large for the person being tested. Estimating $\dot{V}O_2max$ from the final stage of a maximal GXT has a standard error of the estimate (SEE; this reflects the variation or accuracy of a prediction) of about 3 ml · kg^{-1} · min^{-1} (52).

As discussed in chapter 6, formulas may be used to estimate oxygen consumption from the stage reached in a GXT. In general, these formulas reasonably estimate $\dot{V}O_2$ if the GXT is suited to the individual. However, if the increments in the GXT stages are too large relative to the person's CRF, or if the time spent at each stage is too short, the person might not reach the steady-state oxygen requirement associated with that stage (46). Selection of test protocol, including the stage duration and the progression (i.e., MET increase per stage) must be considered. Failure to achieve the oxygen requirement for a GXT stage results in overestimating $\dot{V}O_2$ at each stage of the test, with the overestimation growing larger with each stage. The inability to reach the oxygen requirement is a common problem with people who are less fit (e.g., cardiac patients). This inability suggests that more conservative (i.e., smaller increments between stages) GXT protocols should be used to allow these individuals to reach the oxygen demand at each stage. In contrast, shorter stages and larger increments between stages in a GXT can be used if the purpose of the test is to screen for ECG abnormalities in a clinical setting (rather than to estimate $\dot{V}O_2$max). In addition, changes in a participant's CRF over time can be determined by periodically using the same GXT.

Maximal Exercise Tests

Considerations related to supervision of maximal testing have been discussed previously; ACSM notes maximal testing in health and fitness testing is often not feasible and thus submaximal testing is used (3). This section provides background on maximal testing. No one GXT protocol is appropriate for all people. The durations, starting points, and increments between stages vary from person to person. A duration of 8 to 12 minutes has been suggested to be a target duration for a maximal GXT (26). Young, active people; sedentary people with no health issues; and people with questionable health status should start at 6, 4, and 2 METs, respectively. The same three groups should increase by 2 to 3, 1 to 2, and 0.5 to 1 METs, respectively, for progressive stages of the test. Customized protocols also can be considered with athletic populations. For example, in one research study the treadmill protocol was individualized based on each subject's 10-kilometer race pace, starting 2 mph below race pace, increasing 1 mph every 3 minutes until running at 1 mph above race pace, at which time treadmill grade was increased 2% every 2 minutes until fatigue (28). Maximal exercise testing in children may be conducted in clinical settings to evaluate signs or symptoms related to abnormal responses to exercise, to assess functional capacity or evaluate prognosis, or to provide baseline for rehabilitation (51). Guidance on clinical pediatric stress testing is beyond the scope of this textbook; additional information on protocols and special considerations can be found elsewhere (51).

Oxygen consumption increases with each stage of the GXT until it reaches its upper limit. Measurement of oxygen consumption is described in chapter 4 and requires computer-controlled equipment to measure oxygen consumption, carbon dioxide production, and volume of air exhaled. During a GXT, $\dot{V}O_2$ increases with increasing work until $\dot{V}O_2$max is reached. At that point, $\dot{V}O_2$ does not increase when the test moves to the next stage. To verify that a test provides a maximal effort, various criteria have been applied (3):

- $\dot{V}O_2$max plateaus with increased workload.
- HR does not increase with increasing workload.
- Postexercise blood lactate is greater than 8 mmol · L^{-1}.

- Peak respiratory exchange ratio (RER) is greater than 1.10.
- An RPE of >17 (on the 6-20 Borg scale) or >7 (on the 0-10 scale) has been suggested to confirm maximal effort. (See Research Insight *Criteria for $\dot{V}O_2$max* in chapter 4 for additional background.)

Without more sophisticated equipment for measurement of $\dot{V}O_2$ (as found in clinical, research, and advanced testing centers), estimations can be made based on HR or workload achieved as discussed in chapter 6.

Submaximal Tests to Estimate Cardiorespiratory Fitness

The submaximal test usually provides the HR and BP responses to various intensities of work ranging from light intensity up to a predetermined point (usually 85% of predicted maximum HR). Submaximal tests can be used to estimate $\dot{V}O_2$max by extrapolating HR to a predicted maximum and then using the linear relationship between HR and oxygen consumption to estimate $\dot{V}O_2$max. Although this estimated maximum is useful for evaluating a person's current CRF status and prescribing or revising exercise, the estimation involves considerable error (±15%). Estimation of $\dot{V}O_2$max from submaximal exercise tests has a SEE of about 5 ml · kg^{-1} · min^{-1} (52). However, submaximal tests are reliable, and changes in HR, BP, and RPE resulting from exercise conditioning make submaximal tests a good mechanism for showing improvements in CRF.

The general format for submaximal exercise testing is as follows:

1. Complete all preliminary items: informed consent, preactivity screening, health history, informed consent, protocol selection, test site preparation, and measurement of resting HR and BP.

2. Estimate maximal heart rate (HRmax = 220 – age) and calculate 85% of HRmax (HRmax × 0.85).

3. Review protocol with participant and ensure the participant is comfortable with the mode of exercise, including setting appropriate seat height if using cycle ergometry (i.e., slight bend in the knee when the foot is at the bottom of the pedal stroke).

4. Have subject complete a brief 2- to 3-minute warm-up at a low intensity.

5. Stages are commonly 3 minutes, with the following activities:
   - 1:30—measure and record HR and BP
   - 2:30—measure and record HR
   - 2:55—ask how participant is doing

RESEARCH INSIGHT

Error Involved in Estimating $\dot{V}O_2$max

Estimating $\dot{V}O_2$max by any of the methods described in this chapter is associated with an inherent error compared with the directly measured $\dot{V}O_2$max. To determine the validity of an exercise test to estimate $\dot{V}O_2$max, investigators must first test large numbers of subjects in the laboratory to measure each subject's $\dot{V}O_2$max. On another day, the investigators may have the subjects complete a distance run for time or a standardized graded treadmill or cycle ergometer test to determine the highest percent grade and speed or work rate that the subject can achieve. That information is then used to develop an equation to predict the measured $\dot{V}O_2$max from the time of the distance run, the last grade and speed achieved on a treadmill test, or the final work rate on the cycle ergometer test.

The predicted value usually will not equal the measured $\dot{V}O_2$max value, and the SEE describes how far off (higher or lower) the predicted value might be from the true value when using the prediction equation. One SEE describes where 68% of the estimates are compared with the true value. If the SEE were 1 ml $\cdot$ kg^{-1} $\cdot$ min^{-1}, then 68% of the predicted $\dot{V}O_2$max values would fall within ±1 ml $\cdot$ kg^{-1} $\cdot$ min^{-1} of the true value. Typically, the SEE is larger than that, approaching 5 ml $\cdot$ kg^{-1} $\cdot$ min^{-1} in some cases (52).

The relatively large standard errors might suggest that these exercise tests have little value, but that is not the case. The tests are reliable, and when the same person takes the same test over time, the change in estimated $\dot{V}O_2$max monitored by the test is a reasonable reflection of improvements in CRF. This can serve as both a motivational and an educational tool when working with fitness clients.

- 3:00—increase exercise level if the HR is less than 85% HRmax

6. Repeat the activities in each subsequent stage of increasing intensity until the participant reaches 85% HRmax. (This assumes there were no reasons for stopping the test prior to that point; see *ACSM's General Indications for Stopping an Exercise Test.*)

7. Adjust workload to a low intensity, and have the participant cool down.

KEY POINT

Submaximal and maximal tests can use the same GXT protocol; however, their criteria for test termination differ. Maximal tests are more effective in identifying ischemic heart disease in clinical settings. Submaximal tests are useful in assessing fitness and are relatively inexpensive to administer. Although the $\dot{V}O_2$max estimated from a submaximal test is not as accurate as that obtained from a maximal test, it is useful in evaluating changes in CRF due to an exercise program.

Submaximal Treadmill Test Protocol

The initial stage and rate of progression of the GXT should be selected using the guidelines mentioned earlier. For the example depicted in figure 8.1, a Balke protocol listed in table 8.4 for normal inactive individuals (3 mph, or 4.8 km $\cdot$ hr^{-1}, 2.5% grade increase every 2 minutes) was used; HR was monitored in the last 30 seconds of each stage. The test was terminated at 85% of the age-predicted maximal HR (using the equation 220 − age). Maximal aerobic power was estimated by extrapolating the HR response to the person's estimated maximal HR. Figure 8.1 presents the results of this test with a graph showing the HR response at each work rate. The HR response is rather flat between the 0% and 5% grades (i.e., initial low-intensity stages). This is not uncommon; perhaps the subject is too excited, or perhaps the stroke volume changes are accounting for the changes in cardiac output at these low work rates. The HR response is usually quite linear between 110 bpm and the subject's 85% HRmax.

To estimate $\dot{V}O_2$max, the procedures of Maritz and colleagues (41) are followed. A line is drawn through the HR points from the 7.5% grade to the final work rate. This line is extended (extrapolated) to the person's estimated maximal HR (183 bpm). A vertical line is dropped from the last point to the baseline to estimate the subject's maximal aerobic power, which in this example is 11.8 METs, or 41.3 ml $\cdot$ kg^{-1} $\cdot$ min^{-1}. Any HR estimation formula (e.g., 220 − age) used to estimate maximal HR has error (SEE of about 10 bpm). Consequently, this possible inaccuracy influences any estimate of maximal oxygen consumption derived from extrapolating HR to an estimated maximal HR. If this person's true (measured) maximal HR is 173 or 193 bpm, the estimated maximal MET level is 11.0 METs or 12.6 METs, respectively.

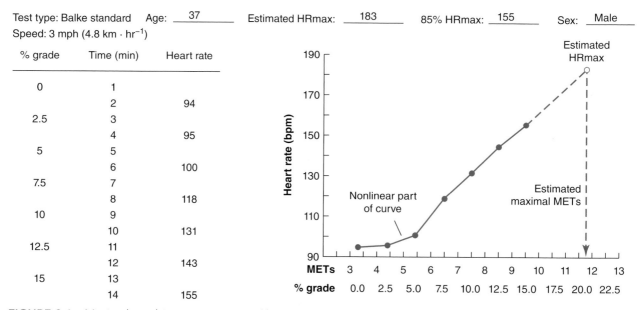

Test type: Balke standard   Age: ___37___   Estimated HRmax: ___183___   85% HRmax: ___155___   Sex: ___Male___
Speed: 3 mph (4.8 km · hr⁻¹)

% grade	Time (min)	Heart rate
0	1	
	2	94
2.5	3	
	4	95
5	5	
	6	100
7.5	7	
	8	118
10	9	
	10	131
12.5	11	
	12	143
15	13	
	14	155

FIGURE 8.1   Maximal aerobic power estimated by measuring the HR response to a submaximal GXT on a treadmill.

Submaximal Cycle Ergometer Test Protocol

Submaximal cycle ergometer protocols have been provided in the *Y's Way to Physical Fitness* (64) and in the *YMCA Fitness Testing and Assessment Manual* (65). These two protocols rely on the linear relationship between HR and work rate ($\dot{V}O_2$) that occurs once an HR of approximately 110 bpm is reached. Both of these protocols require the person to complete one more stage beyond the one that induces an HR of at least 110 bpm (i.e., there must be two stages where the final HR is 110 or above). The line describing the HR–work rate relationship is extrapolated to the person's age-predicted maximal HR (as was done for the treadmill protocol) to estimate the person's $\dot{V}O_2$max. Each test stage lasts 3 minutes unless a person's HR has not yet reached a steady state. Steady state is defined as less than 5 bpm difference between second- and third-minute HR. If steady state is not reached, an extra minute is added to that stage. The pedal rate is maintained at 50 rpm so that, on a Monark cycle ergometer, a 0.5-kilogram increase in load equals 150 kgm · min⁻¹ (25 W). Seat height is adjusted so that the knee is slightly bent (8) when the pedal is at the bottom of the stroke through a revolution. The seat height is recorded for future reference. HR is monitored during the latter half of the second and third minutes of each stage.

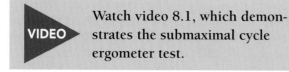

Watch video 8.1, which demonstrates the submaximal cycle ergometer test.

Selection of the initial work rate and the rate of progression on the cycle ergometer should consider body weight, sex, age, and physical activity level. In general,

- absolute $\dot{V}O_2$max (L · min⁻¹) is lower in smaller people,
- women have lower absolute $\dot{V}O_2$max values than men,
- $\dot{V}O_2$max decreases with age, and
- inactivity is associated with low $\dot{V}O_2$max values.

The YMCA tests address body weight, fitness, and so on by starting everyone at 150 kgm · min⁻¹ and using the HR response to that specified work rate to set subsequent stages in the test (see figure 8.2 for one sequencing option [65]; a prior guide from the YMCA uses four sequences based on HR response to the initial 150 kgm · min⁻¹ work rate in ranges of <80 bpm, 80-89 bpm, 90-100 bpm, and >100 bpm [64]). Large or fit subjects would have a low HR response to the initial work rate and would use the most strenuous sequence of work rates (top section in figure 8.2). A small or unfit subject would have a high HR response to the 150 kgm · min⁻¹ work rate and would follow the sequence with the smallest increments in the power output (see bottom section in the figure). Subjects should complete only one additional work rate beyond the one demanding an HR of 110 bpm.

The HR values for the second and third minutes of each work rate are recorded, and directions are followed to estimate $\dot{V}O_2$max in liters per minute. Figure 8.3 presents an example of a test for a 50-year-old woman who weighs 59 kilograms. The stages follow the pattern dictated by the HR response to the initial work rate of 150 kgm · min⁻¹ as presented in figure 8.2. A line is drawn through the last two HR values (i.e., final HR measured for each of the last two stages) and extrapolated to the estimated maximal HR. A vertical line, dropped from the last point of the extrapolated line to the baseline, estimates the subject's maximal work rate to be 750 kgm · min^{-1}. With the formula described earlier (and in chapter 6) for the cycle ergometer, $\dot{V}O_2$max for this woman is estimated to be about 30 ml · kg^{-1} · min^{-1}, or 1.77 L · min^{-1}.

Another way to determine the estimated $\dot{V}O_2$max from the YMCA test is to use the following calculations:

1. Determine the $\dot{V}O_2$ for each of the two workloads within the target range for HR (i.e., final two stages in which the last HR is 110 bpm or higher) using the equation from chapter 6 for leg ergometry:

$$\dot{V}O_2 = (1.8 \times \text{work rate} \div \text{body weight}) + 3.5 + 3.5$$

2. Determine the slope of the line by taking the difference in the $\dot{V}O_2$ for the two stages

(submax 1 [SM1] for the first stage within the target HR range and submax 2 [SM2] for the final stage of the test) divided by the final HR of each of those stages (considered as HR1 and HR2):

$$\text{slope} = (\text{SM2} - \text{SM1}) \div (\text{HR2} - \text{HR1})$$

3. Then calculate the estimated $\dot{V}O_2$max using this equation (estimating HRmax based on age: 220 – age):

$$\dot{V}O_2\text{max} = \text{SM2} + [\text{slope} \times (\text{HRmax} - \text{HR2})]$$

For the prior example of the 50-year-old female (body weight 59 kilograms), these are the calculations for $\dot{V}O_2$ for the final two stages of the test:

$$\dot{V}O_2 \text{ for the work rate of 450: } \dot{V}O_2$$
$$= (1.8 \times 450 \div 59) + 3.5 + 3.5 = 21$$

$$\dot{V}O_2 \text{ for the work rate of 600: } \dot{V}O_2$$
$$= (1.8 \times 600 \div 59) + 3.5 + 3.5 = 25$$

To determine slope:

$$\text{slope} = (25 - 21) \div (154 - 140) = 0.29$$

Estimate $\dot{V}O_2$max, assuming HRmax is 170 (calculated as 220 – age: 220 – 50 = 170):

$$\dot{V}O_2\text{max} = 25 + [0.29 \times (170 - 154)]$$
$$= 30 \text{ ml} \cdot \text{kg}^{-1} \cdot \text{min}^{-1}$$

In contrast to the YMCA test, the Åstrand and Ryhming cycle ergometer test (8) requires the subject to complete only one 6-minute work rate requiring an HR between 125 and 170 bpm. Table 8.5 can be used to estimate $\dot{V}O_2$max from the subject's HR response to one 6-minute work rate (6). HR is measured each minute, with the mean of the final two HRs used to estimate

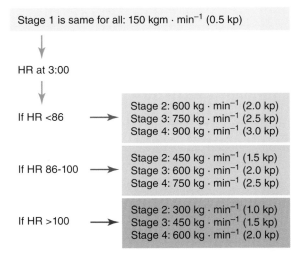

Stage 1 is same for all: 150 kgm · min^{-1} (0.5 kp)

HR at 3:00

If HR <86 → Stage 2: 600 kg · min^{-1} (2.0 kp)
Stage 3: 750 kg · min^{-1} (2.5 kp)
Stage 4: 900 kg · min^{-1} (3.0 kp)

If HR 86-100 → Stage 2: 450 kg · min^{-1} (1.5 kp)
Stage 3: 600 kg · min^{-1} (2.0 kp)
Stage 4: 750 kg · min^{-1} (2.5 kp)

If HR >100 → Stage 2: 300 kg · min^{-1} (1.0 kp)
Stage 3: 450 kg · min^{-1} (1.5 kp)
Stage 4: 600 kg · min^{-1} (2.0 kp)

FIGURE 8.2 Guide for setting power outputs (workloads) on YMCA submaximal cycle ergometer test.

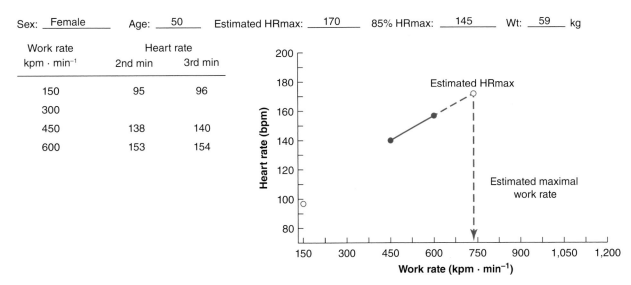

| Sex: Female | Age: 50 | Estimated HRmax: 170 | 85% HRmax: 145 | Wt: 59 kg |

| Work rate | Heart rate | |
kpm · min^{-1}	2nd min	3rd min
150	95	96
300		
450	138	140
600	153	154

FIGURE 8.3 Maximal aerobic power estimated by measuring the HR response to a submaximal GXT on a cycle ergometer using the protocol from the *YMCA Fitness Testing and Assessment Manual*.

Table 8.5 Predicting Maximal Oxygen Uptake From Heart Rate and Workload During a 6-Minute Cycle Ergometer Test

	$\dot{V}O_2MAX$ (L · MIN⁻¹) VALUES FOR WOMEN						$\dot{V}O_2MAX$ (L · MIN⁻¹) VALUES FOR MEN				
HR	300 kgm · min⁻¹	450 kgm · min⁻¹	600 kgm · min⁻¹	750 kgm · min⁻¹	900 kgm · min⁻¹	HR	300 kgm · min⁻¹	600 kgm · min⁻¹	900 kgm · min⁻¹	1,200 kgm · min⁻¹	1,500 kgm · min⁻¹
120	2.6	3.4	4.1	4.8		120	2.2	3.5	4.8		
122	2.5	3.2	3.9	4.7		122	2.2	3.4	4.6		
124	2.4	3.1	3.8	4.5		124	2.1	3.3	4.5	6.0	
126	2.3	3.0	3.6	4.3		126	2.0	3.2	4.4	5.8	
128	2.2	2.8	3.5	4.2	4.8	128	2.0	3.1	4.2	5.6	
130	2.1	2.7	3.4	4.0	4.7	130	1.9	3.0	4.1	5.5	
132	2.0	2.7	3.3	3.9	4.5	132	1.8	2.9	4.0	5.3	
134	2.0	2.6	3.2	3.8	4.4	134	1.8	2.8	3.9	5.2	
136	1.9	2.5	3.1	3.6	4.2	136	1.7	2.7	3.8	5.0	
138	1.8	2.4	3.0	3.5	4.1	138	1.6	2.7	3.7	4.9	
140	1.8	2.4	2.8	3.4	4.0	140	1.6	2.6	3.6	4.8	6.0
142	1.7	2.3	2.8	3.3	3.9	142		2.5	3.5	4.6	5.8
144	1.7	2.2	2.7	3.2	3.8	144		2.5	3.4	4.5	5.7
146	1.6	2.2	2.6	3.2	3.7	146		2.4	3.3	4.4	5.6
148	1.6	2.1	2.6	3.1	3.6	148		2.4	3.2	4.3	5.4
150		2.0	2.5	3.0	3.5	150		2.3	3.2	4.2	5.3
152		2.0	2.5	2.9	3.4	152		2.3	3.1	4.1	5.2
154		2.0	2.4	2.8	3.3	154		2.2	3.0	4.0	5.1
156		1.9	2.3	2.8	3.2	156		2.2	2.9	4.0	5.0
158		1.8	2.3	2.7	3.1	158		2.1	2.9	3.9	4.9
160		1.8	2.2	2.6	3.0	160		2.1	2.8	3.8	4.8
162		1.8	2.2	2.6	3.0	162		2.0	2.8	3.7	4.6
164		1.7	2.1	2.5	2.9	164		2.0	2.7	3.6	4.5
166		1.7	2.1	2.5	2.8	166		1.9	2.7	3.6	4.5
168		1.6	2.0	2.4	2.8	168		1.9	2.6	3.5	4.4
170		1.6	2.0	2.4	2.7	170		1.8	2.6	3.4	4.3

Reprinted by permission from P.-O. Åstrand, *Work Tests with the Bicycle Ergometer* (Varberg, Sweden: Monark Exercise AB, 1979), 24.

$\dot{V}O_2$max (6). A nomogram is also available that allows for determination of $\dot{V}O_2$max if workload and HR are known (3).

If the same 50-year-old woman completed the Åstrand and Ryhming cycle ergometer test at a work rate of 450 kgm · min⁻¹ with a mean HR for the last 2 minutes of the 6-minute test of 140 bpm, then look down the leftmost column of values for women in table 8.5 to an HR of 140, and look across to the second column of values (for a work rate of 450 kgm · min⁻¹). The estimated $\dot{V}O_2$max is 2.4 L · min⁻¹. Because maximal HR decreases with increasing age, however, and the data in table 8.5 were collected on young subjects, I. and P.-O. Åstrand (5, 6) established the following age-correction factors to correct for the lower maximal HR:

Age	Factor
15	1.10
25	1.00
35	0.87
40	0.83
45	0.78
50	0.75
55	0.71
60	0.68
65	0.65

To calculate the corrected $\dot{V}O_2$max, the estimated $\dot{V}O_2$max is multiplied by the appropriate correction factor. For the 50-year-old subject, the correction factor is 0.75, and the corrected $\dot{V}O_2$max is $0.75 \cdot 2.4 \text{ L} \cdot \text{min}^{-1}$ = $1.8 \text{ L} \cdot \text{min}^{-1}$. This value compares well with that estimated by the YMCA protocol. The Åstrand and Ryhming calculations can be completed using formulas developed by Shephard (57).

Submaximal Step-Test Protocol

A multistage step test can be used to estimate $\dot{V}O_2$max and to show changes in CRF resulting from training or detraining. The initial stage and rate of progression of the stages must be suited to the individual. The subject must follow the metronome (4 counts per cycle, i.e., up-up-down-down) and step all the way up and all the way down. Each stage should last at least 2 minutes, with HR monitored in the last 30 seconds of each 2 minutes. Using an HR watch simplifies the process of obtaining an accurate HR measure during a step test.

As in most submaximal GXT protocols, HR is plotted against work rate or $\dot{V}O_2$ for each stage, and a line is drawn through the points to the estimated maximal HR. A vertical line is then drawn to the baseline to estimate the step rate that would have been achieved if the subject had completed a maximal test. Figure 8.4 shows the results of a step test for a sedentary 55-year-old man. His estimated maximal step rate is 40 steps $\cdot$ min^{-1}. The

KEY POINT

A plot of HR responses (at least 110 bpm) to a GXT on a treadmill, cycle ergometer, or bench step can be used to estimate $\dot{V}O_2$max. A line is drawn through the HR values and is extrapolated to the subject's age-predicted estimate of maximal HR. A vertical line is drawn to the x-axis to estimate the work rate and $\dot{V}O_2$ the person would have achieved if the test had been a maximal test.

$\dot{V}O_2$max, calculated with the formula for stepping given in chapter 6, is 7.7 METs, or about 27 ml $\cdot$ kg^{-1} $\cdot$ min^{-1}.

Posttest Procedures

When the test is over, the tester should conduct a cooldown, monitor test variables, and give posttest instructions. Monitoring should continue for 6 to 8 minutes after exercise or longer if measurements of HR and BP have not returned near baseline (26). The tester should also organize the test data.

Posttest Protocol

1. Use an active cool-down procedure to help the participant transition back to rest:
   - Decrease intensity (e.g., grade on treadmill, load on cycle ergometer) and have the participant do an active recovery for 3 minutes.
   - Monitor HR and BP during recovery and transition to sitting rest when the subject feels comfortable.
   - Monitor HR and BP at the end of 1 and 3 minutes of sitting rest.
   - Remove BP cuff and HR monitor when BP and HR are close to pretest values.

2. Provide instructions for showering:
   - The participant should wait about 30 minutes before showering and should move around in the shower and use warm (not hot) water to avoid a potential drop in BP or fainting.
   - Wait for the participant to return from the shower.

3. Have the participant make an appointment to discuss the results of all the fitness tests and to discuss the exercise prescription.

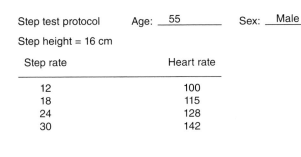

Step test protocol   Age: __55__   Sex: __Male__

Step height = 16 cm

Step rate	Heart rate
12	100
18	115
24	128
30	142

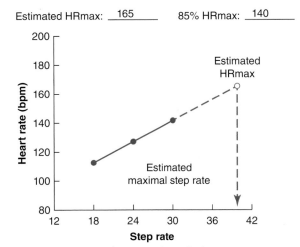

Estimated HRmax: __165__   85% HRmax: __140__

FIGURE 8.4   Maximal aerobic power estimated by measuring HR response to a submaximal graded exercise step test.

Field Tests

A variety of field tests can be used to estimate CRF. They are called *field tests* because they require little equipment, can be done just about anywhere, and use the simple activities of walking and running. Because these tests involve walking or running as quickly as possible over a set distance, they are not recommended at the start of an exercise program. Instead, participants should complete the graduated walking program before taking the walking test and the graduated jogging program before taking the running test. Sample walking and jogging programs are found in chapter 13. The graduated nature of the fitness programs allows participants to start at a low, safe level of activity and gradually improve. It is then appropriate to administer an endurance run test to evaluate fitness status.

Mile Walk Test

A 1-mile (1.6 kilometer) walk test to predict CRF accommodates individuals of different ages and fitness levels. In this test, the person walks as quickly as possible on a measured track, and HR is measured at the end of the mile. For guidance in conducting the test, see *Steps to Administering the Mile Walk Test*. Note that these directions were written for a group setting; however, the test can be used in a one-on-one setting as well.

Estimated $\dot{V}O_2$max (ml · kg^{-1} · min^{-1}) then can be calculated using the data collected in the mile walk test in the following equation:

$$\dot{V}O_2\text{max} = 132.853 - 0.0769 \text{ (weight)} - 0.3877 \text{ (age)} + 6.315 \text{ (sex)} - 3.2649 \text{ (time)} - 0.1565 \text{ (HR)}$$

In this equation, the weight is body weight in pounds, age is in years, sex equals 0 for females and 1 for males, time is in minutes and hundredths of minutes, and HR is in bpm. The formula was developed and validated on men and women ages 30 to 69 years (36), and the SEE is about 5 ml · kg^{-1} · min^{-1} (3, 36).

QUESTION:

What is the CRF of a 25-year-old man (body weight 170 pounds) who walks the mile in 20 minutes and has an immediate postexercise HR of 140 bpm?

ANSWER:

$$\dot{V}O_2\text{max} = 132.853 - 0.0769 \text{ (weight)} - 0.3877 \text{ (age)} + 6.315 \text{ (sex)} - 3.2649 \text{ (time)} - 0.1565 \text{ (HR)}$$

Steps to Administering the Mile Walk Test

Before Test Day

1. Arrange to have the following elements at the test site:
   - A person to start and read the time from a stopwatch
   - A partner with a watch for each walker (perhaps with a sheet to mark off laps)
   - A stopwatch for the timer (with a spare ready)
   - A score sheet or scorecard
2. Explain the purpose of the test (i.e., to determine how quickly the participants can walk 1 mile [1.6 kilometers], which reflects the endurance of the cardiovascular system).
3. Select and mark off (if needed) a level area for the walk.
4. Explain to the participants that they are to walk the mile in the fastest time possible. Only walking is allowed, and the goal is to cover the distance as quickly as possible.

Test Day

1. Participants warm up with dynamic stretching and slow walking.
2. Several people will walk at the same time.
3. Explain the procedure again. Remind the participants not to speed up at the end of the walk but to maintain a fast, steady pace throughout.
4. The timer says, "Ready, go," and starts the stopwatch.
5. Each participant has a partner standing at the start and finish line with a stopwatch.
6. The partner counts the laps and tells the participant at the end of each lap how many more laps to walk.
7. The timer calls out the minutes and seconds as each person finishes the mile walk.
8. The partner listens for the time when the walker finishes the mile and records it (to the nearest second) immediately on a scorecard.
9. The walker takes a 10-second HR immediately after the end of the mile walk, with the partner timing it. Using an HR watch simplifies this measurement.

$$\dot{V}O_2max = 132.853 - 0.0769\,(170) - 0.3877\,(25)$$
$$+ 6.315\,(1) - 3.2649\,(20.0) - 0.1565\,(140)$$

$$\dot{V}O_2max = 29.2\ ml \cdot kg^{-1} \cdot min^{-1}$$

The CRF can be evaluated by comparing that number with the standards presented in table 8.2, which lists percentile values for maximal aerobic power with age and sex considerations. In the example of the 25-year-old man, his maximal oxygen consumption of 29.2 ml $\cdot$ kg^{-1} $\cdot$ min^{-1} is below the 10th percentile, indicating a considerable need for improvement. This low value places him at a much higher risk for heart disease. The percentile values in table 8.2 are not intended to provide reference for comparison, but rather clients are best served by using the value as a reference point for personal change when an exercise program is introduced.

Six-Minute Walk Test

The 6-minute walk test may be used with individuals with reduced CRF, including older adults and those with various conditions such as pulmonary disease (3, 33). The 6-minute walk test is a self-paced test in which the participant is asked to walk as far as possible on a level surface in 6 minutes. Participants can slow down or even stop to rest if necessary, increasing pace or starting again until the 6-minute time has expired. The Senior Fitness Test includes the 6-minute walk test, recommending a

rectangular walking path that is 20 yards by 5 yards with marks every 5 yards (see figure 8.5) (54). The score is the number of yards completed. Normal ranges for men and women between the ages of 60 to 94 years are shown in table 8.6 (54).

Run Test

One of the most common CRF field tests is the 12-minute or 1.5-mile (2.4 kilometers) run popularized by Cooper (17). This test is like the walk test mentioned previously: Participants run as quickly as possible for 12 minutes or for 1.5 mile (2.4 kilometers). This test is based on work by Balke (10), who showed that 10- to 20-minute running tests could be used to estimate $\dot{V}O_2max$. Balke found the optimal duration for the run test to be 15 minutes. The test relies on the relationship between running velocity and the oxygen consumption required to run at that velocity (figure 8.6). The greater the running speed, the greater the oxygen consumption required. The reason for the duration of 12 to 15 minutes is that the running test has to be long enough to diminish the contribution of anaerobic sources of energy to the average velocity. The average velocity that can be maintained in a 5- or 6-minute run overestimates $\dot{V}O_2max$ because anaerobic energy sources contribute substantially to total energy production in a 5-minute run compared with a 12- to 15-minute run. If the run lasts too long, the person is

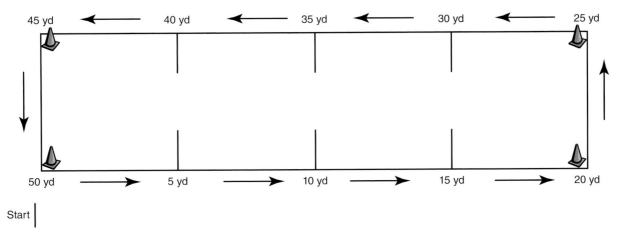

FIGURE 8.5   Setup for 6-minute walk test.
Reprinted by permission from R.E. Rikli and C.J. Jones, *Senior Fitness Manual*, 2nd ed. (Champaign, IL: Human Kinetics, 2013).

Table 8.6   Normal Range of Scores for Men and Women for 6-Minute Walk Test*

	AGE 60-64	AGE 65-69	AGE 70-74	AGE 75-79	AGE 80-84	AGE 85-89	AGE 90-94
Men	610-735	560-700	545-680	470-640	445-605	380-570	305-500
Women	545-660	500-635	480-615	430-585	385-540	340-510	275-440

*"Normal" is defined as the middle 50% of the population; higher scores are considered above average and lower scores below average for the given sex and age; age in years.
Adapted from Rikli and Jones (2013).

not able to maintain a best effort and the estimate will be low (figure 8.7).

The $\dot{V}O_2$ associated with a specific running speed can be calculated from the following formula (see chapter 6 for details; no vertical component is included given the level surface required for this assessment):

$$\dot{V}O_2 = (0.2 \times \text{horizontal velocity}) + 3.5$$

These estimates are reasonable for adults who run the entire 12 minutes or 1.5 miles (2.4 kilometers). The formula underestimates $\dot{V}O_2$max in children because they have a higher oxygen cost of running (22). In contrast, the formula overestimates $\dot{V}O_2$max in trained runners because of their better running economy (21) and in those who walk the test because the net oxygen cost of walking is half that of running (see chapter 6).

QUESTION:

A 20-year-old woman takes the Cooper 12-minute run test following a 15-week walk and jog program and com-

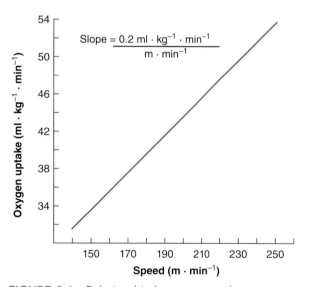

FIGURE 8.6 Relationship between steady-state oxygen consumption and running speed (14).

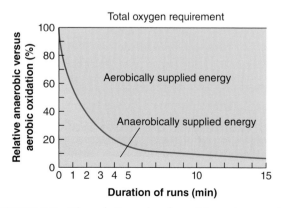

FIGURE 8.7 The relative role of aerobic and anaerobic energy sources in best-effort runs of various durations.

Adapted from Balke (1963).

pletes 6 laps on a 440-yard (402.3 meter) track. What is her estimated $\dot{V}O_2$max?

ANSWER:

$$402.3 \text{ m} \cdot \text{lap}^{-1} \times 6 \text{ laps} = 2{,}414 \text{ m}$$

$$2{,}414 \text{ m} \div 12 \text{ min} = 201 \text{ m} \cdot \text{min}^{-1}$$

$$\dot{V}O_2 = (0.2 \times 201) + 3.5$$

$$\dot{V}O_2 = 40.2 + 3.5 = 43.7 \text{ ml} \cdot \text{kg}^{-1} \cdot \text{min}^{-1}$$

Table 8.2 shows that for this 20-year-old woman, the estimated $\dot{V}O_2$max of 43.7 ml · kg^{-1} · min^{-1} is above the 70th percentile, consistent with good CRF, which should be encouraged. Blair and colleagues (12) found that values of 9 METs (31.5 ml · kg^{-1} · min^{-1}) for women and 10 METs (35 ml · kg^{-1} · min^{-1}) for men were associated with low risks of chronic disease and death from all causes. If people are not at that level, help them make small, systematic progress toward that goal by using the walking and jogging programs in chapter 13.

The advantage of the 12-minute run is that it can be used to regularly evaluate CRF without expensive equipment. It is easily adapted to cyclists and swimmers, who can evaluate their CRF progress by determining how far they can ride or swim in 12 minutes. Although no equations exist that relate cyclists' and swimmers' respective performances to $\dot{V}O_2$max, participants can personally judge their current CRF and improvement attributable to training by monitoring the distance they can cover in 12 minutes.

The 1-mile (1.6 kilometer) run is used in many youth fitness programs (18, 53). These steps can be used for other endurance runs as well (e.g., 1.5-mile [2.4 kilometer] or 12-minute run). Note that *Steps to Administering the Mile Run* is written for a group setting; however, the test can be used in a one-on-one setting as well.

For youth age 10 to 17 years, body mass index and age are considered along with the mile run time to predict $\dot{V}O_2$max (20). The relationship between $\dot{V}O_2$max and the 1-mile run time is curvilinear, with a linear relationship established for times below 11 minutes and no relationship at higher times. Thus, any times above 13 minutes should be set to 13 before using the equation (19). Within the following equations, the MRT is the time it took to complete the mile run in minutes, the age is in years, and the BMI is in kg · m^{-2}. The calculation is as follows for males ($\dot{V}O_2$max in ml · kg^{-1} · min^{-1}):

$$\dot{V}O_2\text{max} = 108.94 - (8.41 \times \text{MRT}) + (0.34 \times \text{MRT}^2) + (0.21 \times \text{age}) - (0.84 \times \text{BMI})$$

And for females (the age adjustment factor is removed; $\dot{V}O_2$max in ml · kg^{-1} · min^{-1}):

$$\dot{V}O_2\text{max} = 108.94 - (8.41 \times \text{MRT}) + (0.34 \times \text{MRT}^2) - (0.84 \times \text{BMI})$$

Steps to Administering the Mile Run

Before Test Day

1. Arrange to have the following elements at the test site:
   - A person to start and read the time from a stopwatch
   - A partner for each runner (perhaps with a sheet to mark off laps)
   - A stopwatch for the tester (with a spare ready)
   - A score sheet or scorecard

2. Explain the purpose of the test (i.e., to determine how quickly participants can run 1 mile [1.6 kilometer], which reflects the endurance of the cardiovascular system).

3. Do not administer the test until participants have had several fitness sessions, including some with running.

4. Have participants practice running at a set submaximal pace for 1 lap, then 2, and so on several times before the test day.

5. Select and mark off (if needed) a level area for the run.

6. Explain to people being tested that they are to run the mile in the fastest time possible. Walking is allowed, but the goal is to cover the distance as quickly as possible.

Test Day

1. Participants warm up with dynamic stretching, walking, and slow jogging.

2. Several people will run at the same time.

3. Explain the procedure again.

4. The timer says, "Ready, go," and starts the stopwatch.

5. Each participant has a partner with a stopwatch.

6. The partner counts the laps and tells the participant at the end of each lap how many more laps to run.

7. The timer calls out the minutes and seconds as the runner finishes the mile run.

8. The partner listens for the time when the runner finishes the mile and records it (to the nearest second) immediately on a scorecard.

9. The runner continues to walk 1 lap after finishing the run.

KEY POINT

A 1-mile (1.6 kilometer) walking test can be used to estimate CRF. The time of the walk and the HR measured at the end of the walk are used to calculate $\dot{V}O_2$max. A 1.5-mile (2.4 kilometer) run test also can be used to estimate CRF. The time to complete the 1.5-mile (2.4 kilometer) run is used to determine average velocity, and a formula is used to calculate $\dot{V}O_2$max. The time for a 1-mile run, along with age and BMI, can be used to estimate $\dot{V}O_2$max for boys and girls ages 10 to 17 years.

Table 8.7 FitnessGram Standards for Aerobic Capacity ($ml \cdot kg^{-1} \cdot min^{-1}$)*

Age (yr)	Boys	Girls
10	40.2	40.2
11	40.2	40.2
12	40.3	40.1
13	41.1	39.7
14	42.5	39.4
15	43.6	39.1
16	44.1	38.9
17	44.2	38.8

*Values listed represent the Healthy Fitness Zone (sufficient fitness if at that level or above).

Adapted from Cooper Institute for Aerobics Research (2017).

This aerobic capacity determination is part of a fitness assessment program for youth called FitnessGram (developed by The Cooper Institute; see www.fitnessgram.net for more information) (19). Performance is criterion-referenced rather than percentile-based standards, so for aerobic capacity, the Healthy Fitness Zone reflects the level of fitness required for low risk of future health problems. Two other levels, Needs Improvement and the Needs Improvement-Health Risk Zone, show elevated levels of risk. See table 8.7 for the FitnessGram values related to aerobic capacity that indicate being in the Healthy Fitness Zone (18).

QUESTION:

An 11-year-old boy completes the 1-mile run with a time of 10 minutes. His body weight is 35 kilograms and height is 138 centimeters. What is his estimated $\dot{V}O_2max$?

ANSWER:

Using the equation, insert the known information. (*Note:* BMI based on his height and weight is 18.4 kg · m^{-2}; steps on how to calculate BMI are found in chapter 11.)

$$\dot{V}O_2max = 108.94 - (8.41 \times 10) + (0.34 \times 10^2) + (0.21 \times 11) - (0.84 \times 18.4)$$

$$\dot{V}O_2max = 45.7 \text{ ml} \cdot \text{kg}^{-1} \cdot \text{min}^{-1}$$

Comparing to norms, he meets the level for being in the Healthy Fitness Zone for the FitnessGram assessment (see table 8.7).

Progressive Aerobic Cardiovascular Endurance Run

An alternative CRF field test is the Progressive Aerobic Cardiovascular Endurance Run, or PACER. This test, developed by Leger and colleagues (38, 39), is a 20-meter shuttle run test done to the sound of a beep as the individual moves between the boundary lines. The speed required at the start is 5.3 mph (8.5 km · hr^{-1}), and it increases 0.3 mph (0.5 km · hr^{-1}) each minute. Three rapid beeps signal progression to the next level, where the time between beeps becomes shorter. The test is terminated when the individual cannot keep up with the beeps, and the number of 20-meter laps completed is used to estimate CRF. The PACER test is part of the fitness testing battery in the FitnessGram, developed by The Cooper Institute (18). In a study of 10- to 15-year-old youth (55), the average $\dot{V}O_2max$ measured (not estimated) on the PACER test was the same as that measured on a standard treadmill test. In addition, no differences were observed in the maximal HR or the RER values, lending additional validity to the PACER test as an excellent indicator of CRF in children. Criterion-referenced standards for CRF have been validated for this test (16). This protocol also has been used to estimate $\dot{V}O_2max$ in adults (44, 58); however, a practice trial may be needed to establish a stable baseline to use as a reference for monitoring changes over time (37). In another version, called the *square shuttle run*, subjects run around a 15-meter square in a gym. Based on directly measured $\dot{V}O_2$ during the run, it has been shown to have good validity and reliability when testing adults (27).

RESEARCH INSIGHT

Can $\dot{V}O_2max$ Be Estimated Without Doing an Exercise Test?

This may seem like a strange question given the focus on exercise testing in this chapter. However, if it were possible, it would allow investigators (primarily epidemiologists) to easily classify large numbers of people into CRF categories (e.g., bottom 20%, middle 20%, and top 20%) and determine if CRF is linked to various chronic diseases. Doing exercise testing on such large populations would be impossible due to time, cost, personnel, and so on.

In one of the earliest investigations, Jackson and colleagues (35) showed that by using the simple variables of age, gender, body fatness or BMI, and self-reported physical activity, $\dot{V}O_2max$ could be estimated with a SEE of approximately 5 ml · kg^{-1} · min^{-1}, an error similar to that observed with field tests and submaximal GXT estimates of $\dot{V}O_2max$. The accuracy of the prediction (SEE of approximately 4-6 ml · kg^{-1} · min^{-1}) has been confirmed in several other studies (29, 32, 42, 60, 61, 63). These models have been useful in placing subjects into fitness categories; however, the prediction is less accurate in the most and least fit subjects (60).

What does this say about doing exercise tests? Even though the SEE is relatively large for field tests and submaximal GXTs, the tests are reliable, and when the same person takes the same test over time, the change in estimated $\dot{V}O_2max$ monitored by the test is a reasonable reflection of improvements in CRF. This can serve as both a motivational and an educational tool when working with fitness clients.

LEARNING AIDS

REVIEW QUESTIONS

1. What is the general relationship between CRF and chronic disease?

2. What is the logical sequence of steps to take leading up to a GXT?

3. You are using the 1-mile (1.6 kilometer) walk test to track CRF over time, but you are not concerned with generating a $\dot{V}O_2max$ value. If you wanted to provide good feedback to your client about fitness improvements being made, what two variables would you measure from this test? What would you expect to happen to them as fitness improves?

4. Why are running tests to estimate $\dot{V}O_2max$ usually done for 12 minutes or so for adults? What would happen to the estimated $\dot{V}O_2max$ value if an all-out 3-minute run test were used?

5. What are some advantages and disadvantages of cycle ergometer tests compared with treadmill tests?

6. Why are clients asked to not eat, smoke, or drink caffeinated beverages in the hours before a submaximal GXT?

7. What is the difference between a submaximal and maximal GXT?

8. If submaximal GXT protocols have an inherent error associated with estimating $\dot{V}O_2max$, why do the test?

9. What investigators would be interested in estimating $\dot{V}O_2max$ without exercise testing?

CASE STUDIES

1. You are contacted by a fitness club to review the test it uses to evaluate CRF in middle-aged participants. The club requires the participants to perform the 1.5-mile (2.4 kilometer) run test during their first exercise session. The club director says he uses this test because, over the past decade, he has developed a good database to track clients. What is your reaction?

2. You conduct the 1-mile (1.6 kilometer) walk test with a 45-year-old male client and record the following information: Time = 15 min, HR = 140 bpm, and weight = 170 pounds. Calculate and evaluate his estimated $\dot{V}O_2max$.

3. A 51-year-old male weighing 80 kilograms completes a submaximal YMCA test, and the following data are obtained. Note that the workload for stage 2 was based on the HR response to the first workload of 150 kgm · min^{-1}, per the YMCA test protocol shown in figure 8.2 (65). Four stages were required in order to achieve the required two workloads with HR of 110 bpm or higher. HR is also steady state for each stage (HR within 5 bpm for measurements at 2 and 3 minutes).

kgm · min^{-1}	HR for min 2	HR for min 3
150	80	84
600	104	108
750	116	120
900	132	128

Estimate the subject's $\dot{V}O_2max$ using the calculations provided within the chapter. Compare the results with the normative values.

4. A 30-year-old woman weighing 54.4 kilograms completes four stages of a submaximal Balke treadmill test at 3 mph (80.4 m · min^{-1}), and the following data are obtained:

% grade	HR
2.5	96
5	120
7.5	135
10	150

Estimate the subject's $\dot{V}O_2$max using the extrapolation method, and express it in $ml \cdot kg^{-1} \cdot min^{-1}$, $L \cdot min^{-1}$, and METs.

Answers to Case Studies

1. Requiring sedentary middle-aged participants to take a maximal, unmonitored test at the beginning of their fitness program is inappropriate. You might suggest the club replace the 1.5-mile (2.4 kilometer) run with the 1-mile (1.6 kilometer) walk test, which should be used after the participants have demonstrated that they can comfortably walk 1 mile.

2. Use the prediction equation described earlier, inserting the measured values:

$$\dot{V}O_2max = 132.853 - 0.0769 \text{ (weight)} - 0.3877 \text{ (age)}$$
$$+ 6.315 \text{ (sex)} - 3.2649 \text{ (time)} - 0.1565 \text{ (HR)}$$

This calculation results in his estimated $\dot{V}O_2$max as $37.8 \ ml \cdot kg^{-1} \cdot min^{-1}$. In terms of group comparisons, his level of CRF is fair for his age group. However, his value indicates that he has a low risk of chronic disease and death from all causes.

3. The HR response used for the calculations must be at 110 bpm or above. Thus, for this example, the calculations will be based on the last two stages. The third workload is the first stage within the required range (referred to as SM1 in the calculations), and the final workload is the second stage within the required range (referred to as SM2 in the calculations). The calculations are as follows:

Determine $\dot{V}O_2$ for the two workloads:

For 750 kgm · min⁻¹:

$$\dot{V}O_2 = (1.8 \times \text{work rate} \div \text{body weight}) + 3.5 + 3.5$$
$$\dot{V}O_2 = (1.8 \times 750 \div 80) + 7$$
$$\dot{V}O_2 = 23.88$$

For 900 kgm · min⁻¹:

$$\dot{V}O_2 = (1.8 \times \text{work rate} \div \text{body weight}) + 3.5 + 3.5$$
$$\dot{V}O_2 = (1.8 \times 900 \div 80) + 7$$
$$\dot{V}O_2 = 27.25$$

Next determine the slope: slope = (SM2 − SM1) ÷ (HR2 − HR1)

$$\text{slope} = (27.25 - 23.88) \div (128 - 120)$$
$$\text{slope} = 0.42$$

Then calculate the estimated $\dot{V}O_2$max:

$$\text{HRmax} = 220 - \text{age}$$
$$\text{HRmax} = 169$$
$$\dot{V}O_2max = SM2 + [\text{slope (HRmax} - HR2)]$$
$$\dot{V}O_2max = 27.25 + [0.42 \times (169 - 128)]$$
$$\dot{V}O_2max = 44.5 \ ml \cdot kg^{-1} \cdot min^{-1}$$

Comparing this to the values in table 8.2, his aerobic capacity is in the 85th to 90th percentile.

4. The HR value of 96 bpm should be ignored, and the remaining HR values should be used. The line is extrapolated to 190 bpm (220 − age), and the vertical line dropped from that point indicates a value of about 16.75% grade, which equals a $\dot{V}O_2$ of about $35.8 \ ml \cdot kg^{-1} \cdot min^{-1}$. This is 10.2 METs, or $1.95 \ L \cdot min^{-1}$.

APPENDIX 8.1: TREADMILL SPEED AND ELEVATION SETTINGS

To calibrate a measuring device is to check its accuracy by comparing it with a known standard and adjusting the device so that it provides an accurate reading. These are suggestions only and should not be viewed as substitutes for the specific procedures recommended by the equipment manufacturers (34). The speed and grade settings on the treadmill must be calibrated because they determine physiological demand and are crucial in estimating CRF. These procedures should be used routinely to maintain test validity and reliability over time. A chart should be posted near each piece of equipment indicating when the calibration was done and by whom.

Calibrating Speed

An easy way to calibrate the speed on any treadmill is to measure the length of the belt and count the number of belt revolutions in a certain amount of time. To calibrate treadmill speed, follow these steps (23):

1. Measure the exact length of the belt in inches (most treadmills in the United States are in English units of measure). This can be done by marking the edge and slowly advancing the belt; alternatively, the manufacturer may have provided the belt length.

2. Place a small piece of tape near the edge of the belt surface.

3. Turn on the treadmill to a given speed by using the speed control.

4. Start your watch as the tape first moves past the fixed point, beginning the count with 0, and count for 1 minute.

5. Calculate the speed in miles per hour:

(Belt length in inches × number of revolutions per minute) ÷ 1.056

Note that dividing by 1.056 will convert inches per minute to miles per hour.

6. Repeat for a number of speeds to ensure accuracy across the speeds used in test protocols. Also, repeat with someone walking on the treadmill to ensure speed is maintained with a weight on the belt.

Calibrating Elevation

Treadmill manuals describe how to calibrate the grade using a simple carpenter's level and a square edge. To calibrate the elevation, follow these steps (23):

1. Use a carpenter's level to make sure that the treadmill is level, and check the zero setting on the grade meter under these conditions (with the treadmill electronics turned on). If the meter does not read zero, adjust the support legs until it is level.

2. Elevate the treadmill so that the percentage grade dial reads 20%. Mark two points at the edge along the length of the treadmill (widely separated from one another) and measure the height of each point above the floor. Then measure the distance between those two points on the floor. Determine grade as follows:

(Height 1 − Height 2) ÷ (distance along the floor)

3. The elevation meter will need to be adjusted if this value does not match 20% (23). Checking at other grades (e.g., 5%, 10%, and 15%) is also recommended (23). Many treadmills have electronic calibration; check with manufacturer's recommendation on making any adjustments (23).

8

APPENDIX 8.2: CALIBRATING THE CYCLE ERGOMETER

To calibrate a measuring device is to check its accuracy by comparing it with a known standard and adjusting the device so that it provides an accurate reading. These are suggestions only and should not be viewed as substitutes for the specific procedures recommended by the equipment manufacturers. The cycle ergometer must be calibrated routinely to ensure that the work rate is accurate. Altering either the pedal rate or the load on the wheel varies the work rate on the mechanically braked cycle ergometer. (*Note:* Many facilities have cycle ergometers with electronic settings; these typically cannot be easily calibrated or adjusted, which limits their use in testing and research settings.) Work equals force times the distance through which the force acts: $w = f \times d$. The kilopond (kp), defined as the force acting on a mass of 1 kilogram at the normal acceleration of gravity, is the proper unit for force. However, the kilopond and the kilogram typically are used interchangeably in exercise testing. The following provides information on calibrating a mechanically braked ergometer; electronically braked ergometers require special equipment (see procedures provided by the manufacturer) (23).

On a mechanically braked cycle ergometer, the force (kilograms of weight on the wheel) is moved through a distance (in meters), so work is expressed in kilogram-meters (kgm). Because work is accomplished over time (e.g., minutes), the activity is referred to as a *work rate* or *power output* ($kgm \cdot min^{-1}$), not a *workload*. On the Monark cycle ergometer, a point on the rim of the wheel travels 6 meters per pedal revolution, so at 50 rpm, the wheel travels $300\ m \cdot min^{-1}$. If a weight of 1 kilogram is hanging from that wheel, the work rate, or power output, is $300\ kgm \cdot min^{-1}$. These simple calculations demonstrate the importance of maintaining a correct pedal rate during the test—if the subject pedals at 60 rpm, the work rate is actually 20% higher (360 versus $300\ kgm \cdot min^{-1}$) than it appears to be. The force setting (resistance on the wheel) also must be carefully set and checked because it tends to drift as the test progresses. It is crucial that the force (resistance) values on the scale are correct. The following four steps outline the procedure for calibrating the Monark cycle ergometer scale (6) (refer to figure 8.8).

1. Disconnect the belt at the spring.

2. Loosen the lock nut and use the adjusting screw on the front of the bike against which the force scale rests so that the vertical mark on the pendulum weight matches with 0 kilopond on the weight scale (see figure 8.8a). The pendulum must be swinging freely. Lock the adjustment screw with the lock nut. To keep the calibration weights from touching the flywheel, it may be easier to elevate the rear of the ergometer (with a 2×4 board on edge), set the zero as described previously, and proceed to the next step.

3. Suspend a 4.0-kilogram weight from the spring so that it is not in contact with the flywheel, and see if the pendulum moves to the 4.0 kilopond mark (see figure 8.8b). If it does not, alter the position or size of the adjusting weight in the pendulum (see figure 8.8c). By loosening the lock screw on the back of the pendulum weight, the adjusting weight can be lowered, raised, or replaced. Check the force scale again and calibrate the ergometer through the range of values used in your tests. If you used the 2×4 to elevate the rear of the ergometer, remove it and reset the zero as described in step 2.

4. Reassemble the cycle ergometer.

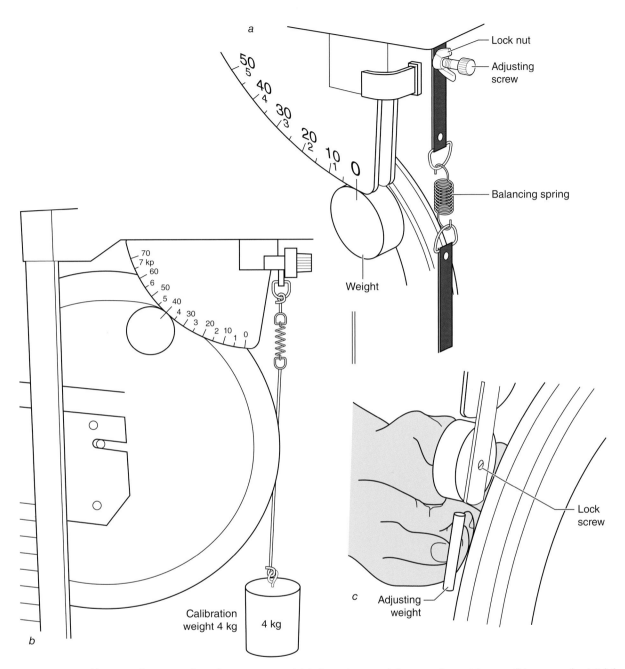

FIGURE 8.8 Calibrating the Monark cycle ergometer. *(a)* Adjust the pendulum to align with zero, *(b)* suspend a 4.0-kilogram weight from the spring, and *(c)* adjust the position or size of the weight in the pendulum.

Adapted by permission from Monark Sports and Medical, *Instruction Manual, Monark Model 818E* (Varberg, Sweden: Monark Exercise AB), 18.

9

Muscular Fitness Assessments

Avery D. Faigenbaum

OBJECTIVES

The reader will be able to do the following:

1. Explain purposes of assessing muscular fitness
2. Discuss precautions that enhance participant safety during muscular fitness assessments
3. Describe various methods of assessing muscular fitness, including repetition maximum tests, push-up tests, the YMCA bench press test, the handgrip strength test, and the vertical jump test
4. Identify methods for standardizing testing protocols to increase accuracy and reproducibility of test results
5. Describe how to interpret the results from various muscular fitness tests
6. Describe how to assess muscular strength and local muscular endurance in older adults
7. Describe safety procedures and precautions for assessing muscular fitness in clients with cardiovascular disease
8. Describe the benefits of, safety for, and precautions for assessing muscular fitness in children and adolescents

9

Muscular fitness is a term that refers to the integrated status of muscular strength (maximal force a muscle or muscle group can generate), local muscular endurance (ability of a muscle to make repeated contractions or to resist muscular fatigue), and muscular power (the rate of performing work) (7, 27, 58). Muscular fitness is important in promoting and maintaining both health- and skill-related components of physical fitness. Accordingly, in the American College of Sports Medicine's (ACSM) position stand on the recommended quantity and quality of exercise to achieve and maintain fitness (32) and in public health recommendations from the U.S. Department of Health and Human Services (HHS) (69) and the World Health Organization (WHO) (74), people are encouraged to participate regularly in muscle-strengthening activities that involve all the major muscle groups. HHS and WHO recommend that resistance training at a moderate or greater intensity, sufficient to develop and maintain muscular fitness, be performed 2 or more days per week as part of a well-rounded exercise program (see chapter 14).

This chapter describes tests commonly used in the health and fitness setting to assess muscular strength, local muscular endurance, and muscular power. Particular emphasis is given to measures of muscular fitness that are valid, reliable, safe, and relatively easy to administer in the fitness setting. Tests that are indicative of a client's health and fitness and those that do not require specialized equipment or sophisticated procedures are highlighted. Assessments of muscular fitness and functional capabilities in special populations, such as older adults, people with cardiovascular disease (CVD), and children or adolescents, are also described.

Preliminary Considerations

Muscular fitness refers to the interrelated parameters of muscular strength, local muscular endurance, and muscular power (see figure 9.1). Since all components of muscular fitness can improve with an appropriately designed resistance training program, this chapter includes assessments for muscular strength, local muscular endurance, and muscular power. Although the effects of resistance training on elements of muscular power typically are associated with athletic performance, assessing and training muscular power can also be worthwhile in general exercise programs that focus on health and fitness (7, 57, 58).

Assessments in this chapter include high-intensity strength and power tests at one end of the assessment scale and low- to moderate-intensity local muscular endurance tests at the other (figure 9.2) (7). High-intensity tests allowing few repetitions (≤3) measure maximal or near-maximal muscular strength and power, whereas those that require a high number of repetitions (>12)

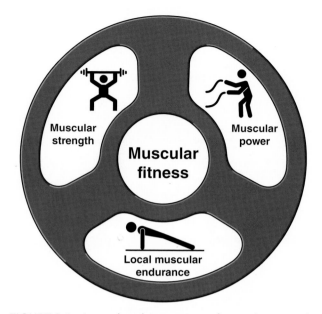

FIGURE 9.1 Interrelated parameters of muscular strength, local muscular endurance, and muscular power.

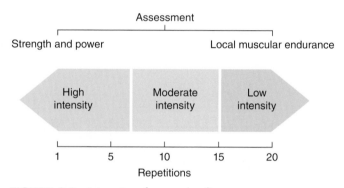

FIGURE 9.2 Intensity of muscular fitness assessments. High-intensity tests allowing few repetitions assess muscular strength and power, whereas tests in which numerous repetitions can be performed assess local muscular endurance.

Adapted from American College of Sports Medicine, *ACSM's Guidelines for Exercise Testing and Prescription*, 11th ed. (Philadelphia, PA: Wolters Kluwer, 2022).

measure local muscular endurance (7). However, the performance of a maximal number of repetitions across a wider range (e.g., 4, 6, or 8 repetitions at a given resistance) also can assess muscular strength (7). Performing tests to assess elements of muscular fitness before commencing exercise training or as part of a fitness screening can provide valuable information about a client's baseline fitness. For example, results from a muscular strength test can be compared with established standards and can help identify weaknesses in certain muscle groups or muscle imbalances that exercise programs could target. The information obtained during baseline muscular fitness assessments also can serve as a basis for designing individualized exercise programs and educating participants about the importance of resistance training. An

RESEARCH INSIGHT

Verbal Encouragement and Strength Performance

Belkhiria and colleagues (10) examined the effects of verbal encouragement on isometric force and associated parameters during a handgrip task. Participants performed a maximal voluntary handgrip contraction under three conditions:

1. With verbal encouragement
2. Without verbal encouragement
3. Self-initiated without concentration and motivation

They found that the maximal voluntary force was highest with verbal encouragement as compared to the other conditions. These findings support the view that motivational and attentional factors can influence maximal voluntary force production, and highlight the potential impact of verbal encouragement and positive feedback on muscular performance during fitness testing.

equally useful application of fitness testing is to motivate participants by evaluating their progress over time. Note that no single test is best for assessing muscular strength, local muscular endurance, and muscular power.

For safety purposes, all participants who undergo fitness testing should first complete a health screening questionnaire and, if necessary, consult with a qualified health care provider for medical clearance or advice on modifying exercise participation. This includes people with known cardiovascular or orthopedic conditions. The ACSM procedures for administering a careful health risk assessment have been described in detail in this textbook (see chapter 2) and elsewhere (7). Recommended steps for muscular fitness testing include the following:

• *Standardization of testing protocols.* People should participate in familiarization (practice) sessions, follow a standardized testing protocol, and perform a proper warm-up in order to obtain a reliable score that can be used to track physiologic adaptations over time (1, 4, 58). Other standardized conditions that promote safe muscular fitness tests that yield valid and reproducible results include reviewing safety measures with each participant and ensuring that the participant uses proper exercise technique throughout the full range of motion (ROM) at a predetermined speed of movement. The same equipment (free weight versus weight machine) should be used for pre- and posttesting, multiple tests should be organized so the same muscle groups are not repeatedly stressed, and the muscular fitness tests should be specific to the training program. Additionally, testers should provide consistent verbal encouragement to ensure accurate muscular performance assessment (10, 52).

• *Familiarization.* To obtain a reliable test score that can be used to track physiological adaptations over time, people should become familiar with the testing equipment and protocol by participating in practice sessions with qualified instruction (30, 58). Without adequate familiarization, strength testing may not provide a stable, reproducible value. A lack of familiarization prior to testing can result in relatively large increases in strength over a short-term training period due to the learning effect. Participants with resistance training experience require little familiarization, but untrained participants may need two or three practice sessions to become familiar with testing procedures and exercise technique.

RESEARCH INSIGHT

Static Stretching and Muscle Performance

Nakamura and colleagues (54) examined time-course changes in maximal isometric muscle strength and explosive muscle strength following three 60-second static stretching interventions of the knee extensors. Participants were sedentary healthy adults. Performance variables were assessed before static stretching and after static stretching at three time intervals (immediately after, 10 minutes after, and 20 minutes after). They found that after a prolonged bout of static stretching maximal isometric muscle strength decreased for 10 minutes after, and impairments in explosive strength were observed at 20 minutes. Fitness professionals should consider the lingering effects of pre-event static stretching on fitness performance when assessing muscular strength and power.

• *Warm-up.* A 5- to 10-minute general warm-up, including low-intensity cardiorespiratory exercise, calisthenics, and several light repetitions of the specific testing exercise, should precede muscular fitness testing. This increases muscle temperature and localized blood flow, and it promotes appropriate cardiovascular responses to exercise (7, 58). Warm-up procedures that include short bouts of higher-intensity dynamic movements for the upper and lower body can be particularly useful when assessing muscular strength and power (31, 48). Prolonged bouts of static stretching are not recommended as the sole warm-up activity prior to strength and power testing (14, 54).

• *Specificity.* Muscular fitness tests are specific to the muscle or muscle group, the type of muscular action (static or dynamic, concentric or eccentric), the speed of muscular action (slow or fast), and the joint angle being tested (58). Accordingly, muscular fitness tests should be similar to the exercises used during the resistance training program.

• *Safety.* Safety measures related to the testing equipment, testing environment and quality of supervision, spotting, and instruction should be employed before testing. Review safety measures with all participants before testing, explain or demonstrate proper technique, and ensure that the environment is comfortable (68-72 °F or 20-22 °C), with humidity less than 60%.

• *Interpretation of results.* The availability of health criteria or normative data should be considered when choosing a test, particularly when classifying a participant's test data, such as when performing a health and fitness screening. However, norms are less of a concern when the test is used primarily to detect improvements in muscular strength, where the absolute strength values (e.g., kilograms lifted) or relative scores (e.g., kilograms lifted per kilogram of body weight) can be compared during repeated testing.

Muscular Strength

Muscular strength refers to the maximal force that can be generated by a specific muscle or muscle group. Tests include static, isokinetic, and dynamic strength assessments as outlined in this section.

Static Strength Testing

Isometric or static strength (constant muscle length during muscle activation) can be measured conveniently with a variety of devices, including cable tensiometers and handgrip dynamometers, which measure strength at one specific point in the ROM. The peak force achieved in such tests is called the *maximum voluntary contraction* (MVC). The handgrip test is widely used by practitioners as an indicator of overall muscle strength (18, 50).

Notably, low handgrip strength has been found to be associated with poor health outcomes including functional disabilities and chronic morbidities in older adults (42, 44). Reference values for maximum grip strength are provided in table 9.1. While different handgrip strength testing protocols are available (49), the ACSM recommends the following procedures for assessing handgrip strength (7):

1. Adjust the handgrip dynamometer so the second joint of the fingers fits snugly over the handle. Set the dynamometer to zero.

2. Stand with feet slightly apart and hold the dynamometer in line with the forearm at the level of the thigh, away from the body with palms facing inward (see figure 9.3).

3. Squeeze the dynamometer as hard as possible without holding the breath. Keep the arm at the side with the palm facing the thigh.

4. Repeat the test at least two times with each hand. Record the highest value attained with each hand to the nearest kilogram.

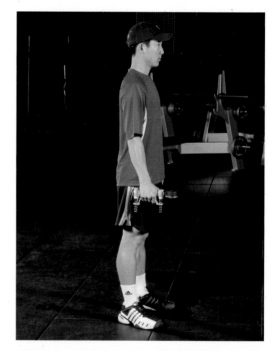

FIGURE 9.3 Handgrip strength test position.

KEY POINT

Handgrip strength is a simple, quick, and inexpensive indicator of general health status and can be used as a screening tool for identifying individuals at risk for muscle weakness and clinically relevant health outcomes.

Table 9.1 Reference Values for Maximum Grip Strength (in Kilograms) for Males and Females for Selected Percentiles

	PERCENTILES													
	5th		10th		25th		50th		75th		90th		95th	
Age (yr)	M	F	M	F	M	F	M	F	M	F	M	F	M	F
6	5	4	6	5	7	6	8	7	9	8	10	10	11	11
7	6	6	7	6	8	8	10	9	11	10	12	12	13	13
8	7	7	8	8	10	9	11	11	13	12	15	14	16	15
9	9	9	10	10	12	11	13	12	16	14	17	16	18	17
10	10	10	12	11	13	13	15	15	18	16	20	18	21	19
11	12	12	14	13	16	15	18	17	21	19	23	21	25	22
12	14	14	16	15	18	17	21	20	24	22	27	24	28	25
13	17	16	19	17	22	19	25	22	28	24	31	26	33	27
14	20	17	22	18	26	21	29	23	33	26	36	28	39	29
15	24	18	26	19	29	22	33	24	38	27	41	29	44	31
16	26	19	28	20	32	22	36	25	41	28	45	30	47	32
17	28	19	30	20	34	22	38	25	43	28	47	31	50	32
18	29	19	31	21	35	23	40	26	45	28	49	31	52	32
19	30	20	32	21	37	23	41	26	46	29	50	31	53	33
20-24	32	20	34	22	38	24	43	27	48	29	52	32	55	34
25-29	34	21	36	22	40	25	45	28	50	30	54	33	57	35
30-34	36	22	38	23	42	25	47	28	52	31	56	34	59	35
35-39	37	22	39	23	43	26	48	28	52	31	57	34	60	36
40-44	37	22	40	23	44	26	48	28	53	31	57	34	60	36
45-49	37	22	39	23	43	25	48	28	53	31	57	34	60	36
50-54	36	21	38	22	42	25	47	28	52	30	56	33	59	35
55-59	34	20	37	22	41	24	46	27	50	30	54	32	57	34
60-64	32	19	35	21	39	23	44	26	48	28	52	31	55	33
65-69	29	17	32	19	36	22	41	25	45	27	49	30	52	31
70-74	25	15	29	18	33	20	38	23	42	25	46	28	49	29
75-79	21	13	24	16	29	19	34	21	38	23	42	26	44	27

Adapted from S.L. Wong, "Grip Strength Reference Values for Canadians Aged 6 to 79: Canadian Health Measures Survey, 2007 to 2013," Statistics Canada, October 19, 2016, https://www150.statcan.gc.ca/n1/pub/82-003-x/2016010/article/14665-eng.pdf.

RESEARCH INSIGHT

Factors Affecting Test-Retest Reliability

Field-based muscular fitness tests have been found to be reliable (or consistent) in participants of varied ages (19). However, for a fitness test to be reliable, the professional conducting the test must be knowledgeable of established testing protocols and familiar with testing equipment (including calibration if required). The demands of the fitness test should be consistent with the health status and exercise history of the individual. Environmental factors such as temperature and humidity can influence the physiological responses to exercise and need to be controlled when fitness testing. Professionals should explain the fitness test protocol clearly, minimize external distractions, and maintain a comfortable environment to maintain the integrity of the testing process.

Isokinetic Testing

Isokinetic testing involves the assessment of maximal muscle tension throughout a range of joint motion at a constant angular velocity (e.g., $60° \cdot \sec^{-1}$). Isokinetic testing devices measure peak rotational force, or torque, and data are obtained with specialized equipment that allows the tester to control the speed of rotation (degrees per second) around various joints (e.g., knee, hip, shoulder, elbow). Although the data collected from isokinetic strength assessments may be useful to health and fitness professionals, the necessary computerized equipment is expensive and therefore limits isokinetic testing almost entirely to rehabilitation and research settings. Consequently, isokinetic strength evaluations may not be practical for most fitness practitioners.

Dynamic Strength Testing

The most common type of strength assessment performed by fitness professionals is dynamic testing, which involves movement of the body (e.g., push-up) or an external load (e.g., bench press). Dynamic testing is typically inexpensive because it does not require specialized equipment. Moreover, dynamic assessments can be performed with a variety of equipment, such as free weights (barbells and dumbbells) or weight-stack machines, and they can test any major muscle or muscle group through a variety of exercises. Exercises typically used for dynamic strength testing in fitness centers include the bench press and leg press.

The gold standard of dynamic strength testing is the 1-repetition maximum (1RM), the heaviest weight that can be lifted only once in a specific exercise using proper form (6, 7). If appropriate testing guidelines are followed, a 1RM test is a reliable measure of maximal strength and can be performed safely in the health and fitness setting with qualified supervision and instruction (7, 33). Although a 1RM can be performed for various upper- and lower-body exercises, multijoint exercises such as the bench press and leg press are typically used for this type of testing. The fitness professional should ensure proper positioning of the client (e.g., grip position and foot stance) and must be readily available to assist in case of a failed repetition. Spotting is particularly important for free-weight exercises such as the bench press and squat. Also, beginners should learn how to exert maximal effort by participating in several familiarization sessions with each strength testing protocol prior to testing. Untrained clients tend to misinterpret submaximal effort for maximal effort due to lack of training experience.

Components of Muscular Fitness Related to Promoting or Maintaining Good Health, Fitness, and Performance

Health Aspects of Muscular Fitness

- Preservation or enhancement of fat-free mass and resting metabolic rate
- Preservation or enhancement of bone mass with aging
- Improved glucose tolerance and insulin sensitivity
- Reduced low-density lipoprotein cholesterol and triglycerides
- Reduced resting blood pressure
- Lowered risk of musculoskeletal injury, including low-back pain
- Improved functional independence and ability to carry out activities of daily living
- Improved balance and decreased risk of falls in older age
- Improved self-esteem and cognitive abilities

Performance Aspects of Muscular Fitness

- Enhanced muscular strength, muscular power, and local muscular endurance
- Enhanced speed and agility
- Improved balance and coordination
- Reduced risk for musculoskeletal injuries
- Improved body composition for various exercise and sport activities
- Improved confidence for performing certain athletic movements
- Improved general and specific sport skills

Adapted from Ratamess (2022); Suchomel, Nimphius, and Stone (2016); Westcott (2012).

Familiarization and the presence of experienced spotters who can recognize potentially hazardous situations (e.g., poor exercise technique) will enhance the safety and reliability of strength testing procedures.

Maximal strength tests also have been shown to be safe and efficacious for clinical populations, including those with coronary heart disease (CHD), breast cancer, and type 2 diabetes (2, 9, 40). Nonetheless, caution should be used when testing older adults, patients with clinical conditions, and people with certain orthopedic concerns (7). In some cases, it may be prudent to perform multiple repetition maximum (RM) testing or delay testing until a qualified health care provider has determined the person to be clinically stable.

Multiple RM tests (e.g., 4RM, 8RM) also can safely and effectively assess muscular strength in healthy adults, although a more conservative approach may be needed for patients with health conditions, such as CVD, pulmonary disease, and diabetes (7). For patients at high risk for or with known disease, the assessment of a 10RM to 15RM that is consistent with resistance training recommendations may be prudent (7). When the purpose of testing is to define an initial training load, multiple RM testing minimizes the potential error compared with extrapolating the exercise intensity as a percentage of 1RM. For example, the maximum weight a person can lift 10 times during testing can be used to identify an appropriate weight load for this number of repetitions performed during training and to provide an index of strength changes over time. It is important that the exercise be performed to failure when performing multiple RM tests.

The procedures for assessing 1RM can be modified to test any given number of repetitions. It is possible to estimate the 1RM when multiple RM tests are used. For example, a 10RM is the most weight a person can lift with proper form for 10 repetitions but not 11. The 10RM weight is approximately 75% of the 1RM weight (34). Although a fair amount of individual variability can be expected when extrapolating 1RM from 10RM, this testing protocol may be desirable in some cases. Also, researchers have developed 1RM prediction equations based on the number of repetitions performed using a submaximal load (e.g., 70%-80% 1RM) (47, 45, 59). When using prediction equations to estimate the 1RM, the prediction accuracy improves as the loads used in multiple RM testing get heavier and closer to the actual 1RM. Because most researchers use the bench press to predict 1RM strength values, the error rate will likely increase if these equations are used with other strength exercises such as the leg press or squat. Regardless of the testing protocol, fitness professionals must communicate with the client to determine a progression pattern of loading that is consistent with the client's capacity. Asking questions (e.g., "Can you lift 5 more pounds?" or "Are you close to your max?"), offering encouragement, and showing concern for the client during the testing session can help to ensure maximal performance.

1RM Testing Procedures

1. Perform a general warm-up of low-intensity aerobic exercise and dynamic movements.

2. Start with a light warm-up set of 5 to 10 submaximal repetitions.

3. After a 1-minute rest, the subject performs 3 to 5 repetitions at approximately 60% to 80% of perceived maximum.

4. The subject attempts a 1RM lift. If the lift is successful, the subject rests for approximately 3 minutes and repeats the test with a heavier load. Note that training experience and exercise type will affect the absolute load increases in subsequent 1RM trials.

5. This process continues until a failed attempt occurs. The goal is to find the 1RM within three to five attempts to avoid excessive fatigue.

6. The 1RM is reported as the weight of the last successfully completed lift with proper exercise technique.

Adapted from Ratamess (2022).

KEY POINT

Muscular strength is best assessed using a resistance that requires maximum or near-maximum resistance with few repetitions. With qualified supervision, proper instruction, verbal encouragement, and technique-driven progression of testing loads, strength testing can be a safe and reliable assessment for individuals with different levels of resistance training experience. An ideal application of strength testing is to evaluate changes in muscular strength over time using standardized testing procedures that ensure valid and reproducible results.

Interpreting Results

It is best to express strength as a ratio of weight lifted during a single or multiple RM test relative to body weight when comparing strength assessments of people who differ in body mass, such as when comparing men and women. The following procedure describes how to determine a strength ratio from a 10RM test:

1. Determine the heaviest weight the client can lift for 10 good repetitions (10RM weight load).
2. Convert the 10RM weight load to a 1RM estimation by dividing the weight load by 0.75.
3. Divide the estimated 1RM by the client's body weight to obtain the strength ratio.

For example, a client who weighs 140 pounds (63.5 kilograms) and completes 10 leg presses with 120 pounds (54.4 kilograms) has an estimated 1RM of 120 ÷ 0.75, or 160 pounds (72.6 kilograms). Their leg press weight ratio is 1.14 (160 ÷ 140).

Normative Data

Normative strength scores for various age and sex categories have been published in *ACSM's Guidelines for Exercise Testing and Prescription* (7). However, most normative data have been derived from a relatively homogeneous sample of subjects using only certain types of resistance training equipment, which limits interpretation of test scores. For example, because equipment design can vary significantly from one manufacturer to another and because of inherent differences in using free weights versus machine weights, strength scores can vary using different testing equipment. Thus, client scores should only be compared with norms generated from tests performed with the same type of equipment. Valid measures of upper-body strength include 1RM values for the bench press, and corresponding indices of lower-body strength include the leg press (7). Future research is needed to provide norms for a variety of resistance training modalities as well as norms for diverse races, ethnicities, and age groups.

Comparing Pretraining and Posttraining

Often, the primary purpose of a muscular fitness test is to evaluate changes in strength over the course of a fitness program. Periodic muscle fitness testing is particularly appealing because it eliminates the need to compare individual data with data provided in normative tables. The frequency of follow-up testing depends on the quality and quantity of exercise training by the client as well as the client's desire and the availability of the fitness staff. When multiple tests are performed over time, useful feedback to the client should include the percentage improvement of RM strength or local muscular endurance (i.e., percentage change between tests). This is obtained by dividing the change in strength (posttraining minus pretraining score) by the pretraining score and multiplying by 100%. For example, if your client performs a 10RM baseline of 40 pounds on the chest press and improves to 60 pounds during follow-up testing, they have demonstrated a 50% strength gain ([(60 − 40) ÷ 40] × 100) on that lift. This information can provide positive reinforcement about the efficacy of the training program. In cases when the client does not improve, recommendations for altering the exercise program can be made based on the client's goals and adherence to the exercise program.

Muscular Power

Muscular power refers to the rate of performing work and is the product of force and velocity. Many physiological and biomechanical factors including muscle fiber type, muscle size, neural activation, energy metabolism, intermuscular coordination, and torque or leverage influence the expression of muscular power (58). While muscular power is vital for many sports or events (e.g., jumping and sprinting) (66), the importance of muscular power for older adults has received increased attention (e.g., fall prevention and crossing a busy intersection) (30, 46, 57). Tests of peak muscular power are explosive and only last a few seconds. Jump tests and medicine ball throws are field-based tests that can be used to assess peak muscular power. The vertical jump test (also called the *counter-movement jump*) is easy to administer and can provide valuable information about lower-body muscular power. The vertical jump can be assessed with a tape measure and chalk or a special testing device with uniformly spaced vanes extending from a vertical beam. See *Vertical Jump Testing Procedures* for ACSM's recommended steps for conducting the vertical jump test (7).

Local Muscular Endurance

Local muscular endurance is the ability of a muscle group to repeatedly contract against a fixed resistance until muscular fatigue is experienced or the ability to maintain a specific percentage of the maximal voluntary contraction (MVC) for a prolonged time (7). Equipment (e.g., free weights or machines) for measuring strength can be used to assess local muscular endurance. In addition, a simple field test such as the maximum number of push-ups that can be performed without rest can be used to evaluate the local muscular endurance of the upper-body muscles (7). This field test can be used either independently or in combination with other methods of strength or endurance assessment, such as RM testing. Tests such as the push-up can screen for muscle weaknesses related to various health indicators. Moreover, the muscles of the upper body are used in many daily activities such as raking or gardening, carrying luggage, or painting. Thus, this test is a practical way to evaluate a client's muscular fitness and can provide useful feedback

Vertical Jump Testing Procedures

1. Explain the purpose of the test and demonstrate proper procedures for assessing standing reach and jump height. Follow appropriate warm-up procedures.

2. Stand with both feet firmly on the ground. Reach up as high as possible along the wall with the dominant hand and make a mark with chalked fingertips at the highest point. Record the distance from the floor to the highest chalk mark. If a commercial testing device is used, measure the reach height with the highest vane that can be touched. (See figure 9.4*a*.)

3. The jump test begins with both feet on the floor without taking a step. Verbally signal the individual to jump as high as possible. Squat down with arms swinging past hips, then explosively reverse direction and jump as high as possible. Touch the wall at the highest point to make a mark with the chalked fingertips, then land safely on the floor. If using a jump testing device, swat the vane with the outstretched dominant arm at the highest point of the jump. Record the jump height to the closest centimeter or half inch. (See figure 9.4*b*.)

4. The vertical jump can be calculated by subtracting the standing reach height from the total jump height. For example, an individual who has a total jump height of 106.5 inches (270.5 centimeters) and a standing reach of 86 inches (218.4 centimeters) has a vertical jump of 20.5 inches (52.1 centimeters). The best of three trials is used for comparison to normative values.

Adapted from American College of Sports Medicine (2022).

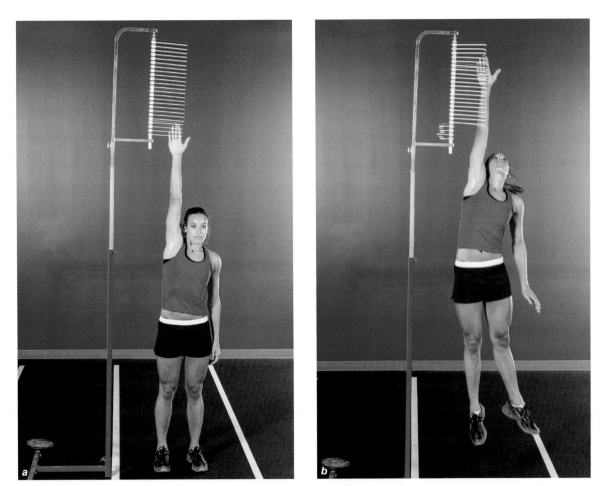

FIGURE 9.4 Vertical jump test (*a*) standing reach to establish baseline and (*b*) max jump height.

RESEARCH INSIGHT

Push-Up Capacity and Cardiovascular Health

While increased aerobic fitness is associated with a lower risk of CVD, Yang and colleagues evaluated the association between push-up capacity and subsequent CVD events in active adult men (mean age 39.6 years) (76). Participants were stratified into 5 groups based on the number of push-ups completed and were followed for 10 years. They found significant negative associations between push-up capacity and cardiovascular events. Men able to perform more than 40 push-ups had a significantly lower incident of cardiovascular events compared with those completing fewer than 10 push-ups. While differences in other CVD risk factors among groups should be considered, these findings suggest that the push-up test can provide useful information to fitness professionals and clinicians.

to the client about how muscular conditioning affects many common activities.

Push-Up Test

The procedures of the push-up test as described by ACSM (7) are presented here and shown in figures 9.5 and 9.6. The push-up test evaluates muscular strength and local muscular endurance of the upper body, including the triceps, deltoid, and pectoral muscles. There are two standard push-up positions: one with the hands and toes in contact with the floor and the other with the hands and knees in contact with the floor (the modified push-up position). Regardless of the push-up position, the hand position should be standardized because varied hand placements elicit varied responses from the pectoralis major and triceps (15). The procedures for administering the test are similar, and either position can be used for men or women because the position should be based on strength, not sex. However, the norms for the standard push-up are for men and the norms for the modified push-up are for women. When women perform the standard push-up and men perform the modified push-up, pre- and posttraining scores can be compared to evaluate improvement over time; however, the table of norms should not be used in these circumstances. As with RM testing, the push-up test should be used with caution when testing older adults and people at heightened cardiac risk.

Push-Up Testing Procedures

1. Explain the purpose of the test to the client: to determine how many push-ups can be completed in order to reflect upper-body local muscular endurance. Demonstrate the test, and allow the client to practice if desired.

2. Inform the client of proper breathing technique: to exhale with the effort, which occurs when pushing away from the floor.

3. The push-up test usually is administered with male clients in the standard down position with hands shoulder-width apart, back straight, and head up, using the toes as the pivotal point. For female clients, the modified knee push-up position often is used, with legs together, lower legs in contact with the mat, ankles plantar flexed, back straight, hands shoulder-width apart, and head up. Some males will need to use the modified position, and some females can use the full-body position.

4. The client must raise the body by straightening the elbows and then return to the down position until the chin touches the mat. The stomach should not touch the mat.

5. For both men and women, the back must be straight at all times and the client must push up to a straight-arm position.

6. Stop the test when the client strains forcibly or is unable to maintain the appropriate exercise technique for two consecutive repetitions. The score is the maximal number of push-ups performed consecutively without rest.

Adapted from American College of Sports Medicine (2022).

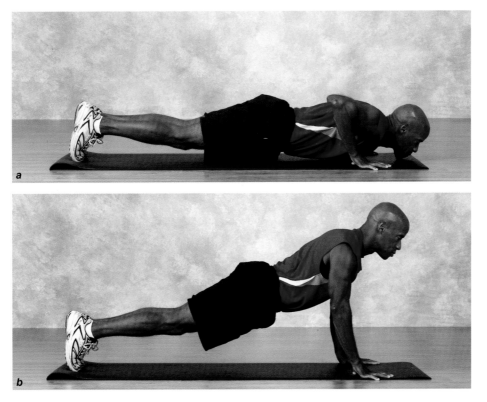

FIGURE 9.5 Proper form for the (a) starting position and (b) finishing position of the standard push-up test, as described by ACSM (7).

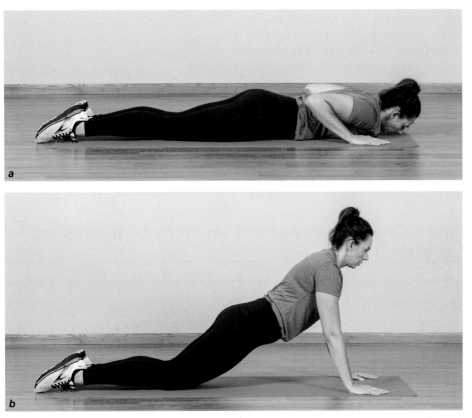

FIGURE 9.6 Proper form for the (a) starting position and (b) finishing position of the modified push-up test, as described by ACSM (7).

The push-up test is a relatively simple, inexpensive method for assessing local muscular endurance, and it can be used for men and women of various ages. Results of the standard push-up test for men and modified push-up test for women can be compared with the standards in table 9.2. As with RM testing, the push-up test can be performed on multiple occasions over time to reliably assess changes in local muscular endurance that occur with training. Finally, very deconditioned people, especially those who are overweight or obese, may find these tests difficult, and poor results obtained during testing may discourage them from exercise participation. Thus, the fitness professional must carefully consider whether these tests are appropriate and likely to yield useful information. In such circumstances where relatively low strength prohibits performance of the test with proper exercise technique, the push-up test is not adequate to assess muscular strength or local muscular endurance.

VIDEO Watch video 9.1, which demonstrates the push-up test.

YMCA Bench Press Test

The push-up test is not the only local muscular endurance test. The fitness professional can adapt resistance training equipment to measure local muscular endurance by selecting an appropriate submaximal level of resistance and measuring the number of repetitions or the duration of static contraction before fatigue. For example, the YMCA bench press test involves performing standardized repetitions at a rate of 30 repetitions per minute to test local muscular endurance of the upper body (63). Men use an 80-pound barbell and women use a 35-pound barbell, and participants are scored by the number of successful repetitions completed. The main disadvantage of the test is that it uses a fixed weight, which favors larger clients over smaller clients. Also,

the fixed weight may be too heavy for deconditioned or older clients to lift repeatedly. On the other hand, the load may be too light for very strong clients, who may perform significantly more repetitions than typically used during training.

Despite these limitations, this test can be used independently or in combination with other tests in the overall assessment of muscular fitness in clients who have experience using free weights. The procedures for this test are summarized in *YMCA Bench Press Test Procedures*, and norms are shown in tables 9.3 and 9.4.

RESEARCH INSIGHT

Muscle Activation Between Push-Up and Bench Press Exercises

Push-ups are a common exercise used in fitness testing and resistance training. Van den Tillar compared the kinematics and upper-body muscle activation between the push-up and bench press exercises over a range of loads in resistance-trained subjects (70). Bench press was performed at 50% to 80% of a predicted 1RM, and push-ups were performed without a weighted vest and with a 10-, 20-, and 30-kilogram weighted vest. No differences in kinematics and muscle activation between the two exercises were reported, and the different loads had the same effect on both push-up and bench press performance. These findings indicate that fitness professionals can use the push-up and bench press exercises interchangeably to activate upper-body musculature, and push-ups with a weighted vest can mimic different loads on the bench press exercise.

Table 9.2 Fitness Categories by Age and Sex for Push-Up Test Using Number Completed

Fitness	20-29 YR		30-39 YR		40-49 YR		50-59 YR		60-69 YR	
	M	F	M	F	M	F	M	F	M	F
Excellent	≥36	≥30	≥30	≥27	≥25	≥24	≥21	≥21	≥18	≥17
Very good	29-35	21-29	22-29	20-26	17-24	15-23	13-20	11-20	11-17	12-16
Good	22-28	15-20	17-21	13-19	13-16	11-14	10-12	7-10	8-10	5-11
Fair	17-21	10-14	12-16	8-12	10-12	5-10	7-9	2-6	5-7	1-4
Needs improvement	≤16	≤9	≤11	≤7	≤9	≤4	≤6	≤1	≤4	≤1

Canadian Standardized Test of Fitness Operations Manual, 3rd ed., Health Canada, 2003. Reproduced with permission from the Minister of Public Works and Government Services Canada, 2011.

YMCA Bench Press Testing Procedures

1. Use a 35-pound straight barbell for women or an 80-pound straight barbell for men. A spotter should be present during the test.

2. Set a metronome to 60 bpm.

3. Have the subject begin with the bar in the down position touching the chest, with the elbows flexed, hands slightly wider than shoulder-width apart, and feet on the floor. A spotter should be available for assistance if needed.

4. Count one repetition when the elbows fully extend. Encourage clients to exhale during the upward phase of each repetition. After each extension, the participant should lower the bar to touch the chest.

5. Instruct the client to complete up or down movements in time to the 60-bpm rhythm, which should be 30 lifts · min^{-1}.

6. The test is terminated when proper lifting technique or cadence cannot be maintained.

7. Count the total number of repetitions completed in good form.

Table 9.3 YMCA Bench Press Norms for Number of Repetitions Completed for Men Using 80 Pounds

Fitness	AGE (YR)					
	18-25	26-35	36-45	46-55	56-65	>65
Excellent	44-64	41-61	36-55	28-47	24-41	20-36
Good	34-41	30-37	26-32	21-25	17-21	12-16
Above average	29-33	26-29	22-25	16-20	12-14	9-10
Average	24-28	21-24	18-21	12-14	9-11	7-8
Below average	20-22	17-20	14-17	9-11	5-8	4-6
Poor	13-17	12-16	9-12	5-8	2-4	2-3
Very poor	<10	≤9	≤6	≤2	≤1	≤1

Adapted from YMCA of the USA (2000).

Table 9.4 YMCA Bench Press Norms for Number of Repetitions Completed for Women Using 35 Pounds

Fitness	AGE (YR)					
	16-25	26-35	36-45	46-55	56-65	>65
Excellent	42-66	40-62	40-62	29-50	24-42	18-30
Good	30-38	29-34	29-34	20-24	17-21	12-16
Above average	25-28	24-28	24-28	14-18	12-14	8-10
Average	20-22	18-22	18-22	10-13	8-10	5-7
Below average	16-18	14-17	14-17	7-9	5-6	3-4
Poor	9-13	9-13	9-13	2-6	2-4	0-2
Very poor	≤6	≤6	≤4	≤1	≤1	0

Adapted from YMCA of the USA (2000).

Watch video 9.2, which demonstrates the YMCA bench press test.

KEY POINT

The most common field measure of upper-body local muscular endurance in the fitness setting is the push-up test. Normative data based on sex and age can be used to assess muscular performance and track improvements over time. The push-up test provides a practical approach for evaluating local muscular endurance, either alone or together with other types of muscular fitness evaluations.

Testing Older Adults

The number of older adults in the United States is expected to increase exponentially over the next several decades. For instance, in 2010 there were 18.6 million U.S. adults age 75 or older, and this number is expected to double by the year 2050 (28). Further, the number of adults age 85 and older is growing the fastest, with numbers expected to reach 19.5 million by 2040 (28). Because people are living longer, it is becoming increasingly important to find ways to extend active, healthy lifestyles and moderate the effects of sarcopenia (low muscle mass), dynapenia (low muscle strength and power), and physical frailty in later years (5, 51, 67). Assessing muscular strength and local muscular endurance as well as other aspects of physical fitness in older adults can reveal physical weaknesses and be used to design exercise programs that improve strength before serious functional limitations occur.

Senior Fitness Test

In response to the need for improved assessment for older adults, Rikli and Jones (60, 61) developed a functional fitness test battery, the Senior Fitness Test (SFT). This test evaluates the key physiological parameters (i.e., strength, endurance, agility, and balance) needed to perform everyday physical activities that are often difficult in later years. The SFT is used by researchers as well as health and fitness professionals who work with older men and women. In addition to evaluating a participant's strengths and identifying areas of physical weakness, data gathered from the SFT can provide evidence of outcome measures to document the effectiveness of an exercise program (62). Test items in the SFT are the 30-second chair stand, 30-second arm curl test, 6-minute walk test,

2-minute step test, chair sit-and-reach test, back-scratch test, 8-foot (2.4 meter) up and go test, and height and weight (62). One of the most popular aspects of the SFT is the 30-second chair stand test (37) (see the *Influence of Seat Height on Chair Stand Performance* Research Insight). This test, as well as others of the SFT, meets scientific standards for reliability and validity, is simple and easy to administer in the field setting, has performance norms for men and women age 60 to 94, and has clinically relevant fitness standards for maintaining physical independence in later years (60, 61). This test also has been shown to correlate well with other strength tests such as the 1RM. The fitness professional can use the SFT to safely and effectively assess functional ability in most older adults.

Before testing, all participants should warm up and follow other preliminary procedures as described earlier. In addition, the following instruction is recommended as a standardization procedure for administering the chair stand test and the arm curl test to all clients:

> Do the best you can on each test item, but never push yourself to a point of overexertion or beyond what you think is safe for you.

30-Second Chair Stand Test

The 30-second chair stand test, which reflects lower-body strength, involves counting the number of times within 30 seconds that the participant can rise to a full stand from a seated position on a chair with a seat height of 17 inches (43 centimeters), with arms folded across the chest (see figure 9.7) (62). Studies have shown that chair stand performance, a common method of assessing lower-body strength in older adults, correlates well with major criterion indicators of lower-body strength, stair-climbing ability, walking speed, and risk of falling, and it has been found to detect normal age-related declines in strength (3, 77). Further, the chair stand has been found to be safe and sensitive in detecting the effects of physical training in older adults (26, 38). Table 9.5 summarizes the normal range of scores of participants age 60 to 94 years. The normal range is defined as the middle 50% of the population tested for each age group, with the lower limits being equivalent to the 25th percentile rank and the upper limits equivalent to the 75th percentile rank within each 5-year age group.

Arm Curl Test

Upper-body function, including arm strength and local muscular endurance, is important in executing many everyday activities such as carrying groceries, lifting a suitcase, and picking up grandchildren. The 30-second single-arm curl test, a measure of upper-body strength and local muscular endurance, determines the number of times a dumbbell (5 pound [2.3 kilogram] dumbbell for women and 8 pound [3.6 kilogram] dumbbell for

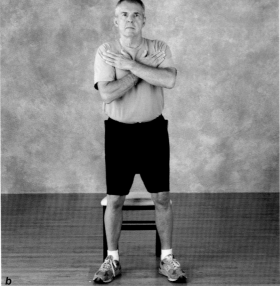

RESEARCH INSIGHT

Influence of Seat Height on Chair Stand Performance

The 30-second chair stand is a useful measure of lower-body strength and performance in seniors. Kuo (41) examined the influence of chair seat height on 30-second chair stand performance in older adults (age 70 ± 6.3 years). Participants performed the test from the standard height of 17 inches (43 centimeters) and from five randomly ordered seat heights from 80% to 120% of each participant's lower-leg length. Analysis of the data revealed that seat height significantly influenced the performance of older adults. The average score for standard conditions was significantly lower than those at 100%, 110%, and 120% conditions. Although a standard seat height of 17 inches (43 centimeters) is recommended for the 30-second chair stand, health and fitness professionals should consider the influence of seat height on performance when interpreting test results.

FIGURE 9.7 The 30-second chair stand test: *(a)* starting position and *(b)* standing position.

men) can be curled through a full ROM in 30 seconds while sitting on a chair with the back straight and feet flat (62). The prescribed protocol includes holding the weight in the dominant hand in a handshake grip at full extension (to the side of the chair) and then supinating during flexion so that the palm of the hand faces the biceps at full flexion (figure 9.8). The score is the total number of arm curls performed in 30 seconds. Studies

Table 9.5 Normal Range of Scores on the 30-Second Chair Stand and 30-Second Arm Curl Tests for Older Adults

	AGE (YR)						
	60-64	65-69	70-74	75-79	80-84	85-89	90-94
Chair stand (number of stands)							
Women	12-17	11-16	10-15	10-15	9-14	8-13	4-11
Men	14-19	12-18	12-17	11-17	10-15	8-14	7-12
Arm curl (number of reps)							
Women	13-19	12-18	12-17	11-17	10-16	10-15	8-13
Men	16-22	15-21	14-21	13-19	13-19	11-17	10-14

Note: Normal is defined as the middle 50% of the population. Participants scoring above or below these ranges would be considered above normal or below normal for their age.

Reprinted by permission from R.E. Rikli and C.J. Jones, *Senior Fitness Test Manual*, 2nd ed. (Champaign, IL: Human Kinetics, 2013), 89-90.

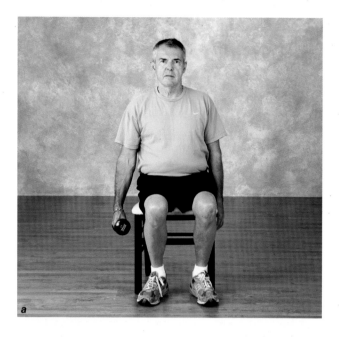

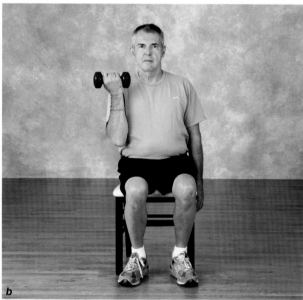

FIGURE 9.8 The 30-second arm curl test: *(a)* starting position and *(b)* full flexion position.

indicate that the 30-second arm curl test is a good predictor of both biceps and overall upper-body strength and local muscular endurance (60). Results obtained from the 30-second arm curl test can be compared with the norms presented in table 9.5.

Testing Clients With Cardiovascular Disease

Progressive resistance training performed 2 days per week improves muscular fitness, prevents and manages a variety of chronic medical conditions, modifies coronary risk factors, and enhances psychosocial well-being for people with CVD, including high BP (hypertension) and CHD (17, 35, 75). Resistance training could benefit most adults living with heart disease and its associated risk factors, including dyslipidemia, hypertension, and pre-diabetes. This is because many adults with and without cardiovascular conditions do not regularly participate in muscular strengthening exercises and lack the physical strength and self-confidence to perform common daily activities that require muscular effort (11, 29, 36). Consequently, authoritative professional medical organizations, including the American Heart Association (AHA) (29), ACSM (7), and American Association of Cardiovascular and Pulmonary Rehabilitation (AACVPR) (64), support resistance training as an adjunct to aerobic exercise in their current recommendations and guidelines for exercise for people with cardiovascular disease.

Moderate-intensity (e.g., 10-15 repetitions) resistance testing and training can be performed safely by cardiac patients deemed low risk (e.g., patients with absence of angina, ST-segment changes on the ECG, or complex ventricular dysrhythmias) (7, 29, 39). Moreover, despite concerns that resistance exercise elicits abnormal cardiovascular pressor responses, such as severely elevated BP in patients with CHD or controlled hypertension, studies have found that strength tests and resistance training in these individuals typically elicit clinically acceptable HR and BP responses (12, 35, 72, 73). Data on the benefits and safety of resistance training in patients with poor left ventricular function, such as those with congestive heart failure, are increasing (7), but additional study is warranted (55). According to ACSM, contraindications for exercise training during cardiac rehabilitation include uncontrolled hypertension (>180/110 mmHg), unstable angina, uncontrolled atrial or ventricular arrhythmias, active myocarditis or pericarditis, uncontrolled diabetes mellitus, and acute systemic illness or fever (7). Also, patients with severe proliferative retinopathy or recent treatments using laser surgery should avoid resistance training (7).

As with graded exercise tests, the risk of a serious cardiac event during strength testing can be minimized by preparticipation screening and close supervision by fitness professionals, particularly those with specialized training and certification regarding people who have special health concerns. When testing patients with known or suspected CHD or hypertension, the fitness professional should do preliminary work to establish appropriate weight loads and instruct the participant on proper lifting techniques. This should include demonstrating proper ROM and speed of movement for each exercise as well as correct breathing patterns to avoid the Valsalva maneuver. The monitoring of resting and recovery BP (e.g., every few minutes) and identification and evaluation of abnormal signs and symptoms should be standard protocol during the initial evaluation of the cardiovascular response during testing. Exaggerated BP responses, clinical signs or symptoms of CHD, or any other abnormal findings as previously described by ACSM that occur during resistance testing or training indicate termination of the activity until further evaluation by a qualified health care provider (7). Because BP measured immediately after exercise tends to underestimate values during contractions, the fitness professional should act conservatively when evaluating cardiovascular responses to testing in this population (24).

Studies have shown no adverse hemodynamic responses in low-risk cardiac patients who perform 1RM or multiple RM testing for upper- and lower-body exercises (12, 24, 75). Moreover, no scientific evidence suggests that 1RM testing is riskier than 10RM testing for low-risk cardiac patients. However, multiple RM testing (e.g., 10RM) is a more conservative and, therefore, sensible approach to testing clients with a history of cardiovascular disease. Thus, multiple RM testing that includes higher repetitions (i.e., 10-15) rather than single or low repetitions is a recommended practice for the fitness professional to assess strength and endurance in people with stable CHD. Regardless of the number of repetitions used during testing, the initial resistance or weight should be moderate to allow the participant to achieve the proper repetition range by working at a level that is fairly light, or somewhat hard (i.e., 11-13 on Borg's 6- to 20-grade rating of perceived exertion scale; see chapters 8 and 13) (7). Furthermore, the procedures for strength assessment previously described in this chapter can be applied safely to clients with a history of known or occult CHD who are clinically stable and to clients with controlled hypertension, diabetes, or other cardiovascular high-risk factors. Careful screening and astute monitoring of abnormal signs or symptoms, such as angina, dizziness, or light-headedness, are paramount to minimize any potential risks while simultaneously maximizing the benefits of resistance testing or training for people with and without known CVD.

Testing Children and Adolescents

Along with cardiorespiratory fitness, flexibility, and body composition, muscular strength is an important component of health-related fitness in children and adolescents (16, 20, 74). Enhancing muscular strength helps young people develop proper posture, reduce the risk of injury, improve body composition, and enhance fundamental movement skills such as kicking, throwing, sprinting, and jumping (43, 65). Assessing muscular strength and local muscular endurance with the push-up test is common in most physical education programs and YMCA recreation programs, whereas maximal load lifting (e.g., 1RM and 10RM) is often used to evaluate training-induced changes in performance in youth sport centers and pediatric research facilities (43).

Although standardized 1RM strength and power testing procedures have been developed for children and adolescents (22, 23), RM testing is time consuming and requires close supervision. Therefore, a standardized field test program, such as the FitnessGram (56), is a time-efficient method for assessing physical fitness in a group or class of school-aged youth. Components of the FitnessGram include body composition, cardiorespiratory fitness, muscular fitness, and flexibility. Performance on field-based tests such as the long jump is strongly associated with upper- and lower-body muscular strength tests in youth (13, 25), although the long jump is not included in the standard FitnessGram assessment (see *Field Tests Versus Repetition Maximum Testing in Children* Research Insight). Normative physical fitness data for children and teenagers are available in the FitnessGram test manual and other resources (56, 68). FitnessGram Healthy Fitness Zone classifications for muscular fitness assessments include those for the curl-up, push-up, modified pull-up, and flexed arm hang. For example, the Healthy Fitness Zone classifications are provided in table 9.6 for the push-up test. For youth, boys and girls follow the same protocol with standard push-ups: from a prone position with hands under or slightly wider than the shoulders, the participant pushes up until the arms are straight; in the down position the elbows are bent at 90 degrees with the upper arm parallel to the floor (56).

Table 9.6 FitnessGram Classifications by Age for Push-Up Assessment*

Age (yr)	Boys	Girls
5	3	3
6	3	3
7	4	4
8	5	5
9	6	6
10	7	7
11	8	7
12	10	7
13	12	7
14	14	7
15	16	7
16	18	7
17	18	7

*Values listed are the start of the Healthy Fitness Zone (sufficient fitness if at that level or above).

Adapted from Cooper Institute for Aerobics Research (2017).

A variety of fitness measures can be used to assess a child's muscular fitness, develop a personalized fitness program, track progress, and motivate participants. While there is no standard age to initiate fitness testing, the appropriate age depends on the nature of the test and the ability of the participants to accept and follow instructions. Generally, when children are ready to participate in sport activities, they are also ready for structured testing and training (20, 65).

Unsupervised or poorly administered strength assessments may not only discourage young people from participating in fitness activities but also result in injury (53). Qualified fitness professionals should demonstrate how to properly perform each exercise, allow the child to practice a few repetitions of each exercise, and offer guidance when necessary. In order to assess muscular strength in a safe and efficacious manner with a focus on proper exercise technique, some youth health and fitness professionals use an approach called *criterion repetition maximum testing (CRM)* instead of RM (21). CRM testing focuses on the quality of the movement and the physical effort needed to perform the lift, which requires testers to carefully assess the technical performance of every repetition. Although all strength testing requires proper exercise technique and qualified supervision, the perception of a CRM as opposed to an RM may help reinforce the importance of proper exercise technique. This approach can be particularly important when testing untrained youth, who may not be aware of the inherent risks associated with resistance training. All participants must understand that the amount of weight lifted or number of repetitions completed is not as important as how the exercise was performed.

When assessing fitness in young people, avoid the pass–fail mentality that may discourage some boys and girls from participating. Instead, refer to the assessment as a *challenge* in which all participants can feel good about their performance and get excited about monitoring their progress. Fitness professionals also should understand that children are not simply miniature adults. Because children are physically and psychologically less mature than adults, evaluating any measure of physical fitness requires special considerations. Fitness professionals should develop a friendly rapport with each child, and the exercise area should be nonthreatening. Most children have limited experience performing at maximum exertion, so fitness professionals should reassure children that they can safely perform exercise at a high exertion. Moreover, positive encouragement can motivate children to help ensure a valid test outcome. Following the strength assessment, cool down afterward with gentle calisthenics and stretching exercises.

RESEARCH INSIGHT

Field Tests Versus Repetition Maximum Testing in Children

Although RM testing has been found to be safe and reliable for assessing muscular strength in children, it may not be practical for large groups when time is limited. Artero and colleagues (8) analyzed the association between isokinetic strength and field-based muscular fitness tests in 126 adolescents. Upper- and lower-body isokinetic strength were measured at preset angular velocities, and muscular fitness was assessed with various field tests, including handgrip strength, arm hang, standing long jump, squat jump, and countermovement jump tests. Analysis of the data found that all field-based tests were significantly associated with isokinetic peak torque and power, but handgrip strength and standing long jump were the most valid field-based muscular fitness tests when compared with isokinetic strength. Health and fitness professionals who work with youth should consider using these field tests to assess muscular fitness when RM testing methods are not feasible.

KEY POINT

Muscular fitness testing is useful for a variety of special populations, including older adults, people at increased cardiovascular risk, and children and adolescents. Although strength tests, particularly those involving maximal exertion, were once thought to evoke unsafe physiological responses in these populations, scientific evidence shows that such tests are safe and can provide valuable information for the resistance training prescription if properly administered and performed. For older adults and people at elevated cardiovascular risk, proper screening by a physician or other qualified health care professional is warranted to promote safe and effective muscular fitness evaluations.

LEARNING AIDS

REVIEW QUESTIONS

1. Define *muscular strength*, *local muscular endurance*, and *muscular power*, and provide examples of different fitness tests that could be used to assess each component of muscular fitness.

2. What would you include in a standardization procedure to improve the safety and reliability of the YMCA bench press test?

3. Describe the warm-up and testing procedures for measuring a 1RM on the leg press exercise for a healthy adult.

4. How would you compare the 1RM strength of two people who differ markedly in body weight?

5. Describe a lower-body and an upper-body muscular fitness test for older adults.

6. How would you assess muscular strength in a low-risk cardiac patient?

7. Develop a test battery that can be used to assess all components of muscular fitness in school-aged youth.

CASE STUDIES

1. A 32-year-old healthy male (height 70 inches [177.8 centimeters], weight 190 pounds [86.2 kilograms]) has been resistance training on weight machines at a fitness center for 2 months. Although he did not have an initial strength assessment when he joined the center, he wants an evaluation of his upper- and lower-body strength. Outline a 1RM testing protocol for this client, and discuss safety procedures. How would you use the test results to provide meaningful feedback to this client?

2. A middle-aged female who recently joined your fitness facility would like to participate in an initial fitness assessment and receive advice about beginning a general fitness program to improve her muscular fitness. She has not participated in a structured exercise program for several years, although she reports that she leads an active lifestyle and often achieves moderate amounts of physical activity throughout the day. Her preparticipation health history questionnaire reveals that she is without signs, symptoms, or diagnosis of any cardiovascular, metabolic, or musculoskeletal conditions. With a classmate playing the role of this client, practice the following procedures presented in this chapter:

   a. Explain, demonstrate, and perform the procedures for the push-up test.

   b. Using the client information just described, explain, demonstrate, and perform the procedures for the 1RM bench press test.

Answers to Case Studies

1. Because this healthy adult has 2 months of resistance training experience, he does not need to participate in familiarization sessions. However, the exercises used for strength testing (e.g., chest press and leg press) should be part of his resistance training program. After a proper warm-up and explanation of testing procedures (e.g., proper exercise technique, full ROM, and predetermined speed of movement), follow standard 1RM testing guidelines. Begin with a light set of 5 to 10 repetitions at 50% perceived maximum. After a 1-minute rest, perform 3 to 5 repetitions at 60% to 80% perceived maximum. Then begin the 1RM tests with a 3-minute rest interval between trials. Continue the process until a failed attempt, ideally within 3 to 5 trials. To determine his relative strength on each exercise, divide the 1RM weight by his body weight. Fitness categories for upper- and lower-body strength are available (7). Percentile values (very poor to superior) can be used to assess his performance and provide meaningful feedback.

2. For this exercise:

   a. Please see pages 204-206 for a summary of the push-up test.

   b. Please see pages 200-202 for a summary of the 1RM test.

   c. Please see *Push-Up Testing Procedures* for a summary of the push-up test.

   d. Please see *1RM Testing Procedures* for a summary of the 1RM test.

Flexibility and Neuromotor Fitness Assessments

Erica M. Taylor

OBJECTIVES

The reader will be able to do the following:

1. List factors that influence flexibility and neuromotor fitness
2. Identify relative flexibility compensations that affect flexibility testing
3. Describe and demonstrate equipment used in assessing flexibility, range of motion, and neuromotor fitness
4. Describe the pros and cons of the sit-and-reach test
5. Recognize when referral to a medical professional is needed
6. Describe simple assessments for neuromotor fitness

10

Flexibility is an important component of overall physical fitness because many activities require good joint motion and muscular extensibility (3). Neuromotor fitness, also called *functional fitness*, is an important component of fitness for health, activities of daily living (ADLs), and participation in physical activity. Additionally, impaired flexibility and poor neuromotor fitness can negatively affect low-back function. The fitness professional likely will come in contact with clients who have a history of or who are currently experiencing low-back pain (LBP), so it is important to be familiar with the relationship between flexibility and LBP. Multiple assessments can be used in addressing flexibility, neuromotor fitness, and related low-back function by fitness professionals and the medical community.

RESEARCH INSIGHT

Low-Back Pain

Low-back pain causes a significant health care burden in the United States and worldwide, and it is the leading cause of years lived with disability globally (46). LBP increases with age, but rates are highest in those 50 to 54 years of age (46). However, approximately 25% of adults have reported LBP within the past 3 months in the United States (18). Due to the rates and global burden of LBP, it is important to understand how flexibility and neuromotor fitness are related to LBP.

As the fitness professional assesses a client, it is essential to consider the factors that may be influencing flexibility and neuromotor fitness. The assessment tools need to be well understood and appropriately applied to create an effective and safe individualized program. In addition, the fitness professional may be in a position to suggest that a client seek medical intervention for LBP or other health issues that are related to flexibility or neuromotor fitness, and the parameters that guide this decision need to be clear. The importance of neuromotor fitness and low-back function in everyday life makes these important areas in which to gain confidence.

Basics of Flexibility and Neuromotor Fitness

Flexibility relates to the ability to bend without breaking; flexion is the act of bending or being bent. In applied anatomy, *flexion* denotes a bending movement that occurs in the sagittal plane as two body segments are brought together (see chapter 3). Flexibility is defined as the capacity to move joints freely through their normal range of motion (ROM). As one assesses the flexibility of a region, all the components influencing the ROM need to be considered, including

- which joints are involved with the motion;
- the shapes and positions of the joints (i.e., correct alignment of joints);
- the muscles, tendons, ligaments, and joint capsules of the involved joints; and
- whether the muscle stretch reflex is being activated in the assessment process.

For example, a person reaching to touch the floor from a standing position flexes both the spine and the hips. The movement pattern that occurs is called the *lumbopelvic rhythm* and is a combination of flexion of the lower intervertebral joints of the spine, lumbosacral motion, and iliofemoral (hip) flexion in varying ratios (12, 29, 61). Therefore, when using the toe-touch test to assess flexibility, all the joints involved, the muscles crossing these joints, and the position of each of these joints must be taken into account.

Consider another example in which hamstring flexibility is assessed with the client lying in the supine position. If the spine is flexed as the leg is lifted, the assessment includes some spine ROM as well as hamstring extensibility. If this assessment is performed quickly, the stretch reflex may be activated and the true length of the hamstring may not be apparent. Sometimes, in an attempt to obtain a greater ROM in an area, the joint is compromised by poor positioning. This can overstretch the ligaments instead of stretching the appropriate muscles, leading to hypermobility of that joint. Awareness of these flexibility components will make the assessment, and the prescription of stretching exercises, more effective.

Having functional ROM at all joints of the musculoskeletal system ensures efficient body movement, which is one reason why flexibility is a key component of physical fitness. Assessing which joints are involved in a particular movement is pivotal in the assessment of flexibility in that region. If a flexibility test involves more than one joint, a person may have a good overall score for ROM but still have stiffness across one of the joints or regions tested. For example, a person may seem flexible because of the ability to easily touch toes from a standing position (see figure 10.1). But which structure is more flexible in the person in figure 10.1a, the hamstrings or low back? Clearly, the hamstrings are more flexible; the back has little curvature in contrast with the spinal curvature in figure 10.1b.

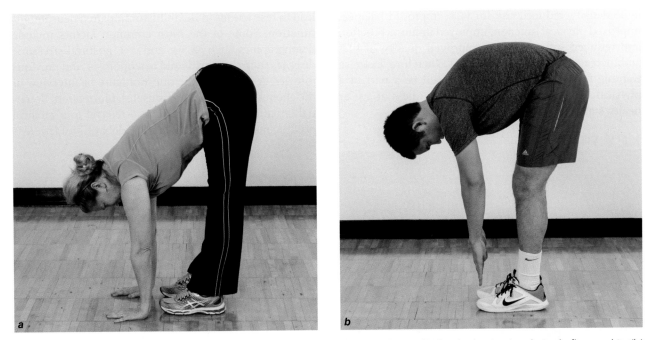

FIGURE 10.1 Relative flexibility demonstrated by the toe-touch test. In (a) the lumbar spine is relatively flat, and in (b) the lumbar spine has a greater curve. The person in (a) has good hamstring flexibility but limited lumbar spine ROM. In (b) the person has good lumbar spine ROM and moderate hamstring flexibility.

According to Sahrmann (76), relative flexibility is demonstrated when a person can touch their toes yet exhibits decreased low-back flexibility. Stiffness across one joint or in one muscle group creates compensatory movements at neighboring joints and muscles. These structures then may have to increase flexibility or become hypermobile to meet the goal of the overall movement. In other words, the body will follow the path of least resistance or the most flexible route to accomplish the overall movement. If the fitness professional prescribes the toe-touch exercise as a low-back stretch for the person in figure 10.1a, it will likely improve hamstring flexibility but not back flexibility because the body will choose the easiest way to get to the floor—using the hamstrings. Caution should be used in interpreting this exercise as a flexibility test due its inclusion of many joints (intervertebral, lumbosacral, and iliofemoral) and relative flexibility when multiple joints are involved.

KEY POINT

Having good ROM at all joints reduces the risk of injury. Noting and addressing relative flexibility compensations can decrease pain and dysfunction.

The neuromuscular system is the network that connects the brain, spinal cord, and nerves to sensory receptors and muscles in the body. The structures of this system work together to coordinate movements in response to the sensory information detected. Balance, coordination, agility, gait, reaction time, and proprioception (i.e., body awareness) are components of neuromotor fitness or neuromotor skills. Essentially all motor tasks performed are orchestrated by the neuromotor system. This aspect of fitness was included in the American College of Sports Medicine's (ACSM) 2011 position stand on guidelines for prescribing exercise (34), and it was also included in the 10th edition of *ACSM's Guidelines for Exercise Testing and Prescription* (4). The prescription guidelines for neuromotor fitness are not as clear as they are for the other fitness components, and are only addressed for older adults and some special populations in the 11th edition of *ACSM's Guidelines for Exercise Testing and Prescription* (5). It is important to understand assessment for neuromotor fitness and prescription for exercises that will improve neuromotor fitness for all due to the potential benefits.

Neuromotor fitness is essential in the performance of ADLs, participation in physical activity, and for general maintenance of health. Research supports the numerous health benefits of good neuromotor fitness and exercises that improve neuromotor fitness. Balance training has been shown to reduce the risk of falls in older adults (57). Reduction in knee pain and faster walking speed have been reported in those with osteoarthritis in the knee after proprioceptive training (50). Physical and mental health benefits have been noted from yoga, qigong, and tai chi (32, 44, 49). These benefits can include improved bone density, reduced risk for falls, improved balance, improved physical function, improved immune function and reduced inflammation, improved quality of life, and increased self-efficacy (32, 44). Therefore, exercise training for neuromotor fitness should be a part of a physical activity plan for all adults regardless of age or health status.

KEY POINT

Neuromotor, or functional, fitness is an important aspect of fitness because essentially all motor tasks performed are orchestrated by the neuromotor system. This system is the network that connects the brain, spinal cord, and nerves to sensory receptors and muscles in the body. The structures of the neuromotor system coordinate movements in response to the sensory information detected. The functions of the neuromotor system are necessary for physical activity participation, performing ADLs, and maintenance of general health.

Factors Affecting Range of Motion and Neuromotor Fitness

When evaluating a client for ROM and neuromotor fitness limitations, it is helpful to consider factors that can lead to restrictions in flexibility or impaired neuromotor function. Some of the most common factors include demographics such as age and sex, postural stressors, diseases such as arthritis and osteoporosis, and previous injuries. A good baseline questionnaire or interview of the client should provide this useful information. Potential situations that may require a referral to a medical professional are discussed in the sidebar *Considerations Related to Referral*.

Age and Sex

Flexibility can be affected by several demographic variables. For example, ROM typically decreases in adulthood; however, it is unknown how much of this diminution is attributable to aging or to the reduction in physical activity related to aging. Overall joint flexibility has been shown to decrease at a rate of 0.6% per year for females and 0.8% for males (seven joints were included in the study) (65). In general, the shoulders and trunk show less flexibility as age advances, while elbow and knee mobility stay relatively stable (65). With age, lumbar spine ROM reduces in flexion, extension, and lateral flexion (48, 64, 65, 79), particularly after age 40 (48). One group of researchers reports that the lower part of the lumbar spine retains its mobility and lordosis, but the middle part flattens and becomes less mobile with age (26). With decreases in muscle mass, changes in the vestibular system, and changes in sight and depth perception, neuromotor fitness is also affected with age (55, 81). Balance, proprioception, and coordination are affected by these changes and can decrease as individuals age (55, 57, 81).

Considerations Related to Referral

While stretching to improve flexibility and exercises to improve neuromotor fitness are recommended in a comprehensive fitness program, for some individuals, referral to a physical therapist or other health care provider is warranted prior to assessment and program development. Medical conditions that limit joint movement, such as osteoarthritis, rheumatoid arthritis, spondylosis, or osteoporosis, can be contraindications for flexibility or neuromotor exercises. These individuals are encouraged to begin a flexibility program, because discomfort or pain from these conditions can be improved or reduced. However, limitations of these conditions may need attention that is beyond the scope of the fitness professional. A recent acute injury, joint inflammation, or significant joint pain are additional reasons to consider a referral before conducting an assessment or prescribing a program to ensure safety of the individual during assessment or within a program. Chapter 15 includes some situations for individuals who experience problems with LBP, report unusual signs or symptoms, or experience other pain that warrant attention from a health care provider. Those who fail to make progress or make slower than expected progress when complying with their program also may need a referral to find the underlying reasons when no signs or symptoms are evident.

Posture

If people do not use the full ROM at a joint, tissues may compensate by shortening. It then becomes difficult to perform some of the movements needed in ADLs. For example, a person sitting at a computer desk several hours each day might develop a greater thoracic curve (i.e., dorsal kyphosis) and rounded shoulders (see figure 10.2*a*). If this posture becomes habitual and no countermeasures are taken to change it, tissue that previously permitted good movement can shorten (37), and correction of this posture may become difficult, if not impossible. A much better posture to assume at a desk is seen in figure 10.2*b*. Additionally, poor core stability and strength negatively affect posture and balance, and they increase the risk of LBP.

Disease

A wide variety of diseases can negatively affect ROM. Two of the most common diseases that have an impact on joint mobility are arthritis and osteoporosis.

Arthritis

Arthritis can have a debilitating effect on ROM because it affects articular cartilage. Articular cartilage, also called *hyaline cartilage*, is avascular (i.e., it does not have a blood supply), which means its healing capability is poor. Because articular cartilage does not repair itself well, fibrocartilage and bony spicules can replace the cartilage, diminishing joint movement (70). Two common types of arthritis are rheumatoid arthritis (RA) and osteoarthritis

(OA). RA occurs more frequently in females than males and can appear any time in life. This autoimmune condition is a chronic inflammatory polyarthritis, an arthritis that affects five or more joints (19). The inflammatory process primarily affects the lining of the joints (synovial membrane). The inflamed synovium leads to erosion of the cartilage and bone, and sometimes joint deformity results, causing joint stiffness and decreased ROM (19). Chronic low-back dysfunction has been associated with RA (10).

OA is a much more prevalent condition, accounting for 90% to 95% of arthritis cases, and it usually begins after the age of 40. OA is a disease of the entire joint involving the cartilage, joint lining, ligaments, and underlying bone (16). The breakdown of these tissues eventually leads to pain and joint stiffness and has a significant impact on the incidence of low-back dysfunction and loss of ROM. The causes of OA are complex and often are the result of both mechanical (injuries or overuse) and cellular (inflammation) events in the affected joint (1, 16). More than 32.5 million people in the United States have OA, with women more likely to have it than men (6, 71). It can occur in any joint, including those in the spine, hands, ankles, feet, hips, and knees, but the knees and the spine are the most commonly affected areas. Arthritis can decrease mobility in the spine if the site is a facet joint (see figure 10.3) that helps guide motion in the spine (70). Facet joint OA is a common cause of low-back dysfunction (35), and it seems to follow lumbar disc degeneration (33) due to the increased forces on the facet joints (see figure

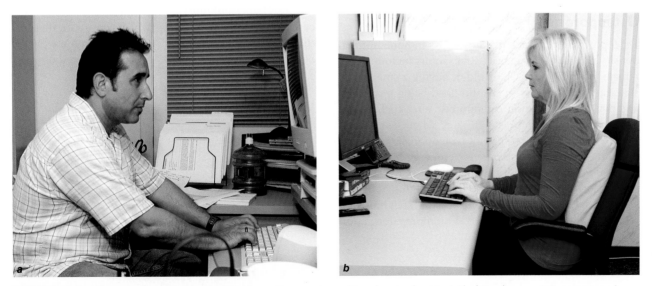

FIGURE 10.2 Connective-tissue structures (e.g., ligaments and tendons) adapt to (a) habitual poor sitting posture (e.g., rounding of the upper back or less lordotic curve in the lumbar region) by lengthening in response to stress. Without an attempt to remove these stresses or to develop counterbalancing ones, poor sitting postures can transfer to poor standing postures. The person in (b) demonstrates a properly balanced sitting posture.

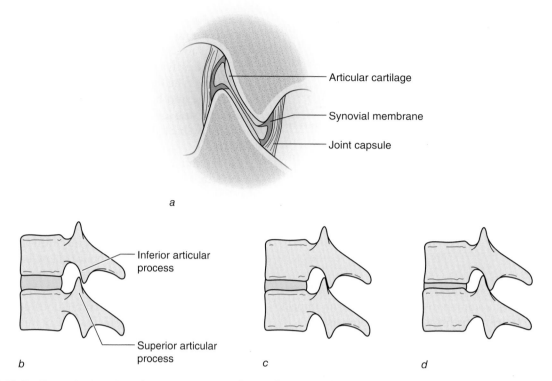

FIGURE 10.3 Posterior junctions between two vertebrae often are referred to as *facet joints*. Facet joints are synovial joints and have articular cartilage, as seen here in the *(a)* sagittal view and *(b)* vertebral column with normal disc thickness. *(c)* Reduction of the disc thickness adds stress to the facet joint. *(d)* Further disc degeneration leads to impingement at the tips of both the superior articulate process and inferior articulate process.

10.3). Articular cartilage is avascular and depends on the diffusion of nutrients from tissue fluid, so further deterioration can result from lack of movement. Thus, it is desirable for people with arthritis to maintain as much movement and ROM as possible.

Osteoporosis

Osteoporosis is characterized by a loss in bone mineral density (BMD) or bone mass. Risk factors include being female, postmenopausal, or older; having a small body size; eating a diet low in calcium; and being physically inactive (47). Common osteoporotic sites include the hip, wrist, and vertebrae—all sites where cancellous bone predominates. In the spine, osteoporosis can cause buckling and compression of vertebrae. A person with this condition may show extreme curves in the spine as well as loss of ROM. Fortunately, cancellous bone can become denser through weight-bearing activities and resistance training. (See chapter 21 for more information on osteoporosis.)

Previous Injury

Previous injury can create either decreased flexibility in injured tissue or increased joint motion (hypermobility). Muscle that has been disrupted due to an injury may show decreased extensibility and loss of endurance and strength (70). For example, a hamstring strain can significantly decrease the capacity of the muscle to lengthen as one reaches to touch the floor. However, ligaments that run bone to bone and guide joint motion can be overstretched if injured and allow too much joint motion (hypermobility) (70). A common example is the case of an inversion ankle sprain. If the sprain disrupts the supporting ligaments sufficiently, the ankle typically becomes more mobile. Some low-back injuries also may

KEY POINT

Factors relating to ROM include age, sex, posture, disease, and injury history. If the ROM of a joint is not used, it may be lost. Although declines in ROM often relate to increased age, some result from a decline in physical activity or from injury. Habitual poor posture also can decrease ROM. Arthritis is a disease of the joints and thus tends to decrease joint ROM. Osteoporosis can reduce spine ROM because of its destructive effect on vertebral bodies. Injury changes the extensibility of soft tissue.

have both immediate and long-term impacts on ROM and can affect overall strength and function even when ROM is not affected. These injuries include herniated discs (all planes of motion possibly limited), spinal stenosis (extension), ankylosing spondylitis (decreased spinal curves), spondylolisthesis (extension), lumbar facet syndrome (usually extension and rotation), muscle strain (can be decreased in any plane) (37), and degenerative disc disease and hypermobility (can have increased or decreased ROM changes) (58). Having a complete history of the client's injuries is ideal in assessing flexibility and neuromotor fitness.

Hip, Knee, Ankle, and Shoulder Flexibility Testing

Flexibility can be assessed at each joint using both quantitative and qualitative approaches. For example, the ROM available at the knee can be measured in degrees with a goniometer or noted in terms of full motion or exhibiting mild, moderate, or significant limitations. Most fitness professionals do not need the specificity of goniometric measures; however, recognizing the extent (i.e., mild, moderate, significant) to which a joint is limited will help identify areas where flexibility is compromised. The fitness professional can then select stretches appropriate for that client's needs. Common joints that should be assessed include the shoulders, elbows, wrists, hips, knees, and ankles. Table 10.1 presents the normal ROM for the major joints. Flexibility can also be considered by investigating the length of specific muscles that cover two joints, such as the hamstrings or hip flexors (iliopsoas). The next section covers tests addressing the flexibility of the hamstrings, hip flexors, iliotibial band (ITB), quadriceps, gastrocnemius, soleus, piriformis, and shoulders. A postural assessment can suggest which muscles may be tight.

Some postural deviations to note are as follows:

- A client with rounded, forward-placed shoulders may have tight pectoralis muscles and limited shoulder motion.
- A client with a posteriorly tilted pelvic girdle may have tight hamstrings.

- A client with an anteriorly tilted pelvic girdle may have tight hip flexors and lumbar musculature.
- A client with overpronated feet or fallen arches may have tight calves and ITBs.

The tight musculature identified through these assessments can be listed in a chart in the client's file to recheck as the fitness program progresses.

Iliofemoral Range of Motion

Some evidence shows that hip muscle imbalance is associated with LBP and dysfunction (68, 69). The muscles crossing the hip joint are sometimes viewed as guy-wires (tensioned cables used to provide stability) because they can limit pelvic motion (see figure 10.4). If any of these guy-wires are too tight, the trunk musculature may have difficulty controlling pelvic position. Because the sacrum (in the pelvis) is the foundation of the 24 vertebrae stacked on it, pelvic positioning plays an important role in the integrity of the spine. For example, tightness in the hip flexors, such as the psoas, can produce an anterior or forward pelvic tilt, and tightness in the hip extensors, such as the hamstrings, can produce a backward or posterior pelvic tilt (see figure 10.4). Thus, if either of these muscle groups is tight, the abdominal muscles are less able to control pelvic positioning. People who cannot control their pelvic positioning with their abdominal muscles are predisposed to LBP, which is one of the reasons why ROM at the iliofemoral joint is important.

Biering-Sorensen's study revealed that weak trunk musculature and poor flexibility of the back and hamstrings were present in those with recurrent or persistent LBP (11). There also may be tightness in the ITB, which can limit thigh adduction. Tightness in the piriformis muscle can limit movement in the transverse plane, but this is a little more complex because such tightness can limit outward or inward rotation of the femur depending on the angle between the hip and the thigh (75). Healthy participants were compared with patients who had LBP in terms of their hip ROM patterns (28). The results suggest an association between hip rotation ROM imbalance (internal and external ROM) and the presence of LBP.

Correct assessment of the musculature crossing the hip is essential to creating an effective flexibility program. The following tests of the ITB, iliopsoas, hamstring,

Table 10.1 Normal Joint Range of Motion

Area	Flexion	Extension	Abduction	Adduction	External rotation	Internal rotation
Shoulder	167°-180°	60°	180°		90°	70°
Hip	140°	15°	30°	25°	90°	70°
Knee	140°	0°			45° max at 90°	35° max at 90°
Ankle	PF 40°-55°	DF 10°-20°				

PF = plantar flexion; DF = dorsiflexion

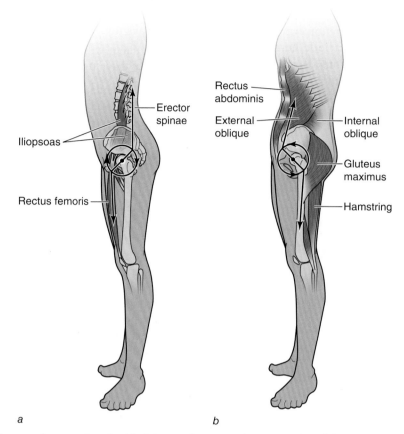

a   b

FIGURE 10.4   The muscles crossing the hip joint can be viewed as guy-wires. If, for example, the erector spinae guy-wires are too tight, (a) they will tend to anteriorly rotate the pelvis. If the hamstring guy-wires are too tight, (b) they will tend to posteriorly rotate the pelvis, making it difficult for the rectus abdominis to control pelvic positioning. Inability to control pelvic positioning with the abdominal musculature predisposes a person to low-back problems.

piriformis, gastrocnemius, soleus, and shoulder girdle musculature can be used in the fitness setting.

Thomas Test

The Thomas test measures tightness in the hip flexors (37), including the iliopsoas, rectus femoris, and ITB

(see figure 10.5). The reliability between testers has been shown to be high for this test (31). The client starts by sitting on the edge of a surface and leaning back to the supine position. The client then brings both knees toward the chest. The left leg is released so that it extends and touches the surface. The left thigh should

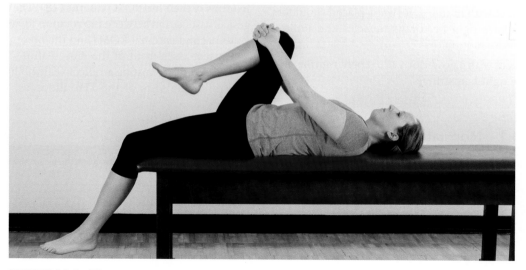

FIGURE 10.5   Thomas test.

remain in contact with the testing surface (37, 53). If it does not, the degree of elevation indicates the tightness of the left hip flexors (iliopsoas). If the knee is bent 70° or less, the rectus femoris is tight. If the left leg abducts or angles outward, the ITB is tight. The pelvic girdle and low back need to remain in a neutral position to avoid a false negative or positive. The low back should be against the surface but not in a posteriorly tilted position.

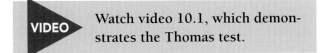

Watch video 10.1, which demonstrates the Thomas test.

Active Knee Extension Test

The active knee extension (AKE) test is a popular assessment that measures tightness of the hamstrings. This test has been shown to have excellent intra- and inter-rater reliability for assessing hamstring length in healthy individuals (38). It requires the use of a goniometer to determine the best measure of joint angle to assess the tightness of the hamstrings. If a goniometer is not available, the ROM can be visually estimated to assess tightness based on the joint angles described here. The test is sometimes referred to the as *90–90 test* because the client lies supine with the hip held at 90° flexion and the knee is also flexed and held at 90° to begin (figure 10.6a). The tester will have to hold the thigh in this position as shown in figure 10.6. The client then actively extends the lower leg. A measure of zero at the knee indicates that the leg moved 90° (i.e., the extended leg is perpendicular to the table, and the lower leg is in line with the thigh); a measure of 10 indicates that the lower leg moved 80°.

A fully extended leg would measure 0°, and a leg extended 10° shy of fully straight (180°) would measure an angle of 10°. Normal angles for the AKE hamstring assessment are 37.7° ± 7.7° (approximately 2/3 fully extended) for males and 25.2° ± 12° (approximately 3/4 fully extended) for females (25).

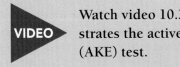

Watch video 10.2, which demonstrates the active knee extension (AKE) test.

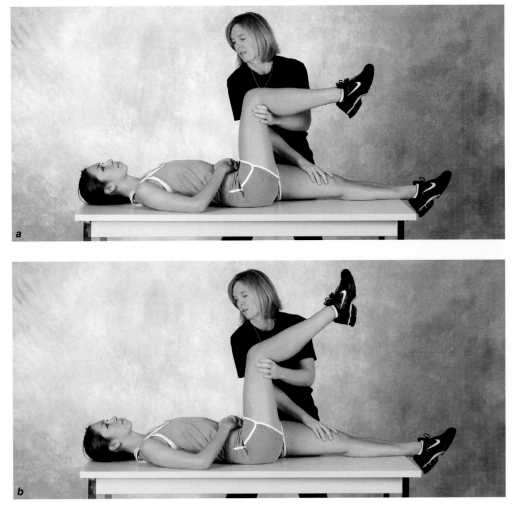

FIGURE 10.6 Active knee extension (AKE) test.

Ober's Test

ITB tightness is common in both the athlete and non-athlete. It frequently contributes to knee dysfunction and is affected by alignment challenges such as over-pronation of the feet. Ober's test is performed to assess ITB tightness. The client is in a side-lying position so that the involved hip is upward. The pelvis is in the neutral position with the hips stacked. The hip is passively extended and then allowed to adduct toward the surface. The test is positive, indicating tightness, if the upper leg remains abducted and does not move toward the table surface (figure 10.7) (37). The client will also likely experience lateral knee pain with a positive test. The inter-rater reliability has been shown to be very high for this test (31).

Piriformis Test

The piriformis muscle is frequently involved in both low-back and hip dysfunctions and can be tested in a supine or seated position. The supine version is typically used in a clinical setting; however, the seated version (figure 10.8) may be easier and ideal to use in the fitness setting.

The seated version is easily performed in a chair. The spine should stay straight with the feet resting on the floor. One leg is lifted, and the ankle is placed on the knee of the other leg as seen in figure 10.8. The tester may help stabilize the client by placing a hand on the knee if needed. The client then leans their body forward at the hips. A tight piriformis can lead to the inability to open or externally rotate the top leg easily. If the test elicits pain, refer the client to a physical therapist for a medical evaluation.

Ely's Test

Ely's test measures quadriceps flexibility, specifically the rectus femoris, and is performed in the prone position (figure 10.9). This test also can be done in a side-lying position. Atamaz and colleagues (7) measured from the heel to the back of the leg and hip as the knee was maximally flexed to document quadriceps flexibility, and they concluded that this measurement of flexibility is reliable. It is important to keep the hips on the surface because a tight rectus femoris may tilt the pelvis anteriorly or laterally, resulting in an inaccurate measurement. This assessment is a passive test, and the fitness professional places one hand on the client's lower back for stability

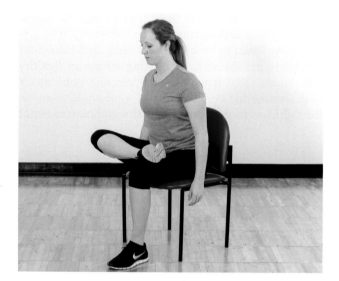

FIGURE 10.8 Piriformis seated test.

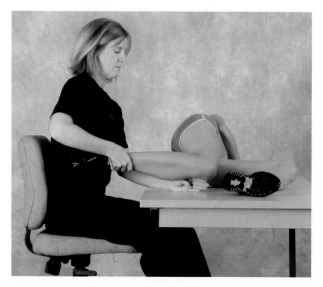

FIGURE 10.7 Ober's test.

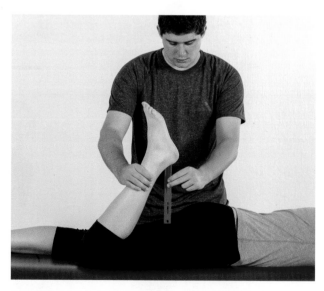

FIGURE 10.9 Prone quadriceps test (Ely's test).

and uses the other hand to move the heel toward the buttocks. Ideally, with sufficient quadriceps flexibility, the heel will be able to touch the posterior leg or buttocks. The distance from the buttocks or leg to the heel can be used as a measurement guide to assess progress in quadriceps flexibility. The test is considered positive for tightness when the heel cannot touch the buttocks, the hips raise up from the table, or the client experiences back or leg pain.

Ankle Range of Motion

ROM at the ankle can be measured with a goniometer, or it can be assessed using active tests that are appropriate for a fitness setting, such as the straight-leg or bent-knee foot raise tests. The gastrocnemius is tested for tightness in the straight-leg test because the muscle crosses both the posterior knee and ankle (figure 10.10). The client stands with their back against the wall and dorsiflexes the foot. The distance from the toe to the floor is measured. The ankle joint needs to move 10° for normal walking without compensations and 15° for running. The test can be adapted (bent-knee foot raise test) to target the soleus by having the client sit straight with feet flat on the floor. The toes are raised while keeping the heel on the surface and the lower leg vertical.

Shoulder Flexibility

A quick test of upper-extremity flexibility is the back-scratch test (figure 10.11). It is relatively easy to perform and document objectively (51). If the fingertips touch, the score is zero. If they do not touch, measure the distance between the fingertips (a negative score); if they overlap, measure by how much (a positive score). Practice two times and then test two times. Stop the test if the client experiences pain. The scores can be compared over time as the fitness program progresses. This assessment is part of the Senior Fitness Test (see normal ranges in table 10.2). The back-scratch test is a flexibility assessment for youth that is part of the FitnessGram (24). Children and adolescents who score in the Healthy Fitness Zone are at a level of fitness that promotes health. The ability for the fingers to touch or overlap meets the Healthy Fitness Zone standard, and the fingertips not touching meets the Needs Improvement classification.

KEY POINT

Flexibility of the hip musculature (ITB, iliopsoas, piriformis, hamstrings) needs to be accurately assessed and addressed. Good ROM at the hip joint is necessary for good biomechanics of the spine (68, 69). Although tightness in the hip flexors is not as common as tightness in the hip extensors, both are important in maintaining a healthy spine. Tightness in the muscles crossing the hip joint may predispose a person to low-back problems (68, 69).

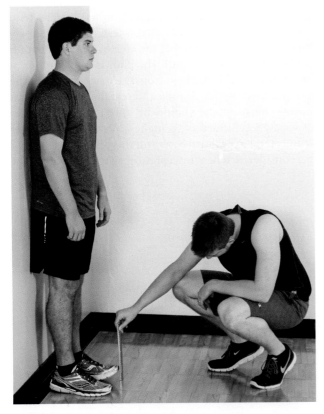

FIGURE 10.10   Straight-leg foot raise test.

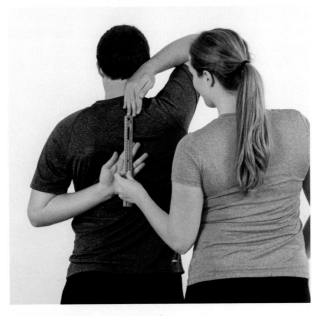

FIGURE 10.11   Back-scratch test.

Table 10.2   Senior Fitness Test Normal Range of Scores for Flexibility Assessments*

MEN							
Test	AGE 60-64	AGE 65-69	AGE 70-74	AGE 75-79	AGE 80-84	AGE 85-89	AGE 90-94
Chair sit-and-reach (inches)	-2.5 to +4.0	-3.0 to +3.0	-3.0 to +3.0	-4.0 to +2.0	-5.5 to +1.5	-5.5 to +0.5	-6.5 to -0.5
Back scratch (inches)	-6.5 to 0	-7.5 to -1.0	-8.0 to -1.0	-9.0 to -2.0	-9.5 to -2.0	-9.5 to -3.0	-10.5 to -4.0

WOMEN							
Test	AGE 60-64	AGE 65-69	AGE 70-74	AGE 75-79	AGE 80-84	AGE 85-89	AGE 90-94
Chair sit-and-reach (inches)	-0.05 to +5.0	-0.5 to +4.5	-1.0 to +4.0	-1.5 to +3.5	-2.0 to +3.0	-2.5 to +2.5	-4.5 to +1.0
Back scratch (inches)	-3.0 to +1.5	-3.5 to +1.5	-4.0 to +1.0	-5.0 to +0.5	-5.5 to 0	-7.0 to -1.0	-8.0 to -1.0

*Normal range of scores reflects the middle 50% for each age group (between 25th and 75th percentiles). Scores above the range listed are considered above normal, and those below the range are considered below normal. Age in years.

Adapted from Rikli and Jones (2013).

Spinal Range of Motion and Low-Back Function

Most movements emanate from or have an impact on the spine. Good spinal mobility and muscle control are essential for normal function without predisposition to LBP. Spinal (intervertebral) ROM is typically assessed using measures done in a physical therapist's office. Some spinal ROM tests can be performed in a fitness center with little equipment. The interaction of the spine and hips in bending forward is termed *lumbopelvic motion*, which can be assessed with overall flexibility tests that include both spine and hip measures, such as the sit-and-reach and toe-touch tests that are more appropriate for the fitness setting. It is important to note that normal lumbar spine extension ROM ranges from 20° to 25° (37) to 6° to 29° (79) because many adults have lost the capacity to extend due to prolonged activities in a flexed posture (i.e., desk work).

Active Extension Test

An active test of spine extension ROM, called the *trunk lift*, was developed by The Cooper Institute for Aerobics Research (23). It is an active test because muscles of the spine (i.e., erector spinae and multifidus) hyperextend the spine (see figure 10.12). In this test, the client slowly lifts the torso by contracting the erector spinae and multifidus muscle groups until the chin is a maximum of 30 centimeters (12 inches) from the mat. Although The Cooper Institute for Aerobics Research did not present norms, most people should be able to raise the chin at least 15 centimeters (6 inches). People with longer trunks tend to perform better on this test, which should be considered when interpreting scores. It should be

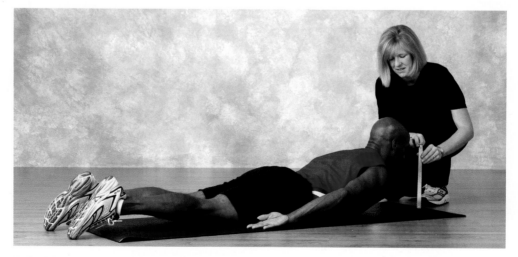

FIGURE 10.12   Active back ROM and strength test.

noted that in addition to ROM, trunk extensor strength contributes to performance in the trunk-lift assessment. This assessment can be included with the FitnessGram assessment for children and adolescents (24). For the trunk lift, ranges are provided that represent the Healthy Fitness Zone, and fitness is considered sufficient if in the zone or above. For boys and girls between the ages of 5 to 9 years of age, 6 to 12 inches is the Healthy Fitness Zone, and for those ages 10 to 17 years of age, the range is 9 to 12 inches (24). Those who score in the Needs Improvement classification (i.e., below those ranges) are considered at increased risk for health problems if fitness in that area is not improved.

 VIDEO Watch video 10.3, which demonstrates the active back ROM and strength test.

Lumbopelvic Rhythm

When a person reaches toward the floor, both the spine and the hips flex. The pattern that occurs is called the *lumbopelvic rhythm* and is a combination of both spine and hip flexion in varying ratios. This pattern can be affected by tightness in both the lower extremities and areas of the spine. A study that analyzed the spine and hip movement during forward bending showed that the lumbar spine had a greater contribution to early bending, the hips and lumbar spine contributed roughly equally to the middle phase, and the hips had a greater contribution to the late phase (29). Therefore, a person with a healthy spine who bends over to touch the floor uses spine flexibility throughout the beginning and middle phases and stretches the hamstrings close to the floor. The participants with a history of LBP tended to use their lumbar range earlier in the forward bending pattern, reaching the end of their lumbar flexibility earlier than those without LBP. The authors suggest that the earlier lumbar spine motion used by those with a history of LBP predisposes them to a higher risk of recurrence because they have an earlier tensile stress to the posterior elements of the spine.

Hamstring tightness has been thought to significantly affect the lumbopelvic rhythm (52). When investigators compared the lumbopelvic patterns and hamstring length in healthy people, it was apparent that flexible hamstrings were associated with a pelvic-dominant pattern and tight hamstrings led to a lumbar-dominant pattern, possibly creating more load on the spine (39), which increases the risk for LBP. The lumbopelvic rhythm during a stooping activity was analyzed in participants with tight hamstrings who performed hamstring stretching exercises (52). The investigators found hamstring stretching exercises increased the ROM of active knee extension significantly, supporting the value in stretching the hamstrings in order to decrease lumbar flexion and increase hip flexion when performing repetitive stoop lifting (52). Hamstring flexibility testing is an important aspect for fitness professionals to include when assessing clients.

KEY POINT

Tight hamstrings can alter the lumbopelvic rhythm and place an increased load on the L5-S1 junction. The principle of relative flexibility is apparent in this situation, with the hamstring tightness creating compensation in the lumbar spine with earlier flexion and an increased load. Improving hamstring flexibility changes this compensation and lessens the load to the posterior elements of the spine, thus decreasing the risk for LBP.

Combined Tests of Range of Motion in Trunk and Hip Flexion

The fingertips-to-floor (or toe-touch) and sit-and-reach tests often have been used under the belief that they measure flexibility in the low back as well as at the hip joint. However, although both can be used to measure hip joint flexibility (i.e., hamstring length), neither effectively measures low-back ROM in conventional use (7, 60, 62).

The toe-touch test is performed with the client standing and bending forward, reaching for the floor with straight legs. As previously noted, this can be performed with little spine motion (figure 10.1). Both the sit-and-reach and the toe touch were found to have moderate validity and acceptable reproducibility (7, 8, 54) as hamstring tests. Several sit-and-reach variations have been found to be reliable (7, 9, 45, 66). These variations include the chair sit-and-reach and the modified back-saver sit-and-reach. These modified versions are often more suitable for older adults and those who have LBP.

Using the sit-and-reach movement pattern as an exercise has been questioned. For example, if the hamstrings are tight and the sitting stretch is performed ballistically, the spine may be obligated to absorb these stresses, and over time these repetitive motions can have serious consequences for low-back function. Moreover, even if the sit-and-reach is done slowly, the static postures resulting during the stretching phase can place high compressive forces on the intervertebral discs (63, 67), and this movement might damage ligaments of the spine, particularly if the hamstrings are tight (14).

Sit-and-Reach Test

A traditional sit-and-reach test requires a solid box about 30 centimeters tall. Fix a meter stick on top of the box so that 26 centimeters of the ruler extend over the front edge of the box toward the client. The 26-centimeter mark should be at the edge of the box. Following a brief warm-up, the client removes their shoes and sits on the floor with their legs stretched out in front with knees straight and feet flat against the front end of the test box. Instruct the client to move forward at the hips at a slow, steady pace, keeping the knees straight. The hands slide up the ruler as far as they can go (figure 10.13a). The client should exhale and drop the head between the arms while reaching to facilitate the best score possible. This position should be held for 2 seconds. Record the result in centimeters, rest, and repeat two times. Chose the best result for the final score (4). Another version requires only a yardstick and a piece of masking tape (36). Place the yardstick on the floor between the client's legs as shown in figure 10.13b. A 12-inch piece of tape is placed at the 15-inch mark perpendicular to the tape measure to guide the distance between the client's feet; heels should be at the inner edges of the tape, which will allow feet to be between 10 to 12 inches apart. As with the traditional box test, the client reaches forward slowly, not bending the knees or bouncing, with hands overlapping or parallel, reaching as far as possible and holding that final position for 2 seconds. Although norms are available for adults (4, 15, 36), questions about validity remain (5). ACSM no longer includes the sit-and-reach test within their *Guidelines* (5) as in the past (4). If the sit-and-reach is used as an indirect measure, tracking the distance reached can be used to gauge progress.

Even though the sit-and-reach test has medical contraindications and a host of factors can affect performance, it still has value as a field test provided that users are aware of its shortcomings. Following are suggestions that can make the sit-and-reach a better test.

- It is argued that the distance reached is not the most valid indicator of performance. The test administrator is better advised to examine the client's quality of movement. Look for the angle of the sacrum (see figure 10.14) and the smoothness of the spinal curve. These relatively simple determinations can make the sit-and-reach a measure of low-back mobility as well as of hamstring length. These and other quality points are delineated in figure 10.14.

- It is recommended that the client extend only one leg during the sit-and-reach test. Although this technique doubles the number of measurements required, the tester will be able to evaluate symmetry. As stated previously, lower-extremity symmetry is desirable with respect to strength and flexibility because imbalance can have an untoward effect on the spine.

- If a sit-and-reach box is used to make measurements, it should be altered to permit passive plantar flexion at the ankle joint; however, normative data are not available for this modification. To alter the standard sit-and-reach box, simply replace the vertical surface under the cantilever extension with a rod at a height of 4 centimeters, which permits plantar flexion into the box but restrains the heel. This adjustment is not necessary if the protocol of Hui and Yuen (45) is followed.

Chair Sit-and-Reach Test

In the chair sit-and-reach, the client sits in a chair about 43 centimeters (17 inches) tall with one foot flat on the ground. The other leg is extended as straight as possible in front of the hip with the heel on the floor and with the foot dorsiflexed. The client reaches to touch the toes, and the distance from the fingertips to the middle toe is measured (figure 10.15). Norms for older adults

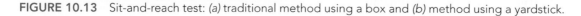

FIGURE 10.13 Sit-and-reach test: *(a)* traditional method using a box and *(b)* method using a yardstick.

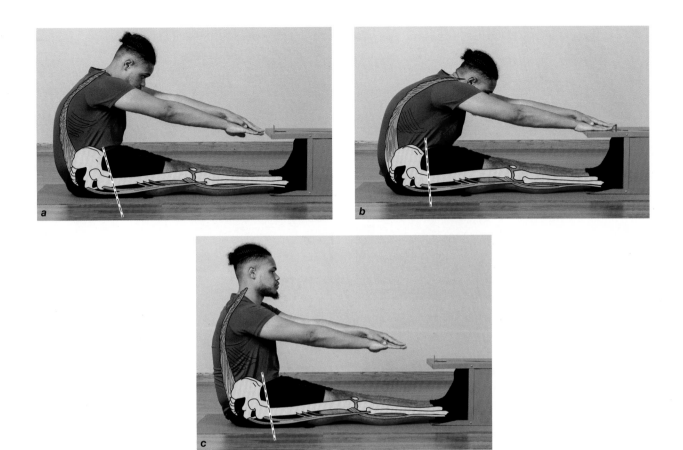

FIGURE 10.14 Sit-and-reach test. Quality points to look for include *(a)* tight hamstrings (note tilt of pelvis), tight low back, and stretched upper back; *(b)* normal length of hamstrings and low back; and *(c)* tight hamstrings (note tilt of pelvis) and tight low back.

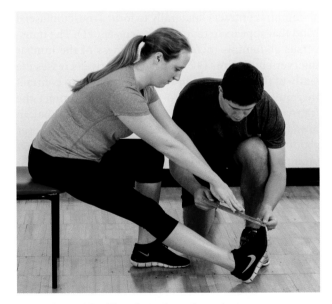

FIGURE 10.15 The chair sit-and-reach test.

are listed in table 10.2 (51, 74) and can help the fitness professional assess the client, set goals, and reassess the client in the future.

Modified Back-Saver Sit-and-Reach Test

The modified back-saver sit-and-reach is a reliable test for low-back and hamstring flexibility (45). There are two versions of the test: a variation with one leg bent while reaching forward (use the same testing procedure as the sit-and-reach test; see figure 10.16*a*) and a variation with only a meter stick and a bench (figure 10.16*b*). The client sits with a single straight leg on a bench and reaches for the toes. The distance reached is the score. Because the ankle is permitted to passively plantar flex, connective-tissue tightness behind the knee, as well as other factors such as sciatic nerve tension, does not affect performance. The back-saver sit-and-reach shown in figure 10.16*a* is also a recommended flexibility assessment used for children and adolescents as part of the FitnessGram assessments (24). As with the trunk-lift test, the scores are classified as meeting the Healthy Fitness Zone or Needs Improvement (see table 10.3).

An important consideration in any of the sit-and-reach tests is foot position. The ankle position for the sit-and-reach tests makes a difference, with higher flexibility scores for the plantar-flexed position (59, 66). Limohn's

229

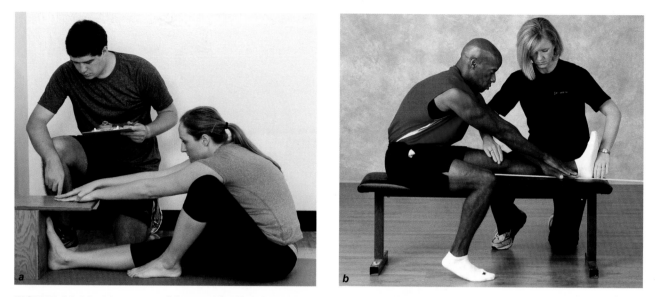

FIGURE 10.16 Variations of the modified back-saver sit-and-reach test: *(a)* one leg bent while reaching forward and *(b)* using meter stick and bench.

Table 10.3 FitnessGram Classifications by Age for Back-Saver Sit-and-Reach (in Inches)*

Age (yr)	Boys	Girls
5	8	9
6	8	9
7	8	9
8	8	9
9	8	9
10	8	9
11	8	10
12	8	10
13	8	10
14	8	10
15	8	12
16	8	12
17	8	12

*Values listed represent the Healthy Fitness Zone (sufficient fitness if at that level or above).

Adapted from Cooper Institute for Aerobics Research (2017).

research (59) suggests that factors such as tightness in the connective-tissue structures located behind the knee and tension on the sciatic nerve can affect performance on the sit-and-reach. More recently, Hui and Yuen (45) reported on a test that also permits plantar flexion of the foot of the tested leg and does not require a sit-and-reach box.

Assessment of Core Stability

The assessment of core stability is important because poor core stability and strength can affect balance and posture and increase the risk for LBP. Because the deep local system of abdominal muscles, the transversus abdominis and multifidus, consists of spine stabilizers, the fitness professional needs to be adept at teaching how to use these muscles and recognizing when they are engaged. The most commonly used technique is the hollowing maneuver or drawing in, which is taught at the beginning of the core exercise program. This is simply drawing in the abdomen or belly button toward the spine. During the drawing-in motion, the transversus abdominis contracts bilaterally to form a musculofascial band that appears to tighten like a corset (41). The transversus abdominis increases the stiffness of the lumbar intervertebral joints (42) and significantly decreases the laxity of the sacroiliac joint (72). The ability to contract the multifidus is related to the ability to contract the transversus abdominis (40). It has been shown that an inward movement (drawing in or hollowing) of the lower abdominal wall when the client is in a supine position produces the most independent activity of the transversus abdominis compared with the other abdominal musculature, and it may be an ideal position to teach transversus abdominis recruitment (80).

The internal oblique and transversus abdominis also can be activated with minimal activity from the rectus abdominis and external oblique in other exercise positions, such as hook lying, bridging, prone lying, four-point kneeling, and wall-support standing with a squat (20, 21, 22). The drawing in or hollowing is effective in engaging the transversus abdominis and multifidus and can be performed in a variety of positions. This exercise should be included even as the program progresses to more advanced levels such as doing exercises on unstable surfaces.

When the drawing-in motion is done correctly, the abdominal region has a scooped or flat appearance. If the client is bracing and recruiting the most superficial muscle, the rectus abdominis, the abdominal region will have a tentlike appearance rather than a scooped-out appearance. The rectus abdominis needs to be recruited for certain core exercises, but with proper involvement of the transversus abdominis and multifidus, the abdominal muscles will not tent.

If clients can recruit the deep abdominal muscles with a drawing-in motion, the fitness professional can use the Sahrmann assessment (see procedures on page 232) and core exercise progression to assess whether clients are strong enough to perform higher-level core exercises (2, 30). It is simple to perform and provides important information about the client's core stability. As the client learns to recruit the transversus abdominis, it is important to pay attention to breathing patterns during these stability exercises. The diaphragm, breathing, and transversus abdominis interact in the control of postural stability (42, 43, 56). It is usually ideal to exhale on the leg lift portion of the exercise.

 VIDEO Watch video 10.4, which demonstrates the Sahrmann assessment.

Once the client can maintain a stable pelvic girdle during the one-leg lift and lower, the next level can be attempted. This second level may be the most revealing of core weakness.

Once clients can control the movement of the spine and pelvic girdle when lifting one leg and then the other, they can challenge themselves by lifting the upper body, extending the arms or legs, holding a weighted ball, or placing the body on a moving object (e.g., a ball or roller), with confidence that the spine will be protected. If the spine and pelvic girdle move out of a neutral spine or imprint position during any of these core exercises, clients should stop the exercise and rest until they are able to control the motion again. They can learn to obtain this neutral spine control in an upright posture for weightlifting and other exercises to provide ideal support to the spine.

Three other exercises that are performed easily in a fitness setting can be used as tests for core stability (78). Figure 10.17 illustrates these tests: the single-leg stance, marching on a ball and holding for 20 seconds, and side plank on the knees. A negative (i.e., no problem) response is the maintenance of a neutral spine without upper- or lower-extremity compensations for the standing and march tests. In the side plank, the quadratus

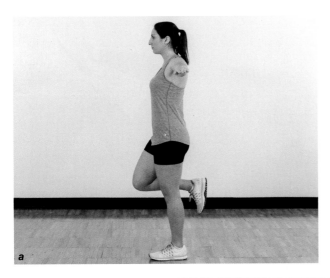

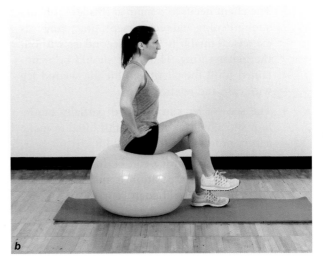

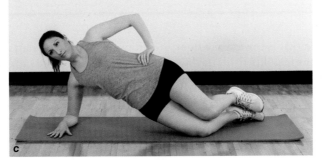

FIGURE 10.17 Supplemental tests for core stability include the *(a)* single-leg stance, *(b)* marching on the ball (hold for 20 seconds and watch for maintenance of neutral spine) (78), and *(c)* side plank (lift the hips off the floor to test for same-side quadratus lumborum strength) (37).

Procedures for Level 1 Sahrmann Assessment

1. The client begins in the supine position with both legs bent and feet on the floor. The spine should be in a neutral position with a normal lordosis. This is the base position from which to progress to all other levels.

2. If the client has difficulty controlling the pelvic girdle and tends to go into an anterior tilt during the first couple exercises, a slight posterior tilt will help protect the spine. This pelvic tilt creates slight flexion of the lumbar spine, with the spine gently pressing into the mat or floor surface. This position is sometimes called *imprint*.

3. A cue is provided to draw in the navel toward the spine in order to activate the deep abdominal musculature.

4. While the navel is maintained in an inward position, the client slowly lifts one foot off the surface without moving the spine.

5. If the deep core musculature cannot control the force of the leg's motion on the spine, the pelvis will shift anteriorly and possibly laterally. The goal of this exercise is to lift and lower one leg and have no motion in the spine.

6. The exercise progresses by lifting and lowering one leg and then the other.

Procedures for Level 2 Sahrmann Assessment

1. The client performs the first level while in an imprint position, holds the first leg in the air, and slowly lifts the second leg off the ground.

2. If the deep core musculature is not able to stabilize the spine, the pelvis will tilt as the psoas contracts to lift the second leg.

3. The client needs to remain at this level of core strengthening and recruitment, practicing this exercise if unable to lift the second leg without the pelvis tilting. This level should be maintained until the client can lift the second leg with ease and control.

4. The second leg can be lifted partially or the foot slid along the ground until lifted to make a safer progression to the full lift.

5. When the second leg can be lifted while the spine and pelvic position is maintained, the upper body can be lifted in a curl or the legs can progress to an alternating toe touch on the floor.

6. This exercise also can be performed on a foam roller for a greater challenge as shown in figure 10.18.

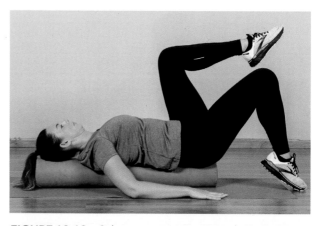

FIGURE 10.18 Sahrmann assessment and core exercise program variation on the foam roller for an additional challenge.

lumborum is tested on the side that is toward the floor. A positive test for weakness is the inability to lift the hips (37). These tests also can be used as strengthening tools.

Assessing Neuromotor Fitness

Several tests can be used to assess aspects of neuromotor fitness with minimal or no equipment. The 4-stage balance test can be used to assess static balance and proprioception. The standing reach test assesses balance and postural control, and the 8-foot up and go test for older adults is used to assess agility and dynamic balance in older adults.

The 4-Stage Balance Test and Unipedal Stance Test

The 4-stage balance test includes a series of standing positions that increase in difficulty (17). The client should be positioned near a wall or fixed object for support in case they lose balance; the tester also should position themselves to help as needed. The client should complete the assessment without shoes; arms can be used to assist with maintaining the position. The client stands with their feet side by side in the first stage and holds this position for as long as possible without assistance or support (figure 10.19a). The tester stops the test if the client cannot maintain the position for at least 10 seconds. If the client maintains balance for at least 10 seconds, they move to stage 2. In the second stage the client will move one foot forward so the instep of the foot is at the big toe of the other foot (figure 10.19b). As with the first stage, the test is terminated if the client cannot maintain the stance for 10 seconds, and the client moves to the next stage if the position is maintained for at least 10 seconds. In stage 3, the forward foot is moved

to the tandem position in which the heel is touching the toes of the other foot (figure 10.19c). If the position is maintained for at least 10 seconds, the client lifts one foot off the floor and maintains that position as long as they are able to do so without moving the feet or requiring support (figure 10.19d). Individuals who cannot maintain the tandem stance for at least 10 seconds are at increased risk for fall and should perform exercises to improve balance.

A related test to consider if the client progressed through the 4-stage balance test is the unipedal stance test. This test is done with arms crossed over the chest, standing on one foot while barefoot and raising the other foot so it is near the ankle of the self-selected stance foot (77). The test is done with eyes open (have client focus on a spot on a facing wall) and eyes closed, repeating

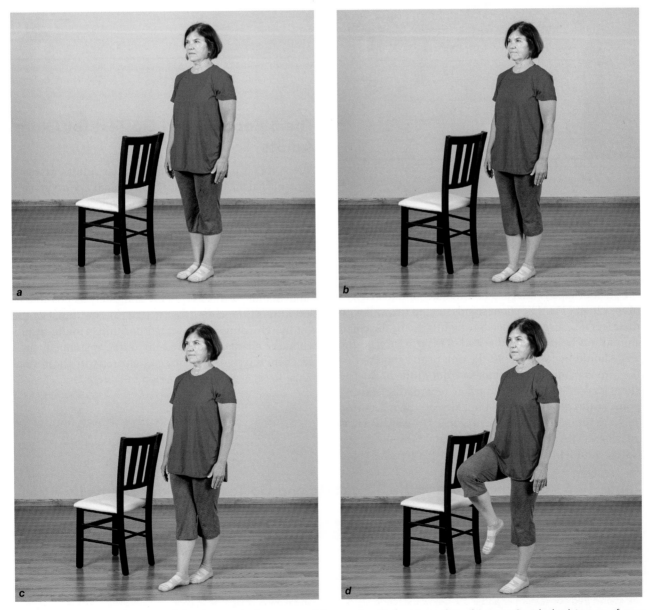

FIGURE 10.19 Each stage of the 4-stage balance test: (a) stage 1 with feet together, (b) stage 2 with the big toe of one foot touching the instep of the other foot, (c) stage 3 with feet tandem, heel to toe, and (d) stage 4 balancing on one foot.

three times for each condition. Record the time for each attempt (to a 45-second maximum) while the client maintains the required position without uncrossing the arms, moving the raised or stance foot, or opening the eyes during the eyes-closed attempts. The tester should position themselves to help as needed. Take the highest (best) score from the eyes-open and eyes-closed trials. These can be compared to data by Springer and colleagues (77), representing the time achieved for a healthy group of volunteers associated with a military medical center. A table adapted from Springer and colleagues (77) is provided for different age groups (table 10.4) (13).

Table 10.4 Unipedal Stance Test Normative Values in Seconds, Best of Three Trials

Age (yr)	Eyes open (best of three trials, time in seconds)	Eyes closed (best of three trials, time in seconds)
18-39	45	15
40-49	42	13
50-59	41	8
60-69	32	4
70-79	22	3
80-99	9	2

Reprinted by permission from B.A. Bushman and A. Robinett, "Neuromotor Exercise Training: Background and Benefits," *ACSM's Health & Fitness Journal* 26, no. 4 (2022): 7.

The Standing Reach Test

The standing reach test should not be performed if the client cannot stand independently for at least 30 seconds without support. The assessment requires that a measuring stick or tape is attached to a wall at shoulder height of the client (27). The client stands next to the wall with their feet next to each other and slightly apart; the client should not be touching the wall. The arm next to the wall should be raised to 90° flexion of the shoulder so the arm is parallel to the floor in front of the body. The client makes a fist, and the tester records the starting point at the position of the knuckles on the measuring stick (figure 10.20a). The client reaches forward as far as possible while maintaining balance and without taking a step or touching the wall (figure 10.20b). The tester

should position themselves to help as needed. The tester records the position of the knuckles on the measuring stick in the extended position and subtracts the starting point to determine the difference. Three successful trials should be completed. Measures can be made in inches or in centimeters and converted to inches to compare to data by Duncan and colleagues (27). A table adapted from Duncan and colleagues is provided for different age groups for the mean of three successful trials (table 10.5) (13).

Table 10.5 Standing Reach Test Averages for Different Age Ranges in Inches, Mean of Three Successful Trials

Age (yr)	Males	Females
20-40	16.7	14.6
41-69	15.0	13.8
70-87	13.2	10.2

Reprinted by permission from B.A. Bushman and A. Robinett, "Neuromotor Exercise Training: Background and Benefits," *ACSM's Health & Fitness Journal* 26, no. 4 (2022): 8.

The 8-Foot Up and Go Test for Older Adults

The 8-foot up and go test for older adults assesses dynamic balance and agility (73). A chair approximately 43 centimeters (17 inches) high is placed against the wall, and a cone is placed 8 feet in front of the chair. The fitness professional uses a stopwatch to time the test. The client begins the test seated in the chair with their hands on their knees and feet flat on the floor (figure 10.21a). The tester gives the "go" command to begin the test. The client stands, walks as quickly and safely as possible to and around the cone (figure 10.21b), and finishes the test by returning to the seated position. Timing begins when the client stands, and the watch is stopped when the client is seated. The time is compared with the normal range for age and sex presented in table 10.6.

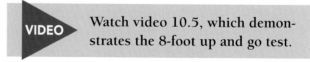

VIDEO ▶ Watch video 10.5, which demonstrates the 8-foot up and go test.

Table 10.6 Classifications for the 8-Foot Up and Go Test for Older Adults by Age in Seconds*

	AGE 60-64	AGE 65-69	AGE 70-74	AGE 75-79	AGE 80-84	AGE 85-89	AGE 90-94
Males	3.8 to 5.6	4.3 to 5.9	4.4 to 6.2	4.6 to 7.2	5.2 to 7.6	5.5 to 8.9	6.2 to 10.0
Females	4.4 to 6.0	4.8 to 6.4	4.9 to 7.1	5.2 to 7.4	5.7 to 8.7	6.2 to 9.6	7.3 to 11.5

*Normal range of scores reflects the middle 50% for each age group (between 25th and 75th percentiles). Scores above the range listed are considered above normal, and those below the range are considered below normal. Age in years.

Adapted from Rikli and Jones (2013).

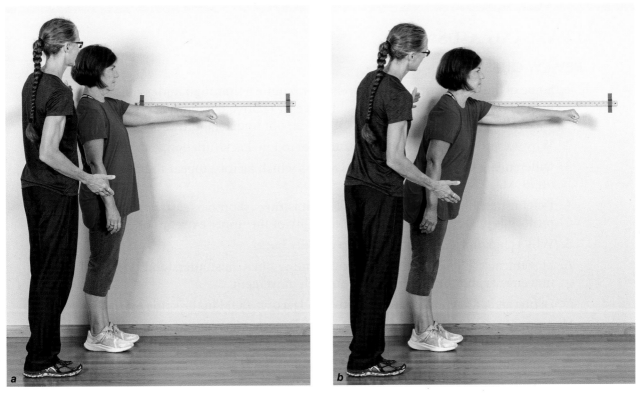

FIGURE 10.20 The beginning point *(a)* and the end measurement point *(b)* of the standing reach test.

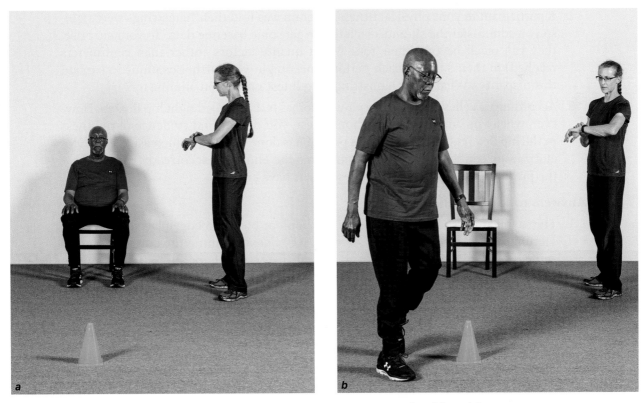

FIGURE 10.21 The start *(a)* and midpoint *(b)* of the 8-foot up and go test for older adults.

LEARNING AIDS

REVIEW QUESTIONS

1. Some of the tests presented in this chapter require a thorough understanding of the nuances of human movement capability (e.g., relative flexibility). Why could it be a mistake to administer these tests if you do not understand these nuances?

2. Why are sitting postures often detrimental to low-back function and flexibility?

3. Differentiate between RA and OA. Discuss which factors appear to have an impact on ROM.

4. Demonstrate flexibility tests for the ITB, hamstrings, iliopsoas, gastrocnemius, soleus, piriformis, quadriceps, and general mobility of the upper extremities.

5. Why is hip mobility important for a healthy back?

6. Movement capability in the lumbar spine is often misunderstood. Describe the movements and the factors that limit each movement.

7. Define and differentiate between active and passive ROM in the spine extension test.

8. A prime reason for using the sit-and-reach test is that it is easy to administer. Discuss the limitations of this test. What are some modifications that can improve the test?

9. What are some simple assessments for neuromotor fitness, and what aspects are examined with each?

CASE STUDIES

1. A participant in your physical fitness program was told their hamstrings were tight, so you administer the sit-and-reach test to get some baseline data. To your surprise, they can reach beyond their toes. What quality factors (other than centimeters reached) in their sit-and-reach performance might you further examine to explain this disparity? What other hamstring length test might you administer?

2. According to a client's record, previous Thomas tests revealed tight hip flexors. However, when you administer the Thomas test, you do not find evidence of tightness in the hip flexors. Assume that this person has done nothing to increase their ROM, and you are confident that you administered the Thomas test correctly. Explain how the previous administrator of the test might have erred.

Answers to Case Studies

1. The sacral angle should be at least 80° (a book or board on edge placed against the sacrum would be snug if the angle were 90°). Next examine the curvature of the spine; it should be smooth with no evident flatness or hypermobility in any one particular area. Discrepancy in arm–leg length might also be a factor (e.g., long arms in relation to legs). You might administer the AKE test to assess hamstring flexibility.

2. Most false positives in the Thomas test result when the client brings the thigh too close to the chest. This can result in excessive posterior rotation of the pelvis, which can make it appear that the hip flexors are tight.

11

Body Composition Assessments

Barbara A. Bushman

OBJECTIVES

The reader will be able to do the following:

1. Discuss how body composition affects health and describe the health implications of various patterns of body-fat distribution
2. Calculate and interpret body mass index
3. Identify common measurement sites for skinfolds and girths
4. Compare and contrast skinfold measurement, hydrostatic weighing, air displacement plethysmography, and bioelectrical impedance analysis as means for estimating body composition
5. Assess body composition using a variety of techniques and describe the advantages and disadvantages of these techniques
6. Calculate target body weight

11

Media are filled with advertisements for programs designed to help people improve their health and fitness. Often the primary focus of these programs is weight loss. A healthy body weight and an appropriate amount of body fat are important aspects of physical fitness. Fitness professionals need to understand the importance of appropriate body composition, become aware of the various means for assessing body fat, and become proficient at estimating body fat through skinfold and girth measurements. As with other aspects of fitness assessment, paying attention to details and gaining experience with the techniques are necessary to become proficient at estimating body fatness. This chapter is meant to assist fitness professionals in acquiring these skills.

Health and Body Composition

Body composition describes the component tissues of the body and is most often used to refer to the relative percentages of fat and fat-free tissues. Fat-free mass (FFM), fat mass (FM), and percent body fat (%BF) are the most frequently reported values in a body composition assessment. *Percent body fat* refers to the percentage of the total body mass that is composed of fat:

$$\%BF = (\text{fat mass} \div \text{body mass}) \times 100$$

Fat-free mass refers to the mass of the fat-free tissues of the body and often is used synonymously with the term *lean body mass*. Body composition is one health-related physical fitness component; consider the ill effects related to excessively low or high body fatness. Various indirect methods are used to estimate body composition, and fitness professionals should understand which one is most appropriate in a given situation and be skilled in the use of such methods. Techniques include calculations reflecting height and weight (body mass index; BMI), measurements of circumference, and estimations of %BF.

Obesity is a condition in which a person has excess adipose tissue, or fat tissue. Based on BMI, obesity is often defined as a value 30 kg · m⁻² or above (7). Although BMI is commonly used, the calculated value only takes into account height and weight and thus should be considered a rough guide because it does not reflect the same degree of fatness in different individuals (27). When looking at BMI for children, absolute BMI is not used, but rather age is considered in addition to height and weight given natural growth and development (11). No universally accepted norms for %BF exist (2). For adults, table 11.1 presents suggested age-based %BFs, with obesity being considered above the ranges listed (22).

Obesity prevalence for adults in the United States has increased over the past 20 years from 30.5% to 41.9% (8). Childhood obesity is a concern for 19.7% of youth

Table 11.1 Age-Based Body-Fat Percentage Standards for Adults (Years of Age)

Men	Recommended range*
18-34 years	8-22
35-55 years	10-25
56 years or older	10-25
Women	**Recommended range***
18-34 years	20-35
35-55 years	23-38
56 years or older	25-38

*Values are %BF levels considered generally healthy.

Based on Ratamess (2014).

between the ages of 2 to 19 (10). In 2019, the estimated annual medical cost of obesity in the United States was nearly $173 billion (8). Obesity has been causally linked with numerous negative health consequences, including coronary artery disease, hypertension, stroke, type 2 diabetes, increased risk of various cancers, osteoarthritis, sleep apnea, and dyslipidemia (11). Obesity, particularly extreme obesity, is linked with higher all-cause mortality (12).

Beyond the amount of body fat, body-fat distribution appears to affect health. Android-type obesity (i.e., male-pattern obesity, apple shape) refers to the excessive storage of fat in the trunk and abdominal areas. Excessive fat in the hips and thighs is labeled gynoid-type obesity (i.e., female-pattern obesity, pear shape). In terms of negative health consequences, android-type obesity appears to be the most dangerous and is closely linked with disease (11). Waist-to-hip ratio (WHR) can be a useful tool for differentiating gynoid-type and android-type obesity. Waist circumference also is used to classify excessive trunk fat. Descriptions of how to take these measurements are presented later in this chapter.

Just as excessive body fat can be unhealthy, too little body fat also can compromise health. Among the many important roles of fat in human health are providing energy, helping with temperature regulation, and cushioning the joints. The minimum level of body fat needed to maintain health differs among individuals and depends on sex and genetics. The %BF thought to be necessary for good health, also known as *essential fat*, is 8% to 12% for women and 3% to 5% for men (22). Infertility, depression, impaired temperature regulation, and early death are among the outcomes of excessive weight loss. Extreme fat loss results from starvation imposed by internal or external forces. Chapter 20 includes background and warning signs of common eating disorders that every fitness professional should understand.

KEY POINT

The prevalence of obesity in the United States is nearly 42% for adults and 20% for children. Significant health consequences (e.g., heart disease, type 2 diabetes) may result from obesity. Disease risk is linked more closely with android-type obesity (apple shape) than with gynoid-type obesity (pear shape). Too little body fat also can lead to negative health outcomes.

Methods for Assessing Body Composition

Numerous techniques have been used to estimate body composition. None of the methods currently used actually measures %BF; the only way to truly measure the volume of fat in the body would be to dissect and chemically analyze tissues in the body (1). The techniques routinely used to estimate %BF are based on the relationship between %BF and other factors that can be measured accurately, such as skinfold thicknesses or underwater weight. Because of the predictable relationship between the measured value and body composition, %BF can be estimated through these indirect methods. Fitness professionals must always remain aware of the limitations of these indirect methods with the understanding that no "gold standard" with accuracy better than 1% exists (1).

Each technique described in the following sections has advantages and disadvantages. With knowledge of these characteristics, the fitness professional can decide wisely when choosing the method for body composition assessment. A comparison of important considerations can be found in table 11.2. For fitness professionals, ease of measurement, relative accuracy, and cost are the primary considerations when choosing a technique. In other situations (for research or clinical applications), the accuracy of the measurement may outweigh other considerations. A review of techniques endorsed by the American Heart Association (AHA) provides greater detail about assessment of body composition (11).

Body Mass Index

A widely used assessment of the appropriateness of a person's weight is the anthropometric calculation of the body mass index (BMI). This value is calculated by dividing the weight in kilograms by height in meters squared. BMI is a quick and easy method for determining if body weight is appropriate for body height. Table 11.3 lists the general adult BMI categories (7). BMI does not differentiate between fat and fat-free weight, which is problematic when testing athletic individuals with a large lean mass. For example, a football linebacker who is 6 feet 2 inches (1.88 meters) and weighs 220 pounds (100 kilograms) is considered overweight according to BMI standards (BMI = 28.3 kg · m^{-2}), when in fact the athlete may have a very low %BF. On the other hand, an inactive person with a similar height and weight is more likely carrying excess adipose tissue.

Although BMI standards are often applied to adults without regard to age, sex, race, or ethnicity, the relationship between BMI and %BF varies among groups (11). The use of BMI to define obesity, along with the relationship between BMI and health outcomes, is an area of ongoing research. Increased cardiometabolic risk is noted at lower BMI for people from some ethnic backgrounds; thus, in one source, overweight has been defined as BMI of 23 to 27.4 kg · m^{-2} and obesity as 27.5 kg · m^{-2} and above for people with South Asian, Chinese, other Asian, Middle Eastern, Black African, or African-Caribbean family backgrounds (18). For incidence of type 2 diabetes, lower thresholds than a BMI of 30.0 kg · m^{-2} for obesity in White populations have been suggested for South Asian (23.9 kg · m^{-2}), Black (28.1 kg · m^{-2}),

Table 11.2 Comparison of Common Body Composition Techniques

	Equipment cost	Time required	Technician expertise	Day-to-day variation	Accuracy
Skinfold measurement	*	**	**	*	**
Hydrostatic weighing	***	***	**	*	***
BIA	* to **	*	*	**	**
Dual-energy X-ray absorptiometry	***	*	***	*	***
Air displacement plethysmography	***	*	*	*	***

* = low; ** = moderate; *** = high.

Note: Comparisons assume client preparation and procedures are fully followed.

Table 11.3 Body Mass Index Classification

Classification	BMI (kg · m⁻²)
Underweight	<18.5
Healthy weight	18.5-24.9
Overweight	25.0-29.9
Obesity	30 and above

Based on CDC (2022).

Chinese (26.9 kg · m⁻²), and Arab (26.6 kg · m⁻²) populations (4). Potential implications of equivalent risk at lower BMI related to prevention and early diagnosis should be considered (4). Even with these limitations in the applicability of BMI, for most adults there is a clear correlation between elevated BMI and negative health consequences (11). In screening situations where estimating body fat is impossible or impractical, BMI can be useful for providing feedback to people about their body weight.

BMI standards for children are age and sex specific (11). BMI percentiles adjusted for age are available for boys and girls, with BMI between the 5th and <85th percentile classified as healthy, between 85th and <95th percentile as overweight, and at or above 95th percentile as obese (11). As with adults, caution should be used in interpretation. BMI-for-age level does not always reflect body fat; children at the BMI-for-age noted for obesity will not necessarily have excess body fat, and those below the obesity classification may have excess body fat (20). Differences in %BF at a given BMI also appear to differ among racial and ethnic groups. For example, at a given BMI, non-Hispanic Black children have a lower %BF than non-Hispanic White or Mexican-American children (20). Thus, rather than viewing BMI-for-age designations as diagnostic, they should be considered part of the assessment of healthy weight that also includes clinical assessment and other considerations related to healthy development (20). Growth charts showing the BMI-for-age percentiles (6) and calculators (9) can be found online.

Girth Measurements

Several girth measurements (body and limb circumferences) are used to either estimate body composition or describe body proportions. Girth measurements provide quick and reliable information. They are sometimes used in equations to predict body composition and also may be used to track changes in body shape and size during weight loss. The major disadvantage is that they provide little information about the fat and fat-free components of the body. For example, a bodybuilder's thigh can have a larger circumference yet less fat than that of a person who is obese. A list of several commonly measured girths follows; refer to ACSM's Guidelines for Exercise Testing and Prescription (2) for additional circumference sites.

- *Waist:* Narrowest part of the torso between the xiphoid process and the umbilicus (note that this is one of several definitions of "waist"; ensure the measurement site selected matches the normative comparisons and that the method is consistently employed [23])
- *Abdomen:* Circumference of the torso at the height of the iliac crest
- *Hips:* Maximal circumference of the buttocks above the gluteal fold
- *Thigh:* Largest circumference of the thigh below the gluteal fold

Waist circumference (WC) can provide valuable information about disease risk (2, 11). WC is a simple tool that reflects body fat distribution (11), and high WC may reveal higher cardiovascular disease risk even in individuals of normal body weight given the relationship between WC and abdominal body fat (21). Many definitions for WC have been documented, including the definition presented previously (which is typically used with the WHR) as well as others, including halfway between the lowest rib and iliac crest, immediately above the iliac crest, at the level of the umbilicus, and 1 centimeter or 1 inch above the umbilicus. When tracking WC over time, it is important to be consistent in the definition applied. The location of the measurement affects the values at which health risk is elevated (11). A WC of greater than 102 centimeters (40 inches) in men or 88 centimeters (35 inches) in women, measured at the midpoint between the lowest rib and iliac crest (11), is included in the list of risk factors for cardiovascular disease by the American College of Sports Medicine (ACSM) (2). ACSM also provides risk criteria when WC is measured at the level of the iliac crest: high risk begins at 90 centimeters (35.5 inches) in women and 100 centimeters (39.5 inches in men) (2).

WHR is a frequently used clinical application of girth measurements. This value is often used to reflect the degree of abdominal, or android-type, obesity. For individuals younger than 60 years of age, a WHR greater than 0.95 for men or 0.86 for women is associated with elevated health risks (2). For men and women 60 to 69 years of age, a WHR of >1.03 and >0.9, respectively, is linked with disease risk (2). Findings have been mixed on the use of ratios, such as WHR, for predicting disease risk, although ratios may be helpful in providing a uniform comparison among populations, a limitation for BMI given differences in values related to disease risk for different ethnic groups (11).

When assessing girths, use the following procedures to standardize the measurements:

- Make sure the measuring tape is horizontal when measuring trunk circumference and is perpendicular to the long axis of the limb when measuring limbs. Use either a mirror or an assistant to help ensure that the tape is placed properly.
- Apply constant pressure to the tape without pinching the skin. Use a tape measure fitted with a handle that indicates the amount of tension exerted.
- When measuring limbs, measure on the right side of the body. Alternatively, measure on both sides and record the values for both right and left.
- Ensure that the person stands erect, relaxed, and with feet together.
- When measuring girths of the trunk, take the measurement after the person exhales and before the next breath begins.

Skinfold Measurements

Measuring skinfold thickness is one of the most frequently performed tests to estimate %BF. This quick, noninvasive, inexpensive method can provide a fairly accurate assessment of %BF. The value obtained by skinfold measurement is typically within 3.5% of the value measured with underwater weighing (22). Skinfold measurement is based on the assumption that, as a person gains adipose tissue, the increase in skinfold thickness is proportional to the additional fat weight in the body.

Because of the widespread use of skinfold measurement, fitness professionals should master the skills involved. Accurately assessing skinfold thickness requires the correct performance of several steps: locating the skinfold site, pinching the skinfold away from the underlying tissue, measuring with the caliper, and choosing the proper equation. The following sections address these aspects.

Watch videos 11.1 through 11.7, which demonstrate skinfold measurements.

Locating the Skinfold Site

Accurate determination of the sites of the skinfold measurement is critical. To increase the accuracy of the measurement, the site should be located and then marked with a washable marker. The mark should include one line that will be aligned with the fold (e.g., will be vertically oriented for a vertical fold) and the other perpendicular to this line to guide where the caliper will be placed on the fold (see figure 11.1). This helps ensure that the calipers are placed in the correct position each time the skinfold is measured. All skinfold measurements should be taken on the right side of the body unless otherwise specified. Refer to table 11.4 and figure 11.2 for some of

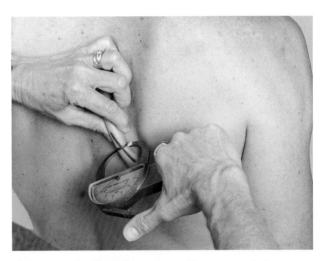

FIGURE 11.1 Skinfold marking of location and placement of caliper.

Table 11.4 Commonly Used Skinfold Sites

Skinfold site	Description
Abdomen	Measure the vertical fold 2 centimeters to the right of and level with the umbilicus. Make sure the head of the caliper is not in the umbilicus.
Chest	Measure a diagonal fold along the natural line of the skin one-half (men) or one-third (women) the distance between the anterior axillary line and the nipple.
Midaxillary	Measure the vertical fold at the level of the xiphoid process on the midaxillary line.
Subscapular	Measure 2 centimeters below the inferior angle of the scapula along the diagonal fold at a 45° angle.
Suprailiac	Measure the diagonal fold in line with the natural angle of the iliac crest. Measure along the anterior axillary line just above the iliac crest.
Thigh	Measure the vertical fold over the quadriceps muscle on the midline of the thigh. Measure half the distance between the top of the patella and the inguinal crease. The leg should be relaxed.
Triceps	Measure the vertical fold over the belly of the triceps muscle. The arm should be relaxed. The specific site is the posterior midline of the upper arm, half the distance between the acromion and olecranon processes.

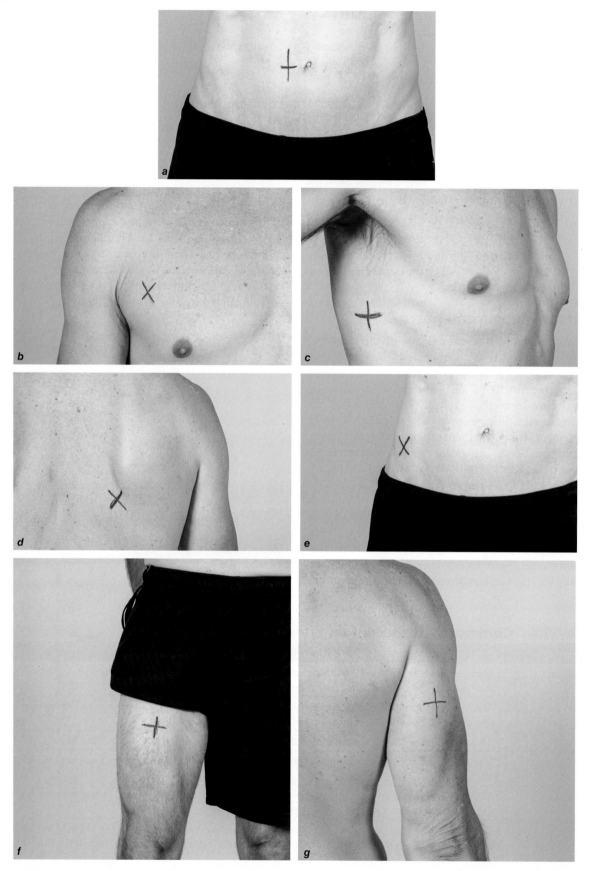

FIGURE 11.2 Common skinfold testing sites include the *(a)* abdomen, *(b)* chest, *(c)* midaxillary, *(d)* subscapular, *(e)* suprailiac, *(f)* thigh, and *(g)* triceps.

the most commonly used measurement sites. For a more complete description of determining skinfold sites, other resources are available (2, 3). Measuring skinfolds immediately after exercise should be avoided because exercise can shift fluid volume, leading to inaccurate results.

Pinching the Skinfold

Once the correct location for the skinfold measurement is determined, the tester gently but firmly pinches and lifts the skinfold away from the underlying muscle in order to measure it. The skinfold should include two layers of skin and the associated subcutaneous fat. The following are guidelines for measuring skinfolds correctly:

1. Place the fingers perpendicular to the skinfold approximately 1 centimeter from the site to be measured.

2. Gently yet firmly pinch the skinfold between the thumb and the first two fingers and lift away from the underlying tissues. Place the jaws of the caliper perpendicular to the skinfold at the measurement site, guided by the mark made on the skin. The jaws of the caliper should be halfway between the bottom and top of the fold. Maintain the pinch while taking the measurement.

3. Read the measurement on the caliper 1 to 2 seconds after the jaws contact the skin.

4. Wait at least 15 seconds before taking a subsequent measurement. To allow time for the fold to return to normal, take one measurement at each site and then repeat measurements. If the second measurement varies by more than 2 millimeters, repeat the measurement. A mean of two values within 2 millimeters of one another will be used in calculations.

Measuring the skinfolds of people who are obese is not recommended given larger prediction errors as well as difficulties in measurement (e.g., jaws of the caliper will not open wide enough to measure the skinfold, difficulty in palpating bone landmarks to determine site location) (14). Instead, use an alternative method for assessing body composition. Girth measurements (e.g., WC, WHR), along with BMI, may be better options for assessing status and tracking progress in these cases.

Measuring With the Caliper

Skinfold thickness is measured with a skinfold caliper. The numerous commercially available calipers vary in price and, potentially, accuracy. Key characteristics to look for when selecting a caliper include consistency in tension that allows for constant pressure over the range of measurement, a clear and precise scale, a sufficiently wide range of measurement, and durability (5). Check calibration with a vernier caliper (high-precision

instrument for linear measures) or calibration blocks; if the value from the skinfold caliper does not match the value set on the vernier caliper, follow the manufacturer's instructions or, if possible, return to the manufacturer for recalibration (14). If the calipers do not measure skinfolds accurately, they will compromise the estimate of body fat.

Choosing the Proper Equation

The use of skinfold measures to estimate %BF is based on the principle that the amount of fat under the skin (subcutaneous fat) is proportional to the total amount of fat in the body (22). Regression equations that take into account specific skinfold measures, sex, and age have been developed to predict body density, which in turn is used to estimate %BF (22). There are general prediction equations to estimate %BF from body density, as well as other equations specific for various ethnic populations, types of athletes, and some patient populations (2). An advantage of general equations is that they can be used to estimate body composition in most people; however, the equations lose accuracy when testing individuals who are dissimilar to those used to develop the equations. These equations are also less accurate for people at either end of the fatness continuum. The advantage of using population-specific equations is that they tend to have higher accuracy when testing people who fit the physical profile of those in the subgroup of interest.

Because sex influences the areas where fat is stored, separate skinfold equations for men (15, 16) and women (16, 17) have been developed. Note that the client's age is used in these equations. This is because the relationship between total body fat and subcutaneous fat changes with age; as a person ages, proportionally less fat is stored subcutaneously. Equations that require three or seven skinfold sites are listed in the sidebar *Equations for Estimating Body Density From Skinfold Thicknesses* (15, 16, 17). These equations allow for calculation of body density, which then must be converted to %BF.

KEY POINT

Skinfold measurements are a quick and relatively accurate method for estimating %BF; however, care must be taken in making these measurements if the values are to be reliable. Girth measurements, including WC, can be useful in assessing risk of visceral or central obesity-related disease, and BMI can be considered for classifying people into overweight and obese categories. The general recommended BMI range is 18.5 to 24.9 kg · m^{-2}.

Equations for Estimating Body Density From Skinfold Thicknesses

Women: Three sites (triceps, suprailiac, and thigh)

$$D_b = 1.0994921 - (0.0009929 \times \text{sum of skinfolds}) \\ + (0.0000023 \times \text{sum of skinfolds}^2) - (0.0001392 \times \text{age in years})$$

Women: Three sites (triceps, suprailiac, and abdominal)

$$D_b = 1.089733 - (0.0009245 \times \text{sum of skinfolds}) \\ + (0.0000025 \times \text{sum of skinfolds}^2) - (0.0000979 \times \text{age in years})$$

Women: Seven sites (triceps, abdominal, suprailiac, thigh, chest, subscapular, and midaxillary)

$$D_b = 1.097 - (0.00046971 \times \text{sum of skinfolds}) \\ + (0.00000056 \times \text{sum of skinfolds}^2) - (0.00012828 \times \text{age in years})$$

Men: Three sites (chest, abdominal, thigh)

$$D_b = 1.10938 - (0.0008267 \times \text{sum of skinfolds}) \\ + (0.0000016 \times \text{sum of skinfolds}^2) - (0.0002574 \times \text{age in years})$$

Men: Three sites (chest, triceps, subscapular)

$$D_b = 1.1125025 - (0.0013125 \times \text{sum of skinfolds}) \\ + (0.0000055 \times \text{sum of skinfolds}^2) - (0.000244 \times \text{age in years})$$

Men: Seven sites (triceps, abdominal, suprailiac, thigh, chest, subscapular, and midaxillary)

$$D_b = 1.112 - (0.00043499 \times \text{sum of skinfolds}) \\ + (0.00000055 \times \text{sum of skinfolds}^2) - (0.00028826 \times \text{age in years})$$

From Jackson and Pollock (1978); Jackson and Pollock (1985); Jackson, Pollock, and Ward (1980).

Densitometry

The density of an object is defined as the ratio of its weight to its volume (density = weight ÷ volume). Two common procedures that estimate body composition based on densitometry are hydrostatic weighing and air displacement plethysmography. The foundation of these techniques is that different types of tissues in the body have different and consistent densities. For example, fat tissue has a density far less than either muscle or bone. Each of these techniques results in the assessment of total body volume and subsequently the calculation of body density.

Once the body density is calculated, it must be converted into %BF. To make this conversion, a two-compartment model is used. In a two-compartment model, all body tissues are classified as either fat or fat free. One of the commonly used equations for this procedure is the Siri equation (24): %BF = (495 ÷ D_b) – 450. In this model, the fat-free portion of the body is composed of all tissues except lipids and is assumed to have a density of $1.1 \text{ kg} \cdot \text{L}^{-1}$. Fat is assumed to have a density of $0.9 \text{ kg} \cdot \text{L}^{-1}$.

Fat density is fairly consistent among individuals; however, in some situations the density of the fat-free body is different from the assumed $1.1 \text{ kg} \cdot \text{L}^{-1}$. If a person's bone density is different from the standard used by Siri, the assumption that the fat-free body density equals $1.1 \text{ kg} \cdot \text{L}^{-1}$ becomes invalid. For example, non-Hispanic Black adults have a higher bone mineral density than Hispanic, non-Hispanic White, and Asian adults (19). Many population-specific equations are available to convert body density into %BF (14). When selecting one of these equations, consider characteristics of the population on which the calculation is based (e.g., age, race, ethnicity, physical activity level), verify the equation has been validated, ensure the accuracy (i.e., standard error of the estimate [SEE] should be between 2.5% and 3.5%), and take care that measurements are done in the same manner as the original study (22). For equations and information on converting body density into %BF for various populations, see *ACSM's Guidelines for Exercise Testing and Prescription* (2). Researchers sometimes use techniques more advanced than two-compartment models. Although these techniques are currently impractical for non-research settings, they are briefly described in the sidebar *Advanced Methods in Body Composition Assessment* at the end of the chapter.

CASE STUDY

Body Composition Assessment Applied

Case Study Contributor: Barbara A. Bushman

Body composition measures have been taken for Tamera, a 33-year-old female who is interested in progressing in her fitness program. She has been active her whole life, engaging in regular aerobic exercise and resistance training. She would like to develop a more focused exercise program and thus has scheduled sessions with a fitness professional. Body composition analysis was conducted as part of baseline assessments. The following measures were taken:

Height: 1.78 meters

Weight: 70.0 kilograms

Waist circumference: 85 centimeters

Skinfold measures:

Site	Measurement #1	Measurement #2	Mean
Triceps	16 mm	14 mm	15 mm
Suprailiac	16 mm	16 mm	16 mm
Thigh	17 mm	19 mm	18 mm

With this data, BMI can be calculated as follows:

$$\text{BMI} = \text{weight in kilograms} \div (\text{height in meters})^2$$
$$\text{BMI} = 70 \div (1.78)^2$$
$$\text{BMI} = 70 \div 3.17$$
$$\text{BMI} = 22.1$$

Tamera's BMI of $22.1 \text{ kg} \cdot \text{m}^{-2}$ is within the healthy weight range for adults. Based on risk-factor levels for cardiovascular disease by the ACSM, her waist circumference is not considered to be a risk factor. Her %BF will be calculated as follows:

1. Measurements were taken at three sites and repeated. The repeated measures are within the required 2 millimeters of one another.

2. The mean of each measurement site is then added together to provide the sum of skinfolds (15 + 16 + 18 = 49).

3. Using the equation for women that has been developed for these three measurement sites (triceps, suprailiac, and thigh), the calculations are as follows for body density (recall her age is 33 years):

$$D_b = 1.0994921 - (0.0009929 \times \text{sum of skinfolds})$$
$$+ (0.0000023 \times \text{sum of skinfolds}^2) - (0.0001392 \times \text{age in years})$$
$$D_b = 1.0994921 - (0.0009929 \times 49) + (0.0000023 \times 49^2)$$
$$- (0.0001392 \times 33)$$
$$D_b = 1.0517687$$

4. Using the general equation for conversion of body density to %BF, the calculations are as follows:

$$\text{%BF} = (495 \div D_b) - 450$$
$$\text{%BF} = (495 \div 1.0517687) - 450$$
$$\text{%BF} = 20.6$$

(continued)

Case Study *(continued)*

Tamera's %BF of 20.6 is within the suggested range for %BF. The fitness professional explains these results to Tamera as follows:

Tamera, the measures that were taken to assess body composition are very encouraging and reflect your consistent hard work with your exercise program. Body mass index, often referred to as BMI, is a calculated value reflecting body weight in relation to height. Your BMI of 22.1 is within the range considered a healthy weight. Since weight carried in the central part of the body around the abdomen is a concern related to health risk, we also measured your waist circumference. This measurement indicates that excessive storage of fat in your trunk or abdomen is not a concern. The final series of measurements, the skinfold pinches, allowed for an assessment of subcutaneous fat, or the fat just under the skin. Subcutaneous fat reflects total body fat. After I completed some calculations that factor in those measures, along with your age, your estimated percent body fat is about 21%. This is an estimate, so we won't get overly focused on the specific number, other than to note that this is within a good range. Thus, your body composition as reflected with BMI, waist circumference, and percent body fat are all within healthy ranges.

Hydrostatic Weighing

Hydrostatic (underwater) weighing is a common means for estimating body composition in research settings and has been used as the criterion method for assessing %BF, although it has been suggested that currently no one universal gold standard exists (1). A criterion method provides the standard against which other methodologies are compared. In hydrostatic weighing, the participant is submerged in a tank of warm water and then exhales fully while technicians record the body mass (figure 11.3). The body mass while submerged and the body mass on land are used to calculate %BF.

Hydrostatic weighing is based on Archimedes' principle, which states that a submerged object is buoyed up by a force equal to the volume of water it displaces. This buoyant force causes the object to weigh less underwater than it does on land. The difference between land mass and underwater mass is used to calculate the volume of the object. Because the density of an object is calculated by dividing mass by volume, body density (D_b) can be calculated using the following formula.

$$D_b = \frac{M}{\frac{(M - M_{UW})}{D_{H_2O}} - RV - GV}$$

In addition to body mass (M) and mass underwater (M_{UW}), the density of the water (D_{H2O}) in the hydrostatic tank, the residual lung volume (RV), and the gastrointestinal air volume (GV) are needed for this calculation. Water density depends on water temperature and is necessary to convert mass into volume; therefore, accurate measurement of the water temperature is essential. Also, this equation corrects for the residual lung volume because any air in the lungs creates an additional buoyant effect that reduces underwater mass. The oxygen dilution technique described by Wilmore is one method for assessing residual lung volume (26). Estimating instead of measuring residual lung volume dramatically decreases the accuracy of hydrostatic weighing. Because sex, age, and height correlate with residual lung volume, it can be estimated with a formula that incorporates the client's age and height (13). Examples of formulas for males and females are shown in the sidebar *Formulas to Calculate Residual Lung Volume From Height and Age*. Because the volume of air trapped in the gastrointestinal tract cannot be measured, an estimate of 0.1 L is typically used.

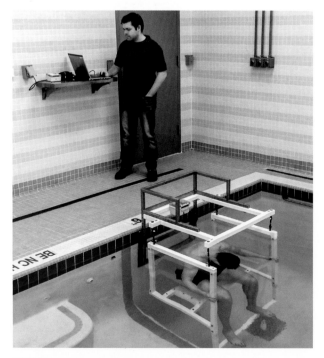

FIGURE 11.3 Hydrostatic weighing.

Photo courtesy of Meghan Perry.

Formulas to Calculate Residual Lung Volume From Height and Age

Females

$$(0.009 \times \text{age in years}) + (0.08128 \times \text{height in inches}) - 3.9 = RV \text{ in L}$$

Males

$$(0.017 \times \text{age in years}) + (0.06858 \times \text{height in inches}) - 3.447 = RV \text{ in L}$$

From Goldman and Becklake (1959).

Hydrostatic weighing accurately estimates body composition for most adults. Major disadvantages to this procedure are the time, expense, and technical expertise required. Also, many people are unable to undergo this procedure because of their discomfort with being underwater. Following are guidelines that will help ensure accurate assessment of body composition with hydrostatic weighing:

- The participant should not eat within 4 hours of testing.
- The participant should urinate and defecate before testing.
- The participant should wear as little clothing as possible. Remove any trapped air bubbles from clothing before weighing.
- Instruct the participant to exhale completely while submerged. (This will take practice for most individuals.)
- The participant should remain as motionless as possible while submerged.
- Perform several (5-10) trials to obtain consistent measurements.
- Measure, rather than estimate, residual volume.

Air Displacement Plethysmography

Another technique for determining %BF that uses the concept of density as the ratio of body mass to body volume is air displacement plethysmography. In this method, the volume of air displaced within a fixed, enclosed chamber is equal to the volume of the object (in this case the person being tested). The Bod Pod is a commercially available air displacement plethysmograph (see figure 11.4). During testing, a computer-controlled diaphragm moves, changing the volume of the chamber. Pressure changes in the chamber are related to the size of the person being measured. By examining the pressure–volume relationship, body volume and, subsequently, body density are calculated (3). Once body density is known, the two-compartment models can be used to estimate %BF.

The primary advantage of air displacement plethysmography compared with hydrostatic weighing is that it is quicker and less anxiety-inducing for many people. The method is considered valid and can be used with a wide range of populations including children, adults, obese individuals, athletes, and those with disabilities (3, 22). The SEE for this technique varies among studies but is typically between 2% and 4% (22). The major disadvantage is the cost of the highly technical equipment needed to make the measurements. A major consideration for obtaining accurate measurements with the Bod Pod is that subjects must dress according to the manufacturer's specifications (i.e., in a tight-fitting swimsuit and swim cap).

Bioelectrical Impedance Analysis

Bioelectrical impedance analysis (BIA) is a simple, quick, noninvasive method that can be used to estimate %BF. This technique is based on the assumption that tissues high in electrolyte-rich water content conduct electrical currents with less resistance than those with little water do (11). Because adipose tissue contains little water, fat impedes the flow of electrical current; muscle, on the other hand, conducts electrical current very well.

BIA requires that a small electrical current be sent through the body. This current is undetectable to the person being tested. Several types of BIA devices are commercially available. Some place electrodes on the hand and foot, some are handheld, and others have contact points for the bottom of the feet and look similar to bathroom scales. Whatever the design of the machine, as the introduced current passes through the body, voltage decreases. This voltage drop (impedance) is used to calculate %BF. Typically, other information such as sex, height, age, and sometimes race are used in conjunction with impedance to predict %BF.

BIA is used in the fitness industry because it is easy, inexpensive, and noninvasive. The accuracy of this technique depends on the type of equipment and equations used; however, a standard error of 1.8% to 6.3% commonly is reported (22). BIA estimates are based on the principle that water makes up 73% of the body's fat-free mass. Thus, hydration status is an important aspect to control; dehydration causes an increase in electrical resistance, which will result in an overestimation of %BF (3). An issue that complicates the application of BIA is that the relationship between impedance and %BF varies among populations. Most devices have programmed equations intended to account for factors that may affect the relationship between water content on body density, including differences between men and women and for

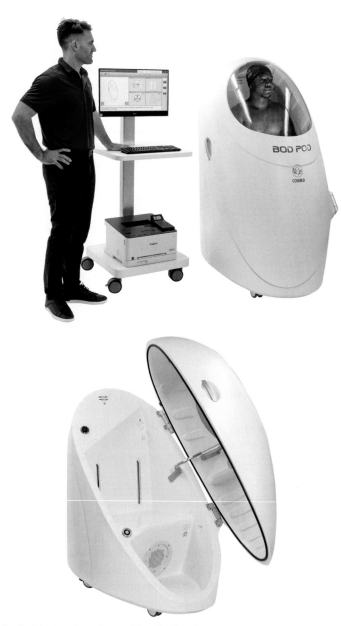

FIGURE 11.4 *(a)* The Bod Pod with the client in position for body composition measurement and *(b)* the interior equipment of the Bod Pod.

Photos courtesy of COSMED USA

age, race or ethnicity, and physical activity status (22). It is recommended that people with pacemakers avoid BIA assessment until the safety of BIA for these individuals has been determined (11).

A person's state of hydration can greatly alter BIA results; therefore, it is essential to follow standardized procedures with this assessment technique (3, 22). Individuals being tested should adhere to the following preparation:

- Do not exercise or use a sauna within 8 hours of the test.
- Avoid use of diuretics (e.g., caffeine, chocolate) (*Note:* Although potentially affecting results, diuretics prescribed by a health care provider should not be stopped for this analysis.)
- Do not consume alcohol for 12 hours and food or drink within 4 hours of the test.
- Void the bladder within 30 minutes of the test.

Other aspects within the testing environment are also key to promote the best results:

- Height and weight must be accurately measured.
- Remove oil and lotions from the skin with alcohol before placing electrodes.
- Place electrodes precisely as directed by the manufacturer of the impedance device. Incorrect electrode placement greatly reduces the accuracy of BIA.
- Note the phase of the menstrual cycle because of its ability to alter hydration levels; females who perceive they are retaining water should not be tested.
- Ensure a neutral temperature, and have the individual rest at that temperature for 15 to 20 minutes to allow skin temperature to stabilize.

Dual-Energy X-Ray Absorptiometry

A technique in clinical settings is dual-energy X-ray absorptiometry (DXA or DEXA). DXA was developed for measuring the density of bones. Although bone density measurement remains the primary use of this methodol-ogy, software has been developed that can estimate total and regional %BF from DXA scans (see figure 11.5). To estimate %BF from DXA, a total-body X-ray is performed with extremely low-dosage energy beams. As the X-rays pass through the subject, the density of all parts of the body is determined. Because fat, bone, and nonbone lean tissue have different densities, these three compartments can be identified (3).

Although DXA requires a full-body X-ray, the radiation exposure is minimal and is only a small fraction of the radiation exposure of a chest X-ray. One unique consideration is the proprietary software used by different manufacturers; differences in DXA software packages may result in varied body fat outcomes, so documentation of software version is important (3). The precision and accuracy (typically between 2% and 3% fat for the SEE) makes this a valuable tool for clinical assessment (3).

This procedure is relatively quick (approximately 15 minutes) and has the potential for accurate results regardless of the age, sex, or race of the subject. The major prohibitive factors for using this procedure are cost and access to the equipment. Because of the radiation exposure involved, DXA equipment is typically housed

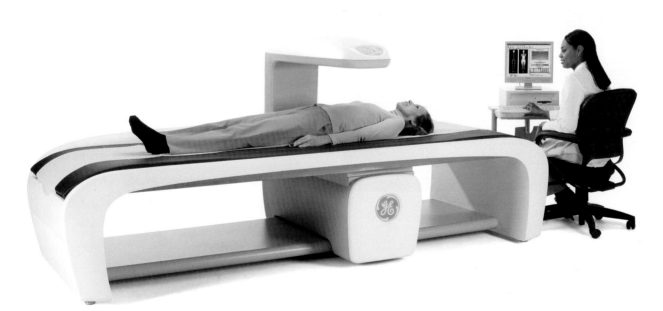

FIGURE 11.5 Dual-energy X-ray absorptiometry.
Courtesy GE Healthcare

in hospitals or clinically oriented research centers. At present, DXA is used most frequently as a research tool and in the clinical assessment of body composition.

Computed Tomography and Magnetic Resonance Imaging

Magnetic resonance imaging (MRI) and computed tomography (CT) also are imaging techniques that provide important information to clinicians and researchers. One of the common uses of these techniques is to determine the amount of fat, particularly deep fat, found in the trunk. Because deep fat (visceral fat) is highly associated with disease, researchers use these techniques to quantify its distribution pattern. CT scans use X-rays to produce images of the fat and nonfat tissues, whereas MRI uses a strong magnetic field. The equipment necessary for this type of imaging is expensive and is found in clinical settings. These techniques provide criterion measurement for regional fat distribution and deep versus superficial fat depots (11).

KEY POINT

Two-compartment models divide the body into fat and fat-free components. Although the Siri two-compartment model is often used, population-specific equations are available to convert body density into %BF. Both hydrostatic weighing and air displacement plethysmography use a two-compartment model. BIA is based on the principle that electrical currents flow more easily through more hydrated tissues (muscle) than through less hydrated tissues (fat). Although BIA is useful in body composition screening, steps should be taken to ensure that the client's hydration is normal at the time of testing. Multicompartment modeling and imaging techniques are used in clinical settings and research to assess body composition.

Calculating Target Body Weight

As shown in table 11.1, proposed healthy %BF ranges are quite different for females and males and cover a wide range. One of the important tasks of fitness professionals is helping clients determine an appropriate weight goal. Once an estimate of %BF has been obtained and %BF goals have been determined, the fitness professional can calculate an appropriate target weight. As discussed in chapter 20, setting reasonable goals for weight loss is a major factor in maintaining compliance. To calculate target body weight, body weight, %BF, and the desired level of body fatness must be known. The following equations can be used for these calculations; note that depending on the desired unit of measure, either pounds or kilograms can be entered into the equations (25):

$$\text{Lean body mass} = \text{body mass}$$
$$\times (1 - \text{current \%BF percentage expressed as a decimal})$$

$$\text{Target body weight} = \text{lean body mass}$$
$$\div (1 - \text{desired \%BF percentage expressed as a decimal})$$

QUESTION:

A 40-year-old woman weighs 155 pounds (70.5 kilograms) and has a %BF of 30. Her goal is to reach 23% body fat. What is her target weight?

ANSWER:

To provide the target weight for the client in pounds:

$$\text{Lean body mass} = 155 \times (1 - 0.30)$$

$$\text{Lean body mass} = 108.5 \text{ pounds}$$

$$\text{Target body weight} = 108.5 \div (1 - 0.23)$$

$$\text{Target body weight} = 140.9 \text{ pounds}$$

This can also be calculated in kilograms:

$$\text{Lean body mass} = 70.5 \times (1 - 0.30)$$

$$\text{Lean body mass} = 49.35 \text{ kilograms}$$

$$\text{Target body weight} = 49.35 \div (1 - 0.23)$$

$$\text{Target body weight} = 64.1 \text{ kilograms}$$

RESEARCH INSIGHT

Advanced Methods in Body Composition Assessment

A disadvantage to using two-compartment models in calculating body composition is the need to make broad generalizations about the composition and density of various body tissues. To avoid this problem, researchers sometimes use models that combine measurements to estimate body composition. Although these techniques still must rely on some basic assumptions about the body's makeup, fewer broad generalizations about its component parts are made. Therefore, these multicompartment models more accurately assess body composition.

An example of a multicompartment model is Siri's three-compartment model, in which the body is divided into fat, water, and solids (protein and mineral) (24). This model requires measuring total body density and total body water. Measurements of total body water typically are determined by having the participant ingest an isotope of hydrogen such as deuterium or tritium. After the ingested isotope spreads through the body's water, a fluid sample (e.g., urine, blood) can be used to calculate total body water. This model is useful in clinical situations when patients have significantly altered body water. Four-component (estimate of mineral is added), five-component, and six-component models also exist (3). Data from these methodologies are used to develop better field methods for assessing body composition in diverse populations. However, the cost, time, and technical expertise required for these processes make them impractical in non-research settings.

LEARNING AIDS

REVIEW QUESTIONS

1. What is the BMI range associated with a healthy weight? What is the BMI range for overweight? For obesity?

2. What are other names for the android-type obesity pattern? What conditions are linked to this obesity pattern?

3. Hydrostatic weighing and air displacement plethysmography use a two-compartment model for body composition. What are the two compartments assumed by this model?

4. Which technique applies a small electrical current to estimate %BF? What are ways to improve the accuracy of this technique?

5. What are important considerations when using skinfold measurements to estimate %BF that will help reduce measurement errors?

6. What are some advantages to using air displacement plethysmography?

7. What body composition technique is also used to measure bone density?

8. Why are multicompartment models of body composition assessment generally limited to research settings?

CASE STUDIES

1. Alexandria is a 30-year-old female who comes into your fitness facility wanting to lose weight. What are appropriate measurements and calculations for a fitness professional to make to assist Alexandria with her goal?

2. Desmond is a 48-year-old male who recently joined your fitness facility. At his initial evaluation you take the following measurements:
   - Height: 70 inches (178 centimeters)
   - Weight: 215 pounds (97.7 kilograms)
   - Hip circumference: 39 inches (99 centimeters)
   - WC: 41 inches (104 centimeters)
   - Skinfolds (in millimeters): chest, 35; abdomen, 49; thigh, 20

   Calculate and interpret Desmond's BMI, WHR, and %BF.

3. Desmond sets his initial %BF goal at 28%. Calculate the target body weight in pounds that will allow Desmond to achieve this goal.

Answers to Case Studies

1. Height, weight, BMI, and waist and hip circumference are appropriate. Percent BF also could be considered.

2. First calculate Desmond's BMI and WHR:

$$\text{BMI} = 97.7 \text{ kg} \div (1.78 \text{ m})^2 = 30.8 \text{ kg} \cdot \text{m}^{-2}, \text{ which is within the obese range.}$$

$$\text{WHR} = 41 \text{ in.} \div 39 \text{ in.} = 1.05, \text{ which is considered high risk.}$$

To calculate %BF, first calculate body density using the three-site formula:

$$D_b = 1.10938 - (0.0008267 \times \text{sum of skinfolds})$$
$$+ (0.0000016 \times \text{sum of skinfolds}^2) - (0.0002574 \times \text{age})$$
$$= 1.10938 - (0.0008267 \times 104) + (0.0000016 \times 104^2)$$
$$- (0.0002574 \times 48) = 1.0283536$$

Next, use the Siri equation to convert the density into %BF:

$$\%\text{BF} = (495 \div D_b) - 450 = (495 \div 1.0283536) - 495 = 31.4\%,$$
$$\text{which is in the obese range.}$$

3. Calculate lean body mass and then target body weight. To provide the target weight for the client in pounds (note 31.4 %BF written as a percentage is 0.314), calculate the following:

$$\text{Lean body mass} = 215 \times (1 - 0.314)$$
$$\text{Lean body mass} = 147.5 \text{ pounds}$$
$$\text{Target body weight} = 147.5 \div (1 - 0.28)$$
$$\text{Target body weight} = 204.9 \text{ pounds}$$

Electrocardiogram (ECG) Assessment

Brittany Overstreet

OBJECTIVES

The reader will be able to do the following:

1. Describe the basic anatomy of the heart
2. Describe the basic electrophysiology of the heart
3. Define *electrocardiogram (ECG)* and identify the standard settings for paper speed and amplitude
4. Identify the basic electrocardiographic complexes and calculate heart rate from ECG rhythm strips
5. Identify normal and abnormal cardiac rhythms and predict the probable effect of the abnormal rhythms on exercise performance
6. Describe electrocardiographic signs and biochemical markers of a heart attack

12

This chapter provides background information on the heart and ECG analysis and how these factors affect exercise testing in the healthy population. This chapter is not intended to be a complete guide to ECG interpretation and cardiovascular medications; several excellent texts on these topics are available (3, 6, 8, 9, 9a).

Structure of the Heart

The heart is a muscular organ composed of four chambers: the right atrium, right ventricle, left atrium, and left ventricle (see figure 12.1). The flow of blood through the heart is directed by pressure differences and valves between the chambers. Venous blood from the lower body is returned to the heart by the inferior vena cava and from the upper body by the superior vena cava, and both empty into the right atrium. From the right atrium, blood passes through the tricuspid valve into the right ventricle. The right ventricle pumps deoxygenated blood through the pulmonary valve into the pulmonary arteries leading to the lungs, where carbon dioxide is eliminated and oxygen is picked up. The oxygen-rich blood is returned to the heart via the pulmonary veins, emptying into the left atrium. From the left atrium, blood passes through the mitral valve into the left ventricle. The left

ventricle pumps oxygenated blood past the aortic valve into the aorta and coronary arteries out to the systemic circuit. The left ventricle, which generates more pressure than the right ventricle in order to overcome vascular resistance from the vessels directly outside the heart, is typically more muscular in a healthy adult heart.

Coronary Arteries

The thick middle layer of the heart, or myocardium, does not receive a significant amount of oxygen directly from blood in the atria or ventricles. To meet the heart's need for nutrients and sustain metabolic activity, oxygenated blood is supplied to the myocardium via the coronary arteries, which lie on the surface of the heart. There are two coronary artery systems (the right and left coronary arteries), which branch off of the aorta. The left main coronary artery follows a course between the left atria and the pulmonary artery and branches off into the left anterior descending and left circumflex arteries (figure 12.2). The left anterior descending artery follows a path along the anterior surface of the heart and lies over the interventricular septum, which separates the right and left ventricles. The left circumflex artery follows the groove between the left atrium and left ventricle on the anterior and lateral surface of the heart. The right coronary artery

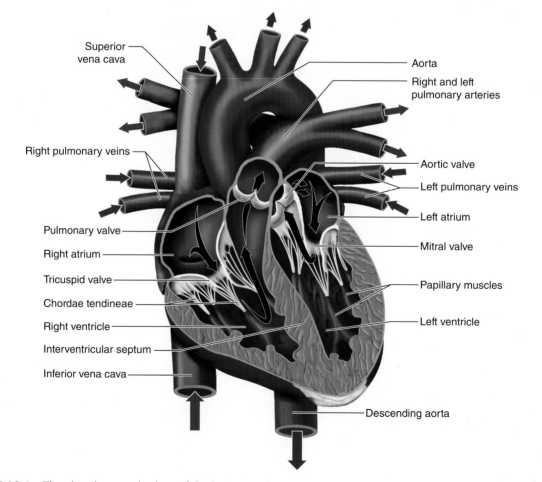

FIGURE 12.1 The chambers and valves of the heart.

follows the groove that separates the atria and ventricles around the posterior surface of the heart and forms the posterior descending artery. Numerous smaller arteries split off the major arteries, becoming smaller and smaller until finally they form the capillaries that transport oxygen to the muscle cells of the heart, where gas exchange occurs.

A major obstruction in any of these coronary arteries results in myocardial ischemia, or reduced blood flow to the myocardium and decreased ability of the heart to pump blood. If the coronary arteries become blocked and the heart muscle does not receive oxygen, a portion of the myocardium might die, which is known as a *myocardial infarction* (MI), or heart attack. Whether it is due to a myocardial infarction or an abnormality within the electrical pathway of the heart, if the ventricles cease to contract in a rhythmic fashion, blood will stop circulating throughout the body and can result in cardiac arrest.

Coronary Veins

Venous drainage of the right ventricle occurs via the anterior cardiac vein, which normally has two or three major branches and eventually empties into the right atrium. The venous drainage of the left ventricle occurs primarily through the anterior interventricular vein, which roughly follows the same path as the left anterior descending artery, eventually forming the coronary sinus and emptying into the right atrium. The primary purpose of the coronary veins is to remove deoxygenated blood from the myocardium and deliver it back to the right atrium for circulation and reoxygenation.

Oxygen Use by the Heart

The myocardium is well adapted to use oxygen to generate adenosine triphosphate (ATP). Approximately 40% of the volume of a myocardial cell is composed of mitochondria, the cellular organelle responsible for producing ATP with oxygen. The oxygen consumption of the heart in a resting person is about 8 to 10 ml · min⁻¹ per 100 grams of myocardium; in comparison, the total resting oxygen consumption for the body is about 0.35 ml · min⁻¹ per 100 grams of body mass (4). Myocardial oxygen consumption can increase six- to sevenfold during heavy exercise in young adults, whereas the total body oxygen consumption can easily increase 12 to 15 times. Heart muscle has a limited capacity to produce energy via anaerobic pathways and depends on the delivery of oxygen to the mitochondria to produce ATP. At rest, the whole body extracts only about 25% of the oxygen present in each 100 milliliters of arterial blood, and the body can meet an increased need for oxygen by simply extracting more from the blood. In contrast, the heart extracts about 75% of the oxygen available in the arterial blood. Consequently, an increase in the oxygen needs of the heart must be met by delivering more blood via the coronary arteries. An adequate oxygen supply to the heart is needed not only to allow the heart to pump blood but also to maintain normal electrical activity, which is covered in the next section.

KEY POINT

The heart is a muscular organ composed of four chambers: the right atrium, the right ventricle, the left atrium, and the left ventricle. The coronary arteries supply the heart muscle (myocardium) with blood, and the heart meets increasing oxygen demands by increasing blood flow.

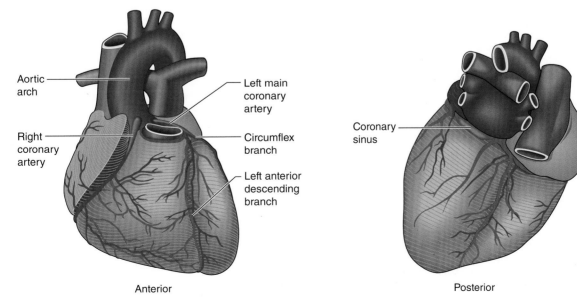

FIGURE 12.2 Coronary blood vessels.

Electrophysiology of the Heart

For cardiac muscle cells to contract they must be stimulated by an impulse from the electrical conduction system of the heart. These electrical signals trigger mechanical activity (contraction) and result in blood being pumped from the heart's chambers to the pulmonary and systemic circuits. At rest, the insides of the myocardial cells are negatively charged and the exteriors are positively charged because the cell membrane is selectively permeable, and the concentrations of certain ions (K^+, Na^+) differ inside and outside of the cells (5). At rest, a higher concentration of Na^+ ions are outside and K^+ ions are inside a cardiac myocyte cell,

resulting in the cell's resting membrane potential. When a cardiac cell is stimulated past a specific threshold, an action potential will occur, resulting in depolarization of the cell. Depolarization occurs as Na^+ ions enter the cell and K^+ ions exit the cell, resulting in the inside of the cell becoming positively charged and the exterior becoming negatively charged. After depolarization, the myocardial cell undergoes repolarization to return to its resting electrical state. During repolarization, Na^+ ions leave the cells and K^+ are returned, resulting in the inside of the cell becoming more negatively charged until it returns to its prestimulated state. The steps leading from rest (complete polarization) to complete stimulation (depolarization) back to rest (repolarization) are shown in figure 12.3.

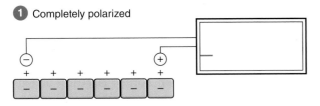

① Completely polarized

The myocardial cells shown on the left are at rest and are completely polarized. Because both of the recording electrodes are surrounded by positive charges, there is no voltage difference between them, and the electrocardiogram (ECG) shown on the right records the isoelectric line (0 mV).

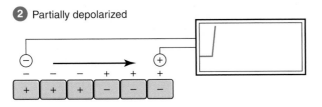

② Partially depolarized

The process of depolarization (positive charges inside the cell and negative charges outside) is spreading from left to right. Because the electrode on the right is surrounded by positive charges, the ECG records a positive deflection. The amplitude of the deflection is proportional to the mass of the myocardium undergoing depolarization.

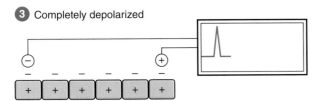

③ Completely depolarized

Depolarization is now complete, and both electrodes are surrounded by negative charges. Because there is no voltage difference between electrodes, the ECG is now recording 0 mV, or the isoelectric potential.

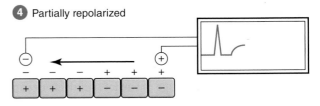

④ Partially repolarized

Repolarization has started from the right and is moving to the left. The ECG shows a positive (upward) deflection, because the right-hand electrode is surrounded by positive charges. Note that repolarization occurs in the opposite direction from depolarization in the human heart, and this is the reason the depolarization and repolarization complexes are both normally positive. If repolarization had started on the left and moved to the right, the ECG deflection would have been negative.

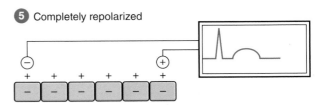

⑤ Completely repolarized

The muscle cells are now completely repolarized, or in the resting state, and the ECG records the isoelectric line. The myocardial cells are now ready to be depolarized again.

FIGURE 12.3   Steps in an electrocardiographic cycle.

Electrodes can be placed across the chest, arms, and legs to measure the electrical activity within the heart. When the myocardial cell is completely polarized or depolarized, the ECG does not record any electrical potential but shows a flat baseline, known as the *isoelectric line*. If a recording electrode is placed on the chest so that the wave of depolarization spreads toward the electrode, the ECG records a positive (upward) deflection above the isoelectric line. If the wave of depolarization spreads away from the recording electrode, a negative (downward) deflection occurs.

A special feature of the heart's electrical conduction system is that it has pacemaker cells that spontaneously fire, without any input from the brain, and control heart rate. In a healthy heart, the sinoatrial (SA) node is the normal pacemaker and is located in the right atrium near the superior vena cava (figure 12.4). As ions slowly move across the cell membrane, causing the resting membrane potential to creep up to the threshold, depolarization spreads from the SA node across the atria. Three tracts within the atria conduct depolarization to the atrioventricular (AV) node. At the AV node, conduction slows to allow the atrial contraction to empty blood into the ventricles before the start of ventricular contraction. The bundle of His is the conduction pathway that connects the AV node with the next step of the electrical pathway, the bundle branches. The right bundle branch splits off the bundle of His and forms ever-smaller branches that serve the right ventricle. The left bundle splits into two major branches that serve the thicker left ventricle. The last part of the electrical conduction system is the Purkinje fibers, which are terminal branches of the bundle branches and form the link between the specialized electrically conductive tissue and the muscle fibers. Small electrical junctions between adjacent cardiac muscle cells, known as *intercalated discs*, allow the electrical impulses to pass from cell to cell with little to no interruption. The intercalated discs allow for coordinated contraction of the ventricular muscle fibers, which is needed for effective pumping of the heart. Because of the conduction pathways and the interconnected myocardial cells, a depolarization of the SA node results in a predictable electrical pattern, coordinated contraction of the heart's muscle cells, and effective pumping of the blood.

KEY POINT

The electrical impulse originates in the SA node, located in the right atrium. From there the electrical impulse spreads to the AV node, the bundle of His, the left and right bundle branches, and the Purkinje fibers. Waves of depolarization then spread from cell to cell throughout the ventricular muscle by passing through the intercalated discs. Any restriction in blood flow to the myocardium could upset the electrical activity of the heart or damage the myocardium.

Interpreting the ECG

The electrocardiogram (ECG) is a graphic recording of the heart's electrical activity. As waves of depolarization travel through the heart, electrical currents spread to the tissues surrounding the heart and then travel throughout the body. If recording electrodes are placed on the skin, small voltage differences between various regions of the body can be detected. Thus, the electrocardiograph is a sensitive voltmeter that records the electrical activity of the heart.

This section on analyzing the ECG may appear to go beyond what a fitness professional needs to know about the topic given that a physician is the person to judge whether an ECG response is normal. However, the fitness professional must be aware of the basic ECG interpretation in order to communicate effectively with the physician, program director, and clinical exercise physiologist.

Systematically evaluating the ECG allows the examiner to determine the heart rate (HR), rhythm, and conduction pathways and to search for signs of ischemia or infarction. Physicians normally evaluate a 12-lead ECG, but in this chapter, a single ECG lead will be reviewed to describe the heart's electrical activity. A commonly used single ECG lead for exercise testing is the CM5, which looks similar to lead V5 on a 12-lead ECG. A 12-lead ECG allows a cardiologist to look at the heart

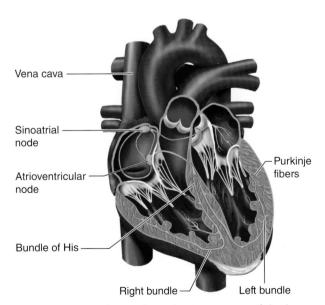

Vena cava

Sinoatrial node

Atrioventricular node

Bundle of His

Right bundle

Purkinje fibers

Left bundle

FIGURE 12.4 Electrical conduction system of the heart. These are the normal pathways used to ensure the rhythmic contraction and relaxation of the heart chambers.

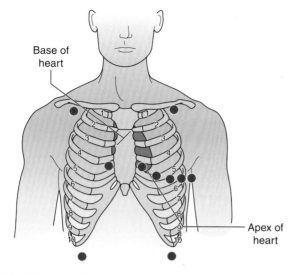

FIGURE 12.5 Electrode placements for a 12-lead ECG.

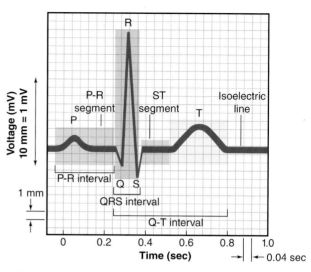

FIGURE 12.6 ECG complex with time and voltage scales.

from 12 different views. (Six-limb leads provide views of the heart from various angles in the frontal plane of the body, and six precordial leads provide views of the heart from various angles in the transverse plane of the body.) These 12 leads are made up of various combinations of 10 electrodes (see figure 12.5). The 12-lead ECG contains much more information than a single ECG lead, and it allows a more detailed picture of the heart's electrical activity. A detailed discussion of 12-lead ECG electrode placement and interpretation is beyond the scope of this chapter. For further information, consult the texts by Dubin (8) or Stein (12).

Time and Voltage

ECG paper markings are standardized to allow measurement of time intervals and voltages. Time is measured on the horizontal axis, and the paper normally moves at 25 mm · sec^{-1}. Most ECG machines can run at 50 or 25 mm · sec^{-1}, so one must know the paper speed when measuring the duration of ECG complexes (see the section Electrocardiographic Wave Forms). ECG paper is marked with a repeating grid (see figure 12.6). Major grid lines are 5 millimeters apart, and at a paper speed of 25 mm · sec^{-1}, 5 millimeters correspond to 0.20 seconds. Minor lines are 1 millimeter apart, and at a paper speed of 25 mm · sec^{-1}, 1 millimeter equals 0.04 seconds. Voltage is measured on the vertical axis, and the standard calibration factor is normally 0.1 millivolt (mV) per millimeter of deflection. Most ECG machines can be adjusted to reduce this factor by 50% or to double it. Knowing the voltage calibration is necessary before evaluating an ECG. All ECG measurements in this chapter refer to a paper speed of 25 mm · sec^{-1} and a voltage calibration of 0.1 mV · mm^{-1}.

KEY POINT

The pattern of electrical activity across the heart is called the *electrocardiogram (ECG)*. The ECG is recorded with an electrocardiograph, and it provides information about the rhythm of the heart. The ECG paper speed is normally 25 mm · sec^{-1}, and at this speed each 1-millimeter mark represents 0.04 seconds. The standard calibration factor is normally 0.1 mV · mm^{-1} of vertical deflection.

Electrocardiographic Wave Forms

The P wave is the graphic representation of atrial depolarization. The normal P wave lasts less than 0.12 seconds and has an amplitude of 0.25 mV or less. In a single cardiac cycle, there should be only one P wave per QRS complex (see description of QRS complex below). The T_a wave is the result of atrial repolarization. It is not normally seen because it occurs during ventricular depolarization, and the larger electrical forces generated by the ventricles hide the T_a wave. The Q wave is the first downward deflection after the P wave, and it signals the start of ventricular depolarization. The R wave is a positive deflection following the Q wave; it results from ventricular depolarization. If there is more than one R wave in a single complex, the second occurrence is called *R'*. The S wave is a negative deflection preceded by Q or R waves, and it is also the result of ventricular depolarization. Collectively, the Q, R, and S waves are referred to as the *QRS complex*. The T wave follows this complex, and it results from ventricular repolarization.

Electrocardiograph Intervals

The R-R interval is the time between successive R waves. When the heart rhythm is regular, the duration of an R-R interval can be used to determine the HR (bpm). If the heart rhythm is irregular, the R-R interval varies and HR must be determined from the number of R waves in a 6-second interval (see figure 12.7).

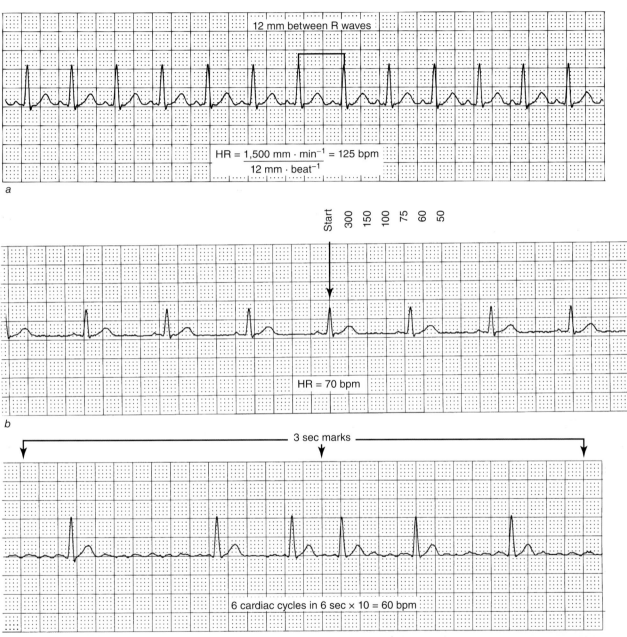

FIGURE 12.7 Three methods of determining HR from the ECG: (a) An approximate HR (bpm) can be determined by dividing 1,500 (60 seconds at 25 mm · sec⁻¹) by the number of millimeters between adjacent R waves. (b) A second method is to begin with an R wave that falls on a thick black line. As you move to the right, count off the next six black lines as 300, 150, 100, 75, 60, and 50. If the next R wave falls on one of these lines, the corresponding number indicates the HR. If the next R wave falls in between two thick black lines, you can estimate the HR by interpolation. (c) A third method is commonly used when the HR is irregular. With this method, you count the number of complete R-R intervals in a 6-second ECG strip and multiply by 10.

The P-P interval is the time between two successive atrial depolarizations. The PR interval is measured from the start of the P wave to the beginning of the QRS complex. The interval is called *PR* even if the first deflection after the P wave is a Q wave. Thus, the PR interval includes the time periods corresponding to atrial depolarization and the delay in the electrical impulse at the AV node. The upper limit for the normal PR interval is 0.20 seconds, or 5 small blocks on the grid of the ECG paper.

The width of the QRS complex depends on the time for depolarization of the ventricles. A normal QRS complex lasts 0.10 seconds, or 2.5 small blocks on the ECG paper, or less. The QT interval is measured from the start of the QRS complex to the end of the T wave and corresponds to the duration of ventricular systole.

Segments and Junctions

The PR segment is measured from the end of the P wave to the beginning of the QRS complex. This segment forms the isoelectric line, or baseline, from which ST segment deviations are measured. The J point is the point at which the S wave ends and the ST segment begins. The ST segment is formed by the isoelectric line between the QRS complex and the T wave. During an exercise test this segment is examined closely for depression or elevation, which may indicate the development of myocardial ischemia or perhaps MI. A description of the process for determining MI and myocardial ischemia can be found later in this chapter. ST segment deviation usually is measured 60 or 80 milliseconds after the J point.

Heart Rhythms

The ECG provides vital information about heart rhythms. Abnormalities in the electrical activity of the heart can be diagnosed from the ECG.

KEY POINT

The P wave signifies atrial depolarization, the QRS complex signifies ventricular depolarization, and the T wave signifies ventricular repolarization. If the rhythm is regular, HR can be determined by dividing 1,500 by the number of millimeters between successive R waves. HR also can be determined by starting with an R wave that falls on a thick black line; counting off the next six black lines as 300, 150, 100, 75, 60, and 50; and determining at which corresponding number the next R wave occurs. If the rhythm is irregular, HR can be determined by counting the number of R-R intervals in a 6-second ECG strip and multiplying by 10.

Sinus Rhythm

Sinus rhythm is the normal rhythm of the heart (see figure 12.8). The HR is 60 to 100 bpm, and the pacemaker is the SA node. In a healthy heart, the presence of a P wave within normal limits (see section on Electrocardiographic Wave Forms) indicates that the SA node is the pacemaker and that the rhythm is, in fact, a sinus rhythm.

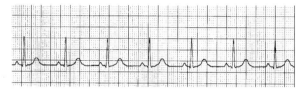

FIGURE 12.8   Normal sinus rhythm. In this example, the HR is 71 bpm.

Sinus Bradycardia

The HR in sinus bradycardia is less than 60 bpm (see figure 12.9). This is a normal rhythm, and it is often seen in conditioned participants and patients taking beta-blockers (see chapter 2 for a full review of medications and their effects on the heart).

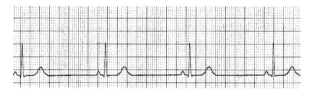

FIGURE 12.9   Sinus bradycardia. In this example, the HR is 35 bpm.

Sinus Tachycardia

Sinus tachycardia (HR >100 bpm) is normally seen during moderate and heavy exercise (see figure 12.10). Thus, exercise-induced sinus tachycardia is perfectly normal. Resting sinus tachycardia may be seen in deconditioned people or in patients who are apprehensive before exercise testing. In these heart rhythms, the SA node still functions as the pacemaker.

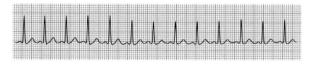

FIGURE 12.10   Sinus tachycardia. In this example, the HR is 125 bpm.

Atrioventricular Conduction Disturbances

Atrioventricular conduction disturbances are caused by a blockage of the electrical impulse at the AV node. The

KEY POINT

If the SA node is pacing the heart, P waves within normal limits should be present. If the HR is between 60 and 100 bpm, the heart is in normal sinus rhythm. Sinus bradycardia is an HR less than 60 bpm, and sinus tachycardia is an HR greater than 100 bpm (normally seen during moderate and heavy exercise).

blockage can be either partial or complete. Disturbances within this area of the heart may result in abnormal P waves or PR intervals.

First-Degree AV Block

When the PR interval exceeds 0.20 seconds and all P waves result in ventricular depolarization (i.e., a 1:1 ratio exists between P wave and QRS complex), a first-degree AV block exists (see figure 12.11). Causes of a first-degree AV block include medications such as digitalis and quinidine, infections, and vagal stimulation.

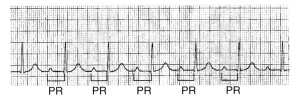

FIGURE 12.11 First-degree AV block. PR marks the prolonged PR interval (0.28 seconds in this example).

Second-Degree AV Block

The distinguishing feature of a second-degree AV block is that some, but not all, P waves result in ventricular depolarization. There are two types of second-degree AV blocks: Mobitz type I and Mobitz type II. Mobitz type I AV block, or Wenckebach AV block, is characterized by a PR interval that progressively lengthens until an atrial depolarization fails to initiate a ventricular depolarization and the QRS complex is skipped (see figure 12.12). This conduction disturbance is seen most commonly after an MI. The site of the block is within the AV node and is probably the result of reversible ischemia.

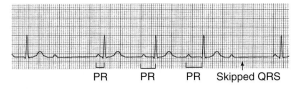

FIGURE 12.12 Mobitz type I (Wenckebach) AV block. The PR interval gradually lengthens until finally a QRS complex is skipped.

Mobitz type II AV block is the more serious of the second-degree AV blocks, and it is characterized by atrial depolarization occasionally not resulting in ventricular depolarization, even though PR intervals remain constant (i.e., do not lengthen; see figure 12.13). The site of the block is beyond the bundle of His, and it is usually the result of irreversible ischemia of the intraventricular conduction system.

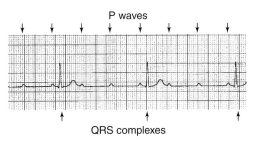

FIGURE 12.13 Mobitz type II AV block. Occasionally, and without lengthening of the PR interval, QRS complexes are skipped.

Third-Degree AV Block

Third-degree AV block, also known as a *complete heart block*, is present when the ventricles contract independently of the atria (see figure 12.14). The PR interval varies and follows no regular pattern. The ventricular pacemaker can be the AV node, the bundle of His, Purkinje fibers, or the ventricular muscle, and it almost always results in a slow ventricular rate of fewer than 50 bpm. A third-degree AV block is considered a relative contraindication to starting a symptom-limited maximal exercise test (1).

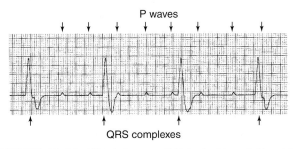

FIGURE 12.14 Third-degree AV block. No relationship exists between the atrial rate (e.g., 94 bpm) and the ventricular rate (e.g., 36 bpm), indicating complete blockage of the AV node.

Arrhythmia

An arrhythmia is an irregular heart rhythm. Arrhythmias often arise when the myocardium becomes hyperexcitable due to a lack of blood flow or the use of stimulants.

Sinus Arrhythmia

Sinus arrhythmia is a sinus rhythm in which the R-R interval varies by more than 10% from beat to beat. In sinus arrhythmia, a P wave precedes each QRS complex, but the QRS complexes are unevenly spaced. Sinus arrhythmia is seen often in highly trained individuals and occasionally in patients taking beta-adrenergic blocking medications. The rhythm may be associated with respiration because HR increases with inspiration and decreases with expiration due to the balance of sympathetic and parasympathetic neural activation.

Premature Atrial Contraction

In premature atrial contractions (PAC), the rhythm is irregular and the R-R interval is short between a normal sinus beat and the premature beat (see figure 12.15). The premature beat originates somewhere other than the sinus node and is known as an *ectopic focus* (an irritable spot on the myocardium that depolarizes on its own). An ectopic focus often is caused by stimulants (e.g., caffeine), antihistamines, diet pills, cold medications (e.g., ephedrine), or nicotine. PACs sometimes are seen before exercise testing in apprehensive participants. They can also occur in insolation or be a frequent occurrence.

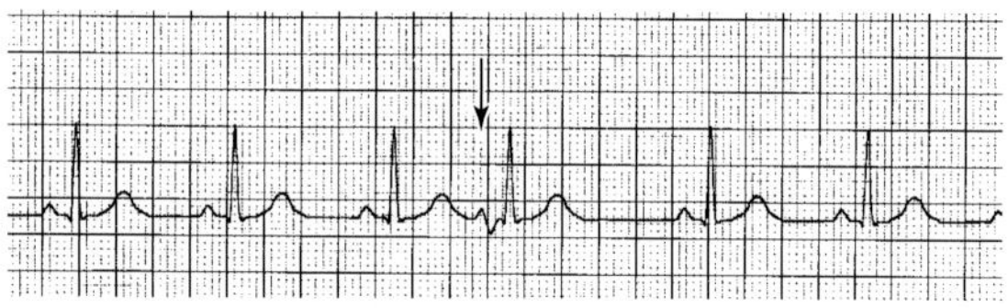

Diphasic P wave

FIGURE 12.15 Premature atrial contraction (PAC). The arrow indicates a premature, diphasic P wave coming from an ectopic focus in the atria.

Atrial Flutter

During atrial flutter, the atrial heart rate is different than the ventricular rate. Typically, the atrial rate is between 200 and 350 bpm, whereas the ventricular response is 60 to 160 bpm. The pacemaker site during atrial flutter is not the SA node but an ectopic focus, so normal P waves are not present. F waves, resembling a sawtooth pattern, may be seen (see figure 12.16). Despite the difference in rates between the atria and ventricles, if the number of F waves between QRS complexes is consistent, the ventricular rhythm may be regular. If the number of F waves varies between QRS complexes, the ventricular rhythm can be irregular. The causes of atrial flutter

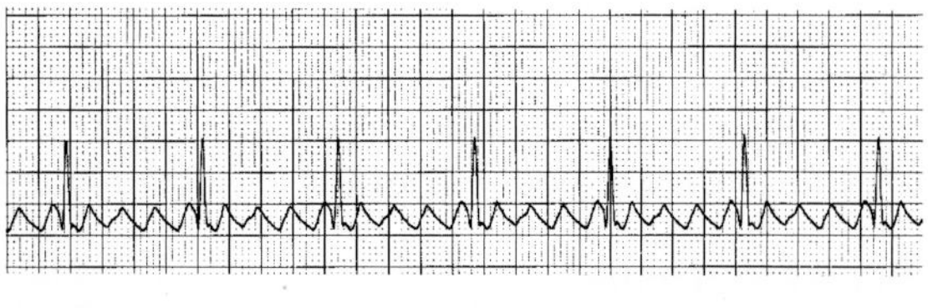

FIGURE 12.16 Atrial flutter. The atrial rate is 200 to 350 bpm (300 bpm in this example), but the ventricular rate is much slower.

include increased sympathetic drive, hypoxia, and congestive heart failure.

Atrial Fibrillation

During atrial fibrillation, the atrial rate is 400 to 700 bpm, while the ventricular rate is usually 60 to 160 bpm and irregular. Multiple pacemaker sites are present in the atria, and P waves cannot be discerned (see figure 12.17). The significance of atrial fibrillation in exercise testing and training lies in its effect on ventricular function. During atrial fibrillation, the atria and ventricles are not coordinated, and the ability of the left ventricle to maintain an adequate cardiac output may be impaired. The causes of atrial fibrillation are essentially the same as those for atrial flutter. Recurrent atrial fibrillation may have little effect on the exercise response of a person with good left ventricular function, but it can cause significant symptoms in a person with poor ventricular function. Another problem with chronic atrial fibrillation is that the blood in the atria can clot and lead to a stroke because there is no concerted pumping action with atrial fibrillation.

FIGURE 12.17 Atrial fibrillation. A jagged baseline and irregularly spaced QRS complexes are seen.

Premature Junctional Contractions

A premature junctional contraction (PJC) results when an ectopic pacemaker in the AV junctional area depolarizes the ventricles. Inverted, or lack of, P waves frequently accompany PJCs as the atrial depolarization proceeds in an abnormal direction (see figure 12.18). This characteristic of PJCs may distinguish them from premature atrial contractions, which frequently have notched or diphasic P waves. If these two conditions cannot be distinguished, the more general term *premature supraventricular contraction* can be used to indicate an ectopic focus above the ventricles.

If the nodal tissue remains in the refractory phase after a PJC, normally conducted waves of depolariza-

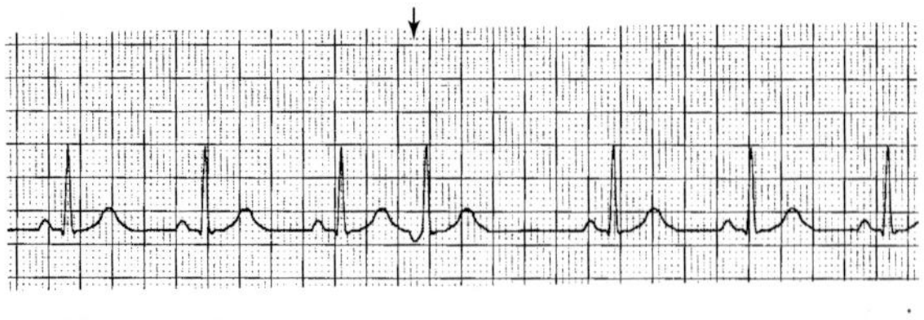

Inverted P wave

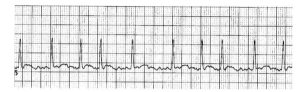

FIGURE 12.18 Premature junctional contraction (PJC). The arrow indicates a premature, inverted P wave coming from the AV node.

tion initiated from the sinus node will not pass into the ventricles and a compensatory pause will develop. PJCs usually result in a QRS complex of normal duration, or they can slightly prolong the QRS complex. They can be caused by catecholamine-type medications, increased parasympathetic tone on the AV node, or damage to the AV node. PJCs are of little consequence unless they occur frequently (more than 4-6 PJCs per minute) or compromise ventricular function (8).

Although supraventricular arrhythmias may concern fitness professionals and patients, Ellestad (9) found that exercise-induced supraventricular arrhythmias do not seem to compromise the long-term prognosis of patients with coronary artery disease (CAD). The significance of the supraventricular arrhythmias lies in the uncoupling of the atria and ventricles and in the resulting effect on the ability of the ventricles to maintain an adequate cardiac output.

Premature Ventricular Contractions

Premature ventricular contractions (PVC) result from an ectopic focus in the His-Purkinje system, which initiates a ventricular contraction. PVCs have a QRS complex that is wide (>0.12 sec) and irregularly shaped (see figure 12.19). They often result in the ventricles being in the refractory phase of depolarization when the normal sinus depolarization wave reaches the ventricle, and a compensatory pause develops. PVCs are among the most common arrhythmias seen with exercise testing and training in patients with CAD. If PVCs have the same shape, they originate from the same site (ectopic focus) and are called *unifocal*. Multiple-shape PVCs that likely originate from multiple sites in the ventricles are called *multifocal* and are much more serious than unifocal PVCs. The rhythm of normal contractions alternating with PVCs is called *bigeminy*; if every third contraction is a PVC, the rhythm is called *trigeminy*. Three or more consecutive PVCs are known as *ventricular tachycardia*. If a single PVC falls on the descending portion of the T wave, the ventricles can be thrown into fibrillation. PVCs adversely affect the prognosis of patients with CAD; generally, the more complex the PVC, the more serious the problem. Ellestad (9) showed that the combination of ST segment depression and PVCs increases the incidence of future cardiac events.

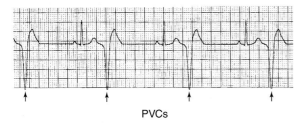

FIGURE 12.19 Premature ventricular contractions (PVC). The arrows indicate PVCs coming from a single ectopic focus in the ventricles (unifocal PVCs).

If a PVC occurs during pulse counting, an individual may report that their heart skipped a beat and therefore may undercount their HR. While an isolated skipped heartbeat does not typically warrant medical attention, if skipped heartbeats occur frequently or in succession, they could increase the risk for an adverse event during exercise. If an individual experiences regular skipped heartbeats, it might be appropriate to decrease the intensity of exercise or even stop the exercise session altogether. Clients should be advised to report the appearance of (or increase in) skipped beats to the fitness professional and their physician, especially if accompanied by symptoms including but not limited to light-headedness or dizziness.

Ventricular Tachycardia

Ventricular tachycardia is present whenever three or more consecutive PVCs occur (see figure 12.20). This situation is an extremely dangerous arrhythmia that can lead to ventricular fibrillation. The HR is usually 100 to 220 bpm, and the heart may be unable to maintain adequate cardiac output during ventricular tachycardia. Ventricular tachycardia can be caused by the same factors that initiate PVCs, and it requires immediate medical attention.

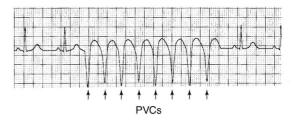
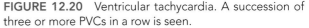

PVCs

FIGURE 12.20 Ventricular tachycardia. A succession of three or more PVCs in a row is seen.

Ventricular Fibrillation

Ventricular fibrillation is a life-threatening rhythm. It requires immediate cardiopulmonary resuscitation (CPR) until a defibrillator can be used to restore a coordinated ventricular contraction; otherwise, death will result. A fibrillating heart contracts in an unorganized, quivering manner, and the heart is unable to maintain significant cardiac output. P waves and QRS complexes are not discernible; instead, the electrical pattern is a fibrillatory wave (see figure 12.21).

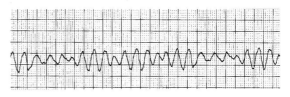

FIGURE 12.21 Ventricular fibrillation. When no P waves or QRS complexes are discernible, the heart contracts in a disorganized, quivering manner.

Automated External Defibrillators

Defibrillators are devices used to treat ventricular fibrillation. They send a momentary electrical shock to the heart, often causing the heart to return to its normal rhythm. Portable, battery-powered devices called *automated external defibrillators*, or AEDs, are available in many settings. The operator applies two surface electrodes to the person's chest. These electrodes are connected to the AED, which has software that determines the person's heart rhythm. If a shockable rhythm is detected, the AED gives a command to stand clear and then signals the operator to deliver a shock by pushing a button. All fitness professionals and health care providers should be certified in adult CPR and AED training. This can be done through organizations such as the American Heart Association and the American Red Cross. Research studies have shown that AEDs result in earlier treatment and greatly improve the chance of survival (2).

Myocardial Ischemia

Myocardial ischemia is a lack of oxygen in the myocardium attributable to inadequate blood flow. Obstruction of the coronary arteries is the most common cause of myocardial ischemia. A coronary artery is significantly obstructed if more than 50% of its diameter is occluded. A 50% reduction in diameter equals a loss of 75% of the arterial lumen (10). An obstructed coronary artery may supply an adequate blood flow at rest, but it probably will be unable to provide enough blood and oxygen during increased demand such as during exercise. Ischemia often, but not always, results in angina pectoris.

Angina pectoris is pain or discomfort caused by temporary, reversible ischemia of the myocardium that does not result in death or infarction of heart muscle. The pain often is located in the center of the chest, but it also can occur in the neck, jaw, or shoulders or can radiate into the arms and hands. Individuals may confuse angina pectoris with musculoskeletal pain and with the discomfort resulting from the sternal incision of coronary artery bypass surgery. Anginal pain generally does not alter with movements of the trunk or arms, whereas such movement can decrease or increase musculoskeletal pain.

Discomfort is probably not angina if the pain changes in quality or intensity when pressure is applied on the affected area (10). While angina is a common symptom of a heart attack for many, men and women may experience heart attack symptoms differently. Specifically, women may not experience angina in their chest at all during a heart attack. Instead, they may experience more subtle symptoms including light-headedness, dizziness, and shortness of breath (2a). Fitness professionals need to be aware of symptoms related to an acute cardiovascular event such as angina and be able to respond appropriately with follow-up questions or emergency protocols if necessary.

Myocardial ischemia can cause ST segment depression on the ECG during an exercise test. ST segment depression usually occurs at a relatively constant rate–pressure product. The rate–pressure product equals HR × SBP (systolic blood pressure), and it is a good estimate of the amount of work the heart is doing. Three types of ST segment depression are recognized: upsloping, horizontal, and downsloping (figure 12.22). Ellestad (9) has shown that the prognostic implications of upsloping and horizontal ST segment depression are roughly similar.

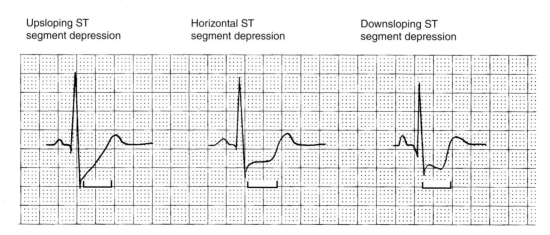

Upsloping ST segment depression   Horizontal ST segment depression   Downsloping ST segment depression

FIGURE 12.22   ST segment depression.

KEY POINT

The ECG can be used to detect disturbances in the electrical conducting system of the heart, such as first-, second-, or third-degree AV block. The ECG can also indicate arrhythmias (abnormal heart rhythms), including sinus arrhythmia, premature beats, ventricular tachycardia, atrial flutter, and atrial fibrillation. Abnormal rhythms may limit exercise performance by decreasing cardiac output. In the case of severe arrhythmias, the fitness professional should terminate the exercise session and obtain immediate medical assistance.

Downsloping ST segment depression, however, affects survival more adversely.

ST segment elevation also can occur during exercise testing. ST segment elevation during an exercise test usually indicates an aneurysm, or a weakened area of noncontracting myocardium or scar tissue.

Myocardial Infarction

If the myocardium is deprived of oxygen for a sufficient length of time, a portion of the myocardium dies; this partial death is called a *myocardial infarction (MI)*. Pain is the hallmark symptom of an MI. It is often very similar to anginal pain, only more severe, and it may be described as a heavy feeling, a squeezing in the chest, or a burning sensation. Other symptoms that may accompany an MI are nausea, sweating, and shortness of breath.

ST segment elevation is often the first ECG sign of an acute MI. Later, pronounced Q waves and T wave flattening or inversion may appear in certain leads. Over time, the ST segment changes subside and the T wave returns to normal (see figure 12.23) (12). Other clinical signs of an acute MI include elevations in cardiac muscle enzymes (serum lactate dehydrogenase and creatine phosphokinase), which leak into the blood after the myocardium is damaged (10).

The Framingham Heart Study demonstrated that up to 25% of MIs may be silent infarctions, meaning that the infarction does not cause sufficient symptoms for the person to seek medical attention (11). These silent infarctions may be recognized later during routine ECG examinations by the presence of significant Q waves in certain leads.

Patients with CAD should be instructed how to differentiate anginal attacks from possible MIs. If an anginal attack occurs, the patient should stop the activity, if any, that precipitated the discomfort and should take a nitroglycerin (NTG) tablet under the tongue. If the anginal discomfort persists after 5 minutes, the patient takes a second sublingual NTG tablet. This procedure is repeated, if needed, one more time. If the pain persists 5 minutes after the third NTG tablet, the patient should seek immediate medical attention (3).

KEY POINT

Inadequate blood flow to the myocardium often, but not always, results in symptoms of chest pain (angina pectoris). ST segment depression or elevation on the ECG can indicate inadequate blood flow (ischemia). Significant Q waves on the ECG can indicate that a portion of the heart muscle has died (MI).

Medications That Affect Heart Rate Response

Fitness professionals do not prescribe medications or deal on a day-to-day basis with people taking all of the medications discussed in chapter 2, but they do encounter participants taking some of them. Often drugs that do not specifically target cardiovascular function still affect the HR response to exercise, such as medications for smoking cessation, bronchodilators for asthma, medications to control blood glucose concentrations, and mood stabilizers such as antidepressants. It is worth noting that some drugs and medications can result in unique changes to the ECG tracing outside of HR and BP. For example, digoxin, a drug prescribed to treat heart failure or atrial fibrillation, can cause ST segment depression and induce other cardiac arrhythmias (9a). Other drugs that may provoke cardiac arrhythmias include nicotine and alcohol (2). A review of medications and their potential effects on exercise responses can be found in chapter 2.

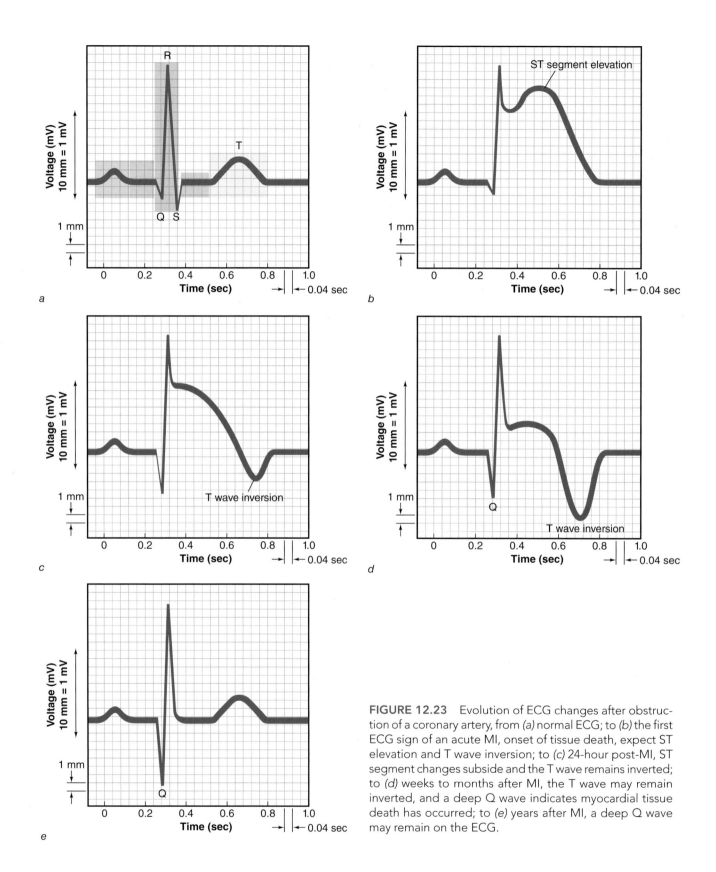

FIGURE 12.23 Evolution of ECG changes after obstruction of a coronary artery, from (a) normal ECG; to (b) the first ECG sign of an acute MI, onset of tissue death, expect ST elevation and T wave inversion; to (c) 24-hour post-MI, ST segment changes subside and the T wave remains inverted; to (d) weeks to months after MI, the T wave may remain inverted, and a deep Q wave indicates myocardial tissue death has occurred; to (e) years after MI, a deep Q wave may remain on the ECG.

LEARNING AIDS

REVIEW QUESTIONS

1. Draw a picture of the heart, and label the four heart chambers, the four heart valves, the pulmonary artery, and the aorta.

2. Name the coronary arteries, and identify to what region of the myocardium they supply blood.

3. Draw the major components of the heart's electrical conducting system, and label the SA node, AV node, bundle of His, left and right bundle branches, and Purkinje fibers.

4. Define the term *electrocardiogram (ECG)*, and give the standard settings for paper speed and amplitude.

5. Identify the electrical event in the heart that corresponds to the P wave, PR segment, QRS complex, and T wave of the ECG.

6. If an individual in normal sinus rhythm has 20 millimeters between two adjacent R waves, what is the HR? If an individual in atrial fibrillation has 11 complete cardiac cycles in a 6-second strip, what is the HR?

7. Describe the following conduction abnormalities: first-degree AV block, second-degree AV block (Mobitz type I and type II), and third-degree AV block.

8. What are the electrocardiographic signs associated with an MI (i.e., heart attack)? What are the symptoms of a heart attack?

CASE STUDIES

1. The following ECG tracing was obtained on a 38-year-old before they participated in a GXT on the treadmill.

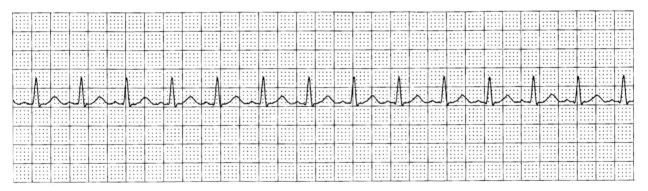

a. Determine the HR (bpm) and the durations of the PR interval, QRS complex, and QT interval (in seconds).

b. What condition does this individual have?

c. What factors might cause this condition?

2. A 75-year-old who reported being light-headed and fatigued came to the emergency room with the following ECG tracing at rest.

   a. What type of arrhythmia does this individual have?

   b. What is the ventricular rate?

3. A 57-year-old participant in your exercise program showed the following ECG tracing while exercising at 3.5 mph on a 6% grade on the treadmill.

   a. What ECG abnormality is shown?

Answers to Case Studies

1. For case study 1:

   a. HR = 1,500 ÷ 12 = 125 bpm

      PR interval duration = 0.12 seconds

      QRS complex duration = 0.08 seconds

      QT interval duration = 0.32 seconds

   b. Sinus tachycardia (HR is >100 bpm).

   c. Common causes of sinus tachycardia are anxiety, nervousness, caffeine, and low fitness.

2. For case study 2:

   a. Atrial fibrillation (jagged baseline with irregularly spaced PVCs).

   b. Ventricular rate = 6 cardiac cycles in a 6-second strip × 10 = 60 bpm.

3. For case study 3:

   a. Trigeminy (every third heartbeat is a PVC).

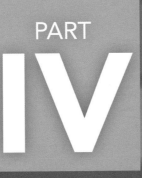

PART

IV

Exercise Prescription

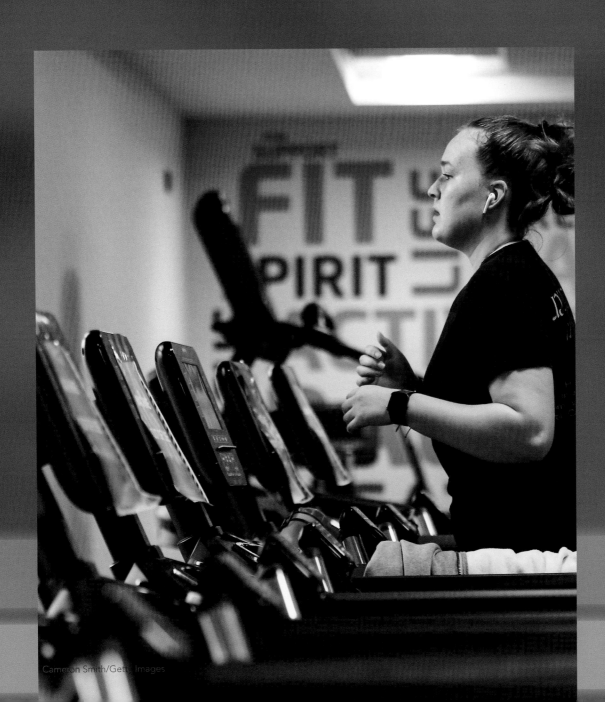

In part IV, guidelines for exercise programming are provided for cardiorespiratory fitness (chapter 13), muscular fitness (chapter 14), and flexibility and neuromotor fitness (chapter 15). Chapter 16 provides examples of how the various components of fitness can be incorporated into a training program. The degree to which a tissue such as bone, skeletal muscle, or cardiac muscle functions depends on the activity to which it is exposed. This statement summarizes the two major principles underlying training programs: overload and specificity.

The principle of overload describes a dynamic characteristic of living creatures: Use increases functional capacity. If a tissue or organ system is required to work against a load to which it is not accustomed, it becomes stronger. The corollary of the overload principle is the principle of reversibility, which indicates that physiological gains are lost when a tissue or organ system is not used. The common adage for this principle is "Use it or lose it." The variables that contribute to overload in an exercise program include intensity, duration, and frequency of exercise. It is the combination of these elements that results in a sufficient volume of exercise or activity to increase the functional capacity of a particular system.

The principle of specificity states that the training effects derived from an exercise program are specific to the exercise performed and the muscles involved. For example, a person who runs for exercise shows little change in the arm muscles. A person who exercises at a low intensity that recruits only slow-twitch muscle fibers will see little or no training effect in the fast-twitch fibers. If muscle fibers are not used, they cannot adapt, and thus they will not become trained. The type of adaptation that occurs as a result of training is specific to the type of training taking place (e.g., aerobic endurance versus heavy resistance training). Running increases the number of capillaries and mitochondria in the muscle fibers involved in the exercise, which makes them more resistant to fatigue. Resistance training causes hypertrophy of the muscles involved due to an increase in the amount of contractile proteins, actin and myosin, in the muscle.

13

Exercise Prescription for Aerobic Fitness

Barbara A. Bushman

OBJECTIVES

The reader will be able to do the following:

1. Characterize the dose of exercise in an exercise prescription and identify means by which a health-related effect might occur

2. Describe the public health recommendation for physical activity

3. Explain the concepts of overload and specificity as they relate to cardiorespiratory fitness (CRF) training programs

4. Describe general guidelines related to CRF programs, including those related to the warm-up and cool-down

5. Develop an exercise prescription with the exercise intensity, duration, and frequency needed to achieve and maintain CRF goals

6. Express exercise intensity in terms of energy production, heart rate, and relative effort

7. Describe the use of *high-intensity interval training (HIIT)*, including how it can be individualized for clients of varying fitness levels

8. Describe the differences between a supervised and an unsupervised program

9. Describe how temperature and humidity, altitude, and pollution affect exercise prescriptions

13

Higher levels of physical activity, exercise, and cardiorespiratory fitness (CRF) are linked to reduced risk of many chronic diseases and death from all causes (43, 31, 52, 70, 72, 71). Within Healthy People 2030 there are 358 measurable public health objectives covering a wide range of topics; a small subset of 23 high-priority core objects, referred to as *leading health indicators*, includes physical activity for adults (i.e., to meet current minimum guidelines for aerobic physical activity and muscle-strengthening activity) (75). This chapter focuses on CRF; figure 13.1 from Myers and colleagues (50) shows that as CRF increases, the risk of death decreases. This figure offers two important takeaways. First, the greatest decrease in risk occurs when moving from the lowest 20% (quintile) of CRF to the next level, and second, the risk continues to decrease with increases in fitness (more is better). The results from this study were consistent with those in the classic study of Blair and colleagues (7), which found that risk levels off at a CRF level of only 9 METs for women and 10 METs for men.

Achieving levels of physical activity and CRF consistent with a lower risk of chronic disease is achievable for most people. This knowledge forms the basis for the public health physical activity recommendations. Consequently, the primary purpose of this chapter is to show how to prescribe physical activity and exercise to improve CRF in adults. Later chapters present additional information on prescribing physical activity and exercise for children, older adults, and people with other conditions or known diseases.

Prescribing Exercise

The fitness professional's desire to know the proper dose of exercise needed to bring about a desired effect (response) closely parallels the physician's need to know the type and quantity of a drug needed to cure a disease. From a medical perspective, there is a difference between what is needed to treat a headache and what is needed to resolve a migraine. In the same way, the dose of phys-

ical activity required to achieve a high level of athletic performance is different from that required to improve a health-related outcome (e.g., lower blood pressure, lower risk of heart disease). Similarities can be drawn between the dose–response relationship for medications and that for exercise, which is shown in figure 13.2 (25). Consider these aspects that apply to both medications and exercise.

- *Potency:* The potency of a drug is a relatively unimportant characteristic in that it makes little difference whether the effective dose is 1 milligram or 100 milligrams as long as the drug can be administered in an appropriate dosage (25). Likewise in exercise prescriptions, walking 4 miles (6.4 kilometers) at a moderate pace is as effective in expending calories as running 2 miles (3.2 kilometers)—see chapter 6.

- *Slope:* The slope of the curve describes how much of an effect comes from a change in dose (25). Some physiological measures (e.g., heart rate and lactate response to a fixed exercise task) change quickly (in days) for a dose of exercise, whereas some health-related effects (e.g., changes in serum cholesterol) are realized only after many months of exercise.

- *Maximal effect:* The maximal effect (efficacy) of a drug varies with the type of drug. For example, morphine can relieve pain of all intensities, whereas aspirin is effective against only mild to moderate pain (25). Similarly, strenuous exercise can increase maximal oxygen consumption (also referred to as *maximal oxygen uptake*, or $\dot{V}O_2$max) and modify risk factors, whereas light to moderate exercise can improve risk factors but cause only a small increase in $\dot{V}O_2$max.

- *Variability:* The effect of a drug varies among and within individuals depending on the circumstances (25). In terms of exercise, gains in $\dot{V}O_2$max attributable to endurance training show considerable variation, even when controlling for the initial $\dot{V}O_2$max (15).

- *Side effect:* No drug produces a single effect (25), and the effects might include adverse (side) effects that

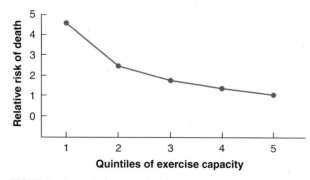

FIGURE 13.1 Relative risk of all-cause mortality to quintiles of exercise capacity (METs) among normal subjects.

Data from Myers et al. (2002).

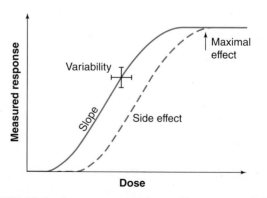

FIGURE 13.2 Representative dose–effect curve with four characterizing parameters.

Adapted from Goodman and Gilman (1975).

limit the usefulness of the drug. For exercise, the side effects may include muscle soreness or an increased risk of injury.

Unlike many drugs, which people stop taking when a disease or condition is resolved, physical activity is needed throughout life to promote its health-related and fitness effects. What factors make up the dose of exercise?

The dose of physical activity and exercise is described using the acronym FITT, which contains the following factors (5):

- *Frequency:* How often an activity is done. This can be expressed in days per week or number of times per day.
- *Intensity:* How hard the activity is. Intensity can be described in terms of %$\dot{V}O_2$max, % maximal heart rate (HR), and rating of perceived exertion (RPE).
- *Time:* The duration of the activity. This is typically expressed as the number of minutes a person engages in the activity.
- *Type:* The mode or kind of activity done.

RESEARCH INSIGHT

Physical Activity and Health Outcomes

With a foundation provided by the first *Physical Activity Guidelines for Americans* in 2008 (72), the second edition in 2018 (74) is based on a scientific report by an advisory committee with nearly 700 pages clearly reviewing the evidence-based recommendations on activity (73). The first sentence of the 2018 *Guidelines* provides a simple but encouraging summary: "Being physically active is one of the most important actions that people of all ages can take to improve their health" (74). The second edition reflects disease prevention benefits as well as other benefits (e.g., sleeping better) (74). The following list provides health benefits associated with regular physical activity that were found by the advisory committee to be rated at moderate or strong levels of evidence (74).

Children and Adolescents

- Improved bone health
- Improved weight status
- Improved cardiorespiratory and muscular fitness
- Improved cardiometabolic health
- Improved cognition
- Reduced risk of depression

Adults and Older Adults

- Lower risk of all-cause and cardiovascular disease mortality
- Lower risk of cardiovascular disease
- Lower risk of hypertension
- Lower risk of type 2 diabetes
- Lower risk of adverse blood lipid profile
- Lower risk of cancers (bladder, breast, colon, endometrium, esophagus, kidney, lung, stomach)
- Improved cognition
- Reduced risk of dementia
- Improved quality of life
- Reduced anxiety and risk of depression
- Improved sleep
- Slowed or reduced weight gain; weight loss; prevention of weight regain after initial weight loss
- Improved bone health
- Improved physical function
- Lower risk of falls and fall-related injuries for older adults

The FITT principle is useful because it allows the major elements of an exercise intervention to be altered to suit a given person. In addition, the product of frequency × intensity × time yields the volume of exercise, which is directly related to health benefits (see the next section for more details). Another element of an exercise prescription, progression, describes the manner in which a person transitions from easier to harder exercise, or increases the duration of activity, over the course of an intervention to continue to provide the necessary level of overload for improvement.

A great deal has been discovered about how much physical activity is needed to achieve a variety of health outcomes. The health-related benefits of physical activity are not dependent on an increase in CRF. That said, an increase in $\dot{V}O_2$max is associated with a decrease in the risk of many chronic diseases and death from all causes. Research studies support the positive effects of physical activity on health and disease. The *Physical Activity and Health Outcomes* Research Insight provides excellent information on the health benefits associated with regular physical activity across the lifespan.

KEY POINT

An exercise dose reflects the interaction of the intensity, frequency, duration, and type of exercise. Many health-related benefits are derived from participation in physical activity and exercise, and within limits, more is better. These benefits are not dependent on an increase in CRF, but there is no question that a higher level of CRF is related to a lower risk of chronic disease.

Short- and Long-Term Responses to Exercise

In addition to understanding the cause-and-effect connection between physical activity and specific outcomes, distinguishing between short-term (acute) and long-term (training) responses is valuable (29, 30). The responses in the days and weeks following the initiation of a dose of exercise can vary substantially, depending on the variable being measured:

- *Rapid responses:* Benefits occur early and plateau.
- *Linear responses:* Gains are made continuously over time.
- *Delayed responses:* Responses occur only after weeks of training.

The need for such distinctions can be seen in figure 13.3 (39), which shows proposed dose–response relationships between physical activity, defined as minutes of exercise per week at 60% to 70% of maximal work capacity, and a variety of physiological responses:

- Blood pressure (BP) and insulin sensitivity are most responsive to exercise, as shown by the curve on the left in figure 13.3.
- Changes in $\dot{V}O_2$max and resting HR are intermediate, as shown by the middle curve in figure 13.3.
- Serum lipid changes such as increases in high-density lipoprotein cholesterol (HDL) are delayed, as shown by the curve on the right in figure 13.3.

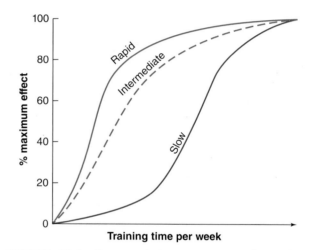

FIGURE 13.3 Proposed dose–response relationships between amount of exercise performed per week at 60% to 70% maximum work capacity and changes in BP and insulin sensitivity (curve on left), which appear most sensitive to exercise; $\dot{V}O_2$max and resting HR, which are parameters of physical fitness (middle curve); and lipid changes, such as increases in HDL (curve on right).

Data from Jennings et al. (1991).

The dose–response relationship of exercise has important implications when exercise is used alone or in concert with medication to control disease. Understanding that some benefits occur immediately (e.g., reduced feelings of anxiety, improved sleep, greater insulin sensitivity, reduced BP) while others take consistent engagement for weeks or months (e.g., increased CRF, sustained reduction in BP) helps give a realistic framework for an exercise program (74). Some improvements require ongoing and consistent engagement in physical activity. To retain benefits, this must be a lifelong commitment.

Public Health Recommendations for Physical Activity

Given the previous discussion, it should be no surprise that it is difficult to provide a single exercise prescription that addresses all the issues related to preventing and treating various diseases. Despite this, there is value in providing a general physical activity recommendation to improve the health status of all adults in the United States. The second edition of *Physical Activity Guidelines for Americans* provides clarity about the roles of moderate versus strenuous (vigorous) exercise in meeting the recommendation, and key guidelines related to aerobic activity include (74) the following:

- Adults should sit less and move more throughout the day. This reflects the concept that some physical activity is better than none.

- People can realize the health-related benefits of physical activity by doing 150 to 300 minutes of moderate-intensity activity per week, 75 to 150 minutes of vigorous-intensity activity per week, or an equivalent combination of the two. Aerobic activity preferably should be spread throughout the week.

- Additional health benefits can be achieved by engaging in activity beyond the equivalent of 300 minutes of moderate-intensity physical activity (i.e., more is better).

In addition, the *Guidelines* recommend muscle-strengthening activities on at least 2 days per week for additional health benefits (5). Muscular fitness programming is discussed in detail in chapter 14.

The health-related gains associated with physical activity are realized when the volume of physical activity is between 500 and 1,000 MET-min · wk^{-1} (74). Volume can be expressed in MET-min · wk^{-1} and is a way to summarize the frequency, intensity, and time of the activities included in CRF training program. *Moderate-intensity activity* is defined as absolute intensities of 3.0 to 5.9 METs or relative intensity of a level of effort of 5 or 6 on a 10-point scale (where 0 is sitting and 10 is maximal effort) (74). *Vigorous-intensity activity* is defined as intensities of 6.0 METs or more in absolute terms, or a relative intensity of an effort level of 7 or 8 on the 10-point scale (74). The use of MET-min · wk^{-1} is helpful to determine the volume for different activities.

- For example, walking at 3 mph (4.8 km · hr^{-1}) requires 3.3 METs, at the low end of the moderate-intensity range. If the person walks at this speed for 30 minutes, an energy expenditure of 99 MET-min (3.3 METs × 30 minutes) is achieved. If done 5 days per week, the weekly volume of activity is 495 MET-min.

- If a person were to jog at 5 mph or 8 km · hr^{-1} (8 METs) for 25 minutes, the volume would be 200 MET-min. If done 3 days per week, the weekly energy expenditure would be 600 MET-min.

- The reality that it takes about twice the time when doing moderate-intensity activity to achieve the same energy expenditure as when doing vigorous-intensity activity leads to the 2:1 ratio when comparing the time it takes to meet the guidelines for these intensities (150 minutes versus 75 minutes).

The duration of each bout of exercise is not specified within the *Physical Activity Guidelines for Americans*. Previously, bouts of activity of at least 10 minutes were required in order to be counted toward the weekly target (72). As new research has been conducted, health benefits have been found resulting from bouts of any length of moderate to vigorous physical activity; this finding is reflected in the current *Physical Activity Guidelines for Americans* (74). Spreading activity throughout the week is recommended (i.e., at least 3 days per week) because this will help reduce the risk of injury and prevent excessive fatigue (74).

KEY POINT

To achieve the physical activity energy expenditure associated with substantial health benefits, either moderate-intensity or vigorous-intensity physical activity can be used. The goal is to achieve between 500 and 1,000 MET-min · wk^{-1} of energy expenditure in physical activity.

General Guidelines for Cardiorespiratory Fitness Programs

As noted in the introduction to part IV, two principles are key to understanding training programs: overload and specificity. To improve CRF, activities that overload the heart and respiratory system need to be used. To overload is to require the organ systems in the body to work against a load to which they are not accustomed. Activities that involve the large muscle groups contracting in a rhythmic and continuous manner can provide overload to the cardiorespiratory system. Activities that involve a small muscle mass or resistance training exercises are less appropriate for gains in CRF because they tend to generate high cardiovascular respiratory loads relative to energy expenditure. Following are some general considerations for the fitness professional to keep in mind when helping someone start a CRF program.

Utilize Test Results

Part III of this book reviews various aspects related to fitness testing. Cardiorespiratory, or aerobic, fitness test results can help establish a baseline of CRF and can be used to compare to others of the same age (i.e., percentile rankings) for a general point of comparison. Given factors such as heredity, percentile rankings may be less meaningful for an individual client than comparing test results over time (see chapter 7 regarding use of percentiles for evaluation of fitness tests). Repeating tests after a period of training allows the fitness professional to gauge the effectiveness of the individual's training program, regardless of where a client may be in comparison to others. Details on tests for CRF are found in chapter 8.

Encourage Regular Participation

Physical activity and exercise must become a valuable part of a person's lifestyle. It should not be done sporadically, nor will doing it for only a few months or years build up a fitness reserve. Gains in CRF accomplished through aerobic activities are lost relatively quickly with inactivity (see chapter 4). Although some benefits of

activity may be immediate (e.g., reduction in feelings of anxiety, reduced BP, improved insulin sensitivity), CRF improvements will take time to develop and require continued physical activity to retain (74). Only people who continue activity as a way of life enjoy its long-term benefits (see chapter 22 for more on how to help clients establish healthy behaviors).

Provide a Variety of Activities

A fitness program often starts with easily quantified activities, such as walking or cycling, so that the proper exercise intensity can be achieved. After establishing a regular routine of physical activity and achieving some gains in fitness, a variety of activities (e.g., games, sports) can be included in the program, with attention on progressing from easier to more difficult activities.

Program for Progression

Given the importance of helping sedentary people become active, the emphasis in any health-related fitness program for such participants should be to start slowly and, when in doubt, do too little rather than too much. The adage "start low and go slow" is appropriate during early stages of an exercise program, to reduce risk of injury or cardiovascular events as well as to promote enjoyment and long-term adherence (5). A 10% increase in the number of minutes per week is a reasonable increase in the quantity of aerobic activity to minimize injury risk. The number of minutes per session and number of days per week should be gradually increased

Walking Program Progression

Guidelines

- Start at a level that feels comfortable.
- Warm up before each session.
- Be aware of aches and pains.
- Progress one stage when comfortable.
- Monitor HR, but do not be concerned about being in the THR zone.
- Walk at least 5 days per week.

Stage	Time (minutes)	Comments
1	10	Walk at a comfortable pace.
2	15	
3	20	Split into two 10-minute walks if needed.
4	25	
5	30	Do two 15-minute walks if preferred.
6	35	
7	40	Do two 20-minute walks if preferred.
8	45	Either continuous or a split plan is an option.

before increasing the intensity (72). For example, sedentary participants who are interested in jogging should begin a training program by walking a distance that they can complete without feeling fatigued or sore. With time, the participants will be able to walk farther and faster without discomfort. After they can walk several miles briskly without stopping, they can gradually work up to jogging continuously during each workout. When the participants are first ready to begin jogging, introduce the interval workout (alternating walking and jogging). As they adapt to the interval workouts, they will be able to gradually increase the amount of jogging while decreasing the distance walked (see the walking and running programs as examples of progression). Use of a target heart rate (THR) range can be incorporated into the program (this will be discussed in greater detail later in the chapter). The importance of gradual progression cannot be overemphasized, whether the client is a child, adult, or older adult (72, 74).

Adhere to Format for a Fitness Workout

The three parts of an exercise session include the warm-up, conditioning phase, and a cool-down (5). The main body of the CRF workout consists of dynamic activities using large muscle groups at an intensity high enough and a duration long enough to accomplish enough total work to specifically overload the cardiorespiratory system. A warm-up is a period that allows the body (i.e., physiology, biomechanics, and bioenergetics) to transition smoothly into the conditioning phase. A warm-up should include activities similar to the conditioning phase but at an intensity that is light to moderate (5). Similarly, a cool-down allows a gradual transition from the intensity of the conditioning phase back toward resting conditions.

There are physiological, psychological, and safety reasons for including the warm-up and cool-down. In general, the warm-up and cool-down should consist of the following:

- Activities similar to those in the main body of the workout but at a lower intensity (e.g., walking, jogging, or cycling below THR)
- Stretching exercises for the muscles involved in the activity with typically dynamic activities included in the warm-up and static stretching as part of the cool-down (5)

These activities help participants ease in to and out of a workout. The duration of the warm-up and cool-down will vary depending on the intensity level of the conditioning phase (5). The greater difference between rest and the intensity of the conditioning phase, the longer the warm-up and cool-down will need to be. In general, a minimum of 5 to 10 minutes should be allowed within an exercise session for the warm-up and 5 to 10 minutes for the cool-down (4).

Running Program Progression

Guidelines
- Complete a walking program first.
- Walk and engage in dynamic stretching before each session.
- Be aware of aches and pains.
- Progress one stage when comfortable.
- Stay at the low end of the THR zone by varying the time of the walk–jog interval or jogging pace. Use of a HR monitor is recommended to keep the HR measurement process as easy and simple as possible.
- Do the program every other day.

Stage	Time (minutes)	Comments
1	20-30	Jog 10 steps, walk 10 steps; repeat 5 times and check HR.
2	20-30	Jog 20 steps, walk 10 steps; repeat 5 times and check HR.
3	20-30	Jog 30 steps, walk 10 steps; repeat 5 times and check HR.
4	20-30	Jog 1 minute, walk 10 steps; repeat 5 times and check HR.
5	20-30	Jog 2 minutes, walk 10 steps; repeat 5 times and check HR.
6	×	Jog 1 lap on a track and check HR. Walk briefly and complete 4-6 laps.
7	×	Jog 2 laps on a track and check HR. Walk briefly and complete 4-6 laps.
8	20-40	Jog continuously and check HR.

Conduct Periodic Fitness Tests

Routine health-related fitness testing to determine a participant's progress can be motivational and may help alter programs that are not achieving desired results. The fitness professional can help by setting realistic goals for the next testing session when discussing test results. A general target might be a 10% improvement in 3 months in the test scores that need to change. Once the person has reached a desirable fitness level, the goal is to maintain that level.

KEY POINT

Following appropriate screening and fitness testing, an exercise program to promote CRF should be encouraged for life. The program should provide a variety of activities that use large muscle groups and overload the cardiorespiratory system, and the participant should start slowly and progress gradually to higher levels of work. The workout should have a warm-up and a cool-down, including stretching exercises. Periodic CRF tests can be used to adjust the exercise prescription to achieve client goals.

Formulating the Exercise Prescription

The CRF training effect depends on the degree to which the systems are overloaded; that is, it depends on the following variables in the FITT principle: frequency, intensity, time (duration), and type of exercise. The interaction of intensity (low to high), duration (short to long), and frequency (seldom to often) should result in a total energy expenditure (volume of exercise) of 500 to 1,000 MET-min · wk^{-1} (74). For 150 minutes of moderate-intensity activity, this is approximately 1,000 kcal · wk^{-1} (22).

Frequency

The recommended frequency of exercise is higher for moderate-intensity exercise (≥5 days per week) than vigorous-intensity exercise (≥3 days per week) in order to achieve the recommended volume of exercise. Figure 13.4 shows that improvements in CRF increase with the frequency of vigorous exercise sessions, with two sessions being the minimum and the gains in CRF leveling off after three to four sessions per week (53, 54). Gains in CRF can be achieved in 2 days per week, but the intensity has to be higher than a program with 3 days per week, and weight-loss goals might be difficult to achieve (53). Figure 13.4 shows that exercising for more than

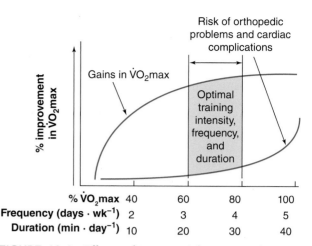

FIGURE 13.4 Effects of increased frequency, duration, and intensity of exercise on $\dot{V}O_2$max.

4 days per week at a vigorous intensity seems to be too much for previously sedentary people, resulting in more dropouts and injuries and less psychological adjustment to the exercise (13, 53). This figure demonstrates the increasing risk of orthopedic problems attributable to exercise sessions that are too long or conducted too many times per week. The probability of cardiac complications increases with exercise intensity beyond that recommended for improving CRF.

Intensity

How hard a person has to work to sufficiently overload the cardiovascular and respiratory systems to increase CRF differs for each client given individual fitness status and goals. This section includes various methods to express and apply exercise intensity to provide an appropriate level of overload for a client.

• *Percentage of maximal oxygen consumption (%$\dot{V}O_2$max)*: Across a broad range of CRF levels, many physiological responses are normalized (i.e., made similar between individuals) when the intensity of exercise is expressed as a percentage of $\dot{V}O_2$max (%$\dot{V}O_2$max). This approach has been used extensively to develop exercise guidelines, as can be seen in ACSM's *Guidelines for Exercise Testing and Prescription* and the ACSM position stand "Quantity and quality of exercise for developing and maintaining cardiorespiratory, musculoskeletal, and neuromotor fitness in apparently healthy adults: Guidance for prescribing exercise" (5, 22).

• *Percentage of oxygen uptake reserve (%$\dot{V}O_2$R)* (3, 4): This method may better place individuals at similar intensity levels above rest (46). $\dot{V}O_2$R is calculated by subtracting 1 MET (3.5 ml · kg^{-1} · min^{-1}) from the subject's $\dot{V}O_2$max. One MET (or 3.5 ml · kg^{-1} · min^{-1}) reflects $\dot{V}O_2$rest. When calculating $\dot{V}O_2$R, the units of measure for max and rest must be the same (i.e., ml · kg^{-1} · min^{-1}). For example, if a client's $\dot{V}O_2$max is 35 ml · kg^{-1} · min^{-1}, the $\dot{V}O_2R$ is $35 - 3.5$ ml · kg^{-1} · min^{-1} = 31.5 ml · kg^{-1} · min^{-1}. When calculating a particular %$\dot{V}O_2R$, first calculate $\dot{V}O_2R$ by subtracting $\dot{V}O_2$rest from the $\dot{V}O_2$max, multiply that value by the desired intensity (percentage expressed as a decimal), and then add $\dot{V}O_2$rest:

$$\%\dot{V}O_2R = [(\dot{V}O_2max - \dot{V}O_2rest) \times \%] + \dot{V}O_2rest$$

Given that $\dot{V}O_2$rest is assumed to be 3.5 ml · kg^{-1} · min^{-1} (1 MET), the equation can be simplified as the following:

$$\%\dot{V}O_2R = [(\dot{V}O_2max - 3.5) \times \%] + 3.5$$

For instance, if the target intensity for that client is 60%$\dot{V}O_2R$, the calculations would be as follows:

$$60\% \dot{V}O_2R = [(35 - 3.5) \times 0.60] + 3.5$$
$$60\% \dot{V}O_2R = [(31.5) \times 0.60] + 3.5$$
$$60\% \dot{V}O_2R = 18.9 + 3.5$$
$$60\% \dot{V}O_2R = 22.4 \text{ ml} \cdot \text{kg}^{-1} \cdot \text{min}^{-1}$$

The %$\dot{V}O_2R$ equals the HR response when HR is expressed as a percentage of the heart rate reserve (HRR), as discussed next (66, 67). This relationship is further explored in the sidebar *Differences in %$\dot{V}O_2$max and %$\dot{V}O_2R$.*

- *Percentage of HRR (%HRR):* The HRR is calculated by subtracting resting HR from maximal HR. The %HRR

Differences in %$\dot{V}O_2$max and %$\dot{V}O_2R$

For many years, %HRR was believed to be linked to %$\dot{V}O_2$max on a one-to-one basis; that is, 60% HRR = 60% $\dot{V}O_2$max. However, Swain and colleagues (66, 67) pointed out that although this is the case when fit people exercise vigorously, it is not the case for low intensities of exercise. In comparing a range of HR that takes resting HR into consideration (i.e., HRR) but not doing so with $\dot{V}O_2$, an error is introduced. Swain and Luetholtz provide a theoretical comparison: one individual with a 5-MET capacity (low CRF) and another individual with a 20-MET capacity (high CRF) (66). At rest (i.e., 1 MET), the individual with a 5-MET capacity would be at 20% of their $\dot{V}O_2$max (1 MET ÷ 5 METs), whereas the individual with a 20-MET capacity would be at 5% (1 MET ÷ 20 METs). As exercise intensity increases and approaches maximal levels, this difference will be less (i.e., the difference between %HRR and %$\dot{V}O_2$max is inversely proportional to exercise intensity). The difference is also of greater impact for individuals with lower fitness (i.e., difference between %HRR and %$\dot{V}O_2$max is inversely proportional to fitness level) (66). An advantage of expressing exercise intensity as %$\dot{V}O_2R$ is the numerical match to %HRR across the fitness continuum (i.e., 60% $\dot{V}O_2R$ = 60% HRR).

Differences in the percentage ranges for $\dot{V}O_2$max are most apparent at the lower intensity levels, especially for low CRF, as shown in this table:

Intensity	%$\dot{V}O_2$max relative to maximal aerobic capacity in METs		
	20 METs	10 METs	5 METs
Very light	<34	<37	<44
Light	34-42	37-45	44-51
Moderate	43-61	46-63	52-67
Vigorous	62-90	64-90	68-91
Near-maximal to maximal	≥91	≥91	≥92

Adapted by permission from C.E. Garber, B. Blissmer, M.R. Deschenes, et al., "Quantity and Quality of Exercise for Developing and Maintaining Cardiorespiratory, Musculoskeletal, and Neuromotor Fitness in Apparently Healthy Adults: Guidance for Prescribing Exercise," *Medicine and Science in Sports and Exercise* 43, no.7 (2011): 1334-1359.

As can be seen looking across the various fitness levels in each row, the percentage of max is very similar at the high intensity levels (e.g., near-maximal to maximal is at or above 91% or 92%) but differences emerge at lower intensity levels. For the lower fitness level (i.e., 5 METs), the very light intensity is 44% $\dot{V}O_2$max, whereas average or higher fitness levels (i.e., 10 METs or 20 METs) would be at only 34% or 37% $\dot{V}O_2$max. The differences are relatively small between individuals of average or high CRF, compared to what is observed for those with lower CRF, especially at lower intensity levels.

is a percentage of the difference between resting and maximal HR and is calculated by subtracting resting HR from maximal HR, multiplying by the desired percentage (percentage expressed as a decimal), and then adding resting HR:

$$\%HRR = [(HRmax - HRrest) \times \%] + HRrest$$

A 20-year-old man has a target exercise intensity of 60% HRR. If he has a maximal HR of 200 bpm and a resting HR of 60 bpm, for a target intensity set at 60%HRR, the calculations would be as follows:

$$60\%HRR = [(200 - 60) \times 0.60] + 60$$

$$60\%HRR = 144 \text{ bpm}$$

- *Percentage of maximal HR (%HRmax):* Because of the linear relationship between HR (above 110 bpm) and $\dot{V}O_2$ during dynamic exercise, investigators and clinicians have long used a simple percentage of maximal HR (%HRmax) to estimate $\%\dot{V}O_2$max in setting exercise intensity. This method may be useful when a resting HR is not available.

- *Rating of perceived exertion (RPE):* The RPE is not viewed as a substitute for prescribing exercise intensity by HR but can be used to refine or modify a prescribed intensity (3). The RPE may not consistently translate to the same intensity for different modes of exercise, so do not expect the RPE to exactly match a %HRmax or %HRR (4).

Table 13.1 shows the categories of exercise intensity as noted within the ACSM position stand (22) and current ACSM *Guidelines* (5). Intensities range from very light to maximal. In the Physical Activity Guidelines Advisory Committee Scientific Report, three absolute intensity categories are outlined (73):

1. *Light-intensity activity defined as non-sedentary waking behavior:* <3 METs
2. *Moderate-intensity activity:* 3.0 to 5.9 METs
3. *Vigorous-intensity activity:* 6 METs or more

Absolute intensity does not take into account an individual's CRF, so relative values are typically used within an exercise prescription. The RPE values are based on the Borg RPE scale (8). Ranges for $\%\dot{V}O_2R$, %HRR, %HRmax, and $\%\dot{V}O_2$max are listed along with the absolute exercise intensities (in METs) for each of the intensity classifications. Table 13.1 allows the fitness professional to classify data on exercise intensity, whether they are expressed in oxygen consumption, HR, or RPE.

A broad range of exercise intensities can be used to achieve CRF goals. Highly trained individuals will exercise at the top end of the range of vigorous and even to maximal levels (5). In contrast, those who are moderately trained may find 70% to 80% $\dot{V}O_2$max to be an adequate stimulus for improvement in CRF (5). Lower intensity levels (i.e., moderate range) are more suitable for people who are deconditioned, and for some with very low levels of CRF, even light intensity can provide opportunity for improvement in CRF. This reflects the need to have a good understanding of an individual's current CRF when determining an appropriate intensity. For individuals starting an exercise program, moderate-intensity physical activity is valuable given it can be carried out long enough to achieve health-related benefits and perhaps gains in CRF. Although the range of intensities reflecting moderate and vigorous is quite broad, the fitness

Table 13.1 Classification of Physical Activity Intensity

Intensity	%HRR or %$\dot{V}O_2$R	%HRmax	%$\dot{V}O_2$max	RPE (6-20 RPE scale)	Absolute intensity in METs
Very light	<30	<57	<37	Very light <9	<2.0
Light	30-39	57-63	37-45	Very light to fairly light 9-11	2-2.9
Moderate	40-59	64-76	46-63	Fairly light to somewhat hard 12-13	3-5.9
Vigorous	60-89	77-95	64-90	Somewhat hard to very hard 14-17	6-8.7
Near-maximal to maximal	≥90	≥96	≥91	Very hard ≥18	≥8.8

%$\dot{V}O_2$R = percentage of oxygen uptake reserve, %HRR = percentage of heart rate reserve, %HRmax = percentage of maximal heart rate, RPE = Borg rating of perceived exertion 6-20 scale, %$\dot{V}O_2$max = percentage of maximal oxygen consumption

Adapted by permission from C.E. Garber, B. Blissmer, M.R. Deschenes, et al., "Quantity and Quality of Exercise for Developing and Maintaining Cardiorespiratory, Musculoskeletal, and Neuromotor Fitness in Apparently Healthy Adults: Guidance for Prescribing Exercise," *Medicine and Science in Sports and Exercise* 43, no. 7 (2011): 1334-1359.

professional will need to individualize and narrow the recommended range of intensity based on many factors including current CRF, age, health status, medical concerns, and goals. The following may be considered as general guidelines rather than strict parameters:

- For the average, apparently healthy sedentary person, an appropriate range of exercise intensities at which to begin is within 40% to 60% HRR.
- For adults who are physically active and at the high end of the fitness scale, intensities greater than 80% HRR may be required for CRF improvements.
- For most people who are cleared to participate in a structured exercise program, progression over time to an intensity within the range of 60% to 80% HRR likely will provide a suitable target exercise intensity.

Figure 13.4 shows that exercise at the high end of the scale has been associated with more orthopedic problems and cardiac complications (13, 33). Exercise intensity must be balanced against duration so that the person can exercise long enough to expend 500 to 1,000 MET-min · wk^{-1}, the higher volume being consistent with greater improvements in CRF and greater reductions in chronic disease risk factors (72, 71). If the exercise intensity is too high, the person may not be able to exercise long enough to achieve the desired energy expenditure.

Time (Duration)

How many minutes of exercise should a person do per session? Figure 13.4 shows that improvements in $\dot{V}O_2$max increase with the duration of the exercise session. However, the optimal duration of an exercise session depends on the intensity. The total work or volume of exercise accomplished in a session is the most important variable determining CRF gains once the minimal intensity threshold is achieved (4). If the goal were to accomplish 300 kcal of total work in an exercise session in which the participant works at 10 kcal · min^{-1} (2 liters of O_2 per minute), the duration of the session would have to be 30 minutes. If the person were working at half that intensity, 5 kcal · min^{-1}, the duration would have to be twice as long. A half hour of exercise can be accomplished in many ways—for example, one 30-minute session or separated into shorter sessions such as two 15-minute sessions or three 10-minute sessions. Figure 13.4 also shows that when the duration of hard exercise (75% $\dot{V}O_2$max) exceeds 30 minutes, the risk of orthopedic injury increases (53).

Type (Mode)

A wide range of activities can be used to promote improvements in CRF. For individuals who are starting out at lower levels of fitness, activities such as walking, easy cycling, or water aerobics may be selected (5). More vigorous activities, such as jogging, running, rowing, spinning, and elliptical exercise, may be considered for those with at least an average level of CRF and who are regularly active (5). These activities require minimal skill. In contrast, other modes of exercise will require the participant to have a certain skill level to be able to perform the activity at an appropriate intensity (e.g., swimming, cross country skiing, or skating) (5). Recreational sports provide a great variety of options for those who regularly engage in aerobic activities and have a good CRF; examples include hiking, racquet sports, soccer, and other team sports (5). Thus, the fitness professional must carefully work with their client to select activities that are within the skill level, as well as the fitness level, of the client. Additionally, finding activities that are easily accessible and the client enjoys will help promote adherence to an exercise program (see chapter 22 for ways to help participants make a lifelong habit of activity).

KEY POINT

CRF improves across a broad range of exercise intensities. The intensity threshold for a training effect is lower (<60% HRR) for people who are sedentary, and it is higher (>80% HRR) for people who are physically active and have high CRF. A general range of training intensity to work toward over time for the average person is approximately 60% to 80% HRR. The duration of an exercise session should balance the exercise intensity to result in an energy expenditure of 500 to 1,000 MET-min · wk^{-1}, the higher volume being consistent with greater improvements in health benefits and CRF. The optimal frequency of training, based on improvement in CRF and a low risk of injuries, is 3 to 4 days a week for exercise intensities rated as hard. Selection of the type of activity should take into account both current CRF and skill level of the client.

Program Design

Designing an exercise program for a particular client requires consideration of many factors. This section focuses on methods to determine appropriate exercise intensity.

Metabolic Load

The most direct way to determine target exercise intensity is to use a percentage of the measured maximal oxygen consumption. A typical range of exercise intensities associated with improved CRF in people who are ready to move from moderate-intensity physical activity to a vigorous-intensity exercise program is 60% to 80% $\dot{V}O_2$max. Take note of the overlap in the range of moderate to vigorous intensity. The advantage of measuring oxygen consumption to determine exercise intensity is that the method is based on the criterion test for CRF—maximal oxygen consumption. The major disadvantages are the expense and difficulty of measuring oxygen consumption for each person and trying to suit specific fitness activities to meet the specific metabolic demand for each person.

QUESTION:

A 33-year-old male, with a body weight of 75 kilograms, completes a maximal graded exercise test (GXT), and his $\dot{V}O_2$max is 45 ml · kg^{-1} · min^{-1} or 12.9 METs. Consulting the normative chart in chapter 8, the percentile for his aerobic fitness is around the 60th percentile. At what exercise intensities should he work to be at 60% to 80% $\dot{V}O_2$max (upper moderate category to middle range of the vigorous category)?

ANSWER:

60% of 45 ml · kg^{-1} · min^{-1} = 27 ml · kg^{-1} · min^{-1}

80% of 45 ml · kg^{-1} · min^{-1} = 36 ml · kg^{-1} · min^{-1}

60% of 12.9 METs = 7.7 METs

80% of 12.9 METs = 10.3 METs

Consequently, he should use activities that require the following:

27 to 36 ml · kg^{-1} · min^{-1}
7.7 to 10.3 METs

When these exercise intensity values are known, appropriate exercises can be selected from tables listing the energy costs of various activities (e.g., Compendium of Physical Activities is discussed in chapter 6). However, this is a cumbersome method for prescribing exercise. Calculations can be used to determine walking or running, cycling, and stepping workloads as described in *Using Metabolic Calculations Within Exercise Prescription*. This can be helpful in providing a starting point for an exercise prescription. However, this does not take into consideration the effect that environmental (e.g., heat, humidity, altitude, cold, pollution), dietary (e.g., hydration state), and other variables have on a person's response to some absolute exercise intensity. The ability of participants to complete a workout depends on their physiological responses and perception of effort rather than only the metabolic cost of the activity itself. Fortunately, by using HR values that are approximately equal to 60% to 80% $\dot{V}O_2$max, it is possible to formulate an exercise prescription that takes many of these factors into consideration. These HR values form the THR range, which is discussed in the next section.

Using Metabolic Calculations Within Exercise Prescription

In chapter 6 calculations to determine energy expenditure for various activities (walking, running, leg and arm ergometry, and stepping) are discussed. These equations also can be used to determine a target workload. In this scenario, the $\dot{V}O_2$ is known and an aspect of the activity in question is to be determined (e.g., treadmill speed or grade, resistance on the flywheel of an ergometer, the step rate or step height).

Return to the example of the client with a $\dot{V}O_2$max of 45 ml · kg^{-1} · min^{-1} for whom 60% $\dot{V}O_2$max was calculated to be 27 ml · kg^{-1} · min^{-1}. If exercising on a treadmill two aspects of the work must be stipulated: speed and grade. With a level treadmill, he would be running at a speed of 4.4 mph, as shown in the following calculations:

$$\dot{V}O_2 = (0.2 \text{ ml} \cdot \text{kg}^{-1} \cdot \text{min}^{-1} \times \text{horizontal velocity})$$
$$+ (0.9 \text{ ml} \cdot \text{kg}^{-1} \cdot \text{min}^{-1} \times \text{vertical velocity}) + 3.5 \text{ ml} \cdot \text{kg}^{-1} \cdot \text{min}^{-1}$$

Or more simply:

$$\dot{V}O_2 = (0.2 \times \text{speed}) + (0.9 \times \text{speed} \times \text{grade}) + 3.5$$

Insert the known values for $\dot{V}O_2$ and grade:

$$27 = (0.2 \times \text{speed}) + (0.9 \times \text{speed} \times 0) + 3.5$$

$$27 = (0.2 \times \text{speed}) + (0) + 3.5 \text{ [subtract 3.5 from both sides of the equation]}$$

$$23.5 = 0.2 \times \text{speed [divide both sides of the equation by 0.2]}$$

$$117.5 = \text{speed}$$

Speed is in m · min^{-1}, so to express in mph divide by 26.8. Thus the running pace will be 4.4 mph.

A similar series of calculations for the 80% $\dot{V}O_2$max would result in a treadmill speed of 6.1 mph (calculated speed of 162.5 m · min^{-1} is divided by 26.8 to express in mph) with no grade on the treadmill. If the client would prefer a slower running pace at this upper intensity, calculations can determine the grade required to match this intensity. For example, if the client feels comfortable with 5.0 mph (134 m · min^{-1}), determine the grade as follows:

$$\dot{V}O_2 = (0.2 \times speed) + (0.9 \times speed \times grade) + 3.5$$

Enter what is known/desired for $\dot{V}O_2$ and speed:

$$36 = (0.2 \times 134) + (0.9 \times 134 \times grade) + 3.5 \text{ [multiply values within parentheses]}$$

$$36 = 26.8 + (120.6 \times grade) + 3.5 \text{ [subtract 26.8 and 3.5 from both sides]}$$

$$5.7 = 120.6 \times grade \text{ [divide both sides by 120.6]}$$

$$0.05 = grade$$

Thus, a grade of 5% if running at 5 mph also would provide a work rate at 80% $\dot{V}O_2$max.

A similar process can be followed for use with cycling (leg or arm); equations for each are included in chapter 6. The following shows calculations for 60% $\dot{V}O_2$max intensity with leg ergometry (recall the client's body weight is 75 kilograms):

$$\dot{V}O_2 = (1.8 \times work\ rate\ in\ kgm \cdot min^{-1} \div body\ weight\ in\ kg) + 3.5 + 3.5$$

Enter the known values of $\dot{V}O_2$ and body weight:

$$27 = (1.8 \times work\ rate \div 75) + 3.5 + 3.5 \text{ [subtract 7 (3.5 + 3.5) from both sides of the equation]}$$

$$20 = 1.8 \times work\ rate \div 75 \text{ [divide both sides by 1.8 and multiply both sides by 75]}$$

$$833 = work\ rate$$

If exercising on a Monark leg ergometer (distance per revolution is 6 m· rev^{-1}) at 60 rpm, the kilogram resistance on the flywheel will be 2.3 kilograms. This is calculated using the equation including the three components of work rate:

$$kgm \cdot min^{-1} = 6\ m \times 60\ rpm \times kg$$

For this example:

$$833 = 6 \times 60 \times kg \text{ [divide both sides by 6 × 60]}$$

$$2.3 = kilograms$$

For stepping on a 0.25-meter step, here is the equation for calculating stepping rate for 60% $\dot{V}O_2$max:

$$\dot{V}O_2\ (ml \cdot kg^{-1} \cdot min^{-1})$$
$$= (0.2 \times step\ rate) + (1.8 \times 1.33 \times step\ rate \times step\ height\ in\ meters) + 3.5\ ml \cdot kg^{-1} \cdot min^{-1}$$

Enter the known values:

$$27 = (0.2 \times step\ rate) + (1.8 \times 1.33 \times step\ rate \times 0.25) + 3.5$$
$$\text{[subtract 3.5 from both sides of the equation and multiply values within parentheses]}$$

$$23.5 = (0.2 \times step\ rate) + (0.60 \times step\ rate) \text{ [add these together]}$$

$$23.5 = (0.8 \times step\ rate)$$

$$29 = steps$$

The fitness professional can use this information as a starting point that can be refined with the use of HR and RPE within the exercise prescription.

Target Heart Rate

As described in chapters 4 and 8, HR increases linearly with the metabolic load. When HR is monitored at each stage of a maximal GXT, HR then can be plotted on a graph against the $\dot{V}O_2$ (or MET) equivalents of each stage of the test. The fitness professional determines the THR range by taking the percentages of $\dot{V}O_2max$ (%$\dot{V}O_2max$) at which the person should train and finding what the HR responses were at those points. Figure 13.5 shows this method being used for a subject with a functional capacity of 10.5 METs. Work rates of 60% to 80% of maximal METs demanded HR responses of 132 to 156 bpm. The HR values become the intensity guide for the subject and represent the THR range (3).

In contrast to this direct method of graphing the relationship between $\dot{V}O_2max$ and HR, two other methods can be used to estimate an appropriate THR: the HRR method and the %HRmax method.

Heart Rate Reserve Method

The HRR method of determining THR range was made popular by Karvonen (42). HRR is the difference between resting and maximal HR. For a maximal HR of 200 bpm and a resting HR of 60 bpm, the HRR is 140 bpm (200 − 60 = 140). As shown in figure 13.6, the percentage of the HRR equals the percentage of $\dot{V}O_2R$ across the range of exercise intensities (66, 67). For participants with average to high levels of CRF, %HRR approximately equals %$\dot{V}O_2max$; this is not the case for those with lower CRF or at low intensities, as described in *Differences in %$\dot{V}O_2max$ and %$\dot{V}O_2R$.*

QUESTION:

A 40-year-old male participant has a measured maximal HR of 175 bpm and a resting HR of 75 bpm. What is his THR range as calculated by the HRR method?

ANSWER:

$$HRR = 175 \text{ bpm} - 75 \text{ bpm} = 100 \text{ bpm}$$

$$60\% \text{ of } 100 \text{ bpm} = 60 \text{ bpm,}$$
$$\text{and } 80\% \text{ of } 100 \text{ bpm} = 80 \text{ bpm}$$

$$60 \text{ bpm} + 75 \text{ bpm} = 135 \text{ bpm for } 60\% \dot{V}O_2R$$

$$80 \text{ bpm} + 75 \text{ bpm} = 155 \text{ bpm for } 80\% \dot{V}O_2R$$

The advantages of using this procedure to determine exercise intensity are that the recommended THR is between the person's resting and maximal HRs and the %HRR equals the %$\dot{V}O_2R$ across the entire range of CRF. Although the resting HR varies and can be influenced by factors such as caffeine, lack of sleep, dehydration, emotional state, and training, this variation does not introduce serious errors into calculating the THR by the HRR method (28). Consider the following example.

QUESTION:

The 40-year-old subject mentioned previously participates in an endurance training program, and his resting HR decreases by 10 bpm. Because maximal HR (175 bpm) is not affected by training, what happens to his THR range?

ANSWER:

$$HRR = 175 \text{ bpm} - 65 \text{ bpm} = 110 \text{ bpm}$$

$$60\% \text{ of } 110 \text{ bpm} = 66 \text{ bpm} + 65 \text{ bpm} = 131 \text{ bpm}$$

$$80\% \text{ of } 110 \text{ bpm} = 88 \text{ bpm} + 65 \text{ bpm} = 153 \text{ bpm}$$

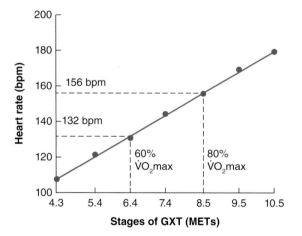

FIGURE 13.5 Direct method of determining the THR zone when maximal aerobic power (functional capacity) is measured during a GXT.

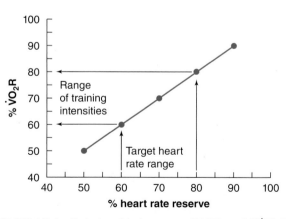

FIGURE 13.6 Relationship between %HRR and %$\dot{V}O_2R$.
Adapted from Swain et al. (1998).

Consequently, the change in resting HR had only a minimal effect on the THR range.

Percentage of Maximal Heart Rate Method

Another method of determining THR range is to use a fixed percentage of the %HRmax. The advantage of this method is its simplicity and the fact that it has been validated across many populations (33, 45, 64). Figure 13.7 shows the relationship between %HRmax and %$\dot{V}O_2$max.

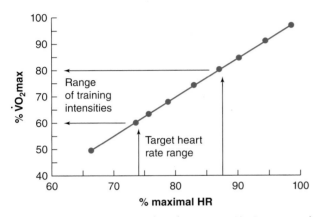

FIGURE 13.7 Relationship between %HRmax and %$\dot{V}O_2$max.

Adapted from Londeree and Ames (1976).

The %HRmax and %$\dot{V}O_2$max are linearly related, and %HRmax can be used to estimate the metabolic load in training programs. A general target of 70% to 85% HRmax equals approximately 55% to 75% $\dot{V}O_2$max and results in an intensity prescription that is slightly more conservative than that generated by the HRR method when 60% to 80% of HRR is used. For a similar calculated THR, a range of 75% to 90% HRmax can be used. The fitness professional must keep in mind that these ranges are guides and the intensity selected for a given client may be higher or lower depending on age, health status, current activity, and goals. The following example shows how to use the %HRmax method to calculate the THR range.

QUESTION:

How can a THR range be calculated if the resting HR is unknown? Use the data from the 40-year-old subject mentioned previously, who had a measured maximal HR of 175 bpm.

ANSWER:

Take 70% and 85% of the maximal HR:

70% of 175 bpm = 122 bpm

85% of 175 bpm = 149 bpm

These values are slightly more conservative than those calculated using the HRR method described earlier. If 75% to 90% HRmax is used, the outcome is a range of 131 to 158 bpm, which is more like the values calculated using the HRR methods (135-155 bpm). These slight differences underscore that the THR ranges are general guides to help a participant achieve a desired intensity. Table 13.2 shows the general relationship between %$\dot{V}O_2$max and %HRmax across the range of exercise intensities from 50% to 85% $\dot{V}O_2$max. Using this table can be helpful in making intensity recommendations by using the %HRmax method.

Table 13.2 Relationship of %HRmax and %$\dot{V}O_2$max

%$\dot{V}O_2$max	%HRmax
50	66
55	70
60	74
65	77
70	81
75	85
80	88
85	92

Adapted from Londeree and Ames (1976).

Threshold

As mentioned earlier, the intensity of exercise that provides an adequate stimulus for cardiorespiratory improvement varies with activity level and age and generally spans the range from moderate- to vigorous-intensity exercise. In a systematic review of the literature, Swain and Franklin sought to clarify the low end of the threshold range. They found that the threshold for improvement in $\dot{V}O_2$max was only 30% HRR for people with $\dot{V}O_2$max values less than 40 ml · kg^{-1} · min^{-1} and only 46% HRR for people with higher $\dot{V}O_2$max values; however, higher intensities more effectively increased $\dot{V}O_2$max (65). Consequently, for much of the population, target intensity falls in the following ranges:

- 60% to 80% of HRR and $\dot{V}O_2$R
- 75% to 90% of HRmax

Threshold levels will vary based on the participant's characteristics. For example, an older sedentary individual will have a much lower threshold than a younger, fit person. The middle of the range (70% HRR, 70% $\dot{V}O_2$max, or 80% HRmax) is an average training intensity and is generally appropriate for the typical apparently healthy person who wishes to be involved in a regular fitness program. Participating in activities at these intensities constitutes an overload on the cardiorespiratory system, resulting in adaptation over time. The fitness professional will need to develop a progression that fits client characteristics and goals. Note that all values are given as ranges; some clients may begin below the ranges and others at the lower or higher ends of the ranges. Individualization is key.

Maximal Heart Rate

The methods for determining exercise intensity use HRmax, and although a measured HRmax (from a maximal GXT) is most accurate, this is not typically available. If HRmax cannot be measured, any estimation must consider the effect of age. Previously, HRmax had been estimated by subtracting age in years from 220. However, this formula tends to overestimate HRmax for younger adults and underestimates HRmax for older adults. Tanaka, Monahan, and Seals (68) evaluated the validity of the classic formula of 220 – age for estimating HRmax. They analyzed 351 published studies and cross-validated these findings with a well-controlled laboratory study. They found almost identical results for both studies: HRmax = 208 – (0.7 × age). This new formula yields HRmax values that are 6 bpm lower for 20-year-olds and 6 bpm higher for 60-year-olds. Although the new formula yields better estimates of HRmax on average, the investigators emphasize that the estimated HRmax for a given individual is still associated with an SD (standard deviation) of 10 bpm. Other equations are also available, including this estimate by Gellish and colleagues (23): HRmax = 207 – (0.7 × age). This is associated with a SD of 5 to 8 bpm (23).

Any estimate of HRmax is a potential source of error for both the HRR and the %HRmax methods of calculating a THR. For example, given that 1 SD of this estimate of HRmax is about 10 bpm, a 45-year-old's true HRmax may statistically be anywhere between 145 and 205 bpm (3 SD, which reflects 99.7% of data assuming a normal distribution) rather than the estimated 175. However, 68% (1 SD) of the population would be between 165 and 185 bpm. If the HRmax is known (e.g., from a GXT), the fitness professional should use this measured HRmax to determine THR rather than using the estimate with its potential error (45). Estimating HRmax is another reason for using caution when relying solely on the THR range as an indicator of exercise intensity. The potential for error exists both in the estimate of HRmax and in the equations in which various percentages of HRmax are used to predict %$\dot{V}O_2$max. The intensity levels should only be considered as guidelines (see the sidebar *Error Involved in Estimating Intensity From HR*).

Progression Using THR and RPE

The concept of an intensity threshold provides the basis for regular fitness workouts. The THR can be used as an intensity guide for large muscle–group, continuous, whole-body activities such as walking, running, swimming, rowing, cycling, skiing, and dancing. With improvements in CRF, clients will be able to increase the work rate and/or duration of their exercise sessions.

The THR range associated with moderate- to vigorous-intensity activity is 40% to 89% HRR; for people who are less active and have more risk factors, lower THR ranges can be used. For example, moderate-intensity activity, equal to only 40% to 59% HRR, typically are within the capabilities of most people and carry a low risk of injury or complications (72). That is why it is the best starting place for most sedentary deconditioned people. Further, many clients may wish to continue doing moderate-intensity activity and not move to vigorous-intensity activity because it suits them and they can work it into

Error Involved in Estimating Intensity From HR

The two HR methods (%HRR and %HRmax) for estimating exercise intensity are simply guidelines to use in an exercise program, and small differences between methods highlight this. Both approaches must be used as guides rather than set absolute values because, as for any prediction equation, an error is involved in estimating the %$\dot{V}O_2$max value. For example, when HR is 81% HRmax, it is estimated that a person is at 70% $\dot{V}O_2$max (see table 13.2). In reality, 68% (1 SD) of the true values are between 64% and 76% $\dot{V}O_2$max for that HR value, and there is no way to know exactly where in that range any individual is (44). Because of this uncertainty, the calculated THR values should be used as guidelines in helping clients increase or maintain CRF. The fitness professional needs other indicators of exercise intensity to compensate for some of the inherent uncertainty in the THR prescription (see later in this chapter).

their schedule. More active people with fewer risk factors can use the upper end of the THR range. The THR can be divided by 6 to provide the desired 10-second THR if a person is taking a manual HR (e.g., palpating the radial pulse). Given the wide availability of technology, many individuals will prefer to use a HR monitor to keep track of HR during exercise rather than stopping to palpate pulse. By checking HR regularly during an exercise session, intensity can be adjusted higher or lower to allow HR to be in the THR range. Using the THR to set exercise intensity has many advantages:

- It has a built-in individualized progression (i.e., as people increase their fitness, they have to work harder to achieve the THR).

- It accounts for environmental conditions (e.g., a person decreases the intensity while working in hot temperatures).

- It is easily determined, learned, and monitored.

These recommendations are appropriate for most people, but individuals differ in terms of the threshold needed for a training effect, the rate of adaptation to the training, and how exercise feels to them. The fitness professional also may use subjective judgment based on observations of the person exercising to determine whether the intensity should be higher or lower. If the work is so easy that the person experiences little or no increase in ventilation and can work without effort, the intensity should be increased. At the other extreme, if a person shows signs of working very hard and is still unable to reach THR, a lower intensity should be chosen. In this case, the top part of the THR range might be above the person's true HRmax because the formula to determine maximal HR based on age only roughly estimates the true value. The fitness professional should not rely on the THR as the only method of judging whether the participant is exercising at the correct intensity; attention should be paid to other signs and symptoms of overexertion. The Borg RPE scale might be useful in this regard.

The Borg RPE scale that is used to indicate the subjective sensation of effort experienced during a GXT (see chapter 8) can be used in prescribing exercise for the apparently healthy person (8). The RPE for the various intensity levels is shown in table 13.1. In *Physical Activity Guidelines for Americans*, a 10-point relative intensity (level-of-effort) scale was recommended, with 5 or 6 being moderate intensity and 7 or 8 being vigorous intensity (72, 74). The RPE or relative intensity scale is not a substitute for prescribing exercise intensity by HR (4). However, if the HRmax is not known and the THR range is perceived as too low or too high, a relative rating can estimate the overall effort experienced by the person,

and the exercise intensity then can be adjusted accordingly. Further, as a participant becomes accustomed to the physical sensations experienced when exercising at the THR range, the need to frequently measure the pulse rate will decrease.

Interval Training

The various guidelines presented thus far have focused on moderate to vigorous aerobic activity that is done in a continuous fashion. When done at a moderate intensity, this has been referred to as moderate-intensity continuous training (MICT). In the past 10 years, the number of research articles focused on high-intensity interval training (HIIT) has dramatically increased. Although descriptions and protocols for HIIT are numerous, a general description is episodic short bouts of high-intensity exercise separated by short periods of recovery at a lower intensity (12). HIIT protocols have been divided into three categories based on the intensity of the intervals (12):

1. Intensities greater than $\dot{V}O_2max$ (also referred to as *sprint interval training*, or SIT)

2. Near-maximal interval training as shown by 90% to 100% of HRmax or $\dot{V}O_2max$

3. Vigorous aerobic intensity as shown by 60% to 89% $\dot{V}O_2R$ or 64% to 90% $\dot{V}O_2max$

The work-to-rest ratio is a key aspect of HIIT training, reflecting the duration and intensity of the work periods, the durations and intensity of the recovery or rest periods, and how many total intervals (work:rest) are to be performed (20). An example is a 4 × 4 protocol including four intervals of 4 minutes at an intensity of 85% to 95% peak HR with 3 minutes of recovery between intervals at about 70% peak HR (49). As shown in the example, this training can be customized by changing intensity of the work period and/or rest period, duration of the work period and/or rest period, and/or number of work:rest repetitions (which will affect total time). Other aspects include selection of exercise mode and weekly frequency.

HIIT training focuses on the intensity within an exercise session and thus may be appealing in lowering the exercise volume and time required (20). HIIT has the potential to improve CRF as well as promote improvement in various risk factors including insulin sensitivity, BP, and body composition; the improvement in risk factors is similar to that observed with MICT and is more likely to be seen in adults who are overweight or obese (12). The use of HIIT within various populations, including clinical applications, is a rapidly expanding area of research and appears to be a safe and viable option with appropriate screening and monitoring (20, 69). For example, interval training is included in a joint position statement by the European Association for Cardiovascular Prevention and Rehabilitation, the American Association of Cardiovascular and Pulmonary Rehabilitation, and the Canadian Association of Cardiac Rehabilitation; this position statement highlights improvements in aerobic capacity and various aspects of cardiorespiratory function (49).

Although studies have shown benefits, the position statement recommends further research on the feasibility, long-term effects, and safety aspects (49). As with any training program, the fitness professional must carefully check for any contraindications to exercise (see chapter 2) and review the health screening questionnaire. As noted, intensity is a key feature. Given that the intensity is relative to an individual's peak aerobic capacity and peak HR, actual activities will differ based on a person's fitness (40). An individual with a high level of fitness may be running for the work interval while an individual with lower fitness may be walking; both would experience the same relative exercise stress. (40). A wide range of relative intensities can be used for the work interval. For example, in a study comparing continuous and interval walking for individuals with type 2 diabetes, the interval walking alternated between fast walking (above target of 70% peak energy expenditure rate) and slow walking (41). Adjusting the intensity within the work interval allows for individualization of HIIT for a wide range of clients and abilities.

KEY POINT

The exercise intensity for a CRF training effect can be described in a variety of ways: $\dot{V}O_2R$ (HRR), %HRmax, and with a relative intensity scale. Continuous or interval training can be considered within a program to improve CRF.

When Moderate-Intensity Exercise May Be Hard

The *Physical Activity Guidelines for Americans* (74) recommend 150 min · wk⁻¹ or more of moderate-intensity (3-5.9 METs) physical activity. The fitness professional must recognize that the range of 3 to 5.9 METs may be moderate exercise for some but hard exercise for others. Figure 13.8 shows that the relative intensity for a fixed exercise varies considerably across the range of $\dot{V}O_2$max values (38, 71). Consequently, some people with low $\dot{V}O_2$max values would function in the intensity range consistent with achieving gains in $\dot{V}O_2$max, whereas those with higher CRF values would not. This example emphasizes the need to consider the THR range and RPE when following recommendations that specify absolute exercise intensities (e.g., METs).

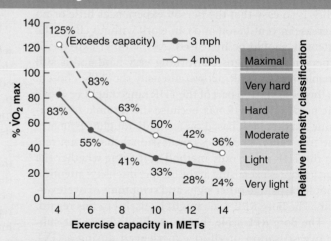

FIGURE 13.8 Relative exercise intensity for walking at 3.0 mph (4.8 km · hr⁻¹ or 3.3 METs) and 4.0 mph (6.4 km · hr⁻¹ or 5.0 METs) expressed as a percent of $\dot{V}O_2$max for adults with an exercise capacity ranging from 4 to 14 METs.

From U.S. Department of Health and Human Services (DHHS), *Physical Activity Guidelines Advisory Committee Report 2008*, Fig, D.1, (2008), D-7.

Putting Together an Individualized Prescription

Determining a starting intensity for each client will differ. Consider the following individual, a 35-year-old male who wants to start to be active following an annual physical during which his physician recommended the value of physical activity:

Weight: 100 kilograms

Height: 1.80 meters

Resting BP: 142/86

Resting HR: 80 bpm

Cholesterol: 198 mg/dL (total)

Activity level: Sedentary—desk/office job

Medication: Mevacor (Lovastatin)

Estimated $\dot{V}O_2$max from submax bike test: 33.0 ml $\cdot$ kg^{-1} $\cdot$ min^{-1}

Risk factors (see table 2.2) include the following: BMI (over 30 kg $\cdot$ m^{-2} with a calculated BMI of 30.9 kg $\cdot$ m^{-2}), BP (both SBP and DBP are in the hypertensive range), lipids (the medication is a statin, which is a lipid-lowering medication), and physical inactivity. His estimated $\dot{V}O_2$max is in the 15th percentile (see table 8.2), and he is not currently active.

How should an initial exercise intensity be determined?

Some aspects that provide a framework for determining a starting intensity are the client's current level of fitness (very low in comparison to other males of his age) and activity (sedentary job and no current activity program). When starting an exercise program, recall the adage "Start low, and go slow." Looking at table 13.1, a focus on the lower aspect of the moderate-intensity range would be a reasonable starting point: 40% to 50% HRR or $\dot{V}O_2$R.

Because a measured maximal HR is not available, an estimate can be calculated using this equation: HRmax = 207 − (0.7 × age). With an estimated HRmax of 182 bpm and a known HRrest of 80 bpm, the 40% to 50% HRR range would be 121 to 131 bpm. Workload guidance could be provided by a similar range of 40% to 50% $\dot{V}O_2$R (calculated to be 15.3-18.2 ml $\cdot$ kg^{-1} $\cdot$ min^{-1}). Using the metabolic equations (see sidebar *Using Metabolic Calculations Within Exercise Prescription*), work rate information can be provided for the treadmill, the ergometer, or stair climbing. Additionally, because the HRmax was estimated and thus may under- or overestimate the client's actual HRmax, adding a relative intensity recommendation (e.g., a level 5 or 6 on a 10-point scale) would be recommended.

In determining the frequency and duration, the fitness professional must work with the client to explore what time limitations may be in place and what steps can be taken to provide scheduled time for activity. Reflecting on "Start low, go slow," a reasonable first week might include 10 minutes per day on at least 3 days of the week. Adding time to each session, or adding days per week, should be continued until reaching at least 30 minutes on at least 5 days per week. At that point, duration can be continued to be increased or, to continue to provide an overload if time is a limiting factor, a slight decrease in time while increasing the intensity is another way to progress the program (followed by a gradual increase in time at the higher intensity level). No one prescription or method of progression is recommended. The fitness professional must work with the client within the framework of current fitness and activity status, along with realities of life and work responsibilities, to develop a program that can be part of their life, for their life.

Exercise Programming to Reach Goals

Certain general recommendations can be made for anyone wanting to begin a fitness program. Although the fitness professional might wish to have each client undergo a complete testing protocol before beginning exercise, that may not be possible. In addition, people without known health problems who follow these general guidelines can begin to exercise at low risk. The coronary heart disease (CHD) risks of continuing not to exercise are greater than those of beginning a moderate-intensity exercise program, so not requiring a fitness test prior to beginning to exercise is of benefit. Figure 13.9 summarizes general recommendations for achieving health, fitness, and performance goals. On the left side, the focus on health is the starting place for most sedentary deconditioned individuals (72). Picture a continuum from this entry point toward the level needed for fitness. No structural barrier exists between what is needed for health and what is needed for fitness. The high end of moderate intensity (59% HRR) is similar to the low end of vigorous intensity (60% HRR); think of the two categories as a continuum to realize many of the same benefits. The fitness professional's challenge is to match the starting point to the client's status and progress the client through a program in a manner that is safe and consistent with the client's goals, which may change as fitness improves. On the right side of figure 13.9, the level of training for performance requires a progression beyond the levels for health and fitness.

Exercise recommendations for people who are regularly active and have achieved a reasonable level of physical fitness tend to be associated with less risk, and these participants require less supervision. People who become fit can simply continue their program using the guidelines in the middle box of figure 13.9. As fitness improves, higher absolute intensities of exercise (e.g., faster jogging speeds) will be needed for the HR to stay in the THR range. Some people in this group may want to focus on performance, in contrast to health and fitness, as the primary goal. A wide variety of programs, activities, races, and competitions are available to address the needs of this group.

Training for competition demands more than the training intensity needed for health and fitness. As figure 13.9 shows, people interested in performance who work at the top end of the THR range, exercise 5 to 7 or more times each week, and exercise for longer than 60 minutes each exercise session are doing much more than those interested in fitness, and it should be no surprise that they tend to experience more injuries (72). Carefully progressed training programs with appropriate periodization should be applied to lower risk of overtraining (see chapter 16 for a discussion of overtraining syndrome) and lower the risk of overuse injuries.

Exercise Prescriptions Using Complete Graded Exercise Test Results

In many situations, the exercise recommendations are based on general information about the people involved (e.g., age, estimated CRF from submaximal test). In other situations, potential participants have had a general medical exam or a maximal GXT with appropriate monitoring of HR, BP, and possibly electrocardiogram (ECG) responses. Fitness professionals can make exercise recommendations using information about the person's functional capacity and cardiovascular responses to graded exercise. The fitness professional is not generally involved in the clinical evaluation of a GXT, but understanding the procedures used to make clinical judgments clearly enhances communication with the program director, exercise physiologist, and physician. The following information on using GXTs for exercise prescription and programming is within this framework.

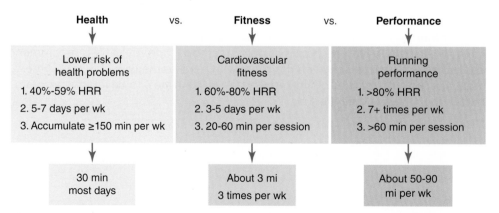

Health	vs.	Fitness	vs.	Performance
Lower risk of health problems		Cardiovascular fitness		Running performance
1. 40%-59% HRR		1. 60%-80% HRR		1. >80% HRR
2. 5-7 days per wk		2. 3-5 days per wk		2. 7+ times per wk
3. Accumulate ≥150 min per wk		3. 20-60 min per session		3. >60 min per session
30 min most days		About 3 mi 3 times per wk		About 50-90 mi per wk

FIGURE 13.9 Contrasting recommendations for achieving health, fitness, and performance goals.

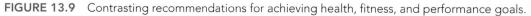

Using Graded Exercise Tests for Exercise Prescription and Programming

Analyzing a Graded Exercise Test for Exercise Prescription

1. Analyze the person's history and list the known risk factors for CHD; also, identify those factors that might have a direct bearing on the exercise program, such as orthopedic problems, previous physical activity, and current interests.

2. Determine if the functional capacity is a true maximum or if it is limited by a sign or symptom. Express the functional capacity in METs, and record the highest HR and RPE achieved without significant signs or symptoms.

3. If ECG was monitored, itemize the person's ECG changes as indicated by the physician.

4. Examine the HR and BP responses to see if they are normal.

5. List the symptoms reported at each stage.

6. List the reasons why the test was stopped (e.g., ECG changes, falling SBP, fatigue).

Designing an Exercise Program From a Graded Exercise Test

1. Given the overall response to the GXT, decide to either refer for additional medical care or initiate an exercise program.

2. Identify the THR range and approximate MET intensities of selected activities needed to be within that THR range.

3. Specify the frequency and duration of activity needed to meet the goals of increased CRF and weight loss.

4. Recommend that the person (a) participate in either a supervised or an unsupervised program, (b) be monitored or unmonitored, and (c) do group or individual activities.

5. Select a variety of activities at the appropriate MET level that allow the person to achieve THR. Consider environmental factors, medication, and any physical limitations of the participant when making this recommendation.

Program Selection

Exercise program options include exercising alone, in small groups, in fitness clubs, and in clinically oriented settings. The fitness professional must consider a variety of factors before recommending participation in a supervised or an unsupervised program.

Supervised Program

The risk factors, the response to the GXT, the health and activity history, and personal preference influence the type of program in which a client should participate. Generally, the higher the risk, the more important it is that the person participate in a supervised program. People at high risk for CHD and those who have diseases such as diabetes, hypertension, asthma, and CHD should be encouraged to participate under supervision, at least at the beginning of an exercise program. The personnel in the supervised program are trained to provide the necessary instruction in the appropriate activities, to help monitor the participant's response to the activity, to provide encouragement, and to administer appropriate first aid or emergency care.

Supervised programs run the gamut from those conducted within a hospital for patients with CHD and other diseases to programs conducted in fitness clubs for people at low risk for CHD. In general, as a person moves along the continuum from inpatient to outpatient, less formal monitoring is required. In addition, the background and training of the personnel tend to vary. Exercise programs aimed at maintaining the fitness level of CHD patients who have gone through a hospital-based program have medical personnel and emergency equipment appropriate for the population being served. Supervised fitness programs for the apparently healthy have a fitness professional who can focus more on the appropriate exercise and other lifestyle behaviors needed to improve health.

The supervised program offers a socially supportive environment for people to become and stay active. This is important, given the difficulty of changing lifestyle behaviors (see chapter 22). The group program allows for more variety in activities (e.g., group games) and reduces the chance of boredom. For the program to be effective in the long run, the program leader should try to wean the participants from the group in a way that encourages them to maintain their activity patterns when they are no longer in the program.

Unsupervised Program

Despite the risks just described, the many people at risk for or already having CHD have limited access to exercise programs within healthcare settings (18). Reasons for this include the limited number of supervised programs, the level of interest of the participant and physician in such programs, and the financial resources required to participate in such programs.

Participation in an unsupervised exercise program requires the fitness professional or physician (see chapter 2 for more on medical clearance) to clearly communicate how to begin and maintain the exercise program. The emphasis in beginning an unsupervised exercise program is on low to moderate intensity (i.e., 40%-50% $\dot{V}O_2R$), because the threshold for a training effect is lower in deconditioned people. The goal is to increase the duration of the activity, with exercise frequency approaching every day. This reduces the chance of muscular, skeletal, or cardiovascular problems caused by the exercise intensity and increases muscle function with the expenditure of a relatively large number of calories. In addition, the regularity of the exercise program encourages a positive habit. As with all programs, individualization is foundational to promoting safety and efficacy of the exercise program. The outcome of such programs results in participants being able to conduct their daily affairs with more comfort and sets the stage for people who would like to exercise at higher levels.

KEY POINT

Exercise recommendations for the general public emphasize moderate intensity (40%-59% HRR) and regular participation. Exercise performed at 60% to 80% HRR for 20 to 40 minutes 3 or 4 days per week increases and maintains CRF. Exercise recommendations for very fit individuals emphasize the top end of the training intensity (>80% $\dot{V}O_2R$) and frequent (almost daily) participation. The potential for injury is greater for such performance-driven workouts. For people who undergo a comprehensive diagnostic GXT with ECG monitoring, all test results are used to select an optimal and safe exercise prescription. Participants with multiple risk factors for CHD and those with existing diseases benefit from participating in a supervised program. For individuals who participate in an unsupervised program, clear communication about the exercise prescription and safety concerns is vital.

Updating the Exercise Program

During participation in an aerobic training program, the capacity for work increases. The best sign of this is that the recommended exercise is no longer sufficient to reach THR; clearly the person is adapting to the exercise. Taking the HR during a regular activity session provides a sound basis for upgrading the intensity or duration of the exercise session.

The exercise program, including the THR, should be updated periodically. This is particularly important for those with a lower initial level of fitness and a greater number of risk factors. In a clinical environment, a person who has a low functional capacity because of heart disease, orthopedic limitations, or chronic inactivity has difficulty reaching a true maximum on a first treadmill test. Further, individuals starting an exercise program often will experience the greatest improvements in the shortest time during the fitness program. This person benefits from frequent retesting because the test allows progress (or the lack thereof) to be monitored, and it may give new information that influences the exercise prescription. In contrast, an established exerciser, for whom smaller, more gradual changes would be expected, might benefit from retesting less frequently (e.g., annually or semiannually).

If the client has had a change in medication that influences the HR response to exercise, the exercise program must be reevaluated, especially if the exercise prescription was originally based on the initial HR response. These issues are found more in clinical rehabilitation programs, but as Exercise is Medicine initiatives (www.exerciseismedicine.org) are enacted, fitness professionals will have to become more aware of how to help patients make a transition to fitness facilities. See the sidebar *Exercise is Medicine and the Fitness Professional* for more on this initiative. Background information on various medication categories is found in chapter 2.

APPLICATION POINT

Exercise is Medicine and the Fitness Professional

Exercise is Medicine is an initiative "to make physical activity assessment and promotion a standard in clinical care, connecting health care with evidence-based physical activity resources for people everywhere and of all abilities" (17). Fitness professionals with appropriate credentials and background are key within the initiative because patients can be referred to them for exercise programming (18). Developing a relationship with health care providers is a potential opportunity for the fitness professional to be part of the promotion of exercise.

Environmental Concerns

THR is used to indicate the proper exercise intensity in health-related fitness programs. However, environmental factors such as heat, humidity, pollution, and altitude can elevate HR and RPE during an exercise session, which may shorten the session and reduce the participant's chance of expending sufficient calories to meet energy balance goals. This section discusses the effects of various environmental factors on the exercise prescription and what the fitness professional can do about them.

Heat and Humidity

Chapter 4 describes the increases in body temperature that occur with exercise, the mechanisms of heat loss called into play, and the benefits of becoming acclimatized to the heat. Core temperature (37 °C, or 98.6 °F) is within a few degrees of a value that could lead to death by heat injury. As described in chapter 23, to prevent a progression from the least to the most serious heat injury, people should recognize and attend to a series of stages from heat cramps to heatstroke. Preventing the problem in the first place is a better approach than treating the problem after it has occurred.

Each of the following factors influences susceptibility to heat injury and can alter the HR and metabolic responses to exercise (55):

- *Fitness:* Fit people have a lower risk of heat injury (2, 24), can tolerate more work in the heat (16), and acclimatize to heat faster (10).

- *Acclimatization:* Exercising for 7 to 14 days in the heat increases the capacity to sweat, initiates sweating at a lower body temperature, and reduces salt loss. Body temperature and HR responses are lower during exercise, and the chance of salt depletion is reduced (2, 4, 10).

- *Hydration:* Inadequate hydration reduces sweat rate and increases the chance of heat injury (2, 10, 61, 62). See *Sweating and Fluid Intake* for insights on ensuring adequate fluid intake (6) and additional information in chapter 5 on hydration.

- *Environmental temperature:* Exercising in temperatures greater than skin temperature results in a heat gain by convection and radiation. Evaporation of sweat must compensate for this gain if body temperature is to remain at a safe level.

- *Clothing:* As much skin surface as possible should be exposed in order to encourage evaporation, although the skin should be protected from the sun by using sunblock. Materials should be chosen that wick sweat to the surface for evaporation; materials impermeable to water increase the risk of heat injury and should be avoided.

- *Humidity (water vapor pressure):* Evaporation of sweat depends on the water vapor pressure gradient

Sweating and Fluid Intake

Prolonged exercise in the heat will result in more sweat loss than is replaced by fluids. Paying attention to fluid consumption before, during, and after activity in the following ways is recommended.

- Starting off with a normal level of hydration is the goal at the start of exercise. Consuming 5 to 7 milliliters of water or sport beverage per kilogram body weight at least 4 hours prior to exercise is recommended (60).

- During exercise it is more difficult to provide specific recommendations because many factors have an impact on hydration such as clothing, intensity of the activity, length of the activity, training status, heat acclimatization, and genetic factors (60). Monitoring body-weight changes can provide some insight, and postactivity body weight should be no more than 2% below preactivity body weight (60). For longer activity sessions, sport drinks, which contain carbohydrate (6%-8% carbohydrate) and electrolytes, may be helpful. The sodium in sport drinks can help encourage fluid consumption by stimulating thirst (60).

- Following an activity session, the goal is to replace fluid and electrolytes. Normal hydration typically can be restored with normal meals and snacks, along with a sufficient volume of water (60). Inclusion of items with sodium can stimulate thirst and help with fluid retention (60).

Thus, fluid intake is important but should not exceed sweat losses. Exercise-associated hyponatremia can occur when too much fluid is consumed, resulting in the lowering of plasma sodium concentration (60). Symptoms include headache, vomiting, confusion, and disorientation, and, with extreme cases, can result in seizure, coma, and death (60). Thus, balance is needed to ensure adequate, but not excessive, amounts of fluid are consumed.

between skin and environment. In warm and hot environments, relative humidity is a good index of the water vapor pressure, with a lower relative humidity facilitating the evaporation of sweat.

- *Metabolic rate:* During times of high heat and humidity, decreasing the exercise intensity decreases the heat load as well as the strain on the physiological systems that must deal with it.

- *Wind:* Wind places more air molecules in contact with the skin and can influence heat loss in two ways: If there is a temperature gradient for heat loss between the skin and the air, wind will increase the rate of heat loss by convection. In a similar manner, wind increases the rate of evaporation, assuming the air can accept moisture.

Recommendations for Fitness

Members of a fitness program should be educated about all of the heat-related factors just mentioned. The fitness professional might suggest the following:

- Learning about the symptoms of heat illness (e.g., cramps, light-headedness) and how to deal with them (see chapter 23)
- Exercising in the cooler parts of the day to avoid heat gain from the sun or from building or road surfaces heated by the sun

- Gradually increasing exposure to high heat and humidity over 7 to 14 days to safely acclimatize to the environmental conditions
- Hydrating before, during, and after exercise and weighing in each day to monitor hydration (see chapter 5 for more information on hydration)
- Taking HR measurements several times during the activity and reducing exercise intensity to stay in the THR zone

The last recommendation is very important: HR is a sensitive indicator of dehydration, environmental heat load, and acclimatization, and variation in any of these factors will modify the HR response to any fixed submaximal exercise. It is therefore important for fitness participants to monitor HR regularly and slow down to stay within the THR zone. RPE also can be used in extreme heat to provide an index of the overall physiological strain that the participant is experiencing.

Environmental Heat Stress

Two measures can be helpful in gauging the impact of the environment: heat index and wet-bulb globe temperature (WBGT). Heat index takes into account temperature and relative humidity (moisture in the atmosphere). See figure 13.10 for combinations of temperature and relative

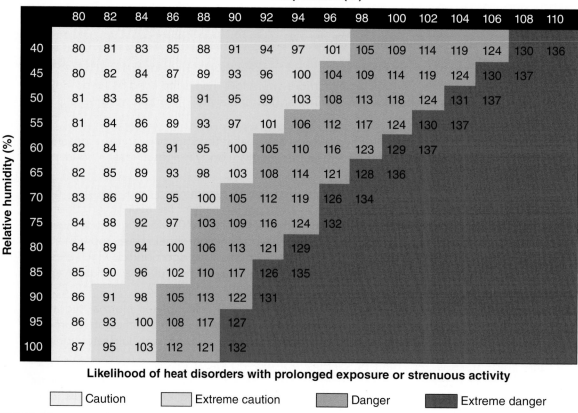

Likelihood of heat disorders with prolonged exposure or strenuous activity

Caution   Extreme caution   Danger   Extreme danger

FIGURE 13.10 Heat index.

From "Heat Forecast Tools, Likelihood of Heat Disorders with Prolonged Exposure or Strenuous Activity," NOAA National Weather Service. Available: https://www.weather.gov/images/safety/heatindexchart-650.jpg.

humidity that warrant caution or avoiding activity due to the likelihood of heat disorders.

In contrast to heat index, which reflects how the temperature feels in a shady area, WBGT takes into account heat stress when in direct sunlight (51). WBGT considers temperature, humidity, and other factors such as solar radiation and wind speed. To do this, three thermometers are used: wet bulb reflects relative humidity, black globe for solar factor, and dry bulb for ambient temperature (51). See figure 13.11 for an example of WBGT equipment.

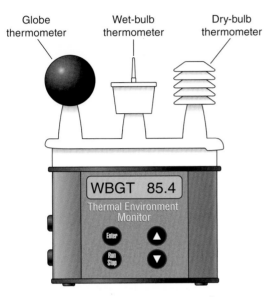

FIGURE 13.11 WBGT equipment example.

From NOAA National Weather Service. Available: www.nws.noaa.gov.

The risk of hyperthermia (heat illness), including exertional heat stroke (EHS), attributable to environmental stress while wearing shorts, socks, shoes, and a T-shirt is rated on the following scale (2):

WBGT exceeds 27.9 °C (>82.1 °F) Extreme risk of hyperthermia; cancel or postpone

WBGT = 25.7 to 27.8 °C (78.1-82.0 °F) Extreme caution; high risk for unfit, nonacclimatized

WBGT = 22.3 to 25.6 °C (72.1-78.0 °F) Extreme caution; risk of hyperthermia increased for all

WBGT = 18.4 to 22.2 °C (65.1-72.0 °F) Caution: moderate risk of hyperthermia; high-risk people should be monitored or not compete

WBGT 10.1 to 18.3 °C (50.1-65.0 °F) Generally safe, but EHS can occur

Heat index and WBGT can be used to promote safety, along with the recognition that activity in hot environments reflect differences in heat acclimatization, fitness, age, intensity and duration of exercise, clothing or uniforms, sleep deprivation, and nutrition (including fluid intake) (2). Additional information on heat illness is provided in chapter 23.

Cold Exposure

Exercising in the cold can create problems if certain precautions are not taken. A WBGT of less than 10 °C (50 °F) is associated with hypothermia. Hypothermia is a decrease in body temperature that occurs when heat loss exceeds heat production, and it is clinically defined as a core temperature below 35 °C (95 °F). In cold air, there is a larger gradient for convective heat loss from the skin; cold air also is dryer (has a low water vapor pressure) and facilitates the evaporation of moisture from the skin to further cool the body. The combined effects can be deadly, as shown in Pugh's report of three deaths during a walking competition of 45 miles (72 kilometers) that was performed in very cold temperatures (56).

Factors related to hypothermia include environmental variables, such as temperature, water vapor pressure, wind, and whether air or water are involved; personal characteristics, such as age and sex; insulating factors, such as clothing and subcutaneous fat; and the capacity for sustained energy production (55). Each of these factors is discussed in the following paragraphs.

Environmental Factors

Conduction, convection, and radiation depend on a temperature gradient between the skin and the environment; the larger the gradient, the greater the rate of heat loss. What surprises many is that the environmental temperature does not have to be below freezing to cause hypothermia. Other environmental factors interact with temperature to facilitate heat loss: wind and water (1).

Windchill Index The rate of heat loss at any given temperature is influenced directly by wind speed. Wind increases the number of cold air molecules coming into contact with the skin, increasing the rate of heat loss. The windchill index indicates the temperature equivalent (under calm air conditions) for any combination of temperature and wind speed (see figure 13.12). This index allows the fitness professional to properly gauge the cold stress associated with a variety of wind velocities and temperatures. Keep in mind that for activities such as running, riding, or cross-country skiing into the wind, the speed of the activity must be added to the wind speed to evaluate the full impact of the windchill. For example, cycling at 20 mph (32 km · hr^{-1}) into calm air at 0 °F (−17.8 °C) has a windchill value of −22 °F (−30.0 °C)! However, wind is not the only factor that can increase the rate of heat loss at any given temperature.

Temperature (°F)

Calm	40	35	30	25	20	15	10	5	0	−5	−10	−15	−20	−25	−30	−35	−40	−45
5	36	31	25	19	13	7	1	−5	−11	−16	−22	−28	−34	−40	−46	−52	−57	−63
10	34	27	21	15	9	3	−4	−10	−16	−22	−28	−35	−41	−47	−53	−59	−66	−72
15	32	25	19	13	6	0	−7	−13	−19	−26	−32	−39	−45	−51	−58	−64	−71	−77
20	30	24	17	11	4	−2	−9	−15	−22	−29	−35	−42	−48	−55	−61	−68	−74	−81
25	29	23	16	9	3	−4	−11	−17	−24	−31	−37	−44	−51	−58	−64	−71	−78	−84
30	28	22	15	8	1	−5	−12	−19	−26	−33	−39	−46	−53	−60	−67	−73	−80	−87
35	28	21	14	7	0	−7	−14	−21	−27	−34	−41	−48	−55	−62	−69	−76	−82	−89
40	27	20	13	6	−1	−8	−15	−22	−29	−36	−43	−50	−57	−64	−71	−78	−84	−91
45	26	19	12	5	−2	−9	−16	−23	−30	−37	−44	−51	−58	−65	−72	−79	−86	−93
50	26	19	12	4	−3	−10	−17	−24	−31	−38	−45	−52	−60	−67	−74	−81	−88	−95
55	25	18	11	4	−3	−11	−18	−25	−32	−39	−46	−54	−61	−68	−75	−82	−89	−97
60	25	17	10	3	−4	−11	−19	−26	−33	−40	−48	−55	−62	−69	−76	−84	−91	−98

Wind (mph)

Frostbite occurs in:	30 min	10 min	5 min

$$\text{Windchill (°F)} = 35.74 + 0.6215T - 35.75(V^{0.16}) + 0.4275T(V^{0.16})$$
$$T = \text{air temperature (°F)} \quad V = \text{wind speed (mph)}$$

FIGURE 13.12 Windchill index.

From NOAA National Weather Service. Available: https://www.weather.gov/safety/cold-wind-chill-chart.

Water   Heat is lost 25 times faster in water than in air of the same temperature. Unlike air, water offers little or no insulation where it meets the skin, so heat is lost rapidly from the body. Movement in cold water increases heat loss from the arms and legs (35), so it is better to stay as still as possible in long-term unplanned immersions or to wear a wetsuit for anticipated activities in cold water.

Personal Characteristics

Both age and sex influence the ability to respond to a cold environment. The fitness professional should give special attention to those at greater risk of hypothermia.

Age   Adults older than 60 years of age may be less responsive to cold stress due to a reduced capacity to vasoconstrict the skin blood vessels and conserve body heat. In addition, from a behavioral standpoint, they respond later to a drop in environmental temperature than younger people. Because of their higher body surface area–to–mass ratios and lower body fat, children may experience a greater drop in body temperature when exposed to the same cold environment as adults (1).

Sex   Sex differences exist in the ability to respond to a cold-water challenge. These are primarily related to sex differences in body fatness, subcutaneous fat, and muscle mass (1). Women generally have greater body fat and thicker subcutaneous fat layer, which provide insulation but have less muscle and higher surface area–to–mass, which promotes heat loss (1).

Insulating Factors

The rate at which heat is lost from the body is related inversely to the insulation between the body and the environment. The insulating quality is related to the thickness of subcutaneous fat, the ability of clothing to trap air, and whether the clothing is wet or dry.

Body Fat   Subcutaneous fat thickness is an excellent indicator of total body insulation per unit surface area through which heat is lost (32). For example, in one report an obese man was able to swim for 7 hours in 16 °C (60.8 °F) water with no change in body temperature, but a thinner man had to leave the water in 30 minutes with a core temperature of 34.5 °C (94.1 °F) (57). For this reason, long-distance swimmers tend to have more body fat than short-distance swimmers; the higher body fatness provides more buoyancy, requiring less energy to swim at any set speed (34).

Clothing   Clothing can extend the natural subcutaneous fat insulation, allowing individuals to endure very cold environments. The insulation quality of clothing is given in clo units, where 1 clo unit is the insulation needed at rest (1 MET) to maintain core temperature when the environmental temperature is 21 °C (70 °F), the relative humidity is 50%, and the air movement is 6 mph (9.7 km · hr⁻¹) (9). As the air temperature falls, clothing with a higher clo value must be worn to maintain core temperature because the gradient between skin and environment is increasing. Figure 13.13 shows the insulation needed at various energy expenditures across a broad range of environmental temperatures, from –60 to 80 °F (–51.1 to 26.7 °C) (9). As energy production increases, insulation must decrease to maintain core temperature. Typically, cold-weather clothing includes three layers: the inner layer, which wicks moisture away from the skin (e.g., lightweight polyester or polypropylene); the middle layer, which provides insulation (e.g., polyester fleece or wool); and the outer layer, which repels wind and rain while still allowing for moisture transfer to the air (1). When clothing is worn in layers, insulation can be removed as needed to maintain core temperature. By following these steps, the sweat rate will be reduced and the clothing will retain more of its insulatingy value.

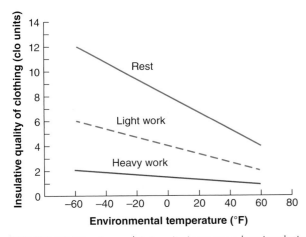

FIGURE 13.13 As work intensity increases, less insulation is needed to maintain core temperature.

Data from Burton and Edholm (1955).

If the clothing becomes wet, its insulating quality decreases because the water can now conduct heat away from the body about 25 times better than air can (35). A primary goal, then, is to avoid wetness caused by either sweat or weather. This problem is exacerbated by the very dry air of the cold environment, which causes a greater evaporation of moisture. When this problem of cold, dry air and wet clothing is coupled with windy conditions, the risk is even greater. The wind not only provides for greater convective heat loss, as described in the windchill section, but it also accelerates evaporation (27).

Energy Production

Energy production can modify the amount of insulation needed to maintain core temperature and prevent hypothermia (see figure 13.13). When male subjects (15%-18% body fat) were immersed in cold water, the drop in body temperature that occurred at rest was prevented when they exercised at an energy expenditure of about 8.5 kcal · min⁻¹ (47, 48). Although being physically fit does not affect the thermoregulatory responses to cold, a fit person can exercise for a longer time at a higher metabolic rate, which can help maintain core temperature (1).

As with heat-related concerns, many factors interact to determine response to cold conditions. With an understanding of environmental factors and individual factors, the fitness professional can reduce the risk of cold injury. Cold-related problems and their treatment are covered in chapter 23.

Air Pollution

Air pollution includes gases and particulates that are products of the combustion of fossil fuels. The smog that results when these pollutants are highly concentrated can have detrimental effects on health and performance. The gases can affect performance by decreasing the capacity to transport oxygen, increasing airway resistance, and altering the perception of effort required when the eyes burn and the chest hurts.

Physiological responses to these pollutants are related to the amount, or dose, received. Several factors determine the dose:

- Concentration of the pollutant
- Duration of exposure to the pollutant
- Volume of air inhaled

The volume of air inhaled is large during exercise, and this is one reason why physical activity should be curtailed during times of peak pollution (19). The following discussion focuses on the major air pollutants: particulate matter, ozone, sulfur dioxide, and carbon monoxide.

Particulate Matter

Particle pollution is a mix of solids and liquid droplets (76). Fine particles (major sources include motor vehicles, power plants, wood burning, and other combustion processes) and coarse particles (sources include grinding operations and dust from roads) are of concern because any particle less than 10 micrometers can get into the lungs (76). Focus has been directed on the very small particles because of their potential to promote pulmonary infection and to cross the epithelium to enter the blood circulation (21). Fine-particle pollution elevates BP in people with preexisting cardiovascular disease and may contribute to an increased risk of cardiac mortality and morbidity (63, 77). Sensitive groups for particle pollution include those with heart or lung disease, older adults, and children (76).

Ozone

The ozone is a gas found in the air. When in the upper atmosphere, ozone provides a shield from the sun's ultraviolet rays. However, concerns are found when ozone forms near the ground due to the reaction of pollutants (sources include vehicles, power plants, refineries) in sunlight (76). Ozone can affect the body in several ways, including irritating the respiratory system, reducing lung function, aggravating asthma and other chronic lung diseases, and, in some cases, causing permanent lung damage (76). Concern about long-term lung health suggests that it is prudent to avoid heavy exercise during the time of day when ozone and other pollutants are highest (19).

Sulfur Dioxide

Sulfur dioxide (SO_2) is produced when fuels containing sulfur (e.g., coal, oil) are burned (76). Sources include power plants and refineries. SO_2 is removed by the nasal passages, so typically higher levels of activities that result in mouth breathing cause greater health effects (76). Individuals with asthma may experience bronchoconstriction as a result of SO_2. At very high levels even healthy individuals without asthma may experience wheezing, chest tightness, and shortness of breath (76).

Carbon Monoxide

Carbon monoxide (CO) is derived from the burning of fossil fuel (coal, oil, gasoline) and wood as well as from cigarette smoke. CO can bind to hemoglobin (HbCO) and decrease the capacity for oxygen transport. The CO concentration in blood is generally less than 1% in nonsmokers but can be as high as 10% in smokers (59). When a person exercises at about 40% $\dot{V}O_2max$, the HbCO concentration can be as high as 15% before endurance is affected. The cardiovascular system simply has a greater capacity to respond with a larger cardiac output when the oxygen concentration of the blood is reduced during submaximal work (36, 58, 59). This will require a higher HR for the same work rate, and participants need to reduce the intensity of exercise during exposure to CO to stay in the THR range. Because it takes about 2 to 4 hours to remove half the CO from the blood once the exposure has been removed, CO can have a lasting effect on performance (19). Unfortunately, it is difficult to predict what the actual CO concentration will be in any given environment. Because previous exposure to the pollutant must be considered, as well as the length of time and rate of ventilation associated with the current exposure, the following guidelines are provided for exercising in an area with air pollution (59):

- Reduce exposure to the pollutant before exercise because the physiological effects are time and dose dependent.
- Stay away from areas where a high dose of CO may be received: smoking areas, high-traffic areas, and urban environments.
- Do not schedule activities during the times when pollutants are at their highest levels because of traffic: 7 to 10 a.m. and 4 to 7 p.m.

Air Quality Index

The air quality index (AQI) is a measure of air quality for five major air pollutants regulated by the U.S. Clean Air Act: ground-level ozone, particulate matter, carbon monoxide, sulfur dioxide, and nitrogen dioxide. The AQI is shown in figure 13.14 as a color-coded chart with interpretations of what the numerical values mean. This information may be provided in a local community's weather forecast, can be found online at www.airnow.gov, and is available in smartphone apps, including a free version from the American Lung Association. The fitness professional should interpret the AQI information to suit the individual; some people experience symptoms at lower levels of pollution than others do (11).

Effect of Altitude

An increase in altitude decreases the partial pressure of oxygen and reduces the amount of oxygen bound to hemoglobin. As a result, the volume of oxygen carried in each liter of blood decreases. Maximal aerobic power steadily decreases with increasing altitude, so by 2,300 meters (about 7,500 feet), the value is only 88% of that measured at sea level. This means that an activity that demanded 88% of $\dot{V}O_2max$ at sea level now requires 100% of the new $\dot{V}O_2max$.

More than maximal aerobic power is affected by altitude exposure; any submaximal work rate is going to demand a higher HR at altitude compared with sea level (shown in figure 13.15). This is because each liter of blood has less oxygen at altitude, and thus more blood is required to deliver the same quantity of oxygen to the tissues. Consequently, the HR response is elevated at any given submaximal work rate. As with exercising in high heat and humidity, monitoring the THR allows the exerciser to modify the intensity of the activity relative to any additional environmental demand (37). Generally, exercise performance decreases 1.5% to 3.5% for every 300 meters of elevation after 1,500 meters (4).

Acclimatization to altitude is the body's response to the low-oxygen (hypoxic) environment. Initially, ventilation increases as does HR and cardiac output in order

Levels of health concern	Numerical value	Meaning
Good	0–50	Air quality is satisfactory, and air pollution poses little or no risk.
Moderate	51–100	Air quality is acceptable. However, there may be a risk for some people, particularly those who are unusually sensitive to air pollution.
Unhealthy for sensitive groups	101–150	Members of sensitive groups may experience health effects. The general public is less likely to be affected.
Unhealthy	151–200	Some members of the general public may experience health effects; members of sensitive groups may experience more serious health effects.
Very unhealthy	201–300	Health alert: The risk of health effects is increased for everyone.
Hazardous	301+	Health warning of emergency conditions: Everyone is more likely to be affected.

FIGURE 13.14   Color-coded AQI chart.

From AirNow, 2015, *Air Quality Index (AQI) Basics*. Available: www.airnow.gov/aqi/aqi-basics/.

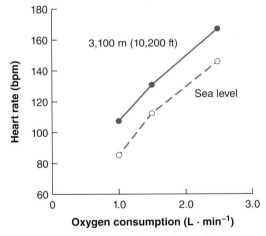

FIGURE 13.15   The effect of altitude on the HR response to submaximal exercise.

Based on Grover et al. (1967).

until 3,000 meters is reached, at which point the increase in sleep location should be limited to 500 meters per night, with a rest day every 3 to 4 days (4). The goal is to gradually acclimatize while avoiding altitude illnesses. It is beyond the scope of this chapter to fully explore acclimatization or to review medical considerations that may arise with ascent to higher altitudes. Other sources are available when working with these situations (4, 14).

KEY POINT

In conditions of high heat and humidity, the exerciser should decrease the work rate to stay in the THR zone. Exercisers should acclimatize to heat over 7 to 14 days to reduce the risk of heat injury. Advise participants to consume fluids before, during, and after exercise and to exercise in the early morning to reduce environmental heat load. When exercising in cold weather, participants should wear clothing in layers and remove layers to minimize sweating and to stay dry. Participants should become aware of the AQI readings in their communities and avoid exercising at times and in places in which air pollution is a problem. When exercising at altitude, participants should decrease work intensity to stay in the THR zone.

to compensate for the lower partial pressure of oxygen (14). Longer-term exposure involves other changes, such as remodeling of smooth muscle in pulmonary arterioles that protects capillaries from damage; increasing secretion of erythropoietin, which brings about gains in red blood cells mass; and even increases in mitochondrial density and myoglobin concentration, among others (14). The time needed to acclimatize varies, and more time is required for additional elevation gains (14). Acclimatization typically involves gradual ascent of 600 meters per day with a rest day every 600 to 1,200 meters

LEARNING AIDS

REVIEW QUESTIONS

1. What do the terms *intensity*, *frequency*, and *duration* mean in describing the dose of physical activity?

2. How might you calculate the volume or amount of physical activity done in a week?

3. Explain the principle of overload.

4. What is the public health recommendation for physical activity for both moderate and vigorous intensities?

5. What is the range of exercise intensities, in %HRR, associated with increasing CRF? Where does moderate-intensity physical activity fit in that range?

6. What is the optimal range of exercise intensities associated with increasing CRF for most people who are cleared to participate in a structured exercise program?

7. What does *progression* mean in terms of helping a person become physically active?

8. What should clients learn to check to help maintain the optimal relative intensity when the environmental temperature and relative humidity are elevated?

9. What is the air quality index (AQI), and how could you obtain information about air quality in your own community?

CASE STUDIES

In the first two case studies, you are given general information about a client, data on risk factors, and the results of an exercise test. Analyze each case, discern the risk factors, and react to the person's responses to the test (whether normal or not). Then, on the basis of your analysis, make some recommendations for the client regarding an exercise program and risk-factor reduction program.

1. Roberto is 36 years old, weighs 96 kilograms, and is 178 centimeters tall. Blood chemistry values indicate that his total cholesterol is 270 mg · dl⁻¹ and HDL-C is 38 mg · dl⁻¹, and his fasting plasma glucose is 99 mg · dl⁻¹. His mother died of a heart attack at the age of 63, and his father had a heart attack at the age of 68. He is sedentary and has engaged in no endurance training since college. The following are the results of a maximal GXT conducted by his physician.

Test: Balke, 3 mph (4.8 km · hr⁻¹); 2.5% Every 2 Minutes

% Grade	METs	SBP (mmHg)	DBP (mmHg)	HR (bpm)	ECG	Symptoms
	Rest	130	84	70	Normal	—
2.5	4.3	142	84	142	Normal	—
5.0	5.4	154	82	150	Normal	—
7.5	6.4	162	82	160	Normal	—
10.0	7.4	174	82	168	Normal	—
12.5	8.5	186	82	176	Normal	—
15.0	9.5	194	82	182	Normal	—
17.5	10.5	198	82	190	Normal	Fatigue

2. Tia is a 35-year-old female, weighs 61.4 kilograms, and is 170 centimeters tall. Blood chemistry values indicate a total cholesterol of 188 mg · dl^{-1} and an HDL-C of 59 mg · dl^{-1}. Her resting BP is 132/78 mmHg. Family history indicates that her father had a nonfatal heart attack at the age of 67. She smoked one pack of cigarettes per day for 10 years but successfully stopped smoking 5 years ago, and her lifestyle is sedentary. She completed the Åstrand and Ryhming cycle ergometer test at a work rate of 300 kgm · min^{-1} with a mean HR for the last two minutes of 136 bpm.

3. You are asked to make a presentation to a group of sedentary faculty members at your school on how to begin a physical activity program to accrue the health-related benefits discussed in this chapter. What guidance would you provide to help them achieve their goals? Discuss the kind of general screening you would recommend (that they could do at the meeting) and how you would instruct them to begin the program (i.e., specifying the frequency, intensity, and time) that ultimately leads to the goal of 150 minutes of moderate-intensity physical activity per week. You can assume that everyone can walk without pain.

Answers to Case Studies

1. If a person has a normal response to a GXT, HR and SBP increase with each stage of the test, whereas the DBP remains the same or decreases slightly. In addition, the ECG shows no concerns. In these cases it can be assumed that the last load achieved on the test represents the true functional capacity (max METs). The GXT presented in this case study is representative of such a test.

   Roberto has a positive family history for CHD (i.e., his mother died of a heart attack before the age of 65). His blood pressure is within the hypertensive range. Plasma glucose is close to but not yet at the level to be considered a positive risk factor. Risk factors include a high BMI (30.3 kg · m^{-2}), a sedentary lifestyle, high BP, and a poor blood lipid profile. His $\dot{V}O_2$max of 10.5 METs is equal to 36.75 ml · kg^{-1} · min^{-1}. This is between the 25th and 30th percentiles for males of his age. Given his current level of activity (i.e., sedentary) and relatively low aerobic fitness, a range of 45% to 55% HRR will be calculated (this is within the moderate intensity level). Roberto has an estimated HRmax of 174 bpm; his measured HR was 16 bpm higher. Given the inherent biological variation in the estimated HRmax, use measured values when they are available. Thus, a THR range of 124 to 136 bpm is an initial target. Similarly, 45% to 55% $\dot{V}O_2$R is calculated, and corresponds to 18.5 to 21.8 ml · kg^{-1} · min^{-1} (5.3-6.2 METs). Engaging in moderate-level intensity, he can emphasize duration initially, and then as he becomes more active, he will be able to increase his intensity. He was referred for nutritional counseling to improve his blood lipid profile.

2. Consulting table 8.5 in chapter 8, Tia's predicted $\dot{V}O_2$max is 1.9 L · min^{-1}, which must account for age by multiplying by the age correction factor of 0.87 for a 35-year-old, resulting in an estimated $\dot{V}O_2$max of 1.65 L · min^{-1} (or 26.9 ml · kg^{-1} · min^{-1}). Tia is in approximately the 30th to 35th percentiles for other females of her age for aerobic capacity.

   Her blood chemistry values are normal, but BP is elevated (just within the hypertensive range). Her family history is negative for CHD. Her HR response to the test is normal and indicates poor CRF. Her maximal aerobic power is related to the sedentary lifestyle. She is congratulated on her success in smoking cessation and encouraged to continue to promote her health with regular physical activity.

The recommended exercise program will focus on moderate-intensity exercise. Since a resting HR was not available, a range of 65% to 75% HRmax is calculated, realizing the limitation of using an estimated HRmax. Using the equation HRmax = 207 – (0.7 × age) results in an estimated HRmax of 182 bpm. A target range of 118 to 136 bpm is provided, along with a level 5 or 6 on a 10-point relative intensity scale. She preferred a walking program because of the scheduling freedom; this is consistent with moderate-intensity physical activity. She was given the walking program in this chapter and was asked to record her HR response to each of the exercise sessions.

3. You might begin by talking about the importance of regular physical activity in reducing the risk of numerous chronic diseases. In addition, you could indicate that the risk associated with regular participation in moderate-intensity physical activity is very low. Have the participants complete one of the simple health screening questionnaires in chapter 2 to help them determine whether they should see their physician before beginning a physical activity program. Next, you might recommend a walking program that begins with short (e.g., 10 minute) bouts of activity done at a comfortable pace each day. Encourage them to gradually increase the number of 10-minute bouts per day until they can do a single 30-minute walk each day. On the other hand, if some wanted to continue to do 10-minute bouts because it fit their schedules, that would be fine. Finally, you might suggest that their weekly goal be at least 150 minutes of walking, but more is better relative to health benefits derived.

Exercise Prescription for Muscular Fitness

Avery D. Faigenbaum

OBJECTIVES

The reader will be able to do the following:

1. Explain the physiological principles of overload, specificity, and progressive resistance and how they relate to exercise programming for developing muscular fitness

2. Describe the following methods of resistance training: isometrics, dynamic constant external resistance (DCER) training, variable resistance training, isokinetics, and plyometrics

3. Describe different modes of resistance training

4. Discuss the health and fitness benefits of resistance training, and understand precautions that enhance participant safety

5. Describe the program variables that are used to design resistance training programs, and discuss how the amount of resistance used, the training volume, the repetition velocity, and the rest intervals between sets and exercises all relate

6. Understand periodization and its application in the design of exercise programs, and discuss how program variables can be organized to achieve long-term goals and avoid overtraining

7. Describe the following methods of resistance training: single set, multiple set, circuit training, superset training, and assisted training

8. Discuss the safety of, benefits of, and recommendations for resistance training for youth, older adults, pregnant women, and people considered to be at elevated cardiovascular risk

14

Traditionally, resistance training was used primarily by adult athletes to enhance sport performance and increase muscle size. Today, resistance training is recognized as a method for enhancing the health and fitness of people of all ages and abilities (5, 41, 146, 154). Resistance training has become a popular method of conditioning in commercial, community, clinical, and corporate health and fitness facilities (55, 123, 147). Current public health guidelines aim to increase participation in resistance training to improve overall health and fitness (149, 158). The World Health Organization now recommends that adults do muscle-strengthening activities at a moderate to greater intensity on 2 or more days per week (158).

Regular resistance training provides a variety of health and fitness benefits that may enhance quality of life while reducing the risk of all-cause mortality and several chronic diseases, including cardiovascular disease, diabetes, and cancer (103, 133, 154). In addition to improving musculoskeletal health (91), participation in resistance training can have favorable effects on body composition (89), cardiometabolic risk factors (7, 29), and mental health (e.g., anxiety and depression) (61, 62, 110). Adequate levels of muscular strength, muscular power, and local muscular endurance are essential for independent living and enable people to perform functional movements and activities of daily living (ADLs) as well as to participate in other physical activities with energy and vigor (81, 119, 152). Resistance training is recommended by professional health, fitness, and medical organizations such as the American Heart Association (AHA), American College of Sports Medicine (ACSM), and National Strength and Conditioning Association (NSCA), and it should be performed by everyone from children to older adults, pregnant women, and patients with chronic disease (5, 41, 69, 146). The effects of resistance training and aerobic training on health and fitness variables are listed in table 14.1.

For fitness professionals, the ability to design safe, effective, and enjoyable resistance training programs for people of all ages, fitness levels, and health conditions is a valuable asset. Since most adults do not report sufficient participation in muscle-strengthening activities (14, 76), continued promotion of resistance exercise with evidence-based approaches is needed to dispel misperceptions, provide reassurance, and increase participation in this type of training. This chapter focuses on principles of resistance training that can be used in designing exercise programs for enhancing muscular fitness in untrained and trained people. Photos and instructions for exercises that target major muscle groups are included in the appendix of this chapter. Guidelines and recommendations for designing advanced resistance training programs for elite athletes are available elsewhere (54, 78).

In this chapter, the term *resistance training* refers to a method of conditioning designed to increase a person's ability to exert or resist force. This term encompasses a wide range of resistive loads (from light weights to plyometric jumps) and a variety of training modalities, including free weights (barbells and dumbbells), weight machines, elastic tubing, medicine balls, stability balls, and body weight. Resistance training should be distinguished from the competitive sports of weightlifting, powerlifting, and bodybuilding. Weightlifting and pow-

Table 14.1 Effects of Aerobic Training and Resistance Training on Health and Fitness Variables

Variable	Aerobic training	Resistance training
Body composition	↓↓ fat mass ↑ bone mass ≠ muscle mass	↑↑↑ muscle mass ↑↑ bone mass ↓ fat mass
Aerobic fitness	↑↑↑ V̇O$_2$max ↑↑↑ submaximal and maximal endurance times	↑ V̇O$_2$max ↑ submaximal and maximal endurance times
Muscular fitness	↑↑↑ capillary and mitochondrial density ↑↑ local muscular endurance ≠ muscular strength and power ↑ functional movements (ADLs)	↑↑↑ muscular strength ↑↑↑ muscular power ↑↑↑ local muscular endurance ↑↑↑ functional movements (ADLs)
Cardiometabolic health	↓↓ resting blood pressure (BP) ↓↓ triglycerides ↑↑ high-density lipoproteins ↓↓ fasting glucose and hemoglobin A1C (A1C) ↑↑ insulin sensitivity	↓ resting BP ↓ triglycerides ↑ high-density lipoproteins ↓↓ fasting glucose and A1C ↑↑ insulin sensitivity
Mental health	↓↓ anxiety and depression ↑↑ cognition	↓↓ anxiety and depression ↑↑ cognition

The number of arrows indicate relative strength of the relationship, either positive (↑) or negative (↓); ≠ means there is no relationship.

erlifting are sports in which athletes attempt to lift maximal amounts of weight, and bodybuilding is a sport in which the goal is to enhance muscle size and symmetry. Although fitness enthusiasts may perform some of the same exercises used by weightlifters, powerlifters, and bodybuilders, the program goals and training regimens are different.

Local muscular endurance refers to the ability of a muscle or muscle group to perform repeated contractions against a submaximal resistance. *Absolute muscular endurance* refers to performing a set with a fixed load for as many repetitions as possible, whereas *relative muscular endurance* is assessed by lifting a specific percentage of the 1-repetition maximum (1RM) for as many repetitions as possible. *Strength* is defined as the maximal force that a muscle or muscle group can generate at a specified velocity, and *power* refers to the rate of performing work and is the product of strength and speed of movement. *Muscular fitness* is a general term that includes local muscular endurance, strength, and power and is related to promoting and maintaining good health and fitness. For ease of discussion, the terms *youth* and *young athletes* are broadly defined in this chapter to include children and adolescents, and the terms *older* and *senior* refer to adults 65 years of age and older.

Principles of Training

A key factor in any resistance training program is appropriate program design. Because the act of resistance training itself does not ensure gains in muscular fitness, the resistance training program needs to be based on sound training principles and must be carefully prescribed in order to maximize training outcomes. Although factors such as initial fitness level, heredity, nutritional status (e.g., dietary protein), health habits (e.g., sleep), and motivation influence the rate and magnitude of the adaptation that occurs, four principles determine the effectiveness of all resistance training programs: progression, regularity, overload, and specificity. These principles of resistance training can be remembered as the PROS.

Principle of Progression

According to the principle of progression, the demands placed on the body must continually and progressively increase over time in order to result in long-term fitness gains. Although it is impossible to improve at the same rate throughout long-term training programs, the systematic manipulation of training variables (e.g., intensity, repetitions, and sets) during the program can limit training plateaus and optimize training adaptations (4). This does not mean that heavier weights should be used in every workout but rather that over time exercise sessions should become more challenging to create a more effective exercise stimulus. Without a more challenging stimulus that is consistent with individual needs, goals, and abilities, the human body has no reason to adapt any further. This principle is particularly important after the first 2 or 3 months of resistance training, when the threshold for training-induced adaptations in conditioned people is higher (4, 102).

The importance of recovery between resistance training workouts should not be underestimated, but the training stimulus should increase at a rate that is compatible with the training-induced adaptations. Beginners can progress relatively quickly, whereas slower rates of improvement are appropriate for people with experience in resistance training. A reasonable guideline for a beginner is to increase the training weight about 5% to 10% and decrease the repetitions (the number of times a movement is completed) by 2 to 4 once a given load can be performed for the desired number of repetitions with proper exercise technique. For example, if an adult female can easily perform 12 repetitions of the chest press using 100 pounds (45 kilograms), she should increase the weight to 110 pounds (50 kilograms) and decrease the repetitions to 8 if she wants to continue to gain muscular strength. Alternatively, she could increase the number of sets (groups of repetitions), increase the number of repetitions, or add another chest exercise (e.g., dumbbell fly) to her routine. The decision on how to progress should be based on the person's training experience and personal goals.

Principle of Regularity

In order to make continual gains in muscular fitness, resistance training must be performed regularly several times per week. Inconsistent training will result in only modest training adaptations, and prolonged inactivity will result in a loss of muscular strength and size. The adage "Use it or lose it" is appropriate for exercise programming because training-induced adaptations cannot be stored. Although adequate recovery is needed between training sessions, the principle of regularity states that long-term gains in muscle strength and performance will be realized only if the program is performed on a regular basis at an appropriate intensity (160).

Principle of Overload

For more than a century, the overload principle has been a tenet of resistance training. The overload principle states that to enhance muscular fitness, the body must exercise at a level beyond that at which it is normally stressed. For example, an adult male who can easily complete 10 repetitions with 20 pounds (9 kilograms) while performing a barbell curl must increase the weight, the repetitions, or the number of sets if he wants to increase his arm strength. If the training stimulus is not increased beyond the level to which the muscles are accustomed, training adaptations will not occur. Overload is typically manipulated by changing the exercise intensity, total repetitions, repetition speed, rest periods, type of exercise, and training volume (4). This process is often referred to as *progressive overload* and is the basis for maximizing long-term training adaptations (4).

Principle of Specificity

The principle of specificity refers to the adaptations that take place as a result of a training program. The adaptations to resistance training are specific to the muscle actions, velocity of movement, exercise range of motion (ROM), muscle groups, energy systems, and intensity and volume involved in training (4, 123). Specificity is often referred to as the *SAID principle*, which stands for specific adaptations to imposed demands. In essence, every muscle or muscle group must be trained to make gains in strength, power, and local muscular endurance. For instance, exercises such as the squat and leg press can enhance lower-body strength, but they will not affect upper-body strength. While the SAID principle is a fundamental concept to consider when designing any resistance training program, the SAID principle becomes even more important when designing advanced resistance training programs due to the specific needs and goals of highly trained individuals (123).

The adaptations that take place in a muscle or muscle group will be as simple or as complex as the stress placed on them. For example, because basketball requires multijoint and multiplanar movements (i.e., in the frontal, sagittal, and transverse planes), basketball players should perform complex exercises that closely mimic the movements and energy demands of their sport. The specificity principle also can be applied to designing resistance training programs for people who want to enhance their ability to perform ADLs such as stair-climbing and house cleaning, which also require multijoint and multiplanar movements. The most effective resistance training programs target specific muscle groups, muscle actions, and energy systems.

KEY POINT

Gains in strength, power, and local muscular endurance will occur only if the overload is greater than that to which the muscle or muscle group is normally accustomed. To make continual gains, training must progress gradually and be performed regularly at an appropriate intensity. The most beneficial resistance training programs are designed to meet individual needs, goals, and abilities.

RESEARCH INSIGHT

Engagement in Resistance Training

Although resistance training offers observable health and fitness benefits, the prevalence of participation in muscle-strengthening activities is low. Rhodes and colleagues aimed to investigate factors that influence participation in resistance training (126). They evaluated research from nine countries that examined correlates or determinants of resistance training in adults. They found that low education levels and poor health status were associated with low participation rates. Intrapersonal factors (e.g., self-efficacy) and interpersonal factors (e.g., program leadership) were associated with participating in resistance training. These findings highlight the importance of targeting vulnerable populations, teaching resistance training skills effectively, and training professionals to design safe, effective, and enjoyable fitness programs in a supportive setting.

Program Design Considerations

As with exercise programs that enhance cardiorespiratory fitness (CRF), resistance training programs should be based on the participant's interests, current fitness level, health needs, clinical status, and personal goals as well as on the principles of resistance training. By assessing the individual needs of each participant and applying principles of training to the program design, safe and effective resistance training programs can be developed for each person. However, because the magnitude of adaptation to a given exercise stimulus varies from person to person, fitness professionals must be aware of interindividual differences and be prepared to alter the program to reduce the risk of injury and to maximize training adaptations.

Health Status

The health status of each person should be assessed before resistance training begins. As discussed in chapter 2, each participant should complete a health and medical questionnaire, and the fitness professional should review it to make decisions about further medical evaluation. Additional questions on the health screening questionnaire (HSQ) regarding past resistance training experiences, previous musculoskeletal injuries, presence of known cardiovascular conditions, and personal goals can also help with designing the resistance training program.

Fitness Level

An important factor to consider when designing resistance training programs is the participant's previous experience with resistance training, or training age. Those who are the least experienced in resistance training tend to have a greater capacity for improvement compared with those who have been resistance training for several years. Although any reasonable program can increase the strength of untrained people, more comprehensive programs are often needed to produce desirable adaptations in trained people (4, 102, 123). Thus, resistance training programs designed for beginners may not be effective for participants who have at least 3 months of experience with resistance training. For example, a 32-year-old person with 2 years of resistance training experience (i.e., a training age of 2 years) may not achieve the same strength gains in a given time as a 25-year-old person who has no experience with resistance training (i.e., a training age of 0 years). The potential for adaptation gradually decreases as training age increases. As people gain experience with resistance training, they need more advanced programs to optimize training-induced adaptations in their muscular fitness (4, 6, 121). Clearly, no single model of resistance exercise will optimize training-induced adaptations in both untrained and trained people.

Therefore, it is reasonable for beginners to start with a general resistance training program and gradually progress to more advanced programs as performance and self-confidence in their ability to perform resistance exercise improve. However, as more advanced training programs are designed, fitness professionals must consider the additional time and effort that are required to make additional gains. For example, people with several years of training experience may need to devote a larger amount of time to training to make relatively small gains. Although athletes may be willing to make this type of commitment for small changes in performance, others may be less willing to devote a large amount of time to resistance training. As such, resistance training program variables can be manipulated to optimize the training response in a time-efficient manner with well-designed sessions that prioritize bilateral, multijoint exercises that target all major muscle groups with full dynamic movements (77).

Because long-term progression in resistance exercise requires a systematic manipulation of the program variables, fitness professionals need to make critical decisions regarding the exercise prescription. These decisions require a solid understanding of training-induced adaptations that take place in both beginners and resist-

ance-trained individuals. Beginners need less variation, but as the program progresses, more variation and more complex training regimens are needed (4, 102, 121).

Training Goals

After the preexercise screening, participants should establish realistic short- and long-term goals. The results of a muscular fitness evaluation (see chapter 9) along with the participant's interests can be used to help set realistic and measurable goals. To improve compliance, these goals ideally are set by the participant with guidance from a knowledgeable fitness professional who can make the experience enjoyable and worthwhile. Typical goals are to increase muscle strength, decrease body fat, and improve physical function. An effort to establish realistic goals and increase confidence to achieve those goals is important because it may help people avoid unrealistic expectations that ultimately can lead to discouragement and poor adherence. Testing fitness periodically and reviewing individualized workout logs can help the fitness professional assess training progress and modify the program. Understanding that resistance training programs designed to improve health and fitness are quite different from training programs designed to enhance sport performance will further promote the development of and adherence to programs suited to a participant's needs.

Types of Resistance Training

Several types of resistance training can be used to enhance muscular fitness. Although each method has advantages and disadvantages, several factors should be considered when selecting one type of training over another or including multiple types of training within a given program. The most common types of resistance training include isometrics, dynamic constant external resistance training, variable resistance training, isokinetics, and plyometrics.

Isometrics

Isometric training, or *static resistance training*, refers to muscle actions in which muscle length does not change. This type of training is usually performed against an immovable object such as a wall, with self-resistance, or with a partner who provides resistance. The concept of isometric training was popularized in the 1950s when Hettinger and Muller reported remarkable gains in muscle strength from this type of static resistance training (73). In contemporary resistance exercise programming, including body-weight isometric training (e.g., planks and wall-sits) and manual- or partner-resisted isometric training (e.g., chest squeeze and lateral raise) is common (123).

An advantage of isometric training is that specialized equipment is not required, and the cost is minimal. Increases in strength and muscle hypertrophy (an increase in size or mass) can occur from this type of training; however, a major limitation is that the strength gains are specific to the joint angle at which the training occurred. For example, if isometric training of the elbow flexors is performed at a joint angle of 90°, muscle strength will increase at this joint angle but not necessarily at other angles. Even though there seems to be about 20° to 30° of carryover on either side of the joint angle, the same isometric exercise must be performed at varying joint angles in order to increase strength throughout the full ROM. Isometric training may help maintain muscle strength and prevent muscle atrophy (a decrease in size or mass) when a limb is immobilized in a cast, but gains in functional strength (e.g., stair-climbing) and motor performance (e.g., sprinting and jumping) as a result of isometric training are unlikely to occur if isometric training takes place only at one joint angle.

Factors such as the duration of contractions, intensity of contractions, and frequency of training can influence the strength gains resulting from isometric training. While experienced lifters may perform isometric training with maximal voluntary contractions for approximately 2 to 6 seconds to increase muscle strength, it is reasonable for others to perform body-weight exercises such as the plank for 20 to 30 seconds and gradually increase the time of contraction or progress to a more challenging exercise (e.g., side plank) (123). Because of the nature of isometric training, it is particularly important to avoid the breath-holding Valsalva maneuver, which reduces venous return to the heart and increases systolic and diastolic BP. During all types of resistance training, regular breathing patterns (i.e., exhalation while lifting and inhalation while lowering) should be encouraged.

Dynamic Constant External Resistance (DCER) Training

Resistance training that involves a lifting and lowering phase is called *dynamic*. Exercises using free weights (e.g., barbells and dumbbells) and weight machines are dynamic because the weight is lifted and lowered through a predetermined ROM. Although the term *isotonic* traditionally was used to describe this type of training, it literally means "constant (*iso*) tension (*tonic*)." Because tension exerted by a muscle as it shortens varies with the mechanical advantage of the joint and the length of the muscle fibers at a particular joint angle, the term *isotonic* does not accurately describe this training method. As shown in figure 14.1, during a barbell curl, the elbow flexors are strongest at approximately 100° and weakest at 60° (elbows fully flexed) and at 180° (elbows fully extended). The same principle applies to other muscle

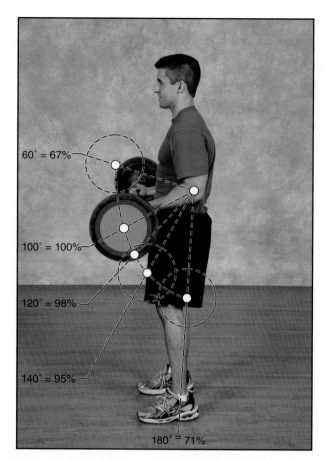

60° = 67%

100° = 100%

120° = 98%

140° = 95%

180° = 71%

FIGURE 14.1 Variation in strength relative to the angle of the elbow flexors during the biceps curl.

groups. DCER better describes resistance training in which the weight does not change during the lifting, or concentric (muscle-shortening) action, and lowering, or eccentric (muscle-lengthening) action (123).

DCER training is the most common method of resistance training for enhancing health and fitness. Endless combinations of sets and repetitions and a variety of training equipment can be used for DCER training. Untrained people should perform each repetition deliberately at a moderate velocity, whereas the performance of various training velocities from unintentionally slow (using heavy loads) to intentionally fast (using power training) will provide the most effective training stimulus for people with resistance training experience (123). Weight machines generally limit the user to fixed planes of motion. However, they are easy to use and are ideal for isolating muscle groups. Free weights (e.g., barbells and dumbbells) are less expensive and can be used for a wide variety of exercises that require greater proprioception, balance, and coordination. Several free-weight exercises (e.g., barbell squat, bench press) require the use of a spotter who can assist the lifter in case of a failed repetition. In addition to improving health and fitness, DCER training is often used to enhance motor performance skills and sport performance. DCER training with free-weight multijoint exercises may produce greater strength–power adaptations, which transfer to athletic performance (144).

During DCER training, the weight lifted does not change throughout the ROM. Because muscle tension can vary significantly during a DCER exercise, the heaviest weight that can be lifted throughout a full ROM is limited by the strength of a muscle at the weakest joint angle (i.e., the sticking point). As a result, DCER exercise provides adequate resistance to stimulate training adaptations in some parts of the movement range but not enough resistance in others. For example, during the barbell bench press, more weight can be lifted during the last part of the exercise than in the first part of the movement, when the barbell is being pressed off the chest. This is a limitation of DCER training that should be recognized when choosing starting weights for beginners or designing more advanced resistance training programs.

In an attempt to overcome the variation in strength across the ROM, mechanical devices that operate through a lever arm or cam have been designed to vary the resistance throughout the ROM of an exercise. These devices, called *variable resistance machines*, became popular in the 1970s and theoretically force the muscle to contract maximally throughout the ROM by varying the resistance to match the exercise strength curve. These machines can be used to train all the major muscle groups, and by automatically changing the resistive force throughout the movement range, they provide proportionally less resistance in weaker segments of the movement and more resistance in stronger segments of the movement. As with all weight machines, variable resistance machines provide a specific movement path. This makes the exercise easier to perform compared with free-weight exercises, which require balance, coordination, and the involvement of stabilizing muscle groups. More recently, individuals with resistance training experience have started to add chains or elastic bands to free-weight exercises to create a type of variable resistance that better matches changes in mechanical load at various joint angles (144).

Isokinetics

The term *isokinetics* refers to muscular actions performed at a constant angular limb velocity. Isokinetic training involves specialized and expensive equipment, and most isokinetic devices are designed to train only single-joint movements. Isokinetic machines generally are not used in fitness centers, but they are used by physical therapists and certified athletic trainers for injury rehabilitation. Unlike other types of resistance training, in isokinetics, the velocity of movement rather than the resistance is controlled. During isokinetic training, any force applied to the isokinetic machine is met with an equal reaction force. Although it is theoretically possible for a muscle to contract maximally through the full ROM of an exercise, this seems unlikely during isokinetic training because of the acceleration at the beginning and deceleration at the end of the ROM.

Isokinetic training studies have generally found that strength gains are specific to the training velocity (123). Isokinetic training at a slow movement velocity (e.g., $60°·sec^{-1}$) will increase strength at that velocity, but strength gains at faster velocities are unlikely to occur. If the purpose of the training program is to increase strength at higher velocities (e.g., for enhanced sport performance), high-speed isokinetic training appears prudent. The best approach may be to perform isokinetic training at slow, intermediate, and fast velocities to develop strength and power at a variety of movement speeds.

Plyometrics

Plyometric training, first known simply as *jump training*, refers to a specialized method of conditioning designed to enable a muscle to reach maximal force in the shortest possible time (22). Unlike an exercise such as the bench press, plyometric training is characterized by quick, powerful movements that involve rapid stretching of a muscle (eccentric muscle action) immediately followed by rapid shortening (concentric muscle action). This type of muscle action, sometimes called *stretch–shortening cycle exercise*, provides a physiological advantage because the muscle force generated during the concentric muscle action is potentiated by the preceding eccentric muscle action (22). Although both muscle actions are important, the amount of time it takes to change direction from the eccentric to the concentric muscle action is a critical factor in plyometric training. This amount of time is the amortization phase and should be as short as possible (<0.1 seconds) in order to maximize training adaptations. Both mechanical factors (i.e., increased stored elastic energy) and neurophysiological factors (i.e., change in the force–velocity relationship of the muscle) contribute to the increased force production resulting from plyometric training (22, 123).

Exercises that involve explosive jumping, skipping, hopping, and throwing can be considered plyometric. Although plyometric exercises often are associated with high-intensity drills such as depth jumps (i.e., jumping from a box to the ground and then immediately jumping up), common activities such as jumping jacks and hopscotch are also plyometric exercises because every time the feet hit the ground, the quadriceps go through a stretch–shortening cycle. Strength and power athletes in sports such as American football, volleyball, and track and field regularly perform plyometric exercises as part of their conditioning program. More recently, this type of training has become popular in exercise classes for youth and older adults with the potential for improving various health- and fitness-related outcomes (41, 105, 151).

Because plyometric exercises can greatly stress muscles, connective tissues, and joints, they need to be carefully prescribed to reduce the likelihood of musculoskeletal injury. In some cases, the risks of performing plyometric exercises outweigh the potential benefits for untrained or overweight people who may lack the strength and coordination to perform the exercises properly. In other cases, plyometrics may be a worthwhile addition to the exercise program of a trained individual who wants to improve physical performance. Clearly, the prescription of plyometric exercises needs to be individualized and based on a person's health history, resistance training experience, and personal goals. Although participants with different levels of physical fitness can benefit from plyometric training, it seems prudent to begin with low-intensity plyometric exercises and gradually progress to higher-intensity drills as technique and performance improve. While rest interval lengths are exercise specific and depend on the intensity, most plyometric studies have used a rest interval length averaging approximately 2 minutes between sets and exercises (123).

Other considerations for plyometric training include proper footwear, adequate space, shock-absorbing landing surfaces (e.g., suspended floor or grass playing field), and training frequency (22). Also, plyometric training should not be considered a standalone training method but rather should be used in combination with other types of conditioning. It seems reasonable to begin plyometric training with 1 to 3 sets of 6 to 10 repetitions of several low-intensity exercises for the upper and lower body twice a week on nonconsecutive days. While a wide variety of plyometric exercises are effective, each repetition should be performed with maximal effort, minimal amortization, and explosive propulsion. Fitness professionals who have experience with plyometric training should provide demonstrations and coaching cues to enhance learning, improve technique, and reduce the likelihood of injury. Additional training guidelines and examples of plyometric drills are available elsewhere (22, 54).

Modes of Resistance Training

Various modes of resistance training can be used to accommodate the needs of young people, adults, and seniors. Provided that the principles of training are adhered to, almost any mode of resistance training can be used to enhance muscular fitness. Some types of equipment are relatively easy to use, while others require balance, coordination, and high levels of skill. The decision to use a certain mode of resistance training should be based on each client's needs, goals, and abilities. The major modes of resistance training are weight machines, free weights (barbells and dumbbells), body-weight exercises, and a broadly defined category of balls, bands, and elastic tubing.

Single-joint exercises such as the biceps curl and leg extension target a specific muscle group and require less skill. Multijoint exercises such as the bench press and squat involve more than one joint or major muscle group and require more balance and coordination. Although both single-joint and multijoint exercises enhance muscular fitness, multijoint exercises are considered to be more effective for increasing muscle strength because they involve a greater amount of muscle mass and therefore enable a heavier weight to be lifted (4, 58, 123). Multijoint exercises also have been shown to have the greatest acute metabolic and anabolic hormonal (e.g., testosterone and growth hormone) response, which could favorably influence resistance training that targets improvements in muscle size and body composition (49, 123). The appendix of this chapter provides examples of resistance training exercises for the major muscle groups. Table 14.2 summarizes the advantages and disadvantages of weight machines, free weights (barbells and dumbbells), body-weight exercises, balls, bands, and elastic tubing.

Weight machines are designed to train all the major muscle groups and can be found in most fitness centers. Both single-joint (e.g., leg extension) and multijoint (e.g., leg press) exercises can be performed on weight machines, which are relatively easy to use because the exercise motion is controlled by the machine and typically occurs in only one anatomical plane. This is particularly important when designing resistance training programs for sedentary or inexperienced participants. Also, several weight-machine exercises such as the lat pull-down and leg curl are difficult to mimic with free

KEY POINT

Various types of resistance training can increase muscular strength, muscular power, and local muscular endurance. The effects of isometric training are generally limited to the joint angle at which the training occurs. DCER training refers to exercises performed throughout a ROM with free weights and weight machines. Isokinetic training occurs at a constant limb velocity with maximal force exerted throughout the ROM of the joint. Plyometric training exploits the muscle cycle of lengthening and shortening to increase speed of movement and muscular power.

Table 14.2   Comparison of Resistance Training Modes

	Weight machines	Free weights	Body weight	Balls and bands*
Cost	High	Low	None	Very low
Portability	Limited	Variable	Excellent	Excellent
Ease of use	Excellent	Variable	Variable	Variable
Muscle isolation	Excellent	Variable	Variable	Variable
Functionality	Limited	Excellent	Excellent	Excellent
Exercise variety	Limited	Excellent	Excellent	Excellent
Space requirements	High	Variable	Low	Low

*Medicine balls, stability balls, and elastic bands.

weights. Weight machines are designed to fit the average adult, so smaller people may not be able to position themselves properly on the equipment. A seat pad or back pad can be used to adjust body position to allow for a better fit. Some companies now manufacture weight machines specifically for children. These machines are smaller versions of adult-sized machines and have weight increments that are appropriate for younger populations.

Free weights are also popular in fitness centers and come in a variety of shapes and sizes. Although it may take longer to master proper exercise technique when using free weights compared with weight machines, free weights have several advantages. For example, proper fit is not an issue with adjustable barbells and dumbbells because one size fits all. Free weights also offer a greater variety of exercises than weight machines because they can be moved in many directions. Another benefit of free weights is that they require the use of stabilizing and assisting muscles to hold the correct body position during an exercise. As such, free-weight training can occur in different planes. This is particularly true with dumbbells because they train each side of the body independently.

In general, free weights allow the participant to train functionally by encouraging different muscle groups to work together while performing exercises that are similar to the participant's chosen sport or activity. If the goal of the program is to improve strength, power, and speed, training with free weights (e.g., weightlifting training) may be advantageous for athletic development (103, 106, 144). However, unlike weight machines, several free-weight exercises require the aid of a spotter who can assist the lifter in case of a failed repetition. Using a spotter is particularly important when performing the bench press. In an epidemiological evaluation of resistance training–related injuries seen in U.S. emergency rooms, a large number of injuries occurred with free weights, and the most common mechanism of injury was weights dropping on the person (80). Accidents such as these underscore the importance of close supervision and an appropriate progression of training loads when training with free weights.

Body-weight exercises such as push-ups, pull-ups, and curl-ups are some of the oldest modes of resistance training. An example of using body weight as a form of resistance is certain forms of yoga that particularly target stability and core strength (i.e., abdominal muscles, lower back, hips). A major advantage of body-weight training is that equipment is not needed and a variety of exercises can be performed. Conversely, a limitation of body-weight training is the difficulty in adjusting the body weight to the individual's strength level. Sedentary or overweight participants may not be strong enough to perform even one push-up or pull-up. In such cases, body-weight exercises not only may be ineffective, but they may have a negative effect on program compliance. Exercise machines that allow people to perform movements that mimic body-weight exercises, such as pull-ups and dips, by using a predetermined percentage of their body weight are available. These machines provide an opportunity for participants of all abilities to incorporate movements similar to body-weight exercises into their resistance training program (see figure 14.2).

Stability balls, medicine balls, and elastic tubing are safe and effective alternatives to weight machines and free weights, provided qualified supervision and instruction are available. The first use of medicine balls dates back almost 3,000 years, and stability balls and elastic tubing have been used by therapists for decades. Now fitness professionals are using balls and bands for resistance training and conditioning. Not only are stability balls, medicine balls, and elastic tubing relatively inexpensive, they can also be used to enhance strength, local muscular endurance, and power. In addition, exercises performed with balls and tubing can challenge proprioception, which carries added benefits, including gains in agility, balance, and coordination.

Stability balls are lightweight, inflatable balls about 18 to 30 inches (45-75 centimeters) in diameter that add elements of balance and coordination to any exercise while

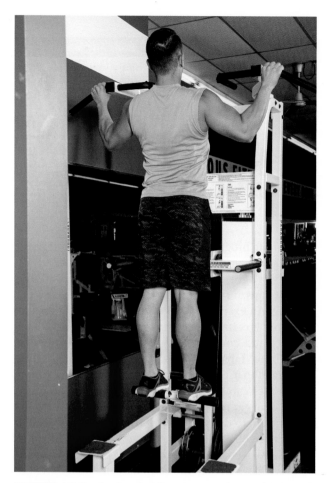

FIGURE 14.2 Assisted pull-up on weight machine.

targeting selected muscle groups. A BOSU ball looks like a stability ball cut in half with a flat platform on one side. Although many exercises can be performed with stability balls and BOSU balls, they are often used to develop core (i.e., abdominal, hip, low back) strength and improve posture. When a participant sits on a stability ball, their feet should be flat on the floor and their knees at a 90° angle. The firmer the ball, the more difficult the exercise will be. Because proper body alignment is crucial when performing an exercise on a stability or BOSU ball, fitness professionals should know how to perform each exercise correctly and when to modify an exercise to meet individual needs and abilities. Many types of exercise programs using stability and BOSU balls can be created to enhance strength, local muscular endurance, flexibility, and balance (59, 139). Figure 14.3a illustrates the performance of a moving plank exercise on a stability ball, and figures 14.3b and 14.3c illustrate the push-up on a BOSU ball.

Medicine balls come in a variety of shapes and sizes (about 2 pounds [1 kilogram] to more than 20 pounds [about 10 kilograms]) and are a safe and effective alternative to free weights and weight machines. Medicine balls have developed over the years and now include core

balls with handles for better gripping and slam balls with ropes attached. In addition to performing squats or chest presses with a medicine ball, participants can use the ball in throwing drills—such as throwing from participant to instructor or slamming the ball on the floor—to enhance upper-body explosive power. High-speed training with medicine balls adds a new dimension to resistance training that can benefit people of all ages. Further, because medicine balls typically require the body to function as a unit instead of as separate parts, they are particularly effective for mimicking natural body positions and movement speeds that occur in daily life and game situations. Progressive medicine-ball training can be used in one-on-one settings or group fitness classes (59, 99). Figure 14.4 illustrates the medicine-ball slam.

Resistance training with an elastic band involves performing an exercise against the force required to stretch the band and then returning it to its unstretched state. The resistance can range from minimal to more than 100 pounds (45.5 kilograms) (136). Bands are usually color-coded based on the amount of resistance they provide. A variety of exercises can be performed by holding the ends of the cord with both hands or attaching one end of the cord to a fixed object. Shorter bands can be placed around the legs to resist lower-body movements (e.g., lateral band walks or side steps). For safety reasons, fitness professionals should ensure that the cord is secured around a body part or to a fixed object before performing any exercise. Also, a band that has rips, cracks, or any defects that weaken the band should not be used. Incorporating exercises with stability balls, medicine balls, and elastic tubing into a workout session can be challenging, motivating, beneficial, and fun. Figure 14.5 illustrates a lateral band walk with an elastic band.

KEY POINT

Weight machines, free weights, body-weight exercises, medicine balls, stability balls, BOSU balls, and elastic bands can be used to enhance muscular fitness. When designing resistance training programs, fitness professionals should evaluate the advantages and disadvantages of each training mode to meet individual needs, goals, and abilities while maximizing participant safety.

Safety Issues

Resistance training programs should be designed by fitness professionals who are knowledgeable about safe and effective training methods. Although all types of exercise have some degree of risk, the chance of injury during resistance training can be reduced by following established training guidelines and safety procedures.

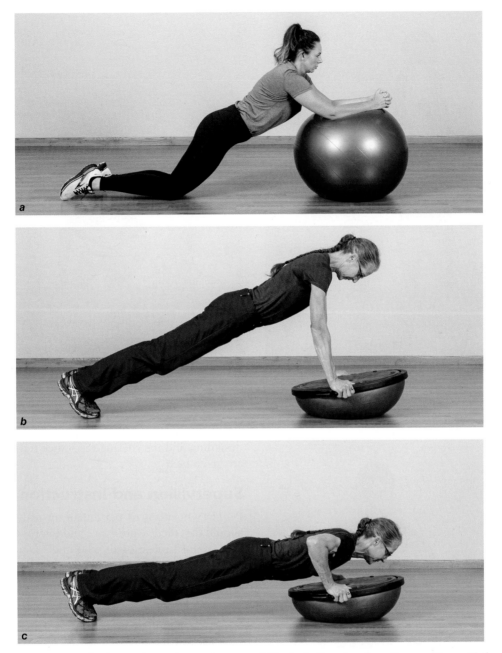

FIGURE 14.3 *(a)* Moving plank (stir the pot) exercise on stability ball: Start in a kneeling position with forearms on the stability ball and the body in a straight line from head to knees, then engage the abdominals and move the forearms in clockwise and counterclockwise circles, allowing the ball to move. BOSU ball push-up exercise (with ball-side down): *(b)* up position with arms extended and *(c)* down position with elbows at 90 degrees.

Without proper supervision and instruction, injuries that require medical attention may occur. An evaluation of resistance training–related injuries presenting to U.S. emergency rooms revealed that 27% of all reported injuries in adults were considered accidental (e.g., dropped weights, improper use of equipment, tripping over equipment) and could have been prevented with strict adherence to safety guidelines (109). A majority of the reported injuries were considered nonaccidental because they resulted from exertion (sprain or strain), overuse, or equipment malfunction (109). Further, these researchers reported that men suffered more trunk injuries than women, whereas women had more foot and leg injuries than men (118). Figure 14.6 illustrates the percentage of resistance training–related injuries at each body part for men and women who presented to U.S. emergency rooms (118). Clearly, people who resistance train should receive instruction on appropriate training loads, exercise guidelines, and equipment use from qualified fitness professionals. General safety recommendations for

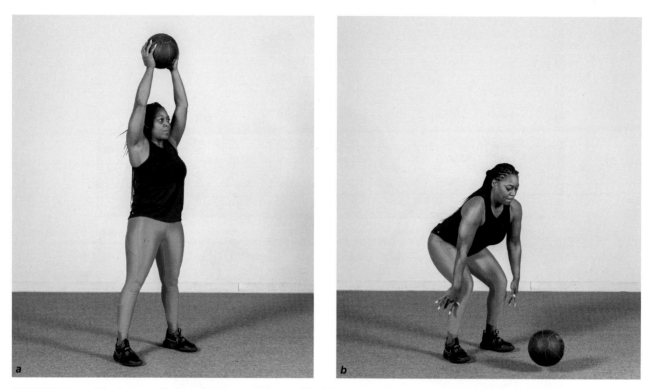

FIGURE 14.4 Medicine-ball slam. *(a)* Start standing tall holding a medicine ball overhead with arms extended. *(b)* Slam the medicine ball to the floor with as much force as possible, pressing the hips back and bending the knees.

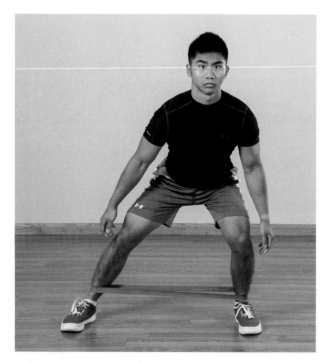

FIGURE 14.5 Lateral band walk with elastic band. Place the band above each ankle, bending the knees slightly and maintaining an athletic standing position, and take a sideways step while keeping the toes pointing forward and feet at least shoulder-width apart. Continue to step laterally for the desired number of repetitions before switching to walk in the opposite direction.

designing and instructing resistance training programs are given next.

Supervision and Instruction

People who want to participate in resistance training should first receive guidance and instruction from qualified fitness professionals who understand principles of resistance training and appreciate the daily variation in strength performance capabilities. Fitness professionals must be well versed in the correct performance of all exercises prescribed and be able to modify exercise form and technique if necessary. A demonstration of an exercise can be particularly effective when providing instruction. They should know which exercises require spotters and should be prepared to offer assistance in case of a failed repetition. When working in a health or fitness facility, the staff should be attentive and should try to position themselves with a clear view of the training center so that they can quickly access people who need assistance. In addition, the fitness staff is responsible for enforcing safety rules (e.g., wear proper footwear, store weights safely, no foolish play in the fitness center) and safe training procedures (e.g., emphasizing proper exercise technique rather than the amount of weight lifted). Not only can fitness professionals enhance the safety of resistance training, but they can help clients maximize gains in muscular fitness when they develop and supervise personalized programs (35, 83, 94, 124).

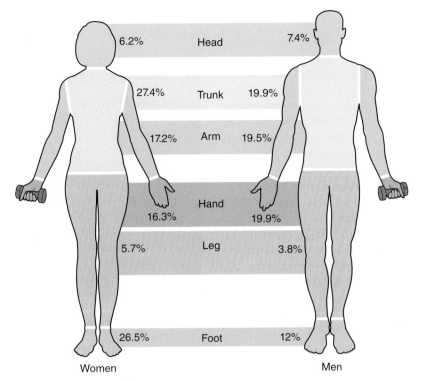

FIGURE 14.6 Percentage of injuries at each body location for men and women.

Based on data from Quatman et al. (2009).

Safety Recommendations for Resistance Training

- Review participants' HSQ before they begin resistance training.
- Select appropriate starting weights and exercises.
- Provide adequate supervision and instruction when necessary.
- Regularly practice emergency procedures.
- Encourage participation in warm-up and cool-down activities.
- Move carefully around the resistance training area, and do not back up without looking first.
- Place an out-of-order sign on broken or malfunctioning equipment, and take the necessary steps to ensure that this equipment is not used by any client until it is completely repaired.
- Use collars on all plate-loaded barbells and dumbbells.
- Be aware of proper spotting procedures, and offer assistance when needed.
- Model appropriate behavior, and do not allow horseplay in the fitness center.
- Demonstrate correct exercise technique, and do not allow participants to train improperly.
- Periodically check all resistance training equipment.
- Ensure the training environment is free of clutter and appropriately maintained.
- Stay up to date with current resistance training guidelines and safety procedures for special populations.

Training Environment

If exercise is to take place in a public, community, work-site, or school-based fitness center, the training area should be well lit and large enough to handle the number of people exercising in the facility at any given time. The facility should be clean, and the equipment should be well maintained. Equipment pads that come in contact with the skin should be cleaned daily, and cables, guide rods, and chains on machines should be checked at least weekly. Equipment should be spaced to allow easy access to each resistance training exercise, and equipment such as free weights and collars should be returned to the proper storage area after each use. Recommended room temperature (68-72 °F, or 20-22 °C) and humidity of less than 60% with adequate airflow should be maintained in the exercise training area (5). Additional recommendations for fitness facility design and layout are available elsewhere (69).

Warm-Up and Cool-Down

Resistance training should be preceded by warm-up activities. A general warm-up increases body and muscle temperature, increases blood flow, and may enhance performance (5). This type of warm-up typically includes 5 to 10 minutes of low- to moderate-intensity aerobic exercise such as slow jogging or stationary cycling. Since the benefits of static stretching as the sole activity during the warm-up have been questioned (10, 20, 95), fitness professionals are incorporating dynamic activities including moderate- to high-intensity hops, skips, and jumps and various movement-based exercises for the upper and lower body into the warm-up period (5, 69). Although a general warm-up can elevate muscle temperature, a well-designed dynamic warm-up can also enhance motor unit excitability, improve kinesthetic awareness, and increase strength and power (10, 95). Although the combination of factors that are responsible for enhancing muscle performance after a dynamic warm-up might be unclear, most factors relate to a neuromuscular phenomenon known as *postactivation potentiation (PAP)* and the more recently termed *postactivation performance enhancement (PAPE)* (16). In this phenomenon, muscular performance is acutely enhanced as a result of prior activity performed at a relatively high intensity.

A specific warm-up involves movements that are similar to the resistance training exercises that are about to be performed. For example, after a general or dynamic warm-up, a lifter could perform a light set of 10 repetitions on the bench press before performing the training set with a heavier weight. It makes sense to prepare physically and mentally for the demands of resistance training by spending about 10 minutes warming up. After a resistance workout, it is a good idea to cool down with general calisthenics and static stretching exercises. A cool-down may reduce the risk of cardiovascular issues (e.g., low BP).

KEY POINT

Qualified supervision and instruction, a safe training environment, sensible training loads, and technique-driven progression will help optimize performance and minimize the risk of injury during resistance training. Fitness professionals should educate participants about safe training procedures and design programs that are consistent with each person's needs and abilities. Dynamic warm-up activities can prepare the body for resistance exercise and enhance strength and power performance.

Resistance Training Guidelines

Although fitness and sports medicine organizations recognize the importance of resistance training for health and fitness (5, 69), no one combination of sets, repetitions, and exercises optimally promotes long-term adaptations in muscular fitness for all people. Rather, many program variables may be altered to achieve desirable outcomes provided that the tenets of resistance exercise are followed. Resistance training programs need to be individualized and based on a person's training history and personal goals.

Many factors must be considered when designing a resistance training program, including the following (49, 123):

- Choice of exercise
- Order of exercise
- Resistance used
- Training volume (total number of sets and repetitions)
- Rest intervals between sets and exercises
- Repetition velocity
- Training frequency

By varying one or more of these variables, endless resistance training programs can be designed. But because different people will respond in various ways to the same resistance training program, decisions must be based on an understanding of exercise science, individual needs, and personal goals. The ACSM's *Guidelines* are summarized in the sidebar *Summary of ACSM's Resistance Training Guidelines for Healthy Adults*.

Summary of ACSM's Resistance Training Guidelines for Healthy Adults

- Include multijoint exercises that involve more than one muscle group.
- Begin with a resistance that allows 8 to 12 repetitions per set (60%-70% 1RM).
- A wide range of repetitions and intensities are effective depending on muscular fitness goals.
- A reasonable rest interval between sets is approximately 2 minutes.
- Perform each exercise with proper technique during the concentric, isometric, and eccentric phases of the repetition.
- Maintain a regular breathing pattern that typically involves exhaling during the lifting phase and inhaling during the lowering phase.
- Train each major muscle group at least 2 nonconsecutive days per week.
- Progressively overload the muscles to create a greater training stimulus if continued gains in muscular fitness are desired.
- Perform a variety of exercises with different types of equipment or body weight.
- Seek instruction from a qualified fitness professional on proper exercise technique and program design.

Adapted from American College of Sports Medicine (2022).

Choice of Exercise

A limitless number of exercises can be used to enhance muscular strength, power, and local muscular endurance (69, 123). Selected exercises should be appropriate for a participant's exercise experience and training goals. Also, the choice of exercises should promote muscle balance across joints and between opposing muscle groups (e.g., quadriceps and hamstrings). Selected weight-machine and free-weight exercises and the primary muscle groups strengthened are listed in table 14.3.

Exercises generally can be classified as single joint (i.e., body-part specific) or multijoint (i.e., structural). Dumbbell biceps curls and leg extensions are examples of single-joint exercises that isolate a specific body part (biceps and quadriceps, respectively), whereas squats and deadlifts are multijoint exercises that involve two or more primary joints. Exercises also can be classified as closed kinetic chain or open kinetic chain. Closed-chain exercises are those in which the distal joint segment is stationary (e.g., squats), whereas open-chain exercises are those in which the terminal joint is free to move (e.g.,

Table 14.3   Selected Weight-Machine and Free-Weight Exercises and the Primary Muscle Groups Strengthened

Weight-machine exercise	Free-weight exercise	Primary muscle groups strengthened
Leg press	Barbell squat	Quadriceps, gluteus maximus
Leg extension	Dumbbell step-up	Quadriceps
Leg curl	Dumbbell Romanian deadlift	Hamstrings
Chest press	Barbell bench press	Pectoralis major
Pec deck	Dumbbell fly	Pectoralis major
Front pull-down	Dumbbell pullover	Latissimus dorsi
Seated rows	Dumbbell one-arm row	Latissimus dorsi
Overhead press	Dumbbell press	Deltoids
Biceps curl	Barbell curl	Biceps
Triceps extension	Lying triceps extension	Triceps

Note: A description of the proper exercise technique for select exercises is available in the appendix of this chapter.

leg extensions). Closed-chain exercises more closely mimic everyday activities and include more functional movement patterns (79).

Single-joint exercises and many machine exercises are often used by people who have limited experience resistance training or who need to correct muscle imbalances. This mode is beneficial in activating specific muscles (e.g., during injury rehabilitation), although long-term research studies comparing gains in muscle size and strength found no additional effects when single-joint exercises were included in a multijoint exercise program (58). With most machines, the path of movement is fixed and therefore the movement is stabilized. Conversely, exercises with free weights require additional muscles to stabilize the movement and therefore are more challenging. Also, bilateral exercises with free weights (e.g., dumbbell lateral raises) might be particularly beneficial for people who need to strengthen a weaker limb. It is important to incorporate multijoint exercises (e.g., lunge, squat, chest press) into a resistance training program to promote the coordinated use of multijoint movements and enhance long-term adaptations (58).

The performance of exercises on unstable surfaces (e.g., stability balls, BOSU balls, and balance pads) has become popular in fitness centers. This type of training has been found to increase core activation and improve balance as well as functional performance in recreationally active people (11). However, force production is reduced when exercises are performed on an unstable surface. Although a multitude of free-weight and body-weight exercises can be performed on unstable surfaces, when participants learn a new exercise, they should become familiar with the movement on a stable surface before progressing to an unstable surface. Additionally, they should start with a light weight so that they can master the technique before adding weight.

Another issue concerning choice of exercise is including exercises for the core musculature. It is not uncommon for beginners to focus on strengthening the chest and biceps and not spend enough time strengthening their abdominals, hips, and lower back. Strengthening the midsection not only may improve force output and enhance body control during free-weight exercises such as the squat, it also may decrease the incidence of low-back pain (30, 129). Notably, low-back pain is the leading worldwide cause of disability, and health care costs attributed to low-back pain are projected to increase in coming decades (71). Thus, prehabilitation exercises for the core muscles should be included in all resistance training programs. In other words, as a preventive health measure, exercises that may be prescribed for the rehabilitation of an injury should be performed even though no injury is present. Exercises such as abdominal curl-ups and back extensions are useful, but they only train the muscles that control trunk flexion and exten-

sion. Free-weight exercises as well as multidirectional exercises that involve rotational movements and diagonal patterns performed with body weight or a medicine ball on a stable or unstable surface can strengthen the core muscles (113). Depending on the needs and goals of the person, other prehabilitation exercises (e.g., internal and external rotation for the rotator cuff) can be incorporated into the exercise session.

Order of Exercise

The order of resistance exercises within a training session may influence training adaptations because strength gains are the largest in the exercises performed at the beginning of the exercise session (111). Traditionally, exercises for large muscle groups are performed before exercises for smaller muscle groups, and multijoint exercises are performed before single-joint exercises. Following this order will allow participants to use heavier weights on the multijoint exercises because fatigue will be less of a factor. It is also helpful to perform more challenging exercises earlier in the workout when the neuromuscular system is less fatigued. However, in some cases (e.g., injury prevention or rehabilitation), it may be appropriate to reverse this order so that the smaller muscle groups are trained first. In general, it seems reasonable to follow the priority system of training in which the exercise order is dictated by the goals of the training program. Also, participants should perform power exercises such as plyometrics before strength exercises so that they can train for maximal power without undue fatigue. An example of a resistance training program is illustrated in the Sample Weekly Resistance Training Log (form 14.1).

Resistance Used

One of the most important variables in designing a resistance training program is the amount of weight used for an exercise (4, 123). Gains in muscular fitness and performance are influenced by the amount of weight lifted, which is highly dependent on program variables such as exercise order, training volume, repetition velocity, and rest-interval length (4, 123). By definition, the amount of weight that can be lifted with proper technique for only 1 repetition is the 1RM. Similarly, the amount of weight that can be lifted with proper technique for 10 but not 11 repetitions is the 10RM. To minimize the risk of injury or residual muscle fatigue, training sets should be performed with proper exercise technique to the point of muscular fatigue but not failure (5, 67, 144).

While gains in muscular fitness can be obtained across a wide spectrum of RM loads, research studies indicate that heavy RM loads (<6RM) have the greatest effect on muscular strength and lighter loads (>10RM) maximize gains in absolute and relative local muscular endurance (4, 90, 130). Gains in muscle hypertrophy can be max-

FORM 14.1 Sample Weekly Resistance Training Log

Date	Monday			Thursday			Comments
	Wt (lb)	Rep	Set	Wt (lb)	Rep	Set	
Goblet squat	20	10	3	20	11	3	Focus on keeping torso upright
Dumbbell step-up	10	8	2	10	10	2	
Lateral band walk	Band	10	2	Band	12	2	
Medicine ball chop	8	10	2	8	12	2	
Dumbbell incline press	10	8	2	10	9	2	
Dumbbell row	10	8	2	10	9	2	Increase weight next week
Dumbbell hip thrust	15	10	2	15	12	2	
Plank variations	Body weight	30 sec	2	Body weight	30 sec	2	Focus on keeping core tight throughout

imized across a wide RM loading range (15, 89, 130). Although untrained people can make significant gains in muscle strength with lighter loads, people with resistance training experience need to train with a heavier resistance to optimize strength gains (4, 19, 121). Relatively light to moderate loads can be used for novice local muscular endurance training, whereas higher-repetition sets (>15 repetitions) are optimal for advanced local muscular endurance training (4).

ACSM recommends novice trainers perform between 8 and 12 repetitions per set to enhance muscular fitness (5). This repetition range translates to a training intensity of approximately 60% to 70% 1RM. However, deconditioned exercisers and older adults should start at a lower intensity (e.g., 40%-50% 1RM) with more repetitions (i.e., 10-15) to reduce the risk of a musculotendinous injury. For trained individuals, ACSM recommends a higher intensity (>80% 1RM) with a greater emphasis on heavier loads (1RM-6RM) to maximize strength performance (5). Training for gains in muscular power is best achieved with light to moderate loads for 3 to 6 repetitions performed as quickly as possible with maximal or near-maximal velocity, avoiding concentric failure (5). A general RM guide for optimizing gains in muscular strength, local muscular endurance, and muscular hypertrophy is presented in figure 14.7. Importantly, fitness professionals should appreciate the importance of systemically varying the RM load over time to avoid training plateaus and reduce the risk of injury.

A percentage of a person's 1RM also can be used to determine the resistance training intensity. If the 1RM on the chest press is 100 pounds (45 kilograms), a training intensity of 70% would be 70 pounds (32 kilograms). It is reasonable for beginners to use a training resistance of approximately 60% to 70% 1RM because they are mostly improving motor performance at this stage (4). As partic-

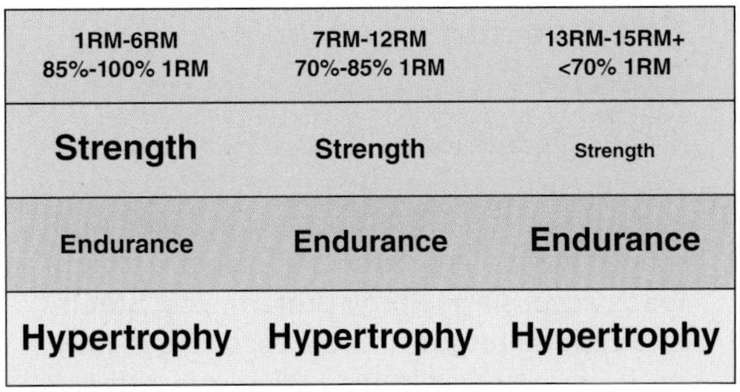

FIGURE 14.7   The RM guide. The use of low repetitions with a heavy load has the greatest effect on strength, whereas the use of high repetitions with a light load has the greatest effect on local muscular endurance. A range of RM loads can be used to maximize muscle hypertrophy.

ipants get stronger and gain training experience, heavier resistances (~80% 1RM) will be needed to optimize gains in muscular strength and local muscular endurance (4, 69). This method of prescribing resistance exercise requires testing the 1RM on all exercises in the training program. In many cases this is not realistic because of the time required to correctly perform 1RM testing on 8 to 10 exercises. Furthermore, maximal resistance testing for small-muscle-group exercises (e.g., biceps curls and lying triceps extensions) typically is not performed.

Fitness professionals also should be knowledgeable about the relationship between the percentage of 1RM and the number of repetitions that can be performed. In general, most people can perform about 10 repetitions using 75% of their 1RM. However, the number of repetitions that can be performed at a given percentage of the 1RM varies with the amount of muscle mass required to perform the exercise. For example, studies have shown that at a given percentage of the 1RM (e.g., 60%), adults can perform more repetitions of an exercise for large muscle groups such as the squat or leg press compared with an exercise for smaller muscle groups such as the arm curl or leg curl (135). Therefore, prescribing a resistance training intensity of 70% of 1RM on all exercises warrants additional consideration because at 70% of the 1RM, a person may be able to perform 20 or more repetitions on a large-muscle-group exercise, which may not be ideal for enhancing muscle strength. If a percentage of the 1RM is used for prescribing resistance training, the prescribed percentage of the 1RM for each exercise may need to vary to maintain a desired training range (e.g., 8RM-10RM). Further, because self-selected resistance exercise intensities tend to be lower than what is recommended (141), fitness professionals need to carefully prescribe the amount of weight used for each exercise to maximize training adaptations.

RESEARCH INSIGHT

Self-Selected Loads in Resistance Exercise

Although the loads used in a resistance training program can be prescribed as a percentage of the 1RM for a target repetition range, individuals often self-select training loads according to their preferences. Steele and colleagues performed a scoping review to examine what loads individuals self-select in resistance training sessions (141). They found that on average individuals self-selected a load equal to 53% of their 1RM. Additionally, individuals did not select heavier loads when prescribed lower repetitions, and vice versa. While 53% 1RM may be sufficient to stimulate muscular strength in novices, it is suboptimal for maximizing strength gains in individuals with resistance training experience. Fitness professionals should provide guidance and instruction on load selection and progression if individuals want to maximize strength performance.

Training Volume

The number of exercises performed per session, the repetitions performed per set with a given weight, and the number of sets performed per exercise all influence the training volume (4). For example, if a participant performs 3 sets of 10 repetitions with 100 pounds (45 kilograms) on the bench press, the training volume for this exercise is 3,000 pounds ($3 \times 10 \times 100 = 3,000$), or about 1,350 kilograms. Altering the training volume can influence neural, hypertrophic, metabolic, and hormonal responses and adaptations to resistance training (4, 119, 121, 123). Although training volume has been widely discussed, it is important to remember that every training session does not need to be characterized by the same number of sets, repetitions, weights, and exercises.

Untrained individuals can make significant improvements in muscular fitness with one set per muscle group per session (5, 6). However, for trained individuals who want to maximize gains a graded dose–response relationship exists between the number of weekly sets per muscle group and gains in muscular strength and hypertrophy (15, 119, 121). The dose–response continuum includes low volume (<5 sets per muscle group), moderate volume (5-9 sets per muscle group), and high volume (≥10 sets per muscle group) weekly training (5). These sets may be for the same exercise or for different exercises affecting the same muscle group. For example, over the course of a week a trained individual could perform 8 sets of squats or 4 sets of squats and 4 sets of leg press. Using different exercises to train the same muscle groups adds variety to the resistance training program and can help keep the training stimulus effective.

When fitness professionals design a resistance training program, they need to consider the person's resistance training status and goals because of the numerous possibilities for program design. It seems reasonable for beginners and very deconditioned people to start with a single-set program of moderate intensity and gradually increase the number of sets depending on personal goals and time available for training. A single-set protocol reduces training time and may therefore increase the likelihood for exercise compliance in people who do not train regularly. However, it is also possible that a multiple-set protocol can be a time-efficient method of training if the program is well designed (77). For example, instead of performing 1 set for each of 12 exercises during every workout, participants can perform 3 sets for each of 4 bilateral, multijoint exercises through a full ROM.

It is important to understand that a dramatic increase in training intensity or volume may increase the risk of overtraining. By gradually varying the sets, repetitions, and number of exercises, the training stimulus will remain effective and therefore the adaptations to the training program will be maximized. Periods of low-volume training can provide a needed variation for people who have been participating in a high-volume conditioning program for a prolonged time.

Rests Between Sets and Exercises

The rest interval between sets and exercises is an important training variable that affects the acute responses and chronic adaptations to resistance training (65, 68). In general, the length of the rest influences energy recovery and the training adaptations that take place. For example, if the primary goal of the program is to increase muscular strength, heavier weights and longer rests (e.g., >2 minutes) are needed, whereas if the goal is local muscular endurance, shorter rests (e.g., <1 minute) are required. Training intensity, training goals, and fitness level will influence the length of the rest interval. For example, it has been shown that the number of repetitions performed is compromised with short rest intervals (<1 minute), whereas performance can be maintained during a multiset protocol when 3- and 5-minute rest intervals are used (125). As previously noted for the other program variables, the same rest interval does not need to be used between all sets and exercises. In addition, fatigue resulting from a previous exercise should be considered when prescribing the rest interval. If time is not a factor, resting >2 minutes between sets is recommended for exercises with heavier loads, which may lead to greater improvements in muscular strength in trained individuals, although a shorter rest interval of 1 to 2 minutes may suffice for untrained individuals (68). Although short rests (<30 seconds between sets and exercises) may not be appropriate for beginners because of the discomfort associated with muscular fatigue, the rests can be shortened gradually over time to provide ample opportunity for the body to tolerate this type of training. For example, circuit training is a type of conditioning that is characterized by relatively short rest intervals between exercise stations.

Repetition Velocity

The velocity or cadence at which a resistance exercise is performed can affect the neural, hypertrophic, and metabolic adaptations to a training program (4, 32, 123). According to the principle of training specificity, gains in muscle strength and performance are specific to the training velocity (49). For example, fast-velocity plyometric training is more likely to enhance speed and power than are slow-velocity exercises on weight machines. However, it is useful to recognize two types of slow-velocity training. Unintentional slow velocities are used when a heavy resistance is lifted and the velocity is slow despite the attempt to exert maximal force. On the other hand, intentional slow velocities are used when a person trains with a submaximal load and purposefully performs the exercise at a slow velocity. Increasing time under tension with intentionally slow velocities results in greater fatigue and less muscle fiber activation (72). Given that concentric force production is lower for an intentionally slower velocity compared with a moderate to fast velocity, lighter loads performed at an intentionally slow velocity may not be optimal for maximizing strength development (32).

Because beginners need to learn how to perform each exercise correctly with a light resistance, it is generally recommended that untrained people perform exercises in a deliberately controlled manner (5). As they gain experience, they may use unintentional slow velocities with a heavier resistance to optimize strength gains or they may use intentional fast velocities to optimize power gains. The intent to maximally accelerate the weight during training is essential for maximizing strength gains in trained people (123). This concept has been termed *compensatory acceleration* and requires the trained person to accelerate the weight maximally throughout the concentric phase of the lift (123). Therefore, participants with resistance training experience can perform a continuum of velocities, from unintentionally slow to intentionally fast, in order to maximize performance adaptations.

Training Frequency

Training frequency typically refers to the number of training sessions per week and is dependent on several factors including training experience, exercise selection, intensity, and volume. In general, a training frequency of at least two sessions per week on nonconsecutive days is recommended for untrained individuals, although improvements in muscular fitness can be made by resistance training only once per week (5). However, the principal driver for muscular fitness improvements in trained people who perform more advanced programs is training volume per muscle group per week (5, 66). While increasing training frequency certainly can increase weekly training volume, many program design options are possible to achieve gains in muscular fitness in trained individuals. For example, trained people who perform a split routine may resistance train four times per week, but they only train each muscle group two times per week; they might train muscles of the lower body on Monday and Thursday and muscles of the upper body on Tuesday and Friday. Although an increase in resistance training experience does not necessitate an increase in training frequency, a higher frequency does allow for greater specialization characterized by more exercises and a higher weekly training volume.

Periodization

Periodization refers to systematic variation in a resistance training program. It is impossible to improve continually at the same rate over long-term training, but properly varying the training variables can limit training plateaus, maximize performance gains, manage fatigue, and reduce the likelihood of overtraining (18, 102). Observable manifestations of overtraining include a plateau or decrease in performance, sleep disturbances, muscle tenderness, and increased risk of infection (64, 100). A resistance training program characterized by excessive frequency, volume, or intensity of training, combined with inadequate rest and recovery, eventually will shift toward overtraining syndrome (for additional information on avoiding overtraining syndrome, see chapter 16). Periodization is a process whereby fitness professionals systematically vary the training stimulus over time in order to keep it effective. Although periodization has been part of sport conditioning programs for many years, the benefits of periodized programs compared with nonperiodized programs for long-term progression continue to be explored in the literature (102, 142, 157).

The concept of periodization, or program variation, is not just for athletes but for people with all levels of training experience who want to enhance their health and fitness. A downfall of many resistance training programs is not regularly changing program variables over time. By periodically changing program variables such as choice of exercise, training weight (resistance), number of sets, rest intervals between sets, or any combination of these, long-term performance gains will be optimized and the risk of overuse injuries may be reduced (4, 102, 157). Moreover, it is reasonable to suggest that people who participate in well-designed periodized programs and continue to improve their health and fitness may be more likely to adhere to an exercise program over the long term (28).

For example, if a person's lower-body routine typically consists of leg presses, leg extensions, and leg curls, performing step-ups and dumbbell lunges on alternate workout days likely will add to the effectiveness and enjoyment of the resistance training program. Further, varying the volume and intensity of training can help to prevent training plateaus, which are common after the first 2 months of training. Many times participants can avoid a strength plateau by varying the training intensity and volume to allow for ample recovery. In the long term, program variation with adequate recovery will result in even greater gains because the body will be challenged to adapt to even greater demands. The underlying concept of periodization is based on the theory that, after a certain time, adaptations to a stimulus will no longer take place unless the stimulus is altered. Periodized resistance training has been shown to be superior to nonperiodized resistance training for promoting long-term training adaptations in muscular strength and power, and therefore fitness professionals should not underestimate the importance of training variety to keep the stimulus challenging and effective (102, 142, 157). In addition, lifestyle factors such as sensible nutrition, proper hydration, and adequate sleep can influence how people adapt to resistance training.

Although many models of periodization exist, the general concept is to prioritize training goals and then develop a long-term plan that varies throughout the year. In general, the overall training plan is divided into time periods called *macrocycles* (about 1 year), *mesocycles* (3-4 months), and *microcycles* (1-4 weeks), with each cycle having a specific goal (e.g., hypertrophy, strength, or power). The classic periodization model is referred to as a *linear model* because the volume and intensity of training gradually change over time (123). For example, at the start of a macrocycle, the training volume may be high and the training intensity may be low. As the year progresses, the volume decreases as the intensity increases.

Although the linear training model was originally designed for weightlifters and track and field athletes who wanted to peak for a specific competition, it can be modified by fitness professionals in order to enhance health and fitness. For example, people who routinely perform the same combination of sets and repetitions may benefit from gradually increasing the weight and decreasing the number of repetitions as strength improves. Notably, this model of training should be applied to the primary exercises that form the foundation of the program. Secondary or assistance exercises may follow a different paradigm depending on the needs and goals of the individual. The classic periodized model is outlined in table 14.4. After the four-phase program is complete, people should be encouraged to participate in recreational activities or low-intensity resistance training to reduce the likelihood of overtraining. This period of unloading or restoration is called *active rest* and typically lasts for 1 to 3 weeks. After active rest, participants can then return to the first phase of their training program with more energy and vigor.

Table 14.4 Sample Linear Periodized Workout for Maximizing Strength Gains in Healthy Adults

	Phase 1 General preparation	Phase 2 Hypertrophy	Phase 3 Strength	Phase 4 Peaking
Intensity	12RM-15RM	8RM-12RM	6RM-8RM	4RM-6RM
Sets	1-2	2	2-3	3
Rest between sets	60-120 seconds	60 seconds	60-120 seconds	120-180 seconds

Note: The workout is for major-muscle-group exercises performed each phase; each phase lasts about 6 to 8 weeks. RM = repetition maximum.

A second model of periodization is referred to as an *undulating (nonlinear) model* because of the daily fluctuations in training volume and intensity. For example, a person may perform 2 sets of 8 to 10 repetitions with a moderate load on Monday, 3 sets of 4 to 6 repetitions with a heavy load on Wednesday, and 1 set of 12 to 15 repetitions with a light load on Friday. The heavy training days will maximally activate the trained musculature, and selected muscle fibers will not be maximally taxed on light and moderate training days. By alternating training intensities, the participant can minimize the risk of overtraining and maximize the potential for maintaining training-induced strength gains. While primary exercises follow a similar periodized scheme, secondary or assistance exercises may follow a different model depending on individual needs and goals. A sample nonlinear periodized workout plan for a trained adult is presented in table 14.5. In addition, fitness professionals should consider a participant's vacation schedule or travel plans when incorporating active rest into the year-long training schedule. Periods of restoration lasting from 1 to 3 weeks will allow for physical and psychological recovery from the resistance training. A detailed review of periodization and specific examples of periodized programs are available elsewhere (4, 18, 69).

KEY POINT

Designing a safe, effective, and enjoyable resistance training program involves an understanding of exercise science along with an appreciation of the art of prescribing exercise while addressing individual needs, concerns, and abilities. The specific exercises, the order of exercises, the resistance used, the number of sets, the rest intervals between sets and exercises, the training velocity, and the training frequency are variables that contribute to the design of a resistance training program. Periodization is the systematic variation of program variables to optimize long-term training adaptations, promote long-term adherence, and reduce the risk of overtraining.

Resistance Training Methods

Many resistance training methods can be used to enhance muscular fitness. Some methods have been scientifically proven to be effective, whereas others are based on anecdotal evidence. The wide variety of methods illustrates the types of programs that can be developed by manipulating program variables. Five of the most common resistance training methods are single set, multiple set, circuit training, supersets, and assisted training.

Single Set

This method of resistance training is one of the oldest and consists of performing a single set of a predetermined number of repetitions (e.g., 8-12) until volitional fatigue. This time-efficient method of resistance training can be an effective method for people who have no resistance training experience or who have not trained for several years. Because the acute adaptations to resistance training (i.e., 6-12 weeks) are primarily due to neuromuscular adaptations (123), a single-set system can be an appropriate method of training for beginners. Trained individuals also can benefit from single-set training with loads ranging from 70% to 85% 1RM, but the strength gains will be suboptimal (6).

Multiple Set

The multiple-set method is an effective training method for enhancing strength and power. This method of training became popular in the 1940s and originally consisted of 3 sets of 10 repetitions with increasing weights. For example, the classic multiple-set protocol used by DeLorme in his pioneering rehabilitation work involved performing the first set of 10 repetitions at 50% of 10RM, the second set of 10 repetitions at 75% of 10RM, and the third set of 10 repetitions at 100% of 10RM (33). Over the years, many multiple-set programs using various combinations of sets and repetitions have been shown to be effective. For example, the pyramid system is a multiple-set system in which the weight increases progressively over several sets so that fewer and fewer repetitions can be performed (see table 14.6). For continued progression in a resistance training program, multiple sets should be used (119). However, to

Table 14.5 Sample Nonlinear Periodized Workout for a Trained Adult

	Monday	Wednesday	Friday
Intensity	8RM-10RM	4RM-6RM	13RM-15RM
Sets	2	3	3
Rest between sets and exercises	2 minutes	3 minutes	1 minute

Note: This plan is for the major-muscle-group exercises performed each day.

Table 14.6 Sample Light-to-Heavy Pyramid Training System

Set number	Repetitions	Intensity (%1RM)
1	10	75
2	8	80
3	6	85

reduce the risk of overtraining, the total number of sets performed per training session should gradually increase. In addition, not all exercises need to be performed for the same number of sets.

Circuit Training

This method of training involves performing a series of resistance exercises with body weight or with a light, moderate, or heavy load in a circuit with minimal rest (about 30 seconds) between exercises. Generally, moderate weights are used (about 60%-80% of 1RM), and 10 to 15 repetitions are performed at 8 to 12 exercise stations. It has become popular to include jumping, sprinting, and agility exercises within a training circuit (e.g., metabolic circuit training). The number of circuits depends on the training experience of the individual as

well as the program design (e.g., exercise choice and intensity). In addition to increasing muscular fitness, circuit training also can improve CRF, decrease total body fat, and increase muscle mass (122). Circuit training performed three times per week with short rest periods between exercises (<30 seconds) tend to result in larger effects (122). Starting with a 1-minute rest between exercises and gradually reducing the rest to the desired range as the body adapts is recommended when a person is beginning circuit training. A sample circuit training program is illustrated in figure 14.8.

Supersets

Superset training (also called *compound sets*) consists of performing successive sets of two or more exercises (for the same muscle group or different muscle groups) with limited or no rest between exercises. For example, after performing a set to volitional fatigue on the bench press, the participant immediately performs a set of dumbbell flys to facilitate chest development. This type of training forces the target muscle group (e.g., pectoralis major) to work longer and harder and is often used to increase muscle hypertrophy and local muscular endurance. Alternatively, the biceps curl exercise can be paired with the triceps push-down as an efficacious and time-efficient alternative to traditional resistance training (127).

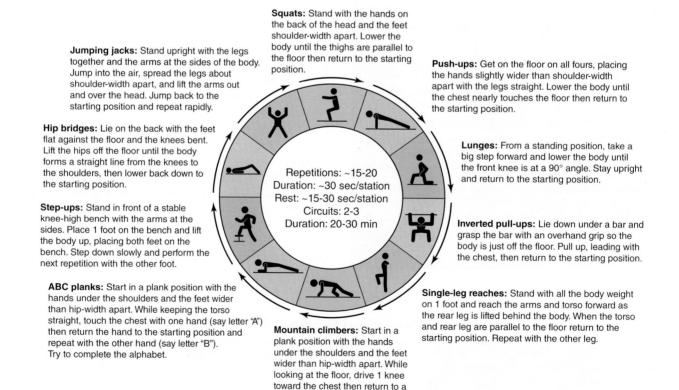

Jumping jacks: Stand upright with the legs together and the arms at the sides of the body. Jump into the air, spread the legs about shoulder-width apart, and lift the arms out and over the head. Jump back to the starting position and repeat rapidly.

Hip bridges: Lie on the back with the feet flat against the floor and the knees bent. Lift the hips off the floor until the body forms a straight line from the knees to the shoulders, then lower back down to the starting position.

Step-ups: Stand in front of a stable knee-high bench with the arms at the sides. Place 1 foot on the bench and lift the body up, placing both feet on the bench. Step down slowly and perform the next repetition with the other foot.

ABC planks: Start in a plank position with the hands under the shoulders and the feet wider than hip-width apart. While keeping the torso straight, touch the chest with one hand (say letter "A") then return the hand to the starting position and repeat with the other hand (say letter "B"). Try to complete the alphabet.

Squats: Stand with the hands on the back of the head and the feet shoulder-width apart. Lower the body until the thighs are parallel to the floor then return to the starting position.

Push-ups: Get on the floor on all fours, placing the hands slightly wider than shoulder-width apart with the legs straight. Lower the body until the chest nearly touches the floor then return to the starting position.

Lunges: From a standing position, take a big step forward and lower the body until the front knee is at a 90° angle. Stay upright and return to the starting position.

Inverted pull-ups: Lie down under a bar and grasp the bar with an overhand grip so the body is just off the floor. Pull up, leading with the chest, then return to the starting position.

Single-leg reaches: Stand with all the body weight on 1 foot and reach the arms and torso forward as the rear leg is lifted behind the body. When the torso and rear leg are parallel to the floor return to the starting position. Repeat with the other leg.

Mountain climbers: Start in a plank position with the hands under the shoulders and the feet wider than hip-width apart. While looking at the floor, drive 1 knee toward the chest then return to a straight-leg position. Repeat with the other leg.

Repetitions: ~15-20
Duration: ~30 sec/station
Rest: ~15-30 sec/station
Circuits: 2-3
Duration: 20-30 min

FIGURE 14.8 Sample program for circuit resistance training.

Assisted Training

As the name implies, this method of training requires the assistance of another person who, after several repetitions of an exercise are performed to volitional fatigue, can provide just enough assistance to allow the lifter to complete 1 to 4 additional forced repetitions. Because muscles are stronger eccentrically than concentrically, assistance may not be needed during the eccentric phase of the forced repetitions, but a spotter should be available to assist in case of a failed repetition. Although this advanced training system will enhance muscular fitness, it is not recommended for beginners because it typically results in muscle soreness and fatigue attributable to the overload placed on the neuromuscular system (123). Other training systems also may result in some muscle soreness, but assisted training increases the likelihood that soreness will result.

KEY POINT

A variety of resistance training methods can be used to enhance strength, power, and local muscular endurance. Although all training methods can be effective, the key is to match the method with the needs, goals, and abilities of each participant for long-term success. The design of the resistance training program will influence the training-induced adaptations that take place.

Resistance Training for Special Populations

Resistance training can be a safe, effective, and beneficial method of conditioning for people of all ages and physical abilities. Although research on resistance training has focused predominantly on healthy adults, a growing body of evidence indicates that children, seniors, pregnant women, and people with certain chronic but stable conditions (e.g., coronary heart disease) can participate safely in resistance training provided that appropriate training guidelines are followed.

Children and Adolescents

Research studies clearly demonstrate that children and adolescents can benefit from resistance training (13, 40, 85, 86). ACSM (5), American Academy of Pediatrics (AAP) (143), Canadian Society for Exercise Physiology (CSEP) (12), NSCA (39), and other international organizations (86) support participation in youth resistance training provided that the program is appropriately designed and supervised. Furthermore, public health recommendations now support regular participation in muscle-strengthening activities for children (149, 158). In addition to increasing muscular fitness, regular participation in a youth resistance training program may improve fundamental movement skills and favorably influence several measurable indexes of health, including body composition, bone mineral density, psychosocial well-being, and metabolic risk factors (26, 27, 56). Further, because many aspiring young athletes who enter sport programs may not be prepared for the demands of training and competition, participation in a preseason conditioning program that includes resistance training may decrease the risk of sport-related injuries (108, 117).

A traditional concern associated with youth resistance training is that it may harm the developing musculoskeletal system. However, observations indicate no evidence of a decrease in stature in young people who participate in resistance training in controlled environments (44, 93). The belief that resistance training is harmful to the immature skeleton of young weight trainers is inconsistent with current findings suggesting that childhood may be the time during which the bone-modeling process responds best to the mechanical loading of weight-bearing physical activities such as jumping and resistance training (60, 148). Children and adolescents are now encouraged to participate daily in 60 minutes or more of physical activity that includes aerobic activities as well as developmentally appropriate muscle-strengthening and bone-strengthening activities (149, 158). Because a certain level of muscular strength is needed to perform fundamental movement skills such as jumping and throwing, resistance training during childhood can help prepare youth for ongoing participation in exercise and sport activities (42, 138).

Another corollary of youth resistance training is its influence on body composition. As the number of overweight young people in the United States and other countries continues to increase (75, 87), the effect of resistance training on body composition has received increased attention (57, 131). Although aerobic exercise is typically prescribed for decreasing body fatness, researchers have reported that resistance training or combined aerobic and resistance training may be beneficial for treating children who are overweight or obese (34, 101, 137). Of interest is the finding that progressive resistance training has been found to significantly increase insulin sensitivity in overweight youth (132, 150), and integrative training programs that include resistance exercise have been found to improve intelligence and cognitive flexibility among overweight and obese children (114). It appears that young people who are overweight or obese enjoy resistance training because it is not aerobically taxing and it gives all participants a chance to experience success and feel good about their performance. Further study is warranted, but the first step in encouraging these youth to exercise may be to increase their confidence in their ability to be physically active, which in turn may lead to an increase in physical activity and a decrease in body fat.

RESEARCH INSIGHT

Benefits of Aerobic and Resistance Training in Adolescents With Obesity

As the prevalence of obesity among youth continues to increase worldwide, effective strategies are needed to treat and manage this condition. Sigal and colleagues (137) examined the effects of 22 weeks of aerobic training, resistance training, or combined training in previously inactive adolescents who were obese. Following the training period, aerobic, resistance, and combined training reduced total body fat and waist circumference in study participants. In participants with the best adherence to the exercise intervention, combined training appeared to offer the greatest benefit. These findings demonstrate that interventions that include resistance training may be most beneficial for youth who are sedentary and obese.

Although there is no minimum age requirement for participating in a youth resistance training program, all children who participate should have the emotional maturity to accept and follow directions and understand the benefits and risks associated with this type of training. In general, if children are ready for organized sport, they are ready for some type of resistance training. As a point of reference, an age range of 5 to 7 years is when many children are involved in sports, and it is reasonable that they could benefit from strength-building activities that are developmentally appropriate (e.g., bear crawls, frog jumps, and one-leg hops) (143). Although some observers may be concerned about the stress that resistance training places on the developing musculoskeletal system, the peak loads associated with high-impact jumping activities may be greater in both duration and magnitude than those resulting from resistance training (47). Further, injury to the epiphyseal plate or growth cartilage has not been reported in any prospective study on youth resistance training (44, 93). Nevertheless, fitness professionals should follow youth resistance training guidelines to decrease the likelihood of an acci-

dent or injury when young people perform resistance exercises (86, 143).

Children should begin resistance training at a level that is commensurate with their physical abilities. No matter how big or strong a child is, adult training programs and philosophies (e.g., "No pain, no gain") should not be imposed on children. The focus of youth resistance training should be on learning proper technique for a variety of exercises in an engaging environment. During each session, fitness professionals should listen to each child's concerns and closely monitor each child's ability to handle the prescribed training weight. Focusing on the physical and mental health needs of each participant and implementing enjoyable and educative exercise interventions with effective pedagogical practices can help maximize participation, enhance training-induced outcomes, and spark an ongoing interest in resistance exercise (45). Various combinations of sets and repetitions and a variety of training modes including child-sized weight machines, free weights, medicine balls, and body-weight exercises have proven to be effective (41, 86).

When working with children, remember that the goal of the program should not be limited to increasing muscle strength. Due to the developmental needs of children and adolescents, programming to promote resistance training skill literacy should be integrated into youth fitness programs. Resistance training skill literacy is an inclusive concept that includes knowledge, understanding, and skill performance that evolves over time to sustain participation in resistance exercise (43). In order to enhance resistance training skill literacy, youth should have an opportunity to learn and practice a variety of resistance exercises in a supportive setting as they apply learned skills in novel situations. Consider the following guidelines for program design when developing resistance training programs for children:

- Parents or legal guardians should complete an HSQ for each child.
- Children with diseases or disabilities should have their exercise program tailored to their condition, symptoms, and functional capacity.
- Qualified instructors should design and supervise youth fitness activities.
- The exercise area should be free of clutter and adequately ventilated.
- Begin with 1 to 2 sets of 8 to 12 repetitions using a light resistance (≤60% 1RM).
- The program can be progressed to 2 to 4 sets of 6 to 12 repetitions with a light to moderate load (≤80% 1RM).
- As resistance training experience increases, youth can be introduced to periodic phases of higher-in-

tensity resistance training (≥80% 1RM), provided the focus is on technical competency.

- Resistance should be increased only when the child can perform the desired number of repetitions with proper exercise technique.
- Include multijoint exercises that are designed to enhance muscular fitness, coordination, and motor skill competency.
- Two or three nonconsecutive training sessions per week are recommended.
- Focus on enhancing resistance training skill literacy in a socially supportive environment.

Seniors

The number of men and women over the age of 65 in the United States is increasing (see chapter 18), and research studies and clinical observations indicate that seniors can benefit from exercise programs that include resistance training (3, 53, 97). Even people over the age of 90 can enhance their muscular fitness through resistance training (48). Regular participation in a resistance training program can help offset the age-related declines in bone, muscle mass, and strength that often make ADLs—such as climbing stairs—more difficult (97, 152).

Further, structured physical activity programs that include resistance training may help counter muscle disuse and reduce the risk of major mobility disability in seniors (97, 112). Bones become more fragile with age, and sedentary behaviors can have a detrimental effect on bone health (98). Advancing age also is associated with a loss of muscle mass (sarcopenia) and a loss of muscular strength and power (dynapenia) (23, 145). Evidence indicates that seniors who resistance train can improve muscle strength, muscle power, gait speed, and balance, which in turn can enhance overall function and reduce the potential for injuries caused by falls (53, 63, 97). Moreover, evidence is emerging of significant psychological and cognitive benefits from regular resistance exercise participation by older adults (21, 24, 104). Fitness professionals should educate seniors on the benefits of resistance training due to the debilitating consequences of disuse-induced muscle atrophy on physical functioning and quality of life (112).

Seniors can adapt readily to resistance training exercises. If the training intensity is adequate, they can make relative gains in strength that are equal to or greater than those of younger people. Of interest is the observation that resistance training trials comparing training intensities show strong resistance training effects in a dose–response manner, with higher-intensity training (70%-79% 1RM) being more effective than lower-intensity training in seniors (19). Research studies using computed tomography (CT) and muscle-biopsy analysis also have reported evidence of muscle hypertrophy in seniors who resistance train, and others have reported that resistance training can increase bone mineral density and improve cardiometabolic health of older adults who resistance train (29, 48, 53, 96, 153). Although both aerobic and resistance exercise are important for seniors, only resistance training can maximize gains in muscle strength, muscle power, and muscle mass. These potential benefits may be particularly important for frail older adults who are at increased risk for falls and osteoporotic fractures (88). However, adults will retain the beneficial effects of resistance training only as long as they continue their exercise program. During prolonged inactivity, adaptive changes in skeletal muscle strength and functional mobility regress toward preexercise levels (25, 70). This is sometimes referred to as the *principle of reversibility*.

Before starting a resistance training program, seniors should undergo preparticipation health screening because many have a variety of known, coexisting medical conditions. In addition, at least during the initial phase of training, fitness professionals should provide instruction and offer assistance as needed. Older adults should begin resistance training at a light intensity (i.e., 40%-50% 1RM) during the first few weeks to allow time for musculoskeletal adaptation and to practice exercise technique (5). Over time, the intensity can increase gradually to 60% to 80% 1RM (5). Older adults may also benefit from power training because this type of exercise offers more potential for improving functional performance and reducing the risk of falling (8, 38). Power training can include exercises with body weight (e.g., jumping) or exercises using light to moderate loading with high velocity (120). While older adults may not be able to perform fast muscle actions at the start of the program, they can begin with slower movements and then progress gradually. Although no specific recommendations exist for neuromotor training, exercises that combine balance, agility, and proprioceptive training (e.g., tai chi, dancing, and ball games) can be effective in reducing and preventing falls in older adults (5, 83, 134). Chapter 15 includes more information on neuromotor exercise training and ways to provide progression. ACSM recommends the following program design considerations for seniors who want to resistance train (5):

- Begin with ≥1 set of 10 to 15 repetitions for each of 8 to 10 exercises involving the major muscle groups.
- Progress to 1 to 3 sets of 8 to 12 repetitions for each exercise.
- Use a rating between moderate (5-6) and vigorous (7-8) on a scale of 0 to 10 for level of physical exertion.
- Use a light to moderate load (30%-60% 1RM) for 6 to 10 repetitions for power training.

- Maintain proper breathing patterns while exercising.
- Perform all exercises within a pain-free ROM.
- Individualize progression of all resistance training activities.
- Gradually incorporate balance, agility, and proprioceptive training into the exercise program.
- Resistance train at least 2 days per week.
- Use behavioral strategies such as social support to enhance adherence.
- Fitness professionals should supervise initial training sessions.

Pregnant Women

Research evidence suggests that regular exercise during a low-risk pregnancy poses little risk to either the mother or the fetus and improves overall maternal fitness and well-being (2, 5, 37, 107). Indeed, regular exercise may reduce the risk of developing conditions associated with pregnancy, including pregnancy-induced hypertension and gestational diabetes mellitus (37, 92, 128). Furthermore, regular physical activity during pregnancy may influence psychological health, reducing feelings of depression and anxiety (37). Participation in a range of aerobic activities appears safe during and after pregnancy, and resistance training may also be beneficial because it enhances muscular fitness, which allows expectant mothers to perform ADLs with greater ease and possibly minimizes low-back pain, which is common during pregnancy (2, 31, 155). Along with moderate-intensity aerobic exercise, resistance training at an appropriate intensity, duration, and frequency may offer significant health value to women with an uncomplicated pregnancy.

Exercise is not advised for all women who are pregnant, especially those who have medical complications. Thus, pregnant women should undergo a medical evaluation with their personal physician or qualified health care provider and ask about activities that may or may not be appropriate during pregnancy. Contraindications for exercise during pregnancy and warning signs to stop exercise during pregnancy are discussed in chapter 19. Fitness professionals must be aware of these contraindications and be watchful for warning signs when working with pregnant clients.

Limited data are available regarding resistance training for pregnant women (9, 115, 116, 155). General guidelines for resistance training are outlined in this chapter, and recommendations for exercising while pregnant are discussed in chapter 19. General exercise recommendations include maintaining adequate hydration, wearing appropriate clothing, and exercising at a comfortable intensity. The ACSM recommends resistance training activities including pelvic floor muscle training (e.g., Kegel exercises) during pregnancy, although the program may need to be modified based on prior resistance exercise experience, physical abilities, and health-related concerns (5). Pregnant women should avoid physical activity on the back after the first trimester and any exercise using the Valsalva maneuver or prolonged isometric contractions. Hot Pilates and hot yoga should be avoided during pregnancy due to the risk of rising core temperature. Exercise movements that involve jumping, a quick change of direction, or possible loss of balance are not recommended (5). Guidelines about exercise and pregnancy in recreational and elite athletes are available from the International Olympic Committee (17). Women should consult with their health care provider to determine when physical activity can be gradually resumed following delivery.

Adults With Heart Disease

Coronary heart disease (CHD) is a leading cause of morbidity and mortality, and individuals with CHD typically have multiple risk factors. Secondary prevention programs are designed to not only control these risk factors but to

RESEARCH INSIGHT

LIFTMOR to Build Strong Bones

Weight-bearing physical activity is an effective strategy for managing osteoporosis, but high-intensity resistance training is not routinely prescribed. The primary aim of the Lifting Intervention for Training Muscle and Osteoporosis Rehabilitation (LIFTMOR) study was to determine the efficacy of bone-targeted high-intensity resistance training for improving bone mineral density in postmenopausal women with low bone mass (153). Participants were randomized either to 8 months of twice-weekly, 30-minute, supervised, high-intensity resistance training (5 sets of 5 repetitions, >85% 1RM) or a home-based, low-intensity exercise program. They found that the high-intensity training program enhanced indices of bone strength and functional performance in postmenopausal women. No fractures or other serious injuries were reported. These findings underscore the potential bone-building benefits of supervised high-intensity resistance training for postmenopausal women.

improve exercise capacity, psychosocial well-being, and quality of life (36, 50). Also, by preventing or delaying the progression of this disease, longevity is likely to increase and yearly health care costs are likely to decrease (36, 50). Cardiac rehabilitation programs traditionally have emphasized aerobic exercise to maintain and improve CRF. However, muscular strength and local muscular endurance are also important to prepare individuals for return to work and leisure activities (50, 51, 82). Many ADLs, as well as most occupational tasks, place demands on the cardiovascular system that closely resemble resistance exercise. Because many cardiac patients are deconditioned and lack the strength and confidence to perform common activities involving muscular effort, adding resistance training to an overall physical activity program provides individuals with an opportunity to restore or gain optimal physiologic, vocational, and psychosocial status (52, 82, 159). The AHA (156), ACSM (5), and American Association of Cardiovascular and Pulmonary Rehabilitation (AACVPR) (140) recommend resistance training as part of a comprehensive cardiac rehabilitation program.

Research indicates that medically stable cardiac patients can safely engage in resistance training provided that the program is appropriately designed and carried out within the prescribed guidelines (1, 5, 46). Regular participation in a resistance training program may favorably affect muscular strength, local muscular endurance, cardiorespiratory endurance, cardiac risk factors, body composition, physical function, and psychosocial well-being. Training-induced gains in muscular strength also can improve vascular function and decrease the rate–pressure product (and associated myocardial demands) during daily activities such as carrying groceries and gardening (82, 156). In general, improving both CRF and muscular fitness can improve a patient's quality of life and help older patients live independently (46, 74, 84).

Before patients begin a resistance training program, a qualified health care provider should review their health and medical history to identify any condition that may exclude participation. Although most low- to moderate-risk patients can participate safely in resistance training, programs for patients with low fitness levels or severe left ventricular dysfunction may be safer in a medically supervised environment. ACSM provides contraindications for inpatient and outpatient cardiac rehabilitations, as noted in chapter 21.

KEY POINT

Resistance training can be a safe and effective component of a comprehensive fitness program for people of all ages and those with medical conditions provided that appropriate guidelines are followed and qualified instruction is available. Despite previous concerns, children, older adults, pregnant women, and patients with heart disease can benefit from participation in a well-designed resistance training program. Participants with medical conditions first should be screened to identify those who may be contraindicated for resistance training, as determined by a qualified health care provider.

All patients entering cardiac rehabilitation should be considered for resistance training, particularly those whose jobs involve manual labor (5). Although patients can begin with elastic bands and light weights (1-5 pounds, or 0.5-2 kilograms), they should progress toward

Program Design for People With Heart Disease

- A physician or other qualified health care provider should review the health and medical history.
- Begin with a light weight, and focus on controlled movements for 10 to 15 repetitions.
- Following initial adaptations, gradually increase the load to 40% to 60% 1RM.
- Perform each exercise initially for 1 set, and progress to 2 or 3 sets as tolerated.
- A perceived exertion rating of 11 to 13 on a scale of 6 to 20 may be used to guide effort.
- Include multijoint exercises that involve more than one muscle group.
- Progress slowly as the individual adapts to the training program.
- Train two to three times per week on nonconsecutive days.
- Maintain regular breathing and avoid straining.
- Stop exercise in the event of any warning signs or symptoms such as dizziness, dysrhythmias, unusual shortness of breath, or anginal discomfort.

a traditional resistance training program in which they lift weights corresponding to an RPE of 11 to 13 on a 6 to 20 scale (40%-60% 1RM) for 10 to 15 repetitions for each exercise (5). ACSM recommends that patients perform 1 to 3 sets of 8 to 10 exercises that focus on the major muscle groups 2 to 3 nonconsecutive days per week (5). Patients should perform warm-up and cool-down activities including dynamic movements and static stretching. Further, patients should maintain a regular breathing pattern and avoid sustained, tight gripping, which may evoke an excessive BP response. The decision to begin a resistance training program should be based on current health status as determined by a qualified health care provider. The guidelines for designing a resistance training program for cardiac patients are the same as those for older adults—namely, patients should start with a light weight and gradually progress as they adapt to the training program. For patients returning to work, exercise training should be specific to the muscle groups and energy systems used for occupational tasks in order to increase physical work capacity, improve safety, and enhance self-efficacy (5).

LEARNING AIDS

REVIEW QUESTIONS

1. What four training principles determine the effectiveness of resistance exercise programs?

2. Distinguish between isometric, concentric, eccentric, and isokinetic muscle actions.

3. What musculoskeletal, cardiorespiratory, metabolic, and mental health outcomes may result from resistance training in adults?

4. List five resistance training systems that can enhance muscular fitness, and provide an example of each method.

5. What are the advantages and disadvantages of resistance training with weight machines, free weights, medicine balls, and body-weight exercises?

6. Discuss the benefits and concerns associated with youth resistance training.

7. What exercises should healthy pregnant women perform, and what exercises should be avoided?

8. What resistance training guidelines are appropriate for low-risk patients with CHD?

9. What resistance training system would be most appropriate for a deconditioned client, for a healthy adult who wants to enhance general fitness, and for a trained person who wants to optimize gains in muscle strength?

CASE STUDIES

1. A 25-year-old male member of your fitness center has been resistance training for 4 months and claims to have made significant gains in strength. He performs 1 set of 12 to 15 repetitions on eight weight machines 2 days per week. However, over the past 6 weeks he has noticed that he is not making the strength gains that he used to. His goal is to get stronger and increase his muscle mass. How would you modify his training program to optimize his desired gains in muscular fitness over the long term?

2. A 48-year-old female currently swims for 45 to 60 minutes, 3 to 4 days per week, at the local recreation center. Although she has been a swimmer for years, she was recently advised by her doctor to participate in weight-bearing physical activities to increase her musculoskeletal strength. She has no previous experience resistance training and is excited about incorporating this type of exercise into her training program. However, she is somewhat concerned about lifting heavy weights and does not want to get hurt. Address her concerns regarding resistance training and modify her current exercise program to optimize gains in musculoskeletal strength.

3. The director of a local assisted living center for seniors wants to offer a new activity class at the facility, and they ask you for guidance and recommendations. In addition to a walking program that is already established, they want you to develop a proposal for a senior resistance training program that not only enhances muscular fitness, but is safe and enjoyable for adults over 65 years of age who have no resistance training experience. The facility does not have weight machines, but it does have several pairs of lightweight (1-5 pounds, or 0.5-2 kilograms) dumbbells and a variety of elastic bands. Discuss program design considerations for seniors that will enhance muscular fitness and reduce the risk of falling.

Answers to Case Studies

1. Because it is not possible to improve at the same rate over long-term training, it is important to vary the resistance training program over time to limit training plateaus and optimize adaptations. By periodically varying the program variables (e.g., choice of exercise, sets, and repetitions), long-term performance gains will be optimized and exercise adherence will be improved. One option for this member is to follow an undulating or nonlinear training program, which is characterized by daily fluctuations in volume and intensity. For example, over time he could progress to 2 or 3 sets of 8 to 10 repetitions with a moderate load on Monday, 3 or 4 sets of 6 repetitions with a heavy load on Wednesday, and 1 or 2 sets of 12 to 15 repetitions with a light load on Friday. In addition, he should seek advice from a fitness professional and learn how to safely incorporate free-weight exercises and other training systems into his program.

2. Although this client should be encouraged to continue swimming, resistance training can offer additional benefits in terms of musculoskeletal strength. A fitness professional should review the potential health and fitness benefits of regular weight-bearing physical activity with the client and should discuss the importance of proper exercise technique and a gradual progression of training weights to avoid injury. This client does not have any resistance training experience, so she should begin with a single set of 8 to 12 repetitions on a variety of single-joint and multi-joint exercises to improve her confidence and exercise compliance. Over time, she should progress to a multiple-set system at a higher training intensity to optimize gains in musculoskeletal strength.

3. Regular resistance training can offer observable health and fitness benefits to older adults; however, the health status of seniors should be assessed before resistance training begins in order to identify any preexisting medical conditions. Also, fitness professionals who have experience working with older populations should be available to provide instruction and assistance as needed. General program design considerations to discuss with the director of this assisted living center include the following:

- Resistance training should begin with minimal resistance during the first few weeks so participants can learn proper exercise technique and have time for musculoskeletal adaptation.

- The resistance, repetitions, or number of sets should be increased gradually to maximize gains in muscular fitness.

- Over time, exercises that reduce the base of support, stress postural muscle groups, and reduce sensory input should be sensibly incorporated into the program to enhance balance, agility, and proprioception.

Further, the importance of exercising in a group setting should be emphasized because social support can enhance exercise adherence in older populations.

APPENDIX 14.1: SELECTED RESISTANCE TRAINING EXERCISES FOR THE MAJOR MUSCLE GROUPS

Leg Press

Prime muscle movers: Quadriceps, gluteus maximus

Exercise technique: The exerciser starts in a sitting position with the knees bent at 90° and the feet placed about shoulder-width apart on the foot pad. The torso should be erect, and the back should be pressed against the back of the seat. The participant extends the legs almost completely (without locking the knees) and then slowly returns to the starting position.

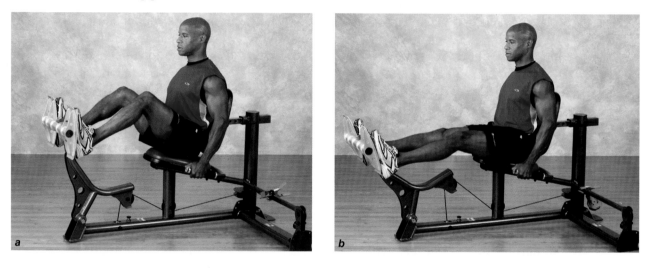

Leg Curl

Prime muscle movers: Hamstrings

Exercise technique: The participant faces the machine with one ankle in front of the pad. After grasping the handles and stabilizing the body, the participant bends the knee to lift the weight. Slowly return to the starting position and repeat the movement. Do not use momentum to complete the lift. After the desired number of repetitions, switch legs.

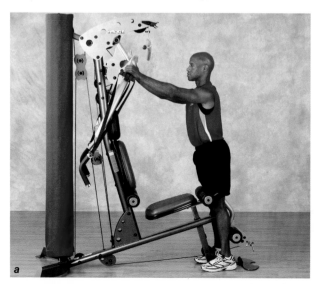
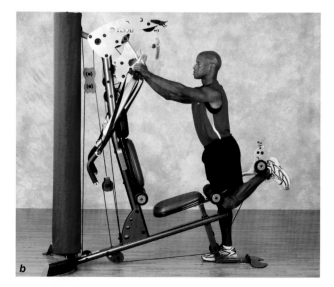

Dumbbell Heel Raise

Prime muscle movers: Gastrocnemius, soleus

Exercise technique: The participant stands, holding a dumbbell in the right hand and placing the left hand on a wall for support. The left foot is lifted off the floor. The participant raises the heel of the right foot as high as possible and then slowly lowers it to the starting position. This exercise should be performed on both sides of the body. The participant should concentrate on keeping the torso and knees straight to avoid upper-leg involvement. To increase the ROM, a 1- to 2-inch (2.5-5.0 centimeter) board or weight plate can be placed under the ball of the exercising foot. If this is too difficult, the exercise can be performed with both feet on the floor or board.

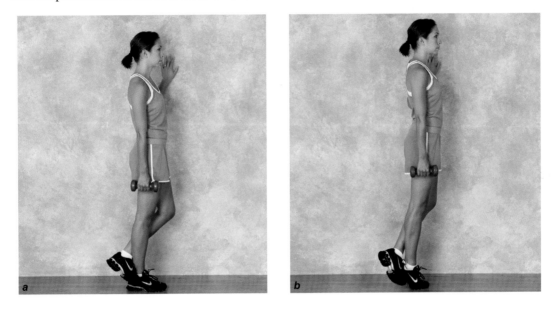

Bench Press

Prime muscle movers: Pectoralis major, anterior deltoid, triceps

Exercise technique: The participant lies flat on the bench and holds the barbell with a wider-than-shoulder-width grip directly above the chest, with thumbs around the bar, arms straight, and feet flat on the floor. The participant slowly lowers the barbell to the chest with elbows about 45° from the body and then presses the barbell back up to the starting position. The barbell should not be bounced on the chest, and a spotter should stand by in case of a failed repetition.

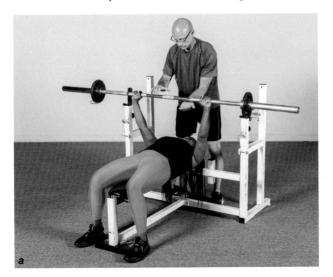
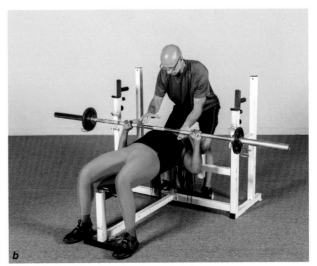

Front Pull-Down

Prime muscle movers: Latissimus dorsi, biceps

Exercise technique: The participant sits on the seat with the arms fully extended, places both knees under the exercise pad, and grips the bar underhand (palms toward the face) using a shoulder-width grip. The participant should lean slightly backward from the waist and maintain this position throughout the duration of the exercise to avoid getting hit by the bar. The bar is pulled down just under the chin and then returned slowly until the arms are fully extended.

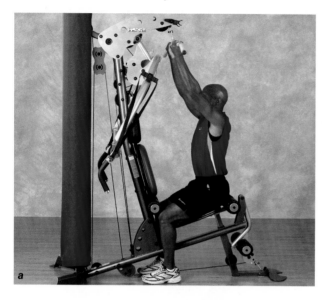 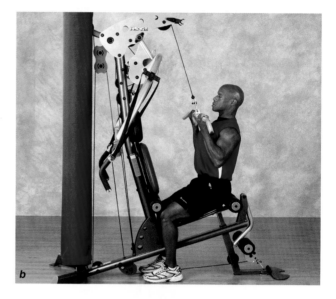

Dumbbell Overhead Press

Prime muscle movers: Deltoids, triceps

Exercise technique: In the standing position, the participant holds a dumbbell in each hand at shoulder level with palms facing forward. The participant presses the weights overhead to a straight-arm position and then slowly returns to the starting position. The participant should not bend or sway the back to complete a repetition.

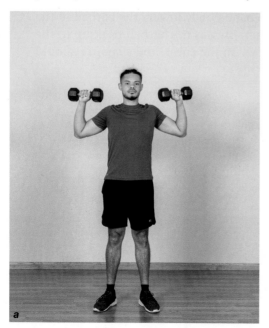 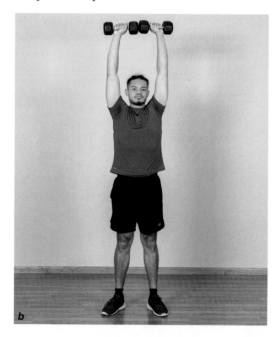

Dumbbell Curl

Prime muscle movers: Biceps

Exercise technique: The participant stands with a dumbbell in each hand (palms facing forward) and the arms at the sides of the body. The participant bends the elbows to bring the weights toward the shoulders and then slowly returns to the starting position. The back should not be bent or swayed to complete a repetition.

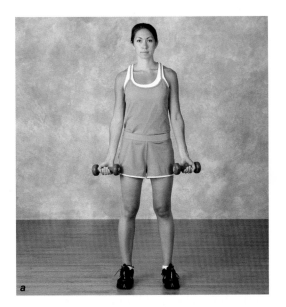
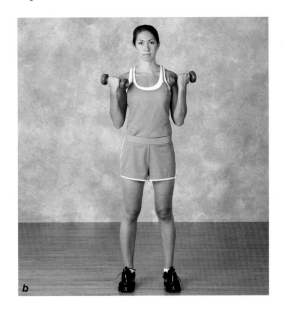

Lying Triceps Extension

Prime muscle movers: Triceps

Exercise technique: The participant lies flat on the back on an exercise bench and holds a dumbbell in each hand with arms straight over the shoulders and palms facing each other. The participant lowers both dumbbells to the side of the head by bending only at the elbows and then slowly returns to the starting position. The upper arm should not be swayed to complete a repetition.

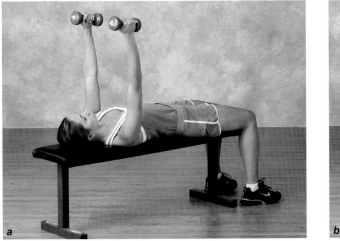
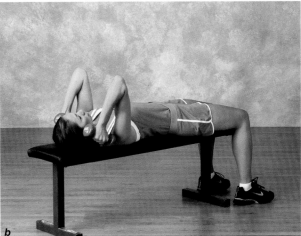

Kneeling Trunk Extension

Prime muscle mover: Erector spinae

Exercise technique: The participant kneels on the floor and supports the body on both hands and knees. The participant extends the right leg backward until it is parallel to the floor, pauses briefly, returns to the starting position, and then extends the left leg backward. To make this exercise more challenging, the participant can raise the left arm parallel to the floor while extending the right leg (and vice versa).

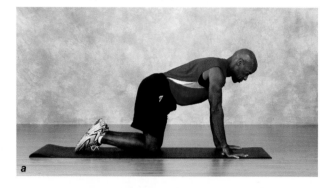 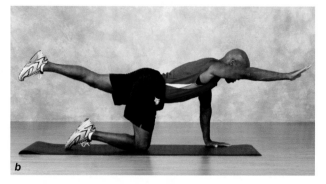

Abdominal Curl

Prime muscle mover: Rectus abdominis

Exercise technique: The participant lies flat on the back with the knees bent, feet about 12 to 15 inches (about 30.5-38.0 centimeters) from the buttocks, and hands placed on the thighs (or across the chest). Leading with the chin, the participant lifts the shoulders and upper back off the mat (about 30°-45°) while moving the hands toward the knees, pauses briefly, and then returns to the starting position. If the hands are placed behind the head, the participant must not pull the head forward with the hands.

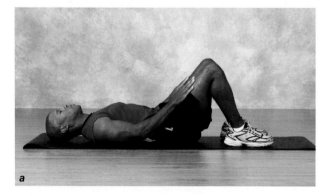 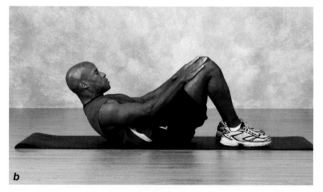

15

Exercise Prescription for Flexibility and Neuromotor Fitness

Erica M. Taylor

OBJECTIVES

The reader will be able to do the following:

1. Describe a motion segment and explain the role of the facet joints
2. Differentiate between functional and structural spinal curves
3. Describe flexibility exercises for the major muscle groups and body regions
4. Describe different methods of stretching
5. Explain why it is important for the trunk muscles to be able to control pelvic positioning
6. Identify the musculature of the local and global stabilizing systems
7. Describe the ideal ways to activate the deep abdominal layers
8. Describe exercises that increase the strength and endurance of muscles that are fundamental to the development of core stability
9. Describe the current recommendations for stretching exercises
10. Describe exercises that can be used to enhance neuromotor fitness

15

Activities of daily living (ADLs) and recreational activities can be significantly affected by flexibility and neuromotor fitness. The capacity to move a joint smoothly through its full range of motion (ROM) allows for more efficient and comfortable movement, and neuromotor fitness is involved in the coordination of all movement. The extensibility of the major muscles crossing the lumbosacral region can have a significant impact on low-back function. The American College of Sports Medicine's (ACSM) recommendations include performing flexibility training at least 2 days per week to increase or maintain the normal ROM at joints (4). A minimum of 2 to 3 days per week also has been recommended to improve or maintain neuromotor fitness (21). Exercises directed at improving flexibility and neuromotor fitness are both diverse and common in the fitness setting.

This chapter covers several aspects of flexibility and neuromotor fitness. Many clients who sign up for fitness training will have either a history of or current low-back dysfunction. Fitness professionals need to be able to design an appropriate individualized program for clients that strengthens the lumbopelvic region and protects it from injury. The ability to create and refine a program that addresses low-back function and flexibility requires an understanding of basic spine anatomy and biomechanics. Additionally, flexibility exercises addressing the major joints and muscles, the current recommendations for stretching, and core stability principles and exercises are presented. Although the recommended prescription is less clear for exercises to support neuromotor fitness, general guidelines supported by research are covered. The chapter closes with a discussion about when to refer a client for a medical consultation.

Anatomy of the Spine

Figure 15.1 depicts the lumbar spine. Appreciating the anatomy of the spine allows for an understanding of low-back pain (LBP). The fundamental unit of the lumbar spine is the motion segment, which consists of two vertebrae and their intervening disc. The bodies of the vertebrae and their intervening disc are sometimes referred to as the *anterior aspect* of the motion segment. The posterior aspect of the motion segment is attached to the anterior aspect by the pedicles, which provide the lateral boundary of the foramen (vertical passageway) for the spinal cord and its nerves. In addition to the transverse and spinous processes, the posterior elements of the vertebrae include the superior and inferior articular processes, and each of their junctions is referred to as a *zygapophyseal joint*, or facet joint. In addition to supporting loads on the spine, the facet joints control the amount and direction of vertebral movement based on their joint surface orientation (53).

The anterior and posterior longitudinal ligaments provide stability for the anterior portion of the motion segments; they run the length of the spine on the anterior and posterior surfaces of the vertebrae bodies as well as the intervertebral discs. All of these ligaments have pain receptors, so a sprain to any of them can signal a back problem. The discs enable each vertebra to be more mobile and distribute forces (figure 15.2). However, with the exception of their periphery, the discs do not have pain receptors. The peripheral receptors can respond if the nucleus of a disc breaks through its normal boundaries (e.g., distends or ruptures its annulus).

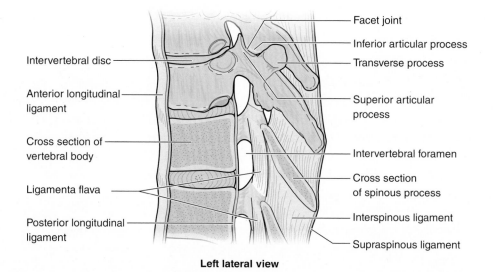

Intervertebral disc

Anterior longitudinal ligament

Cross section of vertebral body

Ligamenta flava

Posterior longitudinal ligament

Facet joint

Inferior articular process

Transverse process

Superior articular process

Intervertebral foramen

Cross section of spinous process

Interspinous ligament

Supraspinous ligament

Left lateral view

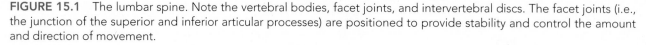

FIGURE 15.1 The lumbar spine. Note the vertebral bodies, facet joints, and intervertebral discs. The facet joints (i.e., the junction of the superior and inferior articular processes) are positioned to provide stability and control the amount and direction of movement.

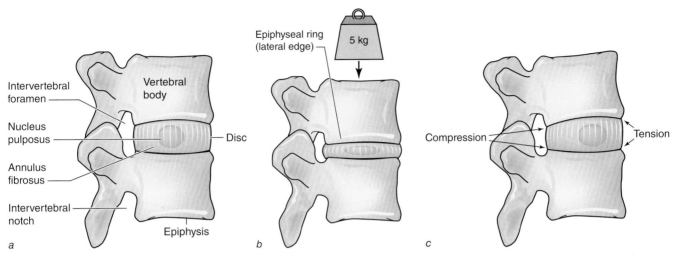

FIGURE 15.2 *(a)* Discs allow flexibility and act as shock absorbers. *(b)* When weight is added (in this case perpendicular to the disc), the force is absorbed in all directions; however, if the external force is applied obliquely, the pressure within the disc is away from the direction of the applied force. *(c)* Compression force is on the side of the bend, and tension is on the opposite side. Spine extension brings compression on the posterior disc and tension on the anterior annulus.

Figures 15.2a and 15.2b adapted from W. Liemohn, *Exercise Prescription and the Back* (New York, NY: McGraw-Hill, 2001).

KEY POINT

The fundamental unit of the spine is the motion segment, which consists of two vertebrae and their intervening disc. The spinal discs absorb shock to the vertebral column by exerting pressure in all directions. Although the facet joints help support loads, one of their primary responsibilities is controlling the amount and direction of spinal movement, such as that seen in rotation. A lack of proper mechanics can compromise the discs, ligaments, facets, and musculature of the spine, causing injury.

This information is important because it is essential to understand and educate clients in the ideal alignment of the spine during exercises to avoid injury. The fitness professional needs to be aware of positions that may compromise the spinal structures. If a disc is diseased or injured, its ability to withstand stress is adversely affected and the motion segment to which it belongs may become unstable.

The disc is avascular (i.e., without a blood supply), and motion in the spine enhances its nutrition (i.e., motion enables the disc to absorb nutrients through the vertebral end plates). It is wise to frequently change positions, altering the loads on the discs and promoting the flow of fluid and nutrition to the disc (68). Discs absorb fluid and become tighter during sleep. The fuller discs permit less movement, which is a reason back injuries

often occur in the morning. Thus, slow warm-ups before strenuous exercise or work are especially important in the morning or following sleep.

Spinal Curves

The curvatures of the spine as viewed from the side are described as a lordotic curve when they are concave and as a kyphotic curve when they are convex. Cervical and lumbar curves are normally lordotic, and the thoracic curve is kyphotic. Exaggerations of these curves are not desirable; for example, an increased anterior (or forward) pelvic tilt increases the lordotic curve in the lumbar area, which increases the stresses on the ligaments, discs, vertebrae, and musculature of the spine (especially L5). A small lumbar lordotic curve is natural and, along with the cervical lordosis and thoracic kyphosis, assists the discs in cushioning compressive forces occurring in the spine during ADLs. The neutral spine concept is based on a balance of these curves. (This concept will be revisited later in a discussion of core exercises.) Factors such as being overweight, wearing high-heeled shoes, and lacking appropriate muscle length or strength can affect the degree of lordosis. Tightness in the hip flexors (i.e., the psoas) can increase the lordotic curve by causing an anterior pelvic tilt; conversely, tightness in the hamstrings can reduce the lordosis (see figure 15.3).

Functional and Structural Curves

Spinal curves may be either functional or structural. Spinal curves are functional if the curve can be removed by assuming a posture that takes away the force respon-

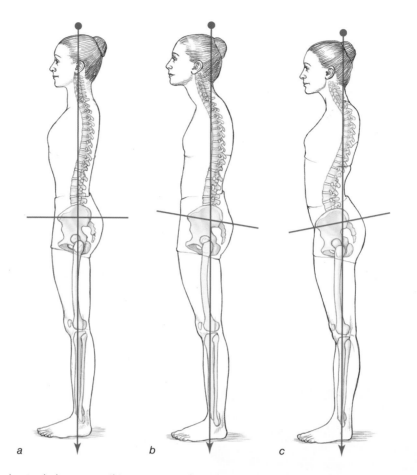

FIGURE 15.3 (*a*) Ideal spinal alignment, (*b*) posterior pelvic tilt with decreased lordosis and forward placement of the head, (*c*) anterior pelvic tilt with increased lordosis.

sible for the curve. A functional curve may be present due to a spasm or tightness of a particular muscle group and will disappear when the client is lying down or bending or when the spasm has dissipated. In contrast, a structural curve is always present independent of the person's position; it is fixed and not flexible. However, a functional curve may eventually become structural if one assumes an unhealthy posture over several years. For example, a person sitting at a desk for many hours each day often assumes a slumping posture during this time, which may result in an increase in thoracic kyphosis and rounded shoulders, a forward head position, and a decrease in the lumbar curve. If this person does not extend the spine or retract the shoulders periodically, the ability to perform these movements may decrease and the poor posture may become structural. A structural curve is not easy to straighten and is associated with a loss of spinal flexibility.

These issues are important when working with a client. If a client has a structural lumbar lordosis or thoracic kyphosis, obtaining an ideal spine position from which to perform both stretching and core exercises

may be difficult or painful. The fitness professional can teach the client to obtain the most comfortable position midway between flexion and extension where there is no pain, or the client may need supportive props such as yoga blocks or pillows to support the structural curve. Gentle stretching exercises to facilitate movement in the restricted direction may help the client obtain a more ideal position in the future.

Scoliosis is another curvature of the spine to consider. When the spine is viewed from the back, ideally a straight vertical line is seen. Scoliosis is noted as a lateral curve of the spine that can occur in any, or multiple, regions of the spine (see figure 15.4). If a lateral curve that might indicate scoliosis is seen, the fitness professional should refer the client to a medical doctor or physical therapist for evaluation and clearance for a fitness program that includes spinal flexibility and core strengthening.

Spinal Movement

When the whole spine moves in any direction, each vertebra contributes motion in a complex pattern of

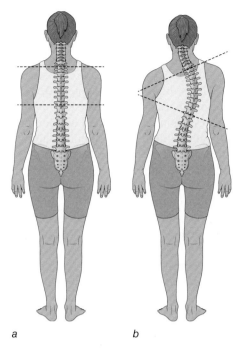

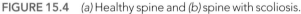

FIGURE 15.4 *(a)* Healthy spine and *(b)* spine with scoliosis.

KEY POINT

> Functional curves can be removed by assuming a posture that reduces the force that caused the curve. Structural curves can develop over several years and are not easily removed. Structural curves increase the difficulty of obtaining the ideal spine position needed for flexibility and core exercises. Helping the client find a comfortable position midway between flexion and extension or providing props such as yoga blocks or pillows to support the structural curve can help.

simultaneous rotation and translation (53). With injury, such as degenerative disc disease, the vertebral motion pattern changes (53) and influences the motion of the whole spine, potentially causing pain and hypermobility (23). There is a region of intervertebral motion around a neutral position that has little restraint from the passive spinal components, similar to the wiggle room between two vertebrae without passive restraint (i.e., ligaments). If too much movement, or wiggle room, is present, it cannot provide a stable base for the attaching muscles. Panjabi (56) termed this region of intervertebral motion that has little resistance from the passive spinal components the *neutral zone*, and it is used to quantify the amount of segmental instability that is present (57,

62, 69). It is thought that the neutral zone is a better measurement of instability than spine ROM (58, 59). If the neutral zone grows larger as disc degeneration or ligamentous injury occurs, there is more laxity or instability in the spine to control, which places more demands on the stabilizing systems. Therefore, it is important to understand how to improve the stability of the spine. The stabilizing system is an interconnected set of the passive, active, and neutral subsystems. The passive system consists of the bony structures, ligaments, joint capsules, discs, and passive portion of the musculotendinous units (55). The active system is composed of the muscles and tendons and is the subject of the core exercises described later in this chapter. The neural subsystem receives and transmits information from and to the other two systems to manage spinal stability. It is also important to recognize that neuromuscular control can be compromised in those with LBP and must be considered in a core stabilization program (32, 35).

Most spinal motions in functional activities and some exercises use some combination of the three planes of motion: sagittal (flexion and extension), frontal or coronal (lateral flexion or side bending), and transverse (rotation) (see chapter 3 for background on planes of motion). Because some of the most forceful stresses on the discs occur during movements that combine bending and rotation, exercises involving these movements should always be done under muscle control. In other words, exercises involving intervertebral movement should not be ballistic (e.g., movements in which momentum plays a major role). If the movement results from momentum rather than muscle control, normal end ROM may be exceeded and connective-tissue structures such as spinal ligaments or discs may be damaged. As mentioned, the spine is particularly vulnerable at the beginning of the day because the discs imbibe tissue fluid while recumbent in sleeping postures, resulting in tighter discs that are more vulnerable to sprain or other injury.

Mechanics of the Spine and the Hip Joint

The muscles crossing the hip joint (hip flexors, hamstrings, iliotibial band [ITB]) can be viewed as guy-wires (tension cables that provide stability) bracing the pelvis. If any of these guy-wires are too tight, the abdominal musculature has difficulty controlling pelvic positioning. Because the sacrum (in the pelvis) is the foundation for the 24 vertebrae stacked on it, pelvic positioning is important to the integrity of the spine. Tightness in the hamstrings can severely affect the ability of the pelvis to tilt anteriorly and thus can diminish pelvic ROM. Tightness of the hip flexors (iliopsoas and rectus femoris) also can be detrimental to low-back function because the pelvic girdle may rest in an anterior tilt, causing increased load to L5-S1 (53). If the length of the iliopsoas is asymmetrical from one side to the other, a pelvic girdle asymmetry may occur, creating a sacroiliac joint dysfunction. A shortened ITB may restrict lower-extremity adduction, and a tightened piriformis also might restrict hip rotatory motion. When healthy participants were compared with LBP patients in terms of their hip ROM (18), an association was observed between hip rotation imbalance (internal and external rotation) and the presence of LBP.

A neutral position of the pelvic girdle and spine is one in which the joints are in an optimal position for performing daily activities and exercise. The person in figure 15.3a is displaying a good neutral spine posture in which the convex curves in the thoracic and sacral areas are balanced by the concave curves in the cervical and lumbar areas. Energy expenditure is minimal because body segments are in balance and forces on the discs are minimized. Figures 15.3b and 15.3c demonstrate altered pelvic positions that change the rest of the spinal curves, placing additional strain on the spinal components. An anteriorly tilted pelvis may be from tight hip flexors or trunk extensors, whereas a posteriorly tilted pelvis may result from tight hamstrings. Both flexibility and core exercises need a neutral spine alignment as a starting point. As mentioned previously, a structural spinal curve may prevent a person from obtaining the ideal neutral spine position; finding a position that is pain free and as close to neutral as possible usually is the best solution. A person who is unable to obtain a neutral position while standing due to tight hamstrings or hip flexors may be able to reach a neutral position in a supine position because the tight hip muscles are in a slack position. Frequently, the first goal of flexibility and spine exercises is to teach clients how to obtain a neutral spine position. It is common for this position to feel foreign to them if they have had poor posture for some time. Consequently, for effective stretching and core strengthening programs, gaining an understanding of what constitutes a neutral spine position is key for clients.

KEY POINT

> The pelvis serves as the foundation for the spine, so the ability of the trunk muscles to control pelvic positioning is essential for maintaining a neutral spine and a healthy back. If either the hip flexors or hip extensors are too tight, posture may be compromised.

Exercise Considerations: Preventive and Therapeutic

ACSM recommends flexibility and core-strengthening exercises (3). As discussed in chapter 10, neuromotor fitness is also important, and exercises to promote neuromotor fitness should be included in a comprehensive fitness program. Although core stability training is often used to train athletes to perform better in their particular sports, it is also emphasized in LBP prevention and in therapeutic programs. Good isometric endurance of the trunk musculature may prevent a first occurrence of LBP (10, 24), and deconditioning of the lumbar extensor musculature is a risk factor for low-back injury and pain (24, 29, 65). The core exercise of drawing in the abdominal muscles, which activates the transversus abdominis and multifidus, has been shown to reduce the 3-year recurrence rate of LBP from 75% to 35% (28). The rationale behind flexibility and strength training for the core are discussed, and suggestions for specific exercise programs are presented.

Core stability is the ability to control the forces across the spine and pelvic girdle while protecting the integrity of the spinal structures. It is the ability to achieve and sustain control of the trunk region at rest and during precise movements (45). The objective of core stability training is to challenge the muscular systems enough to achieve functional stability without excessive load to the spine (46). Two components of core stability are the muscles themselves and neuromuscular control. Core stability results when the passive structures of the spinal column (i.e., the vertebrae, discs, rib cage, pelvis, and all associated connective tissue) are stabilized by the active component (i.e., the neuromuscular component).

Stability can be viewed both from a larger perspective of trunk stability during ADLs (45) and from the stability present at the vertebral segments in the neutral zone (58, 62). Consider whether a client keeps the spine stable while performing a squat, chest press, or plank, or if extra motions are occurring at the spine to compensate for the arm and leg muscular contractions that pull on the spine. Table 15.1 presents a model of spine stability that divides the muscles into local and global musculature; the local muscles are recruited in a coordinated fashion to keep the segments stable, while the global muscles generate torque (T) and control spinal motion during trunk or extremity movement (9). Figure 15.5 presents a cross section of these muscles.

Some extremely small muscles are close to the spinal column, including the intertransversarii mediales, interspinales, and rotatores. These muscles have a high density of muscle spindles (52) and are thought to act as

Table 15.1 Local and Global Core Muscle Divisions

LOCAL MUSCLES (STABILIZATION SYSTEM)		GLOBAL MUSCLES (MOVEMENT SYSTEM)
Primary	**Secondary**	
Transversus abdominis	Internal oblique	Rectus abdominis
Multifidus	Medial fibers of external oblique	Lateral fibers of external oblique
	Quadratus lumborum	Psoas major
	Diaphragm	Erector spinae
	Pelvic floor muscles	Quadratus lumborum
	Iliocostalis and longissimus (lumbar portion)	

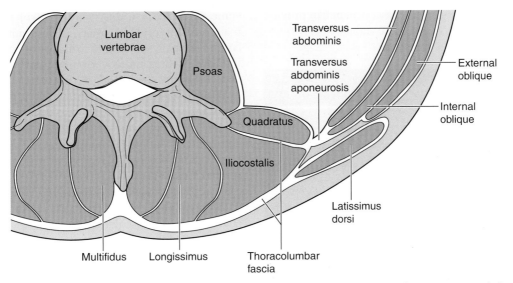

FIGURE 15.5 Cross section of the major trunk muscles, listed in table 15.1, that contribute to core stability. Note the primary and secondary muscles that make up the stabilization system. The global muscles that make up the movement systems are also shown.

vertebral position sensors and maintain core stability by providing feedback on the amount of contraction needed by other muscles (11, 47).

The coordination or neural control of the local and global musculature is important to core stability (2, 12, 31-35). As noted in table 15.1, the local system includes the deeper core muscles of the transversus abdominis, multifidus, and internal oblique, which provide support to the individual segments of the spinal column (58). The global system, including the superficial trunk muscles rectus abdominis and erector spinae, responds to the loads on the spine, maintaining equilibrium (9). If the local musculature is not performing well, the contraction of the global muscles may add loads to the local segments that may cause injury. For example, when a person performs an exercise engaging the latissimus dorsi, such as a pull-down or row, the latissimus dorsi, which originates at the spinous processes of T7-L5, pulls

on the spine, creating a load that must be managed with the local musculature. A person performing any leg lift during a core routine uses the psoas, which originates from and thus pulls on the spine, again creating a load that must be managed by the local system of muscles. These systems need to work in a coordinated fashion to simultaneously perform the movement needed (e.g., bench press, lunge) and protect the spine (12).

When healthy people lift an arm or leg, the transversus abdominis and internal oblique contract before the limb moves (32, 33, 35). Transversus abdominis and internal oblique recruitment is significantly delayed or nonexistent in those with back pain (35). This means there is a good chance that the person with a history of LBP, who is in the fitness setting performing various arm and leg movements during weightlifting or core work, may have a delayed response in the deep stabilizing abdominal muscles. In addition, the psoas (8) and lumbar multifidus atrophy (8, 27, 29, 30) after low-back injury (24), and multifidus recovery is not spontaneous even when pain and disability improve (29). The fitness professional needs to teach the client how to activate the deep local stabilizers (transversus abdominis and multifidus) before suggesting strengthening workouts using the upper and lower extremities. It then would be wise to incorporate cueing of the deep stabilizers during any other fitness exercise to restore this trunk stabilizing component. Healthy participants can change muscle recruitment patterns with a training program that focuses on this neuromuscular control (66). As described in chapter 10, clients can recruit deep abdominal muscles with a drawing motion; the Sahrmann assessment can provide information about the client's core stability.

KEY POINT

The transversus abdominis is controlled independently of the other trunk musculature and should be trained separately from other trunk muscles with hollowing or drawing in. Its function needs to be assessed when beginning a core strengthening program. The transversus abdominis and multifidus are the principal deep core muscles affected by LBP; when atrophied, they predict a high rate of recurrence of LBP and dysfunction. Cueing for use of the deep abdominal muscles with the drawing-in or hollowing motion can be included with any strengthening or flexibility exercise to promote protection of the spine.

Core Muscle Exercises

Table 15.2 presents exercises aimed at recruiting and improving neuromuscular control of the deep spine stabilizers, the transversus abdominis and multifidus, and stabilization exercises aimed at recruiting both the local stabilizers and the global musculature. Address the deep abdominal recruitment exercise progression first (19, 60), and then add the more global exercises.

A variety of abdominal exercises are required to challenge all the abdominal muscles sufficiently (see table 15.2) with minimal stress to the spine (5). Four exercises in particular are appropriate for enhancing spine stability with low loads to the spine (50):

- *Trunk curl:* Progressing with variations noted in table (row 4)

- *Dead bug:* Increasing range of extremities during motion (row 2)
- *Side bridge (plank):* Knee support progressing to foot support, addition of rotation to a prone plank, and transition to the other side bridge (rows 6 and 7)
- *Bird dog:* Beginning with one extremity and then alternating both an arm and opposite leg (26, 50) (row 5)

McGill and colleagues suggest using the side bridge because it produces high activation levels in the quadratus lumborum, which is a significant stabilizer of the spine (49). Because this exercise involves only nominal contraction of the psoas, it does not place much compressive pressure on the intervertebral discs of the lumbar vertebrae; moreover, it emphasizes both strength and endurance (48). Bridging exercises are commonly prescribed for core strengthening. A study investigating trunk muscle activity during the front bridge (plank), supine bridge, and side bridge (plank), all with unilateral and bilateral support, showed that the exercises with bilateral lower-extremity support provided a challenge to the erector spinae and multifidus (22, 54). The bridging exercises with a leg lifted revealed more internal oblique recruitment on the side of the raised leg and an increased challenge to all musculature.

Core stability exercises can be performed on stable (floor) or unstable surfaces (exercise ball, foam roll, BOSU) (table 15.2). In general, exercises performed on an unstable base provide a greater challenge based on core muscle activity (37, 61, 67). A trunk curl on a ball increases rectus abdominis recruitment (67), performing a bridge on an exercise ball increases both internal oblique and multifidus activity, and integrating arm movements increases internal oblique activity (40). Exercises on the ball have been shown to be effective in a core stability training program (64), and foam roller exercises induce greater abdominal recruitment compared with the same exercises done on the floor (41).

Suspension exercises have become a popular core training approach that is in the unstable category. One or both limbs are supported on handle straps at the end of a suspension cable with an overhead anchor point. One study showed that the hip abduction in plank most effectively activated the external oblique, internal oblique, and transversus abdominis (table 15.2), and the hamstring curl most effectively activated the lumbar multifidus (51) while performing these exercises using suspension straps. The authors concluded that this approach is appropriate for healthy young adults.

Table 15.2 Common Core Exercises and Their Progressions

Exercise focus	Level 1	Level 2	Level 3
1. Basic stability progression to recruit transversus abdominis	Drawing in with one leg lifted	Addition of second leg	Addition of a trunk curl
2. Basic stability progression to recruit transversus abdominis with addition of arm and leg motion (dead bug variations)	Toe tapping with the spine held in neutral or imprint position	Arms and legs added as neutral spine is maintained	Addition of a twist
3. Bridge series	Basic bridge	Bridge with leg extension	Bridge with a march
4. Basic trunk curl	Basic trunk curl (twist may be added while keeping the transversus abdominis drawn in)	Supine trunk curl with a ball	Seated ball trunk curl
5. Swimmer exercise and bird dog to recruit multifidus and transversus abdominis	Performed with alternating just the arms or just the legs before adding them together Opposite arm and leg are lifted Pillow may be needed under the abdomen	Progression to quadruped and the ball	Trunk extension on ball Trunk may be lowered and lifted or held Legs may be separated to increase support

(continued)

Table 15.2 Common Core Exercises and Their Progressions *(continued)*

Exercise focus	Level 1	Level 2	Level 3
6. Plank exercises	Plank on the elbows	Plank with full arm extension	Plank with alternating arms and legs
7. Side plank variations	Progressing from knees to feet	Full leg extension in a side plank	Focus change and rotation
8. Unstable surfaces: ball and suspension straps	Dynamic variations of planks	Plank into lower-extremity curl	Suspension exercises
9. Unstable surfaces: BOSU and foam roller	Bridge on BOSU	Side plank on BOSU	Foam roller with one leg lifted at a time into a balance

Exercises to Enhance Flexibility

To improve flexibility, *ACSM Guidelines* (4) suggest the following:

- Stretches should be done at a frequency of 2 to 3 days per week, with daily stretching producing the best results.

- Each stretch should be performed for a total of 60 seconds (10-30 seconds per repetition can be effective), repeated 2 to 4 times. Older adults may benefit from a 30- to 60-second duration with each stretch.

- Stretches can be passive, static (muscle fully relaxed), dynamic (as in actively straightening the leg in a hamstring stretch), ballistic, or contract–relax style as in proprioceptive neuromuscular facilitation (PNF).

- The stretch position should not cause pain or take the joint past the normal ROM; it can be to the point of tightness or slight discomfort.

Precautions for Core Stability Exercises

According to Axler and McGill (5), four exercises are not recommended: the supine bilateral straight-leg raise, bent-leg raise, hanging bent-leg raise, and static cross-knee curl-up. Unfortunately, these are common exercises in the fitness setting. The supine bilateral straight-leg raise appears to be challenging, but the load and shear to the spine can be dangerous, and most people cannot stabilize their spine sufficiently to perform the exercise safely. When performing flexion trunk curls, it is only necessary to lift the shoulder girdle off the exercise surface. It is critical to minimize the role of the hip flexors (i.e., the paired psoas) in any trunk flexion exercise, particularly for people who are less fit. Many people believe that bending the knees reduces the role of the psoas muscles, but this is not so, particularly if the feet are supported (e.g., held by another person). Moreover, the psoas muscles place extreme compressive forces on the discs of the lumbar-motion segments of the vertebral column in activities such as sit-ups or bilateral leg lifts (5, 39). Posterior rotation of the pelvis often is incorporated into abdominal-strengthening exercises, but for someone with disc disease, it is not always appropriate. Posterior rotation of the pelvis typically removes the lumbar lordosis, and such movement can prompt the nucleus of the intervertebral disc to migrate posteriorly. If the disc is damaged, pressure can be placed on the damaged tissue and its pain receptors or even on spinal nerves. Exercisers can place the palm of one hand on the exercise surface under the lumbar lordotic curve (i.e., the small of the back) to provide feedback to maintain the lumbar lordosis.

- It is most effective to perform the flexibility exercises when the muscle temperature has increased through warm-up exercise. It is suggested that flexibility exercises follow cardiorespiratory exercise, resistive exercise, or sports (especially when power and strength are important), or are used as a standalone program. Static stretching exercises may acutely reduce power and strength.

- Suggestions for PNF include a 3- to 6-second light to moderate (20%-75% maximum) volitional muscle contraction with a 10- to 30-second assisted stretch.

Many approaches have been taken to stretching various muscle groups, and a discussion of some recent approaches for the hamstrings is presented next.

Many variations have been suggested as the most efficient way to create more flexible hamstrings. The variables that may be altered are the type of stretch, the duration of the stretch, the repetitions performed in one session, and the number of days per week the stretches are done. Many combinations have been successful in increasing hamstring flexibility:

- 3 days per week, 6 repetitions of 30 seconds, active stretching (6)

- 5 days per week, 6 repetitions of 5 seconds, active stretching (7)

- 5 days per week, 1 repetition of 30 seconds, passive stretching (7) (with more than two times the improvement than the active stretch of 5 seconds previously noted)

- 7 days per week, 2 times a day, 2 repetitions of 30 seconds (15)

- 7 days per week, 2 times a day, 6 repetitions of 10 seconds (15)

- 3 days per week, 15 to 45 seconds per repetition, totaling 120 seconds per day, active or passive (17)

These studies show that some variation is allowed for individual prescription of stretching, ranging from 3 to 7 days per week of active or passive stretching, a stretch duration of 5 to 45 seconds, and a daily duration of 30 to 180 seconds.

These findings differ according to age, as shown in a study that included participants 65 years or older with tight hamstrings who stretched 5 days per week for 6 weeks with a 15-, 30-, or 60-second stretch (20). The group that performed the 60-second stretch had a better outcome at the end of the 6 weeks and improvement that persisted longer than the gains of the other groups. Therefore, one might recommend that adults over the age of 65 stretch for 60 seconds 5 days per week.

Stretches to avoid include the standing toe touch, hurdler stretch, and full-circle neck stretch (figure 15.6). Unfortunately, these are commonly seen in fitness settings.

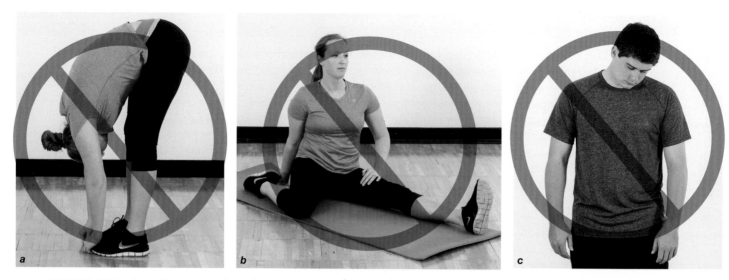

FIGURE 15.6 Stretches to avoid are the *(a)* standing toe touch, *(b)* hurdler stretch, and *(c)* full-circle neck stretch.

Stretching Techniques

- *Static stretching:* In static stretching, the muscle is slowly lengthened to a point where further movement is limited, and the stretch is held for a period of time (e.g., 10-60 seconds).

- *Active stretching:* In active stretching, a position with a muscle in a lengthened position is assumed and held there with no assistance other than the strength of the agonist muscles (the muscles that produce the main action). For example, the quadriceps (agonist) holds the leg straight in the active hamstring (antagonist) stretch. The tension of the agonists in an active stretch helps to relax the muscles being stretched (the antagonists) by reciprocal inhibition.

- *Passive:* A passive stretch is one in which no active muscular contraction occurs in the stretched muscle. An example of this is where a fitness professional holds the leg of a client in a hamstring stretch and gently presses the leg into a stretch as the client is totally relaxed.

- *Ballistic:* This type of stretching uses velocity and a fast, bouncy movement to stretch a muscle or body region. It may be considered, when properly performed, for adults who participate in sports that involve ballistic movements (e.g., basketball) (4). For most, it may not be safe because the forces involved with bouncing may push tissues past a safe length (the end point of normal ROM) where the client can control the movement and prevent injury from occurring.

- *Dynamic:* This type of stretching involves moving while stretching, but it does not include bounding or pushing muscles past their normal ROM. An example of dynamic stretching is arm circles, progressing from smaller to larger as the shoulders warm up.

- *Proprioceptive neuromuscular facilitation (PNF):* PNF includes stretching techniques that are commonly used in the clinical setting. They are aimed at improving active and passive ROM as well as optimizing motor performance and neuromuscular performance. The active PNF stretches common in a fitness setting combine stretching with alternating contraction and relaxation of muscles to improve flexibility.

Stretching Program

When designing a fitness program for a client, it is important to include a general stretching program addressing flexibility of all the major muscle groups. Following are some suggested stretches for most major muscle groups and body regions. It is wise to address all areas of the body in flexibility training. Remember to not take the joint past the normal ROM and to avoid ballistic stretching. The stretch position should not elicit pain. If clients experience pain, refer them to the appropriate medical provider for further evaluation.

Neck Stretches

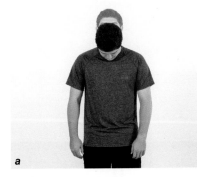
a

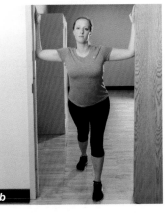
b

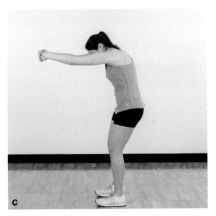
c

Upper-Back and Chest Stretches

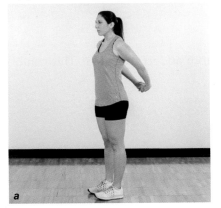
a

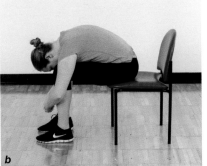
b

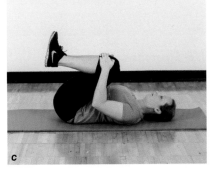
c

Spine Stretches

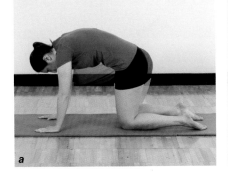
a

b

c

(continued)

Stretching Program *(continued)*

Spine Stretches (continued)

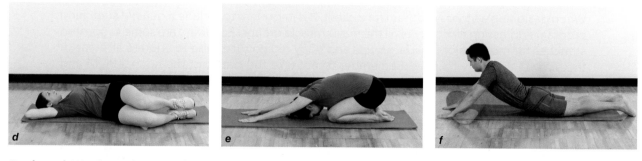

Back and Hip Stretches (Piriformis)

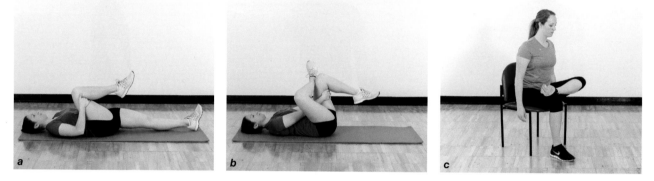

Hamstring Stretches

It is best if the natural lumbar lordosis is maintained to protect the disc from added stress (43). This can be performed with a strap passively or actively extending the leg.

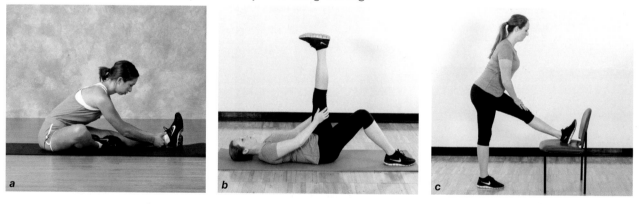

ITB Stretches

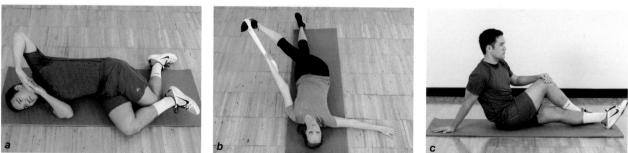

Hip, Thigh (Quadriceps), and Inner Thigh Stretches

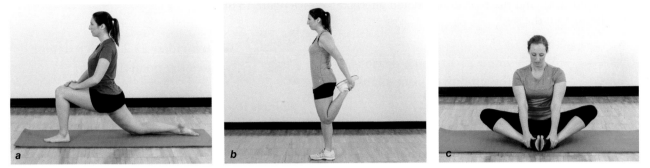

Calf Stretches (Soleus and Gastrocnemius)

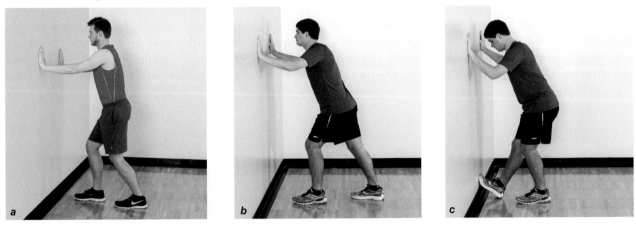

Exercises to Enhance Neuromotor Fitness

Exercises that focus on balance, agility, and proprioception generally are recommended to enhance neuromotor fitness. Although there is not a definitive set of exercise recommendations for improving neuromuscular fitness, ACSM's position stand includes guidelines based on the literature (21). Additionally, ACSM's most recent *Guidelines for Exercise Testing and Prescription* provides recommendations for exercises to promote neuromotor fitness and to reduce risk for older adults at increased risk for falls (4). Research supports that exercises to enhance neuromotor fitness and balance should be performed at least 2 to 3 days per week for sessions of at least 20 to 30 minutes with the goal of 60 minutes or more per week (21). Exercises to target stationary and dynamic balance, agility, and proprioception should be included in a program for neuromotor fitness (14, 21).

Exercises that gradually reduce the base of support and those that reduce sensory input are recommended to improve balance and reduce the risk of falls (14). For example, gradually moving from a two-legged stance to a one-legged stance can improve balance. The exercise can be progressed further by having the client close their eyes

at any stage, which will also improve proprioception. (Be sure to maintain close supervision and be available for support.) Dynamic balance can be improved with dynamic exercises that disrupt the center of gravity, such as lateral or braided side stepping. Tai chi also is recommended for improving neuromotor fitness and reducing the risk for falls (14, 36, 38).

It is important to consider the starting point for clients. The exercises in the chapter are presented for multiple levels of fitness and show how exercises can be progressed as neuromotor fitness improves. In addition to the exercises presented in this section of the chapter, several of the exercises for core muscle stability will also enhance balance. The addition of the stability ball, BOSU, or foam roller for the basic trunk curl, swimmer, and planks will improve balance as well as the level 3 progression for the plank and side plank (see table 15.2).

For example, the up-down prone plank progression can be included in a neuromotor fitness program. In this variation the client begins in a plank position on the forearms and elbows, then raises to the plank in the full-arm extension position one arm at a time. Weight is shifted to one side, and the client pushes up, extends the other arm to finish in the full-arm extension plank, and then returns to the starting plank position one arm at a time (see figure 15.7). The next repetition starts on the opposite side, and the repetitions should alternate sides throughout the set.

 Watch video 15.1, which demonstrates the up-down prone plank.

The push-up with a row improves core stability and is an opposing movement of the up-down plank. Beginners can start without weights in the modified push-up position with the knees slightly apart and hands placed slightly wider apart than with a regular push-up. The client begins in the up position, lowers to the down position, and returns to the up position, where a row is performed with the right arm (see figure 15.8a). Push-ups continue with alternating rows between the right and left sides. The exercise can be progressed by moving

to a full push-up and completing the rows with weights (see figure 15.8b).

 Watch video 15.2, which demonstrates the push-up row.

Multiple levels of exercises to maintain and improve neuromuscular fitness are included in this section so the fitness professional can select activities appropriate to the client's fitness level and can progress their programs as neuromotor fitness improves. An example of a beginner exercise, sit-to-stand, is an ideal exercise to improve stationary balance in those who scored below average on their balance assessments. The client begins seated in a chair with a seat that is approximately 17 inches (43 centimeters) from the ground. The feet should be placed about hip-width apart with the toes pointed

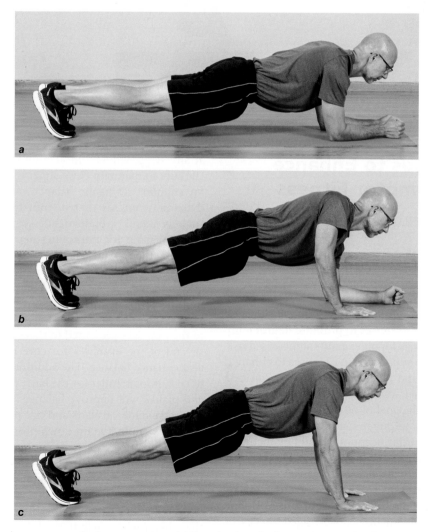

FIGURE 15.7 Up-down prone plank progression. *(a)* Start in the plank position on the forearms and elbows. *(b)* Rise to the plank with full-arm extension position one arm at a time. The client shifts their weight to one side, pushes up so the arm is extended, and repeats on the other side. *(c)* Once in the upright position, the client reverses the process and lowers the body to the starting position *(a)*.

straight forward. The knees should be flexed to slightly less than 90°. The client simply stands to a full upright position and returns to the initial seated position for a repetition. Ideally, the exercise is performed in a chair without arms, and the client stands and sits with their arms held across the chest (see figure 15.9). However, those who need support can use a chair with arms and use one or both arms for support while standing and returning to the seated position. The goal is to work toward 1 to 3 sets of 10 to 12 repetitions.

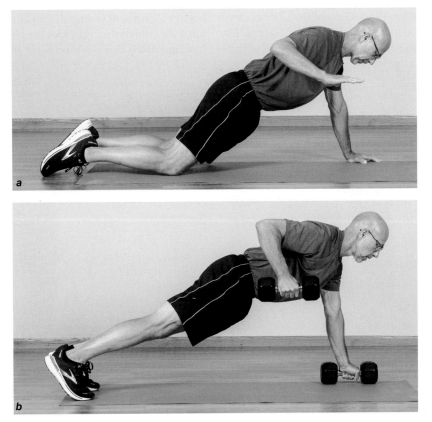

FIGURE 15.8 Push-up with a row. (a) The client completes a row in the up position of a modified push-up without weights, and (b) the client completes a row in the up position of a push-up with dumbbells.

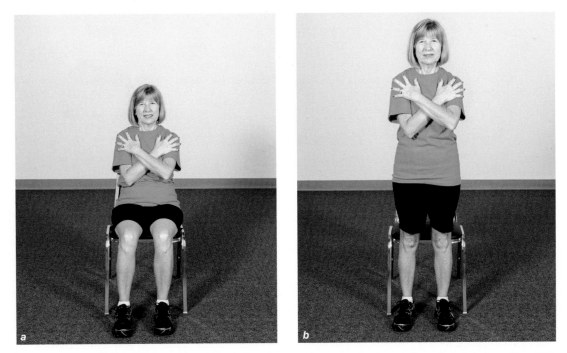

FIGURE 15.9 Sit-to-stand. (a) The client sits with feet hip-width apart, the knees flexed slightly less than 90°, and the arms across the chest, and (b) the client stands.

The single-leg standing balance exercise is another exercise for stationary balance. The client stands next to a fixed object or wall to provide support. Holding to the fixed object with the right hand, the left leg is lifted so the thigh is parallel with the ground and the knee is flexed at a 90° angle (see figure 15.10). Ideally, the client will hold this position for 30 to 45 seconds. Clients can gradually progress to that time frame if necessary. The exercise is performed on the other side to complete the repetition. The exercise can be progressed in various ways including performing it with the eyes closed (improving proprioception) or not holding on to the fixed object (introducing a greater challenge). Ensure appropriate supervision to provide assistance if needed.

Another exercise for balance that can be done without equipment is the tandem standing balance. The exercise begins with the feet together. The client steps forward until the heel of the right foot touches the toes of the left foot and holds this position for a given time period (see figure 15.11). Use the results of the balance assessment

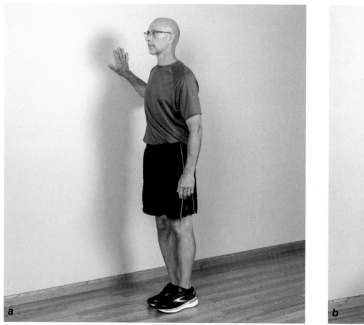
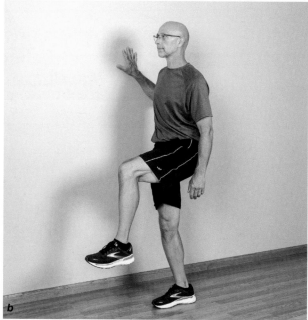

FIGURE 15.10 Single-leg standing balance. *(a)* The client stands next to the fixed object, and *(b)* the client is in the single-leg balance position with the thigh parallel to the floor and the knee flexed at 90°.

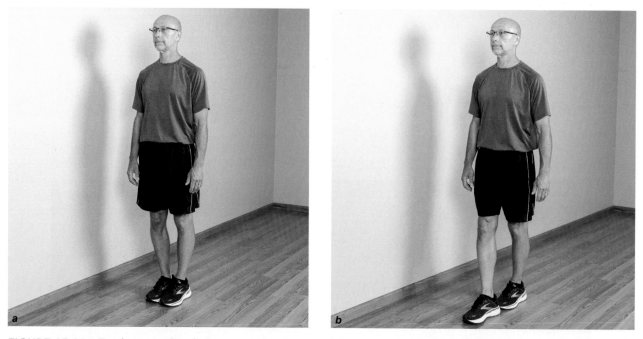

FIGURE 15.11 Tandem standing balance. *(a)* The client stands with the feet together, and *(b)* the client stands in the tandem position.

discussed in chapter 10 to determine the starting duration with the goal of balancing for 30 to 45 seconds. The client returns to the starting point and repeats with the left foot forward to complete each repetition. This exercise also can be performed with the eyes closed and the feet in the tandem position to improve proprioception. To make the activity less challenging, the feet can be in the semi-tandem position with the big toe of one foot touching the side (instep) of the other foot.

An additional progression to the tandem standing balance exercise is the tightrope walk. Instead of return-ing to the starting position, the client walks by placing each foot in front of the other in the tandem position as if walking on a tightrope to improve dynamic balance.

The single-leg forward reach, an exercise for dynamic balance, requires more stability than the previous two exercises. The client stands with the feet together, then flexes the right knee so the foot is behind the body. The client then slowly leans forward, reaching toward the ground with the right arm. The goal is to maintain balance on the left leg while keeping the hips neutral so that the body does not lean to one side. Once the client can no longer maintain balance leaning forward, the client slowly returns to the starting position. It is then repeated on the other side. This exercise can be performed with a lightweight kettlebell as a progression (see figure 15.12).

 Watch video 15.3, which demonstrates the tightrope walk exercise.

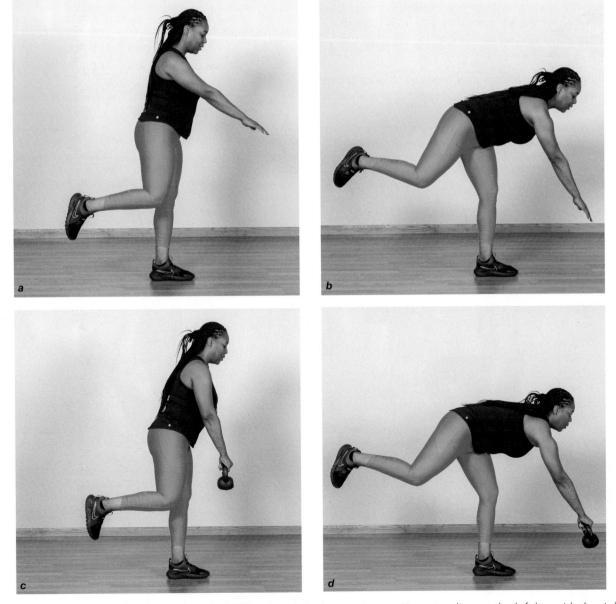

FIGURE 15.12 Single-leg forward reach. *(a)* The client is in the starting position, standing on the left leg with the right knee flexed at 90°, and *(b)* the client is in the reach forward position. *(c)* The client is in the starting position holding a kettlebell, and *(d)* the client is in the reach forward position holding a kettlebell.

VIDEO Watch video 15.4, which demonstrates single-leg forward reach.

The single-leg step also targets dynamic balance. This exercise requires the use of a stable step, such as a plyometric box. The ideal box height should have the client's knee flexed at approximately 90°. The client begins with the right foot fully on the box. The client will have a slight lean as they extend the right leg until the left foot reaches the top of the box. The client returns to the starting position to complete the repetition. The client should perform 10 to 12 repetitions with each leg and work toward being able to complete 1 to 3 sets on each side (see figure 15.13). Lightweight dumbbells can be added to progress the exercise.

 VIDEO Watch video 15.5, which demonstrates the single-leg step up.

Lunges perturb the center of mass and reduce the base of support to improve dynamic balance. Lunges can be performed by lunging forward with one leg, returning to a standing position with feet side by side, and repeating the lunge with the alternate leg. This basic lunge can be progressed to a walking lunge or walking lunge with weights (see figure 15.14). The side step and braided side step are additional exercises for dynamic balance that will disrupt the center of mass. Beginners should start with the side step. This exercise can be progressed by gradually increasing speed and working toward the braided side step (see figure 15.15). Because these exercises include progressively faster movement and changing directions, they will also improve agility.

 VIDEO Watch video 15.6, which demonstrates the walking lunge.

 VIDEO Watch video 15.7, which demonstrates the side step and braided side step.

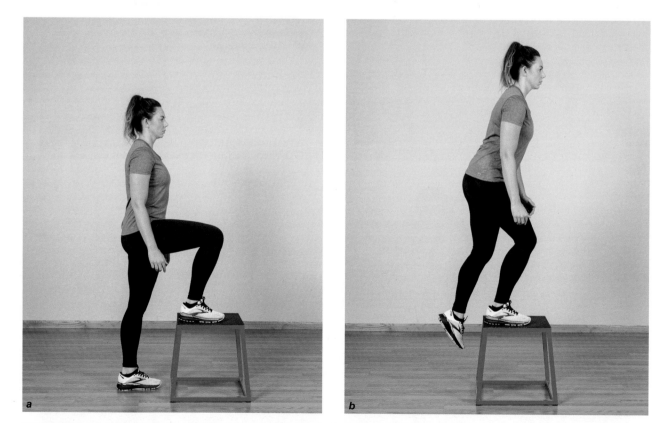

FIGURE 15.13   Single-leg step. *(a)* The client begins with the right foot fully on the box and the knee flexed at approximately 90°, and *(b)* the client moves toward the extended position.

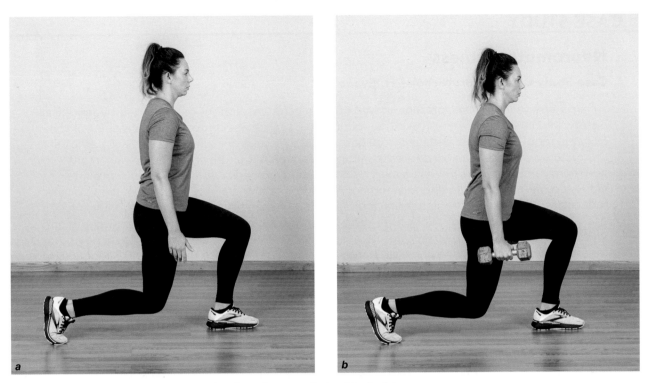

FIGURE 15.14   Walking lunge *(a)* and walking lunge with dumbbells *(b)*.

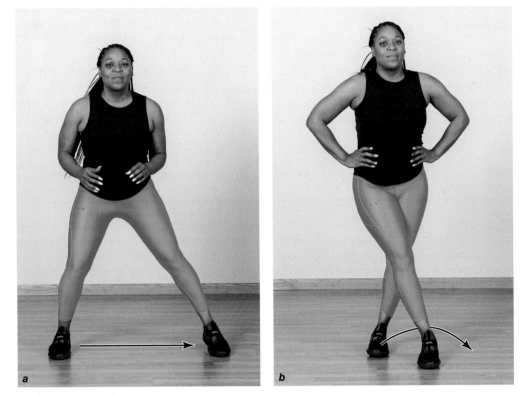

FIGURE 15.15   Side step *(a)* and braided side step *(b)*.

CASE STUDY

Neuromotor Fitness

Case Study Contributor: Nicholas H. Evans

Julian is a 69-year-old male, presenting with no prior cardiorespiratory, metabolic, or neurological history, who intends to begin an exercise routine at a local fitness center after many years of inactivity. He reports that work and family obligations have made it difficult to find time to participate in structured exercise but now desires to improve his overall strength and conditioning in order to feel more confident and safer navigating his home and community environment. Julian expresses increased difficulty transitioning to standing, either from a low chair or sofa or from the floor, and reduced confidence descending stairs and managing uneven terrains (e.g., gravel paths, broken or cracked sidewalks, sand). Along with tests of cardiorespiratory fitness, muscular strength and endurance, and flexibility, a fitness professional at the fitness center performs a series of neuromotor assessments including the unipedal stance test, the standing reach test, and the 8-foot up and go test. The fitness professional documents the following:

Neuromotor assessment	Quantitative observations		Qualitative observations
Single-leg stance (best of 3 trials)	**Eyes open**	**Eyes closed**	• Greater difficulty performing single-leg stance on the left (nondominant) leg. • Participant verbalized concern for falling during eyes-closed condition.
	Left leg: 21.6 seconds Right leg: 42.0 seconds	Left leg: 3.3 seconds Right leg: 8.1 seconds	
Standing reach (mean of 3 trials)	15.6 inches		• Frontal plane view: Observable but subtle body weight shift to the right while forward reaching (weight was not distributed equally between left and right lower limbs).
8-foot up and go (single trial)	8.8 seconds		• On "Go" command, participant required two stand attempts (insufficient forward trunk lean to get body weight over the feet during the first attempt). • Observable shuffled gait while turning left around the cone.

In other fitness testing, based on age and sex, Julian presents with fair cardiorespiratory fitness, poor hamstring flexibility, and average lower-limb strength with a discrepancy between limbs of >15 pounds in favor of the right leg. Considering this information, and assuming no underlying neurological or musculoskeletal pathology, develop a neuromotor training program specifically targeting Julian's goals and movement deficiencies.

Sample Response

Julian demonstrates decreased standing balance and agility performance as evidenced by prolonged 8-foot up and go time and diminished unipedal stance performance, with an emphasis on left leg instability (see chapter 10 for score ranges). Standing reach performance was within normal range; however, Julian favored weight bearing through the right lower limb, indicating development of an abnormal compensatory movement strategy. Disparity in strength between the left and right legs along with hamstring range of motion insufficiency are possible contributors to the observed performance deficits. Along with a targeted flexibility and lower-extremity strength routine (emphasizing muscles involved in left hip and knee stabilization), the following neuromotor training program (performed 2-3 days per week) could be incorporated into Julian's weekly exercise routine to positively affect strength, standing balance, and functional stability.

SAMPLE NEUROMOTOR TRAINING PROGRAM (BEGINNER)			
Category	Exercise	Sets (# circuits)	Time (per exercise)
Agility	Lateral side step (left and right)	3-4	Up to 30 seconds
Stationary balance	Single-leg standing balance (eyes open)		
	Sit-to-stands (no upper extremity support from chair)		
	Semi-tandem stance (with upper extremity diagonal reach)		
	Side plank (from knees)		
Dynamic balance	Single-leg step-ups		
	Forward inline stepping (tightrope walk)		

This program incorporates a combination of activities emphasizing agility and stationary and dynamic balance. The program can be completed as a circuit, with the goal of performing each activity for 30 seconds. During the initial stage of neuromotor training, participant education is critical. An emphasis should be placed on controlled, quality movements, working toward mastery of the movement pattern with little to no maladaptive compensation. The fitness professional likely will need to employ a combination of verbal, visual, and tactile feedback strategies to ensure individuals demonstrate competency at performing each activity prior to working independently. Movement patterns performed poorly will perpetuate suboptimal movement strategies and will impede the development and maintenance of new, more competent movement strategies. Therefore, performing consistent and repetitive movements that break away from the previous compensatory patterns will be necessary for optimizing neuromotor adaptation. For example, during semi-tandem stance, sit-to-stand, and unipedal step-ups, the fitness professional should describe to Julian the importance of maintaining stability on the left lower extremity without defaulting to stabilizing primarily through the right leg. Julian then should perform the exercises while the fitness professional visually inspects the quality of movement and provides verbal and hands-on cueing, as necessary, to ensure proper execution. Once Julian demonstrates comprehension of each exercise and is sufficiently self-aware to make appropriate corrections in the presence of movement deviations, the fitness professional can be reasonably confident that Julian is prepared to work independently. Follow-up neuromotor assessments can be performed at regular intervals to monitor progress and adjust the exercise prescription accordingly.

Pilates, Yoga, Tai Chi, and Aquatic Approaches

Pilates has been incorporated into both fitness settings and physical therapy settings as a core strengthening and flexibility tool (63) and is a good method to develop core stability. Pilates is an exercise method that focuses on core strength, flexibility, and balance in the body. In the early 1900s, Joseph Pilates created a systematic practice of specific exercises coupled with focused breathing patterns that has been refined to integrate current biomechanical principles to protect the spine. It is important to note that one needs proper training to teach Pilates, and a variety of certification programs are available for instructors. The Pilates Method Alliance (PMA) is a professional association with a certification program for Pilates teachers that validates that a PMA-certified Pilates instructor meets entry-level standards for safety and competency. The PMA website is a good place to begin for people who are interested in this training (www.pilatesmethodalliance.org).

Yoga has been recommended for many reasons, including improving flexibility, reducing stress, and reducing pain (63). Some fitness settings offer yoga classes, and the fitness professional may need to determine whether yoga is appropriate for a particular client. Some research points to yoga being a supportive adjunct to other fitness activities. For example, Cramer and colleagues found strong evidence for short-term effectiveness and moderate evidence for long-term effectiveness of yoga for chronic LBP (16). Yoga comes in many forms, such as hot yoga, Hatha yoga, and Vinyasa yoga. More information and additional types of yoga can be found on the Yoga Alliance website (www.yogaalliance.org/LearnAboutYoga/AboutYoga/Typesofyoga). As with Pilates, fitness professionals interested in teaching yoga should seek education and certification in this area. Yoga Alliance is a nonprofit organization that credentials yoga teachers and may be found at www.yogaalliance.org.

Another popular group exercise aimed at flexibility, balance, and control of the spine is tai chi. Tai chi is a good alternative for those age 18 to 70 with long-term LBP (25) and those with chronic conditions of the musculoskeletal system (44). Tai chi is also associated with reduced risk for falls and overall physical function (36, 38). A 2011 study had participants 18 to 70 years of age participate in 18 sessions, each lasting 40 minutes, in a group setting for 10 weeks. Overall functional fitness tests and pain improved for these participants over the 10-week period (42).

Before performing tai chi, Pilates, or yoga the client needs to be able to recruit the deep abdominal musculature stabilizing the lumbosacral region in neutral spine position or slight flexion for any exercise. This capacity for abdominal hollowing or pelvic stability needs to be present without additional cueing from the instructor because these activities frequently occur in a class situation where personal observation of the individual is sometimes missing. The possibility of injury increases if clients who cannot stabilize the lumbosacral region are asked to perform larger movements. The neutral zone needs to be stabilized by the local system before adding a larger challenge from the global muscular system.

Aquatic exercise can be extremely beneficial for clients needing flexibility and core stability training. Some researchers recently investigated spine stabilization exercises in the pool (13). They found that the exercises that maximized trunk muscle activity in the pool were abdominal hollowing and resistance against an exercise ball forward and laterally (holding the ball and pressing into it forward and sideways). For more details about aquatic exercises, contact the United States Water Fitness Association (USWFA), which offers national certifications for water fitness instructors (www.uswfa.com).

A Note About Medical Intervention

It is important for fitness professionals to know when they need to refer a client to a medical professional. A fitness professional spends a lot of time with a client and may have the opportunity to hear concerns that the client has not shared with others. The discussion here is not about emergency situations that occur in a fitness setting but rather when progression is slow or nonexistent or when unusual signs and symptoms are mentioned. Encourage clients to visit a medical professional if they report any of these signs and symptoms related to low-back function: unrelenting pain, pain that does not change with rest or change of position, persistent night pain when younger than 20 years or older than 55 years of age, bilateral leg pain or paresthesia, saddle region (where a person would sit on a saddle) paresthesia, or changes in bowel or bladder control (23). If these are reported, the client should see a medical professional before continuing.

Clients also might comply with a program that has been well designed for them but make slow or nonexistent progress. This may be evident in a lack of progression in specific exercises, no change or an increase in pain, or no change in flexibility. Such cases might be an opportunity to refer the client to a physical therapist to address potential biomechanical and alignment needs. Ahmed and colleagues (1) found that patients with mechanical LBP showed more improvement with lumbar mobilization (manual therapy) and core strengthening combined than with core strengthening alone. The client may need manual therapy or orthotic assessment to support the fitness program. Referral to a physical therapist does not mean the client needs to stop attending the fitness sessions but that the addition of another tool may help the client progress faster and further. The fitness professional should communicate with the medical professional to create a cohesive approach for the client.

LEARNING AIDS

REVIEW QUESTIONS

1. What constitutes a motion segment? What is a function of the facet joints?
2. Describe the difference between a structural and a functional spinal curve.
3. Which muscles are important in controlling pelvic position?
4. Explain the roles of the local and global trunk musculature.
5. Explain why knowing a client's back history is important.
6. Describe the hollowing or drawing-in abdominal exercise and its purpose.
7. Describe the progression from the basic drawing-in abdominal motion to a trunk curl with the feet off the floor, and explain when to take the precaution of stopping the progression.
8. Describe a good exercise for developing each of the following muscles: quadratus lumborum, rectus abdominis, transversus abdominis, and erector spinae.
9. Why is good flexibility important to spinal health?
10. Describe flexibility exercises for the major areas of the body and ACSM's *Guidelines* for performing them.
11. Describe activities that promote neuromotor fitness and aspects that can provide progression within a training program.

CASE STUDIES

1. A fitness professional is using a double-leg-lowering task with a group of relatively fit adults, ostensibly to improve the strength of the abdominal muscles. Discuss the appropriateness or inappropriateness of the exercise.
2. A client shares that his favorite hamstring stretches are the hurdler stretch and toe touch, which he has performed since high school. Should he change this stretching routine?
3. A fitness professional reads a book on Pilates exercises and feels successful in performing them. She decides to teach them to a training client at the next session. Discuss the appropriateness of this decision.
4. A fitness professional is progressing a client through the beginning-level hollowing abdominal exercises and sees a tentlike appearance of the abdominal region. What is occurring, and is this person ready to add global musculature strengthening?

Answers to Case Studies

1. The double-leg-lowering task is not an appropriate core exercise if the legs are taken to the floor. According to Axler and McGill (5), four exercises are not recommended, including the supine bilateral straight-leg raise.

2. The hurdler and toe touch are not safe, effective stretches. The fitness professional can instruct this client in alternative hamstring stretches (see examples in the *Stretching Program* sidebar), explaining that research has revealed more effective ways to address hamstring tightness.

3. A fitness professional should have significant training and certification in an area such as Pilates before accepting the responsibility of teaching these specialized exercise techniques to clients.

4. The tentlike appearance is most likely the rectus abdominis (the most superficial abdominal muscle, which runs superior to inferior on the abdomen) contracting as the hollowing exercise is performed. This client is not ready to progress to the next level because the tenting reveals that the transversus abdominis is not yet activated as the primary abdominal stabilizer. The client should continue to work on recruiting the transversus abdominis in a variety of positions and activities.

Putting Together a Comprehensive Program

Barbara A. Bushman

OBJECTIVES

The reader will be able to do the following:

1. Describe components of a complete exercise program
2. Identify ways to progress an exercise program for a beginner, an intermediate-level exerciser, and an established exerciser
3. Describe the value in repeating assessments at set time points in an exercise program
4. Define *adaptation* and explain what constitutes a minimum training threshold
5. Explain the difference between functional and nonfunctional overreaching
6. Define overtraining syndrome and explain factors that can contribute to this prolonged maladaptation
7. Describe ways to reduce the likelihood of developing overtraining syndrome
8. Identify the components of the Male and Female Athlete Triad
9. Describe the spectrum of concerns reflected in Relative Energy Deficiency in Sport (RED-S)
10. Discuss potential ways to reduce the likelihood of low energy availability

All exercise programs must be individualized based on the person's current health and fitness status, time availability, resources, and future goals. The focus of this chapter is on exercise programs to promote health and fitness rather than programming that might apply to competitive sport or athletic pursuits. A complete program includes aerobic and muscular fitness conditioning, along with flexibility activities and potentially neuromotor exercise training; see table 16.1 for a summary of recommendations from the *Physical Activity Guidelines for Americans* and by the American College of Sports Medicine (ACSM) (3, 31). Assessments related to each of these areas are discussed in chapters 8, 9, and 10, and considerations for exercise prescription are presented in chapters 13, 14, and 15. This chapter addresses how to design an exercise program that includes the recommended fitness components consistent with each individual's needs, abilities, and goals, and with appropriate progression. Although an apparently basic concept, program design requires careful planning and application of sound training principles by the fitness professional. Additionally, the fitness professional must merge the client's background information (e.g., health history, current fitness, assessment results) with realities of the client's life (e.g., work responsibil-

ities, family activities, recreational interests) to provide a workable, realistic, enjoyable, and progressive exercise program. No simple formula or guide can account for all situations. This chapter includes sample programs and other considerations to promote program safety and to continue to build a foundation to allow exercise to become a lifelong habit.

Developing Progressive and Comprehensive Training Programs

When developing a training program, each aspect should be considered independently and then as a part of the comprehensive training program. For example, one client may have been involved with consistent, progressive resistance training for years but rarely engages in any aerobic activities, while another client may be heavily involved in aerobic exercise but has never included resistance training. Neither of these individuals is meeting recommended levels of activity, as noted in the *Physical Activity Guidelines for Americans* (31) or the guidance provided in *ACSM's Guidelines for Exercise*

Table 16.1 Components of a Complete Exercise Program

Component	*Physical Activity Guidelines for Americans*	American College of Sports Medicine
Cardiorespiratory (aerobic) fitness	Include 150 to 300 minutes per week of moderate aerobic activity, or 75 to 150 minutes per week of vigorous aerobic activity, or an equivalent combination of moderate and vigorous activity; additional benefits are possible by increasing beyond the equivalent of 300 minutes of moderate physical activity per week.	Include moderate- and/or vigorous-intensity aerobic exercise on at least 3 days per week (3 to 5 days per week suggested); 30 to 60 minutes per day (150 minutes per week) or more of moderate activity, or 20 to 40 minutes per day (75 minutes per week) or more of vigorous activity, or a combination of the two to reach the recommended volume of continuous or intermittent aerobic exercise involving the major muscle groups.
Muscular fitness	Include muscle-strengthening activities involving the major muscle groups, on 2 or more days per week at a moderate or greater intensity.	For beginners, include resistance training at least 2 days per week, 8 to 12 repetitions, incorporating a variety of exercises (multi- and single-joint, exercise equipment and/or body weight); for more experienced exercisers, weekly volume will determine frequency, and intensity will depend on fitness goals.
Flexibility	No specific guidance is given, other than to note inclusion within a physical activity program; this activity does not count toward meeting aerobic or muscular fitness recommendations.	Include flexibility exercises at least 2 to 3 days per week, with daily noted as most effective, that target each of the major muscle–tendon units.
Neuromotor fitness	Balance and multicomponent physical activity (combining various aspects of physical activity such as balance and aerobic activity) is included for older adults to decrease the risk of falls or injury from a fall.	Including exercises that combine balance, agility, and proprioception is recommended to reduce or prevent falls for older adults.

Adapted from U.S. Department of Health and Human Services (2018); American College of Sports Medicine (2022).

Testing and Prescription (3). The starting point for each component should reflect the client's current status. In the prior example, the first client could continue with resistance training as an established exerciser but would need to approach the aerobic activities as a beginner, while the second individual would continue at a higher level for aerobic activity but gradually introduce resistance training.

Examples of 10-week training programs are provided:

- Table 16.2 is for beginners, who have not been exercising previously.
- Table 16.3 is for intermediate-level exercisers, who have a foundation of aerobic and muscular fitness; there is no set time to move to this level but rather when an individual's program has progressed toward meeting the general standards for the given fitness component with regular training, typically about 3 months.
- Table 16.4 is for established exercisers, who should be meeting recommended levels of activity for the given fitness component and have been doing so consistently.

As these are examples (2), the starting point and progression need to be individualized and adapted to the client's current level of activity and future goals. Being a fitness professional requires the ability to apply science in a planned and practical manner. If a client finds a given week's activities difficult, adjusting aspects of the program (e.g., reducing intensity or volume) or extending the time at a given level will be appropriate from a physiological standpoint to allow for adequate recovery to reduce risks of overtraining or injury and also will promote long-term adherence (i.e., higher self-efficacy, feelings of accomplishment).

Determining a starting point for each component requires a discussion with the client regarding their current activities. Reflecting on the prior couple months will provide insight on the status and focus of an individual's program. Simple assessments (as found in the chapters in part III) also should contribute to developing a picture of the client's status. An example of how to pull together self-reported activity and fitness assessments is found in the case study *Where to Start*.

The sample programs include ranges and options for many aspects such as number of days per week or the intensity of aerobic activity, the types of exercise or number of repetitions per set for resistance training, and various activities selected for flexibility and neuromotor exercises. This underscores the ability to customize a program that fulfills recommendations for activity while still incorporating individual preferences and goals. Rather than being a regimented prescription, the recommendations provided by the *Physical Activity Guidelines for Americans* (31) and ACSM (3), as well as the sample

programs based on these recommendations (2), are general guides that the fitness professional can use to design the optimal program for a client. To gauge progress and to motivate clients, repeat fitness assessments periodically. For those just beginning, who have greater potential for change, assessments may occur every 2 to 3 months, while more established exercisers whose fitness level is more stable may benefit from semiannual or annual testing. Determining which assessments and the timing of those assessments is not by formula, but rather the fitness professional must use good judgment and individualize plans for the client.

Within each of the sample programs, foundational training principles guide the progression. Applying a training stimulus of a sufficient level with regularity allows the targeted physiologic capacity to expand; this is referred to as *adaptation* (1). Adaptation requires a challenge beyond a minimal intensity (i.e., training threshold), thus providing an overload (3). Training is defined as "a process of overload that is used to disturb homeostasis, which results in acute fatigue leading to improvement in performance" (22). What constitutes that minimum threshold depends on many factors, including current fitness level, age, health status, genetics and physiological differences, and general level of physical activity (3). Over time, as adaptations occur and the physiologic capacities increase, the training stimulus needs to be increased because a given workload will be below the training threshold. This is desired and is the reason an exercise program must be progressed (i.e., presenting a new or greater challenge). One of the roles of a fitness professional is to design a program with sufficient, but not excessive, overload to promote improvements in fitness and health. The adage "Start low and go slow" can be applied to progression and is a positive framework to increase the overall workload gradually from where the client is (3). The concept of periodization includes a planned training approach, which is divided into smaller segments or phases of training, allowing for the application of overload along with opportunity for sufficient recovery (for more details on the history, theory, and application of periodization see reference 6). Problems can arise when an imbalance exists between the training stress and adequate recovery (22). Improvement requires overload, but if overload is excessive and time for recovery and adaptation is inadequate, overreaching and even overtraining may result, as discussed in the next section.

Developing the Optimal Training Stimulus

Fitness professionals need to balance sufficient overload for improvement with adequate recovery between work-

Table 16.2 Sample 10-Week Beginner Exercise Program for Adults[a]

Weeks	Aerobic[b]	Resistance	Stretching and neuromotor activities[c]	Comments
1-2	Three days per week; 10 to 20 minutes per day; light intensity (level 3 or 4)	Two days per week; one set, 8 to 12 repetitions of six exercises	Two days per week; 10 minutes of stretching activities with additional option for agility and balance exercises	An easy beginning aerobic activity for a client who is starting an exercise program is walking at a comfortable pace. Target 5 to 10 minutes at a time for the aerobic activity, and on at least 2 days include some stretching after the walk. Optional balance exercises (e.g., single-leg stance) could be included within the warm-up before any fatigue from the walking activity or at another time. For resistance training, beginners should select one exercise for each of the following body areas: hips and legs, chest, back, shoulders, low back, and abdominal muscles. For example, the following activities for an at-home program target each of these areas and can be done with resistance bands and body weight: body-weight squat, band seated chest press, band seated row, band upright row, prone plank, curl-up.
3-4	Three days per week; 20 to 30 minutes per day; light to moderate intensity (level 4 or 5)	Two days per week; one or two sets, 8 to 12 repetitions of six exercises	Two to three days per week; 10 minutes of stretching activities with additional option for agility and balance exercises	Work with the client to develop a habit of activity, which is key for a lifelong approach. The focus for the client in the next couple of weeks is getting comfortable with at least 20 minutes of aerobic exercise at least 3 days per week. Additionally, the client will include stretching, and optional balance exercises, on at least 2 days per week. Stretching activities can be done following the walking sessions or at another time. Balance activities can be done at a separate time or prior to the walking session. The client should continue with the resistance training program from the first 2 weeks. For some, 12 repetitions now may feel easy; if so, add more weight or resistance for 8 repetitions for each set.
5-7	Three or four days per week; 30 to 40 minutes per day; moderate intensity (level 5)	Two days per week; two sets, 8 to 12 repetitions of six exercises	Three days per week; 10 minutes of stretching activities with additional option for agility and balance exercises	For the next three weeks, the focus for the client will be getting comfortable with at least 30 minutes of moderate-level aerobic exercise at least 3 days per week. Continue to include stretching, and optional balance exercises, on 3 days per week. For the resistance training program, the client will complete two sets per exercise. If 12 repetitions now feel easy, add more weight or resistance for 8 repetitions for each set.
8-10	Three or four days per week; 30 to 45 minutes per day; moderate intensity (level 5 or 6)	Two days per week; two sets, 8 to 12 reps of six exercises	Three or more days per week; 10 minutes of stretching activities with additional option for agility and balance exercises	The client will have developed an aerobic and muscular fitness base over the past couple months. For some variety, consider other activities such as biking or swimming, or if preferred, the client can continue with walking. Continue to include stretching, and optional balance exercises, on at least 3 days per week. For the resistance training program, consider trying some other exercises for variety.

[a]All activity sessions should be preceded and followed by a 5- to 10-minute warm-up and cool-down of light- to moderate-intensity activity.

[b]The intensity level is noted on a relative intensity scale from 0 to 10: Level 0 reflects rest, and 10 is maximal effort; moderate intensity is a level of 5 or 6, and vigorous intensity is an effort level of 7 or 8.

[c]Include stretching activities to improve flexibility; also consider including some activities for agility and balance (i.e., neuromotor training).

Adapted by permission from B.A. Bushman, "Adults: Ages 18 to 64," in *ACSM's Complete Guide to Fitness and Health,* 2nd ed., edited by B. Bushman (Champaign, IL: Human Kinetics, 2017), 240.

Table 16.3 Sample 10-Week Intermediate-Level Exercise Program for Adults[a]

Weeks	Aerobic[b]	Resistance	Stretching and neuromotor activities[c]	Comments
1-2	Three or four days per week; 30 to 45 minutes per day; moderate intensity (level 5 or 6)	Two days per week; one or two sets, 8 to 12 repetitions of 8 to 10 different exercises	Two or three days per week; 10 minutes of stretching activities with additional option for agility and balance exercises	At this point, the client should be able to maintain aerobic activity for a longer duration. The total for aerobic activity should increase to a target of 150 minutes per week (moderate-intensity activity). Stretching and optional neuromotor (balance and agility) exercises are included on at least 2 days per week; additional benefits are possible with greater frequency. For resistance training, the client will include exercises for biceps and triceps (in addition to the body areas previously targeted: hips and legs, chest, back, shoulders, low back, and abdominal muscles) and add exercises for the quadriceps and hamstrings in the second week for a total of 10 exercises.
3-5	Three to five days per week; 30 to 50 minutes per day; moderate intensity (level 5 to 6)	Two days per week; one or two sets, 8 to 12 repetitions of 10 different exercises	Two or three days per week, 10 minutes of stretching activities with additional option for agility and balance exercises	The focus for the next 3 weeks is for the client to increase the time spent in aerobic exercise or to increase the intensity, but not both aspects at the same time. For those more comfortable with moderate-intensity activity, 150 or more minutes per week is appropriate. For clients ready to increase intensity (e.g., jogging rather than walking for those who do not have orthopedic or other concerns), cut back the time to 20 to 30 minutes per day to realize the same benefits (note that the target for vigorous-intensity activity is 75 minutes per week). A mix of moderate- and vigorous-intensity activity also can be considered. Continue with the stretching and optional neuromotor exercises and the resistance training program from the prior weeks.
6-10	Three to five days per week; 30 to 60 minutes per day; moderate intensity (level 5 or 6)	Two days per week; two sets, 8 to 12 repetitions of 10 exercises	Two or three days per week, 10 minutes of stretching activities with additional option for agility and balance exercises	For aerobic activity, the client can either increase the time spent per day or increase the number of days per week. Ultimately, the target weekly total is 150 to 200 minutes of moderate-intensity activity or 75 to 100 minutes of vigorous-intensity activity (2 minutes of moderate activity equals 1 minute of vigorous activity) or a combination of moderate and vigorous activity. For stretching and optional neuromotor exercises, consider introducing some new activities to provide variety and challenge. For the resistance training component, select different exercises while still targeting the same muscle groups.

[a]All activity sessions should be preceded and followed by a 5- to 10-minute warm-up and cool-down of light- to moderate-intensity activity.

[b]The intensity level is noted on a relative intensity scale from 0 to 10: Level 0 reflects rest, and 10 is maximal effort; moderate intensity is a level of 5 or 6, and vigorous intensity is an effort level of 7 or 8.

[c]Include stretching activities to improve flexibility. Target all the muscle groups, holding each stretch for 10 to 30 seconds, repeated for a total of 60 seconds. Additionally, consider adding activities for agility and balance (i.e., neuromotor exercises).

Adapted by permission from B.A. Bushman, "Adults: Ages 18 to 64," in *ACSM's Complete Guide to Fitness and Health,* 2nd ed., edited by B. Bushman (Champaign, IL: Human Kinetics, 2017), 241.

Table 16.4 Sample 10-Week Established Exercise Program for Adults[a]

Weeks	Aerobic[b]	Resistance[c]	Stretching and neuromotor activities[d]	Comments
1-2	Five days per week for moderate exercise, 3 days per week for vigorous exercise, or 3 to 5 days per week for a mix of moderate and vigorous exercise	Two days per week; two sets, 8 to 12 repetitions of 10 different exercises	Two or three days per week, minimum; 10 minutes of stretching activities with additional option for agility and balance exercises	For the client to achieve greater benefits, progress the weekly aerobic total to 150 to 300 minutes of moderate-intensity activity or 75 to 150 minutes of vigorous-intensity activity (2 minutes of moderate activity equals 1 minute of vigorous activity) or a combination of moderate and vigorous activity. Stretching and optional neuromotor (balance and agility) exercises are included on at least 2 days per week; additional benefits are possible with greater frequency. Continue with the resistance training program, including hips and legs, chest, back, shoulders, low back, abdominal muscles, triceps, biceps, hamstrings, and quadriceps.
3-4	Two or three days per week of moderate activity and 1 or 2 days of vigorous activity	Two to three days per week; two sets, 8 to 12 repetitions of 10 different exercises	Three days per week, minimum; 10 minutes of stretching activities with additional option for agility and balance exercises	For the next couple weeks, consider mixing up the aerobic activities. Try a new aerobic exercise or change the intensity or duration of an activity. Continue with stretching and optional neuromotor activities on 3 days per week and the resistance training program at least 2 days per week. Consider varying the sets or repetitions, gradually progressing to heavier loads on primary exercises.
5-7	Five days per week for moderate exercise, 3 days per week for vigorous exercise, or 3 to 5 days per week for moderate and vigorous exercise	Two to three days per week; two sets, 8 to 12 repetitions of 10 exercises	Three days per week, minimum; 10 minutes of stretching activities with additional option for agility and balance exercises	Continue with the aerobic training program and with stretching and optional neuromotor activities. For resistance training, consider introducing the client to different exercises and movement patterns that involve pushing, pulling, and squatting. For example, if typically using machines, try a couple new exercises using dumbbells, medicine balls, or kettlebells to provide muscles with a new challenge while maintaining good form when trying new activities.
8-10	Five days per week for moderate exercise, 3 days per week for vigorous exercise, or 3 to 5 days per week for moderate and vigorous exercise	Two to three days per week; three sets, 8 to 10 repetitions of 10 exercises	Three days per week, minimum; 10 minutes of stretching activities with additional option for agility and balance exercises	Continue with the aerobic training program and stretching and optional neuromotor exercises. For resistance training, consider increasing the training intensity or number of sets; the number of repetitions may need to be decreased when adding additional weight.

[a]All activity sessions should be preceded and followed by a 5- to 10-minute warm-up and cool-down of light- to moderate-intensity activity.

[b]The intensity level is noted on a relative intensity scale from 0 to 10: Level 0 reflects rest, and 10 is maximal effort; moderate intensity is a level of 5 or 6, and vigorous intensity is an effort level of 7 or 8.

[c]Note that for experienced exercisers, a range of repetitions and intensities is effective; maximal strength gains are noted by ACSM at a mean training intensity of 80% 1RM and with an emphasis on heavier loads (e.g., 6RM).

[d]Include stretching activities to improve flexibility. Also, consider including some activities for agility and balance (i.e., neuromotor exercises).

Adapted by permission from B.A. Bushman, "Adults: Ages 18 to 64," in *ACSM's Complete Guide to Fitness and Health*, 2nd ed., edited by B. Bushman (Champaign, IL: Human Kinetics, 2017), 242. Additional information in table footnote c from American College of Sports Medicine, *ACSM's Guidelines for Exercise Testing and Prescription*, 11th ed. (Philadelphia: Wolters Kluwer, 2022).

CASE STUDY

Where to Start

Case Study Contributor: Barbara A. Bushman

Following appropriate informed consent and screening, the following fitness tests were conducted for Dedra, a 35-year-old, apparently healthy female (see chapters 8, 9, and 10 for details on the assessments and interpretation of results):

Height: 68 inches (1.73 meters)

Weight: 140 pounds (63.6 kilograms)

Resting heart rate: 64 bpm

Resting blood pressure: 122/78

Estimated $\dot{V}O_2$max from submaximal cycle ergometer test: 36 ml $\cdot$ kg^{-1} $\cdot$ min^{-1}

Push-ups: 11

Sit-and-reach: 14 inches

Dedra reports that she enjoys walking with a group of friends three mornings each week, typically about 45 minutes of brisk walking at a neighborhood park. This has been ongoing for the last 5 years. Weekends include getting away from the city where she lives to hike at some of the state parks nearby. She typically hikes for at least a couple hours. She indicates she has not devoted much time to resistance training or stretching but would like to learn more.

In developing a training program, the fitness professional should consider Dedra's self-reported physical activity along with fitness test results.

- Based on height and weight, her body mass index is 21.3 kg $\cdot$ m^{-2}, which is within what is considered the normal range.
- Her resting blood pressure is also normal.
- Her estimated $\dot{V}O_2$max is at the 75th percentile (upper end of the good range) compared to women of her age.
- For the push-up assessment, completing 11 push-ups is in the middle of the fair range.
- For the sit-and-reach assessment using a yardstick, Dedra was able to reach to 13.5 inches (recall that the feet are placed at a piece of tape located at the 15-inch mark on the yardstick for this assessment). This means she was not able to reach to her feet, indicating there is room for improvement in her overall flexibility.

The test results reflect Dedra's self-reported activity. Her regular walking program and additional weekend hiking activity have allowed her to maintain a good level of aerobic fitness. Compared to the sample programs in this chapter, her level of aerobic activity is best reflected as an established exerciser. Discussions could include additional time devoted to her walking program during the week or potentially introducing new activities to provide variety. Because she is engaging in approximately 225 minutes per week of moderate activity, she is meeting physical activity recommendations. With limited (to no) attention to muscular fitness and stretching, her push-up assessment and sit-and-reach measure support the value of adding these components to her activity program. In addition, including neuromotor training would be of benefit (e.g., balance and agility, which are important for her hiking outings as well as day-to-day activities). For these areas, she will need to start from the beginner level of activity. It is not uncommon for individuals to have a relative imbalance in an activity program where time and attention have been devoted to one or two of the fitness components while the others are lacking.

As Dedra looks to expand her exercise to include resistance training, flexibility, and balance and agility exercises, the fitness professional can promote adherence with various methods of behavior modification as discussed in chapter 22. Although she is established in the maintenance phase of her aerobic training, she will be in the preparation stage for the other areas. Preparation reflects the

(continued)

Case Study *(continued)*

time when plans are made to move into action. Just as Dedra already has personally seen benefits of aerobic conditioning, the fitness professional can provide information on the many benefits of resistance training, stretching, and neuromotor training. For example, the fitness professional can explain that resistance training lowers the risk of several chronic diseases, has favorable effects on body composition and mental health, and is key to being able to participate in physical activities. This also would be a time to dispel myths that resistance training requires heavy weights or that training will result in bulky muscles and instead emphasize the value of muscular fitness in allowing her to fully engage in daily activities and recreational pursuits. Instruction on specific activities will be key to giving Dedra confidence (i.e., self-efficacy) and comfort in expanding her exercise program into these additional areas. Practical strategies to promote motivation could include goal setting, behavior contracts, and hints on time management. Discussing what barriers may be in place for her to begin resistance training, stretching, and activities for balance and agility, along with ways to overcome those barriers, will help her reframe situations that might feel discouraging. For example, she shares that she has some out-of-town travel as part of her job. In the past, continuing with her walking program was relatively easy and she can see that adding stretching and some balance activities would not be difficult, but she questions how to include resistance training. The fitness professional can work with Dedra to develop an on-the-road workout using body-weight exercises, along with resistance bands that can easily be packed to take on the trip. Chapter 22 provides insights and suggestions for fitness professionals on enhancing motivation, monitoring and supporting behavior changes, and helping clients avoid relapse.

outs to allow for optimal training adaptations. Part of successful training is avoiding excessive overload with inadequate recovery. An intense exercise session or an intense training period may result in acute fatigue and even temporary decreases in performance (22). With appropriate recovery (less intense training or active rest), a positive adaptation can result in improved performance (7, 22) (see figure 16.1).

Within the Joint Consensus Statement of the European College of Sports Medicine and ACSM, the term *overreaching* is defined as "an accumulation of training and/or nontraining stress resulting in *short-term* decrement in performance capacity with or without related physiological and psychological signs and symptoms of maladaptation in which restoration of performance capacity may take from several days to several weeks" (22). Short-term overreaching followed by recovery that leads to improved performance has been referred to as *functional overreaching* (22); recovery may take days to weeks. However, if the balance between training and recovery is disrupted such that performance suffers for several weeks or months, the term *nonfunctional overreaching* has been applied. With nonfunctional overreaching, performance will decline, the individual will have decreased vigor and increased fatigue, and hormonal disturbances will occur (22).

The difference between nonfunctional overreaching and overtraining syndrome is not clearly defined. Overtraining syndrome (OTS) has been described as

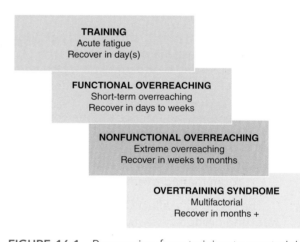

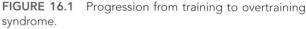

FIGURE 16.1 Progression from training to overtraining syndrome.

Reprinted by permission from B.A. Bushman, "Finding the Balance Between Overload and Recovery," *ACSM's Health & Fitness Journal* 20, no. 1 (2016): 5-8.

"prolonged maladaptation" regarding the individual's response to training (biological, neurochemical, and hormonal) (22). Rather than only being a result of excessive training, other factors such as caloric intake, diet composition (protein or carbohydrate intake), sleep quality, and cognitive effort are potentially involved, leading some to suggest *paradoxical deconditioning syndrome of the athlete* as a more descriptive term to reflect the combination of factors (9). Although research has focused on athletes, others engaging in excessive exercise can experience OTS as well. What constitutes "excessive exercise" is hard to define because many aspects affect an individual's response to training. Diagnosis of OTS is difficult and typically is a diagnosis of exclusion (10). Other medical conditions that may have similarities to OTS include asthma, anemia, hypothyroidism, immunodeficiency, hypocortisolemia, chronic fatigue syndrome, depression, and others (21). Thus, ruling out other causes for decrements in performance is an important step (22). Given that OTS has many potential impacts, combinations of variables have been used in research to monitor for OTS such as hormones, neurotransmitters, metabolites, immunological responses, psychological aspects, and electrocardiographic and electroencephalographic patterns (10). Researchers continue to explore the definitions and methods to study OTS in comparison to functional overreaching and nonfunctional overreaching (32). Although of interest from a research perspective, limited availability of laboratory techniques in training situations along with the lack of a definitive diagnosis present challenges.

As with the individualization needed in program development, each person has a different "tipping point" related to training stress capacity (21). Warning signs include decreased performance even with increased effort and increased perception of effort for the same workout (21). OTS has been compared to an orthopedic injury in its debilitating effects and required time for recovery (22). Thus, focusing on prevention with appropriate periodization within the training program is valuable, as well as attention to other areas, including the following (22):

- *Passive rest:* This includes 1 rest day from the training activity each week; this provides opportunity for recovery and may be a helpful mental time-out from a focused training program.

- *Adequate sleep:* Due to variation between individuals, sleeping for the amount of time that is required to feel wakeful during the day is recommended rather than prescribing a given number of hours of sleep.

- *Nutrition:* Ensure adequate carbohydrate intake, fluid intake, and caloric consumption to meet increased demands of training; also ensure sufficient protein remains in the diet.

Use of training logs and tracking body weight, heart rate (morning or maximal), and sleep, among other aspects, may be of value (21). Morning heart rate may reflect increased catecholamines and increased sympathetic tone and a loss of parasympathetic tone; maximal heart rate also has been used to measure sympathetic and parasympathetic balance (21). Given the variability in responses to training, fitness professionals and coaches need to individualize training programs and maintain accurate records charting performance (19, 22). This will allow for gradual adjustments in training intensity or highlight the need to provide a rest day. The importance of gradual progression, along with the need to individualize training programs given that many factors affect response to a given training load (e.g., age, prior injury, training history, fitness level), cannot be overemphasized (16).

Research in this area has focused on endurance-based training; the potential within strength sports and resistance training has also been examined, although studies have not clearly identified OTS but rather nonfunctional overreaching in which short-term performance loss resolved within days to weeks (5). Caution is still warranted related to extreme conditioning (i.e., high-volume, high-intensity training) and excessive training loads (5), and susceptibility to overtraining is potentially increased with frequent, high-intensity, monotonous resistance training (17). This reinforces the value of periodization within training programs. Fitness professionals should appreciate that overtraining can result from poor programming characterized by frequent high-intensity training sessions without adequate rest and recovery between workouts. From a practical perspective, it is important to consider a person's training experience and all fitness activities regularly performed. Periodized training, which should include periods of less intense training and active rest, can help individuals avoid overtraining and promote long-term gains in muscular fitness (3, 23). Other resources are available regarding periodization (6, 18, 30).

KEY POINT

Training programs should be characterized by an appropriate overload and progression combined with planned periods of rest and recovery. Overreaching is often the first stage of the overtraining syndrome, which is characterized by a decrease in performance and other physical and psychological effects. Adequate rest and recovery between workouts, adequate sleep, and proper nutrition can help individuals avoid overtraining syndrome.

Balancing Activity Level With Nutritional Requirements

For optimal health, active individuals must match caloric intake with expenditure, meeting requirements for not only activities of daily living and growth but also for physical activity, exercise, or sport. Chapter 5 provides background on dietary aspects, including considerations for active individuals. When there is a mismatch between intake and expenditure such that there is low energy availability resulting in energy deficiency, a condition reflecting inadequate intake to support the body's exercise energy needs, health and performance can suffer.

To promote the health benefits of regular physical activity while avoiding health risks of low energy availability, a task force within ACSM focused on women's issues introduced the Female Athlete Triad in 1992 (33). In the first ACSM position stand on the Female Athlete Triad, in 1997, three interrelated components were identified (29):

1. *Disordered eating:* Described as a "wide spectrum of harmful and often ineffective eating behaviors used in attempts to lose weight or achieve a lean appearance." This could range from restriction of food intake to the defined disorders of anorexia nervosa or bulimia nervosa.

2. *Amenorrhea:* Including delayed menstruation by age 16 in a female with secondary sex characteristics (primary amenorrhea) or missing three or more consecutive menstrual cycles after menarche (secondary amenorrhea). (*Note:* The age for primary amenorrhea was reduced from 16 to 15 years of age in the subsequent ACSM position stand given that menarche is occurring earlier [28].)

3. *Osteoporosis:* A disease resulting in low bone mass and deterioration of bone tissue that increases the risk of fracture (potentially presenting with a stress injury to bone).

The initial position stand called for more research on causes, prevalence, treatment, and consequences (29). Although the terminology of "athlete" is used, the Triad can occur not only in individuals participating in sports but also individuals engaging in habitual, strenuous physical activity (28).

In 2007, an updated position stand on the Female Athlete Triad was published in which energy availability, menstrual function, and bone mineral density were viewed along continuums from health to disease (28). This model highlighted the importance of the recognition of subclinical concerns, as well as the spectrum of severity of these disorders, to allow for early recognition and intervention (12). Individuals presenting with one component of the Triad should be assessed for the others (28). For energy availability (defined as dietary energy intake minus exercise energy expenditure), an individual might have optimal (healthy) energy availability or might have reduced or even low energy availability; these latter

two situations could occur with or without disordered eating (see the sidebar *Energy Availability*). The spectrum of menstrual function ranges from eumenorrhea (i.e., menstrual cycles occurring every 28 days, plus or minus 7 days) to amenorrhea (i.e., absence of menstrual cycles for more than 90 days; amenorrhea after menarche is called secondary amenorrhea and a delay in the start of menses after age 15 is called primary amenorrhea), with subclinical menstrual disorders (e.g., oligomenorrhea, or menstrual cycles longer than 35 days) between the two (28). Note that menstrual irregularities or amenorrhea should be evaluated by a physician for other potential medical conditions that may be present (28). Bone health might be optimal, or the individual might have low bone mineral density or, at the most severe, osteoporosis. Adequate energy availability to match daily needs is key in maintaining both reproductive and bone health (28). Movement along the spectrum between health and disease for each of the three components of the Triad occurs at different rates (28). For example, energy availability can be changed quickly, while menstrual status or bone density take longer periods of time (28).

In 2014 the International Olympic Committee (IOC) updated its 2005 consensus statement on the Female Athlete Triad, introducing the term *Relative Energy Deficiency in Sport* (RED-S) (24). This update provided an emerging view of the consequences of low energy availability in which energy deficiency is noted as a cause of impaired function for both females and males related to several physiological functions such as metabolic rate, bone health, immune function, protein synthesis, and cardiovascular health, and menstrual function in females (24). The IOC statement reflects the complex nature of the syndrome and the potential impact on males as well as females (24).

In 2021, the Female and Male Athlete Triad Coalition published a consensus statement that retained the term *Female Athlete Triad* and added a definition of the *Male Athlete Triad* (27). Like the model developed in the ACSM 2007 position stand on the Female Athlete Triad, the Coalition consensus statement discusses three interrelated conditions, each with a spectrum from healthy to unhealthy: energy deficiency/low energy availability, impaired bone health, and suppression of the hypothalamic-pituitary-gonadal axis (27). At the time of the consensus statement, the specific subclinical outcomes for males were less clearly defined and researched (15, 27). The association between energy deficiency/low energy availability and reproductive and bone health for males is being explored; currently, a more severe energy deficiency/low energy availability appears to be required in males compared to females to affect the other aspects of the Triad (27). The Coalition has developed a new model (see figure 16.2) that depicts the continuum for

Energy Availability

Meeting the energy demands of body functions and routine daily activity, as well as those of a training program, can be a challenge. Energy availability is the amount of energy available to perform all body functions after the energy cost of activity and exercise is subtracted and is calculated as dietary energy intake minus exercise energy expenditure normalized to fat-free mass (28). Low energy availability can result due to increased expenditure in exercise without increasing caloric intake, or by decreasing intake below that required (28). This mismatch between what the body needs and what is supplied may occur because of lack of knowledge on nutritional requirements; fitness professionals can promote healthy approaches to nutrition to adequately fuel the body as discussed in chapter 5 (this chapter includes important information on scope of practice related to discussion of nutritional information). Other situations could involve a continuum of disordered eating behaviors all the way to an eating disorder, such as anorexia nervosa or bulimia nervosa, both of which have specific diagnostic criteria per the American Psychiatric Association and can be life-threatening, requiring advanced treatment and medical attention (25). Anorexia nervosa symptoms include extremely restrictive eating, intense and excessive exercise, extreme thinness, intense fear of gaining weight, unwillingness to maintain a healthy weight, distorted body or self-image, and denial of extremely low body weight (26). Bulimia nervosa involves binge eating, often followed by actions to prevent weight gain, including vomiting, laxative or diuretic use, excessive exercise, or a combination of behaviors (26). Additional information on eating disorders is found in chapter 20. Other situations may involve disordered eating, defined as including "restrictive eating, fasting, frequently skipping meals, diet pills, laxatives, diuretics, enemas, overeating, binge-eating and then purging (vomiting)" (28). *Disordered eating* is a descriptive phrase rather than a diagnosis; potential negative impacts of disordered eating on physical and mental health are still present, and seeking treatment is important to avoid detrimental consequences (4).

Some signs of low energy availability include symptoms of the metabolic changes of energy deficiency, such as feeling tired and fatigued, a decrease in athletic performance, problems concentrating, fractures or recurring injuries, and, in women, irregular or missed menstrual periods (14). Active women must realize that losing their menstrual cycle is *not* a normal response to exercise (14). When energy availability is too low, the body must shift energy to focus on "survival," and thus reproduction and growth are compromised, leading to reproductive suppression (e.g., low estrogen and menstrual disturbances for females, reduced testosterone in men) and poor bone health (e.g., stress fractures) (14).

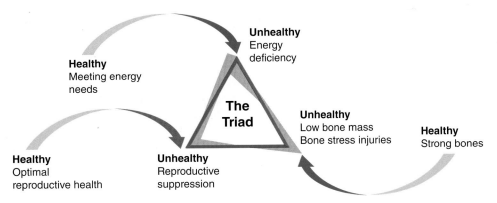

FIGURE 16.2 The Female and Male Athlete Triad model.

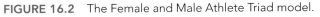

Reprinted by permission of The Female and Male Athlete Triad Coalition: An International Consortium, https://femaleandmaleathletetriad.org/athletes/what-is-the-triad/.

each component of the Triad, ranging from healthy to unhealthy status, for both females and males (14).

Risk factors for developing the Triad include dieting at an early age, disordered eating habits (e.g., skipping meals), dissatisfaction with body type, perfectionism, and the belief that weight or body-fat loss at any cost will improve performance (14). Additionally, for the Female Athlete Triad risks include involvement in sports that favor lean body size or shape, or have weight classes or revealing uniforms, and for the Male Athlete Triad risks include frequent weight cycling, extremely high training volumes, and extreme weight-control behaviors such as vomiting and saunas (14). Fitness professionals must be educated regarding risk factors and be watchful of warning signs that warrant evaluation by a qualified health care provider such as stress fractures, excessive or compulsive exercise behaviors, or, for females, irregular or absent menstrual periods (14).

With an understanding of the potential concerns of the Triad, the fitness professional is in a position to help guide individuals to a realistic body image and to support proper day-to-day nutrition with referral to nutritionists (i.e., Registered Dietitian Nutritionist, or RDN, with expertise in working with disordered eating and eating disorders) and medical professionals as appropriate. A key factor is the metabolic consequences of energy deficiency; this may be due to either excess energy expenditure within a training program or not consuming sufficient calories to match expenditure, or both (14). Low energy availability can occur with inadvertent low energy intake in relation to expenditure or restrictive dieting. The impact is complex and multifactorial, with increased susceptibility to injury or poor bone health in addition to concerns with cardiovascular and neuromuscular function (8). Where appropriate, fitness professionals may educate others on the potential consequences of low energy availability, including fatigue, poor recovery, poor healing, bone loss, and impaired performance. With energy deficiency, the body will focus on immediate needs and reproductive functions will be suppressed, resulting in menstrual disorders such as amenorrhea (11). Research in this area is active and ongoing; for example, researchers with the REFUEL study, a randomized control study looking at the effects of increased energy intake, found that a modest increase in daily caloric intake of 300 to 350 kcal · day^{-1} above baseline energy intake during a 12-month intervention study was beneficial for menstrual recovery (11) but not bone mineral density (the latter potentially limited by the study duration) (13).

Various tools are available on risk assessment and return to play for athletes with one of the Triad disorders. The latter decision should be done by the appropriate health care professional (12, 15, 24); depending which risk assessment tool is used (12, 24), clearance decisions for athletic participation may differ (20). These clearance recommendations are provided for athletes; no specific guidance is currently available related to high-level fitness participation. The unifying message of the Triad and RED-S is the need to ensure that dietary energy intake is sufficient to meet the requirements of general body functions and routine daily activities in addition to the calories expended within a training program. Ensuring adequate energy availability involves increasing caloric intake or reducing expenditure, or both (28). Prevention can be promoted with education (e.g., healthy eating, understanding risks and early warning signs of the Triad) and a positive emphasis on nutrition and health rather than weight to enhance performance (24). Fitness professionals may have opportunities to educate and model positive body images, promoting the health of their clients rather than emphasizing measures of body weight or composition. With expanded understanding of the need to ensure adequate caloric intake to meet daily requirements, fitness professionals can provide supportive environments for clients. If components of the Triad are recognized, the fitness professional should refer the client to a health care provider in their network, including physicians or other health care professionals, a registered dietitian, and, if disordered eating or a defined eating disorder is present, a mental health practitioner (28). See the sidebar *Jenna the Triathlete: Weight Loss, Performance Issues, and Amenorrhea* for a case study.

KEY POINT

The Female and Male Athlete Triad and RED-S both reflect the concerns that can arise from a mismatch between energy intake and total energy requirements. Fitness professionals should be aware of and knowledgeable about the importance of their role in prevention, education, and early recognition.

CASE STUDY

Jenna the Triathlete: Weight Loss, Performance Issues, and Amenorrhea

Case Study Contributor: Carol Otis

Jenna is a 25-year-old triathlete who swims at your facility and often discusses her training with you. Previously, she was involved with a club team, but, desiring to improve her performance, she started working with a new coach who increased her training volume and also advised her to drop "at least 10 pounds to improve her run times." Her training volume increased at least 25%, she limited her caloric intake to 1,200 calories a day, and she started to weigh herself daily as she sought to lose weight. Measuring 5 feet 7 inches, she was at her usual healthy weight around 136 pounds at the start of the season but reports losing 15 to 20 pounds over the past five to six months. She got positive comments from her coach and training partners on her weight loss, and she says she initially felt great after losing the first 10 pounds, describing feeling "lighter" on her runs. But now she weighs about 115 pounds, and her recent two competitions were the worst of the season. She complains of feeling tired all the time when trying to train and feeling irritable, and her menstrual periods, which were always quite regular, suddenly stopped and have been absent the last few months. Training partners have said the loss of her periods shows the new training program is effective. She is frustrated at how she is feeling and performing, and wonders if the menstrual cycle change really is a good training indicator. How would you respond?

As you reflect on the situation, Jenna, who was advised by a new coach to increase training and lose weight, dramatically decreased her caloric intake. She now appears to be in a state of low energy availability in which her performance is declining and her menses stopped. She has symptoms of two of the disorders of Female Athlete Triad and needs intervention now before her health declines further. In situations like this, having relationships with a multidisciplinary referral team of nutritionists, physicians, and mental health professionals who specialize in eating disorders is key.

Initially, you can help her by describing your concerns and referring her for complete evaluation and care. Start by telling her honestly what you observe by using "I" statements. ("I notice that you are losing weight, and you mentioned your periods have stopped. Can we talk about that?"). Explain to her the importance of meeting energy needs with a healthy diet and frequent snacks to fuel training, performance, and recovery. Confirm her suspicion that loss of menses is *not* a normal response to training. Refer her to both a nutritionist for specific dietary guidance and to her health care providers to have her weight and amenorrhea assessed. By recognizing the warning signs of low energy availability and the Triad disorders and by referring someone at risk for evaluation and care, you are helping her recover her energy, health, and performance.

Jenna's experience clearly shows how comments and suggestions from coaches and others to lose weight can unintentionally trigger unhealthy dieting. The resultant low energy availability can lead to medical issues (in this situation, amenorrhea) as well as decrements in performance. The availability of a knowledgeable fitness professional who was approachable was key in allowing Jenna to feel comfortable reaching out and then following up with the referrals. As a result, she stopped weighing herself daily and began adding snacks during training and recovery. She gained a few pounds and developed a healthier eating pattern. She talked to her coach about what she learned about better nutrition, and she slightly decreased her training. She felt comfortable gaining a few pounds. Two months later, she weighed 123 pounds, her training was back on track, and she was meeting with her doctor about her missed menstrual cycles. Early recognition of the warning signs of the Triad and prompt referral can keep someone from developing more serious disorders and help them achieve their performance and health goals.

LEARNING AIDS

REVIEW QUESTIONS

1. What are the components of a complete exercise program? What are recommendations in each of these areas?
2. What should the fitness professional consider when determining the starting point for each of the components of a complete exercise program?
3. List ways that an exercise program can be progressed over time.
4. Describe what *adaptation* means within a training program.
5. What is overtraining syndrome, and how can it be avoided?
6. What are short-term and potential long-term impacts of low energy availability?

CASE STUDIES

1. Tobias, a 40-year-old male, comes to you to discuss his current exercise program, which has focused predominately on muscular fitness. He typically goes to the gym 2 or 3 days each week to use both the free weights and resistance machines. He would like to know what other activities might be beneficial. How would you respond?
2. Samantha is a 28-year-old female; she is a runner who has dreams of someday competing in an Olympic marathon. You have been helping plan her resistance training workouts for the past year, and you notice some disturbing signs: Her weight has decreased dramatically, she is battling stress fractures, her mood is negative and characterized by self-criticism, and her performance times are worse than a few months earlier. What do you do?

Answers to Case Studies

1. Assuming that informed consent and screenings have been completed with no noted health concerns, additional discussion of current activity and future goals can provide important information. You can ask Tobias for additional background on his current and any prior exercise programs. For example, you can discuss the amount of resistance training he is doing, how long has he been engaging in this level of activity, and if he has any concerns with his current resistance training program. Additionally, determining his prior experience (if any) with aerobic activity and flexibility exercises and his interest in expanding his exercise program beyond resistance training is key. You then can decide what fitness assessments will be included. Interpreting the fitness test results, with appreciation for his current activities and future goals, can be used to work with Tobias to create his individualized exercise program.
2. This is a difficult and potentially dangerous situation. At the very least, Samantha is exhibiting signs of poor physical and emotional health. Before you engage Samantha in conversation about your concerns, you need to seek out a support system for assistance and advice. Access your network of nutritionists (i.e., RDN), physicians, and mental health professionals in your area who specialize in working with athletes and in eating disorders. Given that Samantha is already exhibiting diminished health and signs associated with disordered eating, she is likely going to require the assistance of a multidisciplinary team. Begin a dialogue with Samantha by addressing observed concerns; be supportive and provide recommendations within your network of professionals (e.g., RDN, physicians, and mental health professionals).

Special Populations and Conditions

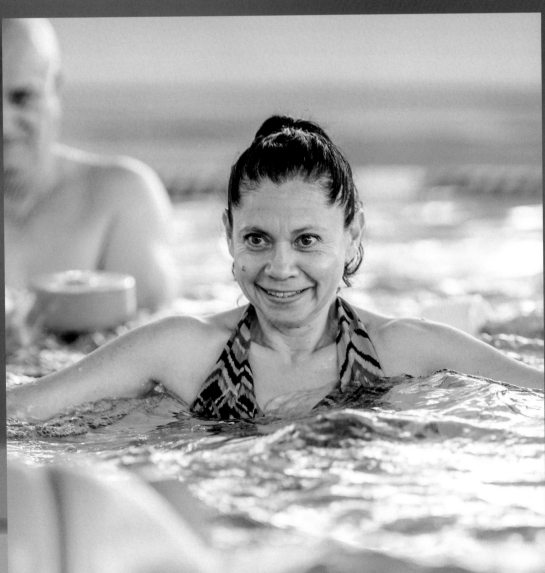

Physical activity has the potential to benefit individuals of all ages and with a variety of health conditions or chronic diseases. Fitness professionals need to understand unique factors that can have a bearing on physical activity and exercise recommendations for a given individual such as age or a health or medical condition. With the understanding of the benefits of physical activity throughout the lifespan, in chapters 17 and 18 the special characteristics for youth and older adults are discussed. Pregnancy is another time in life when physical activity has many potential benefits; chapter 19 provides background on and recommendations to optimize health and safety during pregnancy. Chapter 20 focuses on weight management and the importance of lifestyle habits, including nutrition and physical activity. Chapter 21 provides background on and recommendations to promote safe and effective physical activity (including during clinical supervision, like cardiac or pulmonary rehabilitation programs) for people experiencing health problems including cardiovascular disease, cancer, diabetes, pulmonary disease, and osteoporosis. Any one of these topics could make a complete book in and of itself. The purpose here is to help fitness professionals understand the role of physical activity in the quality of life for all people and to provide general knowledge of and practical guidelines for screening, testing, supervision, and activity modifications for each population.

17

Youth

Avery D. Faigenbaum

OBJECTIVES

The reader will be able to do the following:

1. Discuss public health physical activity guidelines for children and adolescents
2. Describe contemporary trends in youth physical activity
3. Compare the physiological responses to exercise between children and adults
4. Explain the physical, psychosocial, and cognitive benefits of youth physical activity
5. Define fundamental movement skills and explain the concept of a proficiency barrier
6. Design integrative programs that enhance both health- and skill-related physical fitness
7. List strategies to promote ongoing participation in youth fitness programs

17

A compelling body of evidence indicates that ongoing participation in physical activity can offer observable health and fitness benefits to children and adolescents (31, 100). In addition to enhancing cardiorespiratory fitness, increasing muscular strength, and improving metabolic health, well-designed youth fitness and sport programs provide an opportunity for participants to learn skills, make friends, have fun, and feel good about their accomplishments (50, 78). From a developmental perspective, youth who gain confidence and competence in their physical abilities appear more likely to continue participating in exercise and sport activities later in life (33, 41, 90). Fitness professionals should recognize the importance of establishing healthy physical activity behaviors early in life and exposing girls and boys to a variety of physical activities throughout the growing years.

Leading health and fitness organizations recognize the importance of daily physical activity for children and adolescents as part of active transportation, outdoor play, recreational exercise, physical education, and sport activities (2, 92, 100). However, epidemiological reports indicate that contemporary youth are not as active as they should be, a troubling trend that seems to have worsened during the COVID-19 pandemic (3, 43, 69). Technological advances and social media usage have decreased the need to move, physical education is considered expendable in some communities, and the cost of participating in organized sport is a barrier for youth who come from families without extensive financial means (46, 68, 74). The inevitable consequences of physical inactivity during childhood and adolescence on lifelong pathological processes has made clear the urgent need to identify physically inactive youth and design interventions that target exercise deficits before youth become resistant to interventions later in life. Fitness professionals who understand the science of pediatric exercise and genuinely appreciate the physical and psychosocial uniqueness of children and adolescents are in an inimitable position to design and implement youth fitness programs.

This chapter focuses on the importance of physical activity for youth, the essentials of pediatric exercise science, and recommended strategies for designing fitness programs for children and adolescents. In this chapter, the term *children* refers to boys and girls who have not yet developed secondary sex characteristics (e.g., breast development in girls and increased muscle mass in boys) and corresponds roughly up to the age of 11 years in girls and 13 years in boys. The term *adolescence* refers to a period of time between childhood and adulthood and generally includes girls 12 to 18 years of age and boys 14 to 18 years of age. The terms *youth* and *pediatric* are broadly defined to include children and adolescents.

Physical Activity in Youth

The *Physical Activity Guidelines for Americans* emphasizes the importance of regular moderate to vigorous physical activity (MVPA) for children and adolescents and includes the recommendation of a total of 60 minutes or more of MVPA on a daily basis (92). The recommended physical activities include aerobic exercise as well as activities that strengthen muscle and bone (92). Many activities incorporate multiple aspects, as shown in the following examples:

- Games that involve running and chasing (e.g., tag) result in an elevated heart rate (aerobic activity) with weight-bearing movements (bone strengthening).
- Climbing on playground equipment may include all three types of activity with elevation of heart rate (aerobic activity) while climbing and supporting body weight (muscle strengthening and bone strengthening).
- Circuit training exercises including a variety of activities (e.g., jumping jacks, hula hooping, medicine ball throws) promote strengthening of the muscles and bones while also having an aerobic component (i.e., elevation of heart rate).

The recommendation of at least 60 minutes per day is intended to be accumulated over the course of the day. This can be reached with a combination of many shorter periods of time throughout the day, including physical education class, brief activity breaks interspersed throughout the day in the classroom, active transportation to and from school (e.g., walking or biking), play and games at recess, before- and after-school activity programs, organized youth sport, and family activities (e.g., walking the dog, playing at the park or in the backyard). Although greater amounts of physical activity may provide additional benefits, it is important to consider the exercise intensity as well as the mix of health- and skill-related activities (67). Health-related activities require endurance, strength, or flexibility, whereas skill-related activities require agility, balance, coordination, speed, power, and reaction time. Watching children on a playground (figure 17.1) or young athletes on a soccer field supports the premise that both health- and skill-related components of physical fitness are foundational for ongoing participation in a variety of exercise and sport activities throughout the growing years (67).

Despite public health efforts to increase participation in youth physical activity, epidemiological reports indicate that a majority of children and adolescents are not accumulating the recommended amount of MVPA (3,

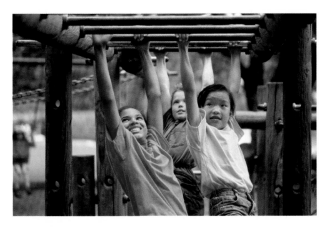

FIGURE 17.1 Children playing on a playground.

Steve Satushek/The Image Bank/Getty Images

KEY POINT

Children and adolescents should be encouraged to participate in at least an average of 60 minutes of moderate to vigorous physical activity (MVPA) daily. In addition to physical education and recess, youth should have regular opportunities to be physically active before and after school. Reducing sedentary behaviors such as watching television and viewing social media can increase the amount of time youth have for physical activity.

17, 43). Self-report data on physical activity suggest that only 24% of youth in the United States participate in 60 minutes of MVPA every day (53), and these findings are consistent with reports from other countries (3). In one global report that used data from 146 countries, less than 20% of 11- to 17-year-old students were sufficiently physically active (43). Notably, the decline and disinterest in physical activity appears to emerge early in life (about 6-8 years of age) (83, 91) and seems to be a consequence

of poor fundamental movement skills and low muscle strength (10, 23, 32). Since a requisite level of muscular strength is needed to run, jump, and skip proficiently (30, 49, 62), weaker youth with poor fundamental movement skills may be less able (and therefore less willing) to engage in active play, recreational exercise, and sport activities with their stronger (and faster) peers.

Although the term *dynapenia* traditionally has been used to describe the loss of muscle strength or power in older adults (19), the construct of dynapenia also can be applied to modern-day youth who are weaker and slower than previous generations (34). Over the past few decades, a decline has been observed in selected field measures of youth muscular fitness in most countries (34). For example, a study of English 10-year-olds found downward trends in the standing long jump, handgrip, sit-ups, and bent arm hang, which were consistent with self-reported declines in physical activity (82). Australian researchers had similar findings, reporting that children and adolescents were jumping 7 centimeters less in 2015 than in 1985 (45). In a large sample of children and adolescents from 31 countries, the rate of improvement in sit-up performance slowed from 1964 to 2000, stabilized until 2010, and declined thereafter (52). Since levels of muscular strength tend to remain relatively stable between childhood and mid-adulthood (39), weaker youth may be less likely to engage in the recommended amount of MVPA and more likely to suffer adverse health consequences associated with dynapenia and unhealthy lifestyle behaviors (34, 71).

Levels of muscular strength are inversely associated with the risk of all-cause mortality and major noncommunicable diseases in adults (64), and it seems weaker youth also are susceptible to the inevitable consequences of muscle disuse and dysfunction (38, 47, 77). Notably, low handgrip strength measured in childhood, young adulthood (28-36 years), and mid-adulthood (38-49 years) has been found to be equally associated with prediabetes or type 2 diabetes, which underscores the importance of exposing youth to strength-building activities early in life and maintaining these behaviors into later life

Fundamental Movement Skills

Fundamental movement skills are often referred to as the building blocks of human movement because they are considered foundational for ongoing participation in more complex exercise and sport activities (5, 49). Fundamental movement skills can be classified into three categories: locomotor (e.g., jumping and running), object control (e.g., catching and throwing), and stability (e.g., balancing and twisting). Youth fitness specialists should integrate developmentally appropriate skill-building activities and games into exercise programs so youth can learn a variety of movement patterns in a supportive setting and reinforce these skills during active play and sport activities.

(38). Without developmentally appropriate interventions that target neuromuscular deficits and spark an ongoing interest in exercise and sport activities, it seems the divergence in performance between less active and more active youth likely will widen throughout this developmental phase of life. The impact of physical inactivity on lifelong pathological processes and associated health care costs highlight the need to focus on prevention and a disease-free state by implementing cost-effective youth physical activity interventions (58, 96).

RESEARCH INSIGHT

The Cost of Youth Physical Inactivity

Public health guidelines suggest that children and adolescents should accumulate on average at least 60 minutes of MVPA daily, yet a vast majority of youth are falling short of this recommendation. Lee and colleagues quantified the economic and health effects of increasing children's physical activity in the United States (58). They estimated that maintaining the current physical activity levels would result in an annual net present value of $1.1 trillion in direct medical costs and $1.7 trillion in lost productivity over the course of their lifetimes. Even modest increases in physical activity could reduce the prevalence of obesity-related health outcomes (e.g., coronary heart disease and type 2 diabetes) and save billions of dollars. The possible savings substantially outweigh the costs of school- and community-based youth physical activity programs.

Unlike adults, children and adolescents are in a constant state of change because they are still growing and maturing. As their developing bodies evolve physically, psychologically, and socially into mature adults,

markers of physical fitness are in a constant state of transformation. Comparing the 100-meter sprint time of an 8-year-old to a 16-year-old supports the premise that physical measures of performance in youth improve over time as a result of growth, maturation, and active play. While differences are observable in physical development among youth of the same chronological age, youth who participate in well-designed fitness programs make even greater gains in physical performance over time. These observations underline a potential synergistic adaptation whereby regular exposure to developmentally appropriate fitness training throughout childhood and adolescence complements naturally occurring adaptations (29).

Responses to Exercise

The acute responses to exercise are different between youth and older populations and can be easily observed when children play with adults. For example, at the same play or exercise intensity, children breathe a little harder and have higher heart rates. Although these physiological differences do not influence the ability of healthy children to participate in various types of MVPA, fitness professionals should be knowledgeable of expected responses to exercise when designing, implementing, and assessing youth fitness programs. The information in figure 17.2 provides a summary of the physiological responses to acute exercise between children and adults.

While resting heart rates between children and adults are similar, at all exercise intensities children exhibit higher heart rates and lower stroke volumes than older populations. Because children have smaller hearts than adults, a lower stroke volume can be expected. The higher heart rates during exercise probably are an attempt to compensate for the smaller ventricular size and lower stroke volume. Cardiac output is a function of heart rate and stroke volume. The heart rate compensation during exercise is unable to account for the lower stroke volume, and therefore children show smaller increases in cardiac output during exercise than adults. Notably, maximal heart rates do not appreciably change during childhood and early adolescence, and it is not uncommon for heart rates to exceed 200 beats per minute during vigorous

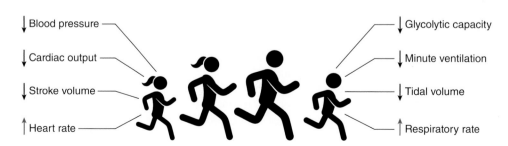

↓ Blood pressure

↓ Cardiac output

↓ Stroke volume

↑ Heart rate

↓ Glycolytic capacity

↓ Minute ventilation

↓ Tidal volume

↑ Respiratory rate

FIGURE 17.2 Comparison of the physiological responses to acute exercise between children and adults.

exercise and sport activities (80). Therefore, the estimation of maximal heart rate from age-based equations is inappropriate for youth (18). If heart rate monitors are used during youth fitness classes, the expected heart rate response to vigorous bouts of exercise should be discussed in advance to avoid any concerns that may arise from high heart rates.

Resting systolic and diastolic blood pressure is lower in healthy children than adults. Since the magnitude of the increase in systolic blood pressure during exercise is related to the value at rest, children tend to have a lower systolic blood pressure during exercise than older populations (80). Diastolic blood pressure remains stable or decreases slightly during exercise. Systolic and diastolic blood pressure are influenced by body composition; youth with higher body-fat percentages tend to have higher blood pressure levels (16).

Children have smaller lungs than adults, and therefore children have a lower tidal volume, which is the amount of air inspired or expired in a single breath. *Respiratory rate* refers to the number of breaths per minute and is higher in children than adults. The total amount of air a person breathes per minute is called *minute ventilation* and is a product of tidal volume and respiratory rate. During vigorous exercise it is normal for children to breathe rapidly because they process a smaller amount of air in absolute terms per minute. Despite a higher breathing frequency during exercise, minute ventilation is lower in children than adults due to the lower tidal volume (80). These are expected responses to physical activity and do not limit exercise performance in healthy children.

In terms of exercise-related differences in anaerobic metabolism, children appear to have a faster rate of intramuscular creatine phosphate resynthesis than adults, which suggests that children are prepared for short bursts (<10 seconds) of high-intensity physical activity (36). However, glycolytic activity appears limited in children as compared to adults; therefore youth should not be expected to perform as well as adults on high-energy activities lasting 30 to 120 seconds. Because of the depressed capacity for glycolytic metabolism, children demonstrate lower levels of blood lactate during submaximal and maximal exercise than adults (9). Although the rate of elimination of lactate after exercise is the same in children and adults, children tend to recover more quickly from physical exertion than adults (36). Different physiological factors related to muscle mass and energy metabolism may explain child–adult differences in recovery. Fitness professionals should be aware of the ability of children to recover more quickly than adults and may need to shorten the length of the rest intervals between sets or bouts of high-intensity exercise when working with youth to maintain interest, maximize exercise time, and improve training outcomes.

RESEARCH INSIGHT

MICE Versus HIIT

Regular participation in aerobic exercise can lead to substantial fitness benefits in children and adolescents, but what type of exercise is best? Cao and colleagues performed a meta-analysis with 17 studies to compare the effects of moderate-intensity continuous exercise (MICE) with high-intensity interval training (HIIT) on cardiorespiratory fitness in healthy youth (14). They found that HIIT was more effective than MICE in improving cardiorespiratory fitness in children and adolescents irrespective of modality or duration. Because HIIT appears to be an effective and time-efficient method of exercise, this type of training may be a worthwhile addition to youth fitness programs.

Peak Oxygen Uptake

The measurement of maximal oxygen uptake ($\dot{V}O_2max$) during a progressive exercise test is considered the single best measure of aerobic fitness and can serve as an important marker of health. Since $\dot{V}O_2max$ is the product of maximal cardiac output and maximal arteriovenous oxygen difference, each system involved in the delivery of oxygen to the working muscles can influence aerobic fitness. A true $\dot{V}O_2max$ requires a plateau in oxygen uptake despite an increase in exercise intensity. Because this plateau is observed infrequently in children and adolescents, the term $\dot{V}O_2peak$ has been introduced to define the highest value recorded during a pediatric exercise test to exhaustion (37). Improvements in $\dot{V}O_2peak$ throughout the growing years are mediated by increases in heart size, lung size, and skeletal muscle mass as well as size-independent factors (80).

Another difference between exercising children and adults involves thermoregulation (70). Children have a larger surface–to–body mass ratio than adults, which allows for a greater heat exchange. If the environmental temperature is lower than body temperature (e.g., swimming in an outdoor pool), children dissipate more heat than adults. Conversely, when the environmental temperature is higher than body temperature (e.g., playing tennis in the summer) less heat will be lost. Children also produce less sweat per gland than adults when exercising in a hot environment. Not only may these differences in thermoregulation affect exercise performance, but poor heat tolerance may increase the risk for heat-related illness in youth when engaged in outdoor sports or other vigorous physical activities (22). Even mild (approximately 1%) hypohydration can reduce children's high-intensity exercise performance in the heat (99). Educational interventions that emphasize adequate fluid intake before, during, and after exercise have been found to improve hydration status and enhance exercise performance in young athletes (54).

Potential Benefits of Youth Physical Activity

Regular participation in physical activity promotes many aspects of health and can offer observable physical, psychosocial, and cognitive benefits to children and adolescents (25, 51, 72). If youth fitness programs are well designed and consistent with the needs, abilities, and interests of the participants, significant improvements in aerobic fitness, muscular strength, motor skills, body composition, skeletal tissue, blood lipids, and cardiometabolic health are possible (40, 65, 78, 100). Further, regular participation in meaningful physical activities can reduce symptoms of anxiety and depression in youth and can offer cognitive effects that can improve academic performance and brain health (26, 48, 56). The potential benefits of youth physical activity are presented in figure 17.3.

Perhaps of equal importance to fitness professionals is the observation that healthy physical activity behaviors that are established early in life tend to carry over into adulthood (39, 90, 93). Youth with high levels of sedentary time tend to remain sedentary as they get older, whereas a high level of physical activity throughout childhood and adolescence predicts a high level of adult physical activity (89, 93). Notably, physically active lifestyles in 3- and 6-year-old boys and girls have been found to significantly predict physical activity along the life span into adulthood (90). In support of these observations, researchers found that cardiorespiratory fitness, muscular strength, and muscular endurance showed moderate tracking from childhood or adolescence to adulthood (41). Collectively, these findings underscore the importance of activating inactive youth early in life and modifying low youth physical fitness levels to reduce the risk of future chronic disease and enhance overall well-being.

Participation in school- and community-based fitness programs can provide opportunities for children and adolescents to become proficient in a range of fundamental movement skills (49, 65). Youth who do not develop and enhance their fundamental movement skills tend to engage in less physical activity and, in turn, develop

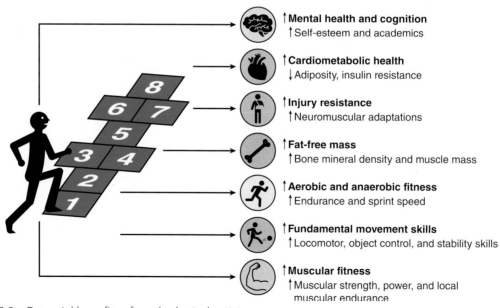

FIGURE 17.3 Potential benefits of youth physical activity.

unhealthy lifestyle behaviors (44, 57, 79). Proficiency in fundamental movement skills does not occur naturally (5). Rather, these skills are learned and developed with qualified fitness instruction and reinforced with practice during active play, recreational exercise, and sport activities. Youth who do not develop the prerequisite movement-skill proficiency may not be able to break through a proficiency barrier that consequently would limit their ability to perform more context-specific skills during exercise and sport activities (23, 73, 86). Due to troubling global trends in levels of fundamental movement skills in today's children (10), fitness professionals should allocate time during exercise sessions for direct learning experiences that target neuromuscular deficiencies with strength- and skill-building activities as part of a long-term approach to physical development (60).

RESEARCH INSIGHT

Identifying a Motor Proficiency Barrier

Several factors can influence children's ongoing participation in MVPA. De Meester and colleagues assessed locomotor skills (e.g., running, jumping, and hopping) and object-control skills (e.g., kicking, catching, and throwing) in 326 children (23). Accelerometers were used to assess daily MVPA. They found that almost 90% of the children with low levels of motor skill competency did not accumulate the recommended amount of MVPA daily. Children with average or high levels of motor skill competency were more likely to attain the MVPA guideline. These findings provide evidence of a proficiency barrier related to motor-skill competence and underscore the importance of targeting improvements in locomotor and object-control skills in youth.

Physical inactivity and muscular weakness at any age predispose individuals to activity-related injuries. Children with the lowest level of habitual physical activity have been found to have the highest risk of injury during physical education classes, recreational activities, and sport (8). Although preparatory conditioning for young athletes is not a novel concept, an important yet sometimes overlooked benefit of well-designed fitness programs is a reduction in injury in youth sport (85, 88). Evidence indicates that injury-reduction training programs that include strength exercises and focus on landing mechanics could reduce the risk of all anterior cruciate ligament (ACL) injuries by half in all athletes and of noncontact ACL injuries by two-thirds in female athletes (76, 97). Without adequate levels of health- and skill-related fitness, it seems less likely that youth will optimize performance gains and more likely that they will experience negative health outcomes (66).

KEY POINT

Integrative youth fitness programs that target neuromuscular deficits and enhance both health- and skill-related components of physical fitness are needed to prevent the accumulation of risk factors and functional limitations that increase the risk of sport-related injuries in young athletes.

In addition to the potential physical benefits of exercise and sport activities, fitness professionals should recognize the positive impact of well-designed exercise programs on youth mental health and cognitive functioning (7, 25, 35). While the relationship between physical inactivity and mental ill-health is complex, it is becoming increasingly evident that low levels of MVPA during childhood and adolescence are associated with increased mental ill-health (i.e., anxiety and depression) and impairments in self-perceptions and psychological well-being (7, 55). Physically inactive youth experience more self-perceived loneliness than active youth and have fewer positive social interactions with fitness professionals (94). Regular exposure to fitness programs with qualified instruction in a supportive setting can provide an opportunity for participants to make friends, overcome challenges, and be more psychologically resilient (6, 35). Moreover, an increasing body of evidence supports the view that single bouts of MVPA and regular exercise training can have a positive impact on academic achievement and classroom behavior in school-age youth (1, 25, 63). Fitness professionals should view MVPA as a mental health–promoting strategy that can boost self-perceptions, promote happiness, and enhance cognitive functioning in youth.

Program Design Considerations

Children and adolescents can enhance their health and fitness with regular participation in well-designed fitness programs that are characterized by qualified instruction, meaningful experiences, and positive social interactions. Viewed from this perspective, the quantitative aspects of promoting youth physical activity (i.e., ≥60 minutes of MVPA daily) should be balanced with the qualitative aspects of having fun, making friends, and learning something new (75). This is where the art and science of designing youth fitness programs come into play because children are active in different ways and for different reasons than adults. An age range of 5 to 7 years is when many children begin to play sports, and it is reasonable that they could also benefit from exercise activities that enhance both health- and skill-related components of physical fitness. Recommendations for youth fitness testing are included in chapters 8 (cardiorespiratory fitness), 9 (muscular fitness), and 10 (flexibility).

While adults often exercise within a predetermined target heart rate range, children tend to be active in short bursts of high-intensity physical activity interspersed with brief rest periods of less-intense activity as needed (81). This does not mean that continuous cycling, swimming, or jogging is not beneficial for youth, but rather that children tend to be intermittently active and prefer to engage in sporadic bouts of MVPA characterized by increases and decreases in exercise intensity. Fitness professionals should not expect children to exercise in the same manner as adults and should recognize the importance of exposing youth to a variety of exercise and sport activities during this developmental phase of life. The key is to create a physically active experience whereby youth enjoy physical activity as they interact positively with others in an aesthetically pleasing and entertaining environment (12). As youth gain confidence and competence in their abilities to move proficiently and acquire the necessary behaviors that support an active lifestyle, they can enhance their physical literacy, which supports ongoing participation in a variety of physical activities throughout the life span (33, 98).

FUNdamental Fitness

Fitness professionals should integrate different types of physical activity into youth fitness programs with active games, exercises, circuit training, and small-sided sport activities. For example, FUNdamental integrative training is a method of conditioning that is designed to enhance both health- and skill-related components of physical fitness with meaningful instruction, deliberate practice, and technique-driven progression (13). As illustrated in figure 17.4, this type of training recognizes the shared importance of strength, skill, and aerobic activities for sustainable participation in exercise and sport (32). With a focus on fun and challenging activities, an integrative fitness circuit of exercises with body weight, medicine balls, battling ropes, and balance boards can pose a moderate to vigorous cardiometabolic stimulus in youth (28). An obstacle course of engaging activities modeled after American Ninja Warrior can challenge a child's agility, speed, and strength (11). In either exam-

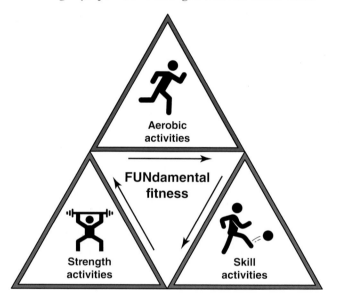

FIGURE 17.4 Interrelated components of FUNdamental fitness.

Adapted from A. Faigenbaum, J. MacDonald, A. Straccioloni, and T. Rial Rebullido, "Making a Strong Case for Prioritizing Muscular Fitness in Youth Physical Activity Guidelines," *Current Sports Medicine Reports* 19 (2020): 530-536.

The Physical Literacy Continuum

The concept of physical literacy is not just about participating in daily bouts of MVPA, but also about being proficient in a range of movement skills with confidence and motivation. Youth who are physically literate enjoy participating in a variety of exercise and sport activities and help others acquire the necessary skills and behaviors that support an active lifestyle. With qualified fitness instruction and leadership, youth can progress along the physical literacy continuum as they demonstrate competence, gain confidence, and interact positively with active peers. Conversely, youth who drop out of exercise or sport programs and lose interest in MVPA can regress along the physical literacy continuum as their confidence and competence to move and play begin to wane (33). Designing a physical activity experience that sparks an ongoing interest in exercise and sport activities requires an understanding of the physical, psychosocial, and cognitive attributes that can hinder or enhance physical literacy along the continuum.

ple, the circuits and courses can range from simple skills that target selected components of fitness to a complete program that targets all components of physical fitness. Sedentary and overweight youth can remain active for 30 minutes or more if the exercises are carefully chosen and if participants have an opportunity to take short breaks as needed (15). As fitness levels improve, the activities can become more challenging and the rest interval between exercise bouts can decrease.

Resistance training has become an important component of youth fitness programs (32, 61, 87). In addition to improving muscular fitness and enhancing motor skill performance, positive outcomes of improved muscular strength in youth include favorable changes in bone mineral density, body composition, cardiometabolic health, and feelings of self-worth (20, 21, 42). Further, evidence supports a link between muscular fitness and physical activity including organized sport in children and adolescents (84). Notably, resistance training in children can enhance strength and performance without training-induced gains in muscle hypertrophy because strength gains during childhood are primarily the result of neuromuscular mechanisms (87). Despite outdated misperceptions associated with strength-building activ-

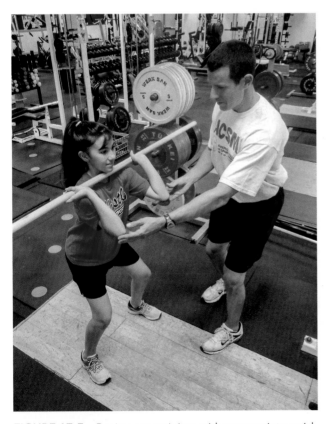

FIGURE 17.5 Resistance training, with appropriate guidance, is an important component of youth fitness programs.

Reprinted by permission from A.D. Faigenbaum and G.D. Myer, "Kids Stuff: Effective Strategies for Developing Young Athletes," *Health and Fitness Journal* 16 (2012): 9-16.

ities, resistance training should be considered an important component of youth fitness programs (figure 17.5). An important first step in encouraging inactive youth to be physically active is to expose them to a type of fitness training that prepares them for the demands of exercise and sport. These recommendations may be particularly important for today's youth, who tend to be weaker and slower than previous generations (34).

Because resistance training is a learned skill, it is important for youth to begin at a level that is consistent with their physical abilities. While children with limited resistance training experience may enjoy strength-building animal-like movements such as crocodile planks, bunny hops, and bear crawls, more advanced resistance exercises with external loads (e.g., dumbbells, barbells, and medicine balls) can be sensibly integrated into the fitness training program over time (27). A light to moderate load (≤60% 1RM) that can be lifted for 1 or 2 sets of 8 to 12 repetitions on a variety of upper- and lower-body exercises appears to be a safe and effective training load for beginners. As resistance training skill literacy improves, youth can be introduced to more complex exercises and periodic phases of lower repetition and higher load (>80% 1RM) training provided progression is based on technical skill competency (59, 61, 87).

The primary aim of youth fitness training is not only to participate in MVPA regularly, but to value the movement experience by promoting feelings of well-being, enhancing self-esteem, and becoming aware of the intrinsic value of active play, exercise, and sport. The importance of creating an environment in which the activities are creative, challenging, and entertaining should not be overlooked, because enjoyment has been found to mediate the effects of youth exercise and sport programs (4, 24, 95). Long-term adherence to youth fitness programs is best when youth are internally driven to do their best, feel good about their performance, and develop positive relationships with peers and fitness professionals. Because a major aim of youth fitness training is for physical activity to become an ongoing lifestyle choice, fitness professionals should strive to increase each child's self-efficacy or self-confidence in their ability to engage in recreational exercise and sport activities. This can be accomplished with clear instructions, visual demonstrations, adequate practice, and meaningful feedback so that youth can develop a sense of mastery of specific skills and movements. Guiding strategies for fitness professionals who work with youth include the following:

- Greet participants by their name when they arrive.
- Ensure a safe exercise environment, and explain safety rules.
- Encourage youth to share ideas, use their imagination, and choose fitness activities.

- Understand that youth are active in different ways and for different reasons than adults.
- Create an environment in which the focus is on cooperation, learning, and fun.
- Design integrative lessons that include skill, strength, and aerobic activities.
- Recognize individual differences, and praise youth for their effort.
- Provide constructive feedback in a positive and supportive manner.
- Support participation in a variety of exercise and sport activities.
- Be a good role model, and lead a healthy lifestyle.

Given the global pandemic of youth physical inactivity and related health care concerns, concerted efforts are needed to activate this generation of children early in life before they become resistant to interventions later in life. Developmentally appropriate fitness interventions clearly are needed in school- and community-based programs that enhance both health- and skill-related components of physical fitness. Fitness professionals should be strong advocates for establishing positive lifestyle behaviors including daily physical activity early in life, and should educate youth, parents, community leaders, and school administrators about the potential physical, psychosocial, and cognitive benefits of daily physical activity.

17

LEARNING AIDS

REVIEW QUESTIONS

1. How much physical activity is recommended for children and adolescents, and how can school-age youth meet this activity goal throughout the week?
2. What are the health- and skill-related components of physical fitness?
3. If an 8-year-old boy was riding a bicycle with his mother, how would the cardio-pulmonary responses differ between the child and the adult if they were bicycling at the same intensity?
4. Describe potential physical, psychosocial, and cognitive benefits of regular physical activity for children and adolescents.
5. What are the three categories of fundamental movement skills, and why are they an important component of youth fitness programs?
6. Discuss the influence of physical literacy on physical activity behaviors during childhood.
7. What is FUNdamental integrative training?
8. List several strategies that can be used to create a meaningful youth physical activity experience.

CASE STUDIES

1. The parents of a 10-year-old girl enrolled their child in an after-school fitness program at a recreation center, but they are concerned that the program includes strength-building activities and think this type of exercise may be inappropriate for young girls. How would you address their concerns?
2. A local school board decided to eliminate physical education from the school day to focus on academics. How would you respond to the school board's decision?
3. A high school soccer player wants to make the varsity team in the fall and asks you for advice about summer conditioning. How would you respond?

Answers to Case Studies

1. Acknowledge the parents' concerns, and assure them that the recreation center is committed to providing safe, effective, and enjoyable fitness activities to all participants. Address any misperceptions associated with youth resistance training, provide clear rationale for including strength-building activities in your youth fitness program, and encourage parents to observe a youth fitness class that includes qualified instruction and technique-driven resistance training. Remind parents that professional health and fitness organizations now support participation in well-designed youth resistance training programs.

2. Quality physical education provides a needed opportunity for all students to engage in a variety of exercise and sport activities in a supportive setting. In addition to noting the expected changes in heart health and muscle strength, underscore the cognitive and psychosocial benefits of engaging in exercise and sport activities, which include improvements in concentration, attention, and classroom behavior. Instead of eliminating physical education, the school board should look for creative ways to incorporate physical activity throughout the school day if their aim is to improve academic performance. The Latin phrase *mens sana in corpore sano* is frequently translated as "a healthy mind in a health body" and can be used to capture the synergy between mental well-being and physical well-being.

3. A well-designed summer conditioning program can enhance physical fitness, improve performance, and reduce the risk of sports-related injuries in young athletes. The program should include strength- and skill-building exercises as well as information on healthy lifestyle behaviors (e.g., adequate sleep and proper nutrition) to optimize training-induced adaptations. Recommend participation in a youth conditioning program with a fitness instructor who understands the essentials of pediatric exercise science and has experience working with young athletes.

Older Adults

NiCole R. Keith

OBJECTIVES

The reader will be able to do the following:

1. Describe the changes in the number of people older than 65 years that will take place during the first six decades of the 21st century, and provide a brief profile of older adults, indicating factors that affect the delivery of fitness-related programs

2. Describe the typical changes in aerobic capacity, strength, body composition, and flexibility that occur with age and the effect of exercise training on each

3. Describe modifications to exercise tests to accommodate limitations that may be observed in some older adults

4. Describe functional tests used to evaluate the components of fitness

5. Explain why it is necessary to address individual differences in older adults regarding exercise prescription

6. Provide current physical activity guidelines for cardiorespiratory fitness, muscular fitness, bone health, flexibility, and balance for older adults

18

A constant theme throughout this text is the importance of physical activity and exercise in leading a healthy life. This message is especially important for older adults, the fastest growing segment of the U.S. population. The baby boom was a period after World War II between 1946 and 1960 when a spike in the birth rate occurred in the United States. Individuals born during this time are now characterized as being older adults. Figure 18.1 shows the changes in the number of people over age 65, projected to the year 2060 (47). The number increases by nearly 50% between 2019 and 2040 because of baby boomers. In addition, because of advances in lifestyle behaviors, hygiene, and medicine over the past century, life expectancy has increased in general and, with it, the number of people living to advanced ages. Historically, aging was a chronological concept that was associated with the number of weeks, months, and years that passed with time. More recently, aging has a more intricate and individualized description that considers not only chronological, but also biological, psychological, and social aspects of aging. Decades of evidence have demonstrated the individual variance in aging patterns based on behavior, and associations are strong between regular physical activity and successful aging (10).

Currently, there are 20 times more people in the 75-to-84 age group and 53 times more people in the 85-plus age group than there were in 1900 (47). These latter age groups already have had a major effect on health care delivery systems, financing of health care, family caregiving for friends and loved ones, and general concerns about quality of life for those contemplating aging. These changes also affect the role of the fitness professional in providing appropriate physical activity and exercise programs to improve and maintain health and fitness in older adults. This chapter summarizes important health and fitness information related to older adults.

Demographic Profile

A variety of demographic and physiological characteristics of the older population (defined as over 65 years of age) affect the planning of fitness facilities, the programming options available, and the kinds of situations to anticipate. The following information, from the 2020 Profile of Older Americans (47), provides some insights into the population as a whole:

- In 2020, widows (8.8 million) outnumbered widowers (2.6 million) in this age group by almost four times.

- The majority live with a spouse or partner; however, as the population ages, the number living alone or in an institution increases.

- In 2019, 22.3% of older adults between the age of 65 to 74 rated their health as fair or poor; this number rose to 29.3% of older adults who were 75 years or older.

- In 2019, 19% of older adults who were 65 years or older reported either having a lot of difficulty with physical functioning or not having the ability to function at all. The link between disability and reported health status is strong. Disabilities interfere with the capacity to carry out activities of daily living (ADLs), such as bathing, dressing, and feeding, and instrumental activities of daily living (IADLs), such as preparing meals, shopping, and doing housework.

- Most older adults have at least one chronic condition, and many have several. These include hypertension (82% of men and 85% of women), arthritis (48%), heart disease (14%), cancer (25%), and diabetes (29%).

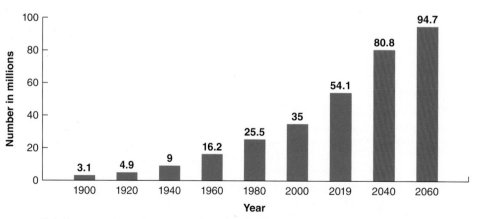

Note: Increments in years are uneven. Green bars (2040 and 2060) indicate projections.

FIGURE 18.1 Number of people (in millions) age 65 years and older from 1900 to 2060 (47). Increments in years are uneven.
From U.S. Department of Health and Human Services (HHS) 2021. Available: https://acl.gov/sites/default/files/aging%20and%20Disability%20In%20America/2020Profileolderamericans.final_.pdf.

This brief demographic profile indicates that fitness programs must address health-screening issues, the need for socialization, joint-protective activities, prevention and treatment of chronic diseases, and pragmatic goals to maintain independent living (11, 37). However, these characteristics (i.e., type and severity of disease, physical limitations, fitness) are not distributed uniformly across the older population, and fitness professionals must attend to individual differences. Considerations related to physical activity and exercise programs for individuals with chronic diseases are addressed in chapter 21.

KEY POINT

The number of older adults in the United States is increasing as the baby boom generation reaches older adulthood. Older participants may present special challenges to fitness professionals because of potential chronic disease conditions and physical activity limitations. Programs must focus on preventing chronic diseases or reducing their progression as well as increasing or maintaining mental and physical health and fitness outcomes to support independent living.

Effects of Aging on Fitness

The decline in physiological function associated with aging is unavoidable; however, some functions decrease more quickly than others. Because each person displays a unique rate of aging that is influenced by behavioral, genetic, and environmental factors (e.g., education, health care, economic status, nutrition, exercise), gerontology, or the combination of aging biology, chronic disease, and health, can be complex (13, 40). Consequently, it is not uncommon to find a person who is intellectually young but physically old, or an active older adult who has the physiological capacity of a sedentary adult who is decades younger.

In general, the common chronic diseases that contribute to mortality in older adults respond to exercise interventions in a positive manner similar to that of younger adults. Endurance training improves blood lipids (linked more to a reduction in body fatness than an increase in exercise), lowers blood pressure to the same degree as shown for younger individuals with hypertension, and improves glucose tolerance and insulin sensitivity (10).

As described earlier in this chapter, the primary fitness components affect one's ability to perform ADLs, IADLs, and work, and engage in recreational pursuits at any age. Although natural changes in these fitness components occur with age, the evidence is overwhelming that regular physical activity and exercise maintain fitness at considerably better levels than does a sedentary lifestyle. The following sections address each fitness component.

Cardiorespiratory Fitness

Figure 18.2 shows that maximal aerobic capacity ($\dot{V}O_2max$) decreases at the rate of about 1% per year in sedentary healthy men after the age of 20 (18, 41). This decrease is due to behaviors such as physical inactivity and poor diet and the resulting weight gain, in addition to the physiological effects of aging (10). Some studies show that this rate of decline is reduced by half in men who maintain a vigorous exercise program (2, 18). The most notable example of this effect of chronic training is from a study that tracked a world-class rower who won a medal in five consecutive Olympics. $\dot{V}O_2max$ was unchanged (approximately 5.9 L · min^{-1}) over that 20-year period when measured in the year leading up to the Olympics, when training was most intense (26). In addition, figure 18.2 shows that the $\dot{V}O_2max$ values of 80-year-old athletes were much higher (average: 38 ml · kg^{-1} · min^{-1}) compared with age-matched untrained individuals (average: 21 ml · kg^{-1} · min^{-1}). In support of continued exercise throughout the life span, the $\dot{V}O_2max$ values of the trained individuals were similar to those of typical untrained people who were several decades younger (41).

In contrast to men, women show a 10% decline per decade independent of activity status (12). However, trained women, as expected, have a higher $\dot{V}O_2max$ at any age compared with their sedentary counterparts (15).

Historically, aging has been associated with a decline in $\dot{V}O_2max$, but more recently, lifestyle factors, including physical inactivity, emotional stressors, and an unhealthy diet, have been identified that may contribute to this decline. More longitudinal research studies focusing on nonathletes are needed to further understand these relationships. Presently, data from lifelong athletes demonstrate that the rate of age-related decline in $\dot{V}O_2max$ may be slowed by a lifetime of vigorous exercise, which produces protective effects for pulmonary and cardiovascular function, blood oxygen transport capacity, skeletal muscle capillary density, and oxidative capacity (48). However, it should be of no surprise that the decrease in $\dot{V}O_2max$ affects endurance performance. Average running speed in distance races decreases about 1% per year, suggesting a link between the decrease in $\dot{V}O_2max$ and performance in distance running. However, a variety of other factors (e.g., running economy, lactate threshold, joint trauma) also might affect running performance (18).

Given that most people experience a decline in $\dot{V}O_2max$ with age means that by the time of older adulthood, the ability to engage in routine physical activities has been compromised for individuals who do not engage

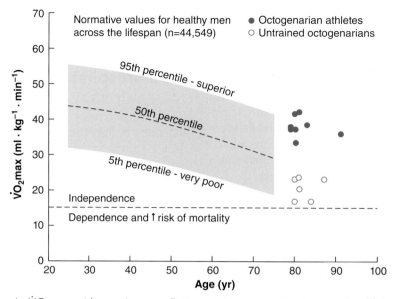

FIGURE 18.2 Change in V̇O₂max with age in men. Data points represent octogenarian lifelong endurance athletes (filled circles) and healthy untrained octogenarians (open circles).

Reprinted by permission from S. Trappe, E. Hayes, A. Galpin, et al., "New Records in Aerobic Power Among Octogenarian Lifelong Endurance Athletes," *Journal of Applied Physiology* 114 (2013): 3-10.

in a high level of endurance activities. This reduced capacity for work can further reduce physical activity, setting up a reciprocal cause and effect that results in lower and lower levels of cardiorespiratory fitness (CRF). Left unchecked, such outcomes may ultimately result in the inability to perform ADLs, which affects quality of life and the ability to live independently (40). Figure 18.2 clearly shows the impact of this decline in V̇O₂max. The dashed line (at a V̇O₂max of 17.5 ml⁻¹ · kg⁻¹ · min⁻¹) represents a threshold for independent living, and all of the untrained octogenarians are just above that value. Also, remember that a V̇O₂max value of 17.5 ml⁻¹ · kg⁻¹ · min⁻¹ is associated with a much higher risk of death—a risk that is reduced 12% for every 3.5 ml⁻¹ · kg⁻¹ · min⁻¹ increase in V̇O₂max (41).

Maximal oxygen uptake (see chapter 4) equals the product of maximal cardiac output (maximal heart rate [HR] × maximal stroke volume [SV]) and maximal oxygen extraction (systemic arteriovenous oxygen difference). Despite the limitations presented by using the equation 220 – age to calculate HR max, formulas used to calculate heart rate reserve (HRR) and maximal HR include calculations that assume HR decreases with age (refer to chapter 13). These decreases are the major contributors to the age-related reduction in maximal cardiac output. The Frank–Starling mechanism (greater stretch of the ventricle due to higher venous return) appears to compensate for the lower maximal HR in middle age and so reduces the magnitude of change in maximal cardiac output, but this mechanism is less effective in old age (10, 18). Maximal oxygen extraction is also lower in less active older adults when compared with younger

sedentary adults, but this decrease is probably attributable more to their level of inactivity and its impact on mitochondrial number than to a true aging effect (i.e., the passing of time).

Endurance training increases V̇O₂max by about 10% to 30% in previously sedentary older adults, an increase similar to that of younger adults (10, 18). The increase in V̇O₂max is due to an increase in both maximal cardiac output and oxygen extraction in older men, but it is due almost entirely to an increase in oxygen extraction in older women. This may be related to the observation that older women show little or no increase in left ventricle mass, end-diastolic volume, or maximal SV after endurance training. The increase in oxygen extraction is due to increases in capillary number and mitochondrial enzymes, which are the same mechanisms as in younger adults (10, 18).

KEY POINT

V̇O₂max decreases about 1% per year in sedentary men and women because of a decrease in both maximal cardiac output and maximal oxygen extraction. Endurance training increases V̇O₂max in older adults just as it does in younger adults. The greater V̇O₂max results from gains in both maximal cardiac output and oxygen extraction in men but is due solely to an increase in oxygen extraction in women.

Muscular Strength and Endurance

Figure 18.3 shows that muscular strength in untrained men begins to decline at about age 30, but the majority of the decrease occurs after age 60, when it falls at a faster rate (24, 33). The loss of strength relates directly to a loss of muscle mass, or sarcopenia, which is attributable primarily to a loss of muscle fibers (motor units) and secondarily to an atrophy of those muscle fibers (primarily type II) that remain. However, the distribution of fiber types is maintained across age, as is strength per cross-sectional area of muscle (10, 18, 24, 33). The pattern is very different in strength-trained men, in that strength was maintained until after age 60.

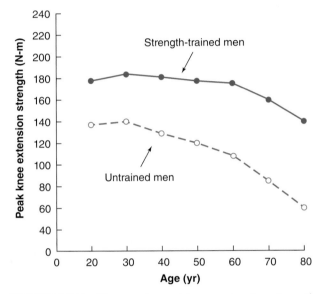

FIGURE 18.3 Changes in peak knee extension strength in trained and untrained men at various ages.

Adapted by permission from W.L. Kenney, J.H. Wilmore, and D.L Costill, *Physiology of Sport and Exercise*, 6th ed. (Champaign, IL: Human Kinetics, 2015), 462.

This loss of strength and muscle mass is not due to aging alone. Figure 18.4 shows computed tomography scans of the upper arm of three 57-year-old men of similar body weights. Note the large differences in the muscle cross-sectional area and subcutaneous fat from the individual who strength trained (on the right) to the individual who swim trained (center) to an untrained individual (on the left). Similar observations were made in a 70-year-old triathlete, in which an MRI scan of his thigh showed little difference in muscle mass compared to a 40-year-old triathlete. In contrast, a 70-year-old sedentary man showed dramatically reduced muscle mass and much more fat (51).

Muscle strength and mass also increase in women as a result of resistance training (21). Although research that has used dose–response models to ascertain whether chronic resistance training yields different skeletal muscle adaptations when men and women are compared is limited, several studies have used the same resistance training protocol to compare men and women (1). However, sex-specific skeletal muscle responses to resistance training remain unclear (32). Additionally, studies have found that generally a dose–response relationship exists between the amount of exercise performed and the gains in muscle strength and mass. This is well-established in both women and men who are older adults (10). While absolute increases in strength are higher in men when compared to women, there is strong evidence that following strength training interventions, relative increases in muscle strength and mass are at least comparable (10, 19, 34, 49). For example, in one comprehensive 12-week intervention study comparing improvements in muscle strength and mass, higher relative strength increases were found in women when compared to men (21).

Clearly, it is important for both men and women to maintain muscle mass throughout adulthood, including older adulthood. Muscle mass is necessary not only for

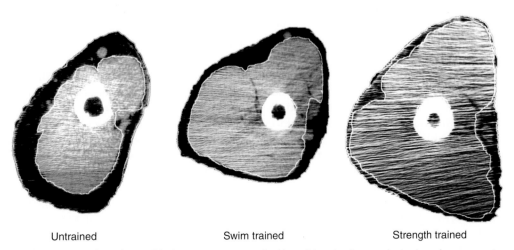

Untrained   Swim trained   Strength trained

FIGURE 18.4 These scans show bone (dark center surrounded by white ring), muscle (striated gray area), and subcutaneous fat (dark perimeter).

Reprinted by permission from W.L. Kenney, J.H. Wilmore, and D.L. Costill, *Physiology of Sport and Exercise*, 6th ed. (Champaign, IL: Human Kinetics, 2015), 463.

preserving the ability to carry out ADLs and IADLs but also for its link to resting metabolic rate (see chapter 20) and the risks of type 2 diabetes, hypertension, and other chronic medical conditions (see chapter 21) (2, 33). Considerable evidence shows that an intense (80% 1-repetition max, 1RM) resistance training program increases both muscle mass and strength in 60- to 96-year-old individuals (10, 14, 17). These training programs result in modest increases in muscle fiber area (10%-30%) but large increases (>100%) in 1RM strength. The disproportionate increase in strength is similar to what is observed when young adults participate in intense resistance training programs and is ascribed to neural adaptations. Additionally, there is evidence that resistance training can increase $\dot{V}O_2$max in this population (16). For some older adults who are frail, resistance training should occur concurrently with aerobic conditioning to promote both neuromuscular and cardiovascular adaptations (10).

KEY POINT

If gone unchecked by physical activity or exercise, muscular strength decreases with age because of a loss of motor units (muscle mass) as well as a reduction in the size of the remaining muscle fibers. Intense resistance training (80% 1RM) can cause large (>100%) increases in strength; this is attributable primarily to neural factors because fiber size increases only 10% to 30%.

Body Composition

Chapters 11 and 20 provide details about health risks, measurement issues, and recommendations for achieving body composition goals. The accumulation of body fat in muscles and other organs such as the liver increases, while subcutaneous fat mass tends to decline in older adults (29). In terms of general aging, body fatness increases from about 16% (males) and 25% (females) in 25-year-olds to 28% (males) and 41% (females) in 75-year-olds. This amounts to a gain of about 22 pounds (10 kilograms) of fat for both groups during that time. Fat-free mass is stable for the untrained human in caloric balance until about age 40 but decreases 3% (males) and 4% (females) per decade between age 40 and 60 and 6% (males) and 10% (females) per decade from age 60 to 80 (18). As mentioned, exercise can play an important role in addressing sarcopenia.

Evidence indicates that the increase in body fat relates to a sedentary lifestyle rather than to an increase in food intake or an aging effect. Cross-sectional and longitudinal studies on older male and female athletes suggest that regular vigorous exercise is associated with maintaining a stable weight during aging (18). However, observations of highly trained athletes indicate that body fatness still increases about 2% per decade. Consequently, vigorous exercise attenuates, but does not prevent, the increase in body fatness that accompanies age. Importantly, when body composition in older adults changes due to exercise, most of the body fat is lost from central stores, which reduces the risk of metabolic and cardiovascular diseases (18). Exercise is also important in dealing with the loss of bone mineral density (BMD) with age, but there is more to that story (see the sidebar *Bone Mineral Density*).

KEY POINT

An increase in body fat with age is attributed more to a decrease in physical activity than to an increase in caloric intake. Vigorous exercise is associated with maintaining a stable body weight and improved bone density with increasing age. Exercise intervention results in the loss of body fat from central stores, which is associated with reduced risk of cardiovascular and metabolic diseases. Exercise intervention also reduces fall risk and development of pro-inflammatory markers as well as being protective for improved sleep and anti-inflammatory markers.

Flexibility

Flexibility is the ability to move a joint through its maximal range of motion (ROM) without injury. Static flexibility is joint ROM in a relaxed muscle, while dynamic flexibility is the maximal ROM performed during movement (22). Flexibility is an important factor related to the ability to carry out ADLs and IADLs as well as to the risk of low-back problems (see chapter 10). Joint motion is influenced by the condition of the muscle, connective tissues, and cartilage associated with the joint. In general, the increase in collagen cross-links in tendons and ligaments and a degradation of articular cartilage contribute to decreased joint ROM with age (10). However, in evaluating the health of a joint, it is difficult to separate aging effects from those associated with chronic inactivity.

While improving flexibility in older adults through performance of a variety of ROM exercises has been demonstrated, it is difficult to provide a general profile of the effect of training on flexibility as was done for

Bone Mineral Density

Almost all of the minerals in humans are housed in the bones. Bone mineral density (BMD), a measure of bone mass, generally decreases with age at about the same rate as the fat-free mass; however, bone loss accelerates in most women who are postmenopausal (18). Generally, higher bone density is associated with better bone strength, which is protective against fractures and falls (36). Higher BMD is also associated with better sleep quality, fewer inflammatory markers, more anti-inflammatory markers, and improved body composition (25, 35). A general recommendation is to maximize BMD through adequate calcium intake and physical activity before age 30 and then reduce the rate of loss from that point in time (3, 6). Hormone levels (estrogen and testosterone), calcium intake, and physical activity affect the rate of loss of BMD. The higher rate of loss after menopause can be prevented by hormone-replacement therapy, but some women may choose not to use this therapy because of an increased risk of coronary heart disease and cancer (10, 28). In addition, there are certain drugs (e.g., bisphosphonates) that can prevent bone loss. Vigorous exercise, calcium intake, and vitamin D are important in maintaining BMD. Older adults need additional calcium (see chapter 5) to help maintain BMD and possibly to realize the full benefits of increased physical activity. The most effective exercise programs for bone health include activities that

- involve a wide variety of muscle groups and movement directions,
- are weight-bearing (e.g., walking, jogging; higher-impact activities are more effective), and
- are muscle strengthening and generally exceed 75% of maximal capacity for both strength and endurance.

Regarding the last point, the fitness professional needs to introduce activity (aerobic and strengthening) in an appropriate and progressive manner to help the client make a smooth and safe transition to higher-intensity activities (6, 10, 11). Further, in older adults with severe osteoporosis, impact-producing exercises and those that involve forward spinal flexion should be avoided (6, 10). Additional information on osteoporosis is found in chapter 21.

$\dot{V}O_2$max and strength due to the variability in the number of subjects, the types of research design, and the methods used to assess flexibility (9, 10, 31, 40). Additionally, the research on ROM exercises to improve flexibility in older adults is limited. Lastly, few studies exist that examine the safety of performing flexibility training in older adults (23). However, general physical activity programs that incorporate stretching exercises, as well as special ROM exercise programs, have been shown to improve flexibility in older adults (10, 37). See the later section on exercise prescription for improving flexibility for more details.

KEY POINT

Possessing adequate flexibility throughout old age contributes to the ability to perform ADLs and IADLs for maintenance of independence. Flexibility can be improved through general programs of physical activity that incorporate stretching exercises, as well as through programs using special ROM exercises.

Special Considerations Regarding Exercise Testing

Age is a risk factor because the likelihood of developing serious conditions that are a threat to health and longevity increases with age. The passage of time allows the consequences of poor health behaviors (e.g., smoking, high-fat diet, physical inactivity) to combine and manifest themselves as major medical problems (e.g., lung cancer, atherosclerosis, glucose intolerance). Consequently, fitness professionals should closely follow the American College of Sports Medicine (ACSM) guidelines for risk classification (3) when developing and implementing training programs for older adults (10).

Risk classification provides guidance for test selection and personnel requirements (see chapter 2). Clearly, with the higher incidence of cardiovascular disease in older age groups, diagnostic exercise testing may be used as part of a medical exam. However, following appropriate screening, standard submaximal CRF tests (see chapter 8) may be used as part of a fitness assessment. Independent of the reason for testing, modifications may be necessary to address certain limitations (3, 11, 12, 38):

INSTRUMENTATION

- A cycle ergometer may be a better choice for those with arthritis of the knee or hip or those with balance problems.

- Tracking cadence may be a problem unless an electronic cycle ergometer is available.

- If a treadmill is used, additional practice may be needed, with emphasis on slow walking speeds.

INTENSITY AND PROGRESSION

As mentioned in chapter 8, for deconditioned people with suspected low $\dot{V}O_2$max values, the initial intensity of a graded exercise test should begin at a light-intensity workload, increments per stage should be small, and it may be necessary to prolong the time (3 versus 2 minutes) per stage so the person can achieve a steady state. See the sidebar *Functional Testing* for alternatives to traditional exercise testing for older adults.

Exercise Prescription

Current levels of physical activity in the United States are far below desired levels; only 32.2% of adults 18 to 44 years of age meet both aerobic and muscular-strengthening guidelines, and the percentage drops considerably for adults 65 years of age or older, with only 12.8% meeting the guidelines (42). Consequently, the general recommendation that adults should participate in moderate-intensity physical activity for at least 150 minutes per week and do muscle-strengthening activity at least 2 days per week is essential for all ages but especially for people who are older adults and positioned to benefit substantially from an increase in physical activity (3,

Functional Testing

A common method used to evaluate the capabilities of older adults involves a series of performance tests that are linked to underlying fitness components. The Senior Fitness Test developed by Rikli and Jones uses a battery of six measures that evaluate upper- and lower-body physical function. The tests included a nationwide sample of independent-living older adults (age 60-94) who provided performance-standard data to support validity and reliability for each measure (31). The following are tests used to evaluate the various functional components:

- *Chair stand:* Number of times within 30 seconds a person can stand from a seated position with arms folded across the chest (assesses lower-body strength)

- *Arm curl:* Number of curls that can be completed in 30 seconds with a 5-pound (2.3 kilogram) dumbbell (women) or 8-pound (3.6 kilogram) dumbbell (men) while the participant is seated (assesses upper-body strength)

- *Six-minute walk:* Number of yards the participant can walk in 6 minutes around a 50-yard (46 meter) course (assesses aerobic endurance)

- *Two-minute step:* Number of full steps the participant can complete in 2 minutes, raising knee to midway between the knee and hip while standing in place, while the opposite foot maintains contact with the ground during each step; this is an alternative to the 6-minute walk

- *Chair sit-and-reach:* Number of inches between extended fingertips and tips of toes when the participant is sitting in a chair with legs extended and hands reaching toward toes (assesses lower-body flexibility)

- *Back scratch:* Number of inches between the extended middle fingers when the participant reaches with one hand over the shoulder and the other hand up the back (assesses upper-body flexibility)

- *Eight-foot up and go:* Number of seconds required to get up from a seated position, walk 8 feet (2.4 meters), turn, and return to the seated position (assesses agility and dynamic balance)

- *Height and weight:* Used to calculate BMI

These tests have been shown to be valid and reliable, and normative data are provided for men and women 60 to 94 years of age (31). These practical tests require limited equipment, are simple to deliver, and can be used to monitor progress over the course of a training program or to document functional decline that might necessitate additional medical attention.

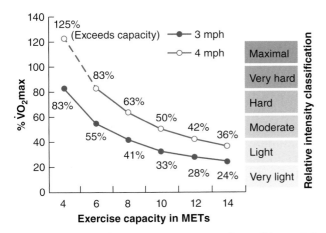

FIGURE 18.5 Relative exercise intensity for walking at 3.0 mph (4.8 km · hr⁻¹ or 3.3 METs) and 4.0 mph (6.4 km · hr⁻¹ or 5.0 METs) expressed as a percent of V̇O₂max for adults with an exercise capacity ranging from 4 to 14 METs.

From U.S. Department of Health and Human Services (DHHS), *Physical Activity Guidelines Advisory Committee Report 2008*, Fig, D.1, (2008), D-7.

10, 27, 46). When working with older adults, the fitness professional needs to consider that levels of activity exertion may vary considerably depending on age and exercise history (see figure 18.5) (44).

Older adults are not all the same, and fitness professionals must treat them as unique individuals. The only thing two 65-year-olds may have in common is their age. They may differ substantially in their health risk (including chronic disease and musculoskeletal limitations), CRF (V̇O₂max), and experience with exercise. Individualization is important when working with any client, and understanding the diversity of older adults' physical capabilities is especially important. Some older adults will have no major medical problems and engage in regular moderate- to vigorous-intensity exercise, while others may be inactive or fall below recommended levels of physical activity. Still others may have a chronic disease (e.g., heart disease, diabetes) or may have limited physical abilities and rely on partial or complete assistance for ADLs. Given the diversity that exists among older adults, it should be no surprise that physical activity recommendations for individuals must be customized to reflect their current health and fitness status as well as their goals and interests. Special considerations related to fitness level may require adaptations if a participant has been inactive or has particular limitations. In some situations where chronic diseases are involved, supervised physical activity may be warranted. Education in gerontology, as well as pathophysiology and pharmacology, is valuable for anyone working with older adults. Fitness professionals along with professionals in other fields (e.g., nursing, physical therapy, therapeutic recreation) may work together to create effective programs for those with physical limitations.

Aerobic Activity for Health and Cardiorespiratory Fitness

Physical activity recommendations for older adults were addressed in the *2008 Physical Activity Guidelines for Americans* (44) as well as the second edition in 2018 (46) and in the 2009 ACSM position stand, "Exercise and Physical Activity for Older Adults" (10). What follows is a summary of those recommendations for health and fitness.

The following physical activity guidelines for older adults are the same as for adults:

- All older adults should move more and sit less; some activity is better than none, and older adults who sit less and participate in any amount of moderate to vigorous physical activity gain some health benefits.

- For substantial health benefits, older adults should do at least 150 minutes per week of moderate-intensity physical activity, 75 minutes per week of vigorous-intensity aerobic activity, or an appropriate combination of both. The total amount of physical activity should be spread throughout the week. On a scale of 0 to 10 for the level of physical exertion, use 5 or 6 for moderate-intensity activity and 7 or 8 for vigorous-intensity activity.

- For additional health benefits, older adults should increase their physical activity beyond the equivalent of 300 minutes per week of moderate-intensity activity.

- Older adults should include muscle-strengthening activities of moderate or greater intensity involving all the major muscle groups on 2 or more days per week.

The following additional guidelines are focused just on older adults:

- As part of their weekly physical activity, older adults should do multicomponent physical activity that includes balance training as well as aerobic and muscle-strengthening activities.

- If older adults cannot do 150 minutes of moderate-intensity activity because of chronic conditions, they should be as active as their abilities and conditions allow.

- Older adults should determine their level of effort for physical activity relative to their level of fitness.

- Older adults with chronic conditions should understand how their conditions affect their ability to do regular physical activity safely.

Consistent with the breadth of these guidelines and the diversity of the older adult population, special attention must be given to progression. The physical activity must be suited to each individual, with an emphasis on a conservative approach for the most deconditioned older adults. Although a formal program of activities aimed at improving CRF should be built on a base of regular moderate-intensity activities, some older individuals may need to begin with light-intensity activities (10). As with any workout, it should begin with a formal warm-up and end with a cool-down during which flexibility exercises can be done.

It is crucial to adapt the activities to the abilities of the group. Those at the high end of the fitness continuum can participate in a wide variety of activities similar to those used for younger adults. Those who have a lower $\dot{V}O_2$max (5-7 METs) can follow exercise routines that would not be too different from those used in a cardiac rehabilitation program (see chapter 21). However, prescribing activities for those at the low end of the func-tional continuum, in whom $\dot{V}O_2$max may be only 2 to 4 METs, demands special creativity and attention to safety. Exercises can be done standing with support, seated on a chair, or in the water (4, 31). Because of the prevalence of joint-related problems, exercise modes should be chosen that do not aggravate the problem. The need for additional assistance with balance and attention to safety regarding the risk of a fall should be incorporated into the routine (see the sidebar *Balance and Falls*).

The general exercise prescription for older adults includes the following (2, 3):

- *Frequency:* Even though the recommendation is given in minutes per week, there is no question that the total volume of activity should be spread over the course of the week and, as mentioned previously, over the course of a day if the person cannot do a single 30-minute bout of moderate-intensity physical activity. Formal vigorous-intensity exercise sessions should be done over the course of 3 to 4 days each week, with a rest day between exercise days.

Balance and Falls

Loss of balance can lead to a fall, with dire consequences. The potential lower bone density in older adults predisposes them to fractures, and about half are unable to return to regular walking after a fracture (40). The ability to maintain balance is influenced by a variety of factors, such as strength; vision and hearing, which influence proprioception; medications; illnesses; flexibility; and environmental hazards (40). Considerable information shows that exercise programs improve balance and reduce falls, but not without exception (10, 37). In older adults at greater risk for falling, the research shows that regular physical activity is safe and reduces the risk of falls. However, due to inadequate research no firm recommendation can be made regarding intensity, frequency, and type of balance exercises (3, 10). That said, successful programs to improve balance include balance training, moderate-intensity strength training, and moderate-intensity aerobic training. Balance exercises may include backward walking, sideways walking, heel walking, toe walking, and standing from a seated position. Following is a progression of difficulty in balance exercises for each of three ways to stress balance (11). Additional background is provided in the neuromotor exercise section in chapter 15. These exercises should be done under supervision until the individual has demonstrated enough control to work independently.

1. *Narrow the base of support:* Stand with feet apart with assistive device; with feet apart without assistive device; with feet together; heel to toe; one-legged stand.
2. *Displace the center of mass:* Turn in a circle; shift weight side to side; step over obstacles; do crossover or sideways walking; move weighted arms to front and side.
3. *Minimize contributions of visual and proprioceptive pathways:* Close eyes with movements mentioned previously; stand on foam or soft surface.

The frequency of balance exercises will vary considerably from several times a day for someone in a rehabilitation setting to 1 day per week for someone who is simply maintaining gains in balance (11). Tai chi exercises may be useful in this regard (45, 46). However, medications, environmental hazards, and vision also must be addressed to reduce the risk of falls (40).

- *Intensity:* Target heart rate (THR) can be used to set the exercise intensity, but use of measured maximal HR is preferred to predicted maximal HR in this calculation. Intensity guidelines are similar to those for younger adults, but the low end of the THR zone should be emphasized at the beginning of the program, and rating of perceived exertion (RPE, or the self-reported status of how hard the exercise feels) or an equivalent relative intensity scale should be used to determine whether the intensity is suitable.

- *Time (duration):* If the client is extremely deconditioned, the exercise sessions should be divided into segments (5-10 minutes) that can be done throughout the day (or within the context of a single class). Some participants may not be able to exercise continuously for 30 minutes.

The National Institute on Aging (NIA) provides information and examples of exercises that address all of the fitness components for this population. You can browse publications by topic under the Health and Aging tab at www.nia.nih.gov/health/exercise-physical-activity.

Muscular Fitness

To achieve muscular strength and endurance, there is again an emphasis on the need for progression. The goal is to slowly and safely help the client progress to strength training exercises at a vigorous level. The exercise prescription for increasing strength in older adults was described in chapter 14 and is highlighted here (3, 10, 46):

- Instruct participants on safety, proper lifting technique, and breathing.
- Individualize progression of all resistance training activities.
- Begin with light intensity (40%-50% 1RM) to allow for adaptation to the activity, and progress to 60% to 80% 1RM. In place of 1RM, a relative scale (0-10) can be used with 5 or 6 for moderate and 7 or 8 for vigorous.
- Participants should perform at least 1 set of 10 to 15 repetitions of 8 to 10 exercises that use the major muscle groups.
- For power training, light to moderate loads are used, 6 to 10 repetitions done with high velocity.
- Participants should exercise at least twice a week on nonconsecutive days.
- Participants should stay within the pain-free ROM.
- Participants should participate in low-impact exercises (5).
- Participants with arthritis should avoid strenuous exercise during acute flareups; gentle movements through ROM and light activity to break up sedentary behavior is appropriate (3). (See the sidebar *Osteoarthritis.*)

Osteoarthritis

Osteoarthritis (OA), a common problem in many older adults, is a degenerative joint disease associated with damage to the articular cartilage that lines joint structures. The swelling and pain associated with OA affect joint ROM and may discourage some individuals from participating in physical activity. A variety of over-the-counter and prescription medications can reduce pain and inflammation. Physical activity is considered to be beneficial with regard to reduction of pain, fatigue, inflammation, and disease activity (3). The focus of aerobic exercise is to improve CRF without worsening joint pain or damage (3). Typically recommended activities include those with low joint stress, such as walking, cycling, swimming, or aquatic exercise (3). Gradual warm-up and flexibility exercises should be included, and the intensity and duration of the endurance exercise program should be matched to current fitness. For example, moderate-intensity aerobic activity (40%-59% HRR) is appropriate for most people with OA, but 30% to 39% HRR might be better for those who are extremely deconditioned. A frequency of 3 to 5 days per week is recommended, with a goal of 150 minutes per week of moderate-intensity activity or 75 minutes per week of vigorous-intensity activity (3). However, a series of short (e.g., 10 minutes) bouts may be better tolerated than one longer bout. Resistance training should begin with an intensity of 50% to 60% 1RM (goal is 60%-80% 1RM) with 8 to 12 repetitions for 1 to 3 sets (3). Flexibility training is particularly important to promote ROM and joint mobility, and balance training should be included given the increased risk of falling when arthritis affects the lower limbs (3).

Flexibility

A flexibility program should involve all joints, with the goal of maintaining their normal ROM. However, few studies compare or contrast various ROM exercises and their flexibility outcomes, and as a result little consensus has been reached on the frequency, duration, or type of exercise (static versus dynamic) to use (3, 10). That said, the results do suggest that flexibility can be increased in major joints by doing ROM exercises specific to the joint (see chapter 15 for more information). Tai chi and yoga programs can be used to achieve and maintain flexibility goals. However, for most people, flexibility goals can be achieved independently following education and practice with a fitness professional or within the context of a regular exercise class. Elements of a flexibility program include the following (3):

- Movements should be performed as a regular part of the warm-up and cool-down, the same as for younger participants.
- Doing flexibility exercises after the warm-up prior to the workout as well as following a cool-down following a workout when the muscles are warm is more effective.
- Static stretches are preferred, although others can be done (10).
- For static stretches, use slow movements through pain-free ROM, with stretches held for 30 to 60 seconds; stretches are held to the point of feeling tightness.
- Stretching should be performed at least 2 days per week.

Psychological Health and Well-Being

This chapter has focused on the fact that regular participation in physical activity is associated with better health (lower risk of chronic diseases and injury) and fitness (cardiovascular function, strength, body composition, and flexibility) during aging. However, regular participation in physical activity also has been shown to improve brain health including cognition, executive function, processing speed, attention, memory, and psychological health and well-being (8, 10, 30, 39, 50). Short-term benefits due to a single exercise session include enhanced cognition, relaxation and improved mood state, enhanced social and cultural integration, and empowerment to be more independent (7, 30, 43). A review of the long-term benefits shows that physical activity (10)

- improves overall psychological well-being (mediated through effects on self-concept and self-esteem),
- decreases risk of clinical depression and anxiety,
- decreases risk of cognitive decline and dementia,
- improves cognitive performance in previously sedentary adults, and
- has a positive impact on quality of life.

This list shows how regular physical activity affects the whole person, leading to a more active and fulfilling life.

LEARNING AIDS

REVIEW QUESTIONS

1. By the year 2040, how many people in the United States will be over the age of 65 compared with the year 2000?
2. Briefly describe the kinds of chronic conditions that exist in older adults that are less common in younger adults.
3. What happens to $\dot{V}O_2$max, muscular strength, and body fatness with age?
4. How might a fitness test for CRF be modified to accommodate limitations present in some older adults?
5. What are some functional tests to evaluate flexibility, muscular fitness, and CRF?
6. Would you implement the same exercise program for all 65-year-old adults? Why or why not?
7. Present the newest physical activity guidelines for older adults that address health and CRF, muscular strength, and flexibility.

8. Consider this statement: "If older adults cannot meet the physical activity guidelines, they should do nothing." Do you agree? Why or why not?

9. Discuss the role that progression plays in implementing physical activity programs for older adults, with specific emphasis on how to manage duration and intensity in deconditioned individuals.

10. What are some psychological benefits that older adults experience as a result of regular participation in physical activity?

CASE STUDIES

1. Darya is a 55-year-old woman who does three workouts every week, with an emphasis on vigorous aerobic exercise in a competitive masters swim class. Her doctor is concerned that her bone density is decreasing in spite of the exercise, and she comes to you for help. What do you recommend to address this concern?

2. Marcy, a 70-year-old woman, has been referred to you for advice. She indicates that she has not been able to comfortably perform her ordinary activities, and she would like your help. What assessments do you use, and what physical activities do you recommend to improve her CRF, muscular fitness, flexibility, and balance to help her regain her confidence in doing routine activities?

3. Osvaldo is a 65-year-old retired occupational therapist who worked with patients in their homes following hospital discharge. He and his wife are very involved in their community, co-coaching a youth soccer team, volunteering with a food pantry and meal home delivery program, and tutoring at a local school. Osvaldo also enjoys gardening to grow vegetables and herbs he uses to cook the traditional Mexican recipes passed down by family members. He had an athletic scholarship throughout college, and when he graduated, he promised himself that the inside of a weight room would never see him again. While he loved the team competition, he hated the tedious workouts his coaches made him do. Since college, Osvaldo has exercised sporadically, has gained 25 pounds, and was found to be prediabetic and prehypertensive at his last physical. Osvaldo has a family history of diabetes and hypertension and has been referred to a Registered Dietitian for nutritional guidance and to you for help with an exercise program. He is willing to begin a regular exercise program and has also specifically asked you for advice on how be more active to avoid diabetes and hypertension. He believes that doing this will help him avoid other negative health outcomes experienced by his family members. Identify positive aspects in Osvaldo's life and how these might affect an exercise program. What goals might he wish to achieve, and how would he define success? Describe how to develop an exercise plan that is enjoyable and sustainable.

Answers to Case Studies

1. Darya is clearly fit, but she needs to add other types of activities to her regular routine to improve bone health. You might recommend that she add a resistance training program that will not only improve bone strength but also her swimming performance. In addition, you might suggest that she add regular walking to her weekly activities to provide some downward loading to the bone that she is not experiencing in her swim workouts.

2. You might begin by using the Senior Fitness Test to obtain some baseline values for the various fitness components. Based on those test results, you should develop a program of activities for Marcy that include walking (graduated in a manner that encourages multiple short walks with plenty of rest), muscle-strengthening activities using either very light dumbbells or low-tension elastic bands (with only a few repetitions in the beginning), and balance-related exercises.

3. Osvaldo is currently healthy, retired from a rewarding career in health care, has support from his family, and is respected and involved in his community. He has many activities he enjoys, including volunteering, cooking, and gardening. He is educated, socially connected, ready to change, and has discretionary time to be active. He has prior personal experience with exercising; being aware of aspects he did not like (i.e., "tedious" workouts) is important when developing a new plan of action (e.g., variety of activities, group classes). Although he has general background related to physical activity with his career in occupational therapy, he is looking for specific guidance related to an exercise program to meet his current goals.

   General goals and marks of success may include lowering body weight, staying free from diabetes and hypertension, continuing with his volunteer activities, incorporating food he grows for healthy eating, identifying physical activity and exercises he enjoys, and continuing to see the dietitian for expert recommendations on healthy eating practices.

   Help Osvaldo determine what modalities of exercise he enjoys outside of the fitness center and how these can become a habit within his weekly schedule (e.g., outdoor cycling, walking outside, and hiking with his wife). For activities within the fitness center, provide options that will provide variety such as use of different methods of resistance training or group exercise classes. In addition, ask him if he would perhaps enjoy the social aspects of workouts that are related to competition, because he enjoys coaching his soccer team and may find similar enjoyment in being a participant.

19

Pregnancy

Barbara A. Bushman

OBJECTIVES

The reader will be able to do the following:

1. Describe the benefits of physical activity and exercise during pregnancy
2. Assess situations that are contraindications for exercise during pregnancy
3. Describe screening tools available to promote safety during exercise and enhanced communication with health care providers
4. Describe changes in anatomy and physiology that occur during pregnancy
5. Describe the fetal responses to maternal exercise
6. List signs or symptoms that warrant stopping exercise and seeking medical advice for pregnant women
7. Describe considerations for exercise testing during pregnancy
8. Describe the general recommendations for physical activity and exercise for healthy women during pregnancy and postpartum

Pregnancy places enormous demands on a woman's body. Concerns about the safety of the fetus and the mother may lead to questions about whether being active during pregnancy is wise. Historically, concerns related to risks of maternal physical activity on the fetus led to limitations related to maternal exercise (29). For example, in 1949, the U.S. Children's Bureau recommended pregnant women without complications could continue housework, gardening, walking up to a mile in short bouts, and swimming occasionally, although sports should be avoided (19). In 1985, the American College of Gynecology issued guidelines for prenatal physical activity that supported the safety of most aerobic activity (with caution for high-impact activities or ballistic movements) but also noted restrictions on duration (i.e., not exceeding 15 minutes of strenuous exercise) and heart rate (i.e., maternal heart rate should not exceed 140 bpm) (1a). Now recommendations encourage women without contraindications to be physically active throughout pregnancy (1, 2, 26) and go further to point out risks of not engaging in prenatal physical activity (26). Research supports the benefits of physical activity related to pregnancy complications for potential prevention and treatment as well as maternal and fetal health (26). The 2019 *Canadian Guideline for Physical Activity throughout Pregnancy* highlights this perspective in the summary statement that suggests that there has been "a foundational shift in our view of prenatal physical activity from a recommended behaviour to improve quality of life, to a specific prescription for physical activity to reduce pregnancy complications and optimize health across the lifespan of two generations" (26).

Moderate-intensity activity done by healthy women during pregnancy has been found to carry a very low risk and without increased risk of low birth weight, preterm delivery, or early pregnancy loss (39, 40). One systematic review and meta-analysis reported that prenatal exercise was associated with 39% decreased odds of high birth weight (macrosomia, or a birth weight greater than 4,000 grams [8.8 pounds]) without increasing the odds of other concerns such as preterm birth, small for gestational age, and intrauterine growth restriction (11). In another analysis, researchers found that exercise reduces the odds of gestational diabetes by 38%, gestational hypertension by 39%, and preeclampsia by 41% (14). Potential benefits, in addition to decreasing risk of gestational diabetes or hypertensive disorders associated with pregnancy, include maintaining physical fitness, decreasing cesarean birth and increasing incidence of vaginal delivery, decreasing excessive weight gain, lowering bodily pain, and preventing postpartum depressive disorders (1). The period of early development is related to long-term health of the child; exercise interventions during pregnancy for women with normal body weight have been found to reduce the risk of childhood obesity by 53% (9).

The *Physical Activity Guidelines for Americans* recommends that women who are pregnant should be under the care of a health care provider who can monitor progress of the pregnancy, including discussion of whether or how physical activity might need to be adjusted during pregnancy and postpartum (39). When no medical reasons to avoid physical activity are present, women can begin or continue light- to moderate-intensity aerobic and muscle-strengthening activities (39). The American College of Obstetricians and Gynecologists (ACOG) notes that the principles of exercise prescription for the general population also apply to pregnant women (1). If there are no medical reasons to limit or avoid exercise, ACOG recommends an exercise program that progresses to at least 20 to 30 minutes per day, on most or all days of the week, noting the necessity of individualization and adjusting if medically indicated (1). Other organizations such as the Canadian Society for Exercise Physiology (CSEP) and the American College of Sports Medicine (ACSM) as well as the *Physical Activity Guidelines for Americans* recommend 150 minutes per week of moderate-intensity aerobic activity spread throughout the week, with daily activity encouraged (2, 26, 39). Inclusion of resistance training and strength conditioning is also promoted (1, 2, 26). Considerations to maximize safety are presented throughout this chapter.

Although exercise is safe and beneficial for most pregnant women, some conditions require a cautious approach to exercise. CSEP provides a prescreening for physical activity to help identify individuals who should seek medical advice before becoming or continuing to be physically active; the screening tool is called the Get Active Questionnaire for Pregnancy (6) (see form 19.1). This tool replaces the previous pre-exercise screening tool, the Physical Activity Readiness Medical Examination for Pregnancy (PARmed-X for Pregnancy), which was found to present barriers related to the length of the form and a required health care provider signature, among other concerns (13). The intent of the Get Active Questionnaire for Pregnancy is to identify the minority of women at risk for contraindications to physical activity that would necessitate further screening (10). Completion of the questionnaire should be done by all women once they become pregnant and desire to be physically active (13). CSEP points out that this screening tool is one step in the overall preparticipation screening process; the responses can help a fitness professional better know their client's health status. If any "yes" answers are given on the Get Active Questionnaire for Pregnancy, a referral to the client's health care provider is recommended, including the use of another CSEP resource, the Health Care Provider Consultation Form for Prenatal Physical Activity (6) (see form 19.2). This consultation form is considered a communication tool rather than a formal medical clearance form.

FORM 19.1   Get Active Questionnaire for Pregnancy

GET ACTIVE QUESTIONNAIRE FOR PREGNANCY   ⊕ CSEP | SCPE

NAME (+ NAME OF PARENT/GUARDIAN IF APPLICABLE) [PLEASE PRINT]:			
TODAY'S DATE (DD/MM/YYYY):	YOUR DUE DATE (DD/MM/YYYY):	NO. OF WEEKS PREGNANT:	AGE:

Physical activity during pregnancy has many health benefits and is generally not risky for you and your baby. But for some conditions, physical activity is not recommended. This questionnaire is to help decide whether you should speak to your Obstetric Health Care Provider (e.g., your physician or midwife) before you begin or continue to be physically active.

Please answer YES or NO to each question to the best of your ability. **If your health changes as your pregnancy progresses you should fill in this questionnaire again.**

1.	In this pregnancy, do you have:		
	a. Mild, moderate or severe respiratory or cardiovascular diseases (e.g., chronic bronchitis)?	Y	N
	b. Epilepsy that is not stable?	Y	N
	c. Type 1 diabetes that is not stable or your blood sugar is outside of target ranges?	Y	N
	d. Thyroid disease that is not stable or your thyroid function is outside of target ranges?	Y	N
	e. An eating disorder(s) or malnutrition?	Y	N
	f. Twins (28 weeks pregnant or later)? Or are you expecting triplets or higher multiple births?	Y	N
	g. Low red blood cell number (anemia) with high levels of fatigue and/or light-headedness?	Y	N
	h. High blood pressure (preeclampsia, gestational hypertension, or chronic hypertension that is not stable)?	Y	N
	i. A baby that is growing slowly (intrauterine growth restriction)?	Y	N
	j. Unexplained bleeding, ruptured membranes or labour before 37 weeks?	Y	N
	k. A placenta that is partially or completely covering the cervix (placenta previa)?	Y	N
	l. Weak cervical tissue (incompetent cervix)?	Y	N
	m. A stitch or tape to reinforce your cervix (cerclage)?	Y	N
2.	In previous pregnancies, have you had:		
	a. Recurrent miscarriages (loss of your baby before 20 weeks gestation two or more times)?	Y	N
	b. Early delivery (before 37 weeks gestation)?	Y	N
3.	Do you have any other medical condition that may affect your ability to be physically active during pregnancy? What is the condition? Specify:	Y	N
4.	Is there any other reason you are concerned about physical activity during pregnancy?		

Go to Page 2 *Describe Your Physical Activity Level*

© Canadian Society for Exercise Physiology (CSEP)

(continued)

FORM 19.1 *(continued)*

Describe Your Physical Activity Level

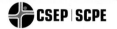

During a typical week, what types of physical activities do you take part in (e.g., swimming, walking, resistance training, yoga)?

_____

_____

_____

During the same week, please describe ON AVERAGE how often and for how long you engage in physical activity of a light, moderate or vigorous intensity. See definitions for intensity below the box.

ON AVERAGE	FREQUENCY (times per week)		INTENSITY (see below for definitions)	DURATION (minutes per session)	
How physically active were you in the **six months before pregnancy**?	☐ 0 ☐ 1-2	☐ 3-4 ☐ 5-7	☐ light ☐ moderate ☐ vigorous	☐ <20 ☐ 20-30	☐ 31-60 ☐ >60
How physically active have you been **during this pregnancy**?	☐ 0 ☐ 1-2	☐ 3-4 ☐ 5-7	☐ light ☐ moderate ☐ vigorous	☐ <20 ☐ 20-30	☐ 31-60 ☐ >60
What are your physical activity goals for the **rest of your pregnancy**?	☐ 0 ☐ 1-2	☐ 3-4 ☐ 5-7	☐ light ☐ moderate ☐ vigorous	☐ <20 ☐ 20-30	☐ 31-60 ☐ >60

Light intensity physical activity: You are moving, but you do not sweat or breathe hard, such as walking to get the mail or light gardening.

Moderate intensity physical activity: Your heart rate goes up and you may sweat or breathe hard. You can talk, but could not sing. Examples include brisk walking.

Vigorous intensity physical activity: Your heart rate goes up substantially, you feel hot and sweaty, and you cannot say more than a few words without pausing to breathe. Examples include fast stationary cycling and running.

General Advice for Being Physically Active During Pregnancy

Follow the advice in the 2019 Canadian Guidelines for Physical Activity throughout Pregnancy: **csepguidelines.ca/pregnancy**

It recommends that pregnant women get at least 150 minutes of moderate-intensity physical activity (resistance training, brisk walking, swimming, gardening), spread over three or more days of the week. **If you are planning to take part in vigorous-intensity physical activity, or be physically active at elevations above 2500 m (8200 feet), then consult with your health care provider.** If you have any questions about physical activity during pregnancy, consult a Qualified Exercise Professional or your health care provider beforehand. This can help ensure that your physical activity is safe and suitable for you.

Declaration

To the best of my knowledge, all of the information I have supplied on this questionnaire is correct. **If my health changes, I will complete this questionnaire again.**

☐ **I answered NO to all questions on Page 1.**
Sign and date the declaration below.
Physical activity is recommended.

I answered YES to one or more questions on Page 1 and I will speak with my health care provider before beginning or continuing physical activity. *The Health Care Provider Consultation Form for Prenatal Physical Activity can be used to start the conversation (**www.csep.ca/getactivequestionnaire-pregnancy**).*

☐ **I have spoken with my health care provider who has recommended that I take part in physical activity during my pregnancy.**
Sign and date the declaration below.

NAME (+ NAME OF PARENT/GUARDIAN IF APPLICABLE) [PLEASE PRINT]:	SIGNATURE (OR SIGNATURE OF PARENT/GUARDIAN IF APPLICABLE):
TODAY'S DATE (DD/MM/YYYY):	TELEPHONE (OPTIONAL):	EMAIL (OPTIONAL):

**FORM 19.2   Health Care Provider Consultation Form
for Prenatal Physical Activity**

HEALTH CARE PROVIDER CONSULTATION FORM FOR PRENATAL PHYSICAL ACTIVITY

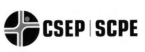

PATIENT NAME:	DUE DATE (DD/MM/YYYY):	TODAY'S DATE (DD/MM/YYYY):

Your patient wishes to begin or continue to be physically active during pregnancy. Your patient answered "Yes" to one or more questions on the Get Active Questionnaire for Pregnancy and has been asked to seek your advice (**www.csep.ca/getactivequestionnaire-pregnancy**).

Physical activity is safe for **most** pregnant individuals and has many health benefits. However, a **small number of patients** may need a thorough evaluation before taking part in physical activity during pregnancy.

The Society of Obstetricians and Gynaecologists of Canada/Canadian Society for Exercise Physiology *2019 Canadian Guideline for Physical Activity throughout Pregnancy* recommends that pregnant women get at least 150 minutes of moderate intensity physical activity each week (see next page or **csepguidelines.ca/pregnancy**). But there are contraindications to this goal for some conditions (see right).

> Specific concern from your patient and/or from a Qualified Exercise Professional:

To ensure that your patient proceeds in the safest way possible, they were advised to consult with you about becoming or continuing to be physically active during pregnancy. Please discuss potential concerns you may have about physical activity with your patient and indicate in the box below any modifications you might recommend:

☐ Unrestricted physical activity based on the *SOGC/CSEP 2019 Canadian Guidelines for Physical Activity throughout Pregnancy.*

☐ Progressive physical activity

  ☐ Recommend avoiding:

  ☐ Recommend including:

☐ Recommend supervision by a Qualified Exercise Professional, if possible.

☐ Refer to a physiotherapist for pain, impairment and/or a pelvic floor assessment.

☐ Other comments:

Absolute contraindications

Pregnant women with these conditions should continue activities of daily living, but not take part in moderate or vigorous physical activity:

☐ ruptured membranes,
☐ premature labour,
☐ unexplained persistent vaginal bleeding,
☐ placenta previa after 28 weeks gestation,
☐ preeclampsia,
☐ incompetent cervix,
☐ intrauterine growth restriction,
☐ high-order multiple pregnancy (e.g. triplets),
☐ uncontrolled Type I diabetes,
☐ uncontrolled hypertension,
☐ uncontrolled thyroid disease,
☐ other serious cardiovascular, respiratory or systemic disorder.

Relative contraindications

Pregnant women with these conditions should discuss advantages and disadvantages of physical activity with you. They should continue physical activity, but modify exercises to reduce intensity and/or duration.

☐ recurrent pregnancy loss,
☐ gestational hypertension,
☐ a history of spontaneous preterm birth,
☐ mild/moderate cardiovascular or respiratory disease,
☐ symptomatic anemia,
☐ malnutrition,
☐ eating disorder,
☐ twin pregnancy after the 28th week,
☐ other significant medical conditions.

Page 1

(continued)

FORM 19.2 *(continued)*

SOGC/CSEP 2019 CANADIAN GUIDELINE FOR PHYSICAL ACTIVITY THROUGHOUT PREGNANCY

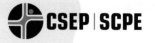

The evidence-based guideline outlines the right amount of physical activity women should get throughout pregnancy to promote maternal, fetal, and neonatal health.

Research shows the health benefits and safety of being active throughout pregnancy for both mother and baby. Physical activity is now seen as a critical part of a healthy pregnancy. Following the guideline can reduce the risk of pregnancy-related illnesses such as depression, by at least 25%, and of developing gestational diabetes, high blood pressure and preeclampsia by 40%.

Pregnant women should get at least 150 minutes of moderate-intensity physical activity each week over at least three days per week. But even if they do not meet that goal, they are encouraged to be active in a variety of ways every day. Please visit **csepguidelines.ca/pregnancy** for more information. The guideline makes six recommendations:

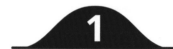

All women without contraindication should be physically active throughout pregnancy. Specific subgroups were examined:

- Women who were previously inactive.
- Women diagnosed with gestational diabetes mellitus.
- Women categorized as overweight or obese (pre-pregnancy body mass index ≥25kg/m^2).

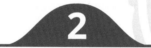

Pregnant women should accumulate at least 150 minutes of moderate-intensity physical activity each week to achieve clinically meaningful health benefits and reductions in pregnancy complications.

Physical activity should be accumulated over a minimum of three days per week; however, being active every day is encouraged.

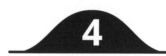

Pregnant women should incorporate a variety of aerobic and resistance training activities to achieve greater benefits. Adding yoga and/or gentle stretching may also be beneficial.

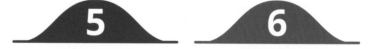

Pelvic floor muscle training (e.g., Kegel exercises) may be performed on a daily basis to reduce the risk of urinary incontinence. Instruction in proper technique is recommended to obtain optimal benefits.

Pregnant women who experience light-headedness, nausea or feel unwell when they exercise flat on their back should modify their exercise position to avoid the supine position.

No. 367-2019 Canadian Guideline for Physical Activity throughout Pregnancy
JOINT SOGC/CSEP CLINICAL PRACTICE GUIDELINE | Volume 40, ISSUE 11, P1528-1537, November 01, 2018

Page 2

Reprinted by permission from "Pre-Screen for Physical Activity in Pregnancy: Get Active Questionnaire for Pregnancy," Canadian Society for Exercise Physiology, accessed October 2022, https://csep.ca/2021/05/27/get-active-questionnaire-for-pregnancy/ Download here: https://csep.ca/wp-content/uploads/2021/05/GAQ_P_HCP_English.pdf.

The Get Active Questionnaire for Pregnancy should be completed again if any health changes occur over time (13). Also, even if all answers to the screening portion are "no," if exercise plans include vigorous-intensity physical activity or will involve activity at higher elevations (above 2,500 meters [8,200 feet]), consultation with a health care provider is recommended (6).

The Health Care Provider Consultation Form for Prenatal Physical Activity supports communication with the health care provider regarding any concerns. This form includes absolute and relative contraindications as noted in the 2019 *Canadian Guideline* (26). Pregnant women with absolute contraindications should not engage in moderate or vigorous activity but typically can continue with activities of daily living (6). Bed rest or restricted activity in pregnancy is not routinely recommended because research has not supported benefits related to preterm birth or preeclampsia; in addition, concerns with bed rest include increased risk of venous thromboembolism, bone demineralization, and deconditioning as well as negative psychosocial effects (1). Relative contraindications are conditions that should be reviewed to consider the pros and cons of exercise. At times modification of exercise may be warranted (frequency, duration, and/or intensity of activity) (6). Re-evaluation if health changes should continue throughout pregnancy. See the case study *Pre-Activity Screening for Pregnancy*.

Anatomic and Physiologic Changes During Pregnancy

An understanding of the changes in anatomy and physiology during pregnancy can be helpful when prescribing physical activity or exercise. For example, low-back pain is reported by a majority of pregnant women. Given the shift in the center of gravity resulting in progressive lordosis due to the weight gain and enlargement of abdomen and breasts associated with pregnancy reinforces the value of core-muscle strengthening to minimize risk of low-back pain (1). Additionally, various hormonal changes that allow the pelvis to open for birth also act globally, resulting in body-wide effects. Connective tissue relaxes, which may lead to laxity of ligaments and instability of joints (21). This change in range of motion may increase the risk of injury (26).

Many physiologic parameters shift to provide a circulatory reserve for pregnant women to sustain both self and fetus, including increases in blood volume, heart rate, stroke volume, and cardiac output and decreases in systemic vascular resistance (1). The magnitude of changes is substantial; for example, by the third trimester, resting heart rate is about 15 bpm higher and cardiac

output has been found to increase by approximately 30% (15). When considering blood flow, ACOG notes that maintaining the supine position during exercise after 20 weeks of gestation may decrease venous return and thus may result in hypotension due to the weight of the uterus on the inferior vena cava (as well as the abdominal aorta) (1). Both ACSM and the *Physical Activity Guidelines for Americans* suggest avoiding supine physical activity after the first trimester (2, 39). The 2019 *Canadian Guideline* recommends that pregnant women who experience light-headedness or nausea or feel unwell when exercising on their back should avoid the supine position by modifying body position (26).

Pulmonary changes include increased oxygen consumption and minute ventilation, along with decreased residual capacity (21). Early in pregnancy there is an increase in sensitivity to carbon dioxide; this increases tidal volume and minute ventilation, helping to create a buffer to protect the fetus (5). By the third trimester, ventilation increases 30% to 50% (15).

During the first trimester the fetus is particularly vulnerable to developmental defects caused by excess heat (5). Temperature regulation is affected by hydration and the environment in which activity occurs, so avoiding dehydration and finding cooler settings are key. Thermoregulation improves throughout pregnancy; for example, a downward shift in body temperature threshold for sweating provides for loss of heat via evaporation at a lower body temperature (5). Increased temperatures that occur with typical exercise have been found to be below hyperthermic levels where congenital abnormalities are concerning (16). To prevent heat stress, pregnant women should ensure they are well hydrated, dress appropriately, and avoid high heat and humidity (1, 2, 26).

Because of the nutritional demands of pregnancy, greater caloric consumption is needed. The daily caloric needs increase over the course of pregnancy; appropriate caloric intake during pregnancy depends on prepregnancy weight, gestational weight gain, and multiple pregnancies (41). Appropriate weight gain is based on prepregnancy body mass index (BMI); gaining weight within recommended ranges promotes health outcomes (38). Ranges vary depending on BMI prior to pregnancy; the Institute of Medicine recommends women with a BMI between 18.5 to 24.9 kg · m^{-2} gain 25 to 35 pounds (11.5-16 kilograms), those who are underweight are recommended to gain more (28-40 pounds [12.5-18 kilograms]), and those who are overweight or obese are recommended to gain less (15-25 pounds [7-11.5 kilograms] or 11-20 pounds [5-9 kilograms], respectively) (8). Physically active women are less likely to exceed recommendations for healthy weight gain (18). This lowers the risk of excessive postpartum weight retention

CASE STUDY

Pre-Activity Screening for Pregnancy

Case Study Contributor: Margie H. Davenport

Case 1: Emma is 29 years of age with her second pregnancy. She has a prepregnancy BMI of 24.9 kg · m^{-2} and has previously experienced one miscarriage. Emma was not engaging in exercise prior to pregnancy, but her friends have encouraged her to join a prenatal fitness class to meet other moms. She is 11 weeks pregnant when she comes to your class for the first time. What do you do?

Upon finding out that Emma is pregnant and wishes to participate in your fitness class, you have her complete the Get Active Questionnaire for Pregnancy. She fills out the top of page 1 with her name, date, due date, number of weeks pregnancy, and age. She answered no to all questions. She indicated that she was not active before or during pregnancy but wishes to engage in moderate-intensity physical activity for 20 to 30 minutes 3 to 4 times per week. Because she did not answer "yes" to any questions, she can sign and date the declaration. Be sure to keep a copy of the signed Get Active Questionnaire for Pregnancy for your records, and advise her that if her health changes during her pregnancy she should fill out the questionnaire again. Emma is able to join your class.

Case 2: Patricia is 43 years of age with her first pregnancy. After becoming pregnant, she was surprised to learn that she was carrying twins! Patricia has always been active and has continued to run during her pregnancy. However, she is currently 32 weeks gestation and is beginning to develop some mild low-back pain. She approached you to develop a pregnancy-specific training program so that she can comfortably continue to run as long as possible during her pregnancy. In your consultation, you provide Patricia with the Get Active Questionnaire for Pregnancy. She fills out the top of page 1 with her name, date, due date, number of weeks pregnant, and age. She answered yes to question 1g (twins and 28 weeks or later). On page 2 Patricia indicated that she was active prior to and during her pregnancy. She wishes to remain active for the rest of her pregnancy.

Since Patricia answered "yes" to one question, she needs to speak to her health care provider before she can start to train with you. Patricia takes the Health Care Provider Consultation Form for Prenatal Physical Activity to her obstetrician to discuss the pros and cons of continuing to be physically active during her pregnancy. After consulting with her midwife they determined that the benefits of physical activity outweigh any potential harms, and unrestricted physical activity following current guidelines is recommended. Patricia checks the box that she consulted with her health care provider and signed and dated the declaration. Be sure to advise her that if her health changes during her pregnancy she should fill out the questionnaire again. Keep the document for your records.

A few weeks later, you assess Patricia's resting blood pressure and discover that it is 142/94 mmHg. Because her blood pressure is elevated, Patricia answers yes on the Get Active Questionnaire for Pregnancy, and you cannot continue with your exercise session. You record on the Health Care Provider Consultation Form for Prenatal Physical Activity that you assessed her blood pressure and found it to be elevated. Patricia takes this form to her obstetrician to discuss the pros and cons of continuing to be physically active during her pregnancy. During this appointment, Patricia is diagnosed with preeclampsia. As a result, she is advised by her obstetrician that she may continue with her normal daily activities (e.g., walking for the mail, light cleaning, dressing) but should not participate in more strenuous exercise for the remainder of her pregnancy.

and future obesity (18). In general, calorie needs due to pregnancy in the first trimester are not increased; approximately 300 to 400 additional calories are needed for later trimesters (41). The nutritional demands of exercise in addition to fetal development must be adequately met by the exercising woman. Adaptations will occur to provide adequate glucose for fetal development, including increases in maternal blood glucose and increases in insulin resistance, allowing for decreased use of glucose in peripheral tissues to allow for glucose availability for fetal use (5). If insulin production does not increase, hyperglycemia can result; see sidebar *Gestational Diabetes* for risk factors and implications of this condition.

Gestational Diabetes

Gestational diabetes is a type of diabetes that develops during pregnancy in women who do not already have diabetes. This affects 2% to 10% of pregnancies in the United States (7) and is thought to be caused by hormonal changes that occur during pregnancy plus genetic and lifestyle factors (27). Overweight and obesity are linked with gestational diabetes because insulin resistance may be present prior to pregnancy (27). Gaining excessive weight during pregnancy also may increase risk (27). Other risk factors include having gestational diabetes during a prior pregnancy, giving birth to a baby who weighed over 9 pounds (4 kilograms), polycystic ovarian syndrome, age older than 25 years of age, and having a family history of type 2 diabetes (7). In addition, risk is higher for African Americans, American Indians, Asians, and Hispanics/Latinas (27). A significant inverse relationship is found between physical activity and risk of gestational diabetes (40). A systemic review and meta-analysis found that exercise reduces the odds of developing gestational diabetes by 38% (14).

During pregnancy, maternal metabolism is altered, including increasing insulin resistance over time to ensure the fetus has an adequate supply of nutrients (23). Local and placental hormones contribute to the insulin resistance, resulting in a slightly elevated blood glucose; this glucose is transported across the placenta to provide needed fuel for the fetus (30). As pregnancy advances, the insulin resistance increases, and if insulin production cannot keep pace, hyperglycemia will result (23).

In the short term, gestational diabetes is associated with increased risk of preterm birth, preeclampsia, cesarean delivery, and macrosomia (30). Babies are at increased risk of hypoglycemia at delivery due to fetal hyperinsulinemia in response to maternal hyperglycemia. Long-term consequences of gestational diabetes for the woman include increased risk of cardiovascular disease and type 2 diabetes; approximately 60% of women with gestational diabetes will develop type 2 diabetes in the future (30). Long-term sequelae for offspring who have been exposed to maternal hyperglycemia include increased risk of obesity and diabetes later in life (23).

The American Diabetes Association points out that lifestyle behavior change is "an essential component of management of gestational diabetes mellitus" (3). The risk of gestational diabetes may be reduced with diet, exercise, and lifestyle counseling (3). An individualized nutritional plan should be developed by a Registered Dietitian Nutritionist (3). Beyond general physical activity recommendations, specific guidance on optimal type, timing, and duration of physical activity has not been determined (37). Findings from a systematic review and meta-analysis suggest that accumulating at least 600 MET-min $\cdot$ week^{-1} of moderate-intensity exercise is needed to achieve at least a 25% reduction in the odds of developing gestational diabetes (14). An example would be 140 minutes of brisk walking.

Fetal Responses to Maternal Exercise

In addition to the impact of exercise on maternal responses, fetal responses also have been studied. Heart rate of the fetus is minimally to moderately changed by maternal exercise (34). Researchers have found that the fetus responds to maternal exercise with a 10 to 30 bpm increase in heart rate during or after exercise compared to baseline (1). Increases in fetal heart rate are thought to be a positive response to compensate for lower oxygen levels due to reduced placental blood flow; to maintain cardiac output, fetal heart rate increases because stroke volume increases are limited (44).

Birth weight is another aspect that has been studied. Both low birth weight and high birth weight are concerning. Based on current research, minimal to no differences have been found between pregnant women who exercise compared with those who did not exercise (1). The likelihood of lower birth weight (200-400 grams [0.4-0.9 pounds] less than comparable controls) was found for women who continued with vigorous exercise, although the risk of fetal growth restriction (when fetal weight is less than 10th percentile for gestational age) was not increased (1). As noted previously, exercise has been found to reduce the odds of high birth weight (greater than 4,000 grams [8.8 pounds]) by 39% without affecting the odds of low birth-weight babies (11). ACOG points out that exercise above 85% capacity (i.e., beyond "vigorous") has not been fully studied (1).

Signs or Symptoms to Stop Exercise

With a focus on long-term engagement in physical activity, pregnant women should be encouraged to adapt or reduce activity levels as needed. Knowledge of signs or symptoms that activity should be stopped and medical advice sought is extremely important (10). Examples of warning signs compiled from several sources (1, 2, 26) include ongoing shortness of breath that does not resolve with rest, dyspnea before exertion, chest pain, regular painful uterine contractions, vaginal bleeding, loss of fluid from the vagina reflecting rupture of membranes, amniotic fluid leakage, ongoing dizziness or faintness that does not resolve with rest, abdominal pain, dizziness, headache, muscle weakness affecting balance, and calf pain or swelling.

Exercise Testing During Pregnancy

Exercise testing has the potential to provide insights on fitness as well as to assess risk for various medical conditions. Current ACSM recommendations suggest that maximal exercise testing should not be performed at any stage of pregnancy and that submaximal exercise testing, if warranted, only should be done under the supervision of a physician following a careful evaluation for contraindications to exercise (2). Ongoing research in this area seeks to establish procedures for exercise testing that promote safety and are adapted for pregnant women. Safety starts with prescreening, including identification of any contraindications (44). Given various adaptations with pregnancy, assessment of resting heart rate, blood pressure, and glucose is recommended (44). Resting heart rate typically increases over the course of pregnancy (i.e., by the third trimester resting heart rate may be 15 to 20 bpm higher than before pregnancy). Thus, typical prescreening cut-offs (e.g., resting heart rate to be below 100 bpm) may need to be reconsidered (44); no formal guidance is available currently. Blood pressure responses will differ over the course of pregnancy. Early in pregnancy blood pressure may be lower (5-10 mmHg drop in systolic and 10-15 mmHg drop in diastolic) and then gradually increases to prepregnancy blood pressure levels after around the 20th week of gestation (44). Pregnancy-specific guidance on pre-exercise blood pressure is not available; given that the diagnosis of pregnancy hypertensive disorders begins at 140 mmHg for systolic and 90 mmHg for diastolic, any resting blood pressure above those values has been sug-

gested as a level at which exercise should not occur and referral for medical assessment be made (44). Attention to hypotension is also warranted given the related risk for dizziness or falls; blood pressure assessment before, during, and after exercise is important (44). Glucose also should be assessed before and after exercise given the risk of hypoglycemia (44).

Warm-ups are recommended to be about 5 minutes (slightly longer than the typical 2-3 minutes of lower-intensity activity before an exercise test) (44). This is not only to prepare the cardiovascular system but also to decrease injury risk due to the increased relaxin during pregnancy, which causes ligaments to become lax around joints (44). Similarly, a 5-minute or longer cool-down has been proposed to decrease the risk of dizziness due to blood pressure dropping quickly if exercise is terminated abruptly (44).

As with all cardiorespiratory exercise testing, there are considerations when selecting the mode of exercise. Although treadmills can incorporate the common activity of walking, balance and fall risk will be higher given changes in the center of gravity, laxity of joints, and the enlarged abdomen (44). Cycle ergometry, although providing a non-weightbearing option, may be uncomfortable because of pelvic girdle pain when sitting on a traditional upright bike seat or may be difficult to adjust if using a recumbent ergometer due to spacing between legs and abdomen (44). Protocol selection should be determined based on the woman's fitness and training status. Given the lack of information available on higher-intensity activity (i.e., over 80% heart rate reserve), exercising in that range requires consultation with a health care provider (44).

Although beyond the scope of a fitness professional, in addition to maternal monitoring, assessment of fetal responses is critical (44). Fetal heart rate is one measurement often used to reflect fetal distress (44). Decreases in fetal heart rate (i.e., fetal bradycardia is considered below 110 bpm) could indicate hypoxemia (e.g., due to reduced uteroplacental blood flow). Increases in heart rate occur normally in response to maternal exercise; abnormally high fetal heart rate is considered over 160 bpm (44).

The prior information on exercise testing has focused on cardiorespiratory assessment. Various assessments have been proposed for other health-related fitness components, including handgrip for muscular strength, five times sit-to-stand test for muscular endurance, and back-scratch test for flexibility (32).

Exercise Prescription During Pregnancy

General recommendations for exercise depend on activity level before pregnancy as well as current status and presence of any concerns or contraindications that would prevent engagement in physical activity. Women who have been active previously are encouraged to continue being physically active throughout pregnancy, with modifications as needed. For women who were not physically active, a gradual progressive program of physical activity is recommended (1, 2). Clinically meaningful reductions in health outcomes (including gestational diabetes, gestational hypertension, and preeclampsia) have been identified with lower than recommended levels of physical activity (14). Thus, women are encouraged to be physically active, even if levels of activity do not meet recommendations (26).

No single program can be applied in all situations; the need to individualize and adapt over time is key. The type, intensity, frequency, and duration of activity should conform to the woman's health, fitness level, and comfort. There are some differences in recommendations among various sources:

• *Duration and frequency:* Some sources reflect a weekly total of 150 minutes or more with activity occurring a minimum of 3 days per week (daily is encouraged) or spread throughout the week (26, 39), while another suggests 20 to 30 minutes per day on most if not all days of the week (1).

• *Intensity:* Moderate-intensity activity is recommended (1, 26, 39), though lower-intensity activity also is beneficial (i.e., even if unable to reach recommended amounts of activity, being active is encouraged) (26). For cautions related to vigorous-intensity activity, see the sidebar *Higher-Level Activity During Pregnancy.* Monitoring intensity can be done with the talk test, which references the ability to maintain a conversation while physically active (if conversation is not possible, intensity should be reduced) (26, 39), or use of perceived exertion (e.g., level 5 or 6 on a 10-point scale, where 0 is sitting and 10 is maximal effort) (39). Although potentially less useful during pregnancy, heart rate ranges for moderate intensity have been reported (data based on low-risk

medically screened pregnant women) for those less than 29 years of age (125-146 bpm) and for those 30 years of age or above (121-141 bpm) (26).

• *Type of activity:* Aerobic conditioning is recommended (1, 2, 26, 39) as is resistance training and muscle-strengthening activities (1, 2, 26). Combining aerobic and resistance training activities has been found to be beneficial for pregnancy outcomes compared to aerobic conditioning alone (26). Yoga and/or stretching are suggested as potentially beneficial (26). To reduce the odds of urinary incontinence, pelvic floor muscle training (e.g., Kegel exercises) may be included daily (26). See the sidebar *Pelvic Floor Training.*

Within these general guidelines, the need to individualize an exercise program and make modifications over time cannot be overemphasized. General safety precautions include the following (1, 2, 26):

• Avoid activity in hot and/or humid environments to avoid heat stress. Hot Pilates and hot yoga are best avoided given the risk associated with rising core temperature.

• Avoid scuba diving given the inability of the pulmonary circulation of the fetus to filter bubble formation.

• Ensure appropriate acclimatization for physical activity at high altitude; seek guidance from an obstetrician with appropriate knowledge and background on potential impacts of high altitude on maternal and fetal well-being. Sources provide slightly different guidance; generally, for those who live at a lower altitude with appropriate acclimatization, physical activity is tolerated up to 6,000 feet (about 1,829 meters).

• Avoid activities that may increase risk of fetal trauma, including physical contact or situations that have a fall risk. Examples include downhill skiing, water skiing, ice hockey, gymnastics, or

Higher-Level Activity During Pregnancy

Less is known about vigorous activity; evidence is lacking on safety or if there are additional benefits beyond those realized with moderate-intensity activity (26). For high-intensity physical activity, a monitored environment has been recommended (26). Other considerations for high-intensity or prolonged activity include ensuring adequate caloric intake to avoid hypoglycemia and considering environmental conditions to avoid excessive heat exposure (26). For highly conditioned aerobic-trained individuals, research studies suggest aerobic fitness will stay the same or even improve slightly if exercise is continued as material symptoms allow (5). Another research focus is in the area of resistance training; researchers highlight the need for more studies examining safety and potential benefits (31). As with many topics, the fitness professional must continue to be an active consumer of scientific, data-driven content.

Pelvic Floor Training

Sidebar Contributor: Tamara Rial

The pelvic floor is comprised of ligaments, fascia, neurovascular structures, and several layers of deep and superficial muscles. The deep pelvic floor muscles (PFM) are mainly comprised of the elevator ani muscles (puborectalis, pubococcygeus, iliococcygeus) and the coccygeus. The PFM provide support to the pelvic organs (bladder, uterus, rectum) while aiding with continence and pelvic stability. Inadequate functioning of the PFM can lead to a variety of conditions known as *pelvic floor disorders*. Pregnancy, birth trauma, and high BMI are well-established risk factors for pelvic floor disorders (22). The pregnancy and postnatal periods are associated with anatomical and physiological changes in the PFM. For example, weight gain during pregnancy can increase intra-abdominal pressure on the pelvic floor–supporting structures and weaken the PFM (33).

Urinary incontinence (UI) is the most common pelvic floor disorder during pregnancy, with an overall prevalence of 41% (25). One year after parturition, UI is present in one-third of women (24). Pelvic floor muscle training (PFMT) is often recommended as a first-line conservative treatment choice for women who develop UI during pregnancy, and it may provide a protective effect for those who are continent (12, 43). High-quality evidence supports PFMT as an effective strategy to reduce the severity of UI symptoms during pregnancy and during the postnatal period (12, 33).

The primary goal of PFMT is to increase muscular strength, muscular power, and local muscular endurance of the PFM. PFMT consists of a cycle of PFM contractions and relaxations done in a progressive and repetitive manner. Since PFMT is a learned skill and technique driven, the first step is to learn how to perform a PFM contraction properly (17). Once this is achieved, the training protocol can progress from submaximal contractions in the supine or seated position to more intense contractions in more challenging body positions (e.g., standing, quadruped) until reaching maximal contractions during functional movements (e.g., squat, lunge). An exercise program for PFMT should be done 3 to 7 times per week, 3 times daily, with 8 to 10 seconds of submaximal or maximal contractions and a rest interval of 6 to 8 seconds for 8 to 10 repetitions (20). Guided breathing and adequate rest between contractions are recommended during each contraction cycle. PFMT can be done during a personal training session, a group fitness class, or as part of a home training routine. A typical PFMT session lasts for 10 to 45 minutes (20).

Technical errors are common during PFMT. Between 30% and 70% of women are unable to perform a PFM contraction correctly (35, 36). These errors can be remembered with the acronym COMMOV (*C*ontraction of *O*ther *M*uscle groups and other *MOV*ements) (28). Examples of COMMOV are contracting the rectus abdominis, the gluteal muscles, and the adductors; performing a pelvic tilt; holding the breath; sucking in; or bulging the abdomen. Verbal instructions have been found to have a positive effect on the performance of PFM contractions during the postpartum period (42). Simple and effective coaching cues to activate the PFM include "squeeze the anus," "prevent the escape of gas," and "squeeze the vaginal muscles you use to hold urine" (4, 17, 42).

PFMT should be considered an integral component of the exercise prescription during pregnancy and the postpartum period. Fitness professionals involved in the design of exercise programs for pregnant women play an important role in educating their clients about PFM and managing modifiable risk factors for urinary incontinence.

Olympic lifts; nonstationary cycling also may have a higher risk of falling. Contact and fall risk are also present in team sports such as soccer or basketball. Consider other activities, such as brisk walking, stationary cycling, swimming, or other aquatic exercise.

- Avoid activities that involve jumping and quick changes in direction due to the increase in joint laxity.
- Avoid breath holding (i.e., Valsalva maneuver) when exercising. (*Note:* The 2019 *Canadian Guideline* recommends avoiding if light-headedness is experienced [26].)

- Seek advice regarding physiotherapy for diastasis recti (visible separation of abdominal muscles), and avoid abdominal strengthening exercises that may worsen the condition.

The fitness professional must be aware, and alert clients to be aware, of reasons to stop activity and seek care from a qualified health care provider. All exercise sessions should include a warm-up and cool-down. In addition, adequate nutrition and hydration should be encouraged. Seek supervision from an obstetric care provider with appropriate background for higher level activities (above recommended levels) or athletic competition (26).

Postpartum Physical Activity

Exercise after pregnancy is important for lifelong health. As with exercise during pregnancy, the exercise program should be individualized. Considerations include mode of delivery (vaginal or cesarean) and whether any medical or surgical complications occurred (1). Because some deconditioning in the initial postpartum time is typical, a gradually progressed program is appropriate.

Physical activity should be part of a healthy postpartum lifestyle considering the many benefits that have been highlighted throughout this book related to fitness and prevention of chronic diseases. Women during postpartum also reap specific benefits. For example, an inverse relationship exists between physical activity during postpartum and reduced symptoms of depression (40). Also, physical activity, along with nutritional modifications, is helpful for achieving and maintaining a healthy body weight postpartum (39).

One other consideration during postpartum is lactation. Aerobic exercise has not been shown to affect milk production, breast milk composition, or infant growth (1, 39). To avoid discomfort of engorged breasts, feeding or expressing milk before exercise can be considered (1). Continued focus on adequate hydration is also recommended (1).

KEY POINT

Exercising during pregnancy is safe and beneficial for most women. Protecting against traumatic impact, heat injury, musculoskeletal injury, and overexertion is the key to planning safe exercise programs for pregnant women.

LEARNING AIDS

REVIEW QUESTIONS

1. What is the current perspective on physical activity during pregnancy?
2. What are potential benefits of physical activity throughout pregnancy for healthy women without contraindications?
3. How does maternal physical activity affect the fetus?
4. What is the difference between absolute and relative contraindications?
5. Provide two examples of how knowledge of anatomic and physiologic changes during pregnancy might affect the choice of physical activities.
6. What are short-term and long-term concerns with gestational diabetes?
7. List signs or symptoms that are considered red flags that should result in stopping the activity and seeking medical advice.
8. What are the general exercise prescription recommendations during pregnancy with regard to type, duration, frequency, and intensity?
9. What are activities that should be avoided during pregnancy?
10. What are benefits of physical activity during postpartum?

CASE STUDIES

1. Lidia is a 31-year-old woman who is pregnant for the second time; her first child is now 3 years of age. She is expecting triplets. She completes the Get Active Questionnaire for Pregnancy, answering "no" to all of the questions except for the question "Are you expecting triplets or higher multiple birth?" Prior to her pregnancy she engaged in a walking program including 45 minutes on 3 days per week. She is interested in maintaining her physical activity. Given her responses on the Get Active Questionnaire for Pregnancy, what would you suggest as the next step?

2. Gabriela is an active, healthy, 32-year-old woman who is pregnant for the first time. She is in her first trimester. Although she has been a runner for years, she has been told by her mother-in-law that she should give up running while pregnant. Her doctor told her that it is perfectly healthy to continue running. What is your advice?

Answers to Case Studies

1. Because Lidia has answered "yes" to one of the questions on the Get Active Questionnaire for Pregnancy form, she should speak with her health care provider. She can be provided a copy of the Health Care Provider Consultation Form for Prenatal Physical Activity, which can be used to start the conversation with her health care provider.

2. Given that Gabriela's physician cleared her to continue running, there is no medical reason to stop running at this point in her pregnancy. However, it is understandable that both Gabriela and her mother-in-law have concerns. The first step is to alleviate fears through education. Give Gabriela background information on the health benefits of remaining active during pregnancy. Also, provide her with the warning signs that she should seek medical help (e.g., vaginal bleeding, dyspnea before exertion). Then encourage her to remain as active as she feels comfortable with during her pregnancy. Talk with her about using a relative exertion rating as a guide to her exercise intensity. Also, acknowledge that the types and intensity of exercise likely will need to change as she gets closer to term. Discuss with her the types of exercise that should be avoided (e.g., supine exercise).

Weight Management

Tanya M. Halliday

OBJECTIVES

The reader will be able to do the following:

1. Define *obesity* and describe its health risks
2. Identify factors that contribute to obesity
3. Describe the role that energy balance plays in weight management
4. Discuss the role of exercise in weight loss and weight maintenance
5. Provide guidelines for caloric intake to facilitate appropriate weight loss
6. Provide healthy guidelines for gaining weight
7. Recognize signs of eating disorders

20

Obesity is characterized by excessive adiposity (fat mass) and is linked to multiple adverse health outcomes including cardiovascular diseases (42), type 2 diabetes (1), several types of cancer (27), multiple other health conditions, and decreased quality of life (17). As a result, the direct and indirect economic costs associated with obesity are estimated at hundreds of billions of dollars (9, 47). In response to rising obesity prevalence and its associated morbidity, mortality, and health care costs, in 2013 the American Medical Association labeled obesity as a disease (2). While this decision was considered controversial at the time, it was made to increase the seriousness with which physicians and other health care professionals treat obesity and to decrease weight bias and stigma that adults with overweight and obesity experience. See the sidebar *Person-First Language* for recommendations on language that minimizes weight stigma.

Person-First Language

The use of person-first language—that is, "people *with* overweight or obesity" rather than "obese people"—is recommended when discussing body weight in order to minimize weight stigma. It may sound awkward to say at first, but person-first language should be used when referring to most medical conditions people have. For example, say "the person *with* a disability" or "the person *with* diabetes," not "the disabled" or "the diabetic."

Defining Obesity

Because of ease of measurement, screening for obesity typically is done through evaluation of a ratio of weight to height, known as body mass index (BMI). While BMI does not directly measure body fat, nor is it a definitive indicator of health status, it is closely related to percent body fat (%BF) evaluated through other methods (see chapter 11). Generally accepted guidelines classify a BMI of 30 kg · m^{-2} or higher as obese (19). The following are subclasses of obesity:

- *Grade 1 obesity:* 30.0 to 34.9 kg · m^{-2}
- *Grade 2 obesity:* 35.0 to 39.9 kg · m^{-2}
- *Grade 3 (extreme) obesity:* 40 kg · m^{-2} or higher

Although standards for classifying obesity from %BF are not universally agreed upon, the American College of Sports Medicine (ACSM) publishes ranges based on age for both men and women (see *ACSM Guidelines for Exercise Testing and Prescription* [28] for specific ranges). Another tool used to screen for obesity is waist circumference (WC; see chapter 11 for more details). Adiposity located in the abdominal region is strongly linked with chronic disease risk; therefore, a WC of ≥102 centimeters (40 inches) in men or ≥88 centimeters (35 inches) in women is used to classify individuals with abdominal obesity (28).

KEY POINT

Obesity is a complex condition associated with many adverse health outcomes. Simple measures are used to screen for obesity, including body mass index and waist circumference.

Increasing Prevalence of Obesity in the United States

In the early 1960s, 13.4% of American adults were obese (i.e., had a BMI ≥30 kg · m^{-2}) (18). National statistics from 2017 to 2020 revealed that obesity has increased significantly to 41.9% (38). Figure 20.1 shows the increasing prevalence of obesity during the past six decades for both men and women. However, it is important to note that racial or ethnic and sociodemographic factors affect obesity prevalence and result in health disparities across segments of the population. For example, obesity prevalence for non-Hispanic Black women is currently 57.9% (38), and adults living at 130% or less of the poverty level have higher rates of obesity than those living at more than 350% of the federal poverty level (38). Because of the rapid changes in obesity prevalence in the past few decades, this trend does not appear to be causally linked solely to genetics, but to a combination of environmental and lifestyle factors and genetic susceptibility.

Potential Causes of Obesity

Obesity is a complex disease with many factors contributing to its development. Figure 20.2 shows that environmental, biological/medical, maternal/developmental, economic, behavioral, psychological, and social influences all influence body weight. Despite the large list of contributors, ultimately, a positive caloric balance—that is, energy intake exceeding energy expenditure—leads to increased body weight. Two broad contributors to obesity are discussed in the following sections: genetics and lifestyle and environmental factors.

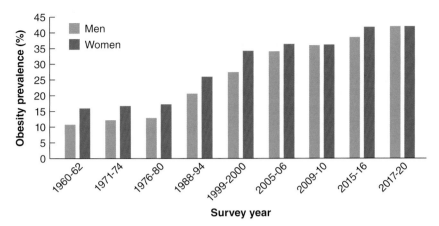

FIGURE 20.1 Prevalence of obesity among American adults.

Data from Fryar, Carroll, and Ogden (2012); National Center for Health Statistics (2021).

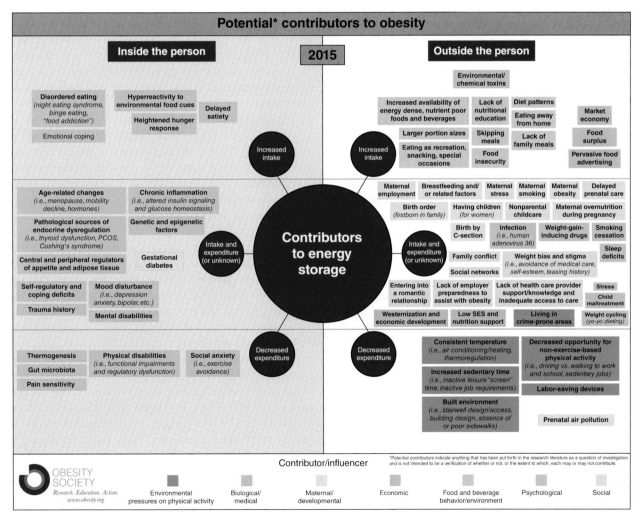

FIGURE 20.2 Potential contributors to obesity.

Potential Contributors to Obesity. © The Obesity Society (The Obesity Society Infographic is freely available to the public for download, use, and distribution at http://www.obesity.org/obesity/resources/facts-about-obesity/infographics/potential-contributors-to-obesity).

Genetics

From a genetic standpoint, obesity typically is classified into two main categories: monogenic, which is more rare, has an earlier onset in life, is more severe, and is due to chromosomal or single-gene defects, or polygenic, which is sometimes referred to as *common obesity* and is the result of hundreds of polymorphisms that ultimately contribute to obesity risk (31). Although estimates vary based on study design, evidence generally suggests that inheritance contributes 40% to 70% of the interindividual variation in obesity (31). In evaluating the genetic influence on obesity, researchers have attempted to differentiate among factors that are genetic and sociocultural. Bouchard and colleagues estimate that approximately 25% of the variance in %BF is attributable to genetics (6). Interestingly, these authors found that inheritance has a larger effect on total fat and deep deposits of adipose tissue than on subcutaneous fat. Additional evidence on the importance of genetics comes from data demonstrating that the BMI of adopted children is more similar to that of their biological parents than to that of their adoptive parents (44). The recent discoveries of genes linked with obesity provide additional evidence that genetic factors help determine the likelihood of being obese and developing diseases that accompany obesity (e.g., type 2 diabetes) (51).

Many genes are linked with obesity, and recently 97 new loci in the human genome were shown to be associated with BMI (29). The expression of each gene depends on environmental factors (e.g., availability of highly caloric, highly palatable foods, as well as social influences); therefore, the genetics of obesity is complex, and much is yet to be learned (31). A negative consequence of the growing knowledge of the genetic link to obesity is that people with many overweight family members may become discouraged and believe that they can do nothing about their weight status. Although genetics can contribute to the development of obesity, a primary reason that people become obese is lifestyle. Loos and Bouchard suggest that only a small percentage of individuals have true genetic obesity that would be present regardless of the environment (30). These authors suggest that the majority of people who develop obesity in modern Western societies (an environment where high-calorie food is abundant and physical activity is not a part of everyday life) might be normal weight or at most overweight in a less obesogenic environment. Fitness professionals must emphasize to clients that genetics may predispose certain people to obesity, but those people still have a great capacity to affect their body weight and fat. For example, a recent study examining health outcomes in pairs of monozygotic twins (i.e., identical twins) who participated in different levels of leisure time physical activity showed that, unsurprisingly, the more active twin had lower body-fat percentage, lower waist circumference, lower liver fat, and higher high-density lipoprotein cholesterol (HDL-C) values than the less active twin (26).

Lifestyle and Environmental

As mentioned previously, given the rapid increase in obesity rates over the years, it is more likely that lifestyle and environmental factors that influence food intake and energy expenditure are the greatest contributors to obesity. While individuals may not be able to do much to change the broader environment in which they live, being aware of how the environment influences behaviors may help fitness professionals devise strategies to improve personal lifestyle habits as well as those of their clients.

Energy Intake

Determining how energy intake has changed over the years is inherently challenging due to the methods available. One strategy is to ask people to report their food intake. However, dietary intake is often underreported because people do not remember all foods that were consumed over a certain time span and are unable to relay portion sizes accurately, and because of social desirability bias (i.e., when a person reports what they think is expected or correct dietary intake rather than actual intake) (41). Another strategy is to use food availability data, such as that reported by the U.S. Department of Agriculture, which can be adjusted for estimated losses due to food spoilage and plate waste (uneaten food). However, this is also not a direct measure of dietary intake. Regardless of the methodology used, data consistently indicate that total energy intake in the United States has increased over recent decades. For instance, national data comparing 1971 with 2000 show that the self-reported daily caloric intake of U.S. adults increased by 168 kcal · day^{-1} for men and 335 kcal · day^{-1} for women (54), whereas estimated intake from food availability data indicates a 23% increase from 1970 to 2010 (15). The increase in caloric intake has been linked to Americans consuming more food away from home; larger portion sizes; and increased salty snacks, caloric soft drinks, and pizza (39, 40). Thus, it is clear that increased caloric intake, which is due in part to greater availability of highly caloric and appetizing foods, has contributed to increased obesity rates.

Energy Expenditure From Physical Activity

In addition to increased caloric intake, daily physical activity is another part of the energy balance equation.

Daily energy expenditure is comprised of basal metabolic rate, which accounts for the majority of energy expenditure; thermic effect of food, which is the energy expenditure associated with food digestion and nutrient absorption; and physical activity, which is the most variable component. Physical activity can consist of activities of daily living (such as walking the family dog or performing housework), commuting (bike commuting expends more energy than driving in a car); work-related physical activity (sitting at a computer or working manual labor); and discretionary physical activity or planned, structured exercise. When examining changes to physical activity energy expenditure over time, it is important to consider these multiple components and how changes to different categories can influence total daily energy expenditure and weight changes over time. For example, Amish adults who live an active life that is similar to what was typical in the late 19th century have much lower rates of obesity compared with the average American (4). Furthermore, data looking at the energy expenditure associated with jobs in the 1960s compared to more recent data show that almost half of the jobs in the 1960s required moderate-intensity physical activity, whereas only about 20% do today (10). This change in occupational energy expenditure requirements represents a decrease of approximately 140 calories per day and helps explain the increased rise of obesity in modern-day society. While it may be assumed that discretionary, or leisure-time, physical activity also has decreased, data from the Centers for Disease Control and Prevention (CDC) indicate that over recent years small increases have been observed in the proportion of adults who report engaging in leisure-time physical activity or meeting the recommendations found in the *Physical Activity Guidelines for Americans* (49). While this is encouraging, the increase has not been sufficient to offset an increased caloric intake and decreases in other components of physical-activity energy expenditure.

Research consistently shows a relationship between low levels of physical activity and an increased likelihood of weight gain and development of obesity (16). For example, women who walk more daily have a lower BMI, WC, and %BF compared with women who are less active (24, 25, 46). Because these are cross-sectional studies, it is impossible to say whether low physical activity leads to obesity or obesity causes people to reduce their activity levels. However, longitudinal data also provide insight into how physical activity influences body weight long term. The longitudinal CARDIA study has shown that adults who maintain active lifestyles over a 20-year period gain significantly less weight and add fewer inches to their waists (22). Similar data exist in large cohort trials from other countries (7, 12, 21), thus strengthen-

ing the evidence base for the role of physical activity in preventing weight gain and obesity. In summarizing the evidence on weight gain prevention, the 2018 *Physical Activity Guidelines for Americans* recommend achieving at least the general level of activity recommended for adults: 150 minutes per week of moderate-intensity physical activity for preventing weight gain, though more may be needed for some individuals (49). Additionally, while muscle-strengthening exercises also are recommended for all adults (two times per week training all major muscle groups), evidence is insufficient regarding the impact of resistance exercise alone on preventing weight regain for recommendations to be made.

KEY POINT

> The prevalence of obesity is high in the United States, with over 40% of adults classified as obese. Both genetics and lifestyle factors contribute to obesity. Fitness professionals must emphasize the capacity clients have to affect body weight, even if genetics may predispose them to obesity. Both energy intake (diet) and energy expenditure (physical activity and exercise) are factors in body-weight management.

Achieving and Maintaining Weight Loss

For adults with overweight and obesity seeking weight loss, the fitness professional first should conduct a complete and thorough health history and fitness assessment (see chapters 2 and 24). If necessary, approval from the client's primary medical care provider should be received prior to exercise testing or prescription. If weight loss is indicated and deemed to be safe, the fitness professional can provide the following guidance, within their professional scope of practice. Overall, achieving weight loss requires creation of a negative energy balance, which can be created through a combination of decreased caloric intake (via dietary changes) and increased energy expenditure (via physical activity).

ACSM recommends that weekly weight-loss goals should target a loss of 1 to 2 pounds (0.45 to 0.9 kilograms) (28). A general guideline is to establish a caloric deficit of 3,500 to 7,000 $kcal \cdot wk^{-1}$ (500-1,000 $kcal \cdot day^{-1}$), which theoretically results in a 1- to 2-pound loss (0.45-0.9 kilogram) of fat each week. (This assumes that 1 pound of fat = 3,500 kcal, though this is not a completely accurate statement. See the sidebar *Is a Pound of Fat Really 3,500 Calories?*)

Is a Pound of Fat Really 3,500 Calories?

While it is true that the energy content of 1 pound (0.45 kilogram) of fat mass is very close to 3,500 kcal (23), weight loss (or gain, for that matter) is not limited to fat mass only. Individuals also experience changes to lean mass, water, and glycogen content with changes in weight. Weight loss will fluctuate with time on a diet, and the 3,500 kcal per pound is an estimate rather than a rule. Many factors come into play regarding energy balance (see figure 20.3). Energy expenditure is not a static but rather a dynamic process (34). As weight is lost, energy needs to maintain that new body weight are also lower, which leads to a blunting of weight loss with a continued energy deficit. A helpful tool for determining rate of weight loss that is based on this dynamic model is the NIH Body Weight Planner (20), found at www.niddk.nih.gov/health-information/weight-management/body-weight-planner. Learners interested in more information on this topic are encouraged to access the article "Rethinking Energy Balance: Facts You Need to Know About Weight Loss and Management" (34). Research continues to provide a greater understanding of energy balance (including how physical activity contributes), and fitness professionals need to seek out evidence-based information in order to support their clients.

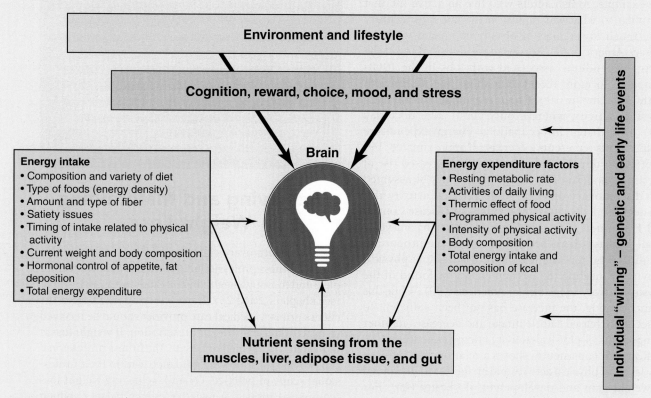

FIGURE 20.3 Key factors regulating and influencing energy balance.

Reprinted by permission from M.M. Manore, "Rethinking Energy Balance: Facts You Need to Know About Weight Loss and Management," *ACSM's Health & Fitness Journal* 19, no. 5 (2015).

Physical Activity and Exercise

Typically, standard testing modes and protocols can be used when testing people with higher body weights (see chapters in part III). As with any client, protocols, intensities, and modality should be determined based on individual fitness, ambulatory capacity, and habitual physical activity. However, the fitness professional should be sure to provide an environment that is comfortable and safe for adults in larger bodies. This includes having chairs that are large enough for clients to sit in, scales with a large enough measurement range, and enough room between exercise equipment machines for clients to move.

Regular physical activity is a strategy to prevent weight regain. It is also a strategy recommended to achieve and maintain weight loss. While at least 150 minutes of moderate-intensity physical activity per week is recommended for general health and prevention of weight gain, participation in this volume of physical activity produces no to minimal weight loss (16). To achieve weight loss, higher volumes of moderate-intensity physical activity are recommended, and a dose–response relationship is observed for increasing levels of physical activity resulting in greater weight loss. It is important for fitness professionals to communicate to their clients the amount of weight loss they can expect for a given amount of physical activity. While individual outcomes vary, in general, the following weight-loss amounts can be expected (16):

- *Physical activity >150 minutes per week:* Modest weight loss of 2 to 3 kilograms
- *Physical activity >225 to 420 minutes per week:* Weight loss of 5 to 7.5 kilograms

Resistance training is recommended within a complete exercise program even though evidence does not support resistance training as effective for weight loss. However, resistance training may maintain or increase lean mass during weight loss, which could prevent reductions in basal metabolic rate.

While weight loss is possible with increased physical activity, results typically are greater when combined with caloric restriction. Pharmacotherapy or bariatric surgery approaches can result in more significant weight loss (see the sidebar *Pharmacological and Surgical Weight Management Options* later in the chapter).

In addition to weight loss, exercise has been shown to be important for weight-loss maintenance. The majority of the scientific evidence on this topic comes from cross-sectional or observation trials and therefore limits researchers' ability to make causal inferences. However, recommendations from ACSM for preventing weight regain following weight loss are for adults to achieve >250 minutes per week of moderate-intensity physical activity (16). Data from the National Weight Control Registry (NWCR) have provided information regarding habits of adults who successfully lose and maintain weight loss, supporting the value of physical activity along with dietary changes (52).

The NWCR was established in 1994 to provide insight into ways that people successfully lose weight and then maintain weight loss (52, 53). Approximately 5,000 people participate in the NWCR, with an average weight loss of 30 kilograms maintained for 5.5 years. About half of these participants used commercial weight-loss programs, whereas the others lost weight without formal guidance. Several interesting details have been gathered from these successful long-term weight-loss maintainers (8):

- The vast majority (>85%) used exercise in their weight-loss programs.
- The most common dietary approach involved choosing a diet low in total calories and low in fat (<25% of calories from fat).
- Most participants weighed themselves frequently to provide feedback on the success of their behaviors.
- A typical exercise routine was 1 hour per day of moderate physical activity (about 420 minutes per week).
- Walking was the most frequently reported exercise (slightly over 80% of participants), while about 29% also used resistance training (only about 8% used resistance training as their only activity).

Additionally, an overwhelming majority (>90%) of NWCR participants report that their weight loss has been associated with higher energy levels, better mobility, improved mood, higher self-confidence, and overall better quality of life (52). For more information on the registry, visit the NWCR website (www.nwcr.ws).

KEY POINT

Engaging in physical activity and exercise can help participants achieve and maintain weight loss, especially when combined with dietary changes. A dose–response relationship exists wherein increasing levels of physical activity result in greater weight loss.

Dietary Aspects

Whether planning individualized programs for weight loss or weight maintenance, it is helpful to know the number of calories the client needs to sustain their current body weight. This can be done by estimating daily caloric need. Daily caloric need is the number of calories a person needs to sustain current body weight, assuming that activity levels remain constant. The resting metabolic rate, thermic effect of food, and energy expended by daily activities determine the daily caloric need (figure 20.4).

Resting metabolic rate (RMR) is the number of calories expended to maintain the body during resting conditions. For most people, RMR is 60% to 70% of their daily caloric need. For people who engage in regular, vigorous exercise, the RMR may account for a smaller proportion of daily caloric need because the energy requirements of exercise account for a larger percentage. RMR can be

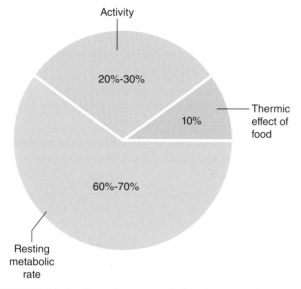

FIGURE 20.4 Contributors to daily caloric need.

measured in a laboratory using indirect calorimetry. To measure RMR accurately, assess the client when they have not eaten for several hours; have not exercised vigorously for the past 12 hours; and have been in a resting, reclined position for 30 minutes (35). Because of the cost of indirect calorimetry and the strict control needed to obtain accurate results, measuring RMR is not always practical; therefore, a number of equations have been developed to predict RMR. These RMR equations are based on the following principles:

- RMR is proportional to body size.
- RMR decreases with age.
- Muscle is more metabolically active than fat.

The larger the body, the more calories needed to sustain it. This relationship is reflected in all RMR equations. In addition to body size, age significantly affects RMR. As a person ages, RMR decreases, meaning that the daily caloric need decreases with age. Generally, RMR equations are sex specific because males often have more fat-free mass than females have, and fat-free mass requires more energy compared with fat tissue.

If a client's fat-free mass is known, the following equation can be used to predict RMR (11). When fat-free mass is known, sex-specific equations are not needed, because a gram of muscle has the same metabolic need whether it resides in a male or female body.

$$\text{RMR (kcal} \cdot \text{day}^{-1})$$
$$= 370 + (21.6 \times \text{fat-free mass in kilograms})$$

When determining daily caloric need, an estimate of the calories burned in physical activity is needed. This assessment requires information about work and leisure activity. Although there are numerous ways to gather information about daily activity, one typical method is an activity log in which the client records work and leisure activity. Once the activity pattern is established, the caloric cost of various activities can be calculated and used to estimate the energy burned in activity (see chapter 6). Estimating this energy is especially important if working with a client who trains extensively (see chapter 16 for concerns that may arise when energy intake is insufficient to meet requirements for daily living and growth as well as for physical activity and exercise). Alternatively, you can estimate daily caloric need by using the methods outlined in the sidebar *Calculating Daily Energy Needs*.

Calculating Daily Energy Needs

The Institute of Medicine recommends the following equations for calculating a person's daily caloric need, or estimated energy requirement (EER) (48). These formulas require the client's age in years, height in meters, weight in kilograms, and level of physical activity (PA).

Adult Man

$$\text{EER} = 661.9 - 9.53(\text{age}) + \text{PA} \times [15.91(\text{weight}) + 539.6(\text{height})]$$

Adult Woman

$$\text{EER} = 354.1 - 6.91(\text{age}) + \text{PA} \times [9.36(\text{weight}) + 726(\text{height})]$$

PA reflects a person's level of daily physical activity. Use the following table to choose the appropriate PA value.

Activity Level	PA Value (Men)	PA Value (Women)
Sedentary: Extremely limited activity	1.0	1.0
Low active: Typical activities of daily living only	1.11	1.12
Active: Regular moderate physical activity	1.25	1.27
Very active: Regular vigorous exercise	1.45	1.45

The smallest part of the daily caloric need comes from the thermic effect of food. This is the energy needed to digest, absorb, transport, and store the food that is eaten. Although this value may vary slightly depending on the food eaten, the thermic effect of food typically accounts for 10% of the daily caloric need (36).

Scope of Practice

It is important to remember that fitness professionals are not Registered Dietitians and as such should not provide medical nutrition therapy to clients (see discussions on scope of practice in chapters 5 and 24). Fitness professionals should only provide information based on established nutrition guidelines, such as the *Dietary Guidelines for Americans* (50). For clients with specialized dietary needs or chronic medical conditions, the fitness professional should refer clients to a Registered Dietitian. Additionally, interventions provided by a Registered Dietitian have been shown to result in greater weight loss than interventions not provided by a Registered Dietitian (37); therefore, these individuals are a valuable member of an interdisciplinary health care team.

Recommended Dietary Changes

The *2020-2025 Dietary Guidelines for Americans* highlights the importance of dietary patterns for health promotion rather than a focus on inclusion or avoidance of any individual foods (50). Healthy weight management–focused diets differ for each individual based on dietary preferences, cultural considerations, budgetary needs, and time and resources available for food procurement and preparation. Therefore, fitness professionals should avoid prescribing set nutrition plans and instead should provide general guidelines based on the above considerations for each client. The core elements of a healthy dietary pattern include all types of vegetables, fruits (especially raw), grains (at least half of which are whole grains), dairy (if tolerated), protein foods (including both animal and plant-based sources), and oils, which are consumed at appropriate calorie levels.

In order to assist clients in creating appropriate caloric reductions, it likely is beneficial for clients to keep food records (see chapter 5) so that current dietary habits and caloric intake can be determined. From there, modifications that are in line with the *Dietary Guidelines for Americans* can be made. Additionally, increasing intake of dietary fiber (such as from vegetables, fruits, and whole grains) and protein may increase satiety, which is important for adherence to caloric reduction. For example, across a day, the following dietary modifications will result in consuming approximately 250 fewer calories per day, 4.6 additional grams of fiber, and 3 additional grams of protein.

- *Breakfast:* Switching from 1.5 cups of whole milk (240 calories) to 1.5 cups of 1% milk (165 calories) in cereal will decrease calories by 75.
- *Morning snack:* Trading a granola bar (190 calories, 2 grams of fiber, 3 grams of protein) for an apple (95 calories, 4.4 grams of fiber) and hard-boiled egg (78 calories, 6 grams of protein) will result in a decrease of 17 calories and an increase of 2.4 grams of fiber and 3 grams of protein.
- *Lunch:* No changes.
- *Dinner:* Reducing the serving size of instant white rice from 1 cup (cooked; 340 calories, 0 grams fiber) to 1/2 cup (cooked; 170 calories, 0 grams fiber) and increasing the serving size of broccoli from 1/2 cup (15 calories, 1.1 grams fiber) to 1 cup (30 calories, 2.2 grams fiber) will result in a reduction of approximately 155 calories and an increase of 2.2 grams of fiber.
- Evening snack: No changes.

Pharmacological and Surgical Weight Management Options

In recent years, new anti-obesity medications have been developed that are classified as *nutrient-stimulated hormone therapies*, which have been shown to be highly effective for weight loss. These include semaglutide (a GLP-1 receptor agonist) and tirzepatide (a combined GIP/GLP-1 receptor agonist), which have been shown in clinical trials to result in weight loss of 12% to 15% body weight. Interested readers are encouraged to read Malik and colleagues (33) for more information. For individuals with extreme obesity (BMI >40 kg · m^{-2}) who have been unsuccessful in previous weight-loss attempts and who have serious comorbid conditions, bariatric surgery may be an option (43). A variety of surgical options exist, but all modify the gastrointestinal system so that food intake is restricted and nutrient uptake is diminished. These procedures often lead to significant weight loss, but they also can have a number of serious side effects (32, 43). These surgeries require major modifications in eating patterns. Once patients recover from surgery, exercise programming is recommended. The dietary planning and exercise programming for these patients should be overseen by medical professionals.

Clearly, this example shows that small changes can add up to significant reductions in caloric intake. With a targeted caloric deficit of 500 calories per day for a client, these modest changes would account for 50% of the reduction, and an exercise prescription could be created to achieve the additional 250-calorie deficit. Additional changes also could be made to result in greater improvements, but large changes from clients' current dietary patterns often are not necessary.

KEY POINT

Daily caloric need reflects the number of calories needed to sustain a current weight and includes the resting metabolic rate, thermic effect of food, and energy expended by daily activities. Equations are available to estimate daily caloric need based on age, height, weight, and level of physical activity. Fitness professionals can promote healthy dietary patterns as provided in the *Dietary Guidelines for Americans*.

Strategies for Gaining Weight

While obesity is common in the United States and many other countries and thus weight loss is a large focus for fitness professionals, some people struggle to increase their body weight. Fitness professionals should encourage these individuals to accumulate fat-free mass rather than all-fat weight. This will necessitate adding resistance training to the exercise routine (see chapter 14). Various nutritional supplements are touted as guaranteed ways to increase muscle mass. However, even those who are training intensely need only about 1.5 grams of protein per kilogram of body weight (see chapter 5 for more information on protein requirements).

The following are tips for increasing weight over time. When individuals continually lose weight or struggle to gain weight, a physician should be consulted about the possibility of underlying conditions.

- Increase caloric intake by 200 to 1,000 kcal · day^{-1} by increasing the meal size, number of meals, or number of between-meal snacks.
- Increase the number of snacks consumed. While the majority should be from nutritious, nutrient-dense foods, clients also should be encouraged to work in some "less healthy" foods that they enjoy and are high in calories.

- Add resistance training to the daily routine. Weight training is an effective means for increasing fat-free mass.
- When training intensely, make sure each day to consume 1.5 grams of protein for each kilogram of body weight.

KEY POINT

Healthy nutritional choices should be part of any plan for weight gain. Additionally, resistance training is recommended to help increase muscle mass.

Eating Disorders and Disordered Eating

Certain conditions exist in which an eating pattern can have a serious negative effect on health. Eating disorders are clinically diagnosed conditions characterized by a persistent disturbance of eating or eating-related behavior that results in the altered consumption or absorption of food that significantly impairs physical health or psychosocial functioning, including even leading to death. Anorexia nervosa, bulimia nervosa, and binge-eating disorder are three of the eating disorders recognized by the American Psychiatric Association (APA) (3). *Disordered eating* refers to subclinical, unhealthy eating patterns that often are the precursors of eating disorders.

The prevalence of anorexia nervosa can be very challenging to determine accurately, because not all people seek treatment for this condition. In the United States, epidemiological studies indicate the prevalence of anorexia as defined by *DSM-5* (*Diagnostic and Statistical Manual of Mental Disorders*, fifth edition) to be 0.0% to 0.05% over a 12-month period, with higher rates in women than in men (up to 0.08% compared to 0.01%) (3) and the prevalence of bulimia nervosa to range from 0.14% to 0.3%, with women having higher rates than men (up to 0.5% compared to 0.1%) (3). However, when evaluating the overall lifetime prevalence of all eating disorders, it is estimated that among females, the lifetime prevalence is 8.6% compared to 4.07% for males, with "other specified feeding or eating disorders" (OSFED) being the most common (14). OSFED is a clinically significant disturbance of eating behavior where the symptoms do not fulfill the criteria for other eating disorders, such as anorexia nervosa or bulimia nervosa (14).

No single mechanism has been identified as the primary cause of disordered eating or eating disorders. It appears that genetic, psychological, and sociocultural factors may predispose a person to these conditions (3). In the United States, these conditions are most common in young women from middle and high socioeconomic environments and in female athletes in sports that emphasize extreme leanness (45). However, it is likely that eating disorders are underdiagnosed in other groups, such as men and people from lower socioeconomic backgrounds (5). It is hypothesized that the social pressure to be thin as well as discomfort with sexual development contribute to unhealthy eating patterns in young women.

In anorexia nervosa, a preoccupation with body weight leads to self-starvation. People with anorexia nervosa typically view themselves as overweight even when their weight is substantially below normal. The APA lists the following criteria for diagnosis of anorexia nervosa (3):

- Restriction of energy intake relative to requirements, leading to significantly low body weight in the context of age, sex, developmental trajectory, and physical health. *Significantly low weight* is defined as a weight that is less than minimally normal or, for children and adolescents, less than that minimally expected.

- Intense fear of gaining weight or of becoming fat, or persistent behavior that interferes with weight gain, even though at a significantly low weight.

- Disturbance in the way in which one's body weight or shape is experienced, undue influence of body weight or shape on self-evaluation, or persistent lack of recognition of the seriousness of the current low body weight.

Note that for individuals who are not underweight by population-based standards (i.e., a BMI of <18.5 kg · m^{-2}), a diagnosis of other specified feeding or eating disorder, such as atypical anorexia nervosa, may be considered if the other criteria are met.

Bulimia nervosa is characterized by recurrent episodes of binge eating, with an episode of binge eating defined as both:

- eating, in a discrete period of time (e.g., within any 20-hour period), an amount of food that is definitely larger than what most individuals would eat in a similar period of time under similar circumstances; and

- a sense of lack of control over eating during the episode (e.g., a feeling that one cannot stop eating or control what or how much one is eating).

Bulimia nervosa is also defined by recurrent inappropriate compensatory behaviors in order to prevent weight gain, such as self-induced vomiting; misuse of laxatives, diuretics, or other medications; fasting; or excessive exercise (3). To meet the diagnostic criteria established by the APA, a person must have engaged in this behavior at least once a week for 3 months. Patients with bulimia nervosa, similar to those with anorexia nervosa, have an impaired body image and fear losing control over their body weight. Both anorexia nervosa and bulimia nervosa should be considered life-threatening disorders.

Binge-eating disorder is characterized by consuming large amounts of food in a short time (3). Unlike bulimia nervosa, binge eating is not associated with purging. Binge episodes often are initiated by emotional or psychological cues (e.g., loneliness, anxiety) rather than by physical hunger. These binges typically occur when the person is alone and may be followed by shame, guilt, and depression. To be clinically diagnosed with binge-eating disorder, a person must engage in at least one binge per week for 3 months (3). The prevalence of binge-eating disorder in the general population has been estimated at 0.44% to 1.2%, with a lifetime prevalence of up to 2.8%, which is also higher in women than men (up to 3.5% compared to 2.0%). In contrast, approximately 30% of obese individuals seeking treatment for weight loss may have this disorder (13).

Recognizing the signs of disordered eating is necessary for successful intervention. Some common signs of disordered eating are listed in the sidebar *Common Symptoms of an Eating Disorder*. Fitness professionals who observe these signs should discuss the issue in a nonconfrontational manner with the client and provide resources and a referral to qualified health care professionals. Successful intervention for eating disorders requires a multidisciplinary approach combining medical, nutritional, and psychological professionals. Knowledge of local support groups or professionals who work with patients who have eating disorders will allow fitness professionals to recommend places for clients to receive help. For additional information and support for dealing with eating disorders, refer to the National Eating Disorders Association (www.nationaleatingdisorders.org) and the National Institute of Mental Health (www.nimh.nih.gov).

KEY POINT

Eating disorders can significantly impair health and may even result in death. Anorexia nervosa, bulimia nervosa, and binge-eating disorder are three eating disorders recognized by the APA. Intervention for eating disorders should be multidisciplinary and should include psychological counseling.

Common Symptoms of an Eating Disorder

Emotional and Behavioral

- In general, behaviors and attitudes that indicate that weight loss, dieting, and control of food are becoming primary concerns
- Preoccupation with weight, food, calories, carbohydrates, fat grams, and dieting
- Refusal to eat certain foods, progressing to restrictions against whole categories of food (e.g., no carbohydrates, etc.)
- Appears uncomfortable eating around others
- Food rituals (e.g., eats only a particular food or food group [e.g., condiments], excessive chewing, doesn't allow foods to touch)
- Skipping meals or taking small portions of food at regular meals
- Any new practices with food or fad diets, including cutting out entire food groups (no sugar, no carbs, no dairy, vegetarianism/veganism)
- Withdrawal from usual friends and activities
- Frequent dieting
- Extreme concern with body size and shape
- Frequent checking in the mirror for perceived flaws in appearance
- Extreme mood swings

Physical

- Noticeable fluctuations in weight, both up and down
- Stomach cramps, other non-specific gastrointestinal complaints (constipation, acid reflux, etc.)
- Menstrual irregularities—missing periods or only having a period while on hormonal contraceptives (this is not considered a "true" period)
- Difficulties concentrating
- Abnormal laboratory findings (anemia, low thyroid and hormone levels, low potassium, low white and red blood cell counts)
- Dizziness, especially upon standing
- Fainting/syncope
- Feeling cold all the time
- Sleep problems
- Cuts and calluses across the top of finger joints (a result of inducing vomiting)
- Dental problems, such as enamel erosion, cavities, and tooth sensitivity
- Dry skin and hair, and brittle nails
- Swelling around area of salivary glands
- Fine hair on body (lanugo)
- Cavities, or discoloration of teeth, from vomiting
- Muscle weakness
- Yellow skin (in context of eating large amounts of carrots)
- Cold, mottled hands and feet or swelling of feet
- Poor wound healing
- Impaired immune functioning

Reprinted by permission from "Warning Signs and Symptoms," NEDA, accessed April 17, 2023, www.nationaleating disorders.org/warning-signs-and-symptoms.

20

LEARNING AIDS

REVIEW QUESTIONS

1. What is the current obesity prevalence for U.S. adults? How does this compare to the past?

2. Why did the American Medical Association decide to classify obesity as a disease? Do you agree or disagree with that decision? Explain your response.

3. Define *positive caloric balance*. Does it lead to weight loss or weight gain?

4. What roles do genetic factors play in the development of obesity?

5. What three factors contribute to the daily caloric need?

6. What is the standard recommendation for daily caloric deficit when attempting weight loss?

7. Why is exercise important for those who are attempting weight loss or maintenance?

8. What is the National Weight Control Registry (NWCR)? What useful information has been obtained from this resource?

9. Explain strategies for healthy weight gain.

10. List the signs of disordered eating.

CASE STUDIES

1. Mr. Fitz is a 46-year-old male who comes to your facility for an initial fitness evaluation. He informs you that the primary motivation for him to come in to see you is because he has gained 30 pounds (13.6 kilograms) over the past 5 years and would like to lose the additional weight. He is 6 feet in height (182.9 centimeters) and currently weighs 220 pounds (100 kilograms). He owns his own florist business, which has expanded over the past several years and has resulted in him being less active due to increased managerial responsibilities involving more computer work. He would like your help to lose weight and also improve his overall fitness. He currently does not participate in any structured exercise.

   a. Calculate his estimated daily energy requirements.

   b. For him to lose approximately 1 pound (0.45 kilograms) a week through dietary changes alone, what caloric intake would be recommended?

   c. Assume Mr. Fitz begins a weekly exercise program in which he will walk (3.5 mph [93.8 m · min^{-1}]) for 30 minutes on 5 days per week. How many additional calories will this expend each day? (*Hint:* See chapter 6.) Describe the contribution this will make to weight loss.

2. Marsha is a 51-year-old female who comes to your fitness facility and expresses interest in purchasing a membership. She is responding to a series of advertisements that your facility is using to attract people interested in weight loss. Following completion of the informed consent and preparticipation screening questionnaire (PARQ+) and health screening questionnaire, you note the following:

   • Based on her self-reported height (5 feet 5 inches [165 centimeters]) and weight (240 pounds [109 kilograms]) her BMI is 40.0 kg · m^{-2}.

   • She has never exercised regularly, has a desk job, and has no active leisure pursuits.

   • It has been more than 3 years since she had a medical examination. At a recent biometric screening event she attended at work, her blood glucose levels were elevated, and she was instructed to follow up with her physician. She has not yet done this. Her blood pressure at the screening event was 148/86. Additionally, there is a history of heart disease on her father's side of the family, and her mother developed type 2 diabetes after menopause.

a. What, if any, medical screening and clearance do you recommend before this client enrolls in your facility's programs?

b. Assuming Marsha has medical clearance from her physician to begin an exercise program, describe steps that Marsha could take to achieve her weight-loss and fitness goals.

3. You have a new client, Kevin. He is a healthy, somewhat active 38-year-old man who is coming to you for advice on exercise and maintaining a healthy weight. Kevin's BMI is 25.5 kg · m^{-2}. He reports that over the past 2 years he has lost more than 75 pounds (34 kilograms) using a commercial weight-loss plan. He is beginning to feel diet burnout, and his weight has crept up 5 pounds (2.3 kilograms) over the past month. What exercise and other lifestyle advice would you provide?

Answers to Case Studies

1. Mr. Fitz's estimated daily energy requirements are as follows:

$$EER = 661.9 - 9.53(age) + PA \times [15.91(weight) + 539.6(height)]$$
$$EER = 661.9 - 9.53(46) + 1.11 \times [15.91(100) + 539.6(1.83)]$$
$$EER = 661.9 - 438 + 1.11 \times (1,591 + 987)$$
$$EER = 661.9 - 438 + 1.11 \times (2,578)$$
$$EER = 661.9 - 438 + 2,862$$
$$EER = 3,086 \text{ kcal} \cdot \text{day}^{-1}$$

a. His target intake is 2,586 kcal · day^{-1} (deficit of 500 kcal · day^{-1}) to lose approximately 1 pound per week in the initial stages of weight loss. Refer the client to a Registered Dietitian for specific dietary advice; small changes and substitutions as described earlier in the chapter can be used to promote the desired caloric deficit.

b. Using the ACSM metabolic equation for walking, the energy expenditure would be approximately 6.4 kcal · min^{-1} × 30 min · day^{-1} = 192 kcal · day^{-1}.

c. If Mr. Fitz engages in this activity 5 days per week, that will add up to 960 kcal · wk^{-1}, which will contribute to weight loss. As weight is lost, Mr. Fitz will require less calories per day to maintain his weight, and thus weight loss will plateau if additional exercise is not added.

2. For the case study of Marsha, consider the following:

a. Because Marsha has extreme (grade 3) obesity, is inactive, has a strong family history of cardiovascular disease and diabetes, and has not undergone a medical examination in several years, and a screening indicated she may have type 2 diabetes and hypertension, medical clearance, including blood work to determine if she has type 2 diabetes and verification of her resting blood pressure, is recommended before beginning an exercise program. The medical examination should reveal any underlying medical conditions that would make it unsafe for Marsha to begin exercising.

b. Assuming medical clearance by her health care provider is in place for Marsha, in addition to accurately measuring height and weight and calculating BMI, you could consider tracking waist circumference if Marsha is interested in that measurement. In place of waist circumference, you also could have her monitor clothing size over time as an informal indication of weight loss (i.e., clothing becomes loose).

A conversation with Marsha is crucial to determine her goals and interests. To increase adherence, close attention should be paid to her willingness to engage in various activities. Attempts should be made to increase lifestyle activity and begin structured exercise. Starting with low levels of activity will be important from both a physiological standpoint as well as in promoting self-efficacy and adherence to an exercise program. A gradual progression, realizing her current activity status (i.e., inactive), must be considered ("start low and go slow," see chapter 16).

Ultimately, a future goal would include exercising 6 days per week with an expenditure of 300 kcal of energy on each of these days. Assuming at that point that Marsha is willing to invest 1 hour a day, 3 days per week, in structured exercise and is willing to exercise on her own on other days, the following exercise program would contribute to a target weight loss of 1 to 2 pounds (0.45-0.9 kilograms) per week. Given that Marsha is inactive now, a gradual progressive program must be included to build up to this level of exercise over time.

The structured exercise should focus on improving cardiorespiratory fitness, strength, and flexibility. On 3 days per week, Marsha could walk on her own or preferably with an exercise partner for 1 hour (could be divided into shorter sessions). This increase in activity will increase her caloric expenditure by approximately 1,800 kcal $\cdot$ wk^{-1}.

Referral to a Registered Dietitian should be made for specific dietary modifications to help make reasonable and achievable dietary goals. While avoiding being too restrictive with diet (e.g., very low-calorie diet), she can target lowering caloric intake (e.g., deficit of 500-750 kcal $\cdot$ day^{-1}), which could be achieved by reducing or eliminating certain high-calorie items from her diet (e.g., packing a lunch lower in calories rather than eating at the deli, avoiding coffee drinks high in calories, using milk rather than cream in coffee, cutting out alcohol, not consuming soda pop or energy drinks).

Overall, the focus needs to be on lifestyle change and feeling better; healthy dietary changes and regular physical activity will need to become habits for a lifetime. The combination of caloric restriction and energy expenditure will support the goal of losing about 1 to 2 pounds (0.45-0.9 kilograms) per week. To better reflect dynamic energy balance, the NIH Body Weight Planner also can be used. Weekly weigh-ins and consultation with you are recommended in order to adjust the exercise program as needed. Additionally, because of Marsha's weight and potential for diabetes diagnosis, you could educate her about additional weight-management options available (pharmacotherapy and surgical options), which she should discuss with her doctor if interested.

3. For the case study of Kevin, do the following:

For Kevin's exercise goals, develop a plan that will allow him to accumulate 300 minutes per week in moderate-intensity exercise. Better yet, given that Kevin is healthy and young, discuss his willingness to spend at least some of his exercise time in vigorous exercise. Determine Kevin's exercise preferences and develop a program that meets aerobic recommendations and also addresses muscular fitness needs (resistance training 2 days per week) and flexibility training during cooldowns from all workouts.

For lifestyle goals, encourage Kevin to eat a well-rounded diet as described in chapter 5. He is at a fairly healthy BMI, so making weight loss a major consideration is unnecessary. However, for a person like Kevin, weight-loss maintenance can be a struggle. Therefore, encouraging him to do the following can be useful:

- Weigh himself each morning.
- Keep a journal of his food intake and exercise.
- Seek out a support system.

In the role as fitness professional, you will be an important part of his support system, but encourage him to seek out friends who can provide additional support and encouragement for his healthy eating and exercise habits.

Chronic Diseases

Barbara A. Bushman

OBJECTIVES

The reader will be able to do the following:

1. Quantify the magnitude of heart disease and stroke, cancer, pulmonary disease, diabetes, and osteoporosis as health problems in the United States and list risk factors for each
2. Describe the atherosclerotic process and the resulting outcome if blood flow becomes obstructed in the arteries of the heart or brain
3. Identify standards for hypertension and blood pressure responses during exercise that should result in test termination
4. Identify the various chronic diseases found in patients attending cardiac rehabilitation programs
5. Describe how exercise is prescribed in cardiac rehabilitation programs
6. Identify ways to decrease the risk of cancer, including the benefit of exercise in cancer prevention
7. Describe exercise considerations for individuals with cancer or for survivors following treatment
8. Define diabetes mellitus and describe the characteristics of type 1 and type 2 diabetes
9. Describe the role that exercise plays in the prevention and treatment of type 2 diabetes
10. Describe special considerations with exercise for clients with diabetes
11. Describe the differences between chronic obstructive lung diseases and restrictive lung diseases
12. Define the underlying physiological complications associated with asthma, emphysema, chronic bronchitis, and cystic fibrosis
13. Explain the dyspnea spiral
14. Describe various laboratory and field tests that can be used to assess a pulmonary patient's ability to exercise
15. Describe how exercise is prescribed in pulmonary rehabilitation programs
16. Describe osteoporosis and its risk factors
17. Describe how exercise is prescribed to promote bone health

21

Chronic diseases are defined by the Centers for Disease Control and Prevention as "conditions that last 1 year or more and require ongoing medical attention or limit activities of daily living or both" (19). In the United States, 6 in 10 adults have a chronic disease and 4 in 10 have two or more chronic diseases (19). Major chronic diseases include heart disease and stroke, cancer, and diabetes. This chapter will briefly review these chronic diseases as well as pulmonary disease and osteoporosis. This is not an all-inclusive list, and this chapter is not intended to be a comprehensive guide. Rather, this chapter provides general overviews of common chronic diseases that may be present in individuals with whom a fitness professional may interact. Other resources are available that provide more detail on various chronic conditions, including recommendations on exercise testing and prescription (6, 7). Fitness professionals need to familiarize themselves with risk factors for and characteristics of chronic diseases present in clients and be aware of precautions and considerations for each disease state to promote safety during physical activity. An awareness of the overlap in risk factors is also valuable (e.g., physical inactivity is a risk factor for heart disease, type 2 diabetes, and many cancers).

Heart Disease and Stroke

Cardiovascular diseases (CVD) are disorders of the heart and blood vessels and include diseases of blood vessels supplying the heart (coronary heart disease), brain (cerebrovascular disease), and arms and legs (peripheral vascular disease) as well as diseases due to rheumatic fever (rheumatic heart disease), malformation of the heart from birth (congenital heart disease), and blood clots that move from the leg veins to the heart and lungs (deep vein thrombosis and pulmonary embolism) (63). Globally, CVDs are the leading cause of death; when looking at deaths due to CVD, 85% resulted from heart attack and stroke (63). Heart attacks and strokes occur when blood flow is blocked to the heart or brain, most commonly because of atherosclerosis; strokes also can be caused by blood clots or bleeding from a blood vessel in the brain (63).

The underlying condition for heart disease and stroke is atherosclerosis, which is a specific type of arteriosclerosis; arteriosclerosis occurs when the arteries become stiff (as opposed to being typically flexible and elastic), restricting blood flow (10, 43). Atherosclerosis is the accumulation of plaque, or fatty deposits, in the arteries and is composed of cholesterol, fatty substances, cellular waste products, calcium, and a clotting material called fibrin (10). When plaque builds up, the wall of the blood vessel thickens, resulting in narrowing, which reduces

blood flow (10). Ischemia is when a lack of blood flow results in decreased oxygen delivery. Plaques also can split open (rupture), triggering the formation of blood clots, which can block blood flow up to 100%. Plaques or blood clots have the potential to break off and travel through the bloodstream, blocking another artery in a different location (57). If an artery is blocked to the heart, a heart attack (i.e., myocardial infarction) occurs; if an artery is blocked to the brain, a stroke occurs (10). Figure 21.1 depicts a normal artery compared to one with blockage due to atherosclerotic plaque.

Injury to the endothelium (inner lining of the artery) appears to be the initial cause of atherosclerosis. Injury may be brought about by physical stresses from turbulent blood flow (e.g., at branching points, especially when coupled with high blood pressure), inflammatory stresses (e.g., cigarette smoking), chemical abnormalities (e.g., elevated cholesterol or high blood glucose), or other causes of inflammation (57). Damage to the lining of arteries resulting from high blood pressure (BP) increases the susceptibility of plaque buildup, which in

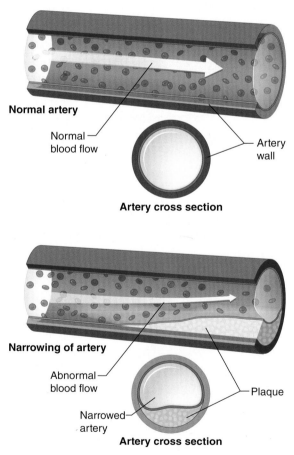

Normal artery

Normal blood flow

Artery wall

Artery cross section

Narrowing of artery

Abnormal blood flow

Narrowed artery

Plaque

Artery cross section

FIGURE 21.1 Normal artery and artery with atherosclerotic plaque buildup.

turn narrows the arteries to the heart and brain (19). Elevated low-density lipoprotein cholesterol (LDL-C) doubles the risk of heart disease; excess cholesterol can build up in the artery walls and thus limit blood flow (19). Diabetes is a chronic disease and is also related to heart disease and stroke because elevated blood glucose can damage blood vessels. Individuals with diabetes are twice as likely to have heart disease or stroke compared to those without diabetes (19). Physical activity is beneficial for each of these concerns, including lowering BP, promoting better lipid profiles, and reducing the risk of type 2 diabetes (60).

According to the Centers for Disease Control and Prevention, heart disease is the top leading cause of death in the United States and stroke is the fifth leading cause of death (19). Coronary heart disease affects about 20.1 million adults in the United States (59). In 2019, strokes were responsible for over 150,000 deaths (59). In an American Heart Association (AHA) update, the number of reported heart attacks per year was over 600,000 plus 200,000 recurrent (repeat) attacks for a total of over 800,000 events; the average age for a first heart attack was 65.6 for males and 72.0 for females (59). Based on incidence data, the AHA notes that an American will have a heart attack approximately every 40 seconds (59). Thus, an understanding of risk factors and a focus on prevention is important.

Risk factors for heart disease and stroke include high BP, high LDL-C, diabetes, smoking and/or secondhand smoke exposure, obesity, unhealthy diet, and physical inactivity (19). In 2022, the AHA released Life's Essential 8, a construct that includes key measures for improving and maintaining cardiovascular health. New to this defi-

nition is the addition of sleep as a component of heart health (34). The eight components include the following:

1. Diet
2. Physical activity
3. Nicotine exposure
4. Body mass index
5. Blood lipids
6. Blood glucose
7. Blood pressure
8. Sleep health

Taken together, with each component scored from 0 to 100 (with 100 representing what is considered optimal or ideal for that metric), a composite cardiovascular health score is generated (34). In an analysis using the AHA Life's Essential 8 score, the overall score for Americans was 64.7; lowest scores were identified for diet, physical activity, and body mass index (BMI) (35). This supports the importance of promoting healthy lifestyle behaviors related to nutrition and physical activity.

KEY POINT

Atherosclerosis can start early in life and leads to blockages in the arteries of the heart, brain, or peripheral muscles. If a blockage occurs in a coronary artery, myocardial ischemia or infarction (heart attack) result. The U.S. population experiences a high prevalence of such health problems.

Hypertension

Hypertension, or high BP, greatly increases the risk of heart disease and stroke. Beginning at 115/75 mmHg, CVD risk doubles for each increment of 20/10 mmHg (22). The definition of what constitutes high BP differs depending on the source and the circumstances under which the BP is measured. The Seventh Report of the Joint National Committee on Prevention, Detection, Evaluation, and Treatment of High Blood Pressure (JNC7) provides the following definitions:

- Hypertension: BP ≥140/90
- Stage 1 hypertension: Systolic blood pressure (SBP) of 140 to 159 mmHg or diastolic blood pressure (DBP) of 90 to 99 mmHg
- Stage 2 hypertension: SBP of ≥160 mmHg and DBP of ≥100 mmHg (22)

In 2017 the AHA and American College of Cardiology (ACC) updated their definition of hypertension to ≥130 mmHg for SBP and ≥80 mmHg for DBP (61). Categories of BP are noted in the table (BP is based on the average of two or more careful readings obtained at rest on two or more occasions) (61):

(continued)

Hypertension (continued)

BP category	SBP (mmHg)		DBP (mmHg)
Normal	<120	And	<80
Elevated	120-129	And	<80
Hypertension stage 1	130-139	Or	80-89
Hypertension stage 2	≥140	Or	≥90

*Individuals with SBP and DBP in two categories should be designated to the higher BP category.

Adapted by permission from P.K. Whelton, R.M. Carey, W.S. Aronow, et al. "CC/AHA/AAPA/ABC/ACPM/AGS/APhA/ASH/ASPC/NMA/PCNA Guideline for the Prevention, Detection, Evaluation, and Management of High Blood Pressure in Adults: A Report of the American College of Cardiology/American Heart Association Task Force on Clinical Practice Guidelines," *Hypertension* 71, no. 6 (2018): e13-e115.

It is estimated that 116 million people in the United States (47.3%) have hypertension (37), defined as a BP of 130/80 or higher. Lifestyle interventions focused on dietary patterns, nutrient intake, and physical activity are recommended for individuals with hypertension (24, 31). Antihypertensive drug treatment guidelines have been developed based on age and other factors (i.e., diabetes, chronic kidney disease); even with medication management, reinforcement of lifestyle interventions is important (31). Nonpharmacological interventions include dietary habits (i.e., heart-healthy diet, reduced intake of sodium and enhanced intake of dietary potassium, moderation in alcohol consumption for those who drink alcohol), weight loss for individuals who are overweight or obese, and increased physical activity (61). Reducing sodium intake has been shown to decrease SBP by 5 to 6 mmHg (61). Obesity is linked to hypertension, and research shows that SBP decreases about 1 mmHg for every 1-kilogram reduction in body weight (61). Physical activity has been shown to provide decreases in SBP of 5 to 8 mmHg for aerobic exercise (90-150 minutes per week at 65%-75% heart rate reserve), 4 mmHg for dynamic resistance exercise (90-150 minutes per week, 50%-80% 1-repetition maximum, 3 sets per exercise, 10 repetitions per set), and 5 mmHg for isometric resistance exercise (4 × 2-minute hand grip with 1 minute rest between exercises, 30%-40% maximum voluntary contraction, 3 sessions per week for 8-10 weeks) (61).

The American College of Sports Medicine (ACSM) recommends that individuals with hypertension that is not controlled or who have stage 2 hypertension should consult with their physician before starting an exercise program (6). In situations where an exercise test is warranted and is conducted for the purpose of developing an exercise prescription, maintaining the current use of antihypertensive medications is preferred (6). Understanding typical responses to medications is important (e.g., suppressed heart rate response with beta-blocker therapy and electrolyte imbalances with diuretic therapy) (6). See chapter 2 for information on common medications and potential impacts on heart rate (HR) and BP.

Exercise recommendations must be made with consideration of various factors, including level of BP control, antihypertensive medications (current status as well as side effects), other diseases that are present, and age (6). Use of both aerobic and resistance exercise is recommended, with daily engagement in aerobic training, resistance training, or a combination of aerobic and resistance training (6). Neuromotor exercise training and flexibility exercises also are recommended 2 to 3 days per week (6).

Fitness professionals need to be aware of special considerations when working with individuals with hypertension. BP response to exercise may be exaggerated even if resting BP is controlled with antihypertensive medications (6). Criteria to terminate an exercise test related to an exaggerated BP response include SBP of >250 mmHg or DBP of >115 mmHg (6). During exercise, a more conservative termination criteria has been suggested, maintaining a lower BP (<220/105 mmHg) (49). Other areas of attention include avoiding the Valsalva maneuver (holding breath while lifting weights) given the potential for elevated BP responses, dizziness, and fainting and ensuring an adequate cool-down following physical activity to avoid postexercise hypotension (drop in BP following exercise) (6).

Cardiac Rehabilitation Programs

Cardiac rehabilitation is a medically supervised secondary prevention program that has a multidisciplinary approach (4). One main aspect of cardiac rehabilitation is supervised exercise; additional areas may include nutrition, medication use, psychological support, and healthy lifestyle choices. Inpatient cardiac rehabilitation incorporates in-hospital assessment, mobilization, evaluation of readiness for physical activity, and development of a comprehensive plan following discharge (6). Educational offerings also are included related to lifestyle and risk factors for heart disease (6). This hospitalization phase is often referred to as Phase I (62) and is typically only a couple of days. Outpatient cardiac rehabilitation (Phase II) includes up to 36 sessions of monitored physical exercise that is individualized based on clinical assessments and exercise testing (62). Phase II is particularly valuable in supporting the development of healthy lifestyle habits. The maintenance phase (Phase III/IV) is intended to continue the lifestyle changes with minimal professional supervision (62) with the hope that these changes will be adopted by the patient for the rest of their lives.

Although benefits have been shown for cardiac rehabilitation programs, over 80% of eligible patients do not participate (58) for a wide variety of reasons including insurance restrictions, location of rehabilitation center, and time of day the program is offered. The potential use of nonclinical or home-based cardiac rehabilitation for low- to moderate-risk patients has been described in a recent scientific statement by major organizations (American Association of Cardiovascular and Pulmonary Rehabilitation, the AHA, and the ACC) as a way to expand opportunities for those with barriers to traditional hospital-based programming (58). This is an area in need of additional study to examine long-term impacts and safety with higher-risk patients, among other aspects of administration of such programs. Cardiac rehabilitation programs may be beneficial for a wide range of conditions, including individuals with current stable angina, a history of myocardial infarction (MI), coronary artery bypass graft surgery (CABG), percutaneous transluminal coronary angioplasty (PTCA) or coronary stenting, heart valve repair or replacement, heart or heart and lung replacement, heart failure, and others (4).

Angina pectoris refers to the pain attributable to ischemia of the heart muscle resulting from an occlusion of one or more of the coronary arteries. The pain occurs when the oxygen requirement of the heart (estimated by the double product, which is calculated by multiplying SBP by HR) exceeds a value that coronary blood flow can meet. The ischemia can be transient and may subside once the oxygen demand of the heart returns to normal. Although the term *chest pain* is often used, angina includes discomfort, often expressed as pressure in the chest. In addition to pain in the chest, discomfort also can occur in the shoulders, arms, neck, jaw, abdomen, or back.

MI patients have heart damage (death of ventricular muscle fibers) caused by the occlusion of one or more of the coronary arteries. The degree to which ventricular function is affected depends on the ventricular muscle mass that is permanently damaged. Individuals who have experienced an MI usually take medications (e.g., beta-blockers) to reduce the work of the heart and to control the irritability of the heart tissue so that dangerous arrhythmias (irregular heartbeats) do not occur. Generally, when these patients engage in regular exercise, they experience a training effect similar to that of people who have not had an MI, allowing them to do more exercise at a higher intensity before they experience anginal pain.

CABG patients have had surgery to bypass one or more blocked coronary arteries. In this procedure, a blood vessel (normally the saphenous vein extracted from the legs or the mammary artery in the chest) is sewn into existing coronary arteries above and below the blockage to reroute the blood flow (see figure 21.2). These patients benefit from systematic exercise training because most are deconditioned before surgery as a result of activity restrictions related to angina.

Some patients undergo an angioplasty procedure, PTCA, to open occluded arteries. In this procedure, the chest is not opened; instead, a balloon-tipped catheter (a long, slender tube) is inserted into the coronary artery, where the balloon is inflated to push the plaque back toward the arterial wall (see figure 21.3). These patients tend not to have as extensive coronary heart disease as those who undergo CABG. To help prevent reocclusion, intracoronary stents often are used to help keep the lumen of the coronary artery open. A stent is composed of a metal mesh that is inserted into the artery on a balloon catheter and positioned in the area of the obstruction. Some stents are designed to slowly release a drug that helps prevent restenosis; these are known as drug-eluting stents. The balloon is first inflated to increase the lumen size, and then it is deflated and pulled back while the stent remains embedded in the artery. Due to the risk of blood clotting in the stent, anticoagulation medication is indicated for a year or longer (41).

KEY POINT

Coronary heart disease may be treated by CABG, angioplasty, or intracoronary stent. Patients who have undergone these procedures, as well as other conditions, are candidates for a hospital-based cardiac rehabilitation program.

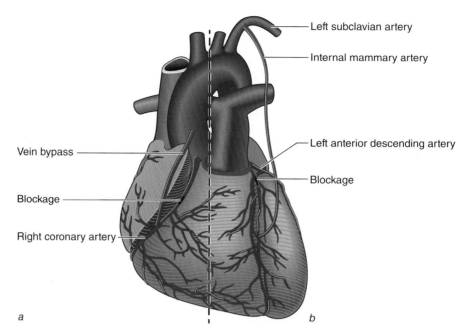

FIGURE 21.2 Coronary artery bypass surgery: *(a)* CABG using saphenous vein and *(b)* CABG using mammary artery. Blood flow is rerouted around the site of obstruction by taking a blood vessel from another part of the body and sewing it to the affected coronary artery, proximal and then distal to the site of the obstruction. Blood vessels typically used in the procedure are the saphenous vein (found in the leg) and the mammary artery located in the chest.

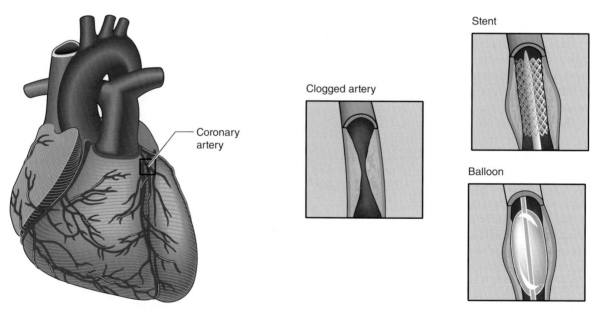

FIGURE 21.3 Percutaneous transluminal coronary angioplasty (PTCA). The cardiologist locates an obstructed section of a coronary artery by injecting a contrast dye into the artery, allowing it to be seen on an X-ray machine. A guide wire is inserted into a femoral artery (or in some cases the brachial artery) and is pushed up to the heart, where it is used to position the balloon catheter at the site of obstruction inside the coronary artery. The balloon is temporarily inflated, increasing the lumen size and capacity for blood flow. The balloon catheter is then deflated and removed. In some cases, a metal stent is placed inside the coronary artery to help keep it open. The stent is expanded by inflation pressure, and it remains inside the patient's artery

Exercise Considerations

With a focus on safety, exercise is not appropriate in some situations. ACSM has described contraindications for inpatient and outpatient cardiac rehabilitations including the following: unstable angina; uncontrolled hypertension (resting SBP of >180 mmHg and/or resting DBP of

>110 mmHg); orthostatic BP drop of 20 mmHg with symptoms; significant aortic stenosis; aortic dissection; acute systemic illness or fever; uncontrolled atrial or ventricular arrhythmias; uncontrolled sinus tachycardia (>120 bpm); uncompensated heart failure; third-degree AV block (without pacemaker); active pericarditis or myocarditis; recent embolism; acute thrombophlebitis; uncontrolled diabetes mellitus; severe orthopedic conditions; and other conditions such as thyroiditis, hypokalemia, or severe psychological disorders (6).

Inpatient programs typically focus on self-care, range of motion, postural changes (i.e., exposure to orthostatic or gravitational stress by sitting or standing), psychological support, and supervised walking while being monitored by electrocardiogram telemetry (6). When entering an outpatient program, a complete medical and surgical history should be reviewed, including recent testing procedures (e.g., electrocardiogram [ECG], stress test), risk factors, and current medications (6). Exercise testing is used to detect and evaluate the severity of coronary heart disease, evaluate physical capacity and effort tolerance before going home, and assessment response to medical therapy and interventions, among others (25). A scientific statement from the AHA provides exercise standards for testing and training (25).

Exercise prescription for outpatient cardiac rehabilitation follows typical recommendations for adults, with some considerations and modifications to reflect clinical status; risk factors; current capacity; threshold level for ischemia, angina, or other adverse events; and other limitations that may be experienced by individuals (6). Aerobic activity is recommended 3 to 5 days per week, resistance training 2 to 3 nonconsecutive days per week, and flexibility at least 2 to 3 days per week (daily is most effective) (6). As with any exercise recommendation, a warm-up and cool-down should be performed during each exercise session, including 5 to 10 minutes of light or very light aerobic activities and dynamic and static stretching (6). For those with angina, the exercise intensity should be at a HR of 10 bpm below the HR where any adverse event was noted (i.e., ECG changes indicating ischemia or other concerns such as arrhythmia). If exercise test results are not available, a rating of perceived exertion (RPE) can be used (<12 on the 6-20 RPE scale for light, 12-13 for somewhat hard, and 14-16 for hard; these correspond to <40% heart rate reserve [HRR], 40%-59% HRR, and 60%-80% HRR, respectively) (6). For more on relative exertion scales, see chapter 8.

Similarly, exercise programming should be adapted for individuals who have experienced a stroke (cerebrovascular accident) based on functional abilities, with a focus on helping the individual regain the ability to engage in activities of daily living; individuals should be medically stable before starting exercise therapy (6). Additional information related to testing and training considerations for individuals with heart disease and stroke, as well as individuals with heart failure, pacemakers or implantable cardioverter defibrillators, cardiac transplantation, and other cardiovascular conditions, is found in other sources (4, 6, 25, 38).

Cancer

In the United States, cancer is the second leading cause of death, with over 600,000 people dying from the disease in 2020 (39). An estimated 40 out of 100 men and 39 out of 100 women will develop cancer at some point in their lives (5). Cancer is a group of diseases that reflect uncontrolled growth and spread of abnormal cells (5). Various factors appear to contribute to an increased risk—some that cannot be modified (e.g., genetic mutations) and others that are potentially modifiable (e.g., tobacco use, physical activity, diet) (5).

Although some aspects cannot be controlled, many steps can be taken to reduce the risk of cancer, including avoiding tobacco use, maintaining a healthy body weight, consuming a healthy diet, avoiding or limiting alcohol, and being physically active (5). Smoking alone causes about 19% of cancers. The other four factors (body weight, diet, alcohol use, physical activity) account for over 18% of cancer cases and nearly 16% of cancer deaths (52). Physical activity and cancer prevention appear to have a linear relationship, with more exercise being beneficial (52). Generally, the 150 to 300 minutes per week as described in the *Physical Activity Guidelines for Americans* is supported, with over 300 minutes per week having potential greater benefit for the prevention of certain cancers (52).

Beyond the benefits of exercise in the prevention of many cancers, exercise is valuable after a cancer diagnosis, during the treatment phase, and into recent posttreatment or long-term survivorship (30). The 5-year relative cancer survival rate is 68% (53); in 2022 over 18 million cancer survivors were reported to be living in the United States (2). Exercise during cancer treatment has been found to be helpful in several aspects of quality of life and in the management of cancer or treatment side effects (e.g., anxiety, depression, physical function, lymphedema) (53). Medical evaluation is a key aspect in the development of a safe and effective exercise plan for individuals undergoing cancer treatment because modifications may be needed based on the type of cancer or issues related to treatment (53). Unique considerations include lymphedema (swelling due to blockage in lymphatic system), bone metastases (cancer spreading to bones), neuropathy (damage or dysfunction of nerves), and an opening in the skin called an *ostomy* (e.g., colostomy connects the colon to an opening in the abdominal wall) (53). Additionally, impacts on the immune system make prevention of infection a priority; fitness profes-

Situations Requiring a Referral During Cancer Treatment

To ensure an exercise program is safe requires attention to how the body responds and any other symptoms. Examples of reasons to refer to the individual's primary care physician include the following:

- Fever or signs of infection
- Extreme or unusual tiredness or unusual muscle weakness
- Irregular heartbeat, palpitations, or chest pain
- Leg pain or cramps, unusual joint pain or bruising, nosebleeds
- Pain not associated with an injury
- Sudden onset of nausea during exercise
- Disorientation, confusion, dizziness, light-headedness, blurred vision, fainting
- Rapid weight loss, severe diarrhea or vomiting
- Flare of lymphedema symptoms
- Change in appearance or feel of the cancer site
- Lump in the breast or groin
- Change in skin color or texture

Adapted from Irwin (2012); National Center on Health, Physical Activity and Disability (n.d.).

sionals need to provide a clean environment and must watch for fever, helping the individual gain medical care to avoid any progression toward serious infection or sepsis (30). Other symptoms that require consultation with the primary care physician include those shown in the sidebar *Situations Requiring a Referral During Cancer Treatment*.

Exercise Considerations

Much of the research related to the benefits of physical activity for individuals diagnosed with cancer is from studies of female breast cancer survivors and male prostate cancer survivors (30). Physical activity needs to be adapted to the type and site of cancer, type of treatments, and side effects (30). For individuals undergoing active treatment, typical exercise may need to be modified both in the short term (e.g., on treatment day or the days following a treatment session) as well as long term (i.e., cumulative effects of treatment may decrease tolerance to exercise) (6, 30).

For survivors following treatment, a gradual progression, rather than trying to return quickly to prediagnosis levels, is the key to a successful exercise plan (30). Allow for sufficient healing time following any surgical procedure. Because cancer can affect any individual regardless of age, and considering survivors are diverse in their health and fitness levels, no one exercise program will fit all situations and therefore should be individualized based on the needs of the patient (6, 30). A generalized exercise prescription for cancer survivors includes aer-

obic activity; resistance training of all the major muscle groups; and stretching, balance, and neuromotor exercises (6). An individualized exercise program should reflect prior exercise experience, current capabilities, and physical limitations due to the type of cancer and treatment procedure (6, 30). The fitness professional must account for many cancer-specific considerations including upper-extremity lymphedema, bone metastases, neuropathy, and presence of an ostomy (6). Exercise recommendations related to cancer types and health outcomes (e.g., fatigue, physical function, anxiety, depressive symptoms) are available based on the 2018 ACSM International Multidisciplinary Roundtable on Physical Activity and Cancer, a meeting that included 40 representatives from 20 organizations around the world (17). Fitness professionals must create customized programs, realizing that each individual's situation will differ. This includes monitoring for poor tolerance to training that necessitates adjusting the exercise dose, even if below recommended training volumes (17). Clearly, an exercise program for an individual cancer survivor must be adapted to address treatment-related side effects, metastatic disease, or other comorbidities (6). An example is shown in the case study, highlighting considerations for an individual following prostate cancer (see the *Prostate Cancer* case study). It is beyond the scope of this chapter to fully discuss all aspects. Excellent resources are available related to the value of physical activity in the cancer journey, along with adaptations to maximize safety when designing an exercise program (6, 17, 48, 53, 55).

CASE STUDY

Prostate Cancer

Case Study Contributor: Kerri Winters-Stone

Wendell is 75 years old. He was diagnosed with prostate cancer 10 years ago and had surgery called a *radical prostatectomy* to remove his prostate gland. The surgery resulted in a small amount of urinary stress incontinence and occasional bowel leakage but no other bothersome symptoms. About 2 years ago, Wendell was put on androgen deprivation therapy (ADT) because lab tests showed his prostate cancer might be coming back, but so far his cancer has not spread to any other distant organs (i.e., no metastases). As a result of the ADT treatment, he has lost some bone density and now has osteopenia in his hip and spine. His blood lipids show an elevated LDL cholesterol and triglycerides and borderline high fasting blood glucose. He has gained 20 pounds (9 kilograms) in the past 2 years but still has a reasonable BMI ($26 \text{ kg} \cdot \text{m}^{-2}$). Wendell's oncologist recommended that he get some regular exercise and cleared him to engage in a low- to moderate-intensity program. When he comes to you Wendell mentions that as soon as he started the ADT treatment, he began to experience hot flushes and night sweats that make it difficult for him to sleep well, causing him to feel tired a lot. He has also noticed that he has difficulty climbing up and down the stairs of his two-story house and it takes him longer to complete household chores. He fell a couple times in the past few months when getting up to go to the bathroom at night, but he only experienced bumps and bruises. He is feeling frustrated that he is not as strong and able as he used to be. His wife is worried about his falls and that he might break a hip. As a former college athlete, Wendell knows he should exercise to get back in shape but is worried about controlling his bladder and his bowels during exercise and does not want to go to a gym. His fatigue makes it difficult for him to be motivated to exercise, and he has not done much in several years. Using your knowledge about exercise in persons with cancer and in older adults, how would you explain how exercise might help with the problems Wendell is experiencing related to his cancer treatment, and how might you advise him on an exercise program that he can stick to?

You can explain to Wendell and his wife that there are solid studies and recommendations that exercise is safe and helpful for persons going through all types of cancer treatment, including ADT. Specifically, you mention that moderate amounts of aerobic and resistance exercise can help reduce his fatigue, restore muscle strength and balance, and help manage his weight and cardiovascular health (lipids and blood glucose). Based on the most recent exercise guidelines, just 30 minutes of moderate-intensity aerobic and resistance training done three times per week can help manage symptoms and side effects. He could do 2 days of walking and 1 day of strengthening exercise per week or do 3 sessions of 15 minutes aerobic exercise plus 15 minutes of strengthening exercise over a week. Given that he has experienced deconditioning with age and his cancer treatment, you encourage him to start slowly and progress gradually because that will increase the chances that he can successfully stick with exercise and work toward a long-term program. You empathize with his concerns about urine and bowel leakage during exercise and let him know that he could exercise safely in his own home, where he could easily access the bathroom and would not be worried about being embarrassed. You might consider taking Wendell through simple functional tests such as a sit-to-stand test, a grip strength test, and a walking or balance test to assess Wendell's exercise capacity and then recommend a beginning at-home program for him. Be sure to assess his environment for safety and fall risk and emphasize functional movements that will help Wendell perform his activities of daily living and household chores more easily. Since he will be exercising on his own at home, have him think about using digital apps or exercising with a friend or his wife to increase enjoyment and accountability. Exercising with a partner or friend also can be safer for older adults than exercising alone, in case an unexpected adverse event occurs.

Diabetes

Diabetes mellitus refers to group of metabolic diseases characterized by hyperglycemia (i.e., elevated plasma glucose). The criteria used to diagnose diabetes are fasting blood glucose levels, the blood glucose response to ingesting a specific amount of carbohydrate (i.e., oral glucose tolerance test), and hemoglobin A1C level (see table 21.1) (9). Hemoglobin A1C (i.e., glycated hemoglobin) is a measure of hemoglobin linking with glucose; greater amounts of glucose in the blood result in a higher percentage of hemoglobin A1C. The lifespan of red blood cells (where hemoglobin is found) is about 2 to 3 months, and thus hemoglobin A1C reflects the average glucose level for that period of time.

The cause of hyperglycemia varies depending on the form of diabetes present, with the most common forms being type 1 and type 2 diabetes (figure 21.4) (9). Type 1 diabetes is characterized by a deficiency of insulin often attributable to an autoimmune destruction of the insulin-producing beta cells located in the pancreas (9). Without insulin, the cells of the body are unable to absorb glucose. In type 2 diabetes, the insulin receptors on the cells of the body become insensitive or resistant to insulin. With type 2 diabetes, although insulin levels may appear normal or elevated, blood glucose is not normalized; this reflects a relative insulin deficiency and an inability to compensate for peripheral insulin resistance (9). In either type 1 or type 2 diabetes, blood glucose levels increase as the glucose is unable to be absorbed from the blood into the cells of the body. Although other forms of diabetes mellitus exist (e.g., gestational diabetes, which is discussed in chapter 19), type 1 and type 2 account for the majority of cases. Regardless of the type, a number of complications may result from diabetes. These complications typically affect the blood vessels and nerves and may include vision impairment, kidney disease, and CVD among others (9). The eco-nomic burden (direct and indirect costs) of diabetes in the United States in 2017 was estimated at $327 billion, an increase of 26% since 2012 after adjusting for inflation due to both increased prevalence and increased cost per individual with diabetes (8).

In the United States, 37.3 million people have diabetes (11.3% of the population), and 8.5 million of them are unaware that they have diabetes (21). Between 90% and 95% of these cases are type 2 diabetes (21). This form of diabetes has both lifestyle and genetic roots that may be modifiable. The risk of type 2 diabetes is increased with age, obesity, and lack of physical activity. Other risk factors include a family history of type 2 diabetes and belonging to certain racial or ethnic groups, including African American, Native American, Hispanic/Latino, and Asian American (9). Type 2 diabetes often

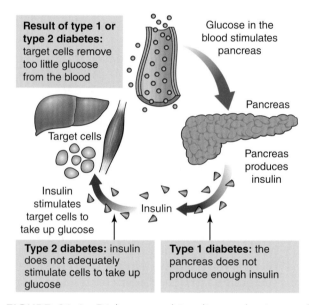

FIGURE 21.4 Diabetes and insulin production and function.

Table 21.1 Criteria for Diagnosis of Prediabetes and Diabetes

Prediabetes	*FPG*: 100 mg · dl⁻¹ (5.6 mmol · L⁻¹) to 125 mg · dl⁻¹ (6.9 mmol · L⁻¹)
	2-hour PG during 75-gram OGTT: 140 mg · dl⁻¹ (7.8 mmol · L⁻¹) to 199 mg · dl⁻¹ (11 mmol · L⁻¹)
	A1C: 5.7%-6.4% (39-47 mmol/mol)
Diabetes	*FPG*: ≥126 mg · dl⁻¹ (7.0 mmol · L⁻¹)
	2-hour PG during OGTT: ≥200 mg · dl⁻¹ (11.1 mmol · L⁻¹)
	Random PG: ≥200 mg · dl⁻¹ (11.1 mmol · L⁻¹) (in patient with symptoms of hyperglycemia or hyperglycemic crisis)
	A1C: ≥6.5% (48 mmol/mol)

FPG = fasting plasma glucose (no caloric intake for at least 8 hours); PG = plasma glucose; OGTT = oral glucose tolerance test using 75-gram glucose load; A1C = hemoglobin A1C

Data from American Diabetes Association (2023).

and frequently coexists with other conditions such as hypertension and dyslipidemia (9). Although type 2 diabetes can appear at any age, the highest rates are seen among people 45 years of age and older (21). However, there is increasing prevalence of type 2 diabetes among children (9).

Type 2 diabetes typically is characterized by insulin resistance, a condition in which the body's insulin receptors no longer respond normally (9). As a result, glucose entry into cells is impaired and hyperglycemia results. Plasma insulin levels of people with type 2 diabetes may be normal, suppressed, or elevated depending on the individual. Regardless, type 2 diabetes is considered a disease of relative insulin deficiency because the insulin available is inadequate to maintain normal glucose concentrations. Although some people with type 2 diabetes can control their disease through exercise and weight loss, others require medications such as oral hypoglycemic agents and possibly insulin injections.

Type 2 diabetes usually develops over time, first appearing as impaired fasting glucose (100-125 mg · dl⁻¹) or impaired glucose tolerance (IGT). IGT is a condition in which the increase in blood glucose after ingestion of a carbohydrate is higher than normal and remains elevated longer than normal. A glucose level of 140 to 199 mg · dl⁻¹ 2 hours after an oral glucose tolerance test indicates IGT. Examples of normal and abnormal blood glucose responses are shown in figure 21.5. A person with either impaired fasting glucose or IGT is classified as having prediabetes (9). Prediabetes is not considered a clinical entity but rather a risk factor for progression to diabetes (9). Without intervention, prediabetes generally

evolves into type 2 diabetes over time. It is estimated that 96 million Americans have prediabetes (21).

Approximately 1.9 million Americans have type 1 diabetes (21). Unlike type 2 diabetes, type 1 diabetes often appears earlier in life. People with type 1 diabetes require exogenous insulin injections as β-cells, which normally produce insulin, are destroyed (9). There are many types of exogenous insulin, and they vary by how rapidly they begin working, their peak time of action, and how long they continue to function (see chapter 2 for insights on insulin types). Some people with type 2 diabetes also require insulin injections depending on their responses to lifestyle modifications and oral medications. More often, individuals with type 2 diabetes take other types of prescription medications to lower blood glucose. Many types of medications are used for this purpose (see chapter 2). For more information on diabetes mellitus, see the websites of the American Diabetes Association (ADA) (www.diabetes.org) and the National Institute of Diabetes and Digestive and Kidney Diseases (NIDDK) (www.niddk.nih.gov/health-information/diabetes).

KEY POINT

Diabetes mellitus is characterized by hyperglycemia (elevated blood glucose). Type 1 diabetes results from a lack of insulin production. Type 2 diabetes, the most common form of diabetes, is characterized by the cells of the body becoming insensitive to insulin. Risk factors for type 2 diabetes include older age, a family history of type 2 diabetes, excess weight, and physical inactivity.

Exercise Considerations

Exercise can provide many benefits to individuals with type 1 or type 2 diabetes. Unfortunately, people with diabetes are less likely to meet recommended levels of physical activity compared their nondiabetic peers (64). Of particular encouragement is that regular exercise has the potential to prevent or delay the development of type 2 diabetes (23). See the *Prediabetes and Lifestyle Modifications* case study, which shows approaches to promoting activity. Although exercise will not prevent or cure type 1 diabetes, exercise should be encouraged in this population as well. Aerobic exercise can lower CVD risk in both type 1 and type 2 diabetes as well as reduce insulin resistance, among many other typical benefits of exercise (23). Resistance training benefits are the same as those for any adult, including improved muscle mass and strength, body composition, physical function, bone

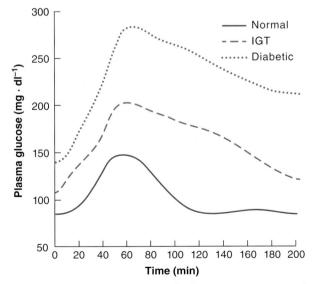

FIGURE 21.5 Comparison of glucose response with carbohydrate ingestion.

CASE STUDY

Prediabetes and Lifestyle Modifications

Case Study Contributor: Sheri R. Colberg

Patrick is 66 years old and has elevated BP levels that are mostly controlled with a combination of antihypertensive medications. A bigger concern is that his recent blood work during a routine annual examination revealed that his A1C (a measure of his average blood glucose over the prior 2-3 months) is 6.2%, which is at the higher end of the prediabetes range (5.7%-6.4%). His current A1C puts him at high risk for developing type 2 diabetes. Both his sister (age 65) and a maternal aunt have type 2 diabetes, so he has a family history of it. At that appointment, his BMI was 37.7 kg · m^{-2} and most of his excess weight is in his abdominal region. His family medicine physician recommended that he "get more exercise and lose some weight" but failed to give him any specific guidance on how to be more active and lose fat weight safely and effectively. In the past, he used to exercise on his own—starting and stopping various commercially available workout programs a handful of times over the past 2 decades. His prior workouts focused on strength, plyometric, cardio, and abs/core work. He knows he needs more help this time since he cannot find the time or motivation to change his lifestyle enough on his own. However, he lives in a small town in a rural area and works long hours with frequent overtime, and his options for getting help are somewhat limited. Plus, although he packs his lunches, he tends to rely on vending machines for sugary snacks throughout his work shift. One benefit of his job is that he is on his feet frequently and takes many steps during each 12-hour shift he works, but his long hours make him feel less like doing anything physically active on his infrequent days off from work. Using your knowledge about exercise in persons with diabetes or prediabetes, especially older adults, how would you explain how exercise and other lifestyle changes might help Patrick lower his A1C and prevent the onset of type 2 diabetes, and how might you advise him on starting an exercise program that he can stick with this time?

You can explain to Patrick that many studies have shown that it is possible to prevent or delay the onset of type 2 diabetes—and even likely reverse prediabetes—with appropriate lifestyle changes, including regular physical activity of various types. You mention that the same guidance related to aerobic and resistance exercise for adults in general can work to manage blood glucose levels and prevent type 2 diabetes. Specifically, mention that he should aim to get at least 150 minutes of moderate aerobic exercise each week but that doing harder (vigorous) exercise may not be advisable unless his BP remains well controlled and he continues to take his BP medications. Let him know that for diabetes prevention, he should try to exercise at least every other day because frequent physical activity helps use stored carbohydrates in muscles (glycogen) and keep insulin sensitivity higher. This means that his body will be better able to appropriately store any carbohydrates that he eats in his "muscle storage tank" for glucose, which will keep his blood glucose levels lower. Lifestyle activity is important both for weight management and diabetes control and prevention, but he also can greatly benefit from doing more structured exercise. Even though Patrick gets plenty of unstructured daily steps at a low intensity while at work (a great activity to use up calories), you also suggest that he take a brisk walk for 15 minutes during some of his breaks during his workdays or a 30-minute walk on his free days to try to reach the goal of 150 minutes per week of moderate aerobic activity. For diabetes prevention, it is equally important for him to do some type of resistance workouts at least 2 days per week—but preferably 3 days per week—and those workouts can be done easily at home, or even at work during breaks, using body-weight exercises. Instruct him on how to do exercises such as wall sits, wall or regular push-ups, lunges, squats, planks, and others, either in a circuit that he repeats two to three times for 20 to 30 minutes total or one at a time as he can fit each one in during the day. Mention that for someone his age, it is also important to stretch regularly and add in some balance exercises (even simple ones such as practicing standing on one leg at a time). As far as other lifestyle changes are concerned, mention that he may want to limit how much candy he consumes from vending machines on workdays, because taking in excess refined sugar and carbohydrates may elevate his risk of developing type 2 diabetes and add on more excess body fat. Encourage him instead to find healthier snack alternatives that may be more filling and less likely to raise his blood glucose, such as an apple and small handful of nuts.

mineral density, BP, lipid profiles, cardiovascular health, and insulin sensitivity (23). For individuals with type 1 diabetes, resistance training appears to help lower the risk of exercise-induced hypoglycemia; if both aerobic and resistance training are included in one workout session, completing resistance training followed by aerobic activity is recommended to help avoid hypoglycemia (23). Flexibility and balance exercises do not carry the same level of impact on glycemic control, but the ADA does note the value in maintaining joint mobility and improved balance and gait, which may be of concern for older adults with diabetes (23).

KEY POINT

Exercise has been shown to be effective in preventing and treating type 2 diabetes. Regardless of the type of diabetes, exercise benefits people with diabetes by improving blood glucose and weight control and by lowering the risk of CVD.

Clients with diabetes are at risk for CVD; thus, screening prior to exercise participation is critical (6, 9). ADA highlights the importance of appropriate assessment of risk factors and a review of health history given that certain conditions may contraindicate exercise (or contraindicate specific exercises); examples of conditions of concern include uncontrolled hypertension, untreated proliferative retinopathy, autonomic neuropathy, peripheral neuropathy, and history of foot ulcers or Charcot foot (9). Expanded background on these conditions and considerations with exercise are found in the ADA Standards of Care in Diabetes (9).

Recommendations related to the need for pre-exercise medical clearance differ between the ADA and ACSM. Based on *ACSM Guidelines*, medical clearance is recommended for all previously sedentary clients with diabetes mellitus to ensure that they can safely perform exercise (6). The ADA position stand specifies pre-exercise medical clearance is unnecessary for asymptomatic individuals with diabetes who are going to do light- or moderate-intensity exercise; ADA does recommend a checkup and potential exercise stress test for individuals with diabetes who want to increase intensity or have other risk factors (23). For individuals who have been engaging in low- or moderate-intensity exercise, a medical clearance to continue is not necessary according to *ACSM Guidelines*, although medical clearance is recommended before beginning vigorous-intensity exercise (6).

Exercise testing (or other ECG stress testing) may not be necessary for individuals with diabetes unless they intend to undertake vigorous-intensity exercise (23). The need for exercise testing before exercise pro-

gramming depends on the person's risk factors and the intensity of the exercise program (6). The decision of whether exercise testing is warranted (including whether ECG or other more advanced assessments are included) should be made in consultation with the client's health care provider.

KEY POINT

Screening clients with diabetes mellitus is important prior to performing any kind of exercise testing. Recommendations on the necessity of medical clearance for those who are sedentary differ between ADA and ACSM. For those who are already active at light or moderate intensity, medical clearance is recommended before engaging in vigorous-intensity exercise. If exercise testing is needed, the type of tests will depend on the client's needs and the intensity of the exercise program.

The goals of exercise programming for clients with diabetes (e.g., increasing aerobic power, reducing disease risk, increasing flexibility, increasing muscular strength and endurance, limiting sedentary time) are similar to those for clients who do not have diabetes, with the exception of increased attention to glucose control to avoid hypoglycemia when glucose levels drop or hyperglycemia when glucose levels are too high. General recommendations based on a position statement by the ADA for exercise for individuals with type 1 or type 2 diabetes are summarized in the sidebar *Exercise Training Recommendations for Individuals With Diabetes*. The ADA recommends regular engagement in aerobic and resistance exercise; as individuals advance their exercise programs, ensuring glycemic control is a key factor to ensure safety (9). In addition to regular exercise, all adults with diabetes should decrease daily sedentary behavior; the ADA recommends interrupting prolonged sitting every 30 minutes to help with blood glucose management (9).

Hypoglycemia is defined as blood glucose below 70 mg · dL^{-1} (3.9 mmol · L^{-1}) of blood (9). Symptoms of hypoglycemia include, but are not limited to the following (9):

- Shakiness
- Irritability
- Confusion
- Tachycardia
- Hunger
- Loss of consciousness
- Seizure

Exercise Training Recommendations for Individuals With Diabetes

An exercise program for individuals with diabetes follows the general guidelines for healthy adults, with some considerations to maximize benefits related to glucose control. This sidebar reflects the position statement of the ADA on physical activity/exercise and diabetes (23). Aerobic activities can be done continuously or may include low-volume high-intensity interval training (HIIT). Safety and efficacy of HIIT for all individuals with diabetes is yet to be determined; for those with more advanced disease, continuous moderate-intensity exercise may be safer. When considering an exercise program that includes HIIT, individuals with diabetes should be clinically stable, have a foundation of regular moderate-intensity exercise, and ideally be supervised. Regular aerobic exercise (3-7 days per week) is particularly valuable, with daily activity of no more than 2 days between exercise sessions to decrease insulin resistance. Progressing to at least 150 minutes per week of moderate-intensity exercise is recommended; for those at a higher fitness level, shorter-duration vigorous-intensity exercise can provide similar benefits.

Resistance training sessions are recommended 2 to 3 times per week. Beginners should start with moderate-intensity resistance training, including 10 to 15 repetitions. For progression, increase resistance with a lower number of repetitions once that initial target number is met consistently. Sessions should include at least 8 to 10 different exercises with 1 to 3 sets.

For flexibility, exercises that focus on all the major muscle–tendon groups are recommended at least 2 to 3 days per week. Balance training for adults 50 years of age and older is recommended 2 to 3 times per week; this is especially valuable for those with peripheral neuropathy (i.e., a complication of diabetes that causes nerve damage, resulting in tingling, pain, and numbness or weakness in the feet and hands). Yoga and tai chi are options that incorporate strength, flexibility, and balance. Increasing movement with unstructured activity (e.g., housework, gardening) throughout the day is also recommended given that even brief bouts of activity improve glucose control and reduce postprandial hyperglycemia (i.e., high blood glucose after a meal).

Hypoglycemia can progress to death (9). Fitness professionals and individuals with diabetes need to be aware of prevention strategies and prepare for treatment if hypoglycemia occurs.

Prevention of hypoglycemia may include adjusting diet and insulin use with exercise, although this will not always be effective and should be done in consultation with the individual's health care provider (9). Exercise-induced hypoglycemia can result due to increases in glucose uptake from peripheral tissues regardless of insulin levels. Individuals should discuss with their health care provider how to modify their insulin dosage and other diabetes medications with exercise, along with carbohydrate intake (23). Changes within a workout might also be considered, such as a brief maximal-intensity sprint before or after moderate-intensity activity, interspersing high-intensity bouts within moderate aerobic exercise, or completing resistance training prior to aerobic exercise (23). *Exercise-induced nocturnal hypoglycemia* refers to hypoglycemia occurring when someone is asleep; hypoglycemia can occur 6 to 15 hours after exercise (potentially extending to 48 hours).

To minimize risk, clients taking insulin should work with their health care provider to reduce basal insulin (i.e., slower-acting insulin that helps to regulate blood glucose levels between meals) and potentially include a bedtime snack (23).

For the immediate treatment of hypoglycemia, carbohydrates must be consumed; pure glucose is preferred, but any carbohydrate will help to elevate blood glucose. Avoid products or foods with fat or protein to treat hypoglycemia (9). If the individual is unable to consume carbohydrate by mouth, glucagon administration is indicated (9). Glucagon comes in various forms (e.g., a powder that is dissolved into a saline solution for injection or intranasal glucagon) (9).

Hyperglycemia with exercise can occur from consuming too much carbohydrate before or during exercise or reducing insulin levels excessively, and some types of exercise can promote hyperglycemia (e.g., sprinting, brief intense exercise, heavy powerlifting) (23). After exercise, a conservative insulin dose may be needed for insulin users (while avoiding too much of a correction that might increase the risk of nocturnal hypoglycemia) or an aerobic cool-down may help to lower blood glucose (23). With hyperglycemia ≥250 mg · dL^{-1}, ketones should be checked; if elevated (≥1.5 mmol · L^{-1}) exercise should be postponed or suspended because glucose levels and ketones may otherwise continue to rise (23).

Awareness of all medications that a client is taking is vital. For individuals using insulin, a deficiency can result in hyperglycemia, while an excess can result in hypoglycemia. Various oral medications for diabetes also can increase the risk of hypoglycemia (e.g., insulin secretagogues that affect the production and secretion of insulin by the pancreas). In addition to pharmacological treatment for diabetes, other medications may affect clients with diabetes. For example, for a client with diabetes who also has hypertension, a beta-blocker may be prescribed. Although this is a medication focused on a BP concern, it also can result in hypoglycemia unawareness (i.e., when a person does not have symptoms of hypoglycemia and thus does not perceive that their blood glucose is low). For more complete information on medications, see chapter 2.

For people who have had diabetes for several years, peripheral neuropathy may be a problem. Damage to the sensory nerves in the feet can lead to ulcerations, and if blood vessels have been damaged, healing can be slow. Thus, prevention of blisters with footwear and breathable socks is important, as is examination of the feet on a regular basis to identify sores early. Non-weight-bearing activities may be better in these situations (6). Diabetic retinopathy is another concern that requires modification of activities to prevent dramatic increases in BP; activities to avoid include vigorous-intensity aerobic or resistance exercise, jumping, jarring, head-down activities, and the Valsalva maneuver (6). Autonomic neuropathy may cause a blunted HR response among other concerns. Individuals with autonomic neuropathy may not be able to perceive angina, so instead, monitor for other signs or symptoms (e.g., unusual shortness of breath). HR and BP should be carefully monitored and likely will be blunted (fail to rise); thus, use of RPE is recommended to set exercise intensity (6). For individuals with nephropathy, exercise can improve physical function and quality of life; programs should be tailored to individual clinical status (6). Additional guidance on working with individuals with diabetes can be found in several sources (6, 9, 23).

Pulmonary Disease

Pulmonary diseases can be subdivided into two major categories. In obstructive pulmonary diseases, the airflow into and out of the lungs is impeded. In restrictive lung diseases, expansion of the lungs is reduced because of conditions involving the chest cavity or parenchyma (lung tissue). Some pulmonary diseases are genetically inherited (e.g., cystic fibrosis), but in other cases a history of cigarette smoking; environmental pollutants; or occupational exposure to silica, coal dust, or asbestos is the primary contributing factor. All pulmonary diseases show a disruption in the exchange of gases between the ambient air and the pulmonary capillary blood. As a result, maximal oxygen consumption ($\dot{V}O_2$max) is reduced, the work of breathing is increased, and the ability to exercise is limited.

Types of Chronic Obstructive Pulmonary Disease

Chronic obstructive pulmonary disease (COPD) causes a reduction in airflow that can dramatically affect a person's ability to perform daily activities. Characteristics of COPD include expiratory flow obstruction and shortness of breath on exertion. There are several types of obstructive pulmonary disease. All of these obstruct airflow, but the underlying reason for obstruction differs for each (12, 16):

- Asthma is caused by bronchial smooth muscle contraction (bronchospasm) and inflammation.
- Chronic bronchitis is caused by long-term inflammation of the bronchi, characterized by chronic productive cough (i.e., producing mucus) not attributable to other causes.
- Emphysema is caused by damage to the alveoli (air sacs in the lungs) and enlargement of those pulmonary structures.

Another obstructive pulmonary disorder is cystic fibrosis, a genetic disorder that results in excessive mucus production in the airways, which hinders ventilation of the lungs.

Asthma

Over 25 million people in the United States have asthma; approximately 20% of those are children under the age of 18 years (18). Asthma is a condition that can reverse itself, and it varies from wheezing and slight breathlessness to severe attacks that may result in suffocation. Causes of asthma include allergic reactions to antigens such as dust, pollen, smoke, and air pollution. Nonspecific factors such as emotional stress and exercise as well as viral infections of the bronchi, sinuses, or tonsils also can result in asthma. In some cases, no specific cause of the asthma can be identified. Treatment involves medications that relax muscles around the airways (bronchodilators) and medications that reduce swelling and mucus in the airways (anti-inflammatories) (15).

What Is Exercise-Induced Bronchoconstriction?

Exercise-induced bronchoconstriction (EIB) is a reactive airway disease that occurs in 40% to 90% of people with asthma and up to 20% of the general population without asthma (26). This airflow obstruction during exercise was previously referred to as *exercise-induced asthma*, but that wording incorrectly suggests exercise causes asthma (14). With this condition, exercise tends to cause the bronchioles to constrict. Some activities may present a higher risk for EIB including activities with longer periods of exercise (i.e., greater than 5-8 minutes) in environments that are cold, have dry air, or involve exposure to chlorinated swimming pools (26). These situations challenge normal lung function due to evaporative water loss, temperature changes, and exposure to irritants (26). Various medications can be used, including oral inhalers. Other strategies to improve exercise tolerance include exercising in warm, moist environments rather than in cold, dry ones. For example, swimming in a warm, humid environment would be less likely to trigger EIB than long-distance running in a cold, dry environment. A warm-up exercise that includes 10 to 15 minutes of vigorous or a combination of vigorous- and light-intensity activities may provide a refractory period in which EIB is lessened (6).

Chronic Bronchitis and Emphysema

In 2018 approximately 9 million adults in the United States reported having chronic bronchitis and 2 million reported having emphysema; approximately 6.6% (16.4 million) reported a diagnosis of any type of COPD, emphysema, or chronic bronchitis (11). Chronic bronchitis and emphysema are not reversible. COPD is the fourth leading cause of death in the United States, accounting for 156,045 deaths in 2018 (11). Bronchitis is characterized by inflammation of the bronchi, the anatomical structures that carry air from the trachea to the lungs. A major symptom of chronic bronchitis is a cough with the production of sputum (i.e., mucus that is coughed up from the respiratory tract); in addition to bringing up mucus, the severe coughing may result in wheezing, chest pain, and shortness of breath (12). Emphysema is characterized by destruction of the alveolar walls and enlargement of air spaces, which reduce lung surface area for gas exchange (12). Symptoms include coughing, shortness of breath, wheezing, and chest tightness (12). Note that the term *dyspnea* is used to describe a feeling of increased effort or chest tightness, often expressed as being "short of breath" or "not getting enough air" (12).

The most common risk factor for both chronic bronchitis and emphysema is cigarette smoking (47). Other risk factors include secondhand smoke, air pollution, chemical fumes or dust from the environment or workplace, or, rarely, a genetic predisposition (alpha-1 antitrypsin deficiency) (47). Unlike acute bronchitis, which typically develops from a respiratory infection and resolves within weeks, chronic bronchitis does not go away, although symptom levels may fluctuate (12).

If the patient is a smoker, the most important treatment for chronic bronchitis and emphysema is to stop smoking. Treatment may involve the administration of a bronchodilator, typically using an inhaler, and corticosteroids to reduce inflammation. In severe cases, with hypoxemia (low level of oxygen in the blood), supplemental oxygen may be prescribed (47). Prevention of respiratory infections with antibiotics may also be part of medical management. Expectorants can help loosen the mucus secretions, enabling the patient to cough them up.

Cystic Fibrosis

Cystic fibrosis is a recessively inherited genetic disorder that affects about 35,000 people in the United States (20). Newborns are typically screened soon after birth for cystic fibrosis (20). Any positive screening is then followed up with further testing; diagnosis is based on excessive chloride concentration in the sweat (i.e., a "sweat test") (44). A gene (cystic fibrosis transmembrane conductance regulator [CFTR] gene) mutates, which affects the CFTR protein that is found in body organs that make mucus (e.g., lungs, liver, pancreas, intestine, as well as sweat glands and cells of the heart and immune system) (44). Mucus is normally slippery and helps protect the linings of various body structures. For individuals with cystic fibrosis, the mucus is thick and sticky, which can block airways and make infections more likely (44). In the lungs, the mucus secretions plug the airways, causing inflammation and chronic bacterial infections. Treatment for cystic fibrosis includes airway clearance techniques to clear mucus from the lungs with special breathing and coughing methods, therapy vests that vibrate, and chest physical therapy (44). Potential medications include antibiotics to treat lung infections, anti-inflammatory medications to reduce inflammation, bronchodilators to open airways, CFTR modulators to improve the function of CFTR protein that is affected by cystic fibrosis, and mucus thinners (44). More information about cystic fibrosis can be found at the Cystic Fibrosis Foundation (www.cff.org).

KEY POINT

COPD reduces the capacity for airflow during respiration. Bronchitis and emphysema are not reversible. Bronchial asthma is an intermittent condition caused by restriction of airways relieved with bronchodilator medications. Cystic fibrosis is a disease that results from a genetic defect and affects many organ systems and areas of the body.

Restrictive Lung Diseases

Restrictive lung diseases have many causes with the common outcome of reduced lung volumes (36). Some causes include pulmonary edema, pulmonary embolism, exposure to inorganic dust (coal workers' pneumoconiosis, silicosis, asbestosis), exposure to organic dust (e.g., farmer's lung), and radiation therapy. Various types of neuromuscular diseases (e.g., muscular dystrophy, amyotrophic lateral sclerosis, polio) also can cause restrictive lung disease as can diseases of the rib cage and spine such as kyphoscoliosis. Obesity can restrict lung expansion because of the abdomen pushing up into the thoracic cavity. In general, people with restrictive lung diseases have reduced residual volume (RV), inspiratory reserve volume (IRV), expiratory reserve volume (ERV), forced vital capacity (FVC), and maximal tidal volume (TV) (see figure 21.6). As the disease advances, respiratory rate will increase to compensate for hypoxemia (36).

KEY POINT

Restrictive lung diseases have numerous causes, but all are characterized by the reduced capacity to expand the lungs. Smaller lung volumes, assessed through pulmonary function testing, typically are observed in people with these diseases.

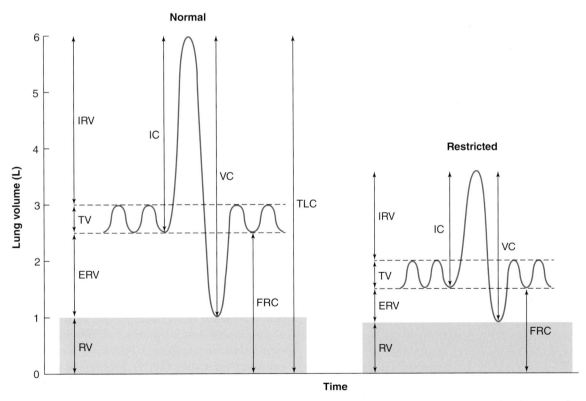

FIGURE 21.6 Lung volumes in a person with restrictive lung disease versus a person with normal pulmonary function. Lung volumes are total lung capacity (TLC), vital capacity (VC), inspiratory capacity (IC), inspiratory reserve volume (IRV), tidal volume (TV), functional residual capacity (FRC), expiratory reserve volume (ERV), and residual volume (RV).

Pulmonary Rehabilitation Programs

Pulmonary rehabilitation programs often are found alongside cardiac rehabilitation programs in many hospitals. Most pulmonary rehabilitation programs focus on people with COPD, although people with other types of respiratory disorders also benefit (3). Like cardiac rehabilitation programs, pulmonary rehabilitation is a comprehensive intervention, including exercise, education, psychological evaluation, nutrition, and behavior change (3).

The goal of a typical pulmonary rehabilitation program is self-care, and to achieve that goal, physicians, nurses, respiratory therapists, exercise specialists, nutritionists, and psychologists work together to address the various manifestations of the disease (13). The pulmonary rehabilitation patient receives education about ways to deal with the disease, including breathing exercises and medical management (13). The American Association of Cardiovascular and Pulmonary Rehabilitation (AACVPR) publishes a detailed description of exercise testing and prescription in its *Guidelines for Pulmonary Rehabilitation Programs* (3).

COPD patients often have other chronic medical conditions, such as cancer and CVD (56), which makes the comprehensive approach of pulmonary rehabilitation especially valuable (3). Although pulmonary rehabilitation typically does not directly improve lung function in most patients, positive outcomes may include symptom relief, exercise tolerance, and health-related quality of life given the focus on treating systemic problems and other health conditions (3). In addition to the cardiorespiratory aspects found with COPD, various skeletal muscle concerns also contribute to exercise intolerance—including reductions in muscle mass and strength, impaired muscle metabolism, atrophy of endurance muscle fibers, and a reduction in muscular endurance (3). To avoid feelings of dyspnea, many patients become progressively more sedentary; this results in further deconditioning and increased dyspnea on exertion. The term *dyspnea spiral* has been used to describe this developing decline (see figure 21.7).

KEY POINT

> Patients with lung diseases can benefit from a comprehensive pulmonary rehabilitation program. Although patients usually demonstrate little improvement in pulmonary function tests, they do improve in their ability to carry out tasks and in other measures of quality of life.

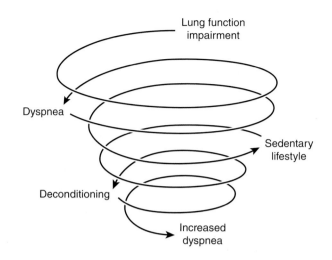

FIGURE 21.7 Dyspnea spiral.

Exercise Considerations

Exercise tests often are administered to assess the patient's ability to exercise. A standard graded exercise test (GXT) on a treadmill or cycle ergometer is typically used, in addition to a timed walk test, arm cycle test, or step test. Monitoring often includes ECG, BP, and perceived exertion, as well as arterial oxygen saturation (SpO_2), symptoms of dyspnea, and expired gases (3). Field tests are commonly used within pulmonary rehabilitation programs to assess functional capacity. One example is the 6-minute walk test, which measures the maximal distance walked in 6 minutes. Some considerations with the 6-minute walk test include whether supplemental oxygen or a walking aid is used (e.g., rollator, which is a rolling walker). Whatever setup is used (e.g., walker with supplemental oxygen source attached) should be used on subsequent testing (3). Another option is a shuttle walk test; two types of shuttle walk tests are used including incremental (outcome is distance covered) and endurance (outcome is time for shuttle walk test). Details on these assessments are available elsewhere, including special considerations for pulmonary patients (3).

In a pulmonary patient, exercise capacity is limited more by the lungs than the cardiovascular system. These patients typically experience hypoxemia (low arterial oxygen content) and dyspnea. Measurements of maximal ventilation rates, obtained during the final minute of an exercise test, also are clinically useful. Maximal ventilation rate is typically 60% to 70% of the maximal voluntary ventilation (MVV), although in COPD patients it may approach 80% to 100%. The Global Initiative for Chronic Obstructive Lung Disease (27) has established criteria to classify the severity of airflow limitation, fol-

Diagnostic Tests to Detect COPD

Within the diagnosis process of an individual with potential COPD (i.e., dyspnea, chronic cough or sputum production, history of repeated lower respiratory tract infections or history of exposure to risk factors), spirometry is used to make a diagnosis (27) (figure 21.8). In COPD the principal measures are forced expiratory volume (FEV$_1$), which reflects the maximum volume of air that can be moved in 1 second (see figure 21.9), and forced vital capacity (FVC), which is the volume of air that can be forcibly breathed out when going from maximal inhalation to maximal exhalation. This FEV$_1$/FVC ratio reflects airflow limitation indicative of COPD when it is <0.70 post-bronchodilator (27). Because of airway obstruction, individuals with COPD have a decreased ability to exhale quickly. Additional tests may include imaging (for differential diagnoses), oximetry and arterial blood gas measures, exercise testing, and assessment of physical activity, among others (27).

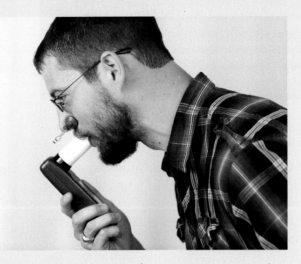

FIGURE 21.8 Pulmonary function testing is used to examine lung volumes and flow parameters.

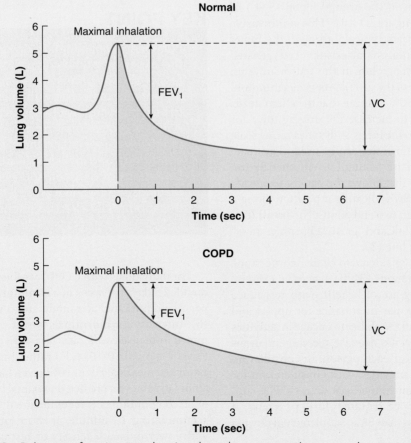

FIGURE 21.9 Pulmonary function test showing the volume-versus-time curves in a normal person and a person with obstructive lung disease. FEV$_1$ = forced expiratory volume in the first second of exhalation; FVC = forced vital capacity.

453

KEY POINT

Spirometry is one of the main clinical tests for COPD, allowing for the determination of airflow limitations. COPD patients demonstrate a reduced ability to exhale quickly because of obstructed airways. Exercise testing of patients with lung diseases, with appropriate monitoring of signs (hypoxemia) and symptoms (dyspnea) to assess the severity of the patient's condition, is beneficial.

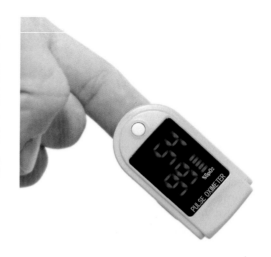

FIGURE 21.10 Portable pulse oximeter used to assess a person's arterial oxygen (O_2) saturation. The finger probe shines a light through the fingertip, and the absorption of light due to the pulsing arterial blood is measured. The number on the bottom of the display shows the percent saturation of hemoglobin in arterial blood (S_aO_2), and the number on the top shows the HR.

© Smikeymikey1 | Dreamstime.com - Oximeter Photo

lowing administration of a bronchodilator, as follows in patients with a FEV_1/FVC <0.70:

- *GOLD 1:* Mild COPD with FEV_1 ≥80% predicted
- *GOLD 2:* Moderate COPD with 50% ≤FEV_1 <80% predicted
- *GOLD 3:* Severe COPD with 30% ≤FEV_1 <50% predicted
- *GOLD 4:* Very severe COPD with FEV_1 <30% predicted

A pulse oximeter is used to assess the percent saturation of hemoglobin in the arterial blood (S_aO_2) of pulmonary patients (figure 21.10). This noninvasive device shines a light beam typically through the finger or earlobe. The absorption characteristics of oxygenated and deoxygenated hemoglobin in the red or infrared region are used to assess the arterial oxygen saturation. Values for S_aO_2 below 90% indicate that the client needs supplemental oxygen to increase the driving force for diffusion of oxygen into the lungs. A dyspnea rating scale (e.g., 0-10 category ratio scale) can be used to evaluate symptoms during exercise testing (3). Another option is a visual analog scale that allows the patient to specify their level of dyspnea by indicating a position along a continuous line between two end points: "no breathlessness" at one end of the line and "greatest breathlessness" at the other end of the line (3).

Exercise training is considered to be the "cornerstone of pulmonary rehabilitation" (3). Both aerobic exercise and resistance training are of benefit, with resistance training being of particular importance for upper- and lower-body strength and the ability to engage in activities of daily living (3). Specific exercise recommendations need to be developed for each person, in consultation with their health care provider, with consideration for oxygen therapy (3). For individuals with COPD, supplemental oxygen may be required during exercise; if oxygen saturation is less than 88%, supplemental oxygen is indicated (6).

KEY POINT

Pulmonary rehabilitation programs involve the expertise of many types of health professionals. The primary goals are to educate patients about dealing with their disease and to help them improve their exercise capacity. A fitness professional in pulmonary rehabilitation must understand the client's medical conditions and physiological limitations. Sensations of dyspnea and pulse oximeter readings are frequently used to determine the appropriate exercise intensity.

For individuals with COPD, aerobic training is recommended 3 days per week at a minimum and up to 5 days per week, preferred at a moderate to vigorous intensity (6). Intensity for individuals with COPD can be determined from peak work rate (50%-80%) or on a ratio scale (level 4-6 on the 0-10 scale) rather than a percentage of estimated maximal HR or HRR given factors that limit the ability to achieve a predicted maximal HR (6). A duration of 20 to 60 minutes is recommended; if not achievable, accumulating 20 minute or more periods of exercise with lower-intensity activity or rest can be substituted until the patient can achieve longer durations. ACSM highlights common types of aerobic exercise including walking, stationary cycling, and upper-body ergometry (6). For muscular strength activity, two to four sets of 8 to 12 repetitions are recommended for strength training (intensity depends on experience level, from 60% to 70% of 1-repetition max [1RM] for those starting to 80% 1RM or more for those who are experienced with resistance training), and two or more sets of 15 to 20 repetitions are recommended for endurance training (intensity less than 50% 1RM) (6). Resistance training should be performed on at least 2 nonconsecutive days per week, and typical modes of resistance exercise can be used, including weight machines, free weights, or body-weight exercises. For flexibility activity, the session duration recommended is to spend 10 to 30 seconds on each static stretch, and 2 to 4 repetitions per exercise; engaging in daily flexibility exercises is most effective, but at a minimum, 2 to 3 days per week is recommended (6).

For individuals with successfully managed asthma, general recommendations on aerobic, resistance, and flexibility exercises apply. However, some considerations are necessary (6):

- Realize the limitations of using predicted maximal HR to develop a target HR given the potential impact of medications used to control asthma.

- Anyone experiencing symptoms should not exercise until symptoms are abated and airway function improves.

- For some, short-acting bronchodilators may be needed to prevent or treat EIB.

- Watch for an asthma attack following exercise.

- Be aware of environmental conditions that can trigger bronchoconstriction such as cold and dry conditions, locations with airborne allergens or pollutants, chlorinated pools, or long-duration or high-intensity exercise.

Osteoporosis

Osteoporosis is a disease that is manifested in low bone density, deterioration of bone tissue, disruption of bone microarchitecture, and reduced bone strength, all of which may lead to bone fracture (33). Osteoporosis is defined by the bone mineral density (BMD) at the hip or lumbar spine being ≤2.5 standard deviations below the mean BMD of a young adult reference population (T-score is calculated) (33). BMD is determined with dual-energy X-ray absorptiometry (DXA) (see figure 11.5 in chapter 11 for an example); sites for DXA measurement include the hip and lumbar spine.

Osteoporosis prevalence in women is higher than in men and higher in older ages (54). Prevalence for osteoporosis at either the neck of the femur or lumbar spine or both in adults ages 50 and older is 19.6% in women and 4.4% in men (54). Similarly, prevalence of low bone mass at one or both of these sites for adults over age 50 was 43.1%, higher in women (51.5%) than men (33.5%) (54).

Bone mass accumulates during childhood and generally peaks in early adult life (50). Although BMD declines somewhat during the middle adult years, the most rapid loss in women occurs in the years around menopause because of the gradual decline in estrogen levels. BMD has been found to decrease 9% to 13% in the first 5 years after menopause (51). Men do not have the same rapid bone loss in their 50s that women experience at menopause, and the rate of bone loss for men and women is the same by age 65 or 70 years (46). Men tend to have fractures later in life than women, while women have a higher lifetime risk, likely due to their smaller bone size and an increased fall risk (1).

Risk factors for osteoporosis include factors that can be changed with lifestyle modifications (e.g., diet and activity) as well as those that cannot be changed (e.g., age, family history). Women are at higher risk than men, and with age, risk increases for both women and men (45). Having a thin or slender frame increases risk as does having a parent with osteoporosis or hip fracture. Low levels of estrogen in women (after menopause, or before menopause due to hormone disorders or high levels of physical activity that disrupt normal menstrual periods) or testosterone in men increase risk. Sometimes osteoporosis results from other medical conditions or is related to use of prescription medications; examples include endocrine disorders, gastrointestinal diseases, certain types of cancer, nutritional deficiencies, and the long-term use of glucocorticoid medications. A diet that is low in calcium and vitamin D increases risk as can heavy chronic alcohol consumption (45). Physical inactivity contributes to bone loss, and poor physical conditioning increases fall risk (45). Thus, because many factors lead to low bone density, people of all ages are at risk of developing osteoporosis.

A risk assessment tool is available that predicts 10-year probabilities of hip fracture and major osteoporotic fracture; the Fracture Risk Assessment Tool (FRAX) is for women and men between the ages of 40 to 90 years who are not currently being treated for osteoporosis with medications (33). Osteoporosis can affect both males and females across all ages and ethnicities. However, older women, particularly White and Asian women, are at the highest risk, while African American and Mexican American women have a lower risk. White men are at higher risk than African American and Mexican American men (45). One in three women and one in five men age 50 or older will experience an osteoporotic fracture in their lifetime (50), so attention to bone health is important for everyone. A general osteoporosis risk check is available from the International Osteoporosis Foundation (https://riskcheck.osteoporosis.foundation/).

Exercise Considerations

Bone mass attained early in life is important for long-term bone health. Genetic factors are a dominant influence, but modifiable factors such as good nutrition (i.e., adequate calcium and vitamin D intake) along with regular exercise (in particular, resistance and high-impact activities) are important for the attainment of optimal peak bone mass (42). The value of such activities is seen in the recommendations for youth in the *Physical Activity Guidelines for Americans* (60). Preschool-aged children, ages 3 to 5 years, are encouraged to include activities like hopping, skipping, jumping, and tumbling to strengthen bones (60). School-aged youth (ages 6-17 years) should include muscle- and bone-strengthening activities in addition to aerobic activities; the *Guidelines* highlight the bone-strengthening activities as "especially important" given the timeline for bone mass gains to maximize peak bone mass (60).

Peak bone mass is obtained by around the age of 30 years, so early adulthood is a continued opportunity to optimize bone mass with activities that provide an overload to the skeleton (i.e., loading in ways to which the bone is unaccustomed) (32). After the age of 40 years, bone mass decreases about 0.5% or more per year; the rate of loss likely is affected by genetics, nutrition, hormone status, and physical activity, in addition to aging (32). Exercise has a potential role in slowing the rate of bone loss rather than in increasing bone mass in middle age and older adulthood (32). Weight-bearing physical activity, activities that involve jumping, and resistance training targeting all major muscles are recommended for adults (32).

The prior recommendations are focused on promoting healthy bones. Potential exercise-related precautions are necessary for individuals with osteoporosis. No specific recommendations exist for exercise testing of people with osteoporosis beyond those for the general population, although ACSM notes some considerations and that the benefits versus the risks of exercise testing must be weighed (6). For individuals with severe kyphosis that limits forward vision or balance, modifications to testing protocols could include using handrail support during treadmill walking and using stationary cycling. Those with compression fractures may find cycle ergometry less painful than walking. Testing muscular strength can be important in designing programs for osteoporotic clients; however, maximal exertion and exercises that involve significant spinal flexion should be avoided because of the risk of compression fractures. Tests of balance and functionality can be useful in designing programs to reduce the risk of falling. Improving functional muscle strength and balance is important in reducing the risk of falls.

Exercise prescription for the osteoporotic client must be individualized based on the severity of disease and the presence of other conditions (6). In general, the exercise prescription should include aerobic activity, exercises that strengthen muscle, flexibility exercises, and activities that improve balance. This combination incorporates cardiovascular health, bone health, and reduced risk of falling. It is common for individuals with osteoporosis to be deconditioned, so initial exercise prescription may involve low-intensity activity and slow progression. Ultimately, clients should attempt to reach the following exercise levels (6):

- *Frequency:* Perform weight-bearing aerobic exercise on 4 to 5 days per week; resistance exercise of 8 to 10 exercises on 1 to 2 days per week (may progress to 2-3 days per week of resistance exercise); and flexibility on 5 to 7 days per week.

- *Intensity:* Perform moderate-intensity aerobic exercise (40%-59% HRR or rating of 3 or 4 on a 0-10 relative exertion scale); adjust resistance so the last two repetitions within a target range of 8 to 12 repetitions are challenging; stretch to the point of tightness.

- *Time:* Begin with 20 minutes per day of aerobic exercise (progress to 30-60 minutes per day); for resistance exercise, begin with one set of 8 to 12 repetitions (may increase to two sets); stretching should involve static stretches held for 10 to 30 seconds and repeated two to four times.

- *Type:* Any aerobic exercise with weight bearing is preferred along with jumping or bench stepping for those with low to moderate risk of fracture; additionally, resistance train with any standard equipment, with a preference for compound movements; perform static stretching.

Activities that involve explosive movement; high-impact loading; or excessive twisting, bending, or compression of the spine should be avoided by people with osteoporosis (6). Clients should be counseled to note any new pain, and this information should be carefully considered in modifying exercise. Exercises that improve balance are valuable for fall prevention and should be included in the exercise program (6).

Metabolic Syndrome

Metabolic syndrome (also called *syndrome X*) is a clustering of risk factors associated with heart disease, diabetes, and stroke. People with metabolic syndrome have a much higher risk for atherosclerotic CVD. Some variation in definitions exists; according to the AHA and National Heart, Lung, and Blood Institute, to be diagnosed with metabolic syndrome, a person must have at least three of the following (28):

- *Abdominal obesity:* Waist circumference ≥102 centimeters (men) or ≥88 centimeters (women)
- *High triglycerides:* ≥150 mg · dl^{-1}, or drug treatment
- *Low high-density lipoprotein cholesterol (HDL-C):* <40 mg · dl^{-1} (men) or <50 mg · dl^{-1} (women), or drug treatment
- *Elevated BP:* ≥130/85 mmHg, or drug treatment
- *Elevated fasting glucose:* ≥100 mg · dl^{-1}, or drug treatment

It is estimated that over a third of American adults have metabolic syndrome (29). Without intervention, chronic disease risk (e.g., heart disease, diabetes) is much higher for these individuals. The approach to control metabolic syndrome depends on the symptoms that are present. Physical activity is commonly recommended because of the positive effect of regular exercise on all characteristics of metabolic syndrome. Achieving a healthy body weight and managing heart disease risk factors are vital for clients with metabolic syndrome.

For individuals with metabolic syndrome who desire to start a low to moderate exercise program, an exercise test is not required but could be helpful (6). If an exercise test is conducted, attention to individual situations is key (e.g., presence of obesity, hypertension, or other condition).

When developing an exercise program, general recommendations apply, with some special considerations (6). Given the clustering of risk factors and potential presence of chronic diseases, the fitness professional should review these and proceed with the most conservative criteria. Progression over time should consider chronic diseases and risk factors.

LEARNING AIDS

REVIEW QUESTIONS

1. List three major chronic diseases in the United States.
2. Define *atherosclerosis*, and list three alterable cardiovascular risk factors that promote the atherosclerotic process.
3. Describe the effects of exercise on people with hypertension. What are special considerations during exercise when working with someone with hypertension?
4. List four patient populations who are commonly referred to cardiac rehabilitation programs.
5. What evidence exists that exercise training can be beneficial for individuals with heart disease or stroke?
6. Outline the recommendations for exercise programming in cardiac rehabilitation in terms of frequency, intensity, duration, and mode.

7. Describe modifiable risk factors to reduce the risk of cancer, including recommendations related to the amount of physical activity per week.

8. Describe how exercise during cancer treatment may be of benefit.

9. Give examples of unique considerations with exercise for cancer survivors.

10. List the two major types of diabetes, including their similarities and differences.

11. What is prediabetes?

12. What are the diagnostic criteria for diabetes?

13. What are exercise recommendations for clients with diabetes?

14. What precautions should be taken to avoid hypoglycemia?

15. What is the major problem in COPD, and what are the physiological consequences of severe COPD?

16. What is the major problem in restrictive lung disease, and what are the physiological consequences of severe restrictive lung disease?

17. Define the underlying problems associated with the following subcategories of COPD: asthma, emphysema, bronchitis, and cystic fibrosis.

18. Identify which of the static lung volumes are decreased in people with restrictive lung disease.

19. Describe how the FEV_1 and FVC are affected in people with COPD.

20. Outline the recommendations for aerobic exercise programming for people with COPD in terms of frequency, intensity, duration, and mode. What are the recommendations for strength training?

21. What is osteoporosis and what are risk factors for osteoporosis?

22. What exercise recommendations for children will help promote good bone development?

23. What precautions should be taken when testing clients with osteoporosis?

24. What is the standard exercise prescription for a person with osteoporosis?

CASE STUDIES

1. Ricardo is a 52-year-old male. He has a sedentary desk job and for recreation plays golf on the weekends. He went to see his cardiologist because he experienced recent fatigue with chest pain on exertion. He has never smoked; he consumes one to two alcoholic drinks on a few days of the week. His medical history reveals a blood cholesterol level of 220 mg · dl^{-1}, a triglyceride level of 195 mg · dl^{-1}, and an HDL-C value of 39 mg · dl^{-1}. Considering his sex, age, symptoms, and risk factors, what do you think is the likelihood he has CVD? What would be a reasonable next step to diagnose the presence or absence of CVD?

2. Aiko is a 61-year-old female. She recently underwent a left heart catheterization, which revealed significant occlusion in the left anterior descending coronary artery and the left circumflex coronary artery. A balloon angioplasty procedure was performed. Approximately 2 weeks later, she performed a GXT with the following results:

   - *Protocol:* Balke (3.3 mph, or 5.3 km · hr^{-1})
   - *Resting:* HR = 72 bpm, BP = 130/72 mmHg
   - *End point:* Stage 3 for 1 minute (approximately 7 METs)
     - HR = 126 bpm, BP = 160/90 mmHg
   - *Reason for termination:* Fatigue
   - No ECG concerns (no ST segment depression), no reported symptoms

Aiko was taking atenolol (a beta-blocker) at the time of her test, and her physician instructed her to continue taking this medication. She was referred to a cardiac rehabilitation center for supervised exercise and risk-factor modification. List some types of exercise that would be appropriate for her. In addition to the mode, be sure to recommend an appropriate frequency, intensity, and duration of exercise.

3. Sofia is a fitness professional who will be working with an individual who recently completed treatment, including chemotherapy, for cancer. What are aspects that Sofia should pay special attention to in order to maximize safety for her client?

4. Tony is a 40-year-old man who, in response to doctor's orders, appears at your medical wellness facility for exercise programming. He recently sought the care of his physician after experiencing fatigue and headaches. Tony's physician ordered a series of tests, including a diagnostic exercise stress test. Here are Tony's test results:

Weight = 265 pounds (120 kilograms)

Cholesterol = 270 mg · dl^{-1}

Fasting glucose = 132 mg · dl^{-1}

Height = 5 feet 9.5 inches (177 centimeters)

LDL-C = 190 mg · dl^{-1}

BP = 148/94 mmHg

Nonsmoker

HDL-C = 32 mg · dl^{-1}

$\dot{V}O_2$max = 22 ml · kg^{-1} · min^{-1}

High stress

Previously inactive

No ischemia with GXT

Tony was diagnosed with type 2 diabetes, placed on medication to lower his cholesterol, and placed on a diuretic to lower his BP. He was told to begin to exercise and lose weight in an attempt to lower his blood glucose.

a. Design a 3-month supervised exercise program for Tony.

b. What are reasonable weight-loss goals for Tony? What recommendations will you make to help him achieve these goals?

c. What additional support systems will you recommend to help Tony achieve success with his exercise and weight-loss goals?

5. Belinda, a 38-year-old woman with asthma, would like to enter your fitness program. What kinds of questions do you ask her during your screening interview?

6. Alex, a 50-year-old man with a history of smoking a pack of cigarettes a day for the past 25 years, enters a hospital complaining of dyspnea. A chest X-ray shows that his lungs are hyperinflated, and spirometry tests show that his FEV$_1$ is only half the normal value. Based on these tests, what type of pulmonary disease does he have, and what is the logical course of treatment?

7. Abigail, a sedentary 52-year-old woman with a family history of osteoporosis, comes to your facility for information on exercise to promote bone health. Her doctor says she is in generally good health and does not have osteoporosis, but there are signs that her bones are weaker than when she was younger (i.e., osteopenia). What type of exercise do you recommend?

Answers to Case Studies

1. Because Ricardo is a 52-year-old male with typical effort-induced angina and an elevated total cholesterol and low HDL-C, he is at risk for CVD. A reasonable next step would be to refer him to his physician for potential graded exercise testing to see if signs or symptoms of CVD occur. If they do, a more definitive diagnostic test such as coronary angiography might be recommended.

2. Aiko's GXT results indicated that her maximal aerobic capacity was 7 METs. Starting off at approximately 50% of this value would result in a target intensity of around 3.5 METs. Suitable exercises include treadmill walking, stationary cycling, and arm cranking. Realize that her maximal HR is low because she is taking a beta-blocker. Thus, exercise could be prescribed based on a relative exertion scale (e.g., level 4 or 5 on a 0-10 scale). Light resistance exercises using dumbbells and elastic bands, as tolerated, also would be acceptable. The resistance should be selected to allow her to perform 12 to 15 repetitions with good form.

3. Given the impact cancer treatment has on the immune system, Sofia needs to ensure a clean environment to prevent infection. A clean environment includes all areas and items the client will encounter, such as showers and locker rooms, exercise equipment, and towels. Other risk-reduction measures include handwashing and avoiding exercise times when the facility is crowded. Sofia should ask the client about symptoms such as fever or chills, and if present, the client should not exercise and should be referred to their health care provider immediately. Sofia should be aware of other situations requiring referral to the client's health care provider (e.g., unusual muscle weakness, pain not associated with injury, and others as discussed in this chapter).

4. Recommend aerobic and resistance training for Tony, as follows:

   Month 1: Begin with 5 days per week of supervised sessions (3 days of aerobic exercise and 2 days of aerobic exercise and resistance training). Although this may seem like a lot of supervised sessions, it is designed to assist with compliance and to help him make the significant lifestyle adjustment. His history indicates he is not likely to exercise without support. Additionally, because he is new to the medication regimen, he needs supervision in case of a hypoglycemic event.

   - *Aerobic component:* Begin with two bouts of walking, 10 minutes each in duration, separated by 5 minutes of stretching. Use relative scale (e.g., 3 on 0-10 scale). If joint pain is an issue, use walking for one bout and select another mode of aerobic activity for the other bout. After the second week, move to 12-minute bouts.

   - *Resistance component:* Select eight multijoint exercises with upper- and lower-body exercises as a part of the workout. Have Tony complete one set of 8 to 12 repetitions during the first month. Do these exercises following his walking bouts on 2 days per week.

   Month 2: Continue with 5 days of supervised exercise, but also encourage him to build activity into his daily life and on his unsupervised days. Focus on building activity into his routine and lifestyle (e.g., parking farther from his office door, taking stairs). Encourage him to download an app to track his steps during the day. On his unsupervised days, encourage him to engage in active leisure activities (e.g., trips to the park, walking at the mall, visiting local outdoor markets).

   - *Aerobic component:* Gradually build up to two bouts of 20 minutes each, separated by 5 minutes of stretching. Use a relative exertion scale (4 or 5 on a 0-10 scale).

   - *Resistance component:* Continue with the same exercises but add a second set.

Month 3: Continue with five supervised sessions per week. If Tony is doing well (no hypoglycemic events and he appears motivated), consider dropping off to three supervised sessions per week. On his days off, set specific exercise goals and have him report his activity.

- *Aerobic component:* Gradually convert his walking to a 30-minute bout followed by a 15-minute bout, separated by 5 minutes of stretching. Use relative exertion scale (5 or 6 on a 0-10 scale).
- *Resistance component:* Same as month 2.

In terms of weight-loss goals, he likely has been given eating recommendations by his health care provider that he can incorporate into his plan. Tony also may work with a Registered Dietitian Nutritionist (RDN). In general, Tony should restrict caloric intake and increase exercise (energy expenditure) to achieve a weekly weight loss of 1 to 2 pounds (0.45-0.9 kilograms). Use strategies outlined in chapter 20 to promote weight loss.

Tony will benefit from building a supportive network. Help him identify friends, family members, coworkers, and so on who will encourage his healthy lifestyle. Encourage him to keep a journal of his eating and exercise. Help him develop strategies to deal with challenges (e.g., travel, time management). Encourage him to monitor his weight and check in with his physician regularly. It will be important to monitor his CVD risk factors. If he makes the suggested changes and follows the medication regimen prescribed by his health care provider, his risk-factor profile should improve.

5. Find out if Belinda has worked with her physician and is currently experiencing any problems with her medication. Additionally, ask if she carries a bronchodilator with her to class, and verify that she knows how to use it when she experiences shortness of breath. Finally, pay special attention to her during the early phases of the class.

6. Alex likely has emphysema and possibly chronic bronchitis, two forms of COPD that commonly result from cigarette smoking. This is shown by his reduced ability to exhale air quickly (decreased FEV_1). The logical course of treatment is a program to help him stop smoking, followed by a pulmonary rehabilitation program to help him regain his ability to exercise so that he can carry out activities of daily living.

7. Abigail will benefit from both weight-bearing aerobic activity and resistance training. To increase her aerobic fitness, protect her against chronic disease, and load her bones, a walking program is appropriate. She should gradually progress to a 30-minute brisk walk on most, preferably all, days of the week. Additionally, she should engage in resistance training 2 to 3 days per week. The program should include upper- and lower-body exercises and focus on areas at high risk for osteoporotic fractures (hip, spine, wrist). Three sets of approximately 70% of 1RM (8-12 repetitions) are appropriate. Suggested exercises include the standing toe raise, leg press, leg extension, leg curl, back extension (use care to avoid hyperextension), bench press, shoulder press, biceps curl, triceps extension, and wrist curl. Additionally, Abigail should consume adequate amounts of calcium and vitamin D (see chapter 5).

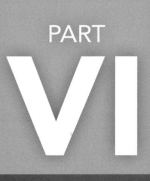

PART

VI

Exercise Programming Considerations

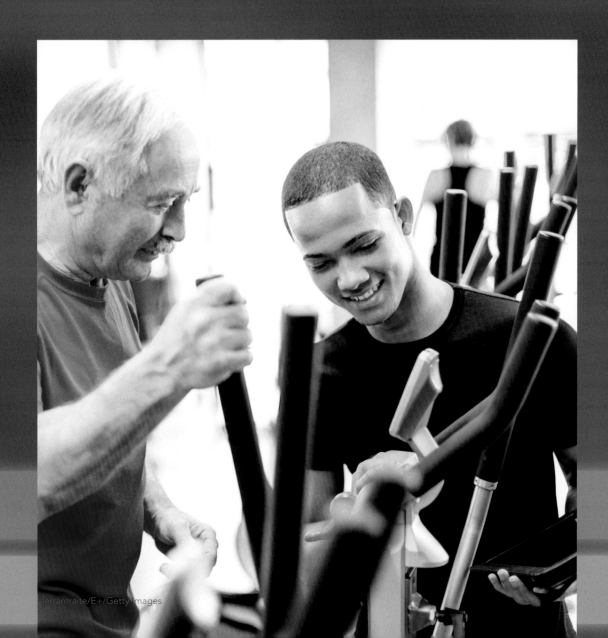

The previous parts of this textbook covered assessment and exercise prescription for components of physical fitness for people with a variety of characteristics and health conditions. This section includes other elements needed for a comprehensive, safe, and effective fitness program. Chapter 22 focuses on how to promote adherence, with insights on ways to motivate people to adopt and maintain a healthy lifestyle. Chapter 23 provides information on the prevention and management of injuries, and safety considerations of which fitness professionals must be aware. Finally, in chapter 24, important legal considerations for fitness professionals are discussed.

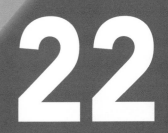

Behavior Modification

Janet Buckworth

Janet Buckworth

OBJECTIVES

The reader will be able to do the following:

1. Describe theories involved in healthy behavior change
2. Discuss the role of motivation in exercise adoption and adherence, and identify behavioral strategies for enhancing motivation
3. Describe at least six strategies that fitness professionals can use to monitor and support behavior change
4. Describe ways to apply relapse prevention to exercise behavior
5. Identify effective communication skills useful in motivating and fostering healthy behavior change
6. Explain the effects of weight bias on the quality and effectiveness of individual interventions

Translating the desire to change a health-related behavior into action is a challenge for most people. They may wish to be more active or to eat a healthier diet but may not have the knowledge, skills, or motivation to make the necessary behavior modifications and stick to them. To help people adopt and maintain a healthier lifestyle, the fitness professional should understand basic principles of behavior change and develop the skills to put those principles into practice.

This chapter begins with a brief description of theoretical models for explaining and predicting human behavior, in particular the transtheoretical model of behavior change (also known as the *stages of change model*) and self-determination theory (SDT). Methods and strategies are presented in the context of behavior change as a process, with suggestions for use based on readiness to change and the promotion of intrinsic motivation. For an excellent review of the transtheoretical model applied to exercise, refer to Kleis and colleagues (10), and for SDT, see Teixeira and colleagues (26). Factors for fitness professionals to consider as they help participants move through each stage of the model are discussed along with strategies for enhancing intrinsic motivation to adopt and maintain healthy behaviors. Additional strategies and suggestions for interventions can be found in *ACSM's Behavioral Aspects of Physical Activity and Exercise* (17) and in *Motivating People to Be Physically Active* by Marcus and Forsyth (14). The last section in this chapter examines communication skills that fitness professionals should possess in order to motivate participants and foster healthy behavior change.

Theories of Behavior Change

Several prominent theories guide strategies for changing health behavior, such as behavior modification, social cognitive theory, SDT, the transtheoretical model of behavior change, and the social ecological model (5). Most theories are based on the assumption that behavior is learned and can be changed by modifying the antecedents (stimuli, cues, thoughts) and consequences (rewards, punishments). A media post listing the benefits of walking during lunch or a memory of enjoying basketball in school while walking past a neighborhood court could cue plans to be more active. A reward could be a certificate presented to the group fitness participant with the best attendance or socializing after playing on a recreational sports team. Social cognitive theory offers the view that behavior is influenced by the dynamic relationships among the person's characteristics, the environment, and the behavior itself. Someone training for a marathon would be more motivated than a novice fitness walker to exercise outside in the rain, but even the most dedicated marathoner would not run in a lightning storm. SDT is a theory of motivation that explains

human behavior with respect to one's motivation for meeting basic needs (competency, autonomy, and relatedness). People may start exercising to lose weight but later train for a road race because they enjoy a sense of accomplishment from running. Social ecological models highlight the dynamic influences of intrapersonal, interpersonal, institutional, community, and public policy on health behaviors. Although effective strategies for behavior change have been developed with these and other theories, most theories of behavior treat change as an all-or-none event. In other words, participants go from being sedentary to being regularly active in response to an intervention.

The transtheoretical model presents change as a dynamic process whereby attitudes, decisions, and actions evolve through stages over time. This model has been applied with some success to promoting exercise (30). The transtheoretical, or stages of change, model can help people think about, decide to begin, take action on, and continue an active lifestyle. SDT has gained popularity as a basis for understanding and promoting healthy behaviors by addressing the continuum of rewarding contingencies from external reinforcement to engagement simply for enjoyment and pleasure.

Transtheoretical Model

The transtheoretical model is a model of intentional behavior modification. Behavior change is a dynamic process that occurs through a series of interrelated stages that are mostly stable but open to change (21). This model emphasizes the individual's motivation, readiness to change, and personal history regarding the target behavior. For example, people who exercised successfully in the past would have more confidence in their ability to exercise again than would people who have been sedentary most of their lives. The problem with most interventions is that they are for people who are prepared to take action (20). According to the transtheoretical model, traditional strategies for participant recruitment will not affect people who are not ready to change. Different strategies must be used to persuade people to consider change and then motivate them to take action. Other approaches will be more effective in supporting adherence to the new behavior.

The transtheoretical model has two key components: stages of change (see the sidebar *Transtheoretical Model Stages of Change*) and attitudes, beliefs, and skills for change (21). By evaluating the participant with respect to these factors, the fitness professional can design individually tailored and stage-specific interventions.

The *how* of behavior change in the transtheoretical model includes attitudes, beliefs, and behavioral skills that change as someone progresses through the stages. These change elements are self-efficacy, decisional balance, and processes of change.

- *Self-efficacy* is confidence in one's ability to engage in a positive behavior or abstain from an undesired behavior. Expectation of success is important in making the decision to change and in maintaining the new behavior. Types of self-efficacy include confidence to accomplish the elements of a task, which is important when beginning a new behavior, and confidence to overcome personal and environmental barriers (coping, time management, and barrier self-efficacy), which is important for adhering to the behavior.

- *Decisional balance* refers to evaluating and monitoring potential gains (pros, benefits) and losses (cons, costs) arising from any decision. Perceived gains increase and perceived losses decrease with respect to the target behavior as the person moves through the stages of change.

- *Processes of change* are strategies used to change behavior. Experiential or cognitive processes are strategies that involve thoughts, attitudes, and awareness. Behavioral processes involve taking specific actions directed toward oneself or the environment. For example, seeking out information about the best exercise for losing weight is a cognitive process, and creating reminders to register for a water aerobics class is a behavioral process.

Self-Determination Theory

Self-determination theory (SDT) is a theory of human motivation developed by Deci and Ryan in the 1980s that has been applied to promoting exercise (2). According to this theory, humans are naturally inclined toward growth and development and have a set of universal psychological needs. Motivation to engage in activities results from the fundamental needs for competency, autonomy, and relatedness. Satisfying these three psychological needs will foster intrinsic motivation and therefore enhance positive behaviors and mental health as well as the persistence of healthy behaviors. SDT is based on the assumption that motivation to engage in a behavior falls on a continuum from extrinsic (avoiding negative consequences or gaining rewards outside of the particular behavior) to intrinsic (engaging in the behavior for enjoyment of the act itself). Behaviors that are more intrinsically motivated have a greater chance of persisting.

For example, two clients may both want to join a high-intensity interval training (HIIT) class, but one wants to lose weight and the other wants to spend time with friends in the class. The *what* is the same, but the *why* is the key to how long each will stick with the class. Losing weight is more extrinsic, and once the weight is lost, so is the reason for participating in the exercise class. Spending time with friends is associated with meeting the basic need for relatedness, and provides ongoing motivation for attending class.

SDT is based on the assumptions that human beings are active in controlling their lives and naturally inclined toward growth and development (2). *Self-determination* describes the motivation for intentional behavior that comes from the person. Motivation stems from efforts to meet the basic psychological needs of autonomy, competence, and relatedness. Deci and Ryan (2) proposed that these needs are universal and vary in terms of self-determination that is intrinsic, in which motive for a task is determined (regulated) by the person, to extrinsic, in which the motive is determined (regulated) by others or outside influences. Thus, behavioral regulation is the degree to which behavior is perceived to be regulated or controlled by oneself. Regulation can be more external, such as joining a swimming class because a physical

---

Transtheoretical Model Stages of Change

1. *Precontemplation:* In this stage, the individual is not seriously thinking about changing an unhealthy behavior in the next 6 months or is denying the need to change.

2. *Contemplation:* The individual is seriously thinking about changing an unhealthy behavior within the next 6 months.

3. *Preparation:* This is a transitional stage in which the individual intends to take action within the next month. Some plans have been made, and the individual tries to determine what to do next.

4. *Action:* This stage is the 6 months following the overt modification of an unhealthy behavior. Motivation and investment in behavior change are sufficient in this stage, but it is the busiest and least stable stage and has the highest risk of relapse.

5. *Maintenance:* Maintenance begins after the individual has successfully adhered to the healthy behavior for 6 months. Self-regulation skills are in place and confidence is strong. The longer someone stays in maintenance, the lower the risk of relapse.

therapist recommended non-weight-bearing exercise, or more internally regulated, such as when someone runs faster simply because it feels good. The more internal the regulation is, the greater the sense of personal choice, or autonomy.

BASIC NEEDS ACCORDING TO SELF-DETERMINATION THEORY

- *Autonomy:* To be the causal agent of one's own life
- *Competence:* To experience mastery
- *Relatedness:* To interact, be connected to, and experience caring for others

Applying Theories to Promote Healthy Behaviors

The transtheoretical model is applied to exercise by matching or targeting the appropriate intervention strategy to the person's physical activity history and readiness for change (21) (see table 22.1). For example, the goal in working with people in the precontemplation stage is to get them to begin thinking about changing their level of physical activity. Discussing information from a health risk assessment (HRA) or fitness test followed by education about personal benefits of physical activity is an appropriate strategy for participants in the precontemplation stage. The goal with people in the contemplation stage is to motivate them and help them prepare to take action. They would benefit from learning about the pros of exercise coupled with accurate, easy-to-understand information about how they can start an exercise program or begin to be more active. Someone in the preparation stage is doing some exercise but realizes that it is not enough and needs help setting up a personalized exercise program. The participant is aware of the benefits of exercise, but barriers must be resolved. Whereas

participants in the contemplation stage may not be ready to set goals, those in the preparation stage are ready to set goals and get a personalized exercise prescription.

Participants in the action stage are participating in regular activity, but exercise is not a habit. They are at a high risk of relapsing into a more familiar, inactive lifestyle. Relapse prevention, which is discussed later, can help keep them on track to the maintenance stage. Movement from the action stage to the maintenance stage reflects a decrease in the risk of relapse and an increase in self-efficacy. Helpful strategies include periodic reevaluations of goals and updates of plans for coping with life events such as travel, inclement weather, or medical events that can disrupt regular exercise.

KEY POINT

The transtheoretical model addresses the dynamic nature of behavior change. Fitness professionals can apply this model by selecting interventions based on characteristics of the participant, environment, and stage of change. Interventions should match the stage the individual is in and address self-efficacy and perceptions of benefits and costs of exercise (see table 22.1). Understanding motivation and using concepts from SDT involves distinguishing between what clients want (i.e., the content of goals or aspirations) and why they want this (i.e., the regulatory reasons). According to SDT, behaviors that meet basic needs are more likely to be sustained. Behaviors that people engage in for less intrinsic reasons are less stable.

Table 22.1 Intervention Strategies for the Stages of Change

Stage of change	Intervention strategies
Precontemplation	Implement a media campaign promoting exercise, educate about personal benefits of exercise, foster values clarification, conduct HRAs and fitness testing
Contemplation	Market benefits of exercise, foster self- and environmental reevaluation, provide clear and specific guidelines for starting an exercise program, be a positive role model, identify social support for exercise
Preparation	Conduct psychosocial and fitness assessments, evaluate supports/benefits and barriers/costs, design personalized exercise prescription, set goals, develop behavioral contracts, teach time management skills
Action	Identify social support for maintaining exercise, set up stimulus control, teach self-reinforcement, implement self-efficacy enhancement strategies, set goals, teach self-monitoring, employ relapse prevention
Maintenance	Encourage new activities with others, reinforce self-regulatory skills, review and revise goals, introduce cross-training, conduct periodic fitness testing

Promoting Exercise in Sedentary and Low-Active Individuals

A variety of strategies and programs can be used to motivate people to consider becoming more active and adopt regular exercise. These approaches are based on understanding the knowledge, attitudes, beliefs, behavioral skills, and environment that foster adoption of a regular exercise program and understanding the person's motivational orientation to exercise. Specific factors related to promoting the adoption of regular exercise are presented next, followed by a review of strategies to market exercise and increase motivation.

Encouraging the Inactive and Unmotivated

People in precontemplation are sedentary and have no plans to start exercising. They may be in this stage because they lack information about the long-term personal consequences of physical inactivity. They also may be demoralized from previous unsuccessful attempts to stick with an exercise program and may have low self-efficacy for exercise. People in the precontemplation stage may feel defensive about their lifestyle because of social pressures to be physically active. They have no personally compelling reasons to change, and the costs of exercising seem to outweigh the benefits. Given these attitudes and beliefs, the clients' perceptions about the benefits of exercise and their ability to change should be strengthened and the costs reduced. Activities to help people develop a personal value for exercise and information about the role of exercise in a healthy lifestyle are useful in moving people to the next stage (14).

Sedentary individuals move to the contemplation stage because of information that is convincing, personal, and timely (13). Contemplators are planning to become more physically active, but they are still ambivalent about changing. For them, the costs of starting to exercise outweigh the perceived benefits. Experiences and information that support the contemplator's desire and motivation to exercise and counter perceived costs and barriers can initiate the move to preparation. Exposure to physically active role models, enhancement of perceived benefits, and strengthening of psychosocial variables such as self-efficacy for exercise are other factors that influence exercise adoption. The cognitive processes of change, such as increasing knowledge about the health benefits of regular exercise and being aware of how one's inactivity affects others, are critical in these early stages of change.

Although initial motivation for starting exercise is often tied to achieving goals that are a consequence of the behavior, such as weight loss or rehabilitation from an injury, many novices exercise primarily because they know they should. Being physically active keeps them from feeling guilty. Behavior that is regulated to avoid guilt through self-imposed pressure can be the spark that gets someone active, but to sustain the behavior, motivation needs to be more self-determined. Linking exercise with improved health or with other highly valued behaviors, such as playing with grandchildren or participating in active hobbies, can move the person to internal regulation.

Influencing Motivation and Action for Exercise Adoption

People in the preparation stage may be doing some exercise but not enough to meet health and fitness guidelines. The fitness professional's goal is to help them become more intrinsically motivated and move to the action stage and adequate regular exercise. The aim is to shift motivation from avoiding guilt at one end of the continuum to exercising because of consistency with personal values or for pleasure at the other end. A thorough assessment of personal, social, and environmental factors that support the person's current level of activity can be particularly useful. A comprehensive assessment can establish physical fitness, motivation, goals, supports, barriers, and other factors to consider when developing a specific plan for change and implementing strategies. Behavioral strategies come into play more as someone begins to move from the preparation stage. Goal setting, behavioral contracts, and time management training are practical strategies to use with participants in the preparation stage, and information from an assessment will help tailor an intervention to the person's needs, characteristics, and situation.

Personal Influences

Individual characteristics that influence the initiation of exercise include demographics, activity history, past experiences, perception of health status, perception of access to facilities, time, enjoyment of exercise, aptitudes, beliefs, self-motivation, and self-efficacy (28). Higher education, higher income, gender (male), and younger age are positively associated with level of physical activity (28). Exercise history is an important factor in current level of physical activity. Past participation is linked with physical activity in supervised exercise programs and in treatment programs for patients with heart disease and obesity (3). Past exercise experience also can influence expectations about exercise and self-efficacy, and high exercise self-efficacy is associated with increased exercise participation.

Motivation is another variable influencing exercise adoption. Motivation depends on expectations for future

Motivational Principles From Self-Determination Theory

Fitness professionals can nurture participants' exercise motivation by setting up exercise tasks to develop a sense of mastery (competence), making sure they have a say in their exercise program (autonomy), and helping them feel connected to others in the exercise setting (relatedness). Teixeira and colleagues published a comprehensive review of SDT-based intervention strategies and concluded that fostering more autonomous forms of motivation can promote enduring exercise (27). Other examples of strategies to foster autonomy—that is, a greater sense of choice and control—include providing information for more informed choices, encouraging choice and self-initiation, and providing options. The fitness professional can make sure that clients on the fence about adopting an active lifestyle know about types of activities available to them (e.g., walking clubs, dance classes, and exercise apps, especially if physical activity opportunities are limited in their communities) and that they understand they are the ones who get to choose what they want to do. Behavior that is consistent with values, goals, culture, and lifestyle is also more intrinsically motivated and likely to be sustained. For example, reframing exercise to be something that fits with a client's priorities, such as supporting the community, can put working on a community garden in a whole new light and shift meaningful physical activity into part of the client's identity.

benefits or outcomes from exercise, such as good health, improved appearance, social outlets, stress management, enjoyment, and opportunities for competition (15). It also varies in degree of self-determination (e.g., autonomy, personal choice); intrinsic motivation is the most self-determined, whereas extrinsic motivation is based on satisfying others or on the consequences of the behavior.

Self-motivation for exercise is the ability to continue an exercise program without the benefit of external reinforcement. Participants high in self-motivation are probably good at goal setting, monitoring exercise progress, and self-reinforcement (24) and are high in intrinsic motivation. People with little self-motivation may need more external reinforcement and encouragement (e.g., group activities and social support) to adopt and adhere to exercise, but even people with high intrinsic motivation can benefit from social support.

Perceived behavioral control is significantly correlated with the intention to exercise (4). If participants believe they have more control over the exercise and have choices about when and how to exercise, they are more likely to begin a program. It follows that participants who set their own goals will have a greater chance of success than if goals are assigned to them (12), and they will be more likely to meet the need for autonomy.

Social Influences

Social support involves comfort, assistance, and information provided by individuals or groups. Practical help, such as providing problem-solving tips or a ride to the fitness facility, can result in tangible benefits to the participant, but emotional support also plays a key role. For example, emotional support (encouragement and expressions of care, concern, and sympathy) could be helpful when a participant is emotionally stressed. Other types of emotional support include esteem support (reassurance of worth, expressions of liking or confidence in the other person), network support (expressions of connection and belonging), and even informational support (information and advice). Exercising with a group also can meet the need for relatedness described by SDT.

RESEARCH INSIGHT

Social Support in Women's Exercise Adherence

Social support plays a big role in exercise adherence, especially for women. In a 12-month social support intervention with sedentary postpartum Latinas, 139 women were randomized to an attention control group or an intervention of walking plus social support (7). Women in the intervention received various types of support, such as practical assistance (e.g., offering childcare or strollers so they could walk with their babies) and emotional support (e.g., encouragement) (7). Women attended weekly sessions for 12 weeks, and physical, psychological, and behavioral variables were measured at baseline, 6 months, and 12 months. The authors found that social support was effective at increasing physical activity during the intervention but not afterward. Beyond support, the environment (e.g., safety) was suggested as a factor in sustaining physical activity in these women.

Social support for exercise from family, friends, and physicians is usually associated with physical activity (28). Spouses appear to provide a consistent, positive influence on exercise participation; in one study of older adults, couples who attended a supervised exercise program together had significantly better adherence to walking 6 months after the program was over compared to non-couples (19). Group factors may be particularly important for older adults and people who are motivated to exercise primarily for social reinforcement.

Environmental Influences

Research has shown that social support, environmental prompts, and convenience are factors in exercise adoption (1). Environments that have easily accessible facilities with few real or perceived barriers make it easier to sustain an exercise program. Posters, emails, texts, self-sticking notes, visibly located exercise equipment, and attractive bike and walking paths are environmental attributes that also serve as cues for exercise.

The convenience of exercise is influenced by the sequence, or chain, of behaviors that must be accomplished for the person to complete each exercise session. The longer and more complicated the behavior chain, the more barriers there are to exercise. For example, the potential for a break in the link is greater if a person must leave work, drive home, gather exercise clothes, drive to a facility, park, sign in, and change clothes to

RESEARCH INSIGHT

Access to Parks, Physical Activity, and Mental Health

Limited access to natural environments has been shown to negatively affect physical and mental health. Researchers examined data collected from 3,652 New York City residents who completed the 2010-2011 Physical Activity and Transit Study (18). They examined how long it took for respondents to walk to the nearest park and frequency of park use for sport, exercise, or physical activity. While park proximity was associated with fewer poor mental health days, this benefit was only found for those not concerned about crime in the park. They concluded that urban dwellers who lived closer to a park had fewer days of mental distress, but the benefits of park proximity may depend on perceived safety. The influence of perceived safety is important for the fitness professional to keep in mind when recommending walking for fitness—location and perceptions make a difference.

walk on a treadmill than if the person walks around the neighborhood first thing in the morning. For many people, exercising in the morning may be easier to stick with than exercising during the day, when numerous demands compete for time.

Researchers and practitioners recognize that the physical environment powerfully influences the level of physical activity in communities. For example, accessible, attractive, and safe places to walk, bike, or run can make physical activity more appealing and convenient. Certainly, workout facilities that are clean, are well ventilated, and have a good selection of equipment and adequate parking will be more enticing to novice exercisers compared with poorly maintained or managed fitness centers.

Marketing and Motivational Strategies for Early Stages of Change

The goal of fitness professionals may be to help people maintain regular exercise, but they may also be called on to promote regular exercise to people who are inconsistently active (i.e., preparation stage) or have not yet considered starting a fitness program (i.e., precontemplation stage). For example, the primary goal of a media campaign may be to capture the attention of inactive people and motivate them to contemplate beginning an exercise program or another healthy behavior. This might involve putting informational prompts at the point of decision to act, such as hanging catchy posters next to elevators encouraging people to take the stairs (9) (see figure 22.1). Bulletin boards, pamphlets, fliers, handouts, websites, and social media with upbeat information about the benefits of exercise and practical suggestions for increasing physical activity also can catch the attention of potential exercisers. Handing out passes at local

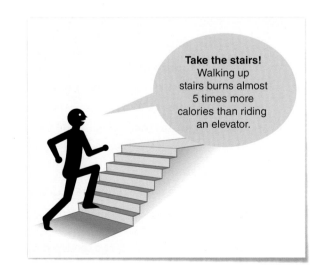

FIGURE 22.1 This sign is an example of a point-of-decision prompt to take the stairs.

471

restaurants for an aerobics class is a proactive form of recruitment. Fun runs and walks supporting charities may motivate people who primarily want to help the organization to begin thinking about exercise for its own sake. Wellness fairs, HRAs, and fitness testing in communities and at work sites also can prompt contemplation and enhance motivation to become more active.

To increase participation in the early stages of behavior change, the fitness professional's role is to provide education about benefits of being physically active, to describe how to exercise sensibly, and to offer encouragement to follow through with a personal exercise program. Specific strategies to increase adoption and early adherence are recommended (1, 5):

• Ask participants about their exercise history. They may need accurate information to dispel myths (e.g., the myth of no pain, no gain) and to develop positive attitudes about exercise.

• Explore ways exercise can benefit them personally. Find out what they think they will get out of being physically active, and provide information and resources about additional benefits.

• Help participants develop knowledge, attitudes, beliefs, and skills to support the behavior change. In addition to providing information and training in self-management skills, the fitness professional may use cognitive restructuring to identify discouraging thoughts and replace them with positive statements (see the sidebar *Cognitive Restructuring: Reframe Negative Statements Into Positive Statements*).

• Bolster the participant's exercise self-efficacy and sense of competency with success-producing learning experiences. Four sources of information contribute to self-efficacy beliefs and can be addressed by the fitness professional:

1. *Mastery experiences:* These experiences include behavioral rehearsal with proper supervision and positive feedback. The fitness professional can make sure participants have chosen activities that are appropriate for their fitness and skill level so they can experience a sense of accomplishment when they exercise. Practical feedback also will help participants be successful and thus feel more confident. Additionally, an increased sense of competency is motivating. Everyone likes to do things they are good at!

2. *Verbal persuasion or self-persuasion:* Suggesting to people that they can succeed in behaviors they have not been successful in previously and giving specific feedback to help enhance their skills and foster success will promote self-efficacy. The fitness professional can provide verbal encouragement and teach participants positive self-talk.

3. *Modeling:* Observing others can serve as a guide to performing a specific behavior. When people see someone successfully doing what they have little confidence to do, they start to expect that they, too, can succeed. The fitness professional can set up situations in which participants see someone like themselves succeed (e.g., post a newspaper story about seniors who now exercise regularly) or watch a peer who has trouble with the task succeed (e.g., point out to a new participant that an established exerciser "also had difficulty jogging 3 miles when they first started the program, but after months of hard work, they reached their goal").

Cognitive Restructuring: Reframe Negative Statements Into Positive Statements

Negative Statements

• I'm never going to get in shape.
• I'm fatter than everyone else in the class.
• I've tried to stay with exercise, and each time I fail.
• There's no time to exercise with my schedule.

Positive Statements

• Change takes time. I didn't get out of shape overnight, and I am making progress bit by bit.
• Everyone has to start somewhere. Other people have worked long and hard to get where they are.
• Every time I begin a new exercise program, I get closer to sticking with it for good.
• I can fit a few minutes in my schedule to be active every day. I don't have to do it all at once.

4. *Interpretations of physiological and emotional responses:* Physiological arousal associated with a behavior can be stressful and contribute to lower self-efficacy for that behavior. The typical increased heart rate, respiration, and muscle tension that occur during exercise may make novices feel anxious or uncomfortable and less confident. The fitness professional can make sure that participants have information about the normal physiological responses to exercise and know how to interpret their physiological responses accurately.

• Clarify expectations, and make sure they are reasonable and realistic. Use guidelines for goal setting to ensure initial successes.

• Identify potential barriers to behavior change and brainstorm with the participant about ways to overcome these barriers. Barriers can be personal (e.g., low exercise self-efficacy), physical (e.g., past injuries), interpersonal (e.g., peer pressure from sedentary friends to engage in sedentary behaviors instead of exercising), or environmental (e.g., inclement weather or lack of a safe place to walk). For example, one person may want to exercise but does not have access to facilities and another person may think they do not have the willpower to stick with a program. The first person would be helped with a home exercise program, whereas the second would benefit from social support and reconsidering discouraging thoughts.

• Foster motivation to adopt and maintain an exercise program. Set up incentives to exercise. Incentives can be tangible (e.g., T-shirts, certificates, water bottles, recognition on a website) or intangible (e.g., sense of competence, enjoyment). Tangible incentives are useful early in a program, but intrinsic motivation is associated with better adherence (23). Offer a variety of incentives, but focus on fostering more intrinsic and self-regulated motivation, such as a sense of accomplishment or enjoyment. Strategies to increase motivation are listed in the sidebar *Motivational Strategies*.

Motivational Strategies

- Provide positive, practical behavioral feedback.
- Encourage group participation and group support to offer the opportunity for social reinforcement, camaraderie, and commitment and to meet the need for relatedness.
- Recruit partners and peers to support the behavioral change.
- Make the program enjoyable.
- When using music, make it upbeat, positive, and matched to the client's preferences.
- Provide a flexible routine to decrease boredom and increase interest and enjoyment. Consider activities such as games and hiking as alternatives to traditional exercise modes to provide a variety of exercise options.
- Provide periodic exercise testing to show progress toward goals, increase a sense of competency, and offer an opportunity for positive reinforcement.
- Use strategies for behavioral change, such as personal goal setting, contracts, and self-management, to foster personal control and perceived competency, and emphasize goals that are meaningful to the participant.
- Chart progress using record cards, graphs, or software applications. Note and record progress daily to give immediate, positive feedback. Encourage self-monitoring.
- Recognize goal achievement in newsletters, on websites, and on bulletin boards. Individual effort increases when that effort is identifiable.
- Set up group or individual competitions.
- Offer lotteries based on individual or group accomplishment of a specific goal. Set a winning criterion (e.g., the first person to walk a certain distance each week for 5 weeks wins) for which the winner is featured in a newsletter or gets money that each participant has contributed. An alternative is to set a criterion (e.g., attending 20 of 24 aerobics classes) for participation in a random drawing.
- Organize teams to train for a charity-sponsored fun walk, run, or bicycle race.

KEY POINT

Individual, social, and environmental factors motivate people to move from not thinking about starting an exercise program to setting up a plan to begin. A variety of strategies can be used, from mass-media campaigns to fitness testing, to motivate people to move from contemplation into the preparation and action stages. Six strategies to facilitate adopting and maintaining exercise are to

1. ask participants about exercise history and use this information to set up a personalized plan;
2. help participants develop knowledge, attitudes, beliefs, and skills to support behavior change;
3. bolster self-efficacy;
4. involve participants in setting clear and realistic goals;
5. identify and address personal and environmental barriers to change; and
6. foster multiple motivators for exercise that have purpose and meaning for participants.

Enhancing Sustained Motivation and Behavioral Adherence

Various strategies have been discussed to illustrate principles of behavior change and to describe ways to market and motivate exercise. Once a participant has started an exercise program (action stage), the fitness professional plays an important role in monitoring and supporting the establishment and maintenance of regular exercise. For example, the fitness professional and the participant should work together to set realistic goals that are consistent with capabilities, values, resources, and needs. Exercise self-efficacy predicts adoption and maintenance, and it can be increased with mastery experiences, which also help meet the need for competency. Thus, initial goals should be challenging but certain to be met, which will foster increased exercise self-efficacy. The fitness professional and participant also should evaluate environmental and social supports and barriers and use this information to determine ways to manage barriers in order to promote the new behavior, enhance coping strategies, and lessen the influence of perceived social and environmental obstacles.

Assessment

Regardless of the intervention, comprehensive fitness and psychosocial assessments are necessary to select and carry out the appropriate strategies of behavior change for participants in the preparation and early action stages. Reassessment should be conducted periodically to evaluate the effectiveness of the plan.

First, the problem must be identified and defined in behavioral terms. For example, the focus on being overweight is shifted to the behaviors—overeating and underexercising—that contributed to weight gain. The fitness professional also can help the participant decide what realistically can be changed and what cannot.

Next, examine past attempts at behavior change. Find out what worked, what did not, and why. This information will be useful in setting goals and identifying high-risk situations (see the section on relapse prevention later in this chapter).

Also, find out if initiation of the behavior change is voluntary or recommended by someone else. This will give a sense of the participant's motivation and commitment to change. Participants who are there because a doctor prescribed exercise may need help finding self-determined motives for exercising. There are many reasons for beginning an exercise program (e.g., health, weight loss, anxiety reduction), but the initial motivation may not be why someone continues to exercise. Most often, people start exercising to achieve an outcome of exercise or to avoid guilt (extrinsic motivation) rather than for personal enjoyment, expression of creativity, or demonstration of mastery (intrinsic motivation). Extrinsic motivation can be useful to get people started, but research has shown that developing intrinsic motivation for exercise is necessary for long-term maintenance. Ask participants what they expect to get out of exercise, and be prepared to pique their interest by presenting additional short- and long-term benefits.

Another useful assessment tool is the decisional balance sheet. The participant lists all short- and long-term consequences, positive and negative, of both changing and not changing the behavior. The participant and the fitness professional then brainstorm ways to avoid or cope with the projected negative consequences of behavior change while also emphasizing and building on perceived benefits.

Self-Monitoring

Part of the assessment process can be accomplished by self-monitoring, in which the participant records information about the target behavior and also indicates thoughts, feelings, and situations before, during, and after the behavior. The participant can identify the internal and external cues and behavioral consequences that inhibit and prompt exercise. Barriers and supports also become evident with self-monitoring. The fitness professional can help the participant develop strategies to cope with the barriers and use the supports. The chain of behaviors encompassing exercise also can be evaluated and weak links identified. For example, if the participant discovers they always skip their 5:30 a.m. aerobics class when they oversleep and do not have time to pack workout clothes before work, suggest that they pack a workout bag the night before. Immediate benefits and reinforcements tailored to individual preferences also can be established at critical links in the chain (e.g., if they pack their workout bag the night before, they can push the snooze button for an extra 10 minutes of sleep the next morning). Tablets, computer programs, calendars, graphs, and charts can be used for self-monitoring as part of the initial assessment and as a way to record progress. Many exercise and diet tracking apps are also available for smartphones and other handheld devices, making self-monitoring more immediate, convenient, and informative than ever.

Time Management

The number one reason most people give for not exercising or for stopping a regular exercise program is lack of time (1). This is an understandable reason, but is the real reason that they do not have enough motivation or enough skills to manage the available time? Though fitness professionals want to be empathetic in response to life's demands, they need to help clients identify the underpinnings of their reason for not becoming or staying active. The fitness professional can help the client identify how time is a barrier and then choose appropriate interventions, such as modification of an exercise schedule or referral to a time management class.

Self-monitoring is an important strategy for getting at the root of the time problem, and a number of electronic tools can reduce the effort in recording daily exercise and diet. When people keep a diary of how they spend their time for at least a week, the payoffs are worth the effort. First, reviewing the diary with the client provides a sense of how much and when discretionary time is available. The goal is to free up blocks of time when the client can be physically active while at the same time accomplishing other necessary tasks. Flexibility in an exercise program (e.g., classes offered at many times, a lunchtime walking group) also can help with time problems. Accumulating several shorter bouts of exercise throughout the day may be another effective strategy. There is evidence for benefits related to bouts of any length of moderate to vigorous activity accumulated throughout the day (29). Additionally, finding patterns in how tasks are organized can reveal ways to be more efficient. For example, fixing lunch the night before can free up 15 to 20 minutes for a brisk walk before work in the morning. Task priorities also can be identified and time blocked out to protect that time from interruptions. For example, setting aside time for social media after studying for an exam can eliminate extra time spent repeatedly settling in where you left off.

Goal Setting

The purpose of goal setting is to accomplish a specific task in a specific time frame. Goals can be as simple and time limited as making a sandwich for lunch and as complicated and encompassing as earning an advanced degree. Goal setting provides a plan of action that focuses and directs activity and emphasizes a clear link between behavior and outcome.

Goals should be behavioral, specific, and measurable. Plans are easier to make if the goal is stated in behavioral terms. For example, a goal of walking 4 days per week for 30 to 45 minutes is easier to implement than a goal to get in shape. Specific, measurable goals make it easier to monitor progress, make adjustments, and know when the goal has been accomplished.

Goals also must be reasonable and realistic. A goal might be achievable, but personal and situational constraints can make it unrealistic. Losing 2 pounds (0.9 kilograms) per week through diet and exercise is reasonable for many people, but it may be almost impossible for the working parent of three who has minimal time for exercise and cooking. Unrealistic goals set the participant up to fail, which can damage self-efficacy and adherence to the program for behavior change. By using information from the assessment and self-monitoring, the fitness professional can help participants set positive, realistic behavioral goals based on their age, sex, fitness, health, interests, exercise history, skills, schedule, and socioenvironmental supports and barriers. Both short-term and long-term goals should be included. Short-term goals mobilize effort and direct present actions, but both short- and long-term goals lead to a more effective plan of action (12).

CHARACTERISTICS OF EFFECTIVE GOALS

- *Behavioral:* Aim for actions, such as lifting weights, rather than outcomes, such as losing weight.
- *Flexible:* Absolute goals can set someone up for a sense of failure if the goal is not met, whereas planning to jog or cycle 4 to 5 days per week, for instance, allows for options to work around the unexpected.
- *Specific:* Make the goal absolutely clear. For example, walking 3 miles (4.8 kilometers) without stopping is much more specific than simply doing cardio.
- *Measurable:* Be able to quantify the goal in miles, minutes, repetitions, and so on.

- *Reasonable:* Goals should be practical and achievable—in other words, are they possible?
- *Realistic:* The outcome should stand a good chance of happening based on the person's circumstances and the amount of effort required.
- *Challenging:* The goal should be difficult enough to be challenging but not overwhelming.
- *Meaningful:* The goals should be important to the participant.
- *Reward for specific accomplishments:* Set up benchmarks with self-rewards, such as going to a theater to see a new movie after completing a yoga course.
- *Have a time frame:* Establish a time frame for short- and long-term goals.
- *Designate the situation:* When, where, and under what conditions will the participant engage in the target behavior?

Reinforcement

Social reinforcement and self-reinforcement are crucial in the action phase, especially because the longer someone has been inactive before starting to exercise, the longer it takes until exercise itself becomes reinforcing. Immediate consequences of exercise can be soreness and fatigue, so external, immediate, positive rewards are necessary for beginners. Monitoring progress is rewarding and can involve charting miles walked or weight lifted after each session or asking for feedback from instructors after a difficult exercise class. Positive reinforcement from others can enhance self-efficacy, especially when feedback comes from people who are important to the participant. Praise is more effective if it is immediate and behaviorally specific (8). "You worked hard in class last week" is not as effective as "You did a great job getting through all the leg lifts today," especially if the participant has been struggling with leg lifts.

Self-reinforcement should involve rewards that are important to the participant. Using special spa soaps and creams only after an aerobic workout and getting tickets to the big game after logging a certain number of miles are rewards that are personalized and self-administered.

Social support can be verbal or tangible, such as transportation to exercise class. It can come from the class instructor, exercise partners, family members, and so on. Significant others must be involved in the exercise plan and educated about the differences between support and nagging. Constructive verbal feedback, praise, encouragement, and positive attention will help a family member stick with exercise, whereas punishing comments, jokes about the person's efforts, and discouraging social comparisons can hinder adherence. Support focuses on what has been accomplished ("You're being consistent in your walking to lose weight. I'm proud of you."), whereas nagging harps on what has not been accomplished ("You should walk faster to lose weight. Why can't you pick up the pace?").

Friends in an exercise program can provide both social support and cues to exercise. They can be positive role models to enhance self-efficacy and part of a buddy system to support the exercise effort. Some participants are more likely to stick with a program if they know someone else is counting on them to be there to work out. Being part of an exercise group also can help participants feel connected to others and support the basic need for relatedness (from SDT).

Behavioral Contracts

Behavioral contracts are written, signed, public agreements to engage in specific goal-directed behaviors,

RESEARCH INSIGHT

Effects of Short-Term Process Goals

Goal setting is an essential strategy for exercise behavior change and adherence, and the importance of short-term process goals for fostering intrinsic motivation and adherence was demonstrated by Wilson and Brookfield (31). They conducted a 6-week intervention based on SDT to examine the impact of goal setting and motivation on adherence. Sixty adult recreational exercisers were randomly assigned to one of three groups: process goal (weekly goals related to behavior, such as maintaining target heart rate or pace), outcome goal (goal to achieve by the end of 6 weeks), and no goal (control group). Intrinsic motivation (interest and enjoyment, perceived choice, and pressure and tension [negative indicator]) was measured at the beginning and end of the intervention and 3 months and 6 months later. The process-goal group had greater increases in interest, enjoyment, and perceived choice and better adherence than the other groups after the intervention and at each follow-up assessment. The outcome-goal group had lower perceived choice and higher pressure and tension than the control group, implying that using only an outcome goal may be detrimental to motivation and success.

and they have been used effectively to increase exercise adherence (1, 3). Contracts should include clear, realistic objectives and deadlines. Developing a contract engages the participant in a way that is motivating, challenging, and public. The public nature of contracts is especially important because public goals are more likely to be met compared with private or semiprivate goals (12). Having the participant make decisions about the nature of the contract fosters a sense of autonomy and can contribute to intrinsic motivation.

Contracts can be set by individuals or groups. The benefits of a group contract include the feeling it gives participants about not wanting to let others down and the desire to be part of a group. Individual contracts, however, can be tailored to the participant's specific situation and goals.

Consequences of meeting and not meeting the contracted goals should be clear and relevant to the participant. Contingency reinforcement can be set up so that the participant agrees to do a low-preference activity (e.g., squats) before a high-preference activity (e.g., sauna). Material and extrinsic reinforcers may be necessary initially but should become limited as natural reinforcers develop, such as social reinforcement. Inherent benefits of exercise, such as enjoyment and a sense of accomplishment, can foster more intrinsic motivation and better adherence, as can fostering a sense of autonomy, relatedness, and mastery through the goal-setting process. A sample behavioral contract for a client starting a walking program is shown in form 22.1.

KEY POINT

Assessment is an important first step in the action stage of behavior change. Self-monitoring is useful in determining the antecedents and consequences of the target behavior as well as the potential costs of and barriers to behavior change. During the maintenance stage, strategies such as goal setting and behavioral contracts must be tailored to the individual and should be reevaluated regularly through assessments and self-monitoring. Some of the variables that influence exercise maintenance are enjoyment, motivation, convenience, exercise intensity, program flexibility, social support, and skills such as self-regulation and self-reinforcement.

Relapse Prevention

Over time, most people experience lapses in absolute adherence to an exercise program. The cyclical nature of long-term adherence to behavior change is addressed by the relapse prevention model (25). The relapse prevention model is based on relapses in alcohol abuse, smoking, and drug abuse; the goal is to decrease a high-frequency, undesired behavior. This model is best applied to voluntary behavior. Although exercise is voluntary, the goal is to increase and maintain a low-frequency, desired behavior. Even so, the concepts and techniques of relapse prevention can be used with exercise adherence (11, 26).

Relapse occurs when people who have been exercising regularly or engaging in other positive health behaviors stop the healthy behavior and go back to the old, unhealthy behavior. It is important to understand the concept of relapse as it applies to exercise because relapse is likely for many people, especially if they do not have many coping skills, such as positive self-talk or good time management. The fitness professional must help participants understand that relapse does not mean failure. Together, they can devise strategies to cope with temporary setbacks in the fitness program and foster an arsenal of coping strategies.

Defining High-Risk Situations

Relapse begins with a high-risk situation that challenges an individual's perceived ability to maintain the desired behavioral change. High-risk situations can be bad weather, stress at work, boredom, fatigue, and social situations. A wedding reception with all their favorite foods can be a high-risk situation for a dieter, and weekend guests can challenge a jogger's motivation to keep up with their afternoon runs. People are predisposed to high-risk situations if they have a lifestyle imbalance in which *shoulds* exceed *wants* (e.g., turning down a ticket to the championship game because the game is played during the only time the pool is open to swim laps that day). This imbalance leads to feelings of deprivation and desires for indulgence. Rationalization, denial, and apparently irrelevant decisions can then occur (11).

Successful coping in a high-risk situation leads to increased self-efficacy and decreased probability of relapse. Not coping or inadequate coping leads to decreased self-efficacy and positive expectations about not maintaining the behavior change (e.g., being able to eat like so-called normal people, having more time to spend with friends). If this leads to a slipup, the abstinence violation effect (or for exercise, the adherence violation effect) occurs in which participants perceive that they have failed. All-or-none thinking, such as the belief that to be a jogger means never skipping a weekend of jogging, makes the participant more susceptible to this effect. Feelings of failure lead to self-blame, lowered self-esteem, guilt, perceived loss of control, increased probability of relapse, and possibly giving up (11).

FORM 22.1   Sample Behavioral Contract

Long-term goal: By <u>June 30</u> I will <u>walk at least 45 minutes at a moderate intensity 5 to 7 days a week.</u>

Baseline (where I am right now): <u>I walk on the treadmill 2 or 3 times a week for 30 minutes.</u>

Benefits of meeting my goal:
1. <u>I will be able to keep up with my family and friends on weekend trips.</u>
2. <u>It will be easier to take the stairs in my building.</u>
3. <u>I will feel like I accomplished something important.</u>

Costs of meeting my goal:
1. <u>I'll have less time with my family and friends.</u>
2. <u>I'll have to plan ahead if I have a busy week.</u>

BARRIERS TO MEETING MY GOAL:	COUNTERMEASURES:
My roommate also uses our treadmill.	Talk to my roommate about setting a schedule.
I get bored walking by myself.	Find interesting podcasts and audiobooks.
It's hard to find 30 minutes each day.	Divide my walks into several shorter bouts.
I'm tired after I get off work.	Walk during lunch or breaks.

To reach my goal, I will do the following (goal-supporting actions, resources, knowledge):

1. <u>Let my roommate and family know what I am trying to accomplish.</u>
2. <u>Find inspiring podcasts to listen to while I walk.</u>
3. <u>Map out safe walking routes at home and at work.</u>
4. <u>Mark days and time in my calendar to walk each week.</u>
5. <u>Find someone at work who will walk with me on our breaks.</u>

When I achieve my goal of <u>walking at least 45 minutes at a moderate intensity 5 to 7 days a week,</u> I will reward myself with <u>a foot massage.</u>

My first short-term behavioral goals for 1 week:

Task/performance: <u>I will walk on the treadmill or outside for 20 minutes after supper 3 to 4 days this week.</u>

Learning: <u>I will find at least three benefits of regular walking for someone my age.</u>

Client: _____ Date: _____

Fitness Professional:_____ Date: _____

Progress reviews (every 2 weeks):

Date: _____

Achievements: _____

Modifications: _____

Fostering Coping Strategies for Exercise

Relapse prevention, as described by Marlatt and Gordon (16), is a method used to identify and deal with high-risk situations. The strategy begins by educating people about the relapse process and enlisting their help as active participants in preventing a relapse. The next step for the fitness professional is determining specific strategies to prevent exercise relapse:

• Identify situations with a high risk of relapse. High-risk situations are those that involve behaviors that are incompatible with exercise, such as overeating, drinking, overworking, or smoking. High-risk situations also can involve relocation, medical events, travel, and inclement weather. Personal high-risk situations can be determined from information gathered during assessment and self-monitoring. The fitness professional should help the participant recognize aspects of the exercise behavior itself, such as intensity, duration, time of day, and location, as well as people, moods, thoughts, and particular situations, that can threaten exercise adherence.

• Revise plans in order to avoid or cope with high-risk situations. Flexible, short-term goals can be adapted to uncontrollable situational demands. Temporarily resetting goals can decrease the sense of noncompliance and increase a sense of control (e.g., "While my weekend guests are here, I will jog 1 day in the morning before they get up instead of trying to jog on both Saturday and Sunday afternoons").

• Improve coping responses by referring participants to classes or webinars covering techniques related to time management, relaxation, assertiveness, stress management, confidence building, and so on.

• Provide realistic expectations of potential outcomes from not exercising so the behavioral consequences of relapse are placed in perspective.

• Encourage participants to expect and plan for potential lapses in an exercise routine. They should plan for some alternative modes of exercise, times of day, places, and so forth. If someone is likely to skip a day of exercise when all the treadmills are in use, suggest the cycle or stair-climber on those days.

• Minimize the tendency to interpret a lapse (e.g., missing one class, not exercising during a business trip) as inevitably leading to a relapse and then defining a relapse as a total failure. Use cognitive restructuring to change the definition of a missed exercise class from "the end of my exercise program" to "a temporary lapse that most exercisers experience."

• Correct a lifestyle imbalance in which *shoulds* outweigh *wants*. Make exercise something participants want to do instead of something they feel they should do. Help them find activities that have purpose and meaning for them. Use positive reinforcement and other strategies to make exercise fun.

KEY POINT

Because missing regular exercise is inevitable for many people, the fitness professional must be prepared to help participants prevent lapses in an exercise routine from ending the exercise program. Strategies such as being flexible in setting and revising goals, realizing that the occasional lapse is just temporary, and building self-confidence and coping skills can help participants deal successfully with a potential relapse.

Health and Fitness Counseling

The fitness professional is called on to provide counseling during assessment, exercise prescription, and ongoing monitoring of exercise programs. More and more professionals are implementing principles of motivational interviewing, such as expressing empathy and fostering self-efficacy in a client-centered, semidirective format (6). Regardless of the approach the fitness professional uses, communication skills are the foundation of effective counseling. Developing good communication skills takes time and focus, so patience is critical to improving listening and understanding. For additional information, see the excellent chapter on health behavior counseling skills by Whiteley and colleagues in the *ACSM Resource Manual* (30) and Rollnick and colleagues' text *Motivational Interviewing in Health Care* (22).

Communication Skills

To be able to communicate well, the fitness professional must be able to listen effectively and respond empathetically. Listening involves being able to accurately discriminate the feeling and meaning of the speaker's message. It is more complicated than simply hearing words. Communication occurs at many levels, and thus fitness professionals should not always assume that what people say is what they mean. The message includes the objective meaning of the words, or the content of the message; however, tone of voice, volume and speed of speech, and nonverbal behavior can change the meaning of a statement. A participant who smiles, makes direct eye contact, and says, "My program is going really well," is not saying the same thing as a person who mumbles the same words and looks away. To enhance understanding of the message, fitness professionals must attend to the verbal and nonverbal as well as overt and covert messages. The fitness professional should pay attention to facial expressions, body language, and tone of voice in addition to listening to the actual words.

The context of the message, determined by social and cultural aspects of the situation, can create noise that will interfere with sending and receiving the message. Noise is also created by personal and social characteristics, ideas, experiences, expectations, and prejudices of the speaker and listener. Barriers to communication occur not only in the context of the message but also in the way a listener responds. Ordering, threatening, criticizing, interpreting, interrupting, interrogating, and diverting (often by humor) are responses that shut off understanding and make the speaker feel dismissed. Backing away, looking around the room, and checking the clock are other obvious ways to shut down communication. Not all times will be good for a conversation, so when approached by a client, the fitness professional should be honest about their schedule and be sure to arrange another time when the client can be given the attention they need and deserve.

Do not automatically assume understanding of what a person is saying. Each person reacts to a communicated message according to personal perceptions of the nature of the message, as well as individual racial, ethnic, educational, and economic characteristics. Conversations between native speakers and those for whom English is a second language especially would benefit from using responsive listening. Aim to clarify communication and confirm with the speaker that their message has been comprehended. One way for a fitness professional to do this is to reflect back what was heard and then ask questions and make statements that respond to the feeling and meaning of the message. Responsive listening lets people know that what they have expressed has been understood, helps build a relationship with them, encourages them to keep talking, and clarifies what they mean.

Characteristics of an Effective Helper

The role of the fitness professional as counselor is to help clients achieve their health-related goals. It is easier to

---

Putting Responsive Listening Into Practice

Participant: I'm the only one in this class who can't get the new boxing routines. *(The fitness professional should observe the tone of voice, eye contact, and posture.)*

Fitness professional: You think the other members of the class catch on before you do. That must be really frustrating. *(The fitness professional paraphrased the participant's statement and interpreted probable underlying feelings. Other feelings could be discouragement or a sense of futility or failure. Responding with an offer to teach the participant the boxing moves might not have addressed an underlying lack of confidence. Responsive listening keeps the communication open so the participant can express what kind of help they want.)*

Participant: Yes, I wonder if I can even do the class. The moves change faster than I can follow them. *(The participant has low self-efficacy for this boxing class. The fitness professional now has more information about the problem and can offer a better solution.)*

Fitness professional: You doubt this is for you because it is so fast paced, but did you know that many of the people in this class started with the Level 1 class? That class teaches all the basic routines at a slower pace and focuses on helping everyone learn the moves. *(The fitness professional acknowledges the participant's beliefs and provides more information to put their perceptions into another context. They are not alone in having trouble getting the routine without some basic training. A beginners' class could provide mastery experiences to increase the participant's self-efficacy.)*

Participant: I've always felt I didn't fit in, but I thought it was just me. Maybe I could try the Level 1 class. *(The fitness professional should observe what the participant said and how they said it to see if the information met the underlying need.)*

Fitness professional: This class was not the right one for you, but the Level 1 class can be a good way for you to learn the boxing moves. We can check the schedule, and I can introduce you to the instructor. *(The fitness professional paraphrases the participant's statement and offers help rather than telling them what to do. This acknowledges the participant's ability to make choices, promoting their autonomy.)*

provide this help when the fitness professional responds to the client with empathy, respect, concreteness, genuineness, and confrontation.

- *Empathy* is an expression of understanding the personal meaning of events and experiences to the participant. It is different from sympathy, which is an attempt to experience another person's feelings. Empathy is also not the same as knowing what the problem is. Knowledge that a client has 28% body fat because they eat fast food every day and do not exercise is different from empathy, whereby the fitness professional has a sense of what it must be like for the client to be overweight and inactive and is able to communicate that understanding in a nonjudgmental manner. Even in situations where a fitness professional may feel unsure of their ability to adequately convey empathy, when the participant perceives the sincere attempt to understand, they will be encouraged to communicate more about the problem. The additional information will help the fitness professional empathize more and will give clues to the underlying nature of the problem so that the fitness professional can come up with a more realistic intervention plan. The effort to understand also communicates to the participant that they are valued as an individual.

- *Respect* is a feeling of positive regard for the participant, includes displaying warm acceptance of the participant's experiences, and places no conditions on that acceptance and warmth. This means not making judgments. It is often hard for the fitness professional to respect a person whose behavior (e.g., smoking, sedentary lifestyle, high-fat diet) shows a lack of self-respect for their body. Prize the person but not necessarily the behavior. When respect is given to another person, that person is supported in developing self-respect.

- *Concreteness* is the ability to help the participant be specific about feelings and goals they are trying to communicate. Reflective listening enables the participant to become more precise in communicating what they experience and want to accomplish, which aids in setting goals.

- *Genuineness* is being authentic and sincere in a relationship with another person. In a helpful relationship, the fitness professional is honest and open with the client. Some self-disclosure is appropriate and can help develop trust, but the goal of the relationship is to help the client, not deal with the fitness professional's personal issues.

- *Confrontation* involves telling the other person that things appear differently from how they are being presented. Respectfully point out incongruities that are observable facts about which the participant may not be consciously aware. Confrontation should be used only after the fitness professional has an established relationship with the client, and it should be directed toward the behavior, not the person.

Other qualities important in effective health counseling are listed in the sidebar *Qualities of an Effective Healthy-Behavior Counselor*.

Weight Bias

Weight bias is the tendency to stereotype and negatively judge an overweight or obese person based on preconceived or unreasoned assumptions and false character traits, such as being lazy, unintelligent, awkward, ugly, or unmotivated. In other words, it is general negativity toward people who are perceived as carrying excess weight.

Currently, more than two-thirds of American adults are overweight or obese. Disturbingly, studies have shown that a significant proportion of health care workers demonstrate bias toward their overweight patients. Given that many of the fitness professional's clients may be overweight or obese, attitudes and beliefs that can harm effective programming must be identified and

Qualities of an Effective Healthy-Behavior Counselor

- Knowledgeable
- Supportive
- Model of healthy behavior
- Trustworthy
- Enthusiastic
- Innovative
- Patient
- Culturally sensitive
- Respectful
- Flexible
- Self-aware
- Able to access material resources and services
- Able to generate expectations of success
- Committed to providing timely, specific feedback
- Capable of providing clear, reasonable instructions and plans
- Sensitive to physical barriers to communication while respectful of the physical limits of someone's personal space
- Aware of personal limitations

addressed. Bias and stigma involve negative attitudes that affect interpersonal interactions and activities in a detrimental way. This can include stereotypes, derogatory names, teasing, and ridicule, although much of bias against obesity can be implicit, or not within conscious awareness. This can lead to weight discrimination, overt forms of weight-based prejudice, and unfair treatment of people who are overweight or obese. This can be seen in environmental barriers, such as examination gowns, tables, chairs, and blood pressure cuffs that are too small, which compound the difficulties associated with adequate health care for people who are obese.

Unfortunately, society promotes the idea that people are responsible for their life situation and get what they deserve. This has changed some since the American Medical Association recognized obesity as a disease, but the belief that weight is a function of personal responsibility and under a person's control is still prevalent. In addition, weight bias can be internalized, and individuals thus engage in self-blame because of their weight. The fitness professional can become sensitive to this bias by first recognizing the complex etiology of obesity, including not just individual behavior but also genetics, biology, the environment, and sociocultural influences (see chapter 20 for more insights). Challenge assumptions that obesity is only the result of eating too much and exercising too little and that the solution is greater motivation. Identify assumptions about someone based on weight regarding health, lifestyle, personality, professional success, character, intelligence, and abilities. Online resources for addressing personal assumptions and bias can be found at the Weight Bias and Stigma resource page of the Rudd Center for Food Policy and Obesity (www.uconnruddcenter.org/weight-bias-stigma).

Ethical Considerations

Promoting healthy behavior change in people who do not want to change presents an ethical dilemma. The fitness professional must weigh the importance of persuading people to behave in ways conducive to good health versus the clients' right to do as they please with their own health as long as it does not impinge on the rights of others. Informed consent theoretically gives participants a free choice after they have been given all the information needed to make a decision. If an unhealthy lifestyle is based on ignorance or incorrect information, the fitness professional should provide the information necessary for an informed choice, not aggravate feelings of guilt or failure. But if someone has chosen an unhealthy lifestyle as a matter of free will, this informed refusal must be accepted, although fitness professionals often have difficulty doing so. Thus, an awareness of personal value preferences is essential in helping others set goals. Consider whose values are to be served by the intervention, and respect clients' choices even if in disagreement with them.

Confidentiality is another ethical concern for the fitness professional. In addition to client information that is clearly confidential, such as medical records, the fitness professional may become aware of other information the participant wants to keep private. Trustworthiness is an important characteristic of an effective helper and reflects an ethical stand. Participants will trust someone who keeps information confidential, treats them with respect, and keeps the relationship professional.

Also, fitness professionals must recognize personal limitations and know when to refer a client to a professional therapist. It is the role of the fitness professional to help people change unhealthy behavior, but marital problems, eating disorders, and affective disorders such as depression are a few examples of areas that should be handled by someone trained to work with these issues. Know and adhere to scope of practice, and help connect participants with the best resources for handling their unique problems.

KEY POINT

Listening to the actual words and the nonverbal message in context is the foundation of good communication skills. To communicate effectively, the fitness professional should practice reflective listening and empathetic responding. Characteristics of an effective helper include empathy, attentiveness, concreteness, genuineness, and respectful confrontation.

22

LEARNING AIDS

REVIEW QUESTIONS

1. What are the five stages of change as applied to exercise? Provide examples of factors fitness professionals must consider when working with clients in each stage.

2. What are the basic human needs according to SDT, and how can participation in a group exercise class help to meet each of these needs?

3. What are strategies fitness professionals can use to target sources of self-efficacy information and to help increase task *and* barrier self-efficacy in a novice exerciser?

4. List the personal, social, and environmental links in a behavioral chain for an overweight woman to participate in a walking program during her lunch hour. Explain how fitness professionals could target the weak links to increase the likelihood of long-term adherence.

5. Explain the benefits of assessing cultural and environmental barriers to exercise adoption.

6. Discuss and give examples of motivational strategies that could be used with participants who are just starting to exercise regularly and those who have been exercising for at least 6 months.

7. Describe the elements of successful goal setting, and write one long-term and one short-term goal for a sedentary older adult who wants to be fit enough to enjoy a vacation at the beach with their grandchildren 4 months from now.

8. Explain the steps in relapse prevention and why each step is important in helping participants stick with an exercise program and resist relapse.

9. Describe the characteristics of an effective helper, and explain how each characteristic is related to good communication skills.

10. Define *weight bias*, and explain how bias toward people who are obese can affect fitness programming.

11. What are examples of weight discrimination in health care and fitness settings?

CASE STUDIES

1. LaTisha is a 35-year-old healthy female who completed her master's degree 10 years ago and has held a mostly sedentary job in downtown Atlanta for the past 7 years. Two years ago, her company shifted to remote work for most employees, and LaTisha has enjoyed not having to dress up for work. LaTisha has never exercised regularly, and working from home increased her sedentary time. She has gained 20 pounds (9 kilograms) over the past year. On her birthday, she decided she was going to take steps to pursue a career path that would allow her to better use her master's degree, although she will no longer be able to work from home. As she started reviewing job openings and preparing for interviews, she panicked when all her professional clothes did not fit. LaTisha knows she needs to be more active to lose weight. She joined your fitness center, and the director referred her to you. What stage of behavior change is LaTisha in? Where is she on the motivation continuum of the self-determination theory? What are your goals for the initial meeting with LaTisha and some strategies you would apply?

2. Taylor is a middle-aged male college professor who joined the walking club in your facility after you conducted his fitness and psychosocial assessment 3 months ago. His long-term goal was to walk around the world (in terms of total miles walked), and his progress has been marked automatically on the walkers' promotional map at the front entrance and on your webpage. His office is two blocks from your facility, and Taylor usually walks on your indoor track before he goes home for the day. You notice his mileage has decreased over the past 2 weeks, and another walker tells you that Taylor said, "I won't make it out of the state thanks to term papers and extra committee work." What stage of behavior change is Taylor in, and what strategies could you use to help him?

3. Your club has sponsored a 10K race every Thanksgiving for the past 5 years, and Marty, a healthy 25-year-old male, has always placed in the top five of his age group.

His younger brother Jim will be in town this Thanksgiving, and they plan to run the 10K together. Marty is determined to beat Jim, so he has been coming into your club at least once a week for the past month to do speed work on the treadmill. However, he's discouraged by his minor increase in speed and the increased tightness in his legs. When you ask Marty about his training program, you discover that he does no resistance training and rarely stretches, but he has doubled his weekly mileage over the past 4 weeks and plans to increase even more to be ready for the race and competition with Jim in 6 weeks. What stage is Marty in, and what strategies could you use to help him?

Answers to Case Studies

1. LaTisha is in the contemplation stage. She is not active but intends to start regular exercise. LaTisha's motivation is extrinsic—to fit in her business clothes again—and she has low exercise self-efficacy. She has not exercised in the past, so you want to educate her about what to expect at the beginning of an exercise program and make sure the prescription is appropriate for her fitness level. Your goal for the initial meeting is to apply motivational interviewing techniques to help her explore other motives besides weight loss that can bolster her commitment. You want to express empathy and optimism to help counter her anxiety about the extra weight and upcoming interviews associated with a career change. Schedule a fitness evaluation to give her a realistic idea of her current fitness level and how much progress she can expect based on a sensible prescription. In setting goals with her, help her to identify how her exercise and dietary behaviors foster weight management, and encourage self-monitoring. Reframe exercise as including activities she might enjoy to help shift her motivation to be more self-determined. Brainstorm about her barriers to exercise and how to counter them. Identify supports, such as friends and family, and ways she could reward herself during the program. Target her low exercise self-efficacy by suggesting several beginners' exercise classes to give her choices and foster mastery. Make sure she gets individual attention and encouragement, especially during the first few weeks.

2. Taylor is in the action stage and is especially susceptible to relapse. Make a point of talking with Taylor the next time he comes in to provide support and education about relapse prevention. Extra work at the end of the term is a high-risk situation for everyone; Taylor is discouraged and at risk of relapse. Talk with him about setting short-term goals that can be readjusted during exams. Help him to make the goals realistic and reachable. Taylor might want to take walk breaks for 10 to 15 minutes during the day as a way to manage stress at work. Praise Taylor for how far he has come and for continuing to walk even with extra demands at work. Help him see that the high-risk situation is time limited, and brainstorm ways he can reward himself for the walking he accomplishes. Recruit veteran walkers to provide support and encouragement.

3. Marty is in the maintenance stage, but his motivation has shifted from intrinsic to extrinsic by focusing on beating his brother Jim in the Thanksgiving race. His relationship with Jim is beyond your role, but you can help him train most effectively for this race. Ask if he has an exercise app you could review together to learn more about his training, or get him to log his miles, speed, and physical and psychological responses over the next week. Find out his experiences with resistance training and stretching to discover why he skips these activities. He might not know their benefits, or he might not enjoy lifting weights and stretching. Invite Marty to a resistance class that has several runners who have benefited from lifting weights. Introduce him to a fast runner who has a balanced training program and can show Marty stretching routines that have helped their running performance.

Injury Prevention and Management

Jenny Moshak

OBJECTIVES

The reader will be able to do the following:

1. Design and implement an emergency action plan (EAP)

2. Describe the signs and symptoms of soft-tissue injuries (sprains, strains, contusions, tendinitis, tendinosis, dislocations, and subluxations), and describe how to provide acute care for injuries

3. Define *delayed-onset muscle soreness (DOMS)* and *exertional rhabdomyolysis*, and explain how to prevent, identify signs and symptoms of, and provide care for these conditions

4. Identify signs, symptoms, and initial proper treatment for bone injuries, wounds, and associated bleeding

5. Provide prevention strategies to deter the occurrence and spread of community-acquired methicillin-resistant *Staphylococcus aureus* (CA-MRSA)

6. Design a safe return to activity program over a 2- to 4-week time frame using the 50/30/20/10 rule for conditioning activities and the FIT rule for strength training activities for those participants returning from injury or scheduled time away from exercise

7. Describe the causes, prevention, and treatment of heat-related disorders and emergencies, and provide guidelines for fluid replacement before and after exercise

8. Explain the causes, prevention, and treatment of cold-related disorders and emergencies, including superficial and deep frostbite and hypothermia

9. Provide direction using the 30–30 rule when lightning poses a threat during outdoor activities

10. Identify and manage diabetic reactions, seizures, and respiratory disorders that occur during exercise participation

11. Identify complications associated with conditioning and the environment related to sickle cell trait (SCT) and exertional sickling, including prevention, recognition of signs and symptoms, and care during an emergent situation

12. Identify the signs and symptoms of a concussion, and determine when to remove a participant from activity

13. Describe the appropriate action and techniques needed in emergency situations, including treating shock, monitoring vital signs, performing cardiopulmonary resuscitation (CPR), clearing airway obstructions, and using an automated external defibrillator (AED) for adults

23

The fitness professional must be prepared to respond in an emergency medical situation and recognize signs and symptoms in order to manage common injuries and conditions to protect the safety, health, and well-being of fitness participants. This chapter discusses injury prevention, injury recognition, and common treatment approaches as well as planning for and handling medical emergencies.

Fitness enhances performance and aids in injury prevention. Improper conditioning is often a cause of sport- and activity-related injuries. Fitness professionals who appropriately develop and implement programs designed to improve flexibility; muscular strength, endurance, and power; balance and proprioception; and cardiorespiratory endurance can help increase performance and decrease the risk of injury.

There are inherent injury risks associated with sport and physical activity. The signs and symptoms of injury often include the following:

- Exquisite point tenderness
- Pain that persists even when the body part is at rest or causes inability to sleep
- Joint pain
- Pain that does not go away after a warm-up
- Swelling or discoloration
- Increased pain with weight-bearing activities or with active movement
- Changes in normal bodily functions

Injury risk in exercise programs may be reduced by assessing the fitness level of the participant, designing a program that gradually increases in intensity and duration, especially during the first 2 to 4 weeks after a period of inactivity, while meeting the participant's goals, and monitoring progress in order to modify the workouts if necessary. Safety regarding external factors such as equipment, facilities, and weather also should be considered. Advanced planning, emergency preparedness, adequate equipment and facilities, and counseling in activity selection can mitigate injury.

Emergency Action Plan

Emergency situations may emerge at any time, and the fitness professional must be prepared when they arise, reflecting this sentiment attributed to author Alan Lakein: "Failing to plan is planning to fail." An emergency action plan (EAP) is a venue-specific written document used to facilitate and organize employee actions during workplace emergencies (see chapter 24 for more details on the legal aspects of EAPs). The EAP must

be functional for all activities, and a professional staff member should be designated as the EAP coordinator to supervise and document the plan. The development and implementation of an EAP, along with personnel training so that employees understand their roles and responsibilities within the plan, will result in the best possible care during an emergency or life-threatening conditions (4, 15, 16, 27, 39). The importance of being prepared when emergencies arise cannot be overemphasized. A client's survival may hinge on the training and preparedness of emergency team members. The American College of Sports Medicine (ACSM) recommends that staff emergency training be conducted at least four times a year (41). The EAP should be reviewed at least once a year with all staff, and agency-determined cardiopulmonary resuscitation (CPR), automated external defibrillators (AED), and first aid recertification must be maintained. It is also critical that staff sustain clear documentation of the EAP, maintain records of staff training, and keep detailed records of any injuries that occur on site (see form 23.1 for a sample EAP). The responsibility of maintaining these records often falls to the EAP coordinator. Following are considerations related to documenting the EAP:

- The EAP should be posted in a public area and kept on file.
- The EAP should be reviewed annually by the staff. Documentation of annual AED and CPR training by personnel, as well as documentation of all fitness professional staff present at the annual review of the EAP, should be recorded and filed.
- Documentation of regular emergency equipment checks and maintenance should be kept on file.

An EAP consists of three components:

1. Trained EAP personnel
2. Communication plan
3. Access to emergency equipment

Trained Personnel

Fitness professionals who are trained to react to emergency situations are essential in a workplace EAP. Fitness professionals should hold certification in CPR with AED, have knowledge of basic first aid and prevention of disease transmission, and be able to implement the EAP.

When forming the emergency team, it is important to develop team members' skills so that they can respond to a variety of situations. If each member is able to act in a wide range of capacities, the team will be better able to respond to situations that arise. This allows the emergency team to function even though certain members may not be present.

FORM 23.1 Sample Emergency Action Plan

Effective: <u>November 2023</u>

Emergency communication: <u>Fixed telephone lines are located in the main office (555-555-0123) and at the front desk (555-555-0121). Supervisors on staff carry cellular telephones.</u>

ROLES OF EMERGENCY TEAM PERSONNEL (FITNESS STAFF TRAINED AND CERTIFIED IN EMERGENCY CARE)

1. Immediate care to the injured participant
2. Activation of emergency medical services (EMS)
   - Call 911 (provide name, location, telephone number, number of people injured, condition of injured, first aid treatment, specific directions, other information as requested).
   - Provide venue directions: <u>Our facility is located at 2000 North Main Street on the corner of Main Street and Central Avenue. The main entrance doors are on the north side of the building off of Main Street. Notify supervisor and other personnel needed to respond to the emergency.</u>
3. Direction of EMS to scene
   - Open appropriate doors.
   - Designate a person to make initial contact with EMS and direct them to the scene.
   - Scene control: Limit scene to first aid providers and move bystanders away from area.
4. Emergency equipment retrieval:
   - <u>Centrally located AED is on the wall next to the main reception desk.</u>
   - <u>A second AED is located on the second floor on the wall between the weight room and multipurpose gymnasium.</u>
   - <u>First aid kits are located at the main reception desk and in the storage closet on the second floor.</u>
5. Following the event: Staff present at the event shall document the incident by completing an injury or accident report of the emergency situation.

ROLES WITHIN THE EMERGENCY TEAM

1. Immediate care of the injured participant
2. Emergency equipment retrieval (e.g., first aid supplies, AED)
3. Activation of EMS
4. Direction of EMS to scene
5. Documentation

Communication Plan

Rapid and effective communication is key to quick delivery of care in emergency situations. Access to a working telephone or other telecommunications device, whether fixed or mobile, should be ensured. The communications system should be checked on a regular basis to guarantee working order. A backup communication plan should be in effect in case the primary communication system fails. The most common method of communication today is a cellular phone; however, it is important to know the location of all workable telephones. Prearranged access to the phones should be established. See the sidebar *Activating Emergency Medical Services* for an example of a facility plan for activating EMS.

Making the Call

- 911 (or local emergency number)
- Additional contacts required by the center (e.g., college campus fitness center may require communication with campus safety unit)

Providing Information

- Name, address, and telephone number of caller
- Specific directions to the emergency scene (e.g., "Come to the south entrance of the facility on Main Street")
- Number of injured people
- Condition of injured people
- First aid treatment initiated by first responder
- Other information as requested by dispatcher

Access to Emergency Equipment

All emergency equipment should be quickly accessible at the facility and stored in a clean, environmentally controlled area. An appropriate number of AEDs should be available and located in areas that allow for a response time of 3 minutes or less (29). Emergency equipment should be checked and calibrated on a regular basis. Personnel should be familiar with the function and operation of each type of emergency equipment and rehearse their use regularly. The emergency equipment should be appropriate for the emergency team personnel's training level and certification.

KEY POINT

The development and implementation of an EAP helps ensure the safety and well-being of fitness participants when an emergency situation arises. Key components of an EAP are a trained staff, a communication plan, and access to working emergency equipment.

Injury Management

The fitness professional should be knowledgeable about common activity-related injuries and may be called on to give initial care. Actual diagnosis and long-term care of injuries is the responsibility of medical professionals. This section provides information to assist in identifying common injuries, administering appropriate acute care, and making referrals to medical personnel.

Managing an injury requires an understanding of the structures involved and the severity of trauma. An acute injury occurs when a force acts on tissue and produces a macrotrauma. A chronic injury occurs over a period of time when repetitive forces produce a microtrauma. Forces involved in the injury process consist of compressive, tensile, and shear. For example, a contusion, or bruise, is caused by a compressive direct force acting on the involved tissue. Damage to a ligament involves a tensile force that pulls the tissue apart, causing a stretch or tear. A blister occurs when a shear force acts in opposite directions on layers of the skin. Some traumatic injuries involve multiple forces and structures. For example, a knee injury that results in tears of the anterior cruciate ligament (ACL), medial collateral ligament (MCL), and meniscus and a bony contusion on the joint surface is an all-too-common complex injury involving multiple structures.

Signs and symptoms associated with an injury often include one or more of the following: swelling, discoloration, pain, instability, muscle spasms, point tenderness, decreased range of motion (ROM), decreased strength, and dysfunction. Some signs and symptoms may manifest immediately, whereas others may take several hours or days to present.

Soft-Tissue Injuries

Common activity-related injuries include the following:

- *Contusion:* Caused by single or multiple forces over time, resulting in bleeding, ecchymosis (black and blue discoloration), and tissue damage of the skin or muscle (e.g., deep thigh bruise)
- *Acute sprain:* Caused by a single tensile force that produces a stretch or tear (partial or complete) of a ligament (e.g., lateral ankle sprain)
- *Chronic sprain:* Occurs from repetitive forces acting on a ligament (e.g., Little League elbow)
- *Muscle or tendon strain:* Involves a tensile force causing an overstretching or partial or complete tear (e.g., hamstring strain)
- *Tendinitis:* Inflammation of a tendon caused by single or repetitive tensile forces (e.g., Achilles tendinitis)

- *Tendinosis:* Degeneration of collagen in a tendon over time (e.g., tennis elbow)
- *Bursitis:* Inflammation caused by compression or friction to a bursa sac (e.g., olecranon bursitis)
- *Dislocation:* When bone is forced out of its normal joint position and remains there until manually or surgically replaced (e.g., shoulder dislocation)
- *Subluxation:* When bone is partially forced out of the joint and spontaneously returns (e.g., patella subluxation)
- *Nerve damage:* Occurs from a compressive or tensile force (e.g., sciatica); signs and symptoms include change in sensation, decrease in strength, numbness, and pain (nerve pain is often described as shooting, aching, sharp, dull, throbbing, tingling, or burning)

Soft-tissue injuries are classified by their severity and dysfunction:

- *Mild or first degree:* Microtearing or stretching of the tissue involving minor tissue damage, mild to moderate pain, minimal swelling, full to limited ROM, and little to no dysfunction.
- *Moderate or second degree:* Partial tearing of the tissue resulting in moderate tissue damage, moderate to severe pain, moderate swelling, limited ROM, and limited function. Muscle spasms may occur around the injury.
- *Severe or third degree:* Major disruption to tissue, often resulting in a complete tear with moderate to severe pain, moderate to severe swelling, and loss of function. Palpable deformity may be present along with muscle spasms in the area.

Fitness professionals are not expected to diagnose the degree of injury, but they should have a basic understanding of the continuum of injuries and be able to provide first aid, including applying common elements of care for injuries.

Protection, rest, ice, compression, and elevation (PRICE principle) are the basis for providing injury care.

PRICE

P—Protection is necessary to avoid further tissue damage when a moderate to severe injury occurs. This requires complete immobilization (stabilizing the injury and the areas above and below) until further evaluation by medical personnel. Items that offer protection include crutches, splints, braces, and arm slings.

R—Rest is necessary to allow damaged tissue to begin the healing process and depends on the severity of injury. It can range from modifying activity, to not using the injured body part, to stopping activity altogether.

I—Ice (cold application) results in an immediate decrease in pain and spasm around the injury. Vasoconstriction of local blood vessels occurs, which may help minimize swelling. Cold applications including ice bags and gel and chemical packs are applied for 20 to 30 minutes. Some individuals cannot tolerate ice directly on the skin due to tissue sensitivity or circulatory impairment. This typically occurs in older adults, young children, or people with systemic disease. In these cases, or when using a cold gel or chemical pack, a barrier such as a towel should be placed between the pack and the skin. Depending on the severity of the injury, ice should be reapplied several times during the first 24 to 72 hours.

C—Compression is applied using an elastic wrap or sleeve to help prevent swelling. The elastic wrap should be applied beginning distal to the injury, completely covering the body part, and extending proximal to the injury site. Compression should be applied firmly but not so tightly that circulation is impaired.

E—Elevation of the injured body part above the heart will maximize the effect of gravity to minimize swelling.

Heat should never be applied to an acute injury. Some chronic injuries such as tendinitis, tendinosis, and bursitis may benefit from heating the area prior to activity, either superficially (e.g., heat pack, warm whirlpool) or deeply (additional dynamic or cardio warm-up time). Heating tissue increases circulation, muscle excitability, tissue elasticity, cellular metabolism, and nerve conduction. Both chronic and subacute injuries can benefit from cold application after activity (5, 38, 39).

KEY POINT

When soft tissues are injured, proper assessment and initial treatment can reduce the possibility of further trauma and can aid in the healing process. Protection, rest, ice, compression, and elevation (PRICE) are the important steps for immediate care of most musculoskeletal and joint injuries.

Delayed-Onset Muscle Soreness

When starting a new exercise program, some participants may encounter an overload condition called *delayed-onset muscle soreness (DOMS)*. DOMS can occur from an activity that places unaccustomed loads on muscle, resulting in microscopic breakdown of muscle tissue that leads to an inflammatory response over several days. This type of soreness is different from acute soreness, which is pain that develops during or immediately after the activity. Delayed soreness typically begins to develop 12 to 24 hours after the exercise has been performed and may produce the greatest pain between 24 and 72 hours after the exercise. Activities that produce an eccentric force, such as running or walking downhill, weightlifting, and jumping, often are associated with DOMS (7, 10). However, anyone participating in a new activity can experience DOMS.

Although pain is usually the most noticeable symptom of DOMS, people may also experience mild swelling in the affected extremities, stiffness, decreased joint ROM, point tenderness, and muscle weakness. When the signs and symptoms become severe, it may be an indication of exertional rhabdomyolysis (see the next section in this chapter).

One of the best ways to prevent or at least reduce the severity of DOMS is to progress slowly—over a 2- to 4-week period in a new exercise program or activity (17). The muscles need time to adapt to new stresses, and this should help minimize the severity of symptoms, although some soreness can be expected. It is also important to allow the muscle time to recover; participating in the same exercises on subsequent days, particularly if exertion is high, is not recommended.

Treatment of DOMS involves decreasing the symptoms. Rest, ice, compression, elevation, along with light massage and nonsteroidal anti-inflammatory drugs (NSAID) may be useful in reducing pain and swelling. Return to activity should be gradual to prevent further muscle damage (10, 17, 21, 22).

KEY POINT

Participants starting a new exercise program often experience DOMS. Muscles should be given an opportunity to adequately recover and adapt to new stresses in order to minimize the pain that accompanies DOMS.

Exertional Rhabdomyolysis

Exertional rhabdomyolysis (ER) is a syndrome that can occur in normal, healthy people following strenuous exercise. Rhabdomyolysis is characterized by skeletal muscle breakdown that subsequently releases its intracellular contents—the muscle protein myoglobin; potassium; and the enzymes creatine kinase, lactate dehydrogenase, serum glutamic oxaloacetic transaminase, and aldolase—into the bloodstream, which is then filtered by the kidneys. This causes electrolyte imbalances that can lead to nausea, vomiting, mental confusion, cardiac arrhythmias, and coma. The myoglobin breaks down into substances that can harm and destroy kidney cells, leading to kidney damage. In severe cases, this syndrome can result in renal failure and sudden death (8, 9, 17, 26, 41, 42, 46).

The National Collegiate Athletic Association (NCAA) states, "Novel overexertion is the single most common cause of exertional rhabdomyolysis (ER) and is characterized as too much, too soon, and too fast" (36). This typically involves strength and conditioning programs that increase in intensity and duration too quickly and do not allow for adequate recovery (42).

The signs and symptoms of ER may initially resemble DOMS; however, the soreness is more severe, and additional signs and symptoms include the following:

- Dark, red, or cola-colored urine
- Decreased urine output
- Severe muscle pain characterized as aching or throbbing, or stiffness
- General weakness, exhaustion, or fatigue
- Abdominal pain
- Nausea or vomiting
- Muscle swelling
- Muscle weakness
- Mental confusion, dizziness, light-headedness
- Irregular heartbeat

Similar to DOMS, the signs and symptoms of ER may take several hours to days to develop. Fitness participants with these signs and symptoms should not participate in activity and should see a physician. Medical clearance is recommended before participation resumes.

Risk factors that can increase the likelihood of ER include the following:

- Being deconditioned
- Exposure to a novel workout regimen
- Hot environmental conditions
- Having hypohydration (the uncompensated loss of body water) or heat-related illness
- Having sickle cell trait (SCT)

Research indicates that there is a relationship between SCT and an increased vulnerability to heat illness and ER (6, 14, 15, 17, 31, 36).

Prevention of ER involves gradually increasing the intensity and duration of exercise programs and preventing hypohydration. Drinking plenty of fluids during and after strenuous exercise will help dilute the urine and enhance the ability of the kidneys to clear large proteins such as myoglobin. A fitness professional should never use strength training or conditioning or the denial of fluid replacement as a form of punishment (14, 15, 17, 36).

KEY POINT

The single most common cause of ER is implementing an exercise program that is too much, too soon, too fast. Using progression when introducing any new activity and emphasizing hydration will help prevent ER. Adequate recovery is essential to protect muscle tissue from excessive breakdown. Exercise should never be used as a form of punishment.

Treating Fractures

Fracture takes place when a break in the continuity of bone tissue occurs. Acute fracture occurs from a direct force that damages the bone, and stress (chronic) fracture results from repetitive forces that progressively injure the bone. The periosteum is affected initially, followed by damage to the cortical bone. Signs and symptoms of a fracture include pain, point tenderness, swelling, and visual or palpable deformity. There may also be muscle spasms and impairment to nearby blood vessels or nerves. A simple (closed) fracture is one that has no open wound, whereas a compound (open) fracture has one or more bones exposed through the soft tissue and skin around it. An acute fracture should be immobilized by splinting the distal and proximal joints to the injured area, and the participant should be referred to a physician. Do not attempt to reduce (push back into place) a fracture. Activate EMS to assist with transport; urgency is a necessity with any skull or spine fracture; compound fracture; or fracture associated with shock, impaired circulation, or nerve damage. A suspected fracture to the skull or spine requires immediate head and neck immobilization until EMS takes over. Table 23.1 gives the possible signs and symptoms and additional procedures to follow when treating a fracture.

KEY POINT

If a fracture is suspected, immobilize the joints above and below the injury, treat for shock, and activate EMS when appropriate. Do not attempt to reduce a fracture.

Treating Wounds and Other Skin Disorders

Wounds are common injuries associated with activity programs. The fitness professional may need to provide emergency treatment for an open wound to control bleeding and prevent infection. Universal precautions are safety measures that prevent exposure to blood, body fluids, and bloodborne pathogens (see the sidebar *Universal Precautions* later in the chapter). Once bleeding is controlled, further care can be given to prevent infection. In minor cases, a thorough cleansing and application of a sterile dressing may be all that is needed. Clean with large amounts of soap and water or sterile

Table 23.1   Fractures and Their Treatment

Signs and symptoms	Care
ACUTE FRACTURE	
Loss of function Deformity or bony deviation Swelling Pain Palpable tenderness Referred pain Crepitus False joint Discoloration (usually becomes apparent later)	**Acute closed fracture:**
	Active EMS if transport is necessary. *Do not* reduce a fracture. Splint the joints above and below the suspected fracture to protect the body part from further injury. Ice can be applied to reduce pain, spasm, and swelling. Treat for shock. (See section on emergency procedures.) Refer to a physician.
	Acute open fracture:
	Activate EMS. Control bleeding and prevent infection by applying a sterile dressing. *Do not* move bones back into place. Follow protocol for closed fracture care.
CHRONIC STRESS FRACTURE	
Pain that increases in intensity and duration Swelling Dysfunction Point tenderness	Remove from activity that causes pain. Refer to a physician.

Based on Anderson and Barnum (2022); Prentice (2020); Prentice (2014).

saline to flush. Use sterile gauze with sterile technique: Begin directly over the wound and sweep, moving away from the injury. Cover with a sterile dressing, and apply moderate pressure until bleeding stops. If bleeding continues, apply more gauze on top of the saturated material. When bleeding stops, cover with topical petroleum-based ointment, a sterile nonadherent dressing, and a bandage. Protect open wounds with a sterile dressing; a covered wound heals faster.

If a wound becomes infected, the infection usually occurs several days later and presents with an increase in pain, heat, redness, swelling, or dysfunction. Refer immediately to a physician. See table 23.2 for additional care for specific wound types.

A wound involving uncontrolled, severe bleeding is a medical emergency. Excessive blood loss can result in shock and lead to death. Internal bleeding, another serious condition, involves bleeding deep within structures of the body, including the chest, abdominal, or pelvic cavities. The fitness professional should treat for shock and alert EMS immediately. Table 23.3 discusses care of severe bleeding.

KEY POINT

The primary steps of treating an open wound are to control bleeding and prevent infection. Clean the wound and keep it covered until it heals.

Staphylococcus Aureus

Staphylococcus aureus, often referred to as *staph*, is a common type of bacteria that lives in our bodies. Plenty of healthy people carry staph without being infected by it. According to the Centers for Disease Control and Prevention (CDC), approximately 30% of the American

Table 23.2 Wounds and Their Treatment

Injury	Signs and symptoms	Care
Abrasion: Scraping of tissues resulting in removal of outermost skin layers and exposure of numerous capillaries	Superficial, reddish, irregular surface Oozing or weeping from underlying capillaries and the clear, yellow liquid, blood serum Dirt, debris, or bacteria may be embedded in tissue	Dirt or debris that is still present after normal cleaning may require gentle scrubbing using sterile technique.
Incision: Cutting of skin resulting in an open wound with cleanly cut edges and exposure of underlying tissues	Smooth edges that may bleed freely	Refer to physician if wound needs suturing (e.g., facial cuts, large or deep wounds).
Laceration: Tearing of skin resulting in an open wound with jagged edges and exposure of underlying tissues	Jagged edges that may bleed freely	Refer to physician if wound needs suturing.
Puncture: Direct penetration of tissues by a pointed object	Small opening that may bleed freely	*Do not* remove object if embedded deeply. Clean wound carefully, moving around the embedded object. Apply sterile dressing and protect the body part. Activate EMS or refer to a physician. Treat for shock.
Blister: Friction causing disruption between epidermis and dermis resulting in fluid accumulation between layers of skin	Superficial redness, heat, and pain Pocket of fluid (clear or bloody) under skin Wound may be open or closed	Apply ice. Soft padding, lubricant, or donut pad may decrease pressure. If the blister opens, treat as an open wound. Both closed and open blisters have potential for infection (if signs of infection, refer to a physician).

Based on Anderson and Barnum (2022); Prentice (2020); Prentice (2014).

Table 23.3 Severe Bleeding and Its Treatment

Injury	Signs and symptoms	Care

Excessive bleeding: External bleeding that results in massive loss of circulating blood volume; often results in shock and can lead to death	External hemorrhage
	• Arterial
	  Color: Bright red
	  Flow: Spurts, bleeding usually profuse
	• Venous
	  Color: Dark red
	  Flow: Steady, oozing
		Activate EMS.
		Elevate the affected part above the heart.
		Put direct pressure over the wound, using a sterile compress if possible.
		Apply a pressure dressing. Use pressure points.
		Treat for shock.

Internal bleeding: Bleeding within deep structures of the body (chest, abdominal, or pelvic cavity) and bleeding of organs contained within these cavities; may result in shock and can lead to death	Generally, no external signs, except when an individual coughs up blood, finds blood in the urine or feces, or experiences the following: • Restlessness • Thirst • Faintness • Anxiety • Cold, clammy skin • Dizziness • Rapid, weak, irregular pulse • Significant fall in blood pressure (BP)	Activate EMS. Treat for shock. Do not give water or food.

Based on Anderson and Barnum (2022); Prentice (2020); Prentice (2014).

population is colonized in the nose with *Staphylococcus aureus*, and approximately 5% of the population is colonized with methicillin-resistant *Staphylococcus aureus* (MRSA) (18). When MRSA is introduced into the body, often through an open wound, it can cause an infection that has become resistant to the antibiotics commonly used to treat ordinary staph infections.

MRSA is most common among people who have weak immune systems and are in hospitals. However, MRSA is also showing up in healthy people who have not been hospitalized or been to outpatient care facilities. This type of MRSA is classified as community-associated MRSA, or CA-MRSA (community-acquired methicillin-resistant *Staphylococcus aureus*), and this is the form fitness professionals may see in fitness settings. CA-MRSA can be contracted through person-to-person contact; sharing of towels or soaps; and improperly cleaned equipment such as mats, pads, whirlpools, and common surfaces (e.g., weight equipment).

Signs and symptoms of CA-MRSA include skin infections. Patients will present with pimples, pustules, or boils that often are mistaken for spider bites. These irritations often are red, swollen, and painful, and they may produce pus. If left untreated, the bacteria can move from the skin, through the bloodstream, to other tissues—the heart, lungs, bones, and joints.

Prevention of CA-MRSA is the responsibility of both the fitness professional and the participant. Maintaining good hygiene and avoiding contact with drainage from skin lesions are the best methods for prevention. Fitness personnel and clients should be educated to do the following:

- Cover any suspicious skin lesions until a medical referral can be made.
- Keep hands clean by washing thoroughly with soap and warm water or routinely using an alcohol-based hand sanitizer.
- Remove sweat-soaked athletic wear, especially when worn in common equipment-use areas such as weight rooms or on cardio equipment.
- Encourage immediate showering following activity.
- People with open wounds, scrapes, or scratches should avoid pools, whirlpools, and common tubs.
- Avoid sharing towels, razors, and daily athletic gear.
- Wash athletic gear and towels after each use in hot water (140 °F or 60 °C). Designate separate laundry bins for collecting soiled laundry and clean laundry.
- Maintain clean facilities and equipment. Equipment routinely should be sanitized and disinfected with a hospital-grade bactericidal and virucidal cleaner.

Care and treatment of CA-MRSA involves the referral of suspicious lesions to a physician for bacterial cultures in order to establish a diagnosis. If a lesion is determined to be contagious, participants must obtain clearance from their physician before being allowed in common-use areas. Cover skin lesions appropriately before participation (35).

Universal Precautions

When treating skin wounds or when exposed to bodily fluids, the fitness professional needs to follow the Occupational Safety and Health Administration (OSHA) universal precautions for safety of the participant and first aid provider. Wear gloves, and when possible, wash hands or use alcohol-based hand sanitizer before donning the gloves. Use a new set of gloves for each patient and wound site. Rewash hands immediately after removing gloves (43).

Hand Washing

1. Wash hands with soap and water.
2. Apply soap and rub for at least 20 seconds.
3. Cover all surfaces.
4. Dry with a fresh paper towel.
5. Use alcohol-based (containing at least 60% alcohol) rub, gel, or foam.
6. Use enough of the product to cover all surfaces.
7. Rub until dry, at least 20 seconds.

Glove Removal

1. Grasp outside of glove with opposite gloved hand and peel off.
2. Hold removed glove in gloved hand.
3. Slide fingers of ungloved hand under remaining glove at wrist.
4. Peel glove off over first glove.
5. Discard gloves in a biohazard waste container.

Based on Centers for Disease Control and Prevention, *Handwashing in Community Settings and Personal Protective Equipment (PPE) Sequence* (United States Department of Labor, 2022).

KEY POINT

Follow OSHA guidelines and universal precautions when dealing with open wounds, bodily fluids, and MRSA.

Medical Referral and Exercise Modification

After initial care and treatment of a moderate to severe injury, fitness professionals should refer the client to a medical professional. Conditions that require immediate attention or activating EMS include bone deformity, uncontrolled pain, suspected fracture, severe bleeding, decreased circulation, nerve damage, and any life-threatening emergencies. Possible indications for a nonemergent referral include pain, swelling, and decreased function.

Upon return to exercise after injury, it is helpful to have instructions from a health care provider indicating any exclusions or modifications in activity. Mild injuries may require modifying activity levels until normal function returns. This may include reducing the intensity and duration of an activity or finding an alternative form of exercise. Exercise in a swimming pool is an effective way to decrease forces from body weight. A runner who experiences pain may be able to run without pain in chest-deep water or in deep water with a vest. Examples of strength training modifications include decreasing the number of sets or amount of weight lifted, using machines to assist accessory muscles with the joint stability required during free-weight exercises, and using resistance bands or body-weight exercises. During the recovery phase, the goal is to find activities the participant can perform safely without compromising the healing process. Maintaining communication with the participant and their health care provider is recommended.

Tragically, 162 high school and NCAA football players died in a 20-year period from 1998 to 2018 during supervised practice or conditioning sessions. The vast majority of cases (94.7%) involved high-intensity aerobic training, and in 36 of the cases the exercise was used as punishment (8).

The Collegiate Strength and Conditioning Coaches Association (CSCCa) and the National Strength and Conditioning Association (NSCA) worked together in

2019 to draft "Joint Consensus Guidelines for Transition Periods: Safe Return to Training Following Inactivity" with the goal of decreasing the incidence of injuries and deaths associated with athletes transitioning from periods of inactivity related to return from injury or scheduled breaks to regular training. The guidelines recommend that transition periods have lower work-to-rest ratios (W:R) (1:4 W:R in week 1; 1:3 W:R in week 2; and 1:2 W:R in weeks 3 and 4) and gradually progress to full intensity using the 50/30/20/10 rule over a 2- to 4-week time frame for conditioning workouts and the FIT (frequency, intensity, volume, and time of rest interval) rule for resistance training (17).

- *50/30/20/10 rule:* The conditioning volume for the first week of a fitness participant returning to activity after time off or an injury is reduced by 50% of the uppermost conditioning volume the participant has experienced prior to time away, with a W:R of 1:4, by 30% with a W:R of 1:3 in week 2, and by 20% and 10% with a W:R of 1:2 in weeks 3 and 4, respectively. See table 23.4 for a basketball conditioning example of the 50/30/20/10 rule.
- *FIT rule:* Sets $\times$ reps $\times$ %1RM as a decimal = IRV units. IRV represents the intensity relative volume. IRV units are the derivation of volume load that includes the percent of 1-repetition maximum (%1RM), and an IRV between 11 and 30 is recommended. The previously described W:R applies to the FIT rule. See table 23.5.

KEY POINT

The 50/30/20/10 rule and the FIT rule over a 2- to 4-week period of time will help ensure the participant's safe return to activity.

Environmental Concerns

Fitness professionals must take into consideration the general health of the population they are working with and the environmental conditions that prevail. The environment can impair performance and contribute to the development of serious medical issues.

Air quality can be a major factor in performance and safety, particularly in urban areas where pollution from factories and motor vehicles may be more prevalent. Extreme temperatures and lightning can prove deadly in some instances. This section examines these concerns and discusses ways to minimize risk to participants.

Air Quality

Fitness professionals need to consider air quality when training participants both outdoors and indoors. The Air Quality Index (AQI) is a daily air quality measurement of outdoor air pollutants calculated by the Environmental Protection Agency (EPA). See chapter 13 for more information about the AQI and recommendations for participation. Also consider that some indoor facilities

Table 23.4 **50/30/20/10 Rule Applied to Basketball Line Drill Conditioning Session With Baseline of 10 Repetitions in 32 Seconds With 1:1.5 W:R**

Week	Reduction in (%)	Repetitions	Intensity (seconds)	Rest time (minutes:seconds)
1	50	5	48	3:12
2	30	7	42	2:06
3	20	8	38	1:16
4	10	9	35	1:10

Based on Caterisano et al. (2019).

Table 23.5 **FIT Rule: Intensity Relative Volume (IRV) Examples for 2- to 4-Week Transition Period From Inactivity**

Example	Sets	Repetitions	%1RM	IRV units	Range level*
1	3	15	0.60	27	Safe
2	3	10	0.65	19.5	Safe
3	5	8	0.70	28	Safe
4	5	6	0.80	24	Safe
5	10	10	0.50	50	Unsafe

*Range level 11-30 IRV units considered safe.

Based on Caterisano et al. (2019).

may have higher levels of dust, mold, or other allergens. Exercise increases exposure to air pollutants due to participants breathing more deeply and rapidly. They take in more air and have a tendency to mouth breathe, bypassing the nasal filtration system. Pollutants or allergens in the air may adversely affect people with asthma, severe allergies, or other breathing problems.

Minimize the risks in these ways:

- Monitor air pollution and allergen levels. Local radio, television, and newspapers often report on daily air quality. Weather apps can provide hour-by-hour updates.
- Exercise should be modified or rescheduled during times of peak pollution or poor air quality. Participants should be advised if the index for certain allergens is high.
- Avoid high-pollution areas such as heavy traffic, industrial, and outdoor smoking areas.
- Exercise indoors on poor air quality days.

KEY POINT

A high pollution index or extreme pollen counts can compromise participants' performance and health. Fitness professionals must be aware of environmental conditions and the sensitivities of the people they are training. Schedule activities for times and places where the participants are unlikely to be affected.

Exertional Heat Illnesses

Exertional heat illnesses are a concern for people who participate in intense and long-duration exercise. This section focuses on exertional heat stroke (EHS), heat exhaustion, and exercise-associated muscle cramps (EAMC). Exertional heat illness usually occurs with one or more of the following: elevation in body core temperature, electrolyte imbalance, and hypohydration. Hypohydration is a deficit of body water caused by dehydration.

Environmental factors that increase the risk of heat illness include ambient air temperature, relative humidity, air motion, and the amount of radiant heat from the sun. When exercising in high temperatures, participants depend on evaporation of sweat for heat loss. High relative humidity inhibits heat loss from the body through evaporation. Intense and long training sessions and the environment can place large heat loads on the body, causing an increase in the core body temperature, or hyperthermia. Even the most highly conditioned athlete can experience a heat-related disorder.

Hypohydration occurs when dehydration, the process of losing body water via sweat, vomiting, or diarrhea, is not combated with adequate fluid replacement. Participants should weigh themselves before and after activity to monitor fluid loss. A water loss up to 2% of body weight is considered safe. A 3% to 5% loss is cause for concern, and more than a 5% loss is considered serious and activity should be suspended until fluid weight is adequately replaced (34). The potential for a cascade effect of fluid loss exists; therefore, it is essential to continually replace fluids lost through sweat and urine excretion.

Fluids lost in the sweating process include electrolytes, essential minerals necessary for nerve and muscle function, body-fluid balance, and other critical processes. The balance of electrolytes is constantly shifting due to fluctuations in fluid intake as well as due to exercise and environmental heat conditions. Salt (NaCl) is an important electrolyte in fluid retention, and loss of salt is evident by a white, chalky film on skin and clothing.

In addition to hypohydration and environmental conditions, certain predisposing factors can contribute to heat illness:

- Being deconditioned
- Incomplete heat acclimatization
- Sudden increase in physical training
- History of heat illness
- History of SCT
- Illness and medications
- Nutritional supplements
- Poor nutrition
- Obesity
- Sleep deprivation
- Age (children and older populations are more susceptible)

EHS is defined as hyperthermia (core body temperature >40.5 °C [105 °F]) associated with central nervous system disturbances and multiple organ system failure (14, 40). It occurs when environmental heat factors (hot and humid weather), internal body heat created by muscle metabolism (exercise), and/or inhibited heat loss (decreased sweating mechanism or evaporation) cause the thermoregulatory system to become overwhelmed. Even though hot, humid weather often is a factor, EHS can occur during intense physical activity in non-extreme environmental conditions. Rectal temperature is the standard used by medical professionals to measure body core temperature and diagnose EHS. This is a life-threatening condition. When a person who has survived EHS is medically cleared to return to activity, exercise should begin in a cool environment and gradually increase in duration, intensity, and heat exposure over a 2- to 4-week, or possibly longer (6-8 week), period using the 50/30/20/10 and FIT rules (17). If any signs and symptoms recur, stop activity and refer to a physician.

Heat exhaustion is the inability to continue exercise associated with any combination of heavy sweating, hypohydration, sodium loss, and energy depletion (14). It occurs most frequently in hot, humid conditions and shares many of the signs and symptoms of EHS; therefore, activating EMS is recommended when either condition is suspected. In heat exhaustion, body core temperature can vary from normal to as high as 40 °C (104 °F). Although heat exhaustion does not always involve elevated core temperature, cooling therapy often will improve the medical status (14, 15, 40). In mild cases, participants should not return to activity for a minimum of 24 to 48 hours. When it is safe to resume activity, a gradual increase in intensity and volume, incorporating the 50/30/20/10 rule and FIT rule over 2 to 4 weeks, is necessary.

EAMC are painful, involuntary muscle contractions that occur during or after intense exercise. They are often called *heat cramps*; however, this is an incorrect term because they are not directly related to an increase in body temperature (14). Possible causes of EAMC are by hypohydration, electrolyte imbalance, fatigue, or a combination of these factors. Although painful, EAMC often responds positively to conservative treatment, and participants can return safely to activity. People who are prone to chronic cramping will benefit from maintaining fluid and salt balance before, during, and after exercise.

Table 23.6 outlines the stages of heat illness, signs and symptoms, and guidelines for immediate care.

Both the fitness professional and the participant should understand preventive measures to decrease the incidence of heat illness. Do the following to prevent heat injury:

- Develop an EAP with understanding of exertional heat illness prevention, recognition, and treatment.
- Through preparticipation screening, identify participants who have a history of exertional heat illness or SCT.
- Acclimatize by gradually increasing activity levels and heat exposure over 7 to 14 days (13).
- Educate participants to match fluid intake with sweat and urine losses to maintain adequate hydration.
- Provide adequate fluids (water or sport electrolyte drink) to replace fluids lost during activity sessions.
- Modify activity in high heat and humidity.
- Plan rest breaks, preferably in a cool or shaded environment, with equipment (e.g., padding, helmets) removed, to match exercise intensity as well as heat and humidity.
- Measure body weight before and after activity to estimate amount of water loss (replenish by consuming 1-1.25 liters [34-42 ounces] of fluid per kilogram of water loss).
- Minimize equipment and clothing if possible.
- Drink sodium-containing fluids to keep urine clear to light yellow.
- Eat a balanced diet and discourage dietary supplements that increase metabolism, cause dehydration, or affect body temperature.
- Get adequate sleep (at least 7 hours) in a cool environment.
- Participants should not exercise if they are febrile (temperature >100.3 °F [38.0 °C]), vomiting, or have diarrhea.

KEY POINT

Modify exercise duration and intensity in hot, humid conditions. Encourage hydration and provide water and rest breaks during activity. The fitness professional must be able to recognize the signs of heat illness and take action.

Cold-Related Problems

Exercising in cold, wet, windy weather can cause problems if precautions are not taken. Considerable heat loss can occur via convective heat loss through the skin and evaporation of skin moisture. Hypothermia occurs when body heat is lost at a faster rate than it is produced and core body temperature drops below 35 °C (95 °F). Peripheral blood vessels in cold areas constrict, which conserves body heat but increases the risk of frostbite. Exercising in cold, damp weather can compound the problem by increasing the rate of evaporation. A high windchill can result in severe loss of body heat even when the air temperature is above freezing (see chapter 13). Additionally, body temperature drops even more quickly in cold water than in air of the same temperature. Table 23.7 describes how to recognize and treat cold-related problems. Cold-related problems are preventable if participants take these precautions:

- Avoid exercising outdoors in extreme cold and wind.
- Modify activity as necessary to prevent overexposure to cold, wet, windy conditions. Consider length of exposure, availability of facilities, and interventions for rewarming if needed. Clothing

Table 23.6 Exertional Heat Illnesses and Their Treatment

Exertional heat illness	Signs and symptoms	Care
Exertional heat stroke (EHS): Hyperthermia (elevated core temperature) causing organ system failure; the most serious form of heat-related illness	High core body temperature (rectal temp >40.5 °C [105 °F]) Central nervous system changes: dizziness, drowsiness, irrational or unusual behavior, confusion, irritability, emotional instability, hysteria, apathy, aggressiveness, delirium, disorientation, staggering, seizures, loss of consciousness, coma Headache Dehydration Weakness Loss of balance and muscle function Prolonged fatigue Hot and wet or dry skin Tachycardia (100-120 bpm) Hypotension Hyperventilation Vomiting Diarrhea	Treat as extreme medical emergency. Activate EMS. Lower core body temperature immediately: • Remove clothes and equipment. • Immerse body in a pool or tub of cold water—*Best method to cool* • If cold tub unavailable, use wet ice towels or body cold-water dousing; however, not as effective in lowering body temp. Monitor vital signs. Maintain airway.
Heat exhaustion: Inability to continue activity due to heavy sweating, dehydration, sodium loss, and energy depletion	Normal or elevated core body temperature (rectal temp 36-40 °C [97-104 °F]) Dehydration Dizziness/fainting Light-headedness Headache Nausea/vomiting Diarrhea or urge to defecate Intestinal cramping Decreased urine output Persistent muscle cramps Fatigue/weakness Profuse sweating Cold, clammy skin Chills Paleness Hyperventilation Thirst	Stop activity. Activate EMS. Move person to a cool or shaded area. Remove equipment and unnecessary clothing. Rapidly cool body by applying ice or ice towels to head, neck, armpits, and groin; use fans and air conditioning if available. Elevate legs. Give cold fluids (if conscious). Monitor vital signs and treat for shock.
Exercise-associated muscle cramps (EAMC): Painful, involuntary muscle contractions	Painful muscle cramping often accompanied by thirst, dehydration, and fatigue Subsides within minutes Profuse sweating White residue on clothing (due to sodium depletion)	Remove from activity. Perform mild stretching. Gently massage or put direct pressure on muscle. Ice the muscle. Replace fluids with a sodium-containing drink (sport drink formula). Return to activity when muscle is functional and no other signs or symptoms of heat illness exist.
Heat syncope: Fainting, dizziness, or excessive loss of strength due to heat	Headache Nausea Weakness Fatigue Dizziness or tunnel vision Pale, sweaty skin Decreased pulse rate	Replace lost fluids. Monitor vitals. Cool the body and place the person in shade. Elevate legs.

Based on Anderson and Barnum (2022); Roberts et al. (2021); Casa, Anderson, Baker, et al. (2012); Casa, Guskiewicz, Anderson, et al. (2012); Casa et al. (2015); National Collegiate Athletic Association (2014-2015); Prentice (2020).

should provide an internal layer that allows sweat evaporation with minimal absorption, a middle layer that provides insulation, and a removable external layer that is wind and water resistant and allows moisture evaporation (11).

- Cover the face, nose, ears, fingers, and head (a large amount of heat is lost when the head is exposed).
- Warm up before exercise and avoid bouts of inactivity.
- Stay dry.
- Avoid swimming or exercising in cold water, particularly when the surrounding air temperature is low.
- Maintain proper hydration and nutrition. Consume fluids even when not thirsty because the normal thirst mechanism is dampened with cold exposure.

KEY POINT

Cold-related problems may be prevented by avoiding exposure to extreme cold, wearing removable layers, warming up before activity, and constantly remaining active.

Lightning

Lightning is a significant weather hazard that may affect all outdoor fitness and sport activities. The fitness professional should have a response plan for lightning that is outlined in all outdoor venues' EAPs and regularly reviewed with personnel. Though the probability of being struck by lightning is low, the odds are significantly greater when a storm is in the area and safety guidelines and precautions are not followed. Weather sources and reports—real-time weather forecasts, commercial

Table 23.7 Cold-Related Problems and Their Treatment

Cold-related problems	Signs and symptoms	Care
Superficial frostbite: Freezing of skin layers and subcutaneous tissue	Skin: Dry, waxy, cold, and firm to the touch; reddening along with white or blue-gray patches Edema Tingling or burning	Remove from cold. Remove jewelry. Slowly rewarm area using water heated to 98-104 °F (37-40 °C). Handle gently and avoid friction or massage. May require medical referral.
Deep frostbite: Freezing of deep tissue, including muscle and bone	Skin: Hard, cold, waxy, and immobile; white, gray, black, or purple Pain: Burning, aching, throbbing, or shooting	Remove from cold exposure. Activate EMS. Protect body part. Remove jewelry from injured body part. Handle gently; avoid friction, rubbing, or massage. Rewarming is best performed in a hospital setting.
Mild hypothermia: Body temperature 37-35 °C (98.6-95.0 °F)	Skin: Pale Shivering Cold extremities Amnesia, lethargy Impaired motor control Excessive urination Typically conscious	Remove from cold. Rewarm with dry clothing, blankets, heating pad (apply only to trunk, armpit, and groin), and warm drinks. Avoid friction massage. Activate EMS if symptoms do not improve quickly.
Moderate to severe hypothermia: Core body temperature 34-32.0 °C (94-90 °F)	Skin: Bluish tinge Impaired neuromuscular function Impaired mental function Slurred speech Reduced respiration and pulse Dilated pupils Decreased BP Cessation of shivering Loss of consciousness Muscle rigidity	Treat as a medical emergency. Activate EMS. Remove from cold. Remove wet clothing. Rewarm with dry clothing, blankets, heating pad (apply only to trunk, armpit, and groin). Monitor vital signs. Treat for shock.

Based on Anderson and Barnum (2022); Cappaert et al. (2008); National Collegiate Athletic Association (2014-2015).

weather-warning services, and lightning monitoring devices—should be checked before outdoor activities and when storm conditions exist (36). Signs of threatening weather include darkening clouds, high winds, thunder, and lightning activity.

Know the location of the closest safe shelter and how long it takes to reach that shelter. A safe shelter is any sturdy building that has metal plumbing, wiring, or both to electrically ground the structure (i.e., not a shed or shack). In the absence of a sturdy building, any vehicle with a hard metal roof (not a convertible car or golf cart) with windows rolled up is considered a safe shelter. If no safe shelter is reachable, look for a dry ditch and instruct clients to crouch with only their feet touching the ground. Minimize body surface area by keeping the feet close together, wrapping the arms around the knees, and lowering the head. *Do not* lie flat. Stay away from tall or individual trees, lone objects (e.g., flagpoles), metal objects (e.g., fences or bleachers), standing pools of water, and open fields. Avoid being the tallest object in a field.

Fitness professionals should be aware of the proximity of lightning in the area. The flash-to-bang method is used to approximate the distance of a lightning strike. Count the seconds from the flash until the bang (thunder) occurs. Divide this number by 5 to determine how far away (in miles) lightning is occurring. When lightning strikes within 6 miles (9.7 kilometers), or 30 seconds from flash to bang, suspend all outdoor activities for 30 minutes. The 30-minute activity suspension clock restarts for each lightning flash or thunder heard within the 6 miles (9.7 kilometers) distance. Table 23.8 explains this 30–30 rule.

People struck by lightning do not carry an electrical charge (36, 45). When caring for a person who has been struck by lightning, employ standard emergency care. First, survey the scene for safety and, because severe weather can arise in any moment, move the victim to a safer location if possible. Activate the EMS system. Treat the person for shock and perform CPR along with AED use, if indicated.

KEY POINT

The fitness professional needs to be aware of severe weather conditions. Outdoor activities should stop and participants should take cover if lightning occurs within 6 miles (9.7 kilometers). Do not resume activities for a minimum of 30 minutes after the last lightning strike.

Medical Conditions

The fitness professional should review each participant's health screening questionnaire (see chapter 2) to identify medical conditions that may become problematic during activity. This section gives a basic understanding of diabetes, hyperventilation, asthma, concussion, and SCT and how to care for these conditions.

Diabetic Reactions

If managed properly, people with diabetes should be able to exercise without complications (see chapter 21). When starting a new exercise program, they should receive medical clearance from their physician, monitor their blood glucose levels more frequently, and gradually progress in the program. Communication between the fitness professional and the participant is vital regarding daily exercise plans. Ideally, 24 to 48 hours' notice of the duration and intensity of the exercise session is helpful to ensure proper preparation by the diabetic participant. Exercise has the potential to lower blood glucose levels; therefore, it must be counterbalanced with an increase in food intake or a decrease in insulin dosage. Blood glucose levels should be monitored immediately before and 15 minutes after activity. Clients should be encouraged to communicate with their physicians regarding their exercise program in order to better manage their diabetes.

The fitness professional should be familiar with the signs and symptoms of diabetic coma and insulin shock (see table 23.9). Diabetic coma occurs when insulin levels drop and the body is unable to metabolize glucose, leading to hyperglycemia. Insulin shock occurs when insulin levels are high and blood glucose is low, leading to hypoglycemia. It is sometimes difficult to differentiate between these two conditions. A person living with diabetes is normally aware of and manages this delicate glucose balance. When the client is in crisis and is conscious

Table 23.8 The 30–30 Rule

Activity criteria	30–30 rule
Suspension of activities	By the time the flash-to-bang count approaches 30 seconds, everyone already should be inside a safe shelter.
Resumption of activities	Wait at least 30 minutes after the last sound (thunder) or observation of lightning before leaving the safe shelter to resume activities. Each time lightning is observed or thunder is heard, reset the 30-minute clock.

Based on Glover (2016); Prentice (2020); Walsh et al. (2013); National Collegiate Athletic Association (2014-2015).

Table 23.9 Diabetic Reactions and Their Treatment

Diabetic reaction	Signs and symptoms	Care
Diabetic coma (hyperglycemia): Loss of consciousness caused by too little insulin; gradual onset	Restlessness and confusion Intense thirst Abdominal cramping and nausea Vomiting Shortness of breath Rapid, weak pulse Sweet, fruity breath Unconsciousness	Activate EMS. If conscious and alert, assist with insulin administration. Treat for shock. Lay person on their side to prevent aspiration of vomitus.
Insulin shock (hypoglycemia): High level of insulin and low glucose levels; rapid onset	Shakiness and anxiety Confusion Pale, cold, clammy skin Profuse sweating Dizziness Rapid HR Intense hunger Nausea Numbness or tingling in face and mouth Headache Aggressive behavior Lack of coordination Seizure Unconsciousness	If conscious, administer sugar (e.g., orange juice, candy). If symptoms do not improve within 15 minutes, activate EMS. If unconscious, activate EMS. Roll the person on their side. If unconscious, administer a glucagon emergency kit, containing an easy-to-use glucagon injection, or glucagon nasal powder. Treat for shock.

Adapted from American Diabetes Association (2018); Anderson and Barnum (2022); Casa and Stearns (2015); Jimenez et al. (2007); National Collegiate Athletic Association (2014-2015); Prentice (2020).

but it is unclear whether diabetic coma or insulin shock is present, give the client a sugar substance (e.g., orange juice, hard candy, honey). If the person is in a diabetic coma, there is little chance of seriously worsening the condition by giving a sugar source. Giving a food or fluid sugar source to an unconscious individual is contraindicated; therefore, administering a glucagon emergency kit, containing an easy-to-use glucagon injection or glucagon nasal powder, is recommended. If symptoms do not resolve rapidly, the fitness professional should activate EMS, monitor vital signs, and treat for shock.

KEY POINT

> Communication between the fitness professional and the participant living with diabetes regarding daily exercise plans is vital. Exercise has the potential to lower blood glucose levels, and therefore it must be counterbalanced with an increase in food intake or a decrease in insulin dosage.

Respiratory Disorders

Hyperventilation can occur with heavy exhalation or rapid breathing, resulting in breathing out too much carbon dioxide (CO_2) and thereby reducing CO_2 levels in the blood. Low CO_2 levels may cause dizziness, faintness, chest pains, and tingling in the feet and hands. Reassuring the person in a calm manner, encouraging a slower breathing rate, and encouraging them to talk often improves the situation. If not, helping the person breathe into a paper bag or into hands cupped over their nose and mouth will help restore CO_2 levels.

Asthma is a condition in which the smooth muscles of the bronchial tubes go into spasm. Edema and inflammation of the mucous lining are triggered by exercise, changes in barometric pressure or temperature, viruses, emotional stress, and noxious odors. The affected person may appear anxious, pale, and sweaty; may cough or wheeze; and may seem short of breath. Hyperventilation may occur, resulting in dizziness, and, because of mucous secretions, the person may try to clear their throat frequently.

The fitness professional should be prepared to handle an asthma attack. Generally, people with asthma know how to care for themselves and carry prescription medication to use before exercising or during an attack. People with asthma benefit from staying hydrated and modifying activity in environmental conditions such as high pollen and ozone warnings. If bronchial spasm is excessive and the participant is unable to breathe adequately, activate EMS.

KEY POINT

Respiratory issues can occur in exercise participation. Recognize that absence of normal breathing is a medical emergency.

Seizures

A seizure is caused by an abnormal electrical event in the brain, which can last a few seconds to several minutes. There are many types of seizures, and signs and symptoms are complex and numerous, ranging from a blank stare with unresponsiveness to convulsions with loss of bodily functions. For the management of seizures, see the sidebar *Care for Seizures*.

Sickle Cell Trait and Exertional Sickling

People with sickle cell trait (SCT) have a genetic condition that involves the inheritance of one gene for sickle hemoglobin and one for normal hemoglobin. The prevalence of SCT is approximately 5% to 10% in African Americans and <0.01% in Caucasians. People of Mediterranean descent (e.g., Italy, Spain, France) also have a higher prevalence (6, 7, 31). The U.S. Preventive Services Task Force recommends screening for SCT in newborns (44). However, many people are unaware that they have SCT or are uncomfortable making their status known to others.

Several risk factors have been identified that contribute to the medical problems associated with people with SCT. These risk factors include hypohydration (the body's state of water deficit), heat, asthma, deconditioning, and high-intensity exercise with little rest and recovery, even in the conditioned athlete. Due to lack of oxygen, exposure to high altitudes from flying, mountain climbing, or visiting a city at higher altitudes puts people with SCT at high risk.

A person with SCT usually can exercise without incidence. However, during intense exertion, exertional sickling can occur. Some of the normally round-shaped red blood cells form the shape of a sickle and are no longer able to carry oxygen. This sickling leads to the obstruction of small blood vessels in muscle or organs. If intense exercise continues, the condition can escalate.

Prevention is the key to avoiding an exertional sickling emergency. Because the fitness professional may not know which clients have SCT, incorporating sound principles of progression for everyone is the best preventive measure. Gradually increase the intensity of workouts, providing adequate time for rest and recovery. Use submaximal fitness testing early in the training

Care for Seizures

Do not place anything in the mouth or attempt to restrain a person having a seizure.

Immediate Care
- Activate EMS.
- Note time of seizure onset.
- Assist the individual to the floor and into a side-lying position.
- Protect the head with soft materials or padding.
- Remove nearby objects.
- Remove glasses and loosen clothing around their neck.

After Seizure
- Open the airway and assess breathing.
- Stay with the individual until fully awake.
- Calmly, tell the person what happened.

Critical Care

For seizures lasting 5 minutes or successive seizures:
- Activate EMS.
- Document length of time and number of seizures.

Based on Anderson and Barnum (2022); Prentice (2020); Prentice (2014).

program; more intense testing can be administered after the participant is better conditioned (see chapter 8). Encourage year-round conditioning that includes appropriate cycles of rest and recovery. Keep participants hydrated, especially in high heat and humidity. Encourage them to avoid high levels of caffeine and supplements containing stimulants. Participants with asthma should be instructed to follow their prescribed medical plan. Exercise during illness should be modified or discouraged. No one should exercise with a fever (temperature of 100.3 °F [38.0 °C] or above).

Exertional sickling is a medical emergency, and the fitness professional must act immediately due to the rapid decline of a participant's medical status. Table 23.10 outlines the signs and symptoms, prevention, and care of exertional sickling.

KEY POINT

> Reduce the risk of exertional sickling by using exercise programs that include appropriate hydration, rest breaks, and a gradual increase in activity. When exertional sickling is suspected, it is a medical emergency—act immediately.

Traumatic Brain Injury

Traumatic brain injury (TBI) occurs when an external mechanical force causes brain dysfunction. A TBI is caused by a bump, blow, or jolt to the head or a penetrating head injury that disrupts the normal function of the brain. Mild TBI may cause temporary dysfunction of brain cells. More serious TBI can result in bruising, torn tissues, bleeding, and other physical damage to the brain that can result in long-term complications or death (25). TBI can result from severe head injuries such as skull fractures, epidural hematomas, or subdural hematomas.

Severe symptoms of a skull fracture, subdural hematoma, or epidural hematoma include bleeding from a head wound, the ears, the nose, or around the eyes; bruising behind the ears (Battle's sign) or around the eyes (raccoon sign); changes in pupils (sizes unequal, not reactive to light); convulsions; drainage of clear or bloody fluid from ears or nose; loss of consciousness; vomiting; slurred speech; and seizures.

Immediate care of severe head injury involves stabilizing the head and neck; checking circulation, airway, and breathing and performing CPR with AED if indicated; controlling bleeding; treating for shock; and activating EMS.

Helmets help prevent or reduce the severity of skull fractures and intracranial hematomas, and experts believe that helmets also can reduce the severity of cerebral concussions. Many sports and fitness activities (American football, ice hockey, lacrosse, softball, baseball, cycling, skateboarding, inline skating, rock climbing, snowboarding, and snow skiing) require or advise the use of helmets (5, 39). Research is showing mouthguards may play a role in concussion reduction, leading the latest "Consensus Statement on Concussion in Sport: The 6th International Conference on Concussion in Sport" to recommend the use of mouthguards in child and adolescent ice hockey (37).

Skull Fracture

The skull provides good protection for the brain; however, a severe impact can fracture the skull. The fracture may be accompanied by concussion or other injury to the brain. Fractures can be simple (a break in the bone without damage to the skin); compound (a splintering of the bone with a break in the skin); or depressed (a crushing of the skull with bone depressed in toward the brain) (16). Skull fractures often lead to subdural or epidural hematomas.

Table 23.10 Exertional Sickling Signs and Symptoms, Prevention, and Care

Signs and symptoms	Prevention	Care
Muscle cramping Muscle weakness and tenderness Pain Swelling Extreme fatigue Inability to catch one's breath Elevated core temperature Slumps to ground during activity	Gradually increase exercise intensity. Allow longer periods of rest and recovery. Modify early exercise testing. Control asthma. Maintain hydration. Avoid caffeine and nutritional stimulants. Modify or stop exercise during illness. No exercise if temperature is above 100.3 °F (38.0 °C).	Stop activity immediately. Activate EMS. Monitor vital signs. Support circulation, airway, breathing (CAB) and begin CPR with AED if indicated. Cool the participant if they are experiencing heat-related illness.

Based on Casa, Anderson, Baker, et al. (2012); Casa, Guskiewicz, Anderson, et al. (2012); Anzalone et al. (2010); Roberts et al. (2021); Harrelson, Fincher, and Robinson (1995).

Subdural Hematoma

A subdural hematoma is bleeding between the skull and the brain. As blood accumulates, pressure on the brain increases, which may occur suddenly or over several days. The bleeding and increased pressure on the brain from a subdural hematoma can be life threatening.

Subdural hematoma is usually caused by a traumatic head injury, such as from a fall or motor vehicle accident. People with a bleeding disorder and people who take blood thinners are more likely to develop a subdural hematoma even from a relatively minor head injury.

Epidural Hematoma

An epidural hematoma is a type of intracranial hematoma that occurs when a blood clot forms between the skull and the dura, the tough covering that surrounds the brain. An epidural hematoma can result from a skull fracture. The jarring of the brain against the sides of the skull can cause shearing (tearing) of the internal lining, tissues, and blood vessels that may result in internal bleeding, bruising, or swelling of the brain (5, 16, 39).

Concussions

The understanding and management of concussions has changed dramatically in recent years. The term *concussion* derives from the Latin term *concutere*, which means to "shake violently." A concussion is a brain injury and is defined as a complex pathophysiological process induced by biomechanical forces (33). It results in a transient disturbance of brain function, encompassing clinical symptoms that may or may not involve loss of consciousness. Concussions also have been referred to as *mild traumatic brain injuries (MTBIs)*; however, it is now widely agreed that concussions are a subset of MTBIs, on the less severe end of the brain injury spectrum, and are generally self-limited in duration and resolution (23, 24, 28, 30, 33).

Concussion may be caused by a blow to the head, face, neck, or body that translates to the brain being shaken. It results in the rapid onset of symptoms, which fall into four categories: physical, cognitive, emotional, and sleep. Common symptoms include headache, dizziness, nausea, mental fog, balance problems, and light and noise sensitivity (for a complete list of symptoms, see table 23.11). Some may appear right away, while others may not be noticed for hours or days after the injury. The damage is functional rather than structural, which is why standard neuroimaging diagnostic studies (e.g., CT scan, X-ray, MRI) often reveal no abnormalities.

If a concussion is suspected, the person should immediately stop participation and see a medical professional trained in the assessment and management of concussions. Controlled cognitive (e.g., reduced screen time) and relative physical rest (allowing for activities of daily living) are the main treatments for a concussion, especially in the first 48 hours. Reinstating noncontact or no-risk-of-fall physical activity after 2 days is now encouraged as long as symptoms do not worsen (37). The fitness professional needs to obtain exercise and activity guidance from the person's medical professional throughout the recovery process along with full return-to-participation clearance before returning to prior fitness activities. If any signs or symptoms exacerbate or recur during activity, stop the activity and refer the participant to their physician.

KEY POINT

If any signs or symptoms of a concussion are present, the participant must cease all activity until evaluated by a medical professional trained in concussion recognition and management, and should not return to activity until cleared medically.

Table 23.11 Concussion Signs and Symptoms

Physical	Cognitive	Emotional	Sleep
Headache	Feels mentally foggy	Irritable	Drowsy
Nausea	Feels slowed down	Sad	Sleeps more than usual
Vomiting	Difficulty concentrating	More emotional	Sleeps less than usual
Balance problems	Difficulty remembering	Nervous	Difficulty falling asleep
Dizziness	Forgetful of recent information and conversations		
Visual problems	Confused about recent events		
Fatigue	Answers questions slowly		
Sensitivity to light	Repeats questions		
Sensitivity to noise			
Numbness, tingling			
Dazed			
Stunned			

Based on Guskiewicz et al. (2004).

Around 80% to 90% of concussion cases resolve in 7 to 10 days. In the other 10% to 20% of cases, symptoms can persist for weeks, months, or even years after the initial injury (23, 28, 30, 33). The original concussion can turn into persistent concussion symptoms, symptoms lasting greater than 4 weeks, leading to post-concussion syndrome (37). This syndrome is simply defined as symptoms and signs of the concussion persisting for weeks to months after the incident.

Basic Life Support and Emergency Procedures

This section addresses the emergency protocols for shock, checking vital signs, CPR with AED, and airway obstruction. Fitness professionals are encouraged to be certified in basic life support, minimally in adult CPR with AED. ACSM and other credentialing bodies may require CPR with AED or a more advanced life support certification depending on the fitness professional's certification. Cardiac emergencies require immediate recognition and activation of EMS, early CPR, and rapid defibrillation.

Shock

When attending to injuries or illnesses, the fitness professional must be aware of the possibility of shock. Shock occurs when the heart is unable to circulate adequate oxygen to vital organs. This may result from trauma involving severe pain or blood loss or may be associated with an allergic reaction, heatstroke, severe infection, poisoning, or severe burns. Although shock most often accompanies severe injury, it may also occur with minor injuries. If untreated, shock can lead to permanent organ damage or death.

A change in vital signs (pulse, respiratory rate, BP, temperature, pupils, skin color) indicates that a person is going into shock. The signs and symptoms of shock can progress over time. Table 23.12 identifies the signs and symptoms of a person going into shock and the immediate care required.

KEY POINT

> The signs and symptoms of shock can develop over time but also can change quickly. It is important to monitor vital signs every 2 to 5 minutes when shock is likely.

Checking Vital Signs

Monitoring vital signs assists in the recognition and care of the injured patient. Vital signs include pulse, respiratory rate, BP, temperature, and color.

- *Check HR:* Use light finger pressure over an artery to monitor pulse rate. The most common sites for checking heart rate (HR) are the carotid, radial, brachial, and femoral pulses. The average HR for an adult is between 60 and 100 bpm.

- *Check breathing:* Normal breathing rates vary from 8 to 20 breaths per minute. A person who takes an occasional breath is not receiving adequate ventilation and is in respiratory distress.

- *Take BP:* Usually BP is taken at the brachial artery with a BP cuff and sphygmomanometer. The following results will help determine the problem:

    - *Normal BP:* <120 mmHg systolic blood pressure (SPB) and <80 mmHg diastolic blood pressure (DBP)

    - *Severe hemorrhage, heart attack:* Marked decrease in BP (20-30 mmHg)

    - *Damage or rupture of vessels in the arterial circuit:* Abnormally high BP (>150 SBP and >90 DBP)

    - *Brain damage:* Increase in SBP with a stable or falling DBP

Table 23.12 Shock Recognition and Treatment

Signs and symptoms	Care
Restless, anxious, fearful, or disoriented Weak, rapid pulse Shallow, irregular breathing Nausea or vomiting Cold, clammy, moist skin Dull, staring eyes with dilated pupils Profuse sweating Dizziness Extreme thirst	Initiate the EAP and call EMS. Check circulation and maintain airway; begin CPR with AED if indicated. Control bleeding, splint fractures, and regulate body temperature. Elevate feet and legs 8-12 inches (20-30 centimeters) unless suspected lower-extremity, head, or neck injury. Keep the person quiet and still. Even if the person complains of thirst, do not give any liquids by mouth. If the person vomits, turn them on their side. If a neck injury is suspected, it must be stabilized before rolling the person. Monitor vital signs every 2 to 5 minutes until EMS arrives.

Based on Anderson and Barnum (2022); Prentice (2020); Prentice (2014).

- *Heart ailment:* Decrease in SBP with an increase in DBP
- *Body temperature:* Normal body temperature is 98.6 °F (37.0 °C). Assess skin quality: Cool, clammy, damp skin suggests shock or heat exhaustion; cool, dry skin indicates exposure to cold air; and hot, dry skin suggests fever or heatstroke.
- *Assess color:* For light-pigmented people, abnormalities include skin, fingernail beds, lips, sclera of eyes, and mucous membranes that are red or flushed, pale or ashen, or bluish. For dark-pigmented people, it is necessary to assess nail beds and inside the lips, mouth, and tongue. Pink is the normal color for these; a bluish or grayish cast is abnormal.

Cardiopulmonary Resuscitation

Current guidelines in CPR training emphasize circulation, airway, and breathing (CAB), stressing the importance of moving the blood in victims of sudden cardiac arrest. Activating EMS and access to an AED are of equal importance. The American Heart Association (AHA) and American Red Cross (ARC) have specific protocols for CPR, depending on certification level (2, 3). The following list is a basic guide to assist the fitness professional in a sudden cardiac emergency:

- Check that the scene is safe to assess the participant.
- Check for responsiveness, pulse, and breathing.
- Activate EMS and retrieve an AED. Location of AEDs should allow for a response time of 3 minutes or less (29). Solicit the help of a bystander if available.
- If no pulse is detected, begin cycles of 30 chest compressions and 2 breaths. For adults, place the heel of the hand on the middle of the chest (lower half of sternum) and compress the chest 2 to 2.4 inches (5-6 centimeters). Allow the chest to recoil completely. Give 30 compressions at a rate of 100 to 120 per minute.
- If there is a pulse and absent or abnormal breathing, give one breath every 5 to 6 seconds. Open the airway using the head-tilt/chin-lift method. If a head or neck injury is suspected, use the jaw-thrust method. Use a barrier or bag mask and other personal protective equipment, when available. Give enough breath for the chest to rise about 1 second, and allow air to exit before giving the next breath. Recheck the pulse every few minutes.
- When the AED arrives ensure cell phones are no closer than 6 feet (1.8 meters) from the victim. Turn AED on and follow audible and visual instructions, placing pads as instructed. Continue CPR while the AED gets set up and analyzes rhythm. If shock is advised, make sure no one is touching the victim. Continue CPR as instructed by the AED until EMS arrives.

Airway Obstruction

Airway obstruction can occur when a foreign object or, in case of an unconscious person, the tongue blocks the airway.

CONSCIOUS PERSON

- If breathing is labored and the person is coughing forcefully, stay with them and encourage continued coughing.
- If the person is unsuccessful in expelling the object or has absent or abnormal breathing, activate EMS and begin the "five and five" approach—five back blows followed by five abdominal thrusts.
  - *Back blows technique:* Place one arm across the victim's chest while standing to the side and slightly behind them. Bend the person forward so that their upper body is parallel to the ground. Firmly strike the victim between the shoulder blades with the heel of your free hand.
  - *Abdominal thrusts technique:* Stand behind the person, wrap your arms around their midsection, and place your fist with the thumb just above their naval. Cover your fist with your other hand. Thrust in and upward until the object is expelled.
- Repeat the sequence until the object dislodges; the person can cough, speak, or breathe; or the person becomes unconscious (3).

UNCONSCIOUS PERSON

- Treat as a cardiac emergency.
  - Activate EMS.
  - Perform CPR.

KEY POINT

Emergency situations can occur at any time. Cardiac emergencies require immediate recognition and activation of EMS, early CPR, and rapid defibrillation. Fitness professionals need to follow the EAP, including routine practice sessions, emergency equipment logistics review, and especially AED locations, and maintain appropriate certification in basic life support to keep up to date with the latest protocols.

LEARNING AIDS

REVIEW QUESTIONS

1. How often should staff be trained in the fitness facility's EAP?

2. How long should ice be applied initially to a suspected sprain?

3. Strength programs that increase in intensity and duration too quickly and do not allow for adequate recovery can result in what serious medical condition?

4. Design a return-to-activity program using the 50/30/20/10 rule for conditioning activities and the FIT rule for strength training activities.

5. Describe how you would splint a suspected fracture to the fibula.

6. What are three ways to prevent the spread of CA-MRSA in a fitness facility?

7. Describe the appropriate technique for cleaning an open wound.

8. Describe the flash-to-bang and 30–30 rule for assessing lightning.

9. List five vital signs to monitor when an emergency occurs.

CASE STUDIES

1. A participant hurts their ankle performing a plyometric exercise. They fall to the ground, are in moderate pain, and are able to partially bear weight. You suspect they have a sprained ankle. Describe how you would give immediate care.

2. You are conducting a boot camp outdoors that meets two times a week for 8 weeks from 5:30 to 6:30 p.m. in Florida beginning June 1. What can you do to prepare for the first class to prevent exertional heat illness in your participants? What recommendations would you give to your participants in an email before the class starts?

3. One of your regular clients comes to you before their weightlifting workout and says that both arms are extremely sore. They challenged their brother to a pull-up contest 2 days ago and now have mild swelling in both biceps, stiffness, decreased ROM at the elbow joint, point tenderness in both forearms and upper arms, and difficulty carrying things. What condition do you suspect they have? What treatment would you provide to help them in order to return to working out?

4. You have been working with a collegiate soccer player on their conditioning during the off-season; however, you have not worked with them for 3 weeks as they recovered from an injury. The last conditioning session you had with them involved running 10 120-yard sprints, each in under 18 seconds with 1:1.5 W:R. What is your plan for getting them back to their prior fitness level safely?

Answers to Case Studies

1. Do the following:
   - *Protection:* Splint the ankle above and below the joint.
   - *Rest:* Discontinue activity.
   - *Ice:* Apply an ice bag for 20 to 30 minutes.
   - *Compression:* Apply an elastic bandage, wrapping from the toes up to the lower leg.
   - *Elevation:* Elevate the ankle above the heart.
   - Refer the participant to a physician.

2. As an instructor, do the following preparation:
   - Screen participants for prior heat illness, SCT, and medications.
   - Provide water and give adequate rest breaks.
   - Monitor the weather and modify activities if heat and humidity are high.
   - Gradually increase the intensity and duration of the activity over a 2-week period for acclimatization.

   Make the following recommendations to participants:
   - Hydrate before class.
   - Monitor urine color for hydration levels.
   - Get plenty of rest (at least 6-8 hours nightly).
   - Minimize clothing.
   - Weigh in before and after class to monitor fluid loss. Replenish fluids by consuming 1 to 1.25 liters (34-42 ounces) of fluid per kilogram of body water loss.

3. The client has DOMS. Give them the following recommendations:
   - No upper-body weight training today. They can work the legs and core.
   - Ice both arms for 20 to 30 minutes.
   - Provide compression with an elastic wrap on both arms.
   - Lightly massage the muscles.
   - Take an over-the-counter NSAID as directed.
   - Return to activity gradually when soreness has subsided.
   - If signs and symptoms worsen, seek medical advice from a physician.

4. Follow the 50/30/20/10 rule to safely return the soccer player to their baseline fitness level over the next 2 to 4 weeks:

Week	# of sprints	Sprint time (sec)	Rest time (sec)
1	5	27	108
2	7	23	69
3	8	22	44
4	9	20	40

Legal
Considerations

JoAnn M. Eickhoff-Shemek

OBJECTIVES

The reader will be able to do the following:

1. Describe why fitness professionals must develop knowledge and skills in the area of legal liability and risk management
2. Distinguish injuries due to (a) risks inherent in the activity, (b) negligence, and (c) product defects
3. Develop a basic understanding of U.S. law and legal system
4. Identify federal laws (e.g., OSHA and ADA) and state laws (e.g., waivers, data privacy, and AEDs) that are applicable to fitness facilities and programs
5. Describe the fault basis of tort liability
6. Define *ordinary negligence* and *gross negligence*
7. List and describe the four elements of negligence that a plaintiff must prove
8. Explain the primary assumption of risk and waiver defenses
9. Identify the four elements of a valid contract
10. Discuss how courts determine duty in negligence cases and why they often rely on the testimony of expert witnesses
11. List and describe situational factors courts will use to help determine the standard of care of a fitness professional
12. Distinguish standards of care and standards of practice from a legal liability perspective
13. Define *risk management* and describe the four steps in the risk management process
14. Develop risk management strategies to help minimize legal liability in the areas of personnel, preactivity health screening, fitness testing and exercise prescription, instruction and supervision, equipment and facilities, and emergency action plans (EAPs)
15. Describe why staff training (upon hiring and on-the-job) is an essential risk management strategy

24

Many physiological and psychological health benefits are associated with regular physical activity. Although these benefits outweigh the risks, risks (e.g., heart attacks, fractured bones, cuts that cause bleeding) do occur, and many people become injured (and sometimes die) each year while participating in physical activity. Unfortunately, in today's litigious society, injured participants do not hesitate to file negligence lawsuits against fitness professionals and their employers. To help minimize injuries and subsequent litigation, fitness professionals must learn the laws that pertain to the field and how to apply the laws to their daily practices. Studies have shown poor adherence by fitness facilities to laws and safety standards and guidelines published by professional organizations (45). This poor adherence is most likely due to a lack of legal and risk management education among fitness professionals. Therefore, the purpose of this chapter is to help fitness professionals gain knowledge and skills in this area.

This chapter covers various legal concerns to help educate fitness professionals about their legal duties and how they can carry out these duties through the development and implementation of risk management strategies. By no means does this chapter cover all of the legal issues relevant to the fitness field. Ideally, fitness professionals will take the opportunity to expand their knowledge with a focused academic course on legal issues. Consulting with legal counsel regarding screenings and other client- and facility-related matters is highly recommended because each situation and case is unique.

Injury Data and Injuries Leading to Litigation

About 11,000 people per day receive treatment in U.S. emergency departments for injuries sustained while participating in sport, recreation, and exercise activities (21). It is unknown how many of these are specifically due to exercise. However, the U.S. Consumer Product Safety Commission's National Electronic Injury Surveillance System (NEISS) tracks injury data resulting from exercise and exercise equipment derived from hospital emergency room visits. As shown in table 24.1, the number of these injuries decreased in 2020, which might be explained by the pandemic when fewer people were exercising. However, at-home exercise injuries that were serious enough for participants to make a visit to the emergency room increased 48% between 2019 and 2020 (48).

Table 24.2 lists selected negligence lawsuits occurring in fitness facilities and the type of injury the plaintiff (injured party) suffered. Negligence lawsuits can be quite costly, with some in the millions of dollars. For

Table 24.1 Exercise and Exercise Equipment Injuries, 2017 to 2021

Year	Number of exercise and exercise equipment injuries*
2017	526,350
2018	498,498
2019	468,315
2020	377,939
2021	409,224

*The total number of injuries reflects estimates based on data obtained from U.S. hospital emergency departments through the NEISS.

Data from NEISS. Available: https://www.cpsc.gov/cgibin/NEISSQuery/home.aspx.

example, in the *Vaid* case, the jury returned a verdict of $14,500,000 in favor of the plaintiffs (89). Plaintiffs often list numerous negligence claims against the defendants (fitness professionals and facilities) in their lawsuits. In the *Baldi-Perry* case, the plaintiff listed 26 and 16 negligence claims against the personal fitness trainer and the facility, respectively (10). In this case, the plaintiff was awarded $1.4 million in monetary damages (54). Fitness professionals should realize that many injuries and subsequent lawsuits can be prevented through risk management, described later in this chapter.

KEY POINT

Several studies have demonstrated that participation in fitness activities and programs can lead to all types of injuries—minor, major, and even death. These injuries can lead to negligence claims and lawsuits against fitness professionals and their employers. To help minimize injuries and subsequent litigation, it is essential that fitness professionals learn the laws that pertain to the field and how to apply them to their practices.

Causes of Injuries and Negligence

Injuries in fitness facilities and programs have many causes. The most common are due to risks inherent in the activity, negligence, and product defects. Risks inherent in the activity are those that happen simply as a result of participation in physical activity—they are no one's fault

Table 24.2 Types of Injuries Leading to Negligence Lawsuits Against Fitness Professionals and Facilities

Type of injury	How the injury occurred	Case
Fractured leg	Kneeling exercise performed by person with spinal cord injury	*Bartlett v. Push to Walk* (11)
Fractured ankle	Fall while performing jump repetitions on a BOSU ball	*Levy v. Town Sports International, Inc.* (61)
Back and neck injuries	Fall during an indoor cycling class when handlebars dislodged	*Stelluti v. Casapenn Enterprises, LLC* (82)
Massive stroke	High-intensity exercise performed on a rowing machine	*Vaid v. Equinox* (89)
Shattered wrist	Fall during a step test	*Covenant Health System v. Barnett and Barnett* (27)
Herniated disc	Injury while performing a squat exercise	*Howard v. Missouri Bone and Joint Center* (56)
Exertional rhabdomyolysis	High-intensity leg workout during first personal training session	*Proffitt v. Global Fitness Holdings, LLC, et al.* (72, 73)
Torn quadriceps	Injury during an indoor cycling class	*Scheck v. Soul Cycle* (79)
Multiple dental injuries	Child's head slammed into a wall after being hit with a ball	*Lotz v. The Claremont Club* (63)
Severe head injuries	Hit head on an exposed exercise machine after falling off a treadmill	*Jimenez v. 24 Hour Fitness* (57)
Traumatic brain injury	A back panel of an exercise machine struck head	*Chavez v. 24 Hour Fitness* (22)
Hip injury requiring surgery	Trip and fall over a weight belt left on the fitness floor	*Crossing-Lyons v. Town Sports International, Inc.* (29)
Cardiac arrest resulting in death	Collapse while playing racquetball	*Miglino v. Bally Total Fitness* (64)

and are inherent in (or inseparable from) the activity. Almost everyone who has participated in physical activity or sport has experienced an injury because of these types of risks. Injuries caused by negligence are due to fault—the fault of a participant (e.g., the participant is careless while lifting weights) or of a fitness professional or facility (e.g., failure to properly instruct and supervise participants, inspect and maintain exercise equipment, and carry out emergency procedures). Injuries also can be caused by product defects. Manufacturers can be found liable if an injury was due to a defect in the exercise equipment. This type of liability is called *product liability*.

This chapter focuses on negligence, the major legal concern facing all fitness professionals and facilities. Negligence is failing to do something that a reasonable, prudent professional would do or doing something that a reasonable, prudent professional would not have done under the same or similar circumstances (34). In other words, negligence can be an act of omission (failure to perform) or commission (improper performance). Unfortunately, negligence lawsuits against fitness professionals and facilities reflect negatively on the profession. To

address this, fitness professionals can learn about their many legal duties toward participants and take steps to adhere to these duties, which will lead to fewer injuries and subsequent negligence claims and lawsuits. To begin this learning process, the next section provides an overview of U.S. law and legal system.

KEY POINT

The most common causes of injuries in fitness programs are risks inherent in the activity, negligence, and product defects. Of these, negligence is the major legal concern facing fitness professionals and facilities. Negligence is the failure to do something that a reasonable, prudent professional would do (omission) or doing something that a reasonable, prudent professional would not have done (commission) under the same or similar circumstances (34).

U.S. Law and the Legal System

This section describes primary and secondary sources of law, criminal versus civil law, trial and appellate courts, tort law, and contract law. It also covers certain federal laws applicable to the fitness profession.

Primary and Secondary Sources of Law

In the United States, law is created from the three branches of government at both the federal and state levels: statutory law from the legislative branch, administrative law from the executive branch, and case law from the judiciary branch. Statutory law is enacted through the legislative process. Examples of federal statutes are the Americans with Disabilities Act (ADA) and Health Insurance Portability and Accountability Act (HIPAA). Examples of state statutes include statutes prohibiting the unauthorized practice of medicine or other allied (or licensed) health professions, data privacy and breach notification statutes, and statutes that require fitness facilities to have an automated external defibrillator (AED). Administrative law is formed by numerous administrative agencies that exist at both the federal and state levels. At the federal level, these include the Food and Drug Administration (FDA), Internal Revenue Service (IRS), and Occupational Safety and Health Administration (OSHA). These agencies enact rules and regulations, investigate potential violations, and impose sanctions (e.g., fines) for any violations. Case law is derived from written court opinions and is sometimes referred to as *common law*. Courts often rely on the written opinions from previous cases to help form an opinion for a current case in which the facts are similar to those in the previous cases. Terms such as *precedent* or *stare decisis* ("to stand by that which is decided") reflect this legal doctrine. Not all litigation results in precedent;

KEY POINT

The law is created from the three branches of government at both the federal and state levels: statutory law from the legislative branch, administrative law from the executive branch, and case law from the judiciary branch. Statutory law is enacted through the legislative process, administrative law is formed by numerous administrative agencies, and case law is derived from written court opinions.

about 95% of negligence cases are settled out of court and therefore never go to trial (95).

In addition to these three primary sources of law (statutory, administrative, and case law), there are many secondary sources of law, including books, treatises (e.g., *Restatement of the Law Third, Torts*), and law review journals. Secondary sources do not reflect the law, but they are helpful for finding primary sources of law or explaining a specific area of law. Both primary and secondary sources of law can be found using electronic legal databases such as Westlaw and Lexis (or Nexis Uni), often available through university libraries.

Criminal Law Versus Civil Law

The law can be categorized into criminal law and civil law. If someone violates a statute, the government can bring criminal charges against that person—the defendant. If the defendants are found guilty, they may have to pay a fine, perform community service, be placed on probation, or go to prison (45). It must be shown that the defendant is guilty beyond a reasonable doubt, meaning 100% guilty of the crime. Fitness professionals could face criminal charges for violating state statutes such as assault and battery, theft, and the unauthorized practice of medicine.

Civil law addresses noncriminal matters and deals primarily with civil disputes between individuals, businesses, organizations, and government agencies (45). For example, when members of a fitness facility are injured while working out in the facility, they can sue the facility for negligence—a civil claim. In this example, the injured member is referred to as the *plaintiff* and the fitness facility is referred to as the *defendant*. Plaintiffs in a civil lawsuit have the burden of proof, so they must prove that the defendant was liable for the injury by the preponderance of the evidence, meaning it was more likely than not (51% or greater) that the negligent conduct of the defendant caused the harm to the plaintiff. Note that the term *liable* is used in civil law rather than the term *guilty*, which is used in criminal law. In civil claims such as negligence, the plaintiff seeks monetary damages from the defendant to compensate for the injury (e.g., medical expenses, lost wages, and pain and suffering). Civil lawsuits also can involve a breach of contract, noncriminal statutory violations, and civil rights violations.

Trial Courts and Appellate Courts

The U.S. court system is made up of trial and appellate courts at the federal, state, and local levels. Trial courts, the lowest courts, are the first to carry out the legal proceedings. At the end of the trial, the judge or a jury renders a decision in favor of one of the parties. Within a given time frame, the losing party can appeal the trial court's decision to a higher court—an appellate court. Appellate courts are made up of an odd number of judges who review the evidence and proceedings of the trial court. An appellate court has several options when forming its opinion about a case. It can remand the case (send it back to trial with instructions), reverse it (disagree with the trial court's decision), affirm it (agree with the trial court's decision), or modify the trial court's decision (19). There are intermediate and supreme (highest) appellate courts at the state and federal levels.

Tort Law and Contract Law

Although many types of law exist, tort law and contract law are most relevant to the fitness field. A tort can be defined as conduct that reflects a legal wrong that causes physical harm, emotional harm, or both (19). Conduct that causes harm can impose civil liability, meaning that defendants can be found liable and, thus, obligated to pay monetary damages to the plaintiff. A contract "is an agreement that can be enforceable in court" (19, p. 349). Contracts are formed when two (or more) parties exchange binding promises. The elements of tort law and contract law are described next, along with their applications to the fitness field.

Tort Law

Tort law can be classified into three levels of fault: intentional, negligence, and strict liability (see figure 24.1). Intentional torts involve conduct that requires the intent to cause harm to another. Examples are assault, battery, false imprisonment, invasion of privacy, and defamation. Although uncommon in fitness facilities, this type of conduct, such as invasion of privacy and defamation, has occurred in fitness facilities by participants and employees (45). This type of conduct also can be considered a

crime (violation of a statute), so the wrongdoer can face both civil claims and criminal charges.

Of the three levels of fault, negligence is the most common in the fitness field and can involve both ordinary negligence and gross negligence. Ordinary negligence is considered careless conduct and, as defined earlier, is the failure to do something (omission) that a reasonable, prudent professional would do or doing something that a reasonable, prudent professional would not have done (commission) given the same or similar circumstances (34). Gross negligence (or reckless, willful, or wanton conduct) goes beyond careless conduct. The *Restatement of Law Third, Torts* states that reckless conduct occurs when "(a) the person knows of the risk of harm created by the conduct or knows facts that make the risk obvious to another in the person's situation, and (b) the precaution that would eliminate or reduce the risk involves burdens that are so slight relative to the magnitude of the risk . . ." (4, p. 13). Courts often refer to gross negligence as the defendant's failure to exercise even slight care/diligence or an extreme departure from the standard of care. For example, in *Bartlett v. Push to Walk* (11), the court found the defendant (an exercise professional) grossly negligent for improper instruction (having a client perform an exercise a second time after experiencing untoward symptoms when performing the same exercise the first time) that caused the plaintiff's injury.

Various forms of strict liability also exist in the fitness field. Two of these are product liability and vicarious liability. Product liability involves a defect in the product (e.g., design defect, manufacturing defect, or marketing defect such as inadequate instructions or warnings). For example, if plaintiffs can show that their injury was due to the manufacturer's defective design of the equipment, the manufacturer could be held strictly liable for the injury. Strict liability is based on public policy (i.e., judicial determination of what is in the best interest of society) rather than fault such as intentional or negligent wrongdoing (19).

Vicarious liability is imposed on employers even if the employer has not been negligent. Under the legal doctrine of *respondeat superior*, employers can be held strictly liable for harm to third parties (e.g., fitness participants) caused by negligent acts of their employees while performing their jobs (19). As demonstrated in the negligence cases described in this chapter, it is common for plaintiffs to name several defendants in their lawsuit. For example, it may be that the personal fitness trainer committed the negligent act, but the plaintiff can name the trainer, facility manager, and owner of the facility as defendants, all of whom could be potentially liable for the plaintiff's injury.

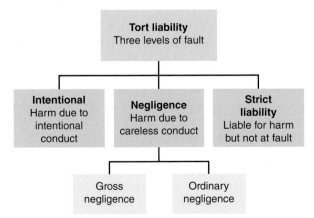

FIGURE 24.1 Fault basis of tort liability.

Reprinted by permission from Law for Fitness Managers and Exercise Professionals, Fitness Law Academy, LLC, Parrish, FL (2020).

KEY POINT

Tort law involves three levels of fault: intentional, or conduct that requires the intent to cause harm to another; negligence, or careless conduct that causes harm to another (ordinary negligence) and reckless conduct that causes harm to another (gross negligence); and strict liability, such as product liability and vicarious liability. Vicarious liability occurs when employers (e.g., fitness facility managers and owners) are held liable for the negligent acts of their employees through a legal doctrine called *respondeat superior*.

Four Elements to Prove Negligence   In a negligence lawsuit, the plaintiff has to prove the following four elements (33):

1. *Duty:* The defendant owed a duty (or standard of care) to the plaintiff.

2. *Breach of duty:* The defendant failed to carry out the duty.

3. *Causation:* The breach of duty was the cause of the harm.

4. *Harm and damages:* A legally recognizable harm occurred to the plaintiff, resulting in damages (losses) to the plaintiff (e.g., medical expenses, lost wages, pain and suffering).

Courts (judges)—not attorneys, juries, plaintiffs, or defendants—determine the first element of duty. The approaches that courts use to determine duty are discussed later. The plaintiff then has to prove that the defendant breached their duty. Therefore, the defendant's conduct becomes a key factor in determining whether there was a breach of duty. If the conduct was consistent with the duty owed, even if the plaintiff was seriously hurt or died, it will be difficult for plaintiffs to prevail with their lawsuit. However, if the defendant's conduct was inconsistent with the duty owed, it will be easier for the plaintiff to show that the defendant breached a duty.

To determine if the breach of duty caused the injury, courts often use the "but for" test: But for the defendant's negligent conduct, would the injury have occurred (4)? Sometimes injuries are caused by reasons other than the negligent conduct of the defendant, such as risks inherent in the activity or the plaintiff's own negligence. A link must exist between the breach of duty and the cause (sometimes referred to as *actual cause*) of the injury. If plaintiffs can show that the breach of duty was the cause of their harm (physical or emotional injury or damage

to their property), monetary damages can be awarded to compensate for the harm. In ordinary negligence cases, these are called *compensatory damages* and can be both economic, such as medical expenses and lost wages, and noneconomic, such as pain, suffering, and loss of consortium (e.g., loss of companionship of a loved one). In gross negligence cases, plaintiffs usually seek compensatory damages as well as punitive damages (additional damages to punish the defendant for reckless conduct).

Defenses Against Negligence   Defendants involved in negligence lawsuits have various defenses they can use to refute (or defend) the negligent claims made against them. The best defense always is to carry out legal duties properly. If the plaintiff cannot prove that the defendant breached a duty, it will be difficult for the plaintiff to win the negligence lawsuit and recover any damages. Two common legally effective defenses, the primary assumption of risk defense and waiver defense, are discussed next. Defenses, sometimes used by defendants, such as (a) it is too costly to adhere to the law, (b) we do not have the staff resources to carry out the law, and (c) ignorance of the law, are not recognized by the law as viable defenses.

The primary assumption of risk defense is always available to defendants after they have been named in a negligence lawsuit. This defense "follows from the plaintiff engaging in risky conduct from which the law implies consent" (70, p. 1213). It is implied that individuals who engage in sport and recreational activities assume the reasonably foreseeable risks inherent in the activity. Risks inherent in the activity are those that are inseparable from the activity and happen because of participation; that is, they cannot be eliminated without changing the nature of the activity. Generally, the law does not allow plaintiffs to seek monetary damages for injuries caused by risks inherent in the activity if the evidence shows three elements: "(1) the plaintiff possessed full subjective understanding, (2) of the presence and nature of the specific risk, and (3) voluntarily chose to encounter the risks" (70, p. 1214).

In determining whether the injury was due to risks inherent in the activity, courts will examine the nature of the activity and the experience of the plaintiff. For example, in *Rutnik v. Colonie Center Court Club, Inc.* (76), a man died from cardiac arrest while participating in a racquetball tournament. The estate of the decedent sued the club for negligence, claiming they failed to carry out certain duties such as emergency procedures. Using primary assumption of risk, the defendants claimed the decedent assumed the risk of a heart attack and, therefore, they were not liable. The appellate court agreed with the defendants, stating that "relieving an owner . . . of a sporting facility from liability for the inherent risk of engaging in sports is justified when the consenting participant is aware of the risks, has an appreciation of the nature of the risks, and voluntarily assumes the risk" (76, p. 452). The court also stated that because the decedent was an experienced racquetball player who had played in many previous tournaments, he must have known and appreciated the risk of cardiac arrest while participating in this strenuous sport. The court found no negligence on the part of the club; that is, they carried out emergency procedures properly. In this case, the primary assumption of risk defense protected the defendants from liability.

In another case, *Corrigan v. Musclemakers, Inc.* (25), primary assumption of risk did not protect the defendants from liability. In this case, a personal trainer placed a woman on a treadmill during her first training session, gave her little or no instruction on how to use the treadmill, and then left her unattended. After a short while, she began to drift back on the belt of the treadmill. She tried to walk faster but instead was thrown from the treadmill, which resulted in her fracturing her ankle. Prior to this incident, she had never been in a fitness facility or on a treadmill. She filed a negligence lawsuit against the defendants (the trainer and the facility), claiming the trainer failed to ensure that she understood how to use the treadmill (i.e., failed to provide proper instruction and supervision). The appellate court stated that the "doctrine of primary assumption of risk . . . may be applied in cases where there is an elevated risk of danger typically in sporting and recreational events" (25, p. 145), but the doctrine was not applicable in this case because fitness activities such as exercising on a treadmill are not the same as sporting and recreational activities. In addition, the court ruled that the risks associated with using the treadmill were not known, understood, and appreciated by the plaintiff, a novice exerciser and treadmill user. Therefore, the plaintiff's injury was not due to risks inherent in the activity but most likely due to the negligence of the trainer, and thus primary assumption of risk was not an effective defense for negligence.

Courts also have considered whether the conduct of defendants increased the risks to the plaintiff over and above those inherent in the activity. If so, the primary assumption of risk defense was ineffective in protecting the defendants. For example, in *Santana v. Women's Workout and Weight Loss Centers, Inc.* (78), a step aerobics instructor increased the risks over and above those inherent in the activity when instructing participants to perform combined exercises (step aerobics with overhead arm-strengthening exercises using a Dyna Band). The plaintiff in this case fell and fractured her ankle, requiring surgery. In *Levy v. Town Sports International, Inc.* (61), a personal fitness trainer increased the risk of harm to the plaintiff by instructing her to perform an advanced exercise (jumping repetitions on a BOSU ball) given her medical condition (osteoporosis). The

plaintiff lost her balance, fell, and fractured her wrist, which required surgery.

Strengthening the Primary Assumption of Risk Defense
Informing participants of the risks inherent in the activity associated with physical activity *may* help strengthen the primary assumption of risk as a defense. Often, a section that informs a participant of these risks (minor, major, life-threatening, and even death) is included in protective legal documents such as waivers (releases of liability) and informed consents. Additional strategies to strengthen the primary assumption of risk defense include the following (45):

- Provide beginner-level fitness programs or classes so that a beginner can receive the necessary instruction and experience to gain knowledge of the activity, an understanding of one's own capabilities, and an appreciation of the potential injuries that can occur so that the beginner can assume the risks inherent in the activity—the requirements needed to establish an effective primary assumption of risk defense.

- Be sure all fitness professionals (e.g., personal fitness trainers, group exercise leaders) are properly trained to teach. For example, they should know how to avoid (a) instructing participants to perform exercises that increase the risks over and above those inherent in the activity, and (b) having participants perform advanced exercises until they are experienced and skilled in performing beginner and intermediate-level exercises.

A waiver (or release of liability) is a defense based on contract law. A waiver, signed by a person before participation, contains a section called an exculpatory clause such as the following that was included in the waiver in *Stelluti v. Casapenn Enterprises, LLC* (82).

WAIVER AND RELEASE FORM

You acknowledge that you have carefully read this "waiver and release" and fully understand that it is a release of liability. **You expressly agree to release and discharge the health club, and all affiliates, employees, agents, representatives, successors, or assigns, from any and all claims or causes of action and you agree to voluntarily give up or waive any right that you may otherwise have to bring a legal action against the club for personal injury or property damage.**

To the extent that statute or case law does not prohibit releases for negligence, this release is also for negligence on the part of the Club, its agents, and employees (82, p. 293).

The trial court, intermediate appellate court, and the New Jersey Supreme Court ruled that the waiver signed by Stellutti was enforceable. The exculpatory clause was effective, absolving the defendant health club from its own negligence. Without this waiver, the health club may have been found liable for its negligent conduct (e.g., negligent instruction) that caused the injury to the plaintiff. Therefore, when individuals sign a waiver, they give up (waive) their civil right to recover any damages due to the ordinary negligence of the defendant. Waivers do not protect defendants against gross negligence or intentional acts, as described later in the chapter.

For the waiver to be effective and enforceable, many factors, described in detail elsewhere (26, 45), must be considered. One important factor is that it must be written properly. It also is important to realize that the validity and enforceability of a waiver varies significantly from state to state. For example, in some states, the language of the exculpatory clause must be explicit for it to be enforceable. In addition, waivers are not enforceable in some states based on court rulings (precedent) or state statutes, such as in Virginia and New York, respectively. Because of the many differences in the requirements for waivers among states, fitness professionals should never adopt a waiver they find in a book or some other source—it must be reviewed and edited by a competent lawyer prior to use. It is important to realize that waivers do nothing to enhance safety—they only provide potential legal liability protection after a lawsuit has been filed.

KEY POINT

Two defenses often used by defendants in negligence cases are primary assumption of risk and waivers. Primary assumption of risk is effective for injuries due to risks inherent in the activity if the plaintiff knows, understands, and appreciates those risks and voluntarily assumes them. The waiver defense can protect (absolve) defendants from their own negligence if the exculpatory clause within the waiver document is enforceable based on state law. Because waiver law is complex and can vary significantly from state to state, fitness professionals must have a competent lawyer prepare (or edit) a waiver prior to use.

Contract Law

Contracts are commonly used in the fitness field. Examples include waivers, informed consents, employment contracts for employees and independent contractors, vendor contracts, membership contracts, and insurance contracts. For a contract to be valid and legally enforceable, it must meet the following four elements (24):

1. *Agreement:* An agreement to form a contract includes an offer and an acceptance.
2. *Consideration:* Any promises made by the parties to the contract must be supported by legally sufficient and bargained-for consideration.
3. *Contractual capacity:* Both parties entering into the contract must have contractual capacity to do so.
4. *Legality:* The purpose of the contract must be to accomplish some goal that is legal and not against public policy.

An agreement occurs when a fitness facility offers a membership to a person and that person accepts. The consideration is the money promised to the fitness facility paid by the member in exchange for programs and services promised by the facility to the member. *Contractual capacity* means that both parties must be capable and competent to form a contract. For example, minors (children under the age of 18) do not have contractual capacity; only adults can sign contracts such as waivers and informed consents. *Legality* refers to the terms within a contract—they must be legal. For instance, waivers are against public policy in some states and therefore do not meet the legality requirement.

If a contract does not meet all four elements, it is considered a voidable contract. An unenforceable contract is one that violates a statute or is against public policy based on a court's ruling (24). In addition, some contracts must be in writing (e.g., contracts involving the sale of goods of $500 or more), and if they are not, they will be unenforceable. If one party fails to meet its contractual obligations, it might be considered a breach of contract and the breaching party may be required by a court to pay compensatory damages to the other party or complete the specific performance as stated in the contract.

Federal Laws Applicable to the Fitness Profession

There are many federal laws that apply to fitness professionals and facilities. This section briefly describes three federal laws: the ADA, OSHA's Bloodborne Pathogens Standard, and the HIPAA Privacy Rule. Additional federal laws are described elsewhere (45). State laws also exist related to many federal laws and, in some cases, the state laws contain more requirements than the federal laws.

The ADA is a federal statute that was enacted in 1990 (6). The purpose of this law is to prohibit discrimination against people with disabilities. The ADA contains five titles and two of these, Title I and Title III, pertain to most fitness facilities and programs and services. Title I prohibits employment discrimination and applies to private employers with 15 or more employees. These employers must provide reasonable accommodations for employees with disabilities. A reasonable accommodation is something that will help employees perform their job without creating an undue burden (significant difficulty or expense) on the employer.

Title III prohibits discrimination in places of public accommodation and commercial facilities. It requires that privately owned or operated places of public accommodation provide access for people with disabilities and make reasonable accommodations with regard to programs and services. Therefore, fitness facilities need to address architectural barriers (e.g., ramps, access to restrooms) and provide programs and services for people with disabilities. Title III requires a reasonable accommodation; that is, facilities do not need to purchase expensive, specialized exercise equipment. However, it is recommended to provide inclusive exercise equipment that can be used by individuals with and without functional limitations and impairments (9). Facilities do need to provide appropriate programs and services for people with disabilities. This may require fitness facilities to have staff members who are qualified to conduct health and fitness assessments and design exercise prescriptions for people with disabilities. One credential that fitness professionals should consider in this regard is the Certified Inclusive Fitness Trainer (CIFT) certification established by the American College of Sports Medicine (ACSM) and the National Center on Health, Physical Activity and Disability (NCHPAD). Monetary penalties for violating Title III are substantial (23).

Title II of the ADA prohibits discrimination by state and federal governments. Fitness professionals working in these settings (e.g., a public university) need to be familiar with the Title II requirements. Both Titles II and III require compliance with the accessibility standards established in the *2010 ADA Standards for Accessible Design* (5), addressing new construction and alterations.

OSHA's Bloodborne Pathogens (BBP) Standard is an administrative law that became effective in March 1992 (13). Exposure to bloodborne pathogens such as the human immunodeficiency virus (HIV) and hepatitis B virus (HBV) can lead to serious illness and death. The major goal of the BBP Standard is to reduce or eliminate occupational exposure to these pathogens that can be transmitted via blood or other potentially infectious materials (OPIM). It specifically applies to employers whose employees could come in contact with blood or OPIM while performing their jobs (e.g., fitness staff members who are responsible for carrying out first aid). This law has numerous requirements, including the establishment of a written exposure control plan (ECP). The ECP needs to include several components such as (a) employee exposure determination (employees expected to be protected), (b) employee training, and (c) record keeping (training records, medical records, incident reporting). OSHA provides a fact sheet that summarizes the BBP Standard (13).

HIPAA protects the use and disclosure of health information by covered entities (e.g., health plans, health care providers) and business associates (e.g., vendors that contract with health plans, health care providers) (97). Covered entities and business associates must comply with three HIPAA rules: (a) Privacy Rule, (b) Security Rule, and (c) Breach Notification Rule. The Privacy Rule requires having safeguards in place to ensure the privacy of protected health information (PHI) (83). The Security Rule requires implementing appropriate administrative, physical, and technical safeguards to ensure the confidentiality, integrity, and security of electronic PHI (84). The Breach Notification Rule requires notifying individuals whose unsecured PHI was breached as well as the Secretary of Health and Human Services (17). The HIPAA rules would not apply to most fitness facilities or programs; however, in some cases, they might. Potential examples include employer-sponsored wellness programs that are considered "group health plan wellness programs" or wellness programs that conduct HIPAA standard transactions such as billing an individual's health insurer for covered services (97). Although most fitness facilities or programs would not need to comply with the HIPAA rules, it may be wise for fitness facilities and professionals to adopt provisions similar to what the HIPAA law requires with regard to PHI. Other laws likely will apply such as the Federal Trade Commission Act (FTCA) and state data privacy, security, and breach notification statutes.

KEY POINT

Many federal laws are applicable to fitness facilities and programs as well as related state laws. Three federal laws were briefly described—the ADA, OSHA's BBP Standard, and HIPAA. With the assistance of legal counsel, fitness facilities and professionals need to develop and implement policies and procedures that reflect the requirements within these laws.

Determining Duty in Negligence Cases

As stated earlier, courts (i.e., judges) determine duty in negligence cases. One of the first things courts consider when determining duty is the relationship that is formed between the plaintiff and defendant. The late Betty van der Smissen, a well-known legal scholar, stated that "the existence of duty is inherent in nearly every situation in which a teacher, coach, recreation leader, fitness specialist, administrator, manager, or executive, et al. might be actively engaged" (90, p. 4). For example, when fitness professionals are teaching or leading exercise programs for participants, an "actively engaged" relationship is formed requiring fitness professionals to carry out certain responsibilities or potential legal duties. A general legal duty of all fitness professionals is to provide reasonably safe exercise programs. *Reasonably safe* means taking precautions (developing and implementing risk management strategies, as discussed later) that will help prevent foreseeable injury risks. Examples of injuries that occurred due to foreseeable injury risks are presented in table 24.2.

Professional Standard of Care

It is likely that courts will hold fitness professionals to a standard of care of a professional, or a professional standard of care. To meet the standard of care, it is essential that fitness professionals possess the knowledge and skills necessary to provide reasonable care and a level of care that is consistent with the knowledge and skills expected of fitness professionals. If their conduct does not meet the standard of care (or duty) owed to the plaintiff, the plaintiff likely will be able to show a breach of duty, as demonstrated in several of the negligence cases described in this chapter.

According to van der Smissen, "If one accepts responsibility for giving leadership to an activity or providing a service, one's performance is measured against the standard of care of a qualified professional **for that situation**" (92, p. 40). The term *qualified professional* in this context means a professional who provides a standard of care that a prudent (competent) professional would provide. In negligence cases, courts will investigate the credentials (e.g., degrees, certifications) and, more importantly, the competence of the professional—that is, what the professional did (or did not do) given the situation. The phrase "for that situation" means that the professional standard of care is determined using three situational factors: the nature of the activity, the type of participants, and the environmental conditions (92). Each of these is described next. Many of the negligence cases described in this chapter involve fitness professionals who failed to carry out duties related to one or more of these three situational factors.

THREE SITUATIONAL FACTORS THAT DETERMINE PROFESSIONAL STANDARD OF CARE

1. *Nature of the activity:* The professional must be aware of the skills and abilities the participant needs to participate safely in the activity (i.e., the fitness professional must possess the necessary knowledge and skills to lead reasonably safe exercise programs).

Fitness professionals must fully understand and apply numerous safety principles when leading any exercise

program. However, professionals who lead complex or advanced exercise programs (e.g., Olympic lifting, high-intensity or extreme conditioning) need to have any additional knowledge and skills necessary to safely teach these programs and know what precautions to take to help minimize injuries.

2. *Type of participants:* The professional must be aware of individual factors of the participants (i.e., awareness of medical conditions that impose increased risks and how to minimize those risks).

Fitness professionals who train people with medical conditions need to possess advanced credentials in the exercise sciences, such as academic coursework and certification in clinical exercise (94). For example, when training participants with medical conditions (e.g., pregnancy, diabetes, hypertension, back problems), fitness professionals need to fully understand any risks the conditions might impose and how to minimize those risks. In addition to advanced credentials in clinical exercise, fitness professionals also should refer to the numerous resources published by professional organizations that address exercise guidelines for all types of medical conditions.

3. *Environmental conditions:* The professional must be aware of any conditions that may increase risks (e.g., heat and humidity, floor surfaces, exercise equipment) and know how to minimize those risks.

Fitness professionals need to have the necessary knowledge, skills, and abilities to lead exercise safely given various environmental conditions. For example, many precautions must be taken to help prevent heat injuries. This would include being familiar with position papers published by professional organizations that describe specific precautions to take to minimize the risk of heat injuries, such as one published by the National Athletic Trainers' Association (20). Fitness professionals should realize that heat injuries do not only occur in athletes. A student, while participating in a jogging class at California State University San Bernardino (CSUSB), suffered a severe heat injury. The case was settled out of court for $39.5 million (69). The environment also includes properly maintaining floor surfaces and exercise equipment (many injuries in fitness facilities are due to slippery floors and poor equipment maintenance) as well as having policies that require participants to return equipment (e.g., exercise balls, dumbbells) to their storage racks to help prevent injuries from tripping and falling.

Adherence to Published Standards of Practice

In addition to the three situational factors just described, courts will consider, as potential evidence of duty (or the standard of care), standards of practice (or best practices) published by various organizations. In recent years, numerous standards of practice (e.g., standards, guidelines, position papers) have been published by both professional organizations (e.g., ACSM, National Strength and Conditioning Association [NSCA], YMCA) and independent organizations such as the American Society for Testing and Materials (ASTM), Consumer Products Safety Commission (CPSC), and manuals published by exercise equipment manufacturers. According to Herbert and Herbert (55), these published standards of practice reflect "benchmark behaviors or actions that are universally exhibited by properly trained and experienced professionals" (pp. 80-81) and should be viewed "as the threshold or minimal acceptable level of service owed to a client, patient, or participant" (pp. 205-206).

Fitness professionals need to develop and implement the standards and guidelines described in these published standards of practice because of the potential legal impact they can have. Expert witnesses, who educate the court as to the duty the defendant owed to the plaintiff in negligence cases, often introduce published standards of practice in their testimony as evidence of the standard of care owed to the plaintiff. Courts often allow these published standards of practice as admissible evidence to help determine duty, as demonstrated in *Elledge v. Richland/Lexington School District Five* appellate court ruling (46):

> Courts have become increasingly appreciative of the value of national safety codes and other guidelines issued by governmental and voluntary associations to assist in applying the standard of care in negligence cases. . . . A safety code ordinarily represents a consensus of opinion . . . and is not introduced as substantive law but most often as illustrative evidence of safety practices or rules generally prevailing in the industry that provides support for expert testimony concerning the proper standard of care (46, pp. 477-478).

Expert witnesses often rely on published standards of practice when providing testimony in negligence cases. For example, two prominent expert witnesses who each have over 30 years of expert witness experience stated, "Not only have we referenced [*ACSM's Health/Fitness Facility Standards and Guidelines*] in our numerous opinions provided in numerous cases, but other prominent standards for fitness facility operation such as those of the NSCA . . . to communicate with courts and juries as to what is appropriate" (93, pp. 20-21). Several legal cases described in this chapter involved published standards of practice introduced as evidence by expert witnesses and were effective in helping the court establish duty or the standard of care.

The proliferation of standards of practice published by professional and independent organizations in recent years makes it impossible to include all of them in this chapter. Therefore, a later section—Strategies to Minimize Legal Liability—only includes selected standards of practice published by the ACSM (77). According to ACSM, *standards* are "minimum requirements that . . . each health/fitness facility must meet to provide a relatively safe environment" (standard statements that reflect requirements use the word *shall*) and *guidelines* are defined as "recommendations that health/fitness operators should consider using to improve the quality of the experience they provide to users" (guideline statements use the word *should*) (77, p. xiii). In NSCA's standards and guidelines (67), a standard is defined as "a required procedure that probably reflects a legal duty . . . for the standard of care" and a guideline is defined as "a recommended operating procedure . . . to further enhance the quality of services provided" (p. 2). NSCA uses the words *must* and *should* in their standard and guideline statements, respectively.

It is often difficult for fitness professionals to know which published standards of practice to follow, especially when inconsistencies exist among them. Therefore, it is best to follow those that are the most safety oriented in their approach as well as those that are the most applicable to their type of facility (45). It is important that fitness professionals do not confuse standards of care (legal duties) and standards of practice (best practices) as shown in figure 24.2. The legal significance is different for each.

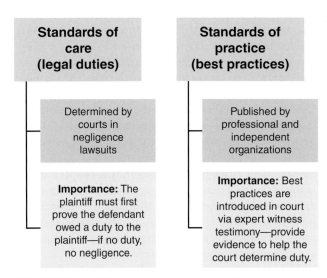

FIGURE 24.2 Distinguishing standards of care and standards of practice.

Reprinted by permission from Law for Fitness Managers and Exercise Professionals, Fitness Law Academy, LLC, Parrish, FL (2020).

KEY POINT

Fitness professionals must understand that they will likely be held to the professional standard of care in a negligence lawsuit against them. This will involve the court investigating the conduct of the professional, often through the testimony and opinions of expert witnesses. If the conduct is consistent with the standard of care, it will be difficult for the plaintiff (injured participant) to prove that the defendants (fitness professional, fitness facility) breached their duty. However, if the conduct is inconsistent with the standard of care, it will be easier for the plaintiff to prove that the defendants breached their duty, which could lead to the defendants being liable for the plaintiff's injury. Whether a fitness professional's conduct meets the professional standard of care likely will be determined by the court examining potential duties related to the nature of the activity, type of participants, and environmental conditions as well as adherence to published standards of practice.

Risk Management

Fitness professionals often are employed in various management positions (e.g., assistant director, personal fitness trainer coordinator, group exercise coordinator) within a facility. In these positions, they perform numerous management functions in areas such as human resource management, financial management, facility management, marketing and promotion, strategic planning, customer service, program and service scheduling, and information technology. However, risk management is one of the most important management functions because it focuses on participant safety. Developing and implementing the risk management strategies, which help ensure the safety of participants, should be the number one priority of all fitness professionals. Risk management strategies provided in this chapter reflect many of the legal duties fitness professionals and facilities have toward their participants. In addition to minimizing injuries and subsequent litigation, risk management has other benefits such as enhancing operational efficiency and improving the quality of services (45).

Risk management is a broad term that reflects an overall goal of many organizations—to reduce accidental losses to help prevent slowed growth, reduced profits, and general interruption of operations (52). Liability losses are one type of these accidental losses. Legal liability exposures, which can lead to liability losses, are situations that (a) create a risk of injury (e.g., a personal fitness trainer who does not possess the knowledge and skills to teach exercise in a safe manner or a facility that does not properly maintain its exercise equipment), or (b) reflect noncompliance with federal and state laws (e.g., facilities that do not comply with the ADA and state data privacy laws) (45). Because this chapter focuses on legal liability in fitness programs and facilities, *risk management* in this context is defined as "a proactive administrative process that will help minimize legal liability exposures facing exercise professionals and fitness facilities" (45, p. 46).

The risk management process involves four steps (45). When assessing legal liability exposures in step 1, fitness professionals need to be aware of the many laws and published standards of practice that apply to the field. To assist in this step, as well as steps 2 through 4, a fitness facility should have a risk management advisory committee that is made up of experts (e.g., legal, medical, insurance) who work with the fitness staff members to develop a comprehensive risk management plan for the facility. Because the law is often complex and varies among jurisdictions, it is essential that fitness professionals consult their risk management experts when making the many decisions involved in the four-step risk management process.

Step 2 involves developing risk management strategies that reflect the laws and published standards of practice identified in step 1. These include (a) loss-prevention strategies (i.e., strategies that help prevent injuries from occurring in the first place, such as providing proper instruction and supervision), (b) loss-reduction strategies (i.e., strategies that help decrease the severity of an injury once it does occur, such as carrying out proper emergency procedures), and (c) strategies that use a contractual transfer of risks (e.g., a waiver transfers the liability risks to the participant who signed it, and the liability insurance provider pays for the damages up to the limits of the policy when a defendant is found liable for negligence).

Some fitness facilities have opted for exposure avoidance strategies. For example, they do not offer certain programs (e.g., high intensity) or equipment (e.g., treadmills, free weights) that can pose increased risks of injury (12, 36, 58). Fitness professionals can minimize the increased risks associated with these types of programs and equipment, but a well-informed, concerted effort is needed to do so.

Step 3 involves the implementation of the risk management plan. Once the risk management strategies are developed as written policies and procedures for staff members to follow (step 2), they can be organized into a risk management policy and procedures manual

(RMPPM). The policies and procedures should be presented in an organized fashion within the manual, divided into sections such as preactivity health screening, equipment inspection and maintenance, emergency action plan (EAP), and so on. Another component of step 3 is staff training, which is necessary so that staff members learn how to carry out the policies and procedures. New employees should receive training upon hiring. Staff members also should receive regular in-service trainings throughout the year. An example of an in-service training is training that includes a review and rehearsal of the EAP.

Step 4, evaluation of the risk management plan, includes two types of evaluation—formative and summative. Formative evaluation is ongoing throughout the year. For example, an evaluation as to whether the EAP was carried out properly should be conducted after every injury. If the EAP was not carried out properly, staff members may need retraining. Summative evaluation involves a formal, annual review of the entire risk management plan. Laws often change, as do published standards of practice, and therefore the risk management advisory committee and the facility's fitness professionals will need to revise and update certain policies and procedures in the RMPPM and then retrain staff members on the changes. For more information on these four important risk management steps, see *Law for Fitness Managers and Exercise Professionals* (45).

Strategies to Minimize Legal Liability

This part of the chapter includes six sections:

1. Personnel
2. Preactivity health screening
3. Fitness testing and exercise prescription
4. Instruction and supervision
5. Equipment and facilities
6. EAPs

Each section provides a brief summary of selected standards of practice published by ACSM (77), followed by important risk management strategies to help minimize legal liability. By no means do these strategies reflect all legal liability exposures that exist.

Personnel

A variety of legal issues can arise with regard to personnel in fitness facilities and programs. This section focuses on hiring credentialed and competent employees; incorporating proper procedures in the hiring, training, and supervision of employees; purchasing both general and professional liability insurance; and legal liability issues involving independent contractors.

SELECTED ACSM STANDARDS AND GUIDELINES RELATED TO PROFESSIONAL STAFF AND INDEPENDENT CONTRACTORS

ACSM provides three standards and four guidelines in this category. Standards #1 and #2 are briefly described.

Standard #1: Health/fitness professionals who have supervisory responsibility and oversight responsibility for the physical activity and exercise training programs, as well as the staff who administer them, shall have appropriate levels of professional education, work experience, and/or certification. Examples of health/fitness professionals who serve in a supervisory role include the fitness director, group exercise director, aquatics director, and program director (77, p. 53).

Under Standard #1, ACSM provides examples of what would be considered appropriate levels of professional education, certification, and work experience for those in supervisory roles. For example, a fitness director should have a 4-year degree in a fitness- or health-related field, certification from a nationally recognized and accredited certification program, and a minimum of 3 years of experience as a fitness professional (77).

Standard #2: Health/fitness professionals who serve in counseling, instruction, and physical activity supervision roles for the facility shall have an appropriate level of professional education, work experience, and/or certification. The primary professional staff and independent contractors who serve in these roles are fitness instructors, group exercise instructors, personal trainers, and health and wellness coaches (77, p. 53).

For example, personal trainers should have a 4-year degree in fitness exercise science, or a related field with 2 years of college education in the field as a minimum, personal trainer certification from a nationally recognized and accredited certification program, and a minimum of 6 months' experience working as a personal trainer fitness instructor (77).

STRATEGY 1: EMPLOYING CREDENTIALED AND COMPETENT PERSONNEL

Fitness professionals who serve in a supervisory role (e.g., manager, owner, fitness director, group exercise coordinator) need to hire credentialed and competent employees. It is important to realize that a credentialed professional (one who possesses a degree/certification) is not necessarily competent to carry out important legal duties (e.g., knows how to apply safe and effective principles of exercise to meet a participant's specific needs).

Several efforts to address the issue of competent professionals have been made in the field, including voluntary or self-regulated efforts, such as the accreditation of certifications through independent agencies such as the National Commission for Certifying Agencies (NCCA), and government-regulated efforts, such as legislative bills proposing licensure in various states. However, many unnecessary injuries and subsequent negligence claims and lawsuits continue to occur in the field. For example, many of the injuries that occurred in the cases described in table 24.2 were caused by fitness professionals and supervisors who were incompetent.

Even though there are no formal education requirements to take personal fitness trainer or group exercise leader accredited certification exams, several states have proposed licensure. However, currently none have become law (45). It is unlikely that states will continue to pursue licensure for personal fitness trainers and group exercise leaders, given the lack of support by ACSM for licensure of nondegree personal trainers working in nonclinical or community settings with apparently healthy clients. However, the ACSM does support licensure for "exercise professionals with at least a bachelor's degree in exercise science and related, accredited certification, assuming these professionals are working with patients and clients with medical conditions that require clinical support" (2, p. 2). As the exercise profession considers pursuing licensure for degreed exercise professionals, challenges will arise, as discussed elsewhere (40, 41, 42).

Whether the field remains self-regulated or is regulated by the government via licensure, the provision of well-designed formal education programs that prepare both credentialed and competent fitness professionals is one of the most important risk management strategies for minimizing injuries and subsequent litigation in the field. Formal education programs to prepare competent personal trainers and group exercise leaders have been described elsewhere (15, 16, 28, 30). Meeting the credentials and experience as recommended by ACSM should serve as baseline requirements when employing fitness professionals. However, employers need to do much more to ensure they are hiring competent employees (e.g., they need to conduct a deep dive to determine their competence during a job interview). Specific interview strategies, such as asking candidates situational-type questions and having them conduct a mock training session, are described elsewhere (45).

STRATEGY 2: HIRE, TRAIN, AND SUPERVISE EMPLOYEES PROPERLY

Fitness professionals who serve in a supervisory role have a duty to use reasonable care in the hiring, training, and supervising of their employees. In addition to vicarious liability, described previously, employers also can face direct liability for failing to properly hire, train, and supervise employees. See table 24.3 for examples of cases involving negligent hiring, training, and supervision. The failure to train employees appears to be the most common claim. Therefore, providing on-the-job (OTJ) training (classroom and practical training) for new hires is an essential risk management strategy. OTJ training strategies include classroom training (e.g., educational sessions that focus on acquiring knowledge of safe principles of exercise) and practical training (e.g., new hires first work under the supervision of a mentor—a credentialed and competent professional who can access a new employee's practical skills). Staff members who are well trained are more likely to carry out their legal duties and risk management responsibilities compared with those who receive little or no training.

Fitness facilities also have been sued for negligent hiring because they did not conduct criminal background checks before hiring employees (45, 66). Under the legal principle of *respondeat superior*, employers generally would not be held liable for an employee who conducts a criminal act (e.g., sexual assault) while on the job because the criminal act would not be within the scope of employment. However, employers do have a responsibility to conduct criminal background checks before hiring employees, especially those who work with vulnerable populations (e.g., children, elderly, people with disabilities) and those who work closely with clients, such as massage therapists and personal fitness trainers.

Table 24.3 Direct Liability Claims Against Fitness Facilities for Failing to Properly Hire, Train, and Supervise Employees

Case	Claims against the facility (employer)
Bartlett v. Push to Walk (11)	Negligent hiring of an exercise professional
Vaid v. Equinox (89)	Negligent retention and supervision of a personal fitness trainer
Lotz v. The Claremont Club (63)	Negligent hiring, training, and supervision of an employee leading a children's activity
Baldi-Perry v. Kaifas and 360 Fitness Center, Inc. (10)	Negligent hiring and training of personal fitness trainers

Additionally, employers have a responsibility to supervise employees serving in these roles. If a fitness supervisor (or any staff member) observes or is made aware of any possible criminal behavior by another staff member or participant, proper steps in consultation with legal counsel need to be taken in a timely fashion.

Failing to properly supervise employees, as shown in table 24.3, also is a direct liability claim made by plaintiffs. For example, in *Vaid v. Equinox* (89), a personal trainer failed to provide proper instruction to a client while using a rowing machine, resulting in the client suffering a massive stroke. The plaintiffs made several claims against the defendant's managers including that they knew the personal trainer used training methods that were too aggressive but allowed him to continue to work as a trainer—an example of improper supervision. Once a supervisor knows of (or observes) inappropriate training methods, corrective action needs to be taken such as retraining. More on proper supervision is described later under Instruction and Supervision.

STRATEGY 3: PURCHASE LIABILITY INSURANCE COVERAGE

If a fitness facility and/or professional is found liable for negligence, liability insurance will pay for the damages up to the limits of the policy. Fitness facilities should have general liability insurance coverage through a commercial general liability (CGL) policy as well as professional liability insurance coverage for staff members who provide professional services.

The need for professional liability insurance coverage and a careful review of any exclusions in an insurance policy is demonstrated in *York Insurance Company v. Houston Wellness Center, Inc.* (96).

The plaintiff in *York* claimed that she was injured due to improper instruction given by an employee on how to use an exercise machine. The fitness club contended that their liability insurance provider had a duty to defend and indemnify the club in this negligence case. However, the insurance company claimed they did not have this duty because of a clause in the CGL policy stating that "this insurance does not apply to 'bodily injury' . . . arising out of the . . . failure to render any service, treatment, advice, or instruction relating to the physical fitness . . . or physical training programs" (96, pp. 904-905). A court ruling agreed with the insurance company. The facility had a CGL policy that specifically excluded professional services such as fitness instruction. If they had also purchased professional liability insurance for their staff members, the outcome of this case might have been different. Fitness facilities should have both general and professional liability insurance policies and should be sure the policies cover all the programs and services they provide. If a facility does not provide professional liability insurance for staff members who provide professional services, these staff members need to purchase their own policy. Fitness professionals can usually purchase professional liability insurance through a low-cost group plan. For example, ACSM members can purchase a professional liability insurance policy through a group plan. In consultation with legal and insurance experts, fitness facilities also should consider purchasing other types of insurance to protect their businesses such as property insurance, loss of business income, and employment practices insurance.

STRATEGY 4: HAVE PROCEDURES IN PLACE FOR INDEPENDENT CONTRACTORS

Fitness facilities often hire independent contractors to provide various services. Several legal concerns are involved when hiring independent contractors; this discussion will focus on a few of these. First, based on IRS tax law, employers do not have a lot of behavioral control over independent contractors. Therefore, it is essential that they hire only credentialed and competent independent contractors. Second, all independent contractors should sign a written contract that specifies the responsibilities of both parties, including a clause stating that the independent contractor must provide proof of having professional liability insurance (the fitness facility's liability insurance does not cover independent contractors—only employees). Third, it is critical that independent contractors do not appear to be employees by their actions or what they wear. For example, they should not wear a shirt with the facility logo. If participants believe that independent contractors are employees, the employer could be held vicariously liable based on a legal principle referred to as *ostensible agency* (45). Therefore, it is recommended that facilities have independent contractors wear a "contractor" badge and inform participants in a membership contract or posted signage that some services are provided by independent contractors.

KEY POINT

Many injuries (and subsequent litigations) that occur in the field are due to the negligent conduct of staff members. Therefore, it is essential to hire credentialed and competent staff members as well as provide them with training and supervision. Additional risk management strategies associated with personnel include conducting criminal background checks before hiring certain staff members, purchasing adequate general and professional liability insurance to cover all programs and services provided by employees, and having several procedures in place when hiring independent contractors.

Preactivity Health Screening

The failure to conduct a preactivity health screening is a common claim made in negligence cases against fitness professionals and facilities, especially when a serious injury has occurred. For example, in the *Baldi-Perry* case, the plaintiff suffered many severe and permanent injuries including herniated discs; surgery to remove, decompress, and fuse discs; and ongoing pain and medical care (10, 54). The jury returned a verdict of $1.4 million in favor of the plaintiff. The following claims related to preactivity health screening were made against the personal trainer, who had a college degree in the field and an accredited certification, and the facility:

AGAINST THE PERSONAL TRAINER

- Failing to consider the plaintiff's prior injuries and physical condition before preparing an exercise routine
- Failing to conduct a health risk appraisal
- Failing to identify the plaintiff as someone with an increased risk of injury
- Failing to evaluate the plaintiff's medical condition before preparing an exercise routine
- Failing to properly evaluate the plaintiff's exercise experience before creating an exercise routine
- Failing to follow industry standards (10)

AGAINST THE FACILITY

- Failing to have trainers who were certified and/or trained to conduct a proper preactivity screening
- Failing to have a medical liaison or medical advisory committee to assist in reviewing physical activity screenings and exercise plans
- Failing to ensure that trainers conducted a health risk appraisal
- Failing to have proper preactivity screening tools in place for its trainers
- Failing to offer appropriate and necessary training to physical trainers
- Failing to follow industry standards (10)

SELECTED ACSM STANDARDS AND GUIDELINES RELATED TO EXERCISE PREPARTICIPATION HEALTH SCREENING

ACSM provides five standards and two guidelines in this category. Standards #1, #3, and #4 are briefly described.

Standard #1: Facility operators shall offer a self-guided or professionally guided exercise preparticipation health screening tool (e.g., preactivity screening questionnaire [PASQ], the Physical Activity Readiness Questionnaire for Everyone [PAR-Q+], and/or health history questionnaire (HHQ) to all new members and prospective users (77, p. 4).

An HHQ is also referred to as a *health screening questionnaire (HSQ)*—the term used in this textbook.

Standard #3: Exercise preparticipation screening tools shall be reviewed by qualified staff (e.g., a qualified health/fitness professional or health care professional), and the results of the review shall be retained on file by the facility for a period of at least one year from the time the tool was reviewed. All health data and related communications shall be kept in such a manner that is private, confidential, and secure (77, p. 4).

Standard #4: If a facility operator is told that a member, user, or prospective member has known cardiovascular, metabolic, or renal disease, or any other self-disclosed medical concern that may affect the individual's ability to exercise safely, medical clearance is recommended before beginning a physical activity program (77, p. 4).

Note: The PASQ, PAR-Q+, and an example of a HHQ (or HSQ) are provided in *ACSM's Health/Fitness Facility Standards and Guidelines* (77) and in chapter 2.

STRATEGY 1: SELECT PREACTIVITY SCREENING TOOLS FOR SELF-GUIDED AND PROFESSIONALLY GUIDED EXERCISE PROGRAMS

Preactivity tools and related policies and procedures need to be established with the assistance of the facility's risk management committee (e.g., medical and legal experts). Once developed, the procedures should be included in the facility's RMPPM. The PAR-Q+ is designed as a self-guided tool. Participants complete the questionnaire on their own and then follow the recommendations provided in the tool (e.g., seek the advice from a qualified exercise professional or consult with their physician) before beginning or resuming a physical activity program. The PASQ is designed to be used in professionally guided programs (39). A fitness professional, with credentials such as a degree in the field and an accredited certification, interprets the health data obtained and then decides if the individual needs to obtain medical clearance prior to beginning an exercise program. The PASQ was developed after ACSM published its revised screening criteria in 2015 (74). The PASQ and related forms (e.g., PASQ interpretation form and medical clearance form) are available to use or adapt (see the Fitness Law Academy website).

The PAR-Q+ and the PASQ are best used as screening tools for all new members upon joining a fitness facility or for new participants when joining an exercise program. An HSQ (also referred to as a *medical history questionnaire*) obtains additional health information (e.g., medical conditions, prescribed medications, recent surgeries) beyond the PAR-Q+ and PASQ. An HSQ should be used by professionals leading individual programs (e.g., personal fitness trainers) or group exercise programs for people with medical conditions. The information obtained from an HSQ is used to (a) determine the need for medical clearance, (b) select proper exercise testing protocols, and (c) design proper exercise prescriptions. The criteria that warrant the need for medical clearance should be determined in consultation with the facility's medical advisers (or medical advisory committee).

Additional preactivity screening policies and procedures should include, as stated in ACSM Standard #3, how long the fitness facilities/professionals should retain preactivity screening forms and how they will be kept private, confidential, and secure. Additionally, policies and procedures should be developed for individuals who refuse to participate in the preactivity health screening procedures. In consultation with legal counsel, managers of facilities and programs may want to have the participant sign a refusal form. An example of such a form is provided elsewhere (45).

STRATEGY 2: HAVE ONLY CREDENTIALED AND COMPETENT FITNESS PROFESSIONALS INTERPRET DATA FROM SCREENING TOOLS USED IN PROFESSIONALLY GUIDED PROGRAMS

To comply with the ACSM Standard #3, only a qualified health/fitness professional or health care professional should review preparticipation tools (77). Individuals who interpret data obtained from a screening tool and are not qualified to do so may be practicing outside their scope of practice (discussed later in this chapter). They likely would not possess the necessary knowledge and skills to meet the professional standard of care. As described previously, the standard of care is determined from three situational factors, with one of these being the "type of participants"—meaning the professional needs to design and deliver an exercise program given the individual's medical conditions. This process begins with proper review and interpretation of the health data obtained on a screening tool, which is essential to help prevent negligence claims.

STRATEGY 3: DEVELOP PROCEDURES FOR OBTAINING MEDICAL CLEARANCE FOR PROFESSIONALLY GUIDED PROGRAMS

For individuals who need to obtain medical clearance, it is unlikely that physicians or other health care providers will respond to such requests from fitness professionals in a timely fashion. Therefore, it is recommended to have individuals take or send the facility's medical clearance form (and a copy of their completed screening tool attached) directly to their physician. This approach does not require having the individual sign a medical release because the exercise professional is not disclosing PHI to a third party. However, a medical release would need to be signed by a patient of the physician before that physician would disclose any of that patient's PHI to a fitness professional (e.g., graded exercise test or lipid profile results). A copy of a HIPAA-compliant medical release form is available elsewhere (45). Once physicians receive the medical clearance form, they decide if their patient needs to have a medical evaluation before completing and signing the medical clearance form.

Fitness facilities can provide a list of physicians in the area who are accepting new patients for individuals who do not have a physician. Also, it is best to have a fitness professional on duty during all operating hours who can administer preactivity screening procedures (review and interpret the screening questionnaire and make decisions regarding medical clearance) so that a new participant experiences minimal delays.

KEY POINT

Preactivity screening is essential to help ensure the safety of participants. Risk management strategies include selecting and using appropriate screening tools for both self-guided and professionally guided programs, as well as having only credentialed and competent fitness professionals review and interpret data from the screening tool and make decisions regarding the need for medical clearance.

Fitness Testing and Exercise Prescription

This section focuses on health-related fitness testing (conducted in fitness facilities) versus clinical exercise testing (conducted in clinical settings for diagnostic purposes). Exercise prescription is also discussed with a special emphasis on scope of practice. (See the sidebar *Exercise Prescription and Scope of Practice.*)

Failing to follow proper fitness testing protocols has been a negligence claim in various lawsuits. For example, in *Howard v. Missouri Bone and Joint Center* (56), the plaintiff claimed that an athletic trainer failed to conduct a proper evaluation (i.e., a squat lift assessment) before designing a workout plan as required by the facility's protocol. The jury returned a verdict in favor of the plaintiff,

Exercise Prescription and Scope of Practice

Fitness professionals should always stay within their scope of practice when designing and delivering exercise programs. It is important to understand the difference between legal and professional scope of practice as follows:

LEGAL SCOPE OF PRACTICE

The legal scope of practice is defined within the context of licensed health care professions such as the following:

> *Scope of practice* is defined as the activities that an individual health care practitioner is permitted to perform within a specific profession. Those activities should be based on appropriate education, training, and experience. Scope of practice is established by the practice act of the specific practitioner's board, and the rules adopted pursuant to that act (47, p. 8).

The legal scope of practice is defined in state statutes for other licensed professionals, such as lawyers, counselors, and massage therapists.

PROFESSIONAL SCOPE OF PRACTICE

The professional scope of practice is applicable to all professions and vocations that require special knowledge, skills, and training, such as fitness professionals. Fitness professionals should practice within their education, training, experience, and practical skills to stay within their professional scope of practice (45). The legal scope of practice is not applicable to fitness professionals except for licensed clinical exercise physiologists in the state of Louisiana. This Louisiana state licensing statute includes several sections such as definitions, powers and duties of the board, and qualifications for licensure.

POTENTIAL LEGAL CONSEQUENCES FOR PRACTICING OUTSIDE ONE'S SCOPE

Criminal Charges

Fitness professionals whose conduct crosses over the line into a licensed profession can face criminal charges for violation of a state statute for practicing medicine or some other licensed profession (e.g., dietetics, physical therapy). No harm is needed to prove the violation, only the conduct. For example, the state of Florida has a law titled Unlicensed Practice of a Health Care Profession (Fla. Stat. § 456.065) that describes various penalties including "cease and desist notice" or even felony charges.

Negligence Claims and Lawsuits

As previously described, if a plaintiff's harm is caused by a fitness professional's breach of duty (or standard of care), the fitness professional can be found liable for negligence. When designing and delivering exercise programs for apparently healthy adults, courts likely will require fitness professionals to meet the standard of care of a qualified (competent) fitness professional. When designing and delivering exercise programs for individuals with medical conditions, courts likely will require fitness professionals to meet a standard of care equivalent to fitness professionals who have appropriate knowledge and skills in clinical exercise.

which was upheld by the appellate court. In *Covenant Health System v. Barnett* (27), the plaintiff claimed the employees of the facility negligently failed to have anyone observe her while performing a 3-minute step test. The court ruled that Covenant's failure to observe and attend to the plaintiff while performing the test breached the standard of care as established by *ACSM's Guidelines for Exercise Testing and Prescription*—likely the eighth edition that was current at the time (87).

Failing to design and deliver proper exercise prescriptions can lead to negligence lawsuits. To understand the importance of practicing within one's scope, fitness professionals need to first obtain formal education and practical training to work with apparently healthy individuals and then obtain advanced formal education and practical training to work with clinical populations. Many negligence cases have occurred in which fitness professionals did not possess the necessary knowledge and skills to safely lead exercise programs for apparently healthy adults.

For example, in *Proffitt v. Global Fitness Holdings, LLC, et al.* (72, 73) and *Mimms v. Ruthless Training Concepts, LLC* (65), both plaintiffs, after their first workout with a personal trainer, were diagnosed with exertional rhabdomyolysis (ER) that resulted in permanent injuries and disabilities. Their workouts included high-intensity exercises (e.g., numerous bouts of continuous squatting and leg exercises) in short periods of time with little or no rest. Both lawsuits included many ordinary and gross negligence claims against the defendants, including failure to assess the health and fitness status of the client, design an exercise program within the client's fitness capacity, respond to the client's complaints of fatigue, and warn of known risks and dangers. The *Proffitt* case was settled for $75,000 awarded to the plaintiff, and in *Mimms*, the plaintiff was awarded $300,000 in damages. An expert witness in Mimms introduced ACSM's position stand *Progression Models in Resistance Training for Healthy Adults* (3) as part of the evidence to show that the plaintiff did not follow these safety recommendations (a breach of duty) with regard to progression and rest periods between sets. It was evident that the personal trainers in these cases did not possess the necessary knowledge and skills to meet the professional standard of care.

In other negligence cases, fitness professionals did not have the advanced knowledge and skills to safely lead exercise programs for people with medical conditions. For example, in *Baldi-Perry* (10), previously described, the personal fitness trainer did not appear to have the necessary knowledge and skills to understand the precautions that needed to be taken before prescribing an exercise program for a client with known back and neck problems. In *Levy v. Town Sports International, Inc.* (61), previously described, the personal fitness trainer did not appear to know what precautions were needed to prevent the injury that occurred to a client with osteoporosis. In this case, the court considered situational factors: (a) the nature of the activity (jumping repetition on a BOSU ball) and (b) type of participant (client with osteoporosis) to determine the standard of care (duty) of the personal fitness trainer. Fitness professionals who practice within their scope know when it is necessary to make a referral (e.g., when they do not have the advanced knowledge and skills to work with individuals with medical conditions).

SELECTED ACSM STANDARDS RELATED TO FITNESS TESTING AND EXERCISE PRESCRIPTION

In addition to ACSM Standards #1 and #2 listed earlier under Professional Staff and Independent Contractors for Health/Fitness Facilities, ACSM provides the following guideline under this same category:

> *Guideline #1*: Facility operators should consider having health/fitness professionals who have the appropriate level of professional education and/or certification conduct assessments with and prescribe physical activity for individuals with special needs (77, p. 58).

Note: Under this guideline the following three clinical certifications are listed, all of which require a degree in the field and hundreds of hours of practical experience to be eligible to sit for the certification examination: (a) Clinical Exercise Physiologist (ACSM), (b) Medical Exercise Specialist (American Council on Exercise), and (c) Certified Cardiac Rehabilitation Professional (American Association of Cardiovascular and Pulmonary Rehabilitation).

STRATEGY 1: DEVELOP A FITNESS TESTING MANUAL THAT DESCRIBES FITNESS TESTING PROTOCOLS AND SAFETY PROCEDURES

This manual can serve as an excellent training tool for all fitness professionals involved in fitness testing. In addition to including descriptions of testing protocols, it should describe the many safety procedures that need to be in place. The following is a brief list of these safety procedures. A more complete list is available elsewhere (38, 62).

- *Pretest administration:* Inspections and calibration of testing equipment, written EAP in place, preactivity screening and medical clearance procedures completed, general information and instructions sent to participants, selection and modification of protocols based on each participant's health and fitness status
- *Test administration:* Completion of informed consent, proper warm-up and instruction for participants—explain and demonstrate each test; close supervision of participants at all times, continually monitoring untoward signs and symptoms
- *Posttest administration:* Proper cool-down and posttest instructions for participants, explain results to participants, retain and keep all participant data private and secure

STRATEGY 2: DEVELOP SCOPE OF PRACTICE GUIDELINES TO HELP AVOID NEGLIGENCE CLAIMS AND LAWSUITS

As described previously, fitness professionals who do not have formal education and practical training likely will not be able to meet the standard of care, even when working with apparently healthy adults. To meet the standard of care when working with individuals who have medical conditions, fitness professionals should have advanced education and practical training. Fitness facilities should prepare written scope of practice guidelines that specify the credentials and competence needed for those who work with apparently healthy adults as well as those who work with clinical populations. For example, those who work with clinical populations should have, as a minimum, a degree in the field and professional certification. Recommendations by Warburton and colleagues (94) also should be considered. In addition, it is recommended that fitness facilities consult with their medical and legal advisers when developing their written scope of practice guidelines.

STRATEGY 3: DEVELOP SCOPE OF PRACTICE GUIDELINES TO HELP AVOID CRIMINAL CHARGES

A fitness professional's conduct must not cross over the line into a license practice such as medicine, counseling, and dietetics. For example, diagnosing and treating a medical condition would be considered practicing medicine without a license. Providing individual advice regarding personal problems (e.g., relationships, drugs, alcohol) or nutrition would be practicing counseling and dietetics, respectively, without a license. Written scope of practice guidelines should describe why (from a legal perspective) fitness professionals should avoid certain conduct that can lead to criminal charges and how to make proper referrals when participants bring up medical, counseling, and nutrition topics.

Regarding nutrition advice that fitness professionals often provide, it is recommended to establish written scope of practice guidelines reflected in state statutes. For example, an Ohio statute describes the following types of general nonmedical nutrition information that unlicensed nutrition educators can provide (75).

- Principles of good nutrition and food preparation
- Foods to include in the normal daily diet
- Essential nutrients needed by the body
- Recommended amounts of the essential nutrients
- Actions of nutrients on the body
- Effects of deficiencies or excesses of nutrients
- Food and supplements that are good sources of essential nutrients

The *Ohio Board of Dietetics v. Brown* (68) is a good example of a violation of state statutes with regard to nutritional advice. In this case, the defendant performed nutritional assessments and recommended nutritional supplements to people for the purpose of treating specific complaints and ailments. The court ruled that the defendant was not licensed to practice dietetics in the state of Ohio and was engaged in the practice of dietetics as defined by the Ohio statute (75). This statute describes the scope of practice of licensed dietitians that includes conducting individual nutritional assessments and counseling.

In another case, *Del Castillo v. Secretary, Florida Department of Health* (31), the defendant had a health coaching business. Clients completed a health history form including dietary health questions and were provided with dietary advice such as taking supplements. Following a cease-and-desist order, Del Castillo subsequently claimed the Florida Department of Health had violated her constitutional free speech rights. A federal court ruled in favor of the Department, stating that *professional speech* is in a unique category of speech exempt from First Amendment principles and that states may regulate professional conduct, even though the conduct incidentally involves speech.

STRATEGY 4: PROVIDE SCOPE OF PRACTICE TRAINING FOR ALL FITNESS PROFESSIONALS

OTJ training of fitness professionals should include definitions of legal and professional scope of practice as well as the facility's scope of practice guidelines. When covering the scope of practice guidelines, it will be helpful to cover cases, such as those described earlier, involving negligence lawsuits and criminal charges. This will help fitness professionals understand why it is essential to practice within their scope of practice and how courts determine the standard of care. Resources such as the following also should be discussed in OTJ training programs:

- *Drawing the Line: Understanding the Scope of Practice Among Registered Dietitian Nutritionists and Exercise Professionals* (59)
- Government resources regarding supplements: (a) Office of Dietary Supplements (https://ods.od.nih.gov) and (b) National Center for Complementary and Integrative Health—Dietary and Herbal Supplements (https://nccih.nih.gov/health/supplements)

OTJ training also can include role-playing activities to help fitness professionals develop proper interpersonal communication skills when participants bring up issues such as medical conditions, personal problems, and nutrition (45). For example, prior to the training, have fitness professionals submit a list of questions their participants often ask. During the training, one fitness professional plays the role of the fitness professional and another plays the role of a participant. The participant asks a question and the professional responds. The group critiques the fitness professional's response to evaluate if it was consistent with the facility's scope of practice guidelines. If it was not, have the group share answers that reflect the guidelines. The leader of the training then would provide feedback to help clarify any misunderstanding of the scope of practice guidelines.

KEY POINT

A variety of risk management strategies can be developed and implemented to minimize liability exposures associated with fitness testing and exercise prescription. Perhaps the most important strategies involve establishing written scope of practice guidelines describing the credentials and competence that fitness professionals need to properly carry out fitness testing and exercise prescription activities for both apparently healthy individuals and those with medical conditions. Additionally, training programs are needed so that fitness professionals understand the distinction between legal and professional scope of practice and how practicing outside one's scope of practice can lead to negligence claims and lawsuits and criminal charges.

Instruction and Supervision

Fitness facilities and professionals have a duty to provide a reasonably safe environment for all participants. This includes providing proper fitness instruction in personal fitness training and group exercise programs and proper supervision of the facility. According to the late Betty van der Smissen, the "lack of or inadequate supervision is the most common allegation of negligence" (91, p. 163). She defined "supervision" as specific, general, and transitional. Specific supervision occurs when a supervisor is directly supervising an individual or small group in an instructional format, such as a personal fitness trainer or group exercise leader. General supervision occurs when a supervisor is responsible for overseeing activities going on in a facility, such as a fitness floor supervisor. Finally, transitional supervision occurs when a supervisor changes from general to specific supervision while supervising an area, such as a fitness floor supervisor who provides individual instruction to a participant on how to use a piece of exercise equipment and then transitions back to general supervision of the area.

Numerous negligence cases involving improper fitness instruction and facility supervision have occurred. Some of these cases involving negligent instruction of fitness professionals are described in this chapter (e.g., *Baldi-Perry, Bartlett, Vaid, Corrigan, Santana, Levy, Prof-*

fitt, and *Mimms*). Often, in these cases, injuries resulted from fitness professionals having their participants perform an unsafe exercise or a high-intensity training (HIT) routine. (See the sidebar *Distinguishing HIT and HIIT*.)

Many injuries and subsequent lawsuits have occurred in popular group exercise programs such as yoga, kickboxing, boot camp, and indoor cycling (45). Most often the injuries were due to the instructor lacking the knowledge and skills needed to properly teach exercise. For example, indoor cycling participants have suffered ER, especially following their first class. These cases and the following case emphasize the importance of offering beginner exercise classes taught by competent instructors. In *Scheck v. Soul Cycle* (79), the plaintiff was injured in his first class due to the instructor failing to inform the plaintiff on how to use the cycle properly, as specified in the Soul Cycle manual. He suffered a torn quadriceps muscle in his right leg. Although the defendant claimed that the plaintiff assumed the risk, the court ruled that indoor cycling was not a sporting activity and that the plaintiff was a novice and, thus, did not fully understand and appreciate the risks inherent in the activity. The instructor created a situation (i.e., failed to provide proper instruction) that increased the risks over and above those inherent in the activity.

SELECTED ACSM STANDARDS AND GUIDELINES RELATED TO INSTRUCTION AND SUPERVISION

ACSM provides two standards and four guidelines under Member Orientation, Education, and Supervision. Standards #1 and #2 and Guideline #4 are briefly described.

> *Standard #1:* Once a new member or prospective user has completed a preparticipation screening process, facility operators shall then offer the new member or prospective user a general orientation to the facility (77, p. 29).

> *Standard #2:* Facilities shall provide a means by which members and users who are engaged in a physical activity program within the facility can obtain assistance and/or guidance with their efforts (77, p. 29).

> *Guideline #4:* Staffed facilities should provide professional health/fitness staff to supervise the fitness floor, particularly during peak usage periods, or when there are a large number of older adults or members with special needs using the facility (77, p. 31).

Distinguishing HIT and HIIT

It is important to distinguish between high-intensity training (HIT) or extreme conditioning programs (ECPs) and high-intensity interval training (HIIT) from safety and legal liability perspectives. The injuries that occurred in the high-intensity exercise cases described in this chapter resulted primarily from sustained high-intensity exercise (HIT), such as continuous high-intensity exercise with little or no recovery intervals, and not from high-intensity interval training (HIIT) that incorporates recovery intervals. HIT injuries, such as ER, have occurred with both resistance training and cardiovascular activities, indicating that the type of activity made no difference regarding the risk of injury. Plaintiffs who suffered from ER (or other high-intensity injuries) have been awarded significant monetary damages in their negligence lawsuits (45). In recent years, HIIT programs have become popular and have been rated as one of the top fitness trends (88).

PRECAUTIONS FOR HIIT PROGRAMS

A key safety feature of HIIT is the recovery interval, which, most often, is an active recovery period performed at a light to moderate intensity level. High-volume exercises without adequate recovery intervals can "prompt early fatigue, additional oxidative stress, less resistance to subsequent exercise strain, greater perception of effort, and unsafe movement execution leading to acute injury . . ." (12, p. 384). To help ensure the safety of individuals participating in a body weight/resistance HIIT program, it is essential to first determine if they can perform the exercises properly and safely. Certain body weight/resistance exercises require precise technique and/or considerable skill, balance, and strength for them to be safely executed. For individuals participating in cardiovascular HIIT programs, it will be important to first determine if they have safely progressed to a continuous moderate to vigorous intensity level of exercise. Therefore, in addition to obtaining a medical history (and medical clearance if needed), exercise professionals need to make these determinations prior to instructing HIIT programs. Of course, the HIIT program must be individually designed. If the HIIT program is taught in a group exercise class, not all participants should have the exact same prescription for the high-intensity interval, and the recovery interval may vary as well. HIIT programs for clinical populations have been reported to be safe and effective, but there are important guidelines for fitness professionals to follow (37, 85) when providing these programs. See also the September/October 2021 issue of ACSM's *Health & Fitness Journal* titled "Special Issue on HIIT & Chronic Disease."

Reprinted by permission from Law for Fitness Managers and Exercise Professionals, Fitness Law Academy, LLC, Parrish, FL (2020).

ACSM also provides eight standards and four guidelines under Health/Fitness Facility Operations. Standard #4 and Guideline #1 are briefly described.

Standard #4: A facility that offers youth services or programs shall provide evidence that it complies with all applicable state and local laws and regulations pertaining to their supervision (77, p. 65).

Guideline #1: Facilities that are staffed during operating hours should have a manager on duty (MOD) or supervisor of duty (SOD) schedule that specifies which professional staff person has supervisory responsibility overseeing all operating activities during the hours that the facility is open (77, p. 71).

STRATEGY 1: PROVIDE A GENERAL ORIENTATION TO THE FITNESS FACILITY AND EQUIPMENT FOR ALL NEW PARTICIPANTS

Providing new participants with an orientation that focuses on fitness safety is an important risk management strategy. For example, the orientation should include information on how to use the exercise equipment and any facilities such as swimming pools and saunas. The staff member leading the orientation should give demonstrations on selected pieces of equipment, pointing out posted warning labels and instructional placards as well as explaining the importance of seeking assistance from staff members on the proper use of equipment. As they go through the orientation, participants should be informed of posted safety policies that all participants should follow and other signage posted throughout the facility (e.g., warning or caution signage in saunas and steam rooms, location of emergency equipment such as AED and first aid kit, and exits and evacuation routes). Additionally, they should receive information (e.g., handout) that describes basic principles of safe exercise. Negligence lawsuits have occurred because participants were not taught basic principles of safe exercise, such as proper cool-downs and the concept of blood pooling (1). Lastly, the orientation should promote the facility's programs and services that might best meet the individual's needs and interests.

A case that clearly demonstrates the importance of providing instruction on the proper and safe use of exercise equipment is *Thomas v. Sport City, Inc.* (86). The plaintiff was injured while using a hack squat machine at the defendant's facility. He thought he had properly engaged the hook to secure the weights, but he had not and the rack of weights (180 pounds [81.6 kilograms]) fell, fracturing his ankle and crushing his foot. Thomas claimed that Sport City failed to instruct and supervise him on the proper use of the hack squat machine, but the court ruled that he did know how to use the machine. He testified that he was an experienced, sophisticated user of the machine and that if he had properly secured the hook, the carriage would not have fallen. Therefore, the failure of the club to instruct and supervise was not the cause of the plaintiff's injury, but his own carelessness (negligence) was. The club was not found negligent in this case. However, the court made the following statement with regard to a fitness professional's duty to instruct: "Members of health clubs are owed a duty of reasonable care to protect them from injury on the premises" and "this duty includes a general responsibility to ensure that their members know how to use gym equipment" (86, p. 1157), and the failure to instruct or supervise the plaintiff on proper use of the machine normally would be a breach of duty because the machine could easily cause injury.

STRATEGY 2: HAVE ALL FITNESS PROFESSIONALS WHO LEAD EXERCISE PROGRAMS PREPARE WRITTEN LESSON PLANS AND LESSON PLAN EVALUATIONS

Training programs for fitness professionals should include instruction on how to prepare written lesson plans and lesson plan evaluations. Templates of these forms are available elsewhere (45) and can be downloaded to use or adapt (see the Fitness Law Academy website). The lesson plan template reflects basic components of a proper exercise program (18). Written documentation can provide evidence that proper instruction took place and, thus, help refute negligence claims and lawsuits made against defendants (instructors, trainers, coaches, and their employers). Preparing lesson plans also can help prevent injuries from occurring in the first place. For example, due to a high number of ER injuries occurring in collegiate strength and conditioning programs, the NCAA chief medical officer published

five guiding principles for strength and conditioning coaches and other athletic personnel to follow. The fifth guiding principle specifies that all strength and conditioning workouts should "(a) be documented in writing, (b) reflect the progression, technique, and intentional increases in volume, intensity, mode, and duration of the physical activity, and (c) be available for review by athletic departments" (81, p. 1).

Supervisors of fitness programs should review written lesson plans prepared by fitness professionals, especially for new hires during their probationary period, and then provide feedback based on the review. Lesson plan evaluations can provide (a) a mechanism for fitness instructors to reflect or self-evaluate each class or session and (b) evidence of situations that occurred during a class or session. For example, if a participant complains about shoulder pain and the instructor recommended the participant seek medical evaluation, the date of the complaint and recommendation is recorded on the lesson plan evaluation. If later this participant claims she suffered a shoulder injury while working out at the facility, this document may provide a helpful defense.

STRATEGY 3: CONDUCT JOB PERFORMANCE APPRAISALS OF ALL FITNESS PROFESSIONALS

In addition to training fitness professionals as discussed earlier, fitness supervisors should conduct regular job performance appraisals that include direct observation and evaluation of fitness staff members while performing their jobs. After a performance appraisal, fitness supervisors should discuss the results of the appraisal with the staff member (e.g., group exercise leader, personal fitness trainer) and design an action plan to address any areas in which the staff member needs improvement, especially those areas that focus on participant safety. A sample performance appraisal tool (PAT) for group exercise leaders is described and available elsewhere (45).

Improper instruction in the cases described in this chapter often was due to fitness professionals not having adequate formal education and training, as well as the failure of fitness supervisors to observe, evaluate, and correct their job performance. When fitness professionals do not possess the necessary knowledge and skills to design and deliver safe and effective exercise programs, they subject themselves and their employers to the possibility of negligence claims and lawsuits. To meet the standard of care (legal duty), as determined by a court, fitness professionals must obtain the competence to properly lead exercise programs.

STRATEGY 4: PROVIDE FITNESS STAFF SUPERVISION DURING ALL OPERATING HOURS

Fitness facilities should have continual staff supervision during all operational hours. A designated manager (e.g., a manager on duty, or MOD) who has overall responsibility for any situation that might come up, such as a medical emergency, should be on duty at all times. Fitness facilities should have a job description for fitness professionals who serve in this important role. Training of MODs should include how to provide proper supervision of the facility and how to handle and document any number of situations that might arise in a facility. For example, if an employee of a 24-Hour Fitness Club had received proper training, a death of a woman could have been prevented. This woman was found dead in the club's steam room at 7:45 a.m. the day after she had entered the club (60). The manager informed investigators that the closing employee did not make sure that everyone had exited the club the night before.

When situations do arise, the MOD should prepare written documentation (e.g., complete incident and injury reports). Incident reports document all types of situations (e.g., equipment or facility issues, inappropriate behavior of participants, member complaints). Injury reports, described later, document injuries after they occur. These reports should be submitted immediately to management so that managers can provide the proper follow-up regarding the situation. If situations are handled and documented properly and in a timely fashion, the potential for liability problems to arise decreases. Unsupervised or partially supervised fitness facilities should consider numerous risk management strategies, which are described elsewhere (45).

STRATEGY 5: PROVIDE PROPER SUPERVISION OF ALL YOUTH PROGRAMS

All youth programs should be adequately supervised by responsible and well-trained individuals. In *Lotz v. Claremont Club* (63), a 10-year-old boy was injured while playing dodgeball under the supervision of an employee of the facility. His head was slammed into a wall after being hit with a ball, causing multiple dental injuries. The plaintiffs alleged both negligence and gross negligence on the part of the Club for failing to properly hire, train, and supervise the employee. The instruction and supervision provided by the employee was improper for a variety of reasons (e.g., youth supervisors were not to have children participate in dodgeball per the Club's policy). The appellate court stated that neither the waiver defense nor the primary assumption of risk defense protected the defendants. The conduct of the youth instructor (a) was considered grossly negligent and (b) increased the risks of injury beyond those inherent in the activity.

As mentioned previously, criminal background checks should be performed before hiring employees and volunteers who supervise youth programs or services (e.g., physical activity or sport programs and childcare services). Also, it is essential that fitness facilities follow all applicable laws; for example, ACSM standards require

that facilities that offer youth services or programs provide evidence that it complies with all applicable state and local laws and regulations pertaining to their supervision (77).

KEY POINT

The failure to provide proper instruction and supervision are common negligence claims made by plaintiffs. To help minimize these types of claims, fitness facilities should (a) provide an orientation for new participants to show them how to use the equipment and facility and inform them of important safety policies, (b) hire and train competent fitness staff members and evaluate their job performance (including direct observation of their teaching) to help ensure they are leading safe and effective programs, and (c) make sure all programs and services are properly supervised during all operating hours.

Equipment and Facilities

Fitness facilities and professionals have numerous legal duties and risk management responsibilities regarding exercise equipment and the facility. For example, negligent claims related to exercise equipment can include the failure to properly (a) purchase and lease equipment; (b) install equipment; (c) maintain equipment; (d) post warning signage; (e) clean and disinfect equipment; (f) remove equipment from use when in need of repair, after an injury, and after a manufacturer's recall; and (g) comply with published standards of practice. Each of these are described in detail elsewhere (45), but this chapter will briefly address risk management strategies regarding installation and maintenance of exercise equipment in accordance with the manufacturer's specifications.

Negligence claims related to fitness facilities can include the failure to properly (a) comply with federal regulations (e.g., post OSHA and ADA signage) and state statutes (e.g., comply with consumer protection laws such as membership contract requirements and deceptive trade practices); (b) protect participant safety and security; (c) conduct regular inspections of the facility premises and equipment; (d) maintain and clean facilities such as saunas, steam rooms, hot tubs, locker rooms, and shower areas; and (e) keep individual data private and secure. Each of these is described in detail elsewhere (45), but this chapter will focus briefly on participant physical safety and security, regular inspections, and data privacy and security.

Negligence claims and lawsuits against fitness professionals and facilities are quite common in this area, but sometimes the plaintiff is also negligent as in *Thomas v.*

Sport City, Inc. (86), described previously. Sometimes the manufacturer may be held strictly liable (i.e., product liability) for a defect in equipment design, manufacturing, or marketing (failure to warn). In *Thomas* the plaintiff claimed that the hack squat machine had a design defect, but he was unable to prove that a design defect existed, so the manufacturer was not held liable for his injury.

SELECTED ACSM STANDARDS AND GUIDELINES RELATED TO EQUIPMENT AND FACILITIES

ACSM provides eight standards and four guidelines under Standards for Health/Fitness Facility Operating Practices. Standard #8 is briefly described.

> *Standard #8:* Facilities shall properly secure physical and electronic data concerning its employees and potential, present, and future members so as to protect against a data breach and the release of their personal information (77, p. 65).

ACSM also provides five guidelines under Guidelines for Health/Fitness Facility Equipment; no standards are in place. Guideline #2 is briefly described.

> *Guideline #2:* Facility operators should have a preventive maintenance program for their fitness equipment, including showing when the scheduled work was performed. It is recommended that all preventive maintenance of fitness equipment be done in accordance with the manufacturer's recommendations (77, p. 99).

Note: It is recommended that fitness facilities and professionals follow the NSCA standards and guidelines under Facility and Equipment Setup, Inspection, Maintenance, Repair and Signage (67). Four standards and four guidelines address many of the legal liability exposures described in exercise equipment injury cases such as improper installation, inspection, and maintenance.

Additionally, ACSM provides five standards under Standards for Signage in Health/Fitness Facilities. Standards #1 and #5 are briefly described.

> *Standard #1:* Facility operators shall post proper caution, danger, and warning signage in conspicuous locations where facility staff know, or should know, that existing conditions and situations warrant such signage (77, p. 107).

> *Standard #5:* All cautionary, danger, and warning signage shall have the required signal icon, signal word, signal color, and layout as specified in ASTM F1749 (77, p. 107).

STRATEGY 1: INSTALL EXERCISE EQUIPMENT PROPERLY ACCORDING TO THE MANUFACTURER'S SPECIFICATIONS

Manufacturers of exercise equipment publish an owner's manual for each piece of equipment. Fitness professionals need to follow the information provided in these manuals, including specifications related to installation, spacing, user safety precautions, warning and caution signage, cleaning, inspections, and maintenance. Other published standards of practice also might apply; for instance, the ASTM standard titled Standard Specification for Motorized Treadmills, F2115-18, requires 2 meters (79.2 inches) of space behind treadmills and 0.5 meters (19.5 inches) on each side of the treadmill (8).

The importance of treadmill spacing was a key issue in *Jimenez v. 24 Hour Fitness* (57). In this case, Etelvina Jimenez fell backward off a moving treadmill and sustained severe head injuries when her head hit the exposed steel foot of an exercise machine placed only 3 feet and 10 inches (1.2 meters) behind the treadmill. Upon joining 24 Hour Fitness, Jimenez signed a waiver. The plaintiffs, Etelvina and Pedro Jimenez, filed a negligence lawsuit claiming that 24 Hour Fitness was grossly negligent because the treadmill was not set up as specified in the manufacturer's specifications. The defendant filed a motion for summary judgment based on the waiver Etelvina signed. The trial court granted the motion. However, the appellate court reversed the trial court's ruling based, in part, on the testimony of an expert witness for the plaintiffs. The court stated that 24 Hour Fitness did not provide a 6-foot (1.8 meters) safety zone, a standard practice in the industry, and their "failure to provide the *minimum* safety zone was an extreme departure from the ordinary standard of conduct . . ." (57, p. 237).

Regarding warning labels, ASTM Standard F1749 (7)—Standard Specification for Fitness Equipment and Fitness Facility Signage and Labels—provides specifications for warning labels including the signal icon (triangle) and signal word (warning) appearing at the top of the warning label. This ASTM standard also provides hazard classifications that are noted by signal words according to the relative seriousness of the potential hazards as follows:

> *DANGER*—Indicates an imminently hazardous situation, which, if not avoided, will result in death or serious injury . . .

> *WARNING**—Indicates a potentially hazardous situation, which, if not avoided, could result in death or serious injury.

> *CAUTION*—Indicates a potentially hazardous situation, which, if not avoided, may result in minor or moderate injury . . . (7, p. 2).

Note: Exercise equipment requires *warning labels* because it is potentially hazardous. Using exercise equipment can result in serious injury as demonstrated in the exercise equipment injuries and lawsuits described in this chapter.

Exercise equipment warning labels are provided by the manufacturer and are placed on the equipment in a location as specified in the owner's manual. In addition to warning labels, facilities should consider posting instructional placards on or near each piece of equipment.

Because it is difficult to place a warning label on certain equipment such as dumbbells, kettlebells, and resistance bands, facilities should consider posting a sign (using a proper warning signal icon and signal word as described in ASTM F1749) that describes the warnings as specified in the owner's manual in the area where this equipment is stored. ASTM F1749 also provides a Fitness Facility Safety sign that is to be posted in the facility. This sign informs users of several safety precautions to follow when using the exercise equipment.

STRATEGY 2: MAINTAIN EXERCISE EQUIPMENT PROPERLY ACCORDING TO THE MANUFACTURER'S SPECIFICATIONS

It is essential to maintain all exercise equipment (including equipment such as exercise balls and resistance bands) based on the specifications provided in the owner's manual and to record and retain documentation that proper maintenance was conducted. The defendant in *Chavez v. 24 Hour Fitness* (22) failed to carry out both of these responsibilities. In this case, Stacey Chavez was injured when the back panel of a FreeMotion cable crossover machine (cross-trainer) struck her in the head. She suffered a traumatic brain injury. She and her husband claimed that 24 Hour Fitness was grossly negligent because they failed to properly maintain the cross-trainer in accordance with the specifications set forth in the owner's manual. The trial court ruled that the waiver was enforceable stating that the defendant's conduct reflected ordinary negligence. The appellate court reversed the trial court's ruling, stating that 24 Hour Fitness was grossly negligent based on the following evidence: (a) expert witnesses provided evidence that the machine was not maintained according to the specifications in the owner's manual and (b) testimony of 24 Hour Fitness managers whereby one testified he did not know if the facility's technicians were required to be familiar with the specifications and if such manuals were even on hand and another testified that the preventive maintenance chart was blank and therefore did not know if the maintenance was performed. The court stated the absence of such notations indicated that no maintenance was done—24 Hour Fitness failed to exercise even scant care, and their conduct was an extreme departure from the ordinary standard of conduct. Due to the defendant's gross negligence, the waiver was unenforceable.

Another case, *Grebing v. 24 Hour Fitness* (51), demonstrates the importance of having evidence that maintenance was conducted. The plaintiff claimed she was injured on a low row machine due to the defendant's negligence to maintain the machine properly. However, the court ruled that the defendant was not liable given evidence that the facility took several measures to maintain their equipment.

STRATEGY 3: CONDUCT DAILY INSPECTIONS OF THE FACILITY AND EQUIPMENT TO MEET THE LEGAL DUTIES TOWARD INVITEES

Facility participants (members, program participants, and guests) would be classified as invitees. An invitee is defined as follows:

> An invitee is a person who goes on the premises with the express or implied invitation of the occupant . . . for their mutual advantage; and to him, the duty owed is that of reasonable and ordinary care, which includes the prior discovery of reasonably discoverable conditions of the premises that may be unreasonably dangerous, and correction thereof or a warning to the invitee of the danger (35, p. 837).

A mutually beneficial relationship exists between an invitee and the land owner or occupier (e.g., the owner of a facility receives a monetary benefit from the fees that a member pays, and the member receives all the benefits that the membership provides). The duties the land owner owes toward invitees are to (a) regularly inspect the premises, both inside and outside, including all equipment and facilities, and (b) upon inspection of any reasonably dangerous conditions warn the invitee of the danger (e.g., post signage) or correct the condition. For example, if inspection of an exercise machine reveals that it is not functioning properly, there is a duty to warn of the danger (e.g., post a sign on the machine), repair the machine, or remove it from use.

The duty to inspect is demonstrated in *Goynias v. Spa Health Clubs, Inc.* (50). The plaintiff in this case was injured from a fall on a wet, slippery floor in the locker area. The duty is to maintain safe conditions and to warn individuals of potentially unsafe conditions that are found with reasonable inspection and supervision. In another case involving a member who suffered an injury requiring hip surgery when she tripped over a weight belt that was left on the floor, the court stated that a business owner "has a duty to guard against any dangerous conditions that the owner knows about or should have discovered; and to conduct reasonable inspections to discover latent dangerous conditions . . ." (29, p. 1). Employees who conduct the daily inspections should be well trained and have an inspection checklist that is completed and then kept as documentary evidence that the inspections took place.

STRATEGY 4: DEVELOP POLICIES AND PROCEDURES TO KEEP INDIVIDUAL DATA PRIVATE AND SECURE

As previously discussed, federal laws (HIPAA and the FTCA) require that individual data be kept private and secure. States have data breach laws that define personally identifiable information (PII) (71). Various sections within these state statutes include definitions, notices of security breaches, and enforcement. For selected definitions included in a Florida statute, see *Selected Definitions From Florida Statute: Security of Confidential Personal Information*. Violations can be costly; in Florida, security breaches can cost $1,000 each day for the first 30 days, with significant additional costs thereafter (80).

Because data breaches are common and can be costly for violating federal and state laws, fitness facilities and professionals who obtain participant PII electronically (e.g., via email, websites, fitness trackers, virtual fitness programs, biometric scans) need to be aware of and follow these laws. It is recommended to (a) consult with a cybersecurity lawyer to help ensure compliance with data privacy and security laws, (b) hire or consult with a data security analyst to help ensure that procedures are in place to keep PII private and secure, and (c) pur-

chase cyber security insurance that will cover incidents such as data breaches. For more information on legal considerations related to virtual fitness programs (a top industry trend [88]), other sources are available (43, 44).

KEY POINT

Fitness facilities and professionals have many legal duties related to exercise equipment and the facility. These include installing and maintaining exercise equipment according to the manufacturer's specifications in the owner's manual as well as regular inspections of the facility premises (both inside and outside) and all exercise equipment. Given the duty owed to invitees (participants), any dangerous condition found on inspection must be corrected or a warning must be posted. Systems should be in place to keep individual data private and secure.

Emergency Action Plans (EAPs)

All of the risk management strategies presented thus far focus on preventing injuries from occurring in the first place, referred to as *loss-prevention strategies*. This

Selected Definitions From Florida Statute: Security of Confidential Personal Information

Breach of security—unauthorized access of data in electronic form containing personal information

Covered entity—sole proprietorship, partnership, corporation, trust, estate, cooperative, association, or other commercial entity that acquires, maintains, stores, or uses personal information . . .

Personal information means either of the following:

a. An individual's first name or first initial and last name in combination with any one or more of the following data elements for that individual:

(I) A social security number;

(II) A driver license or identification card number;

(III) A financial account number or credit or debit card number, in combination with any required security code . . . necessary to permit access to an individual's financial account;

(IV) Any information regarding an individual's medical history, mental or physical condition, or medical treatment or diagnosis by a health care professional; or

(V) An individual's health insurance policy number

b. A username or email address, in combination with a password or security question and answer that would permit access to an online account

Security of Confidential Personal Information, FL Stat § 501.171 (2019). Available: https://www.flsenate.gov/Laws/Statutes/2019/501.171.

section will address loss-reduction strategies—actions that mitigate a medical emergency once it has occurred. Negligence claims and lawsuits continue to occur in this area, even though published standards of practice requiring facilities to have an EAP have existed for many years. A variety of factors need to be considered when developing an EAP, as reflected in the following risk management strategies. It is best to designate a professional fitness staff member to serve as the facility's EAP coordinator and to have a medical liaison or adviser who can be directly involved with this effort. Although this section focuses on having a written medical emergency EAP, fitness facilities also should have in place a written evacuation EAP that addresses natural disasters, fires, and threats of violence such as an active shooter (45).

SELECTED ACSM STANDARDS AND GUIDELINES RELATED TO EMERGENCY ACTION PLANS

ACSM provides eight standards and two guidelines under Emergency Planning and Policies. Standards #1, #4, and #5 are briefly described.

Standard #1: Facility operators must have written emergency response policies and procedures, which shall be reviewed regularly and physically rehearsed at least twice annually. These policies shall enable staff to respond to basic first-aid situations and emergency events in an appropriate and timely manner (77, p. 39).

Standard #4: In addition to complying with all applicable federal, state, and local requirements relating to automated external defibrillators (AEDs), all facilities (i.e., staffed and unstaffed) shall have as part of their written emergency response policies and procedures a public access defibrillation (PAD) program in accordance with generally accepted practice (77, p. 39).

Standard #5: AEDs in a facility shall be located to allow time from collapse, caused by cardiac arrest, to defibrillation of three to five minutes or less. A three-minute response time can be used to help determine how many AEDs are needed and where to place them (77, p. 39).

ACSM also provides the following standard (Standard #3) under Standards for Health/Fitness Facility Professional Staff and Independent Contractors.

Standard #3: Health/fitness professionals engaged in pre-activity screening or prescribing, instructing, monitoring, or supervising of physical activity programs for facility members and users shall have current automated external defibrillation and cardiopulmonary resuscitation (AED and CPR) certification from an organization qualified to provide such certification. A CPR or AED certification should include a hands-on practical skills assessment (77, p. 53).

State Laws

Fitness facilities and professionals need to be aware of and comply with state laws regarding medical emergencies. For example, Wisconsin has a statute (49) that requires each fitness center to have an employee with current first-aid and CPR certifications through the American Heart Association (AHA) or the American Red Cross (ARC). Several states require fitness facilities to keep an AED on site (45, 77). The provisions within these state statutes vary and, therefore, it is essential to consult with legal counsel to help ensure compliance with their requirements. For example, the AED statute in California (53) contains specific requirements that fitness facilities must comply with to avoid civil liability.

All states have Good Samaritan statutes. These laws are based on public policy to encourage volunteers to render aid to individuals in peril. They protect volunteers from ordinary negligence but not gross negligence. Employees of a fitness facility may believe that they have a choice whether to render aid (like a volunteer does in the public domain) to an injured fitness facility participant based on Good Samaritan laws. However, that is not the case—they have a duty to render aid due to the relationship that is formed between the facility and the facility participants. This aid may only include calling emergency medical services (EMS). However, it is essential to be aware of and follow requirements specified in applicable laws (e.g., state AED statutes) and standards of practice published by professional organizations.

AED Cases

One of the issues that comes up in many of the AED cases involving fitness facilities is if the fitness facility had a legal duty to use an AED, based on requirements specified in AED statutes specific to fitness facilities. The general answer is no, but other statute requirements (or other state AED statutes) may be relevant. Three cases will be described—two occurring in New York involving a New York statute (New York General Business Law § 627-a that requires health clubs with 50 or more members to maintain an AED on site and, during all staffed business hours, to have a person trained and certified to use the device) and the other case in Texas involving a Texas AED law (Chapter 779 of the Texas Health and Safety Code).

In *Miglino v. Bally Total Fitness of Greater N.Y., Inc.* (64), Gregory Miglino alleged that the health club failed to use an AED on his father as required by the state's statute. After his father collapsed while playing racquetball, an AED was brought to the area where his father was located, but it was not used. EMS arrived 7 minutes after the collapse and administered shocks with an AED to no avail. His father was pronounced deceased about an hour later at the hospital. The court denied the defendant's motion to dismiss the case stating that New York's AED statute did require health clubs to use an AED if necessary. The defendant questioned the court's ruling and interpretation of the statute. Upon appeal, the Court of Appeals (64) stated that the statute does not specify a requirement to use an AED and that it cannot be implied that it does. Lawmakers would need to expressly state this intent in the statute to impose such a duty on health club owners. The ruling (no duty to use an AED based on New York's statute) was affirmed in a later case in 2020—*Hamlin v. PFNY, LLC* (179 A.D.3d 1027).

In *Dinero v. Aspen Athletic Club* (32), two AEDs were brought to the victim but neither were functioning properly. The victim never regained consciousness. The court denied the defendant's motion for summary judgment because the health club failed to maintain an operable AED as required by the New York AED statute. This statute states that health clubs are classified as a public access defibrillator provider (PADP), which requires, among other things, to maintain and test the AED according to applicable standards of the manufacturer and any appropriate government agency. This case demonstrates the importance of fitness facilities being aware of and following all the requirements within AED statutes.

A Texas case demonstrates the importance of being aware of and following state AED statutes that are not specific to health clubs but may apply to health clubs. In *Boggus obo Casey v. Texas Racquet & Spa, Inc.* (14), John Casey suffered cardiac arrest while participating in a cycling class. One employee called 911, and another began CPR. Although an AED was located nearby, no one used it. EMS defibrillated Casey, but he suffered severe brain damage. In her complaint, Ginny Boggus (Casey's wife) alleged that the club failed to (a) properly train its employees on the use of the AED and (b) comply with Chapter 779 of the Texas Health and Safety Code. Chapter 779 requires entities that acquire an AED to ensure that users are trained. The appellate court disagreed with the trial court's ruling granting the defendant's motion for summary judgment. The appellate court ruled that

the fitness club failed to train its employees on the use of an AED as required by Chapter 779. The case was remanded for further proceedings.

STRATEGY 1: PREPARE A WRITTEN MEDICAL EMERGENCY ACTION PLAN

The first step is to assemble a planning team headed up by a designated professional staff member who can serve as the facility's EAP coordinator. The team should consist of facility managers, members of the facility's risk management advisory committee (legal, medical, insurance experts), and local first responders including EMS personnel. In addition to leading the development of the facility's written EAP, the EAP coordinator has numerous responsibilities that should be specified in a job description, such as training MODs and all staff members on the facility's EAP policies and procedures. The following are responsibilities of the planning team when preparing a written medical EAP:

1. In consultation with legal counsel, review applicable laws (e.g., OSHA regulations, state first-aid and AED statutes) and standards of practice published by professional organizations. In *Miglino* and other cases, courts have considered as evidence in determining duty standards of practice published by the AHA and ACSM regarding AEDs in fitness facilities (45). It is essential that the EAP reflects all the requirements in applicable laws as well as published standards of practice (e.g., staff members have current AED and CPR certifications and are well trained on how to carry out the EAP in a timely fashion).

2. Establish effective "internal" and "external" communication systems. An internal communication system should address the following questions: "(a) how will the first staff member responding to the scene inform other staff members and the MOD of the emergency, (b) how do procedures differ based on the location of the emergency, (c) who will contact EMS, if necessary, and what will be said, and (d) if the first responder (or MOD) on the scene determines the need for an AED or first-aid kit, how and to whom is this communicated so that the AED is delivered in a timely fashion" (45, p. 472). Facilities should have signage posted indicating where AEDs are located. Development of an external communication should involve local first responders who can help ensure the facility's EAP includes effective communication with EMS on arrival (e.g., if more than one entrance, which entrance will EMS use and who on the staff will direct them to the location of the victim).

3. Develop contingency plans for each type of medical emergency. Written contingency plans should be developed for each type of medical emergency: (a)

minor injuries such as a sprained ankle, (b) serious injuries such as a bone fracture, (c) injuries that cause major bleeding, and (d) life-threatening events. It is best to summarize each contingency plan into a flowchart that can clearly depict the steps that staff members (e.g., those first on the scene), front desk staff members, and the MOD should follow.

STRATEGY 2: PROVIDE QUALITY STAFF TRAINING TO HELP ENSURE THE EAP WILL BE CARRIED OUT PROPERLY AND IN A TIMELY FASHION

First, staff members who have responsibilities to carry out the EAP should maintain current certifications in first aid, CPR, and AED. It is also recommended to have a staff member, perhaps the EAP coordinator, be a certified instructor in these areas who can provide recertification classes for staff members as OTJ in-service trainings. Additionally, it is critical that staff members review and rehearse the EAP at least two times a year, as recommended by ACSM (77). Other professional organizations have recommended staff EAP trainings be held four times per year (45). However, the actual number needed should be determined by managers and EAP coordinators assessing the competence of staff members during and after each training drill or rehearsal. If staff members have not demonstrated competence (e.g., cannot retrieve and be ready to use an AED on a victim within 3 minutes), additional training is needed.

STRATEGY 3: ESTABLISH POSTEMERGENCY PROCEDURES

After a medical emergency, the MOD should complete an Injury Report such as the sample provided in form 24.1. The Injury Report should be developed by the EAP planning team including legal, medical, and insurance experts who serve on the facility's risk management advisory committee. In addition to completing an Injury Report the MOD should gather and record any evidence, such as photographs of any equipment and conditions involved in the incident and interviews with witnesses who can describe the "what, how, and when" regarding the incident. This evidence may be helpful in defending any future negligence lawsuits against staff members and the facility. Several additional postemergency procedures are described elsewhere (45) and include following up with the victim and evaluating the staff's performance after every incident (e.g., whether they carried out the EAP properly). Also, the facility's legal counsel and insurance provider may require that a copy of the Injury Report be sent to them immediately after the incident.

KEY POINT

Numerous negligence cases against fitness facilities have occurred for failing to have or properly carry out an EAP. A variety of factors need to be considered when preparing an effective EAP. Each facility should first assemble a planning team and designate a professional staff member as the EAP coordinator. Other members of the planning team include facility managers, legal counsel, insurance providers, and local first responders such as EMS. Once the EAP is written, fitness facilities should provide in-service trainings for staff members that include drills or rehearsals two to four times a year as required or recommended by professional organizations or required in state AED statutes. The EAP coordinator (or others in leadership positions) have many responsibilities such as formally assessing the competence of employees during the trainings and conducting important post-emergency procedures.

Record Keeping and Documentation of Evidence

Reference to various documents (e.g., waivers, informed consents) was made throughout this chapter. These documents should be stored in a secure place because they can provide valuable evidence in the event of a claim or lawsuit. For example, if the fitness facility has retained a copy of the waiver signed by a member, it will provide evidence that can help protect the facility if that member files a negligence lawsuit against the facility. Other record keeping can help provide evidence that a fitness facility and its staff members properly carried out their legal duties. For example, if a facility keeps records documenting maintenance of exercise equipment, it will be difficult for a plaintiff to prove that the facility failed to carry out this duty. If a plaintiff cannot prove that a defendant breached their duty, it will be difficult for the plaintiff to prevail in a negligence lawsuit. It also is important to have duplicate copies of records (written or electronic) stored at another location in case the original is lost or destroyed. Fitness facilities and professionals should seek legal counsel regarding how long records need to be kept.

FORM 24.1 Sample Facility Injury Report

BASIC INFORMATION

Today's date: _____

Facility: Name and location: _____

Employee's name (completing report): _____

Position: _____

Phone number: _____

Email: _____

INJURY INFORMATION

Date: _____

Time: _____

Location: _____

Body part(s) injured: _____

Description of injury: _____

Cause of injury: _____

Care provided: _____

Were emergency medical services contacted?_____

If yes, include EMS personnel and/or police name and contact information.

Name	Contact information
1. _____	_____
2. _____	_____
3. _____	_____

INJURED PARTY

Name: _____

Address: _____

Phone number: _____

Email: _____

Date of birth, if known: _____

Relationship to facility (member, participant, spectator, or staff): _____

WITNESS INFORMATION

(If eyewitnesses were interviewed, attach their written statements.)

Name	Address	Contact
1. _____	_____	_____
2. _____	_____	_____
3. _____	_____	_____
4. _____	_____	_____
5. _____	_____	_____

(continued)

FORM 24.1 *(continued)*

Additional comments such as the following that are relevant to the injury:

a. Comments from victim, if available:

b. Comments of staff member (first responder) and MOD:

c. Description of photos (attached to this report) taken, if applicable:

d. Other:

Signature: _____ (MOD) Date: _____
Signature: _____ (facility manager) Date: _____

FOLLOW-UP WITH VICTIM OR VICTIM'S EMERGENCY CONTACT

Employee conducting follow-up: _____ Date: _____
Victim's name or emergency contact's name: _____
Comments: _____
_____
_____
_____

Reprinted by permission from Law for Fitness Managers and Exercise Professionals, Fitness Law Academy, LLC, Parrish, FL (2020).

Record-Keeping Tips

Keeping records can provide evidence that legal duties were carried out properly. Examples include the following:

- Credentials of staff members (e.g., degrees, current certifications)
- Criminal background checks of personnel
- Staff training meetings (e.g., dates, staff members attending, content covered)
- Preactivity screening forms (e.g., screening tools, medical clearance forms)
- Waivers and informed consents
- Written scope of practice guidelines for staff members
- Facility orientations for participants (e.g., dates, participants attending, content covered)
- Fitness testing data and exercise prescriptions
- Lesson plans and lesson plan evaluations
- Job performance evaluations of staff members
- Facility and equipment inspections
- Facility and equipment maintenance records
- Written EAP and injury reports
- Completed incident reports
- Written exposure control plan (OSHA's Bloodborne Pathogens Standard)

LEARNING AIDS

REVIEW QUESTIONS

1. Describe the causes and types of injuries that can occur while participating in physical activity.
2. Describe the three primary sources of law, and give an example of each.
3. Define the following legal terms: *stare decisis*, *respondeat superior*, *compensatory damages*, *punitive damages*, and *exculpatory clause*.
4. Define the following risk management terms: *loss-prevention strategies*, *loss-reduction strategies*, *contractual transfer of risks*, *general liability insurance*, and *professional liability insurance*.
5. Describe the type of conduct that would be considered ordinary negligence and gross negligence, and list cases described in this chapter in which the defendants were liable for gross negligence.
6. Explain why the primary assumption of risk was an ineffective defense in the *Corrigan* and *Santana* cases.
7. Describe why fitness facilities and professionals should have a competent lawyer review and edit a waiver before having participants sign it.
8. Discuss how courts determine the standard of care of an exercise professional in negligence cases.
9. Explain how a fitness professional could possess credentials (e.g., degree, certification) but not be competent. Then describe why it is essential from a legal perspective that fitness professionals are competent.
10. Describe the difference between legal and professional scope of practice and legal cases involving each.

11. List and describe the legal duties that fitness facilities and professionals have toward invitees.

12. Explain the precautions that need to be taken prior to having individuals participate in high-intensity interval training (HIIT) programs.

13. Using case examples, discuss why it is essential to follow exercise equipment installation and maintenance specifications in manuals published by equipment manufacturers.

14. List federal and state laws involving protected health information (PHI) and personally identifiable information (PII).

15. Describe laws and published standards of practice that require EAP staff training.

CASE STUDY

Upon joining World's Best Gym (WBG) located in Virginia, Mr. Smith requested an orientation on how to use the gym's exercise equipment. Mr. Smith, a 30-year-old commercial airline pilot, knew that regular exercise would help him maintain and improve health-related factors that are evaluated annually during his medical flight exam. After he signed a membership contract and a separate document titled Waiver and Release of Liability, he was told that instead of an orientation he should sign up for personal fitness training sessions, which he did. His personal fitness trainer, Bill—an employee of WBG—did not conduct any preactivity screening procedures, nor did he conduct any assessments to determine Mr. Smith's fitness levels. However, Mr. Smith did inform Bill that he had not worked out in years.

Bill did not have any formal education or supervised practical experiences (e.g., an internship) in exercise science prior to becoming a personal fitness trainer at WBG. He possessed a personal trainer certification that was accredited by a nationally recognized accrediting agency, which was the only credential necessary to become a trainer at WBG. Bill's only experience in the field was that he had been a former collegiate football player and thus was familiar with the strength and conditioning program he participated in for many years.

During the first training session, Bill had Mr. Smith perform numerous bouts of strenuous exercises—repeated sets and fast repetitions of squats and other exercises using the quadriceps with little or no rest between sets. As the session continued, Mr. Smith became very fatigued, showing obvious signs and symptoms of overexertion. He requested several breaks during the workout. However, Bill told Mr. Smith that he did not need a break and that he could handle the high-intensity workout because he was young. He said to Mr. Smith, "No pain, no gain," and pushed Mr. Smith to continue performing the strenuous exercises.

After the workout, Mr. Smith went home exhausted, experiencing extreme fatigue. That night and the next day, Mr. Smith was in severe pain and noticed his urine was dark brown. He went to the emergency room and was immediately hospitalized with a diagnosis of severe exertional rhabdomyolysis and a creatine kinase (CK) level that was extremely high. The medical specialists (a nephrologist and a rheumatologist) had never seen such a severe case of exertional rhabdomyolysis in someone like Mr. Smith who had no other underlying medical conditions.

Mr. Smith ended up in the hospital for 8 days, receiving various treatments including kidney dialysis. Although he had several weeks of physical therapy, his injury resulted in a 35% loss of muscle tissue in both quadriceps and permanent disability. It is unlikely that he will be able to obtain his medical certificate (clearance) ever again, which is necessary for him to retain his pilot's license.

Mr. Smith's lawyer has filed a negligence lawsuit against the personal fitness trainer and WBG seeking damages of $1 million to cover medical expenses, future medical expenses, pain and suffering, lost wages, and future lost wages. Note that WBG has a commercial general liability (CGL) policy but does not have professional liability coverage for any of its employees. Bill also had not purchased any professional liability insurance on his own. The CGL contains an exclusion clause stating it "does not cover any bodily injury that occurred from providing instruction or advice relating to physical fitness or training programs."

1. What negligence claims will Mr. Smith and his lawyer likely file against WBG and the personal fitness trainer?

2. How will the court determine the duties owed to Mr. Smith, the plaintiff in this case?

3. Describe how Bill's conduct would be considered outside his scope of practice.

4. WBG likely will use the waiver and primary assumption of risk as defenses. Will these defenses be effective in protecting WBG? Why or why not?

5. What risk management strategies should WBG have implemented that might have prevented Mr. Smith's injury?

6. Why is it likely that the personal trainer and WBG will be found liable and will have to pay the damages?

Answers to Case Study

1. WBG failed to do the following:

- Hire qualified and competent personal fitness trainers
- Provide adequate training for their personal fitness trainers
- Perform adequate supervision of their personal fitness trainers

The personal fitness trainer failed to do the following:

- Conduct a preactivity screening
- Assess fitness levels to evaluate the client's capacity prior to exercise
- Design an exercise program within the client's safe capacity
- Properly instruct and supervise the client
- Recognize signs and symptoms of overexertion
- Grant the client's repeated requests for a break throughout the session

2. The court can determine duty in several ways in this case. First, the court likely will consider the relationship formed between WBG and Mr. Smith. Given this relationship, a general legal duty exists to provide reasonably safe programs and services, which requires taking steps to prevent foreseeable injury risks. It is likely that an expert witness will testify in this case against the defendants (the personal trainer and WBG). Expert witnesses educate the court as to the standard of care (or duty) that the defendants owed to the plaintiff given the situation. They consider the factors that make up the professional standard of care (nature of the activity, type of participants, and environmental conditions) as well as standards of practice published by professional organizations when judging the conduct of the defendants. An expert witness in this case will be able to show that Bill (the trainer) did not meet the requirements for (a) the nature of the activity (e.g., he did not have the knowledge and skills to take the necessary precautions, such as progression—a basic principle of safe exercise, prior to prescribing a high-intensity workout) and (b) the type of participant (e.g., Bill did not consider the type of client that Mr.

Smith was—a novice who was sedentary—when designing and delivering his first exercise session). Additionally, an expert witness will be able to show that Bill and WBG breached their duty when they failed to follow standards and guidelines published by professional organizations that, for example, require or recommend preactivity screening.

3. Practicing outside one's scope of practice can occur two ways. Fitness professionals whose conduct crosses over the line into a licensed profession can face criminal charges for violation of a state statute for practicing medicine or some other licensed profession (e.g., dietetics, counseling). No harm is needed to prove the violation, only the conduct.

   If a fitness professional's conduct does not meet the professional standard of care (e.g., does not meet situational factors as described in the answer to question 2) or adhere to best practices described in standards of practice published by professional organizations, and the conduct caused harm to a participant, the fitness professional can be found liable for negligence.

   The second one is applicable in this case—the personal trainer's conduct was negligent (his breach of several duties, more likely than not, caused the injuries to Mr. Smith), and, thus, he did not meet the standard of care of an exercise professional.

4. Neither the waiver nor primary assumption of risk will be effective in protecting the defendants in this case. Though Mr. Smith signed a waiver and release of liability, waivers are against public policy in Virginia for personal injury and, therefore, are unenforceable. It is unlikely that the primary assumption of risk will protect the defendants because this defense is effective for injuries due to risks inherent in the activity only. The primary assumption of risk defense requires that the plaintiff knows, understands, and appreciates the risks inherent in the activity and voluntarily assumes them. Because Mr. Smith was a novice, it is unlikely that he knew, understood, and appreciated these risks of any exercise program, let alone the risks associated with high-intensity exercise.

5. WBG could have implemented several risk management strategies to prevent the injuries and subsequent litigation that occurred in this case. WBG should not assume that a personal trainer who has an accredited certification is competent, nor should they assume a former collegiate athlete is competent to be a personal trainer. WBG should require formal education and training for their trainers—either provided internally or externally by credentialed, competent, and experienced instructors. WBG should have evaluated Bill's knowledge and skills prior to hiring him to help ensure he could meet the requirements that make up the professional standard of care and practices set forth in published standards of practice. Shortly after hiring Bill, WBG should have conducted a performance appraisal to evaluate his on-the-job performance. Bill's improper instruction could have been addressed in this appraisal along with inappropriate statements such as "No pain, no gain," which perpetuate a myth of exercise. In addition, WBG should have professional liability insurance to cover their trainers or require that their trainers purchase this coverage on their own.

6. Yes, it is likely that both defendants—the personal trainer and WBG (through the legal doctrine *respondeat superior*)—will be liable for negligence (they breached several duties, which likely caused the injuries to the plaintiff). Neither had purchased professional liability insurance coverage to pay out the damages regarding negligent conduct of an exercise professional. The CGL policy also contained an exclusion clause stating it "does not cover any bodily injury that occurred from providing instruction or advice relating to physical fitness or training programs." Therefore, it is likely that both defendants will have to pay out the monetary damages to the plaintiff as awarded by the court (judge) or jury.

GLOSSARY

1-repetition maximum (1RM)—The heaviest weight that can be lifted only once using good form.

abduction—Movement at a joint around its anteroposterior axis that moves the distal body segment away from the midline of the body, such as moving the hip and leg out to the side.

abrasion—Scraping of tissues that removes the outermost layers of skin and exposes numerous capillaries.

absolute intensity—Can be expressed in a number of ways: kcal of energy produced per minute (kcal · min^{-1}); milliliters of oxygen consumed per kilogram of body weight per minute (ml · kg^{-1} · min^{-1}); or METs, where 1 MET is taken as resting metabolic rate and is equal to 3.5 ml · kg^{-1} · min^{-1}.

acceptable macronutrient distribution range (AMDR)—The percentages of calories from carbohydrate, fat, and protein that are thought to promote good health.

actin—The thin contractile filament of the sarcomere to which myosin binds to release the energy in the activated crossbridges, leading to sarcomere shortening.

adaptation—Expansion of a physiologic capacity in response to a regularly applied training stimulus.

adduction—Movement at a joint around its anteroposterior axis that moves the distal body segment toward the midline of the body, such as moving the hip and leg back in from the abducted position.

adenosine triphosphate (ATP)—The final product of the breakdown of carbohydrate, fat, and protein; a molecule that the cell can use as an energy source for biological work.

adequate intake (AI)—The amount of a nutrient considered adequate, although insufficient data exist to establish an RDA.

adipose tissue—Tissue composed of fat cells.

administrative law—A primary source of law (from the executive branch of the government) that is formed by numerous administrative agencies that exist at both the federal and state levels.

aerobic energy—When oxygen is used to help supply energy (ATP) to a person who is working.

agility—Ability to start, stop, and move the body quickly in different directions.

agonist—A muscle that is very effective in causing a certain joint movement; also called the *prime mover*. Also, for medications (drugs), a chemical that activates a receptor to produce a biological response.

air displacement plethysmography—Method of assessing body composition that estimates body density from body volume and body weight.

airway obstruction—Blockage of the airway that can be caused by a foreign object. Swelling is secondary to direct trauma or allergic reaction.

amenorrhea—Delayed menstruation by age 15 in a female with secondary sex characteristics (primary amenorrhea) or missing three or more consecutive menstrual cycles after menarche (secondary amenorrhea).

amino acids—Nitrogen-containing building blocks for proteins that can be used for energy.

amortization phase—Time between the eccentric and concentric phases of a muscle action.

amphiarthrodial joint—A joint that allows only slight movement in all directions; also called the *cartilaginous joint*.

anaerobic energy—Energy (ATP) supplied without oxygen required. Creatine phosphate and glycolysis supply ATP without using oxygen.

android-type obesity—Obesity in which the trunk and abdomen store a disproportionate amount of fat.

aneurysm—A spindle-shaped or saclike bulging of the wall of a blood-filled vein, artery, or ventricle.

angina pectoris—Severe cardiac pain or discomfort that may radiate to the jaw, arms, or legs. Angina is caused by myocardial ischemia.

angular momentum—The quantity of rotation. Angular momentum is the product of rotational inertia and angular velocity.

anorexia nervosa—An eating disorder in which a preoccupation with body weight leads to self-starvation.

antagonist—A muscle that causes movement at a joint in a direction opposite to that of the joint's agonist (*prime mover*). Also, for medications (drugs), a chemical that blocks a receptor to produce a biological response.

anticoagulants—Drugs that prevent blood clotting.

antihypertensives—Drugs that lower blood pressure.

antioxidant vitamins—Substances that attach to free radicals and diminish their effects. Antioxidants are touted as effective in decreasing the risk of cardiovascular disease and cancer, which is not supported by research.

aortic valve—Heart valve located between the aorta and the left ventricle.

aponeuroses—Broad, flat, tendinous sheaths attaching muscles to one another.

arterioles—Blood vessels between the artery and the capillary that are involved in the regulation of blood flow and blood pressure.

arteriovenous oxygen difference—Volume of oxygen extraction; calculated by subtracting the oxygen content of mixed venous blood (as it returns to the heart) from the oxygen content of the arterial blood.

arthritis—Inflammation of a joint.

articular capsule—A ligamentous structure that encloses a diarthrodial joint.

articular cartilage—Cartilage covering bone surfaces that articulate (meet or come into contact) with other bone surfaces.

atherosclerosis—A form of arteriosclerosis in which fatty substances are deposited in the inner walls of the arteries.

atrial fibrillation—The atrial rate is 400 to 700 bpm, whereas the ventricular rate is 60 to 160 bpm; P waves cannot be seen on the ECG.

atrial flutter—The atrial rate is 200 to 350 bpm, whereas the ventricular rate is 60 to 160 bpm; ECG shows a sawtooth pattern between QRS complexes.

atrioventricular (AV) node—The origin of the bundle of His in the right atrium of the heart. Normal electrical activity of the heart passes through the AV node before depolarization of the ventricles.

atrophy—A reduction in muscle fiber size.

avascular—Without a blood supply.

balance—Ability to maintain a certain posture or to move without falling.

ballistic movement—A rapid movement with three phases: an initial concentric action by agonist muscles to begin movement, a coasting phase, and a deceleration by the eccentric action of the antagonist muscles.

bariatric surgery—A surgical procedure designed to help with weight loss. These surgeries alter the gastrointestinal system to restrict food intake and nutrient uptake.

baroreceptors—Receptors that monitor arterial blood pressure.

behavioral contracts—Written, signed, public agreements to engage in specific goal-directed activities. Contracts include a designated time frame and clear consequences of meeting and not meeting the agreed-upon objectives.

bench stepping—A graded exercise test that can be used for both submaximal and maximal testing to evaluate cardiorespiratory fitness. The height of the bench and the number of steps per minute determine the intensity of the effort. Bench stepping is also a popular conditioning exercise.

beta-adrenergic blocking medications (beta-blockers)—Drugs that block receptors that respond to catecholamines (epinephrine and norepinephrine); they slow heart rate and some can lower blood pressure.

beta-adrenergic receptors—Receptors in the heart and lungs that respond to catecholamines (epinephrine and norepinephrine).

beta-carotene—A precursor of vitamin A and an important antioxidant.

binge-eating disorder—An eating disorder characterized by consuming large amounts of food in a short time.

bioelectrical impedance analysis (BIA)—Method of body composition assessment based on the electrical conductivity of various tissues in the body.

blister—When friction causes disruption between epidermis and dermis, it results in fluid accumulation between the layers of skin.

bodybuilding—A competitive sport in which the primary goal is to enhance muscular size, symmetry, and definition.

body composition—Description of the tissues that make up the body; typically refers to the relative percentages of fat and nonfat tissues in the body.

body-fat distribution (fat patterning)—Pattern of fat accumulation that often is inherited.

body mass index (BMI)—Measure of the relationship between height and weight; calculated by dividing weight in kilograms by height in meters squared.

bone mineral density (BMD)—Amount of bone mineral per unit area. Typically measured with dual-energy X-ray absorptiometry (DXA) and used for clinical diagnosis of osteoporosis.

bronchodilators—Drugs that dilate the bronchioles, providing relief from an asthma attack.

bulimia nervosa—An eating disorder characterized by consuming large amounts of food followed by food purging.

bundle branch—Bundle of nerve fibers between both ventricles of the heart; conducts impulses.

bundle of His—Conduction pathway that connects the AV node with bundle branches in the ventricles.

bursae—Fibrous sacs lined with synovial membrane that contain a small quantity of synovial fluid. Bursae are found between tendon and bone, between skin and bone, and between muscle and muscle. Their function is to facilitate movement without friction between these surfaces.

calcium channel blockers (CCBs)—Medications that act by blocking the entry of calcium into the cell; used to treat angina, arrhythmias, and hypertension.

caloric equivalent of oxygen—Approximately 5 kcal of energy is produced per liter of oxygen consumed (5 kcal · L^{-1}).

carbohydrate—An essential nutrient composed of carbon, hydrogen, and oxygen that is an energy source for the body.

carbohydrate loading—Increasing carbohydrate intake and decreasing activity in the days preceding competition.

carbon monoxide (CO)—A pollutant derived from the incomplete combustion of fossil fuels; binds to hemoglobin to reduce oxygen transport and thus reduce maximal aerobic power.

cardiac arrest—Failure of the heart to circulate blood effectively because the ventricles cease to contract in a rhythmic fashion.

cardiac output (Q̇)—The volume of blood pumped by the heart per minute; calculated by multiplying heart rate (bpm) by stroke volume (ml · beat^{-1}).

cardiopulmonary resuscitation (CPR)—Established procedures to restore breathing and blood circulation.

cardiorespiratory fitness (CRF)—The ability of the circulatory and respiratory systems to supply oxygen to muscles during dynamic exercise involving a large muscle mass.

case law—A primary source of law (from the judicial branch of government) that is derived from written court opinions at both the federal and state levels.

cholesterol—A fatty substance in which carbon, hydrogen, and oxygen atoms are arranged in rings; may be deposited in the arterial walls, contributing to atherosclerosis.

chronic obstructive pulmonary disease (COPD)—Diseases that obstruct the flow of air in the airways of the lung.

communication—Interaction, often verbal, to share information and emotions.

complex carbohydrate—Polysaccharides formed by combining three or more sugar molecules. Polysaccharides include starches and fiber and are found in high numbers in rice, pasta, and whole-grain breads.

concentric action—Type of muscle contraction in which the muscle shortens. This shortening pulls the points of attachment on each bone closer to each other, causing movement at the joint.

conduction—Heat-exchange mechanism in which heat is lost from warmer to cooler objects in direct contact with each other.

convection—Special case of conduction related to heat loss. Heat is transferred to air or water in direct contact with the skin; warm air or water is less dense and rises, carrying heat away from the body.

coordination—Ability to perform a task that integrates movements of the body and various parts of the body.

core stability—The ability to control the forces across the spine and pelvic girdle while protecting the integrity of the spinal structures, or the ability to achieve and sustain control of the trunk region at rest and during precise movements.

coronary angiography—A diagnostic procedure in which a flexible guide wire is inserted into a coronary artery, and a catheter is then passed over it. A radiographic contrast dye is then injected into the artery to reveal any potential blockages.

coronary arteries—Blood vessels that supply the heart muscle.

coronary artery bypass graft (CABG)—Procedure in which arteries or veins are sutured above and below a blocked coronary artery to restore adequate blood flow to that portion of the myocardium.

coronary heart disease (CHD)—Atherosclerosis of the coronary arteries. Also called *coronary artery disease (CAD)*.

criterion method—Method used as the gold standard, or the method against which other methods are compared.

crossbridge—Part of myosin filament that binds to actin, releasing energy that results in shortening of the sarcomere.

cross-training—An alternative training mode that is outside of the athlete's competition sport or could include various fitness components within an exercise program or session.

cycle ergometer—A one-wheeled stationary cycle with adjustable resistance used as a work task for exercise testing or conditioning.

daily caloric need—The number of calories a person needs to sustain current body weight, assuming that activity levels remain constant.

daily values (DVs)—Indicate the percentage of daily recommended levels of nutrients that are contained in a food. DVs are based on a calorie intake of 2,000 kcal · day^{-1}.

DASH diet—The DASH (Dietary Approaches to Stop Hypertension) diet was originally designed to help people control their BP. This diet is characterized by sodium restriction; an emphasis on vegetables, fruits, low-fat milk products, whole grains, and lean meats; and elimination or minimization of added sugars and processed meats.

deep frostbite—Freezing of deep tissue, including muscle and bone.

defendant—The individual or entity whom the plaintiff (injured party) is suing in a civil law case, such as in a negligence lawsuit, or the individual or entity who is accused of committing a crime (violating a statute) in a criminal law case.

delayed-onset muscle soreness (DOMS)—Soreness experienced when one engages in an activity that places unaccustomed loads on muscle, resulting in microscopic breakdown of muscle tissue that leads to an inflammatory response over several days.

diabetes mellitus—Group of metabolic diseases characterized by high blood glucose concentrations.

diabetic coma—Loss of consciousness caused by too little insulin and extremely high levels of blood glucose.

diaphysis—The shaft of a long bone.

diarthrodial joint—A freely moving joint characterized by its synovial membrane and capsular ligament; also called a *synovial joint*.

diastolic blood pressure (DBP)—The pressure blood exerts on the vessel walls during the resting portion of the cardiac cycle, measured in millimeters of mercury by a sphygmomanometer.

dietary fiber—Substances found in plants that cannot be broken down by the human digestive system.

dietary reference intake (DRI)—Set of values used to evaluate dietary intake.

digitalis—A drug that augments the contraction of the heart muscle and slows the rate of conduction of cardiac impulses through the AV node.

disc—Located between vertebrae; acts as a shock absorber and frequently is involved in low-back pain.

disordered eating—Unhealthy eating pattern that can in some cases be a precursor to eating disorders.

diuretics—Drugs that increase urine production, thereby ridding the body of excess fluid and electrolytes.

dose—The quantity (intensity, frequency, and duration) of exercise needed to bring about a response (e.g., lower resting blood pressure). Also, for medications (drugs), it refers to the quantity of a drug that is taken.

double product—See *rate–pressure product*.

duration—The length of time for a fitness workout or a bout of physical activity.

dynamic testing—Strength assessment that involves movement of the body (e.g., push-up) or an external load (e.g., bench press).

dyspnea—Difficult or labored breathing beyond what is expected for the intensity of work. The exercise test or activity should be stopped.

dyspnea rating scale—An instrument used to rate the severity of a patient's symptoms of shortness of breath.

eating disorders—Clinical eating patterns that result in severe negative health consequences.

eccentric action—Type of muscle action that occurs when a muscle under tension lengthens. The muscle generates force, but it is inadequate to overcome the force it is working against. Controls speed of movement caused by another force.

ectopic focus—An irritated portion of the myocardium or electrical conducting system; gives rise to extra heartbeats that do not originate from the SA node.

effect—The desired response resulting from exercise training (e.g., lower resting blood pressure).

ejection fraction—The fraction of the end diastolic volume (EDV) ejected per beat (stroke volume divided by EDV).

elasticity—Ability of ligaments and tendons to lengthen passively and return to their resting length.

electrocardiogram (ECG)—Graphic recording of the electrical activity of the heart. The ECG is obtained with the electrocardiograph.

embolism—Sudden obstruction of a blood vessel by a solid body such as a clot carried in the bloodstream.

emergency action plan (EAP)—A written plan used to facilitate and organize employee actions during workplace emergencies.

emergency medical services (EMS)—A system designed to handle medical emergencies; 911 or other community emergency numbers.

empathy—Identification with the thoughts or feelings of another person and the effective communication that the other person's feelings are understood.

end-diastolic volume (EDV)—The volume of blood in the heart just before ventricular contraction; a measure of the stretch of the ventricle.

endothelial cells—Cells that form the interior lining of the blood vessels, heart, and lymphatic vessels.

epimysium—The connective-tissue sheath surrounding a muscle.

epiphyseal plates—The sites of ossification in long bones.

epiphyses—The ends of long bones.

ergogenic aids—Substances taken in hopes of improving athletic performance.

essential amino acids—The nine amino acids that the body cannot synthesize and therefore must be ingested.

essential fat—The minimum amount of body fat needed for good health.

evaporation—Conversion of water from liquid to gas by means of heat, as in evaporation of sweat; results in the loss of 580 kcal for each liter of sweat evaporated.

excessive bleeding—External bleeding that results in massive loss of circulating blood volumes; often results in shock and can lead to death.

excess postexercise oxygen consumption (EPOC)—The amount of oxygen used during recovery from work that exceeds the amount needed for rest. Previously referred to as *oxygen debt* and *oxygen repayment*.

exculpatory clause—A clause within a waiver (prospective release) that can absolve (protect) defendants from their ordinary negligence.

exercise—A subset of physical activity that is planned, structured, and repetitive and is meant to improve or maintain physical fitness.

exercise-associated muscle cramps (EAMC)—Painful, involuntary muscle contractions.

exercise-induced bronchoconstriction—A reactive airway disease in which exercise tends to cause the bronchioles to constrict.

exercise tests—A series of tests that evaluate prospective exercise participants' current level of fitness and commonly include cardiorespiratory fitness, muscular strength and endurance, body composition, and flexibility.

exertional heat stroke (EHS)—Most severe form of heat-related injury, with body temperature above 41.1 °C (106 °F); treat as medical emergency.

extension—Movement of a joint around its mediolateral axis that generally increases the angle between the body segments, such as straightening the elbow.

external rotation—Movement of a joint around its longitudinal axis away from the midline of the body in the anatomical position, such as rotating the hip and leg so the toes point out to the side.

facet joint—Junction of the superior and inferior articular processes of the vertebrae.

fascicles—Bundles of muscle fibers surrounded by perimysium.

fast glycolytic fiber—See *type IIx fiber*.

fast oxidative-glycolytic fiber—See *type IIa fiber*.

fat—Non-water-soluble substance composed of hydrogen, oxygen, and carbon that serves a variety of functions in the body, including energy production.

fat-free mass (FFM)—Weight of the nonfat tissues of the body.

fat mass (FM)—The mass of the fat tissues in the body.

Female and Male Athlete Triad—Interrelated conditions including energy deficiency/low energy availability, impaired bone health, and suppression of the hypothalamic-pituitary-gonadal axis; these conditions exist on a continuum from health to unhealthy.

first-degree AV block—The delayed transmission of impulses from atria to ventricles (in excess of 0.20 seconds).

flexibility—The ability to move a joint through its full range of motion (ROM) without discomfort or pain.

flexion—Movement of a joint around its mediolateral axis that generally decreases the angle between the body segments, such as bending the elbow.

force arm (FA)—Perpendicular distance from the axis of rotation to the direction of the application of the force causing movement.

forced expiratory volume (FEV$_1$)—The maximal amount of air that can be forcibly exhaled in 1 second, as measured by spirometry; this variable is used to diagnose COPD.

free radicals—Molecules or fragments of molecules formed during metabolic processes that are highly reactive and can damage cellular components.

frequency—Refers to the number of days per week that physical activity is done.

functional capacity—Maximal oxygen uptake, expressed in milliliters of oxygen per kilogram of body weight per minute, or in METs.

functional curve—Spinal curve (e.g., lordotic curve) that can be removed by assuming different postures.

functional overreaching—Training and nontraining stress that results in a short-term decrement in performance that can be restored in days to weeks and results in improved performance.

glucose—A simple sugar that is a vital energy source in the human body.

glycemic index—A rating system used to indicate how rapidly a food causes blood glucose to rise.

glycemic load—A value that reflects the quality and quantity of carbohydrate in a given food.

glycogen—The storage form of carbohydrate in the human body.

glycolysis—The metabolic pathway producing ATP from the anaerobic breakdown of glucose. This short-term source of ATP is important in all-out activities lasting less than 2 minutes.

goal setting—Goals are desired tasks to accomplish in a specific amount of time; they provide direction and foster persistence in the search for task strategies. Effective goal setting includes establishing objectives that can be measured, concretely defined, and practically achieved.

graded exercise test (GXT)—A multistage test that determines a person's physiological responses to various intensities of exercise.

gynoid-type obesity—Obesity in which a disproportionate amount of fat is stored in the hips and thighs.

health—Being alive with no major health problems. Also called *apparently healthy*.

health-related fitness—Refers to muscular strength and endurance, cardiorespiratory fitness, flexibility, and body composition.

Healthy Mediterranean-Style Eating Pattern—Patterns vary somewhat based on region but generally emphasize grains (particularly whole grains), fruits, vegetables, olive oil, and nuts. More monounsaturated fatty acids than saturated fatty acids are consumed in this pattern.

Healthy U.S.-Style Eating Pattern—A dietary approach based on the previously used USDA Food Patterns and the DASH diet. This approach suggests daily amounts that people should consume from five major food groups (vegetables, fruits, grains, dairy products, and protein) and limited sodium intake.

Healthy Vegetarian-Style Eating Pattern—A balanced dietary approach to consuming a healthy diet without meat.

heart rate (HR)—The number of heart beats per minute.

heat exhaustion—Inability to continue activity due to heavy sweating, dehydration, sodium loss, and energy depletion.

heat syncope—Fainting or excessive loss of strength due to heat exposure.

hemoglobin A1C—Also called *glycosylated hemoglobin* or *glycated hemoglobin*, hemoglobin A1C is a form of hemoglobin that is typically found in low concentrations but exists in higher concentrations when blood glucose is constantly higher than normal.

high-density lipoprotein cholesterol (HDL-C)—This form of cholesterol protects against the development of coronary heart disease (CHD) by transporting cholesterol to the liver, where it is eliminated. Thus, low levels of HDL-C are related to a high risk of CHD.

high-intensity interval training (HIIT)—A type of training that uses short bursts of maximal (or supramaximal) activity followed by recovery intervals; also known as *anaerobic interval training*.

high-risk situation—An event, thought, or interaction that challenges a person's perceived ability to maintain a desired behavioral change.

hydrostatic weighing—Method of assessing body composition based on Archimedes' principle; also called *underwater weighing*. Hydrostatic weighing is often used as the criterion method for assessing percent body fat.

hyperglycemia—Blood glucose concentrations above normal.

hypertension—High blood pressure typically defined as systolic blood pressure of 130 mmHg or higher or diastolic blood pressure of 80 mmHg or higher.

hyperthermia—An elevation of the core temperature; if unchecked, it can lead to heat exhaustion or heatstroke and death.

hypertrophy—An enlargement in muscle fiber size.

hyperventilation—A level of ventilation beyond that needed to maintain the arterial carbon dioxide level; can be initiated by a sudden increase in the hydrogen ion concentration attributable to lactic acid production during a progressive exercise test.

hypoglycemia—Low blood glucose level.

hypohydration—Body water deficit greater than normal daily fluctuation.

hypotension—Low blood pressure.

hypothermia—Below-normal body temperature.

hypoxemia—Abnormally low oxygen content in the arterial blood but not total anoxia.

impaired fasting glucose—A fasting blood glucose level between 100 and 125 mg · dl^{-1}; commonly considered a precursor to the development of diabetes.

impaired glucose tolerance (IGT)—A condition in which the body does not normally process glucose; often an intermediate step before the development of type 2 diabetes.

incision—Cutting of skin resulting in an open wound with cleanly cut edges and exposure of underlying tissues.

indirect calorimetry—Estimating energy production on the basis of oxygen consumption.

informed consent—A procedure used to obtain a person's voluntary permission to participate in a program. Informed consent requires a description of the procedures to be used as well as the potential benefits and risks and written consent of the participant.

insulin resistance—A condition in which the body's insulin receptors no longer respond normally to insulin.

insulin shock—A medical condition that results from a high level of insulin and low blood glucose levels.

intensity—Describes the rate of work (e.g., how much energy is being expended per minute) or the degree of effort required to carry out the task (percent of maximal heart rate).

intercalated discs—Junctions between adjacent cardiac muscle cells that allow electrical impulses to pass from cell to cell.

internal bleeding—Bleeding within deep structures of the body (chest, abdominal, or pelvic cavity) and bleeding of organs contained within these cavities; may result in shock and can lead to death.

internal rotation—Movement of a joint around its longitudinal axis toward the midline of the body in the anatomical position, such as rotating the hip and leg so the toes point inward.

interval training—A type of training that alternates periods of exercise with periods of recovery.

intracoronary stent—A device placed within the lumen of the artery to keep the artery open.

iron-deficiency anemia—A condition characterized by a decreased amount of hemoglobin in red blood cells and a resultant decrease in the ability of the blood to transport oxygen.

isokinetic testing—The assessment of maximal muscle tension throughout a range of joint motion at a constant angular velocity (e.g., 60° · sec^{-1}).

isometric action—A muscle action in which the muscle length is unchanged; the muscle exerts a force that counteracts an opposing force. Isometric action is also called *static action*.

isometric training—Refers to resistance training programs designed to use immovable objects such as a wall or a weight machine loaded with a heavy weight. These programs, also called *static resistance training*, focus on the use of isometric muscle actions.

joint cavity—The space between bones enclosed by the synovial membrane and articular cartilage.

J point—On an ECG, the point at which the S wave ends and the ST segment begins.

kyphotic curve—Describes the condition of kyphosis, a convex curvature of the spine (e.g., the thoracic curve).

laceration—Tearing of skin resulting in an open wound with jagged edges and exposure of underlying tissues.

lactate threshold (LT)—The point during a GXT at which the blood lactate concentration suddenly increases; a good indicator of the highest sustainable work rate. Also called the *anaerobic threshold*.

lean body mass—Term often used synonymously with *fat-free mass*.

legal liability exposures—Situations that create a risk of injury or reflect noncompliance with federal and state laws.

ligament—The connective tissue that attaches bone to bone.

lipoproteins—Large molecules responsible for transporting fat in the blood.

local muscular endurance—The ability of a muscle or muscle group to perform repeated contractions against a submaximal resistance.

lordotic curve—Describes the condition of lordosis; a forward, concave curve of the lumbar spine when the spine is viewed from the side.

low-back pain (LBP)—Strong discomfort in the low back, often caused by lack of muscular endurance and flexibility in the midtrunk region or improper posture or lifting.

low-density lipoprotein cholesterol (LDL-C)—The form of cholesterol that is responsible for the buildup of plaque in the inner walls of the arteries (atherosclerosis). Thus, high levels of LDL-C are related to a high risk of coronary heart disease.

lumen—The open space inside a structure such as an artery or intestine.

macrocycle—A phase of training that lasts about 1 year.

malnutrition—A diet in which underconsumption, overconsumption, or unbalanced consumption of nutrients leads to disease or increased susceptibility to disease.

maximal aerobic power or **maximal oxygen uptake ($\dot{V}O_2$max)**—The maximal rate at which oxygen can be used by the body during maximal work; related directly to the maximal capacity of the heart to deliver blood to the muscles. Expressed in $L \cdot min^{-1}$ or $ml \cdot kg^{-1} \cdot min^{-1}$.

maximum voluntary contraction (MVC)—Maximum amount of force that can be elicited during a single repetition.

medical release—A document that is signed by a person that grants permission to release that person's private medical information to a third party. For example, a medical release form can be signed by a client so the personal fitness trainer can obtain medical information such as stress test results, cholesterol, and so on from the client's physician.

menisci—Partial, semilunar-shaped discs between the femur and the tibia at the knee.

mesocycle—A phase of training that lasts for several months.

microcycle—A phase of training that lasts about 1 week.

minerals—Inorganic atoms or ions that serve a variety of functions in the human body.

mitochondria—Cellular organelles responsible for generating energy (ATP) through aerobic metabolism.

mitral valve—Heart valve located between the left atrium and left ventricle.

Mobitz type I AV block—On an ECG, the PR interval progressively increases until the P wave is not followed by a QRS complex; this pattern repeats. The site of the block is within the AV node.

Mobitz type II AV block— On an ECG, multiple P waves per QRS present in a routine ratio (e.g., 2:1, 3:1, 4:1). Common sites of the block are within the bundle of His and/or bundle branches.

moderate intensity—Refers to an absolute intensity of 3 to 5.9 METs and a relative intensity of 40% to 59% $\dot{V}O_2$max.

monounsaturated fatty acids—Fat that has a single double bond between carbon atoms in the fatty acid chain. Examples are olive and canola oils.

motion segment—Fundamental unit of the lumbar spine; made up of two vertebrae and their intervening disc.

motor unit—The functional unit of muscular action that includes a motor nerve and the muscle fibers that its branches innervate.

muscle fiber—Muscle cell. Contains myofibrils that are composed of sarcomeres; uses chemical energy of ATP

to generate tension, which, when greater than the resistance, results in movement.

muscle group—A group of specific muscles that are responsible for the same action at the same joint.

muscular endurance—The ability of the muscle to perform repetitive contractions or sustain a contraction over a prolonged period of time.

muscular fitness—Describes the integrated status of muscular strength, muscular endurance, and power.

muscular strength—The ability of muscle to generate the maximum amount of force.

myocardial infarction (MI)—Death of a section of heart tissue in which the blood supply has been cut off; commonly called a *heart attack*.

myocardial ischemia—A lack of blood flow to the heart tissue.

myocardium—The middle layer of the heart wall; involuntary, striated muscle innervated by autonomic nerves.

myofibril—Component inside muscle fibers that is composed of a long string of sarcomeres.

myosin—The thick contractile filament in sarcomeres that can bind actin and split ATP to generate crossbridge movement and develop tension.

negative health—Negative health is associated with morbidity (incidence of disease) and premature mortality.

negligence—The failure to do something that a reasonable, prudent professional would do or doing something that a reasonable, prudent professional would not have done under the same or similar circumstances.

nicotine gum—Gum containing nicotine that is used for smoking cessation. Nicotine is absorbed through the oral mucosa, providing sufficient plasma nicotine concentrations to curb the craving to smoke.

nitrates—A class of medications used to treat angina pectoris, or chest pain.

nonfunctional overreaching—Training and nontraining stress that results in impaired performance for weeks or months.

nutrient—A substance that the body requires for the maintenance, growth, and repair of tissues.

nutrient density—The amount of essential nutrients in a food compared with the calories it contains.

obesity—Condition in which a person has an excessive accumulation of fat tissue; also may be classified by the relationship between weight and height.

oligomenorrhea—Irregular menses.

oral antiglycemic agents—Medications used to treat diabetes mellitus.

ossification—The replacement of cartilage by bone.

osteoarthritis (OA)—Most common form of arthritis (90%-95% of all cases); affects joints whose articular cartilage is damaged or injured.

osteoporosis—A disease characterized by a decrease in the total amount of bone mineral and a decrease in the strength of the remaining bone.

overload—Placing greater than usual demands on some part of the body (e.g., picking up more weight than usual overloads the muscle involved). Chronic overloading leads to increased function.

overtraining syndrome—Maladaptation due to excessive training along with other factors that results in a decrease in performance despite increased effort and perception of effort.

overweight—Condition in which a person is above the recommended weight-to-height range but is below obesity levels.

oxygen consumption ($\dot{V}O_2$)—The rate at which oxygen is used during a specific intensity of an activity; oxygen uptake.

oxygen deficit—The difference between the steady-state oxygen requirement of a physical activity and the measured oxygen uptake during the first minutes of work.

ozone—An active form of oxygen formed in reaction to UV light and as an emission from internal combustion engines; exposure can decrease lung function.

percent body fat (%BF)—Percentage of the total weight composed of fat tissue; calculated by dividing fat mass by total weight and multiplying by 100.

percentage of heart rate reserve (%HRR)—The heart rate reserve is calculated by subtracting resting heart rate from maximal heart rate. The %HRR is a percentage of the difference between resting and maximal heart rate and is calculated by subtracting resting heart rate from maximal heart rate, multiplying by the desired percentage expressed as a decimal, and then adding resting heart rate.

percentage of maximal HR (%HRmax)—Heart rate expressed as a simple percentage of the maximal heart rate.

percentage of maximal oxygen uptake (%$\dot{V}O_2$max)—Ratio of submaximal oxygen uptake to maximal oxygen uptake, multiplied by 100 to express as a percentage. Also called *percentage of maximal oxygen consumption*.

percentage of oxygen uptake reserve (%$\dot{V}O_2$R)—$\dot{V}O_2$R is calculated by subtracting 1 MET ($3.5 \text{ ml} \cdot \text{kg}^{-1} \cdot \text{min}^{-1}$) from the subject's $\dot{V}O_2$max. When calculating a particular %$\dot{V}O_2$R, first calculate $\dot{V}O_2$R by subtracting $3.5 \text{ ml} \cdot \text{kg}^{-1} \cdot \text{min}^{-1}$ (1 MET) from the $\dot{V}O_2$max, then multiply that value by the desired intensity (percentage expressed as a decimal), and then add $3.5 \text{ ml} \cdot \text{kg}^{-1} \cdot \text{min}^{-1}$ (1 MET).

percutaneous transluminal coronary angioplasty (PTCA)—A surgical procedure in which a flexible guide wire is inserted into a partially blocked coronary artery, and then a catheter with an inflatable balloon near the tip is passed over the guide wire. The balloon is inflated and then deflated and removed in order to open the coronary artery.

performance—The ability to perform a task or sport at a desired level.

perimysium—The connective tissue surrounding fasciculi within a muscle.

periodization—A process of varying the training stimulus to promote long-term fitness gains and to avoid overtraining.

periosteum—The connective tissue surrounding all bone surfaces except the articulating surfaces.

peripheral vascular disease—A disease characterized by blockages in the peripheral arteries.

phosphocreatine (PC)—A high-energy phosphate compound that represents the primary immediate anaerobic source of ATP at the onset of exercise. PC is important in all-out activities lasting a few seconds.

phospholipids—Fatty compounds that are essential constituents of cell membranes.

physical activity—Any bodily movement produced by skeletal muscle that results in energy expenditure; associated with occupation, leisure time, household chores, sport, and so on.

physical fitness—A set of health- or skill-related attributes that people have or achieve relating to their ability to perform physical activity.

plaintiff—The injured party who is seeking damages to recover from a personal injury (or property loss) caused by the conduct of the defendant in a civil law case, such as negligence.

polyunsaturated fatty acid—Fat that has two or more double bonds between carbon atoms in the fatty acid chain. Examples are fish, corn, soybean, and peanut oils.

positive caloric balance—When more calories are consumed than are expended, resulting in weight gain.

positive health—Optimal quality of life, including social, mental, spiritual, and physical fitness components; capacity to enjoy life and withstand challenges, not just the avoidance of disease.

power—Ability to exert muscular strength quickly.

powerlifting—A competitive sport in which athletes attempt to lift maximal amounts of weight in the squat, deadlift, and bench press.

PR interval—The time interval between the beginning of the P wave and the QRS complex. The upper normal limit is 0.2 seconds. This segment is normally used as the isoelectric baseline.

PR segment—Forms the isoelectric line, or baseline, from which ST segment deviations are measured.

prediabetes—A condition in which a person has impaired fasting glucose or impaired glucose tolerance. Without treatment, prediabetes typically evolves into type 2 diabetes.

premature atrial contraction (PAC)—On an ECG, the rhythm is irregular and the R-R interval is short; the origin of the beat is somewhere other than the SA node.

premature junctional contraction (PJC)—On an ECG, the ectopic pacemaker in the AV junctional area causes a QRS complex; frequently seen with inverted P waves.

premature ventricular contraction (PVC)—Wide, bizarrely shaped QRS complex originating from an ectopic focus in the ventricles. The QRS interval lasts longer than 0.12 seconds, and the T wave is usually in the opposite direction.

prevalence—The percentage of a population that has a particular characteristic. For example, obesity prevalence is calculated by dividing the number of people classified as obese by the total number of people.

PRICE principle—The suggested treatment for minor sprains and strains: protection, rest, ice, compression, and elevation.

primary amenorrhea—The absence of menarche (i.e., first menses) in girls age 15 or older.

primary assumption of risk—A legal theory in which a plaintiff is generally not allowed to seek damages for an injury that was due to risks inherent in the activity as long as the plaintiff knew, understood, and appreciated those risks and voluntarily assumed them.

principle of reversibility—A corollary to the principle of overload; loss of a training effect with disuse.

product defects—Various types of defects in exercise equipment (e.g., design, manufacturing, marketing) that can lead to injury.

product liability—A type of liability imposed on a manufacturer for a defect (design, manufacturing, or marketing) in a product that is considered unreasonably dangerous to the user.

protein—Nutrients composed of amino acids that serve a variety of functions in the human body.

pulmonary function testing—Procedures used to test the capacity of the respiratory system to move air into or out of the lungs.

pulmonary valve—A set of three crescent-shaped flaps at the opening of the pulmonary artery; also called the *pulmonary semilunar valve*.

pulmonary ventilation—The number of liters of air inhaled or exhaled per minute.

pulse oximeter—Device used to measure the percent saturation of hemoglobin in the arterial blood.

puncture—Direct penetration of tissues by a pointed object.

Purkinje fibers—The fibers found beneath the endocardium of the heart; the impulse-conducting network of the heart.

P wave—On an ECG, a small positive deflection preceding a QRS complex, indicating atrial depolarization. The P wave is normally less than 0.12 seconds in duration, with an amplitude of 0.25 mV or less.

QRS complex—The largest complex on an ECG, indicating a depolarization of the left ventricle and normally lasting less than 0.1 seconds.

QT interval—The time interval from the beginning of the QRS complex to the end of the T wave. The QT interval reflects the electrical systole of the cardiac cycle.

Q wave—The initial negative deflection of the QRS complex on an ECG.

radiation—The process of heat exchange from the surface of one object to another that depends on a temperature gradient but does not require direct contact between objects; for example, heat loss from the sun to the earth.

rate–pressure product—The product of heart rate and systolic blood pressure; indicative of the oxygen requirement of the heart during exercise. Training lowers the rate–pressure product at rest and during submaximal work. Also called the *double product*.

rating of perceived exertion (RPE)—Borg's scale used to quantify the subjective feeling of physical effort. The original scale was from 6 to 20; a revised ratio scale is from 0 to 10.

recommended dietary allowance (RDA)—The amount of a nutrient found to be adequate for approximately 97% of the population.

recruitment—Stimulation of additional motor units to increase the strength of a muscle action.

reinforcement—Positive reinforcement involves adding something positive to increase the frequency of the target behavior. Negative reinforcement also increases the frequency of the desired behavior, but it is the removal of something negative, such as losing weight because of a regular walking program. Reinforcement can be administered by oneself (self-reinforcement) or by other people (social reinforcement).

relapse prevention—Way to identify and successfully deal with high-risk situations by educating the client about the relapse process and using a variety of strategies to foster an effective coping response.

Relative Energy Deficiency in Sport (RED-S)—Syndrome in which energy deficiency causes impaired function related to metabolic rate, menstrual function, bone health, immune function, protein synthesis, and cardiovascular health.

relative humidity—A measure of the relative wetness of the air; the ratio of the amount of water vapor in the air to the maximum the air can hold at that temperature times 100 to express as a percentage. High relative humidity in a warm environment helps determine the potential for losing heat by evaporation.

relative intensity—Describes the degree of effort required to expend energy and is influenced by the person's maximal aerobic capacity or cardiorespiratory fitness ($\dot{V}O_2max$). Relative intensity can be expressed as a percentage of $\dot{V}O_2max$ or a percentage of maximal heart rate (HRmax).

repetition—One complete movement of an exercise, which typically consists of a concentric (lifting) and eccentric (lowering) phase.

repetition maximum (RM)—The maximum amount of weight that can be lifted for a predetermined number of repetitions with proper exercise technique. For example, 5RM is the most weight that can be lifted five but not six times.

resistance arm (RA)—Perpendicular distance from the axis of rotation to the direction of the application of the force resisting movement.

resistance force (R)—The opposing force that is resisting another force.

resistance training—A method of exercise designed to enhance musculoskeletal strength, power, and local muscular endurance. Resistance training encompasses a wide range of training modalities, including weight machines, free weights, medicine balls, elastic cords, and body weight.

respiratory quotient (RQ) or respiratory exchange ratio (R)—The ratio of the volume of carbon dioxide produced to the volume of oxygen used during a given time ($\dot{V}CO_2 \div \dot{V}O_2$).

respondeat superior—A legal doctrine that imposes vicarious liability (a form of strict liability) upon an employer for the negligent acts of its employees while performing their job responsibilities.

resting membrane potential—The difference in electrical potential across the selectively permeable membrane when the cell is not stimulated, resulting in a higher concentration of Na^+ ions outside, and K^+ ions inside, the cell.

resting metabolic rate (RMR)—Number of calories needed to sustain the body under normal resting conditions.

restrictive lung diseases—Diseases that restrict a person's ability to expand the lungs.

rhabdomyolysis—A syndrome characterized by skeletal muscle degeneration and muscle enzyme leakage that can occur in normal, healthy people following strenuous exercise.

rheumatoid arthritis (RA)—Debilitating arthritis of unknown cause that can affect a few joints (pauciarticular) or many joints (polyarticular).

risk factor—A characteristic, sign, symptom, or test score that is associated with increased probability of developing a health problem. For example, people with hypertension have increased risk of developing coronary heart disease.

risk management—A proactive administrative process that involves four steps: (a) assessment of legal liability exposures, (b) development of risk management strategies, (c) implementation of the risk management plan, and (d) evaluation of the risk management plan. The major goal of risk management is to minimize injuries and subsequent litigation.

risks inherent in the activity—Injury risks that exist during participation in sport or physical activity that are no one's fault; they just happen and are inseparable from the activity.

rotational inertia—Reluctance to rotate; proportional to the mass and distribution of the mass around the axis.

R-R interval—The time interval from the peak of the QRS of one cardiac cycle to the peak of the QRS of the next cycle.

R wave—The positive deflection of the QRS complex in the ECG.

sarcomeres—The basic units of muscle contraction. They contain actin and myosin; tension develops as the myosin crossbridges pull the actin toward the center of the sarcomere.

sarcopenia—Loss of muscle mass often associated with aging.

sarcoplasmic reticulum (SR)—The network of membranes that surround the myofibril; stores calcium needed for muscle contraction.

saturation pressure—Water vapor pressure that exists at a particular temperature when the air is saturated with water.

sciatic nerve—Nerve originating in the sacral area; it is involved in low-back problems that can result in loss of feeling and control in the legs.

scoliosis—An abnormal lateral curvature of the spine.

scope of practice—Activities performed by fitness professionals while carrying out their responsibilities that are within the limitations (or boundaries) of their education, training, certifications, and experiences.

secondary amenorrhea—A lack of menses for 3 or more consecutive months occurring in females after menarche.

secondary prevention—Steps taken to prevent the recurrence of a heart attack.

second-degree AV block—On an ECG, some but not all P waves precede the QRS complex and result in ventricular depolarization.

self-determination theory (SDT)—A theory of human motivation that assumes humans are naturally inclined toward growth and development and have a set of basic psychological needs that are universal.

set—A group of repetitions performed without stopping.

sickle cell trait (SCT)—A genetic condition that involves the inheritance of one gene for sickle hemoglobin and one for normal hemoglobin.

simple sugars—Monosaccharides and disaccharides, such as glucose, fructose, and sucrose. These forms of carbohydrate provide the majority of calories in candy, soft drinks, and fruit drinks.

sinoatrial (SA) node—A mass of tissue in the right atrium of the heart, near the vena cava, that initiates the heartbeat.

sinus arrhythmia—A normal variant in sinus rhythm in which the R-R interval varies by more than 10% per beat.

sinus bradycardia—Normal heart rhythm and sequence, with a slow heart rate (below 60 bpm at rest). Sinus bradycardia may indicate a high level of fitness or a mental illness such as depression.

sinus rhythm—The normal timing and sequence of the cardiac events, with the sinus node as a pacemaker; resting rate is between 60 and 100 bpm.

sinus tachycardia—The normal heart rhythm and sequence, with a fast heart rate (above 100 bpm at rest). Sinus tachycardia may indicate illness or stress.

skill-related (performance-related) fitness—Refers to agility, balance, coordination, speed, power, and reaction time that are linked to games, sport, dance, and so on.

sliding-filament theory—The theory that muscular tension is generated when the actin in the sarcomere slides over the myosin because of the action of the myosin crossbridges.

slow oxidative fiber—See *type I fiber*.

specificity—The principle that states that training effects derived from an exercise program are specific to the exercise done (endurance versus strength training) and the types of muscle fibers involved.

speed—The ability to move the whole body quickly.

sphygmomanometer—A blood pressure measurement instrument.

stability—The ease with which balance is maintained.

standard deviation (SD)—A measure of the deviation from the mean (average) value generalized to the population. One SD above and below the mean includes about 68% of the population, 2 SD includes about 95%, and 3 SD includes about 99% of the population. For example, if the mean $\dot{V}O_2$max = 25 ml · kg^{-1} · min^{-1} and SD = 3 ml · kg^{-1} · min^{-1}, it would be expected that 68% of the population would have $\dot{V}O_2$max values between 22 (25 – 3) and 28 (25 + 3) ml · kg^{-1} · min^{-1}, 95% of the population to be between 19 and 31 ml · kg^{-1} · min^{-1}, and almost all of the population to be between 16 and 34 ml · kg^{-1} · min^{-1}. The standard error of estimate (SEE) is used to indicate the SD of any estimate derived for a prediction formula.

Staphylococcus aureus—Common type of bacteria that lives on the human body and may cause an infection if it enters the skin through a cut or sore.

statutory law—A primary source of law (from the legislative branch of government) that is enacted through the legislative process at both the federal and state levels.

steady-state oxygen requirement—When the oxygen uptake levels off during submaximal work so that the oxygen uptake value represents the steady-state oxygen (ATP) requirement for the activity.

strength—The maximal force a muscle or muscle group can generate at a specified velocity.

strength training—See *resistance training*.

strict liability—A type of tort liability based on public policy (i.e., judicial determination of what is in the best interest of society) rather than fault such as intentional or negligent wrongdoing.

stroke—A vascular accident (embolism, hemorrhage, or thrombosis) in the brain, often resulting in sudden loss of body function.

stroke volume (SV)—The volume of blood pumped by the heart per minute.

structural curve—Curve that cannot be removed in normal movement because of chronically shortened musculotendinous units or ligaments.

ST segment—The part of the ECG between the end of the QRS complex and the beginning of the T wave. Depression below (or elevation above) the isoelectric line indicates ischemia.

ST segment depression—When the ST segment of the ECG is depressed below the baseline; may signify myocardial ischemia.

ST segment elevation—When the ST segment of the ECG is elevated above the baseline; may signify the early (acute) stages of a myocardial infarction.

submaximal—Less than maximal (e.g., an exercise that can be performed with less than maximal effort).

sulfur dioxide (SO_2)—A pollutant that can cause bronchoconstriction in people with asthma.

superficial frostbite—Freezing of skin layers and subcutaneous tissue.

S wave—Negative wave (preceded by Q or R waves) of the QRS complex in the ECG.

sweating—The process of moisture coming through the pores of the skin from the sweat glands, usually as a result of heat, exertion, or emotion.

synarthrodial joint—Immovable joint.

synovial membrane—The inner lining of the joint capsule; secretes synovial fluid into the joint cavity.

systolic blood pressure (SBP)—The pressure exerted on the vessel walls during ventricular contraction, measured in millimeters of mercury by a sphygmomanometer.

tachycardia—Heart rate greater than 100 bpm at rest. Tachycardia may be seen in deconditioned people or people who are apprehensive about a situation (e.g., an exercise test).

talocrural joint—Ankle joint.

target heart rate (THR)—The heart rate recommended for fitness workouts.

tendon—A band of tough, inelastic, fibrous connective tissue that attaches muscle to bone.

tetanic contraction—In contrast to a muscle twitch, this is a smooth, sustained muscle contraction associated with a high frequency of stimulation.

thermic effect of food—The energy needed to digest, absorb, transport, and store the food that is eaten.

third-degree AV block—On an ECG, the QRS appears independently, the PR interval varies with no regular pattern, and heart rate is typically less than 45 bpm.

threshold—The minimum level needed for a desired effect; often used to refer to the minimum level of exercise intensity needed for improving cardiorespiratory fitness.

tolerable upper intake level (UL)—The highest intake of a nutrient believed to pose no health risk.

torque (*T*)—The effect produced by a force causing rotation; the product of the force and length of the force arm.

total cholesterol—The sum of all forms of cholesterol in the bloodstream. Because LDL-C is usually the primary factor in the total amount, a high level of total cholesterol is also a risk factor for coronary heart disease.

total work—The amount of work accomplished during a workout.

training threshold—The minimum intensity required to provide an overload to allow for adaptation.

trans fat (trans-fatty acid)—Hydrogenated fat created to be solid at room temperature and to be used in cooking. Consuming this type of fat lowers HDL-C and raises LDL-C.

transfer of angular momentum—Angular momentum can be transferred from one body segment to another by stabilizing the initial moving part at a joint.

transtheoretical model—A general model of intentional behavior change in which behavior change is seen as a dynamic process that occurs through a series of interrelated stages. Basic concepts emphasize the person's motivational readiness to change, the cognitive and behavioral strategies for changing behavior, self-efficacy, and the evaluation of the pros and cons of the new behavior.

transverse tubule—Connects the sarcolemma (muscle membrane) to the sarcoplasmic reticulum; action potentials move down the transverse tubule to cause the sarcoplasmic reticulum to release calcium to initiate muscle contraction. Also referred to as *T-tubule*.

traumatic brain injury (TBI)—Brain dysfunction resulting from an external mechanical force.

treadmill—A machine with a moving belt that can be adjusted for speed and grade, allowing a person to walk or run in place. Treadmills are used extensively for exercise testing and training.

tricuspid valve—A valve located between the right atrium and right ventricle of the heart.

triglycerides—The primary storage form of fat in the human body.

tropomyosin—A protein (part of the thin filament) that regulates muscle contraction; works with troponin.

troponin—A protein (part of the thin filament) that can bind the calcium released from the sarcoplasmic reticulum; works with tropomyosin to allow the myosin crossbridge to interact with actin and initiate crossbridge movement.

T wave—On an ECG, the wave that follows the QRS complex and represents ventricular repolarization.

two-compartment model—Model that divides the body into fat and fat-free components.

type 1 diabetes—Type of diabetes mellitus in which insulin is not produced. It is caused by damage to the beta cells of the pancreas.

type 2 diabetes—Type of diabetes mellitus in which the insulin receptors lose their sensitivity to insulin.

type I (slow oxidative) fiber—A muscle fiber that contracts slowly and generates a small amount of tension, with most of the energy coming from aerobic processes; active in light to moderate activities and possesses great endurance.

type IIa (fast oxidative-glycolytic) fiber—A muscle fiber that contracts quickly, can produce energy aerobically, and generates great tension; adds to the tension of type I fibers as exercise intensity increases.

type IIx (fast glycolytic) fiber—A muscle fiber that contracts quickly and generates great tension; produces energy by anaerobic metabolism and fatigues quickly.

universal precautions—Safety measures taken to prevent exposure to blood or other body fluids.

ventilatory threshold (VT)—The intensity of work at which the rate of ventilation increases sharply during a GXT.

ventricular fibrillation—The heart contracts in an unorganized, quivering manner, with no discernible P waves or QRS complexes on the ECG; requires immediate emergency attention.

ventricular tachycardia—An extremely dangerous condition in which three or more consecutive PVCs occur. Ventricular tachycardia may degenerate into ventricular fibrillation.

vigorous intensity—Refers to an absolute intensity of 6 or more METs and a relative intensity of 60% to 84% $\dot{V}O_2$max.

vital capacity (VC)—The greatest amount of air that can be exhaled after a maximal inspiration.

vitamins—Organic substances essential to the normal functioning of the human body. They may be subdivided into fat soluble and water soluble.

volume—Refers to the total amount of energy expended or work accomplished in an aerobic activity; equals the product of the absolute intensity, frequency, and time. In resistance training it is the product of the sets, repetitions, and weight lifted.

waist-to-hip ratio (WHR)—Waist circumference divided by hip circumference; often used as an indicator of android-type obesity.

waiver—A protective legal document, also referred to as a *release of liability*, that contains an exculpatory clause and is signed by a participant before participation in sport or physical activity.

water vapor pressure gradient—The difference between the water vapor pressure in the air and the water vapor pressure of sweat on the body; the greater the gradient (or difference between the two), the easier it is to evaporate sweat and cool the body.

weightlifting—A competitive sport in which athletes attempt to lift maximal amounts of weight in the snatch and the clean and jerk.

windchill index—Indicates the temperature equivalent (under calm air conditions) for any combination of temperature and wind speed.

Z line—Connective-tissue elements that mark the beginning and end of the sarcomere.

REFERENCES

Chapter 1

1. American College of Sports Medicine (ACSM). 1975. *Guidelines for graded exercise testing and exercise prescription.* Philadelphia: Lea & Febiger.

2. American College of Sports Medicine (ACSM). 1978. The recommended quality and quantity of exercise for developing and maintaining fitness in healthy adults. *Medicine & Science in Sports & Exercise* 10:vii-x.

3. American College of Sports Medicine (ACSM). 1990. Position stand: The recommended quantity and quality of exercise for developing and maintaining cardiorespiratory and muscular fitness in healthy adults. *Medicine & Science in Sports & Exercise* 22:265-274.

4. American College of Sports Medicine (ACSM). 2022. *ACSM's guidelines for exercise testing and prescription.* 11th ed. Philadelphia: Wolters Kluwer.

5. American Heart Association (AHA). 1972. *Exercise testing and training of apparently healthy individuals: A handbook for physicians.* New York: Author.

6. American Heart Association (AHA). 2014. Women and cardiovascular diseases—statistical fact sheet. www.heart.org/idc/groups/heart-public/@wcm/@sop/@smd/documents/downloadable/ucm_319576.pdf.

7. Arena R., M. Sagner, and C.J. Lavie. 2017. Healthy living: The universal and timeless medicine for healthspan. *Progress in Cardiovascular Diseases* 59:419-421.

8. Artero, E.G., D. Lee, C.J. Lavie, V. España-Romero, X. Sui, T.S. Church, and S.N. Blair. 2012. Effects of muscular strength on cardiovascular risk factors and prognosis. *Journal of Cardiopulmonary Rehabilitation and Prevention* 32:351-358.

9. Bouchard, C., R.J. Shephard, and T. Stephens. 1994. *Physical activity, fitness, and health.* Champaign, IL: Human Kinetics.

10. Bouchard, C., R.J. Shephard, T. Stephens, J.R. Sutton, and B.D. McPherson. 1990. *Exercise, fitness, and health.* Champaign, IL: Human Kinetics.

11. Caspersen, C.J., K.E. Powell, and G.M. Christenson. 1985. Physical activity, exercise, and physical fitness: Definitions and distinctions for health-related research. *Public Health Reports* 100:126-131.

12. Church, T.S., M.J. LaMonte, C.E. Barlow, and S.N. Blair. 2005. Cardiorespiratory fitness and body mass index as predictors of cardiovascular disease mortality among men with diabetes. *Archives of Internal Medicine* 165:2114-2120.

13. Erlichman, J., A.L. Kerbey, and W.P.T. James. 2002. Physical activity and its impact on health outcomes. Paper 2: Prevention of unhealthy weight gain and obesity by physical activity: An analysis of the evidence. *Obesity Reviews* 3:273-287.

14. Farrell, S.W., L. Braun, C.E. Barlow, Y.J. Cheng, and S.N. Blair. 2002. The relation of body mass index, cardiorespiratory fitness, and all-cause mortality in women. *Obesity Research* 10:417-423.

15. Fletcher, G.F., S.N. Blair, J. Blumenthal, C.J. Caspersen, B. Chaitman, S. Epstein, H. Falls, E.S. Sivarajan Froelicher, V.F. Froelicher, and I.L. Pina. 1992. American Heart Association statement on exercise. *Circulation* 86:340-344.

16. Fryar C.D., M.D. Carroll, and J. Afful. 2020. Prevalence of overweight, obesity, and severe obesity amount adults aged 20 and over: United States, 1960-1962 through 2017-2018. National Center for Health Statistics. www.cdc.gov/nchs/data/hestat/obesity-adult-17-18/obesity-adult.htm.

17. Golding, L.A., C.R. Myers, and W.E. Sinning. 1973. *The Y's Way to Physical Fitness.* Emmaus, PA: Rodale Press.

18. Harris, C.D., K.B. Watson, S.A. Carlson, J.E. Fulton, J.M. Dorn, and L. Elam-Evans. 2013. Adult participation in aerobic and muscle-strengthening physical activities—United States, 2011. *Morbidity and Mortality Weekly Report* 62(17): 326-331.

19. Haskell, W.L. 1985. Physical activity and health: Need to define the required stimulus. *American Journal of Cardiology* 55:4D-9D.

20. Haskell, W.L. 1994. Dose–response issues from a biological perspective. In *Physical activity, fitness and health*, ed. C. Bouchard, R.J. Shephard, and T. Stephens, 1030-1039. Champaign, IL: Human Kinetics.

21. Haskell, W.L., I.M. Lee, R.R. Pate, K.E. Powell, S.N. Blair, B.A. Franklin, C.A. Macera, G.W. Heath, and P.D. Thompson. 2007. Physical activity and public health: Updated recommendation for adults from the American College of Sports Medicine and the American Heart Association. *Medicine & Science in Sports & Exercise* 39:1423-1434.

22. Heron, M. Deaths: Leading causes for 2019. *National Vital Statistics Reports* 70(9): 1-114.

23. Institute of Medicine (IOM). 2002. *Dietary reference intakes for energy, carbohydrates, fiber, fat, fatty acids, cholesterol, proteins, and amino acids.* Washington, DC: National Academy of Sciences.

24. Jones, W.H.S. 1953. *Regimen (Hippocrates).* Cambridge, MA: Harvard University Press.

25. Lee, C.D., S.N. Blair, and A.S. Jackson. 1999. Cardiorespiratory fitness, body composition, and all-cause and cardiovascular disease mortality in men. *American Journal of Clinical Nutrition* 69:373-380.

26. Mokdad, A.H., J.S. Marks, D.F. Stroup, and J.L. Gerberding. 2004. Actual causes of death in the United States, 2000. *Journal of the American Medical Association* 291:1238-1245.

27. Mokdad, A.H., J.S. Marks, D.F. Stroup, and J.L. Gerberding. 2005. Correction: Actual causes of death in the United States, 2000. *Journal of the American Medical Association* 293:293-294.

28. National Center for Health Statistics. 2022. Leading causes of death. www.cdc.gov/nchs/fastats/leading-causes-of-death.htm.

29. Paffenbarger, R.S.J., A.L. Wing, and R.T. Hyde. 1978. Physical activity as an index of heart attack risk in college alumni. *American Journal of Epidemiology* 108:161-175.

30. Pate, R.R., M. Pratt, S.N. Blair, W.L. Haskell, C.A. Marcera, and C. Bouchard. 1995. Physical activity and public health: A recommendation from the Centers for Disease Control and Prevention and the American College of Sports Medicine. *Journal of the American Medical Association* 273:402-407.

31. Physical Activity Guidelines Advisory Committee. 2018 Physical Activity Guidelines Advisory Committee scientific report. 2018. https://health.gov/our-work/nutrition-physical-activity/physical-activity-guidelines/current-guidelines/scientific-report.

32. Pilar, M.R., A.A. Eyler, S. Moreland-Russell, and R.C. Brownson. 2020. Actual causes of death in relation to media, policy, and funding attention: Examining public health priorities. *Frontiers in Public Health* 8. https://doi.org/10.3389/fpubh.2020.00279.

33. Rankinen, T., and C. Bouchard. 2007. Genetic differences in the relationships among physical activity, fitness, and health. In *Physical activity and health*, ed. C. Bouchard, S.N. Blair, and W.L. Haskell. Champaign, IL: Human Kinetics.

34. Ruiz, J.R., X. Sui, F. Lobelo, S. Lee, J.R. Morrow, A.W. Jackson, J.R. Hébert, C.E. Matthews, M. Sjöström, and S.N. Blair. 2009. Muscular strength and adiposity as predictors of adulthood cancer mortality in men. *Cancer Epidemiology Biomarkers Prevention* 18:1468-1476.

35. Saris, W.H.M., S.N. Blair, M.A. Van Baak, S.B. Eaton, P.S. Davies, L. DiPietro, M. Fogelholm, A. Rissanen, D. Schoeller, B. Swinburn, A. Tremblay, K.R. Westerterp, and H. Wyatt. 2003. How much physical activity is enough to prevent unhealthy weight gain? Outcomes of the IASO 1st Stock Conference and consensus statement. *Obesity Reviews* 4:101-114.

36. Sui, X., M.J. LaMonte, J.N. Laditka, J.W. Hardin, N. Chase, S.P. Hooker, and S.N. Blair. 2007. Cardiorespiratory fitness and adiposity as mortality predictors in older adults. *Journal of the American Medical Association* 298:2507-2516.

37. Swain, D.P., and B.A. Franklin. 2006. Comparison of cardioprotective benefits of vigorous versus moderate intensity aerobic exercise. *American Journal of Cardiology* 97:141-147.

38. U.S. Department of Health and Human Services (HHS). 1996. *Physical activity and health: A report of the Surgeon General*. Washington, DC: Author.

39. U.S. Department of Health and Human Services (HHS). 2008. *2008 Physical Activity Guidelines for Americans*. www.health.gov/paguidelines/guidelines/default.aspx.

40. U.S. Department of Health and Human Services (HHS). 2008. *Physical Activity Guidelines Advisory Committee report 2008*. https://health.gov/sites/default/files/2019-10/CommitteeReport_7.pdf.

41. U.S. Department of Health and Human Services (HHS). 2018. *Physical Activity Guidelines for Americans*. 2nd ed. https://health.gov/our-work/nutrition-physical-activity/physical-activity-guidelines/current-guidelines.

42. U.S. Department of Health and Human Services (HHS). 2022. Heart disease and African Americans. http://minorityhealth.hhs.gov/omh/browse.aspx?lvl=4&lvlid=19.

43. U.S. Department of Health and Human Services (HHS). n.d. Healthy People 2030: Physical activity. Accessed December 2022. https://health.gov/healthypeople/objectives-and-data/browse-objectives/physical-activity.

44. U.S. Department of Health and Human Services (HHS) and U.S. Department of Agriculture (USDA). 2020. *Dietary guidelines for Americans, 2020-2025*. https://DietaryGuidelines.gov.

45. U.S. Department of Health, Education, and Welfare. 1979. *Healthy people: The Surgeon General's report on health promotion and disease prevention*. Washington, DC: U.S. GPO.

46. World Health Organization (WHO). 1946. Preamble to the Constitution of the World Health Organization as adopted by the International Health Conference, New York, 19 June-22 July.

Chapter 2

1. Abd, T.T., and T.A. Jacobson. 2011. Statin-induced myopathy: A review and update. *Expert Opinion on Drug Safety* 10(3): 373-387. https://doi.org/10.1517/14740338.2011.540568.

2. Akil, H., R. Baldessarini, and C. Beattie. 2001. *Goodman and Gilman's: The Pharmacological Basis of Therapeutics*. 10th ed. New York: McGraw-Hill.

3. Alderman, C.P. 1996. Adverse effects of the angiotensin-converting enzyme inhibitors. *Annals of Pharmacotherapy* 30(1):55-61.

4. American Association for Cardiovascular and Pulmonary Rehabilitation (AACVPR). 2013. *Guidelines for cardiac rehabilitation and secondary prevention programs*. 5th ed. Champaign, IL: Human Kinetics.

5. American College of Sports Medicine (ACSM). 2016. *ACSM's resource manual for guidelines for exercise testing and prescription*. 8th ed. Philadelphia: Lippincott Williams and Wilkins.

6. American College of Sports Medicine (ACSM). 2019. *ACSM's health/fitness facility standards and guidelines*. 5th ed. Champaign, IL: Human Kinetics.

7. American College of Sports Medicine (ACSM). 2022. *ACSM's fitness assessment manual*. 6th ed. Philadelphia: Wolters Kluwer.

8. American College of Sports Medicine (ACSM). 2022. *ACSM's guidelines for exercise testing and prescription*. 11th ed. Philadelphia: Wolters Kluwer.

9. American College of Sports Medicine (ACSM) and American Heart Association (AHA). 1998. ACSM/AHA joint position statement: Recommendations for cardiovascular screening, staffing, and emergency policies at health/fitness facilities. *Medicine & Science in Sports & Exercise* 30:1009-1018.

10. American College of Sports Medicine (ACSM) and American Heart Association (AHA). 2007. Exercise and acute cardiovascular events: Placing the risks into perspective. *Medicine & Science in Sports & Exercise* 39:886-897.

11. American Hospital Formulary Service. 2015. Drug information 2015. Bethesda, MD: American Society of Hospital Pharmacists.

12. Cadwallader, A.B., X. De La Torre, A. Tieri, and F. Botrè. 2010. The abuse of diuretics as performance-enhancing drugs and masking agents in sport doping: Pharmacology, toxicology and analysis. *British Journal of Pharmacology* 161(1):1-16.

13. Cahalin, L.P., and H.S. Sadowsky. 2001. Pulmonary medications. In *Essentials of cardiopulmonary physical therapy*, ed. E.A. Hillegass and H.S. Sadowsky, 587-607. 2nd ed. Philadelphia: Saunders.

14. Canadian Society for Exercise Physiology (CSEP). 2012. Canadian fitness safety standards and recommended guidelines .http://eparmed-x.appspot.com/?locale=en#pub/parmedx.

15. Chick, T., A. Halperin, and E. Gacek. 1988. The effect of antihypertensive medications on exercise performance. *Medicine & Science in Sports & Exercise* 20(5):447-454.

16. Cooper, C.B. 2009. Chronic obstructive pulmonary disease. In *ACSM's exercise management for persons with chronic diseases and disabilities*, ed. J.L. Durstine, G. Moore, P. Painter, and S. Roberts, 129-135. Champaign, IL: Human Kinetics.

17. Coutinho, M., H. Gerstein, Y. Wang, and S. Yusuf. 1999. The relationship between glucose and incident cardiovascular events: A metaregression analysis of published data from 20 studies of 95,783 individuals followed for 12.4 years. *Diabetes Care* 22:233-240.

18. Department of Veterans Affairs Department of Defense. 2022. VA/DoD clinical practice guideline for the management of major depressive disorder. www.healthquality.va.gov/guidelines/MH/mdd/.

19. Eickhoff-Shemek, J.M., and A.C. Craig. 2017. Putting the new ACSM pre-activity health screening guidelines into practice. *ACSM's Health & Fitness Journal* 21(3):11-21.

20. Eickhoff-Shemek, J., D.L. Herbert, and D. Connaughton. 2009. *Risk management for health/fitness professionals*. Philadelphia: Lippincott Williams & Wilkins.

21. Eickhoff-Shemek, J.M., B.J. Zabawa, P.R. Fenaroli. 2020. *Law for fitness managers and exercise professionals*. Parrish, FL: Fitness Law Academy.

22. Fitness Law Academy. 2021. Forms and documents. www.fitnesslawacademy.com/forms-and-documents.

23. Fletcher, G., G. Balady, S. Blair, J. Blumenthal, C. Caspersen, B. Chaitman, S. Epstein, E. Froelicher, V. Froelicher, I. Pina, and M. Pollock. 1996. Statement on exercise: Benefits and recommendations for physical activity programs for all Americans. *Circulation* 94:857-862.

24. Fletcher, G.F., P. Ades, P. Kligfield, R. Arena, et al. 2013. Exercise standards for testing and training: A scientific statement from the American Heart Association. *Circulation* 128:873-934.

25. Ford, E. 2005. Risks for all-cause mortality, cardiovascular disease, and diabetes associated with the metabolic syndrome: A summary of the evidence. *Diabetes Care* 28:1769-1778.

26. Framingham Heart Study. n.d. Cardiovascular disease (10-year risk). www.framinghamheartstudy.org/fhs-risk-functions/cardiovascular-disease-10-year-risk/

27. Franke, W. 2005. Covering all bases: Working with new clients. *ACSM's Health and Fitness Journal* 9:13-16.

28. Franke, W. 2013. Risk classification: Is it safe for your client to exercise? *ACSM's Health and Fitness Journal* 17:16-22.

29. Franklin B.A., P.D. Thompson, S.S. Al-Zaiti, C.M. Albert, M-F. Hivert, B.D. Levine, F. Lobelo, et al. 2020. Exercise-related acute cardiovascular events and potential deleterious adaptations following long-term exercise training: Placing the risks into perspective-an update. *Circulation*, 141:e705-e736.

30. Gibbons, R., G. Balady, J. Bricker, B. Chaitman, G. Fletcher, V. Froelicher, D. Mark, et al. 2002. ACC/AHA 2002 guideline update to exercise testing: Summary article. A report of the American College of Cardiology/American Heart Association task force on practice guidelines (committee to update the 1997 exercise testing guidelines). *Journal of the American College of Cardiology* 40:1531-1540.

31. Global Initiative for Chronic Obstructive Lung Disease. 2021. https://goldcopd.org/.

32. Goff, D., D. Lloyd-Jones, G. Bennett, C. O'Donnell, S. Coady, and J. Robinson. 2014. 2013 ACC/AHA guideline on the assessment of cardiovascular risk. *Journal of the American College of Cardiology* 63:2935-2959.

33. Goodman, J., S. Thomas, and J. Burr. 2011. Evidence-based risk assessment and recommendations for exercise testing and physical activity clearance in apparently healthy individuals. *Applied Physiology, Nutrition, and Metabolism* 36:S14-S32.

34. Grundy, S., R. Pasternak, P. Greenland, S. Smith Jr., and V. Fuster. 1999. Assessment of cardiovascular risk by use of multiple-risk-factor assessment equations: A statement for healthcare professionals from the American Heart Association and the American College of Cardiology. *Circulation* 100:1481-1492.

35. Haskell, W. 2019. Guidelines for physical activity and health in the United States: Evolution over 50 years. *ACSM's Health & Fitness Journal* 23(5):5-8.

36. Health Insurance Portability and Accountability Act (HIPAA), Subtitle F Section 1171 4(a). August 21, 1996. Public Law 104-191, 104th Congress.

37. Koester Qualters, W. 2014. Diagnostic procedures for cardiovascular disease. In *ACSM's resource manual for guidelines for exercise testing and prescription*, ed. J.K. Ehrman, 382-396. 7th ed. Baltimore: Lippincott Williams & Wilkins.

38. Li, T., J. Rana, J. Manson, W. Willett, M. Stampfer, G. Colditz, and F.B. Hu. 2006. Obesity as compared with physical activity in predicting risk of coronary heart disease in women. *Circulation* 113:499-506.

39. Lu, Y., K. Hajifathalian, M. Ezzati, M. Woodward, E. Rimm, and G. Danaei. 2014. Metabolic mediators of the effects of body-mass index, overweight, and obesity on coronary heart disease and stroke: A pooled analysis of 97 prospective cohorts with 1.8 million participants. *Lancet* 383:970-983.

40. MacGowan, G.A., D. O'Callaghan, and J.H. Horgan. 1992. The effects of verapamil on training in patients with ischemic heart disease. *Chest* 101(2):411-415.

41. Magal, M., D. Riebe. 2016. Preparticipation Health Screening Recommendations: What exercise professionals need to know. *ACSM's Health and Fitness Journal* 20(3):22-27.

42. National Library of Medicine. n.d. DailyMed. Accessed October 2022. https://dailymed.nlm.nih.gov/dailymed/index.cfm.

43. Niedfeldt, M.W. 2002. Managing hypertension in athletes and physically active patients. *American Family Physician* 66(3):445-453.

44. Opie, L.H. 1997. Pharmacological differences between calcium antagonists. *European Heart Journal* 18 Suppl A:A71-9.

45. PAR-Q+ Collaboration: The Physical Activity Readiness Questionnaire for Everyone. 2022. https://eparmedx.com/.

46. Prapavessis, H., L. Cameron, J.C. Baldi, S. Robinson, K. Borrie, T. Harper, et al. 2007. The effects of exercise and nicotine replacement therapy on smoking rates in women. *Addictive Behaviors* 13(6):612-632.

47. Riebe, D., B. Franklin, P. Thompson, et al. 2015. Updating ACSM's Recommendations for Exercise Preparticipation Health Screening. *Medicine & Science in Sports & Exercise* 47:2473-79.

48. Roush, G.C., R. Kaur, and M.E. Ernst. 2013. Diuretics. *Journal of Cardiovascular Pharmacology and Therapeutics* 19(1):5-13.

49. Schatzberg, A.F., and C.B. Nemeroff. 2017. *The American Psychiatric Association Publishing textbook of psychopharmacology*. Arlington, VA: American Psychiatric Association Publishing.

50. Standards of care in diabetes—2023: Pharmacologic approaches to glycemic treatment. *Diabetes Care* 2023;46(Supplement_1):S140–S157.

51. Stone, N., J. Robinson, A. Lichtenstein, et al. 2013. 2013 ACC/AHA guideline on the treatment of blood cholesterol to reduce atherosclerotic cardiovascular risk in adults. *Circulation* 129:S1-S45.

52. Teo, K., S. Ounpuu, S. Hawken, M. Pandey, V. Valentin, D. Hunt, et al. 2006. Tobacco use and risk of myocardial infarction in 52 countries in the INTERHEART study: A case-control study. *Lancet* 368:647-658.

53. Thompson, P., B. Franklin, and G. Balady. 2007. Exercise and acute cardiovascular events placing the risks into perspective: A scientific statement from the American Heart Association Council on Nutrition, Physical Activity, and Metabolism and the Council on Clinical Cardiology. *Circulation* 115:2358-2368.

54. Thompson, P.D., A.L. Baggish, B. Franklin, C. Jaworski, and D. Riebe. 2020. American College of Sports Medicine expert consensus statement to update recommendations for screening, staffing, and emergency policies to prevent cardiovascular events at health fitness facilities. *Current Sports Medicine Reports* 19(6):223-231.

55. U.S. Department of Veterans Affairs. 2017. VA/DoD Clinical practice guideline for the management of type 2 diabetes mellitus. www.healthquality.va.gov/guidelines/CD/diabetes/VADoDDMCPGFinal508.pdf.

56. U.S. Department of Veterans Affairs. 2020. Diagnosis and management of hypertension (HTN) in primary care. www.healthquality.va.gov/guidelines/CD/htn/.

57. Wadgave U., and L. Nagesh. 2016. Nicotine replacement therapy: An overview. *International Journal of Health Science* 10(3):425-435.

58. Warburton, D.E., S.S. Bredin, V.K. Jamnik, and N. Gledhill. 2011. Validation of the PAR-Q+ and ePARmed-X+. *Health and Fitness Journal of Canada* 4:38-46.

59. Warburton, D.E., V.K. Jamnik, S.S. Bredin, and N. Gledhill. 2011. The Physical Activity Readiness Questionnaire for Everyone (PAR-Q+) and electronic Physical Activity Readiness Medical Examination (ePARmed-X+). *Health and Fitness Journal of Canada* 4:3-17.

60. Wilson, P., R. D'Agostino, D. Levy, A. Belanger, H. Silbershatz, and W. Kannel. 1998. Prediction of coronary heart disease using risk factor categories. *Circulation* 97:1837-1847.

61. Wright, A.D., and M.E. Penny. 1980. Beta blockers and hypoglycemia. *Diabetes Care* 3(1):204-205.

62. Yusuf, S., S. Hawken, S. Ounpuu, L. Bautist, M. Franzosi, P. Commerford, and INTERHEART Study Investigators. 2005. Obesity and the risk of myocardial infarction in 27,000 participants from 52 countries: A case-control study. *Lancet* 366:1640-1649.

Chapter 3

1. Burkett, B. 2010. *Sport mechanics for coaches*. 3rd ed. Champaign, IL: Human Kinetics.

2. Floyd, R.T. 2021. *Manual of structural kinesiology*. 21st ed. Boston: McGraw-Hill Higher Education.

3. Hall, S. 2019. *Basic biomechanics*. 8th ed. Boston: McGraw-Hill.

4. Hamill, J., K. Knutzen, and T.R. Derrick. 2021. *Biomechanical basis of human movement*. 5th ed. Philadelphia: Lippincott Williams & Wilkins.

5. Hay, J.G., and J.G. Reid. 1988. *Anatomy, mechanics and human motion*. 2nd ed. Englewood Cliffs, NJ: Prentice Hall.

6. Levine, D., J. Richard, and M.W. Whittle. 2012. *Whittle's gait analysis*. 5th ed. New York: Churchill Livingstone.

7. Standring, S., ed. 2020. *Gray's anatomy: The anatomical basis of clinical practice*. 42nd ed. New York: Churchill Livingstone.

Chapter 4

1. Achten, J., and A.E. Jeukendrup. 2004. Optimizing fat oxidation through exercise and diet. *Nutrition* 20(7-8):716-727.

2. Åstrand, P.-O. 1952. *Experimental studies of physical working capacity in relation to sex and age*. Copenhagen: Ejnar Munksgaard.

3. Åstrand, P.-O., K. Rodahl, H.A. Dahl, and S.B. Strømme. 2003. *Textbook of work physiology*. 4th ed. Champaign, IL: Human Kinetics.

4. Bassett Jr., D.R. 1994. Skeletal muscle characteristics: Relationships to cardiovascular risk factors. *Medicine & Science in Sports & Exercise* 26:957-966.

5. Bassett, D.R., and E.T. Howley. 1997. Maximal oxygen uptake: Classical versus contemporary viewpoints. *Medicine & Science in Sports & Exercise* 29:591-603.

6. Bassett, D.R., and E.T. Howley. 2000. Limiting factors for maximal oxygen uptake and determinants of endurance performance. *Medicine & Science in Sports & Exercise* 32:70-84.

7. Bouchard, C., R. Lesage, G. Lortie, J. Simoneau, P. Hamel, M. Boulay, L. Perusse, G. Theriault, and C. Leblanc. 1986. Aerobic performance in brothers, dizygotic and monozygotic twins. *Medicine & Science in Sports & Exercise* 18:639-646.

8. Brooks, G.A. 1985. Anaerobic threshold: Review of the concept, and directions for future research. *Medicine & Science in Sports & Exercise* 17:22-31.

9. Carter, R., D.E. Watenpaugh, W.L. Wasmund, S.L. Wasmund, and M.L. Smith. 1999. Muscle pump and central command during recovery from exercise in humans. *Journal of Applied Physiology* 87(4):1463-1469.

10. Cheung, K., P.A. Hume, and L. Maxwell. 2003. Delayed onset muscle soreness: Treatment strategies and performance factors. *Sports Medicine* 33(2):145-164.

11. Claytor, R.P. 1985. Selected cardiovascular, sympathoadrenal, and metabolic responses to one-leg exercise training. PhD diss., University of Tennessee, Knoxville.

12. Coggan, A.R., and E.F. Coyle. 1991. Carbohydrate ingestion during prolonged exercise: Effects on metabolism and performance. *Exercise and Sport Sciences Reviews* 19:1-40.

13. Costill, D.L. 1988. Carbohydrates for exercise: Dietary demands of optimal performance. *International Journal of Sports Medicine* 9:1-18.

14. Covert, C.A, M.P. Alexander, J.J. Petronis, and D.S. Davis. 2010. Comparison of ballistic and static stretching on hamstring muscle length using an equal stretching dose. *Journal of Strength and Conditioning Research* 24(11):3008-3014.

15. Coyle, E.F. 1988. Detraining and retention of training induced adaptations. In *Resource manual for guidelines for exercise testing and prescription*, ed. S.N. Blair, P. Painter, R.R. Pate, L.K. Smith, and C.B. Taylor, 83-89. Philadelphia: Lea & Febiger.

16. Coyle, E.F., M.K. Hemmert, and A.R. Coggan. 1986. Effects of detraining on cardiovascular responses to exercise: Role of blood volume. *Journal of Applied Physiology* 60:95-99.

17. Coyle, E.F., W.H. Martin III, S.A. Bloomfield, O.H. Lowry, and J.O. Holloszy. 1985. Effects of detraining on responses to submaximal exercise. *Journal of Applied Physiology* 59:853-859.

18. Coyle, E.F., W.H. Martin III, D.R. Sinacore, M.J. Joyner, J.M. Hagberg, and J.O. Holloszy. 1984. Time course of loss of adaptation after stopping prolonged intense endurance training. *Journal of Applied Physiology* 57:1857-1864.

19. Cureton, K.J., P.B. Sparling, B.W. Evans, S.M. Johnson, U.D. Kong, and J.W. Purvis. 1978. Effect of experimental alterations in excess weight on aerobic capacity and distance-running performance. *Medicine and Science in Sports* 10:194-199.

20. Davis, J.H. 1985. Anaerobic threshold: Review of the concept and directions for future research. *Medicine & Science in Sports & Exercise* 17:6-18.

21. Day, J.R., H.B. Rossiter, E.M. Coats, A. Skasick, and B.J. Whipp. 2003. The maximally attainable $\dot{V}O_2$ during exercise in humans: The peak vs. maximal issue. *Journal of Applied Physiology* 95:1901-1907.

22. Dupuy, O., W. Douzi, D. Theurot, L. Bosquet, and B. Dugué. 2018. An evidence-based approach for choosing post-exercise recovery techniques to reduce markers of muscle damage, soreness, fatigue, and inflammation: A systematic review with meta-analysis. *Frontiers in Physiology* 9(403):1-15.

23. Ehrman, J.K., D.J. Kerrigan, S.J. Keteyian. 2018. *Advanced exercise physiology: Essential concepts and applications*. Champaign, IL: Human Kinetics.

24. Ekblom, B., P.-O. Åstrand, B. Saltin, J. Stenberg, and B. Wallstrom. 1968. Effect of training on circulatory response to exercise. *Journal of Applied Physiology* 24:518-528.

25. Faulkner, J.A., D.E. Roberts, R.L. Elk, and J. Conway. 1971. Cardiovascular responses to submaximum and maximum effort cycling and running. *Journal of Applied Physiology* 30:457-461.

26. Fleck, S.J., and L.S. Dean. 1987. Resistance-training experience and the pressor response during resistance exercise. *Journal of Applied Physiology* 63:116-120.

27. Foster, C., E. Kuffel, N. Bradley, R.A. Battista, G. Wright, J.P. Porcari, A. Lucia, and J.J. deKoning. 2007. $\dot{V}O_2$max during successive maximal efforts. *European Journal of Applied Physiology* 102:67-72.

28. Fradkin, A.J., T.R. Zazryn, and J.M. Smoliga. 2010. Effects of warming-up on physical performance: A systematic review with meta-analysis. *Journal of Strength and Conditioning Research* 24(1):140-148.

29. Franklin, B.A. 1985. Exercise testing, training, and arm ergometry. *Sports Medicine* 2:100-119.

30. Gisolfi, C., and C.B. Wenger. 1984. Temperature regulation during exercise: Old concepts, new ideas. *Exercise and Sport Sciences Reviews* 12:339-372.

31. Gledhill, N., D. Cox, and R. Jamnik. 1994. Endurance athletes' stroke volume does not plateau: Major advantage is diastolic function. *Medicine & Science in Sports & Exercise* 26:1116-1121.

32. Haff, G.G., and N.T. Triplett, eds. 2016. *Essentials of strength training and conditioning*. 4th ed. Champaign, IL: Human Kinetics.

33. Hamilton, M.T., and F.W. Booth. 2000. Skeletal muscle adaptation to exercise: A century of progress. *Journal of Applied Physiology* 88:327-331.

34. Hargreaves, M., and L.L. Spriet. 2020. Skeletal muscle energy metabolism during exercise. *Nature Metabolism* 2:817-828.

35. Hawkins, M.N., P.B. Raven, P.G. Snell, J. Stray-Gundersen, and B.D. Levine. 2007. Maximal oxygen uptake as a parametric measure of cardiorespiratory capacity. *Medicine & Science in Sports & Exercise* 39:103-107.

36. Helge, J.W., P.W. Watt, E.A. Richter, M.J. Rennie, and B. Kiens. 2001. Fat utilization during exercise: Adaptation to a fat-rich diet increases utilization of plasma fatty acids and very low density lipoprotein-triacylglycerol in humans. *Journal of Physiology* 537(3):1009-1020.

37. Hickson, R.C., H.A. Bomze, and J.O. Holloszy. 1977. Linear increase in aerobic power induced by a strenuous program of endurance exercise. *Journal of Applied Physiology: Respiratory, Environmental and Exercise Physiology* 42:372-376.

38. Hickson, R.C., H.A. Bomze, and J.O. Holloszy. 1978. Faster adjustment of O_2 uptake to the energy requirement of exercise in the trained state. *Journal of Applied Physiology: Respiratory, Environmental and Exercise Physiology* 44:877-881.

39. Hickson, R.C., C. Foster, M.L. Pollock, T.M. Galassi, and S. Rich. 1985. Reduced training intensities and loss of aerobic power, endurance, and cardiac growth. *Journal of Applied Physiology* 58:492-499.

40. Hickson, R.C., C. Kanakis Jr., J.R. Davis, A.M. Moore, and S. Rich. 1982. Reduced training duration effects on aerobic power, endurance, and cardiac growth. *Journal of Applied Physiology* 53:225-229.

41. Hickson, R.C., and M.A. Rosenkoetter. 1981. Reduced training frequencies and maintenance of increased aerobic power. *Medicine & Science in Sports & Exercise* 13:13-16.

42. Hody, S., J.-L. Croisier, T. Bury, B. Rogister, and P. Leprince. 2019. Eccentric muscle contractions: Risks and benefits. *Frontiers in Physiology* 10:536.

43. Holloszy, J.O., and E.F. Coyle. 1984. Adaptations of skeletal muscle to endurance exercise and their metabolic consequences. *Journal of Applied Physiology: Respiratory, Environmental and Exercise Physiology* 56:831-838.

44. Hotfiel, T., J. Freiwald, M.W. Hoppe, C. Luteer, R. Forst, C. Grim, W. Bloch, M. Hüttel, R. Heiss. 2018. Advances in delayed-onset muscle soreness DOMS: Part 1 pathogenesis and diagnostics. *Sportverl Sportschad* 32:243-250.

45. Howley, E.T. 1980. Effect of altitude on physical performance. In *Encyclopedia of physical education, fitness, and sports: Training, environment, nutrition, and fitness*, ed. G.A. Stull and T.K. Cureton, 177-187. Salt Lake City: Brighton.

46. Howley, E.T., D.R. Bassett Jr., and H.G. Welch. 1995. Criteria for maximal oxygen uptake—Review and commentary. *Medicine & Science in Sports & Exercise* 24:1055-1058.

47. Hughes, D.C., S. Ellefsen, and K. Baar. 2018. Adaptations to endurance and strength training. *Cold Springs Harbor Perspectives in Medicine* 8:a029769.

48. Hultman, E. 1967. Physiological role of muscle glycogen in man, with special reference to exercise. *Circulation Research* 20-21(Suppl. 1):99-114.

49. Issekutz, B., N.C. Birkhead, and K. Rodahl. 1962. The use of respiratory quotients in assessment of aerobic power capacity. *Journal of Applied Physiology* 17:47-50.

50. Jeukendrup, A., and J. Achten. 2001. Fatmax: A new concept to optimize fat oxidation during exercise? *European Journal of Sport Science* 1(5):1-5.

51. Kasch, F.W., J.L. Boyer, S.P. Van Camp, L.S. Verity, and J.P. Wallace. 1990. The effects of physical activity and inactivity on aerobic power in older men (a longitudinal study). *Physician and Sportsmedicine* 18(4):73-83.

52. Kasch, F.W., J.P. Wallace, and S.P. Van Camp. 1985. Effects of 18 years of endurance exercise on the physical work capacity of older men. *Journal of Cardiopulmonary Rehabilitation* 5:308-312.

53. Kasch, F.W., J.P. Wallace, S.P. Van Camp, and L.S. Verity. 1988. A longitudinal study of cardiovascular stability in active men aged 45 to 65 yrs. *Physician and Sportsmedicine* 16(1):117-126.

54. Katch, F.I., and W.D. McArdle. 1977. *Nutrition and weight control.* Boston: Houghton Mifflin.

55. Kenney, W.L., J.H. Wilmore, D.L. Costill. 2021. *Physiology of sport and exercise.* 8th ed. Champaign, IL: Human Kinetics.

56. Kraemer, W.J., S.J. Fleck, M.R Deschenes. 2021. *Exercise physiology: Integrating theory and application.* 3rd ed. Philadelphia: Wolters Kluwer.

57. Lind, A.R., and G.W. McNicol. 1967. Muscular factors which determine the cardiovascular responses to sustained and rhythmic exercise. *Canadian Medical Association Journal* 96:706-713.

58. Lum, D., and T.M Barbosa. 2019. Brief review: Effects of isometric strength training on strength and dynamic performance. *International Journal of Sports Medicine* 40(6):363-375.

59. MacDougall, J.D., D. Tuxen, D.G. Sale, J.R. Moroz, and J.R. Sutton. 1985. Arterial blood-pressure response to heavy resistance exercise. *Journal of Applied Physiology* 58:785-790.

60. Maughan, R.J., and S.M. Shirreffs. 2019. Muscle cramping during exercise: Causes, solutions, and questions remaining. *Sports Medicine* 49(Suppl. 2):S115-S124.

61. McArdle, W.D., F.I. Katch, and V.L. Katch. 2023. *Exercise physiology: Nutrition, energy, and human performance.* 9th ed. Philadelphia: Wolters Kluwer.

62. McArdle, W.D., F.I. Katch, and G.S. Pechar. 1973. Comparison of continuous and discontinuous treadmill and bicycle tests for max $\dot{V}O_2$. *Medicine and Science in Sports* 5(3):156-160.

63. McArdle, W.D., and J.R. Magel. 1970. Physical work capacity and maximum oxygen uptake in treadmill and bicycle exercise. *Medicine and Science in Sports* 2(3):118-123.

64. Menzies, P., C. Menzies, L. McIntyre, P. Paterson, J. Wilson, and O.J. Kemi. 2010. Blood lactate clearance during active recovery after an intense running bout depends on the intensity of the active recovery. *Journal of Sports Sciences* 28(9):975-982.

65. Montoye, H.J., T. Ayen, F. Nagle, and E.T. Howley. 1986. The oxygen requirement for horizontal and grade walking on a motor-driven treadmill. *Medicine & Science in Sports & Exercise* 17:640-645.

66. Murray, B., and C. Rosenbloom. 2018. Fundamentals of glycogen metabolism for coaches and athletes. *Nutrition Reviews* 76(4):243-259.

67. Nagle, F.J., B. Balke, G. Baptista, J. Alleyia, and E. Howley. 1971. Compatibility of progressive treadmill, bicycle, and step tests based on oxygen-uptake responses. *Medicine and Science in Sports* 3:149-154.

68. Oranchuk, D.J., A.G. Storey, A.R. Nelson, and J.B. Cronin. 2018. Isometric training and long-term adaptations: Effects of muscle length, intensity, and intent: A systematic review. *Scandinavian Journal of Medicine and Science in Sports* 29:484-503.

69. Page, P. 2012. Current concepts in muscle stretching for exercise and rehabilitation. *The International Journal of Sports Physical Therapy* 7(1):109-119.

70. Powers, S., S. Dodd, R. Deason, R. Byrd, and T. McKnight. 1983. Ventilatory threshold, running economy, and distance-running performance of trained athletes. *Research Quarterly for Exercise and Sport* 54:179-182.

71. Powers, S., E. Howley, and J. Quindry. 2024. *Exercise physiology: Theory and application to fitness and performance.* 12th ed. New York: McGraw-Hill.

72. Powers, S., W. Riley, and E. Howley. 1980. A comparison of fat metabolism in trained men and women during prolonged aerobic work. *Research Quarterly for Exercise and Sport* 52:427-431.

73. Powers, S.K., S. Dodd, and R.E. Beadle. 1985. Oxygen-uptake kinetics in trained athletes differing in $\dot{V}O_2$max. *European Journal of Applied Physiology* 54:306-308.

74. Raven, P.B., D.H. Wasserman, W.G. Squires Jr., and T.D. Murray. 2013. *Exercise physiology: An integrated approach.* Belmont, CA: Wadsworth Cengage Learning.

75. Rossiter, H.B., J.M. Kowalchuk, and B.J. Whipp. 2006. A test to establish maximal oxygen uptake despite no plateau in the O_2 uptake response to ramp incremental exercise. *Journal of Applied Physiology* 100:764-770.

76. Rowell, L.B. 1969. Circulation. *Medicine and Science in Sports* 1:15-22.

77. Rowell, L.B. 1986. *Human circulation-regulation during physical stress.* New York: Oxford University Press.

78. Sale, D.G. 1987. Influence of exercise and training on motor unit activation. *Exercise and Sport Sciences Reviews* 15:95-151.

79. Saltin, B. 1969. Physiological effects of physical conditioning. *Medicine and Science in Sports* 1:50-56.

80. Saltin, B., and P.D. Gollnick. 1983. Skeletal muscle adaptability: Significance for metabolism and performance. In *Handbook of physiology*, ed. L.D. Peachey, R.H. Adrian, and S.R. Geiger, 555-631. Baltimore: Williams & Wilkins.

81. Saltin, B., J. Henriksson, E. Nygaard, P. Anderson, and E. Jansson. 1977. Fiber types and metabolic potentials of skeletal muscles in sedentary man and endurance runners. *Annals of the New York Academy of Science* 301:3-29.

82. Saltin, B., and L. Hermansen. 1966. Esophageal, rectal, and muscle temperature during exercise. *Journal of Applied Physiology* 21:1757-1762.

83. Schwade, J., C.G. Blomqvist, and W. Shapiro. 1977. A comparison of the response to arm and leg work in patients with ischemic heart disease. *American Heart Journal* 94:203-208.

84. Sherman, W.M. 1983. Carbohydrates, muscle glycogen, and muscle glycogen supercompensation. In *Ergogenic*

aids in sports, ed. M.H. Williams, 3-26. Champaign, IL: Human Kinetics.

85. Smith, D.L., S.A. Plowman, M.J. Ormsbee. 2023. *Exercise physiology for health, fitness, and performance.* 6th ed. Philadelphia: Wolters Kluwer.

86. Spriet, L.L. 2014. New insights into the interaction of carbohydrate and fat metabolism during exercise. *Sports Medicine* 44(Suppl. 1):S87-S96.

87. Spriet, L.L., and R.K. Randell. 2020. Regulation of fat metabolism during exercise. *Sports Science Exchange* 33(205):1-6.

88. Taylor, H.L., E.R. Buskirk, and A. Henschel. 1955. Maximal oxygen intake as an objective measure of cardiorespiratory performance. *Journal of Applied Physiology* 8:73-80.

89. Widmaier, E.P., H. Raff, and K.T. Strang. 2014. *Vander's human physiology.* 13th ed. New York: McGraw-Hill.

90. Zhou, B., R.K. Conlee, R. Jensen, G.W. Fellingham, J.D. George, and A.G. Fisher. 2011. Stroke volume does not plateau during graded exercise in elite male distance runners. *Medicine & Science in Sports & Exercise* 33:1849-1854.

Chapter 5

1. Academy of Nutrition and Dietetics. n.d. Academy of Nutrition and Dietetics. Accessed October 2022. www.eatright.org.

2. Academy of Nutrition and Dietetics. n.d. Nutrition care process. Accessed October 2022. www.eatrightpro.org/practice/quality-management/nutrition-care-process.

3. Academy of Nutrition and Dietetics. 2017. Sports Nutrition, ed. C. Karpinski and C.A. Rosenbloom. 6th ed. Chicago: The Academy of Nutrition and Dietetics.

4. Accreditation Council for Education in Nutrition and Dietetics of the Academy of Nutrition and Dietetics. n.d. Accreditation Council for Education in Nutrition and Dietetics of the Academy of Nutrition and Dietetics. Accessed October 2022. www.eatrightpro.org/acend.

5. American Heart Association. n.d. American Heart Association. Accessed October 2022. www.heart.org/

6. Australian Institute for Sport. n.d. Supplements. Accessed October 2022. www.ais.gov.au/nutrition/supplements.

7. Banned Substances Control Group. n.d. Banned substances control group. Accessed October 2022. www.bscg.org/.

8. Burke, L.M., L.M. Castell, D.J. Casa, G.L. Close, R.J.S. Costa, B. Desbrow, S.L. Halson, et al. 2019. International Association of Athletics Federations Consensus Statement 2019: Nutrition for Athletics. *International Journal of Sport Nutrition and Exercise Metabolism* 29(2):73-84.

9. Centers for Disease Control and Prevention. n.d. Prevention of heart disease. Accessed October 2022. www.cdc.gov/heartdisease/prevention.htm.

10. Commission on Dietetic Registration. n.d. Commission on Dietetic Registration. Accessed October 2022. www.cdrnet.org/.

11. De Souza, M.J., A. Nattiv, E. Joy, M. Misra, N.I. Williams, R.J. Mallinson, J.C. Gibbs, M. Olmsted, M. Goolsby, and G. Matheson. 2014. 2014 Female Athlete Triad Coalition Consensus Statement on treatment and return to play of the female athlete triad: 1st International Conference held in San Francisco, California, May 2012 and 2nd International Conference held in Indianapolis, Indiana, May 2013. *British Journal of Sports Medicine* 48(4):289-289.

12. Informed Choice. n.d. Informed Choice. Accessed October 2022. www.informed-choice.org/.

13. Institute of Medicine. 2005. *Dietary Reference Intakes for Water, Potassium, Sodium, Chloride, and Sulfate.* Washington, DC: National Academies Press.

14. Institute of Medicine, Food and Board Nutrition. 2005. *Dietary reference intakes for energy, carbohydrate, fiber, fat, fatty acids, cholesterol, protein, and amino acids (macronutrients).* Washington, DC: National Academies Press.

15. Kim, J. 2019. Nutritional supplement for athletic performance: Based on Australian Institute of Sport sports supplement framework. *Exercise Science* 28:211-220.

16. Kruskall, L.J., M.M. Manore, J.M. Eikhoff-Shemek, and J.K. Ehrman. 2017. Understanding the scope of practice among registered dietitian nutritionists and exercise professionals. *ACSMs Health & Fitness Journal* 21(1):23-32.

17. Lichtenstein, A.H., L.J. Appel, M. Vadiveloo, F.B. Hu, P.M. Kris-Etherton, C.M. Rebholz, F.M. Sacks, A.N. Thorndike, L. Van Horn, and J. Wylie-Rosett. 2021. 2021 dietary guidance to improve cardiovascular health: A scientific statement from the American Heart Association. *Circulation* 144(23):e472-e487.

18. Maughan, R.J., L.M. Burke, J. Dvorak, D.E. Larson-Meyer, P. Peeling, S.M. Phillips, E.S. Rawson, et al. 2018. IOC consensus statement: Dietary supplements and the high-performance athlete. *British Journal of Sports Medicine* 52(7):439.

19. Mountjoy, M., J.K. Sundgot-Borgen, L.M. Burke, K.E. Ackerman, C. Blauwet, N. Constantini, C. Lebrun, et al. 2018. IOC consensus statement on relative energy deficiency in sport (RED-S): 2018 update. *British Journal of Sports Medicine* 52(11):687-697.

20. National Center for Complementary and Integrative Health. n.d. Antioxidants: In depth. Accessed October 2022. www.nccih.nih.gov/health/antioxidants-in-depth.

21. National Heart, Lung, and Blood Institute. n.d. DASH eating plan. Accessed October 2022. www.nhlbi.nih.gov/education/dash-eating-plan.

22. National Institutes of Health. n.d. Nutrient recommendations: Dietary reference intakes. Accessed October 2022. https://ods.od.nih.gov/HealthInformation/Dietary_Reference_Intakes.aspx.

23. Sawka, M.N., L.M. Burke, E.R. Eichner, R.J. Maughan, S.J. Montain, and N.S. Stachenfeld. 2007. American College of Sports Medicine position stand. Exercise and fluid replacement. *Medicine & Science in Sports & Exercise* 39(2):377-90.

24. Thomas, D.T., K.A. Erdman, and L.M. Burke. 2016. Position of the Academy of Nutrition and Dietetics, Dietitians of Canada, and the American College of Sports Medicine: Nutrition and athletic performance. *Journal of the Academy of Nutrition and Dietetics* 116(3):501-28.

25. Thompson, J.L., M.M. Manore, and L.A. Vaughan. 2020. *The science of nutrition.* Vol. 5. Upper Saddle River, NJ: Pearson Education.

26. United States Department of Agriculture. 2022. MyPlate plan. www.choosemyplate.gov/resources/MyPlatePlan.

27. United States Department of Agriculture. n.d. USDA Choose MyPlate. www.choosemyplate.gov.

28. University of Sydney. n.d. Glycemic index research and GI news. https://glycemicindex.com/.

29. U.S. Anti-Doping Agency. n.d. *Supplement 411.* Accessed October 2022. www.usada.org/substances/supplement-411.

30. U.S. Anti-Doping Agency. n.d. U.S. Anti-Doping Agency. Accessed October 2022. www.usada.org/.

31. U.S. Department of Health and Human Services and U.S. Department of Agriculture. 2020. *2020-2025 dietary guidelines for Americans*. Accessed October 2022. https://health.gov/our-work/nutrition-physical-activity/dietary-guidelines.

32. U.S. Food and Drug Administration. n.d. Changes to the nutrition facts label. Accessed October 2022. www.fda.gov/Food/GuidanceRegulation/GuidanceDocumentsRegulatoryInformation/LabelingNutrition/ucm385663.htm.

33. U.S. Food and Drug Administration. n.d. Label claims for food & dietary supplements. www.fda.gov/food/food-labeling-nutrition/label-claims-food-dietary-supplements.

34. U.S. Food and Drug Administration. 2022. How to understand and use the nutrition facts label. Accessed October 2022. www.fda.gov/Food/IngredientsPackagingLabeling/LabelingNutrition/ucm274593.htm#overview.

35. Whitney, E., and S. Rady Rolfes. *Understanding nutrition*. 16th ed. Boston: Cengage.

36. World Anti-Doping Agency. n.d. *World Anti-Doping Agency*. Accessed October 2022. www.wada-ama.org/.

Chapter 6

1. Ainsworth, B.E., W.L. Haskell, S.D. Herrmann, N. Meckes, D.R. Bassett Jr., C. Tudor-Locke, J.L. Greer, J. Vezina, M.C. Whitt-Glover, and A.S. Leon. 2011. Compendium of Physical Activities: A second update of codes and MET values. *Medicine & Science in Sports & Exercise* 43(8): 1575-1581.

2. Ainsworth, B.E., W.L. Haskell, S.D. Herrmann, N. Meckes, D.R. Bassett Jr., C. Tudor-Locke, J.L. Greer, J. Vezina, M.C. Whitt-Glover, and A.S. Leon. Compendium of Physical Activities tracking guide. Healthy Lifestyles Research Center, College of Nursing & Health Innovation, Arizona State University. Accessed July 2022. https://sites.google.com/site/compendiumofphysicalactivities.

3. American College of Sports Medicine. (ACSM). 1980. *Guidelines for graded exercise testing and exercise prescription*. 2nd ed. Philadelphia: Lea & Febiger.

4. American College of Sports Medicine. (ACSM). 2006. *ACSM's guidelines for exercise testing and prescription*. 7th ed. Baltimore: Lippincott Williams & Wilkins.

5. American College of Sports Medicine. (ACSM). 2022. *ACSM's guidelines for exercise testing and prescription*. 11th ed. Philadelphia: Wolters Kluwer

6. Åstrand, P.-O. 1979. *Work tests with the bicycle ergometer*. Verberg, Sweden: Monark-Crescent AB.

7. Åstrand, P.-O., and K. Rodahl. 1986. *Textbook of work physiology*. 3rd ed. New York: McGraw-Hill.

8. Balke, B. 1963. A simple field test for assessment of physical fitness. In *Civil Aeromedical Research Institute report*, 63-66. Oklahoma City: Civil Aeromedical Research Institute.

9. Balke, B., and R.W. Ware. 1959. An experimental study of "physical fitness" of Air Force personnel. *Armed Forces Medical Journal* 10:675-688.

10. Bassett Jr., D.R., M.D. Giese, F.J. Nagle, A. Ward, D.M. Raab, and B. Balke. 1985. Aerobic requirements of overground versus treadmill running. *Medicine & Science in Sports & Exercise* 17:477-481.

11. Bransford, D.R., and E.T. Howley. 1977. The oxygen cost of running in trained and untrained men and women. *Medicine and Science in Sports* 9:41-44.

12. Bubb, W.J., A.D. Martin, and E.T. Howley. 1985. Predicting oxygen uptake during level walking at speeds of 80 to 130 meters per minute. *Journal of Cardiac Rehabilitation* 5(10): 462-465.

13. Bushman, B.A. 2020. Metabolic calculations in action: Part 1. *ACSM's Health & Fitness Journal* 24(3): 6-10. https://journals.lww.com/acsm-healthfitness/Fulltext/2020/05000/Metabolic_Calculations_in_Action__Part_1.5.aspx.

14. Bushman, B.A. 2020. Metabolic calculations in action: Part 2. *ACSM's Health & Fitness Journal* 24(4): 5-8.

15. Daniels, J.T. 1985. A physiologist's view of running economy. *Medicine & Science in Sports & Exercise* 17:332-338.

16. Dill, D.B. 1965. Oxygen cost of horizontal and grade walking and running on the treadmill. *Journal of Applied Physiology* 20:19-22.

17. Foster, C., A.J. Crowe, E. Daines, M. Dumit, M.A. Green, S. Lettau, N.N. Thompson, and J. Weymier. 1996. Predicting functional capacity during treadmill testing independent of exercise protocol. *Medicine & Science in Sports & Exercise* 6:752-756.

18. Foster, C., A.S. Jackson, M.L. Pollock, M.M. Taylor, J. Hare, S.M. Sennett, J.L. Rod, M. Sarwar, and D.H. Schmidt. 1984. Generalized equations for predicting functional capacity from treadmill performance. *American Heart Journal* 107:1229-1234.

19. Franklin, B.A. 1985. Exercise testing, training, and arm ergometry. *Sports Medicine* 2:100-119.

20. Haskell, W.L., W. Savin, N. Oldridge, and R. DeBusk. 1982. Factors influencing estimated oxygen uptake during exercise testing soon after myocardial infarction. *American Journal of Cardiology* 50:299-304.

21. Howley, E.T., and M.E. Glover. 1974. The caloric costs of running and walking 1 mile for men and women. *Medicine and Science in Sports* 6:235-237.

22. Knoebel, L.K. 1984. Energy metabolism. In *Physiology*, 5th ed., ed. E. Selkurt, 635-650. Boston: Little, Brown.

23. Lee, J-M., Y. Kim, and G.J. Welk. 2014. Validity of consumer-based physical activity monitors. *Medicine & Science in Sports & Exercise* 46:1840-1848.

24. Ludlow, L.W., and P.G. Weyand. 2016. Energy expenditure during level human walking: Seeking a simple and accurate predictive solution. *Journal of Applied Physiology* 120:481-494.

25. Margaria, R., P. Cerretelli, P. Aghemo, and J. Sassi. 1963. Energy cost of running. *Journal of Applied Physiology* 18:367-370.

26. McConnell, T.R., and B.A. Clark. 1987. Prediction of maximal oxygen consumption during handrail-supported treadmill exercise. *Journal of Cardiopulmonary Rehabilitation* 7:324-331.

27. Montoye, H.J., T. Ayen, F. Nagle, and E.T. Howley. 1986. The oxygen requirement for horizontal and grade walking on a motor-driven treadmill. *Medicine & Science in Sports & Exercise* 17:640-645.

28. Nagle, F.J., B. Balke, G. Baptista, J. Alleyia, and E. Howley. 1971. Compatibility of progressive treadmill, bicycle, and step tests based on oxygen-uptake responses. *Medicine and Science in Sport* 3:149-154.

29. Nagle, F.J., B. Balke, and J.P. Naughton. 1965. Gradational step tests for assessing work capacity. *Journal of Applied Physiology* 20:745-748.

30. Shei, R.-J., I.G. Holder, A.S. Oumsang, B.A. Paris, and H.L. Paris. 2022. Wearable activity trackers—advanced technology or advanced marketing? *European Journal of Applied Physiology* 21:1-16.

31. Storer, T.W., J.A. Davis, and V.J. Caiozzo. 1990. Accurate prediction of $\dot{V}O_2$max in cycle ergometry. *Medicine & Science in Sports & Exercise* 22:704-712.

32. U.S. Department of Health and Human Services. 2018. *Physical Activity Guidelines for Americans*, 2nd ed. https://health.gov/our-work/nutrition-physical-activity/physical-activity-guidelines/current-guidelines.

Chapter 7

1. American College of Sports Medicine (ACSM). 2022. *ACSM's guidelines for exercise testing and prescription.* 11th ed. Philadelphia: Wolters Kluwer.

2. American Heart Association and American Medical Association. n.d. Target: BP; Measure accurately. Accessed February 2023. https://targetbp.org/blood-pressure-improvement-program/control-bp/measure-accurately/

3. Balady, G.J., B. Chaitman, D. Driscoll, C. Foster, E. Froelicher, N. Gordon, R. Pate, et al. 1998. AHA/ACSM joint position statement: Recommendations on cardiovascular screening, staffing, and emergency policies at health/fitness facilities. *Medicine & Science in Sports & Exercise* 30(6):1009-1018.

4. Cooper Institute for Aerobics Research. 2017. *FitnessGram test administration manual.* 5th ed. Champaign, IL: Human Kinetics.

5. Eickhoff-Shemek, J.M. 2022. Establishing safety policies and procedures for fitness assessments: A major responsibility of fitness facility managers. *ACSM's Health & Fitness Journal* 26(5):100-102.

6. Garber, C.E., B. Blissmer, M.R. Deschenes, B.A. Franklin, M.J. Lamonte, I.-.M Lee, D.C. Nieman, and D.P. Swain. 2011. Quantity and quality of exercise for developing and maintaining cardiorespiratory, musculoskeletal, and neuromotor fitness in apparently healthy adults: Guidance for prescribing exercise. *Medicine & Science in Sports & Exercise* 43(7):1334-1359.

7. Rimmer, J.H. 2014. A focus and pathway to inclusive physical activity for people with disabilities. *Elevate Health* 4(15). https://health.gov/sites/default/files/2020-09/2014-october_elevate_health.pdf.

8. U.S. Department of Health and Human Services. 2018. *Physical Activity Guidelines for Americans.* 2nd ed. https://health.gov/our-work/nutrition-physical-activity/physical-activity-guidelines/current-guidelines.

Chapter 8

1. American College of Sports Medicine (ACSM). 2006. *ACSM's guidelines for exercise testing and prescription.* 7th ed. Philadelphia: Lippincott Williams & Wilkins.

2. American College of Sports Medicine (ACSM). 2022. *ACSM's fitness assessment manual.* 6th ed. Philadelphia: Wolters Kluwer.

3. American College of Sports Medicine (ACSM). 2022. *ACSM's guidelines for exercise testing and prescription.* 11th ed. Philadelphia: Wolters Kluwer

4. Andani, R., and Y.S. Khan. 2021. Anatomy, head and neck: Carotid sinus. National Library of Medicine. www.ncbi.nlm.nih.gov/books/NBK554378/.

5. Åstrand, I. 1960. Aerobic work capacity in men and women with special reference to age. *Acta Physiologica Scandinavica* 49(Suppl. 169):1-92.

6. Åstrand, P.-O. 1979. *Work tests with the bicycle ergometer.* Varberg, Sweden: Monark-Crescent AB.

7. Åstrand, P.-O. 1984. Principles of ergometry and their implications in sport practice. *International Journal of Sports Medicine* 5:102-105.

8. Åstrand, P.-O., and I. Ryhming. 1954. A nomogram for calculation of aerobic capacity (physical fitness) from pulse rate during submaximal work. *Journal of Applied Physiology* 7:218-221.

9. Åstrand, P.-O., and B. Saltin. 1961. Maximal oxygen uptake and heart rate in various types of muscular activity. *Journal of Applied Physiology* 16:977-981.

10. Balke, B. 1963. A simple field test for assessment of physical fitness. In *Civil Aeromedical Research Institute report*, 63-66. Oklahoma City: Civil Aeromedical Research Institute.

11. Balke, B. 1970. *Advanced exercise procedures for evaluation of the cardiovascular system.* Milton, WI: Burdick.

12. Blair, S.N., H.W. Kohl III, R.S. Paffenbarger Jr., D.G. Clark, K.H. Cooper, and L.W. Gibbons. 1989. Physical fitness and all-cause mortality. *Journal of the American Medical Association* 262:2395-2401.

13. Borg, G. 1998. *Borg's perceived exertion and pain scales.* Champaign, IL: Human Kinetics.

14. Bransford, D.R., and E.T. Howley. 1977. The oxygen cost of running in trained and untrained men and women. *Medicine and Science in Sports* 9:41-44.

15. Bruce, R.A. 1972. Multistage treadmill test of submaximal and maximal exercise. In *Exercise testing and training of apparently healthy individuals: A handbook for physicians*, ed. American Heart Association, 32-34. New York: American Heart Association.

16. Chun, D.M., C.B. Corbin, and R.P. Pangrazi. 2000. Validation of criterion-referenced standards for the mile run and progressive aerobic cardiovascular endurance tests. *Research Quarterly for Exercise and Sport* 71:125-134.

17. Cooper, K.H. 1977. *The aerobics way.* New York: Bantam Books.

18. Cooper Institute for Aerobics Research. 2017. *FitnessGram test administration manual.* 5th ed. Champaign, IL: Human Kinetics.

19. Cureton, K.J., S.A. Plowman, and M.T. Mahar. 2013. Aerobic capacity assessments. In *FitnessGram/ActivityGram reference guide*, ed. S.A. Plowman and M.D. Meredith, 4th ed., 6-1-6-22. Dallas: The Cooper Institute.

20. Cureton, K.J., M.A. Sloninger, J.P. O'Bannon, D.M. Black, and W.P. McCormack. 1995. A generalized equation for prediction of VO2peak from 1-mile run/walk performance. *Medicine & Science in Sports & Exercise* 27(3):445-451.

21. Daniels, J.T. 1985. A physiologist's view of running economy. *Medicine & Science in Sports & Exercise* 17:332-338.

22. Daniels, J., N. Oldridge, F. Nagle, and B. White. 1978. Differences and changes in $\dot{V}O_2$ among young runners 10-18 years of age. *Medicine and Science in Sports* 10:200-203.

23. Drake, S.M. 2014. Preparation for exercise testing. In *ACSM's resource manual for guidelines for exercise testing and prescription*, ed. D.P. Swain, 7th ed., 324-334. Baltimore: Lippincott Williams & Wilkins.

24. Ellestad, M. 1994. *Stress testing: Principles and practice.* Philadelphia: Davis.

25. Falco, M. 2021. Check the calibration of your sphyg. American Diagnostic Corporation. www.adctoday.com/blog/check-calibration-your-sphyg.

26. Fletcher G.F., P.A. Ades, P. Kligfield, R. Arena, G.J. Balady, V.A. Bittner, L.A. Coke, J.L. Fleg, D.E. Forman, T.C. Gerber, M. Gulati, K. Madan, J. Rhodes, P.D. Thompson, M.A. Williams, on behalf of the American Heart Association Exercise, Cardiac Rehabilitation, and Prevention Committee of the Council on Clinical Cardiology, Council on Nutrition, Physical Activity and Metabolism, Council on Cardiovascular and Stroke Nursing, and Council on Epidemiology and Prevention. 2013. Exercise standards for testing and training: A scientific statement from the American Heart Association. *Circulation* 128:873-934.

27. Flouris, A.D., G.S. Metsios, K. Famisis, N. Geladas, and Y. Koutedakis. 2010. Prediction of $\dot{V}O_2$max from a new field test based on portable indirect calorimetry. *Journal of Science and Medicine in Sport* 13:70-73.

28. Flynn, M.G., K.K. Carroll, H.L. Hall, B.A. Bushman, P.G. Brolinson, C.A. Weideman. 1998. Cross training: Indices of training stress and performance. *Medicine & Science in Sports & Exercise* 30(2): 294-300.

29. George, J.D., W.J. Stone, and L.N. Burkett. 1997. Nonexercise $\dot{V}O_2$max estimation for physically active college students. *Medicine & Science in Sports & Exercise* 29:415-423.

30. Golding, L.A. 2004. Convincing adults to exercise. *ACSM's Health & Fitness Journal* 8(6):7-11.

31. Hagberg, J.M., J.P. Mullin, M.D. Giese, and E. Spitznagel. 1981. Effect of pedaling rate on submaximal exercise responses of competitive cyclists. *Journal of Applied Physiology* 51:447-451.

32. Heil, D.P., P.S. Freedson, L.E. Ahlquist, J. Price, and J.M. Rippe. 1995. Nonexercise regression models to estimate peak oxygen consumption. *Medicine & Science in Sports & Exercise* 27:599-606.

33. Holland, A.E., M.A. Spruit, T. Troosters, M.A. Puhan, et al. 2014. An official European Respiratory Society/American Thoracic Society technical standard: Field walking tests in chronic respiratory disease. *European Respiratory Journal* 44(6):1428-46.

34. Howley, E.T. 1988. The exercise testing laboratory. In *Resource manual for guidelines for exercise testing and prescription*, ed. S.N. Blair, P. Painter, R.R. Pate, L.K. Smith, and C.B. Taylor, 406-413. Philadelphia: Lea & Febiger.

35. Jackson, A.S., S.N. Blair, M.T. Mahar, L.T. Wier, R.M. Ross, and J.E. Stuteville. Prediction of functional aerobic capacity without exercise testing. *Medicine & Science in Sports & Exercise* 22:863-870.

36. Kline, G.M., J.P. Porcari, R. Hintermeister, P.S. Freedson, A. Ward, R.F. McCarron, J. Ross, and J.M. Rippe. 1987. Estimation of $\dot{V}O_2$max from a 1-mile track walk, gender, age, and body weight. *Medicine & Science in Sports & Exercise* 19:253-259.

37. Lamb, K.L., and L. Rogers. 2007. A reappraisal of the reliability of the 20 m multistage shuttle run test. *European Journal of Applied Physiology* 100:287-292.

38. Leger, L.A., and J. Lambert. 1982. A maximal multistage 20 m shuttle run test to predict $\dot{V}O_2$max. *European Journal of Applied Physiology* 49:1-12.

39. Leger, L.A., D. Mercier, C. Gadoury, and J. Lambert. 1982. The multistage 20-meter shuttle run test for aerobic fitness. *Journal of Sport Science* 6:93-101.

40. Marchese, R.M., and Z. Geiger. 2022. Anatomy, shoulder and upper limb, forearm radial artery. National Library of Medicine. www.ncbi.nlm.nih.gov/books/NBK546626/.

41. Maritz, J.S., J.F. Morrison, J. Peter, N.B. Strydom, and C.H. Wyndham. 1961. A practical method of estimating an individual's maximal oxygen uptake. *Ergonomics* 4:97-122.

42. Matthews, C.E., D.P. Heil, P.S. Freedson, and H. Pastides. 1999. Classification of cardiorespiratory fitness without exercise testing. *Medicine & Science in Sports & Exercise* 31:486-493.

43. McArdle, W.D., F.I. Katch, and G.S. Pechar. 1973. Comparison of continuous and discontinuous treadmill and bicycle tests for max $\dot{V}O_2$. *Medicine and Science in Sports* 5(3):156-160.

44. McNaughton, L., P. Hall, and D. Cooley. 1998. Validation of several methods of estimating maximal oxygen uptake in young men. *Perceptual and Motor Skills* 87:575-584.

45. Montoye, H.J., and T. Ayen. 1986. Body-size adjustment for oxygen requirement in treadmill walking. *Research Quarterly for Exercise and Sport* 57:82-84.

46. Montoye, H.J., T. Ayen, F. Nagle, and E.T. Howley. 1985. The oxygen requirement for horizontal and grade walking on a motor-driven treadmill. *Medicine & Science in Sports & Exercise* 17:640-645.

47. Morris, D.C. 1990. The carotid pulse. In *Clinical methods: The history, physical, and laboratory examinations*, ed. H.K. Walker, W.D. Hall, and J.W. Hurst, 3rd ed. Boston: Butterworths. https://www.ncbi.nlm.nih.gov/books/NBK312/.

48. Muntner P., D. Shimbo, R.M. Carey, J.B. Charleston, T. Gaillard, S. Misra, G.M. Myers, G. Ogedegbe, J.E. Schwartz, R.R. Townsend, E.M. Urbina, A.J. Viera, W.B. White, and J.T. Wright Jr. on behalf of the American Heart Association Council on Hypertension; Council on Cardiovascular Disease in the Young; Council on Cardiovascular and Stroke Nursing; Council on Cardiovascular Radiology and Intervention; Council on Clinical Cardiology; and Council on Quality of Care and Outcomes Research. 2019. Measurement of blood pressure in humans: A scientific statement from the American Heart Association. *Hypertension* 73:e35-e66. https://doi.org/10.1161/HYP.0000000000000087.

49. Myers, J., D.E. Forman, G.J. Balady, B.A. Franklin, J. Nelson-Worel, B.-J. Martin, W.G. Herbert, et al., on behalf of the American Heart Association Subcommittee on Exercise, Cardiac Rehabilitation, and Prevention of the Council on Clinical Cardiology, Council on Lifestyle and Cardiometabolic Health, Council on Epidemiology and Prevention, and Council on Cardiovascular and Stroke Nursing. 2014. Supervision of exercise testing by nonphysicians: A scientific statement from the American Heart Association. *Circulation* 130:1014-1027.

50. Naughton, J.P., and R. Haider. 1973. Methods of exercise testing. In *Exercise testing and exercise training in coronary heart disease*, ed. J.P. Naughton, H.R. Hellerstein, and L.C. Mohler, 79-91. New York: Academic Press.

51. Paridon, S.M., B.S. Alpert, S.R. Boas, M.E. Cabrera, L.L. Cabrera, S.R. Daniels, T.R. Kimball, and et al. 2006. Clinical stress testing in the pediatric age group: A statement from the American Heart Association Council on Cardiovascular Disease in the Youth, Committee on Atherosclerosis, Hypertension, and Obesity in Youth. *Circulation* 113:1905-1920.

52. Pollock, M.L., and J.H. Wilmore. 1990. *Exercise in health and disease.* 2nd ed. Philadelphia: Saunders.

53. President's Council on Physical Fitness and Sports. 2002. *President's Challenge Physical Activity and Fitness Award Program*. Washington, DC: Author.

54. Rikli, R.E., and C.J. Jones. 2013. *Senior fitness test manual*. 2nd ed. Champaign IL: Human Kinetics.

55. Scott, S.N., D.L. Thompson, and D.P. Coe. 2013. The ability of the PACER to elicit peak exercise response in youth. *Medicine & Science in Sports & Exercise* 45:1139-1143.

56. Sharman, J.E., and A. LaGerche. 2014. Exercise blood pressure: Clinical relevance and correct measurement. *Journal of Human Hypertension* 29(6):351-358.

57. Shephard, R.J. 1970. Computer programs for solution of the Åstrand nomogram and the calculation of body surface area. *Journal of Sports Medicine and Physical Fitness* 10:206-210.

58. Strickland, M.K., S.R. Petersen, and M. Bouffard. 2003. Prediction of maximal aerobic power from the 20 m multistage shuttle run test. *Canadian Journal of Applied Physiology* 28:272-282.

59. U.S. Department of Health and Human Services. 2018. *Physical activity guidelines for Americans*. 2nd ed. https://health.gov/our-work/nutrition-physical-activity/physical-activity-guidelines/current-guidelines.

60. Weir, L.T., A.S. Jackson, G.W. Ayers, and B. Arenare. 2006. Nonexercise models for estimating $\dot{V}O_2$max with waist girth, percent fat, or BMI. *Medicine & Science in Sports & Exercise* 38:555-561.

61. Whaley, M.H., L.A. Kaminsky, G.B. Dwyer, and L.H. Getchell. 1995. Failure of predicted $\dot{V}O_2$peak to discriminate physical fitness in epidemiological studies. *Medicine & Science in Sports & Exercise* 27:85-91.

62. Whelton P., R. Carey, W. Aronow, et al. 2018. 2017 ACC/AHA/AAPA/ABC/ACPM/AGS/APhA/ASH/ASPC/NMA/PCNA guideline for the prevention, detection, evaluation, and management of high blood pressure in adults: Executive summary. *Journal of the American College of Cardiology* 71(19):2199-2269. https://doi.org/10.1016/j.jacc.2017.11.005.

63. Williford, H.N., M. Scharff-Olson, N. Wang, D.L. Blessing, F.H. Smith, and W.J. Duey. 1996. Cross-validation of nonexercise predictions of $\dot{V}O_2$peak in women. *Medicine & Science in Sports & Exercise* 28:926-930.

64. YMCA of the USA. 1989. *Y's way to physical fitness*. 3rd ed. L.A. Golding, C.R Myers, W.E. Sinning, editors. Champaign, IL: Human Kinetics.

65. YMCA of the USA. 2000. *YMCA fitness testing and assessment manual*. 4th ed. L.A Golding, editor. Champaign, IL: Human Kinetics.

Chapter 9

1. Abad, C., M. Prado, C. Ugrinowitsch, V. Tricoli, and R. Barroso. 2011. Combination of general and specific warm-ups improves leg-press one repetition maximum compared with specific warm-up in trained individuals. *Journal of Strength and Conditioning Research* 25:2242-2245.

2. Abdul-Hameed, U., P. Rangra, M.Y. Shareef, and M.E. Hussain. 2012. Reliability of 1-repetition maximum estimation for upper and lower body muscular strength measurement in untrained middle-aged type 2 diabetic patients. *Asian Journal of Sports Medicine* 3:267-273.

3. Alcazar, J., J. Losa-Reyna, C. Rodriguez-Lopez, A. Alfaro-Acha, L. Rodriguez-Mañas, I. Ara, F. García-García, and L. Alegre. 2018. The sit-to-stand muscle power test: An easy, inexpensive and portable procedure to assess muscle power in older people. *Experimental Gerontology* 112:38-43.

4. Amarante do Nascimento, M., R. Januário, A. Gerage, J. Mayhew, F. Cheche Pina, and E. Cyrino. 2013. Familiarization and reliability of one-repetition maximum strength testing in older women. *Journal of Strength and Conditioning Research* 27:1636-1642.

5. American College of Sports Medicine (ACSM). 2009. Exercise and physical activity for older adults. *Medicine & Science in Sports & Exercise* 41:1510-1530.

6. American College of Sports Medicine (ACSM). 2009. Progression models in resistance training for healthy adults. *Medicine & Science in Sports & Exercise* 41:687-708.

7. American College of Sports Medicine (ACSM). 2022. *ACSM's guidelines for exercise testing and prescription*. 11th ed. Baltimore: Lippincott Williams & Wilkins.

8. Artero, E., V. España-Romero, J. Castro-Piñero, J. Ruiz, D. Jiménez-Pavón, V. Aparicio, M. Gatto-Cardia, P. Baena, G. Vicente-Rodríguez, M.J. Castillo, and F.B. Ortega. 2012. Criterion-related validity of field-based muscular fitness tests in youth. *Journal of Sports Medicine and Physical Fitness* 52:263-272.

9. Barnard, K., K. Adams, A. Swank, E. Mann, and D. Denny. 1999. Injuries and muscle soreness during the one-repetition maximum assessment in a cardiac rehabilitation population. *Journal of Cardiopulmonary Rehabilitation* 19:52-58.

10. Belkhiria, C., G. De Marco, and T. Driss. 2018. Effects of verbal encouragement on force and electromyographic activations during exercise. *Journal of Sports Medicine and Physical Fitness* 58:750-757.

11. Bennie, J., K. De Cocker, J. Smith, and G. Wiesner. 2020. The epidemiology of muscle-strengthening exercise in Europe: A 28-country comparison including 280,605 adults. *PLoS One*. 15:e0242220.

12. Caruso, F., R. Arena, S. Phillips, J. Bonjorno, R. Mendes, V. Arakelian, D. Bassi, C. Nogi, and A. Borghi-Silva. 2015. Resistance exercise training improves heart rate variability and muscle performance: A randomized controlled trial in coronary artery disease patients. *European Journal of Physical and Rehabilitative Medicine* 51:281-289.

13. Castro-Piñero, J., F.B. Ortega, E.G. Artero, M.J. Girela-Rejón, J. Mora, M. Sjöström, and J.R. Ruiz. 2010. Assessing muscular strength in youth: Usefulness of standing long jump as a general index of muscular fitness. *Journal of Strength and Conditioning Research* 24:1810-1817.

14. Chaabene, H., D. Behm, Y. Negra, U. Granacher. 2019. Acute effects of static stretching on muscle strength and power: An attempt to clarify previous caveats. *Frontiers in Physiology* 10:1468.

15. Cogley, R., T. Archambault, J. Fibeger, M. Koverman, J. Youdas, and J. Hollman. 2005. Comparison of muscle activation using various hand positions during the push-up exercise. *Journal of Strength and Conditioning Research* 19:628-633.

16. Conkle, J. 2020. *Physical best: Physical education for lifelong health and fitness*. Champaign, IL: Human Kinetics.

17. Cornelissen, V., R. Fagard, E. Coeckelberghs, and L. Vanhees. 2011. Impact of resistance training on blood pressure and other cardiovascular risk factors: A meta-analysis of randomized, controlled trials. *Hypertension* 58:950-958.

18. Cronin, J., T. Lawton, N. Harris, A. Kilding, and D. McMaster. 2017. A brief review of handgrip strength and sport

performance. *Journal of Strength and Conditioning Research* 31:3187-3217.

19. Cuenca-Garcia, M., N. Marin-Jimenez, A. Perez-Bey, D. Sánchez-Oliva, D. Camiletti-Moiron, I. Alvarez-Gallardo, F. Ortega, and J. Castro-Piñero. 2022. Reliability of field-based fitness tests in adults: A systematic review. *Sports Medicine* 52:1961-1979.

20. Faigenbaum, A., R. Lloyd, and J. Oliver. 2020. *Essentials of youth fitness.* Champaign, IL: Human Kinetics.

21. Faigenbaum, A., and J. McFarland. 2014. Criterion repetition maximum testing. *Strength and Conditioning Journal* 36:88-91.

22. Faigenbaum, A., J. McFarland, R. Herman, F. Naclerio, N.A. Ratamess, J. Kang, and G. Myer. 2013. Reliability of the one-repetition-maximum power clean test in adolescent athletes. *Journal of Strength and Conditioning Research* 26:432-437.

23. Faigenbaum, A., L. Milliken, and W. Westcott. 2003. Maximal strength testing in healthy children. *Journal of Strength and Conditioning Research* 17:162-166.

24. Featherstone, J.F., R. Holly, and E. Amsterdam. 1993. Physiologic responses to weightlifting in coronary artery disease. *American Journal of Cardiology* 71:287-292.

25. Fernandez-Santos, J., J. Ruiz, D. Cohen, J. Gonzalez-Montesinos, and J. Castro-Piñero. 2015. Reliability and validity of tests to assess lower-body muscular power in children. *Journal of Strength and Conditioning Research.* 29:2277-2285.

26. Filipović, T., M. Lazović, A. Backović, A. Filipović, A. Ignjatović, S. Dimitrijević, and K. Gopćević. 2021. A 12-week exercise program improves functional status in postmenopausal osteoporotic women: Randomized controlled study. *European Journal of Physical and Rehabilitation Medicine* 57(1):120-130.

27. Fleck, S., and W. Kraemer. 2014. *Designing resistance training programs.* 4th ed. Champaign, IL: Human Kinetics.

28. Fleg, J., D. Forman, K. Berra, V. Bittner, J. Blumenthal, M. Chen, S. Cheng, D. Kitzman, M. Maurer, M. Rich, W. Shen, M. Williams, S. Zieman, and American Heart Association Committees on Older Populations and Exercise Cardiac Rehabilitation and Prevention of the Council on Clinical Cardiology, Council on Cardiovascular and Stroke Nursing, and Council on Lifestyle and Cardiometabolic Health. 2013. Secondary prevention of atherosclerotic cardiovascular disease in older adults: A scientific statement from the American Heart Association. *Circulation* 128:2422-2446.

29. Fletcher, G., P.A. Ades, P. Kligfield, R. Arena, G.J. Balady, V.A. Bittner, L.A. Coke, J.L. Fleg, D.E. Forman, T.C. Gerber, M. Gulati, K. Madan, J. Rhodes, P.D. Thompson, M.A. Williams, and American Heart Association Exercise, Cardiac Rehabilitation, and Prevention Committee of the Council on Clinical Cardiology, Council on Nutrition, Physical Activity and Metabolism, Council on Cardiovascular and Stroke Nursing, and Council on Epidemiology and Prevention. 2013. Exercise standards for testing and training: A scientific statement from the American Heart Association. *Circulation* 128:873-934.

30. Fragala, M., E. Cadore, S. Dorgo, M. Izquierdo, W. Kraemer, M. Peterson., and E. Ryan. 2019. Resistance training for older adults: Position statement from the National Strength and Conditioning Association. *Journal of Strength and Conditioning Research* 33:2019-2052.

31. Fukuda, D. 2019. *Assessments for sport and athletic performance.* Champaign, IL: Human Kinetics.

32. Garber, C., B. Blissmer, M.R. Deschenes, B.A. Franklin, M.J. Lamonte, I. Lee, D.C. Nieman, D.P. Swain, and American College of Sports Medicine (ACSM). 2011. American College of Sports Medicine position stand. Quantity and quality of exercise for developing and maintaining cardiorespiratory, musculoskeletal, and neuromotor fitness in apparently healthy adults: Guidance for prescribing exercise. *Medicine & Science in Sports & Exercise* 43:1334-1359.

33. Grgic, J., B. Lazinica, B. Schoenfeld,, and Z. Pedisic. 2020. Test-retest reliability of the one-repetition maximum (1RM) strength assessment: A systematic review. *Sports Medicine Open* 6:31.

34. Haff, G., and N. Triplett. 2016. *Essentials of strength training and conditioning.* Champaign, IL: Human Kinetics

35. Hollings, M., Y. Mavros, J. Freeston, and M. Fiatarone Singh. 2017. The effect of progressive resistance training on aerobic fitness and strength in adults with coronary heart disease: A systematic review and meta-analysis of randomised controlled trials. *European Journal of Preventive Cardiology* 24:1242-1259.

36. Hyde, E., G. Whitfield, J. Omura, J. Fulton, and S. Carlson. 2021. Trends in meeting the physical activity guidelines: Muscle-strengthening alone and combined with aerobic activity, United States, 1998-2018. *Journal of Physical Activity and Health* 18:S37-S44.

37. Jones, C.J., R.E. Rikli, and B.C. Beam. 1999. A 30 s chair-stand test as a measure of lower body strength in community residing older adults. *Research Quarterly for Exercise and Sports* 70:113-119.

38. Kerr, A., A. Clark, E. Cooke, P. Rowe, and V. Pomeroy. 2017. Functional strength training and movement performance therapy produce analogous improvement in sit-to-stand early after stroke: Early-phase randomised controlled trial. *Physiotherapy* 103:259-265.

39. Kirkman, D., D. Lee, and S. Carbone. 2022. Resistance exercise for cardiac rehabilitation. *Progress in Cardiovascular Disease* 70:66-72.

40. Klassen, O., M. Schmidt, C. Ulrich, A. Schneeweiss, K. Potthoff, K. Steindorf, and J. Wiskemann. 2017. Muscle strength in breast cancer patients receiving different treatment regimes. *Journal of Cachexia Sarcopenia and Muscle* 8:305-316.

41. Kuo, L. 2013. The influence of chair seat height on the performance of community-dwelling older adults' 30-second chair stand test. *Aging Clinical and Experimental Research* 25:305-309.

42. Leong, D., K. Teo, S. Rangarajan, A. Lopez-Jaramillo, A. Avezum, P. Orlandini, S. Seron, et al. 2015. Prognostic value of grip strength: findings from the Prospective Urban Rural Epidemiology (PURE) study. *Lancet* 386:266-273.

43. Lloyd, R., A. Faigenbaum, M. Stone, J. Oliver, I. Jeffreys, J.A. Moody, C. Brewer, K. Pierce, T. McCambridge, R. Howard, L. Herrington, B. Hainline, L. Micheli, R. Jaques, W. Kraemer, M. McBride, T. Best, D. Chu, B. Alvar, and G. Myer. 2014. Position statement on youth resistance training: The 2014 International Consensus. *British Journal of Sports Medicine* 48:498-505.

44. Lu, Y., G. Li, P. Ferrari, H. Freisling, Y. Qiao, L. Wu, L. Shao, and C. Ke, 2022. Associations of handgrip strength

with morbidity and all-cause mortality of cardiometabolic multimorbidity. *BMC Medical* 20:191.

45. Macht, J., M. Abel, D. Mullineaux, and J. Yates. 2016. Development of 1RM prediction equations for bench press in moderately trained men. *Journal of Strength and Conditioning Research* 30:2901-2906.

46. Martins, A., O. Fernandes, A. Pereira, R. Oliveira, F. Alderete Goñi, N. Leite, and J. Brito. 2022. The effects of high-speed resistance training on health outcomes in independent older adults: A systematic review and meta-analysis. *International Journal of Environmental Research and Public Health* 19:5390.

47. Mayhew, J., B. Johnson, M. Lamonte, D. Lauber, and W. Kemmler. 2008. Accuracy of prediction equations for determining one-repetition maximum bench press in women before and after resistance training. *Journal of Strength and Conditioning Research* 22:1570-1577.

48. McCrary, J., B. Ackermann., and M. Halaki. 2015. A systematic review of the effects of upper body warm-up on performance and injury. *British Journal of Sports Medicine* 49:935-942.

49. McGrath, R., P. Cawthon, B. Clark, R. Fielding, J. Lang, and G. Tomkinson. 2022. Recommendations for reducing heterogeneity in handgrip strength protocols. *Journal of Frailty and Aging* 11:143-150.

50. McGrath, R., W. Kraemer., S. Snih, and M. Peterson. 2018. Handgrip strength and health in aging adults. *Sports Medicine* 48:1993-2000.

51. Mcleod, J., T. Stokes, and S. Phillips. 2019. Resistance exercise training as a primary countermeasure to age-related chronic disease. *Frontiers in Physiology* 10:645.

52. Miller, W., S. Jeon, M. Kang, J. Song, and X. Ye. 2021. Does performance-related information augment the maximal isometric force in the elbow flexors? *Applied Psychophysiology and Biofeedback* 46:91-101.

53. Myer, G., C. Quatman, J. Khoury, E. Wall, and T.E. Hewett. 2009. Youth versus adult "weightlifting" injuries presenting to United States emergency rooms: Accidental versus nonaccidental injury mechanisms. *Journal of Strength and Conditioning Research* 23:2054-2060.

54. Nakamura, M., Y. Suzuki, R. Yoshida, K. Kasahara, Y. Murakami, T. Hirono, S. Nishishita, K. Takeuchi, and A. Konrad. 2022. The time-course changes in knee flexion range of motion, muscle strength, and rate of force development after static stretching. *Frontiers in Physiology* 13:917661.

55. Patti, A., L. Merlo, M. Ambrosetti, and P. Sarto. 2021. Exercise-based cardiac rehabilitation programs in heart failure patients. *Heart Failure Clinics* 17:263-271.

56. Plowman, S., and M. Meredith (Eds.). 2013. *FitnessGram/ActivityGram reference guide.* 4th ed. Dallas: The Cooper Institute.

57. Radaelli, R., G. Trajano, S. Freitas, M. Izquierdo, E. Cadore, and R. Pinto. 2023. Power training prescription in older individuals: Is it safe and effective to promote neuromuscular functional improvements? *Sports Medicine* 53:569-576

58. Ratamess, N. 2022. *ACSM's foundations of strength training and conditioning.* 2nd ed. Philadelphia: Wolters Kluwer.

59. Reynolds, J., T. Gordon, and R. Robergs. 2006. Prediction of one repetition maximum strength from multiple repetition maximum testing and anthropometry. *Journal of Strength and Conditioning Research* 20:584-592.

60. Rikli, R.E., and C.J. Jones. 1999. Development and validation of a functional fitness test for community residing older adults. *Journal of Aging and Physical Activity* 7:129-161.

61. Rikli, R., and C.J. Jones. 2013. Development and validation of criterion-referenced clinically relevant fitness standards for maintaining physical independence in later years. *Gerontologist* 53:255-267.

62. Rikli, R.E., and C.J. Jones. 2013. *Senior fitness test manual.* 2nd ed. Champaign, IL: Human Kinetics.

63. Ronai, P. 2020. The YMCA bench press test. *ACSM Health and Fitness Journal* 24:33-36.

64. Squires, R., L. Kaminsky, J. Porcari, J. Ruff, P. Savage, and W. Williams. 2018. Progression of exercise training in early outpatient cardiac rehabilitation: An official statement for the American Association of Cardiovascular and Pulmonary Rehabilitation. *Journal of Cardiopulmonary Rehabilitation and Prevention* 38:139-146.

65. Stricker, P., A. Faigenbaum, T. McCambridge, and the Council on Sports Medicine and Fitness. 2020. Resistance training for children and adolescents. *Pediatrics* 145:e20201011.

66. Suchomel, T., S. Nimphius, and M. Stone. 2016. The importance of muscular strength in athletic performance. *Sports Medicine* 46:1419-1449.

67. Tessier, A., S. Wing, E. Rahme, J. Morais, and S. Chevalier. 2019. Physical function-derived cut-points for the diagnosis of sarcopenia and dynapenia from the Canadian longitudinal study on aging. *Journal of Cachexia Sarcopenia and Muscle* 10:985-999.

68. Tomkinson, G., K. Carver, F. Atkinson, N. Daniell, L. Lewis, J. Fitzgerald, J. Lang, and F. Ortega. 2018. European normative values for physical fitness in children and adolescents aged 9-17 years: Results from 2779165 Eurofit performances representing 30 countries. *British Journal of Sports Medicine* 52:1445-14563.

69. United States Department of Health and Human Services (HHS). 2018. *Physical activity guidelines for Americans.* 2nd ed. Washington, DC: Author.

70. van den Tillaar, R. 2019. Comparison of kinematics and muscle activation between push-up and bench press. *Sports Medicine International Open* 3:E74-E81.

71. Westcott, W.L. 2012. Resistance training is medicine: Effects of strength training on health. *Current Sports Medicine Reports* 11:209-216.

72. Williams, M., W. Haskell, P. Ades, E. Amsterdam, V. Bittner, B. Franklin, M. Gulanick, S. Laing, K. Stewart, American Heart Association Council on Clinical Cardiology, and American Heart Association Council on Nutrition, Physical Activity, and Metabolism. Resistance exercise in individuals with and without cardiovascular disease: 2007 update: A scientific statement from the American Heart Association Council on Clinical Cardiology and Council on Nutrition, Physical Activity, and Metabolism. *Circulation* 116:572-584.

73. Wise, F.M., and J.M. Patrick. 2011. Resistance exercise in cardiac rehabilitation. *Clinical Rehabilitation* 25:1059-1065.

74. World Health Organization (WHO). 2020. *WHO guidelines on physical activity and sedentary behaviour.* Geneva: Author.

75. Yamamoto, S., K. Hotta, E. Ota, R. Mori, and A. Matsunaga. 2016. Effects of resistance training on muscle strength, exercise capacity, and mobility in middle-aged and elderly patients with coronary artery disease: A meta-analysis. *Journal of Cardiology* 68:125-34.

76. Yang, J., C. Christophi, A. Farioli, D. Baur, S. Moffatt, T. Zollinger, and S. Kales. 2019. Association between push-up exercise capacity and future cardiovascular events among active adult men. *JAMA Network Open* 2:e188341.

77. Yee, X., Y. Ng, J. Allen, A. Latib, E. Tay, H. Bakar, C. Ho, W. Koh, H. Kwek, and L. Tay. 2021. Performance on sit-to-stand tests in relation to measures of functional fitness and sarcopenia diagnosis in community-dwelling older adults. *European Review of Aging and Physical Activity* 18(1):1.

78. YMCA of the USA. 2000. *YMCA fitness testing and assessment manual*. 4th ed. L.A Golding, editor. Champaign, IL: Human Kinetics.

Chapter 10

1. Aigner, T., J. Rose, J. Martin, and J. Buckwalter. 2004. Aging theories of primary osteoarthritis: From epidemiology to molecular biology. *Rejuvenation Research* 7:134-145.

2. Akuthota, V., and S.F. Nadler. 2004. Core strengthening. *Archives of Physical Medicine and Rehabilitation* 85:S86-S92.

3. American College of Sports Medicine (ACSM). 2011. *ACSM's complete guide to fitness and health*. Champaign, IL: Human Kinetics.

4. American College of Sports Medicine (ACSM). 2018. *ACSM's guidelines for exercise testing and prescription*. 10th ed. Philadelphia: Lippincott Williams & Wilkins.

5. American College of Sports Medicine (ACSM). 2022. *ACSM's guidelines for exercise testing and prescription*. 11th ed. Philadelphia: Wolters Kluwer.

6. Arthritis Foundation. 2022. Arthritis facts. Accessed October 2022. www.arthritis.org.

7. Atamaz, F., B. Ozcaldiran, S. Ozdedeli, K. Capaci, and B. Durmaz. 2011. Interobserver and intraobserver reliability in lower-limb flexibility measurements. *Journal of Sports Medicine and Physical Fitness* 51:689-694.

8. Ayala, F., P. Sainz de Baranda, M. De Ste. Croix, F. and F. Santonja. 2012. Reproducibility and criterion-related validity of the sit and reach test and toe touch test for estimating hamstring flexibility in recreationally active young adults. *Physical Therapy in Sport* 13:219-226.

9. Baltaci, G., N. Un, V. Tunay, A. Besler, and S. Gerceker. 2003. Comparison of three different sit and reach tests for measurement of hamstring flexibility in female university students. *British Journal of Sports Medicine* 37:59-61.

10. Baykara, R.A., Z. Bozgeyik, O. Akgul, and S. Ozgocmen. 2013. Low back pain in patients with rheumatoid arthritis: Clinical characteristics and impact of low back pain on functional ability and health related quality of life. *Journal of Back and Musculoskeletal Rehabilitation* 26:367-374.

11. Biering-Sorensen, F. 1984. Physical measurements as risk indicators for low-back trouble over a one-year period. *Spine* 9:106-119.

12. Burton, A.K., K.M. Tillotson, and J.D.G. Troup. 1989. Variation in lumbar sagittal mobility with low-back trouble. *Spine* 14:584-590.

13. Bushman, B.A., and A. Robinett. 2022. Neuromotor exercise training: Background and benefits. *ACSM's Health & Fitness Journal* 26(4):5-9.

14. Caillet, R. 1988. *Low back pain syndrome*. Philadelphia: Davis.

15. Canadian Society for Exercise Physiology (CSEP). 2013. *CSEP physical activity training for health (CSEP-PATH) resource manual*. Ottawa: Canadian Society for Exercise Physiology.

16. Centers for Disease Control and Prevention (CDC). 2020. Osteoarthritis. Accessed October 2022. www.cdc.gov/arthritis/basics/osteoarthritis.htm.

17. Centers for Disease Control and Prevention (CDC). 2021. 4-stage balance test. https://www.cdc.gov/steadi/materials.html.

18. Centers for Disease Control and Prevention (CDC). 2022. Acute low back pain. https://www.cdc.gov/acute-pain/low-back-pain/index.html.

19. Centers for Disease Control and Prevention (CDC). 2022. Rheumatoid arthritis. Accessed October 2022. www.cdc.gov/arthritis/types/rheumatoid-arthritis.html.

20. Chanthapetch, P., R. Kanlayanaphotporn, C. Gaogasigam, and A. Chiradejnant. 2009. Abdominal muscle activity during abdominal hollowing in four starting positions. *Manual Therapy* 14:642-646.

21. Cho, M. 2013. The effects of modified wall squat exercises on average adults' deep abdominal muscle thickness and lumbar stability. *Journal of Physical Therapy Science* 25:689-692.

22. Cho, M. 2015. The effects of bridge exercise with the abdominal drawing-in maneuver on an unstable surface on the abdominal muscle thickness of healthy adults. *Journal of Physical Therapy Science* 27:255-257.

23. Cooper Institute for Aerobics Research. 1992. *The prudent FitnessGram*. Dallas: Author.

24. Cooper Institute for Aerobics Research. 2017. *FitnessGram test administration manual*. 5th ed. Champaign, IL: Human Kinetics.

25. Corkery, M., H. Briscoe, N. Ciccone, G. Foglia, P. Johnson, S. Kinsman, L. Legere, B. Lum, and P.K. Canavan. 2007. Establishing normal values for lower extremity muscle length in college-age students. *Physical Therapy in Sport* 8:66-74.

26. Dreischarf, M., L. Albiol, A. Rohlmann, E. Pries, M. Bashkuev, T. Zander, G. Duda, C. Druschel, P. Strube, M. Putzier, and H. Schmidt. 2014. Age-related loss of lumbar spinal lordosis and mobility—A study of 323 asymptomatic volunteers. *PLoS ONE* 9(12): e116186.

27. Duncan, P.W., D.K. Weiner, J. Chandler, S. Studenski. 1990. Functional reach: A new clinical measure of balance. *Journal of Gerontology* 45(6):M192-197.

28. Ellison, J.B., S.J. Rose, and S.A. Sahrmann. 1990. Patterns of hip rotation range of motion—A comparison between healthy subjects and patients with low-back pain. *Physical Therapy* 70:537-541.

29. Esola, M.A., P.W. McClure, G.K. Fitzgerald, and S. Siegler. 1996. Analysis of lumbar spine and hip motion during forward bending in subjects with and without a history of low back pain. *Spine* 21:71-78.

30. Faries, M.D., and M. Greenwood. 2007. Core training: Stabilizing the confusion. *Strength and Conditioning Journal* 29:10-25.

31. Ferber, R., K.D. Kendall, and L. McElroy. 2010. Normative and critical criteria for iliotibial band and iliopsoas muscle flexibility. *Journal of Athletic Training* 45:344-348.

32. Fishman, L.M. 2021. Yoga and bone health. *Orthopaedic Nursing*. 40:169-170.

33. Fujiwara, A., K. Tamai, M. Yamato, H.S. An, H. Yoshida, K. Saotome, and A. Kurihashi. 1999. The relationship between facet joint osteoarthritis and disc degeneration of

the lumbar spine: An MRI study. *European Spine Journal* 8:396-401.

34. Garber, C.E., B. Blissmer, M.R. Deschenes, B.A. Franklin, M.J. Lamonte, I.-M. Lee, D.C. Nieman, and D.P. Swain. 2011. Quantity and quality of exercise for developing and maintaining cardiorespiratory, musculoskeletal, and neuromotor fitness in apparently healthy adults: Guidance for prescribing exercise. *Medicine & Science in Sports & Exercise* 43(7):1334-1359.

35. Gellhorn, A.C., J.N. Katz, and P. Suri. 2013. Osteoarthritis of the spine: The facet joints. *Nature Reviews Rheumatology* 9:216-224.

36. Golding, L.A. and C.R. Myers. 1989. *Y's way to physical fitness: The complete guide to fitness testing and instruction.* Champaign, IL: Human Kinetics.

37. Gulick, D. 2009. *Ortho notes: Clinical examination pocket guide.* Philadelphia: F.A. Davis Company.

38. Hamid, M.S.A., M.R.M. Ali, and A. Yusof. 2013. Interrater and intrarater reliability of the active knee extension (AKE) test among healthy adults. *Journal of Physical Therapy Science* 25:957-961.

39. Hasebe, K., K. Sairyo, Y. Hada, A. Dezawa, Y. Okubo, K. Kaneoka, and Y. Nakamura. 2014. Spino-pelvic rhythm with forward trunk bending in normal subjects without low back pain. *European Journal of Orthopaedic Surgery and Traumatology* 24(Suppl. 1):S193-199.

40. Hides, J., W. Stanton, M.D. Mendis, and M. Sexton. 2011. The relationship of transversus abdominis and lumbar multifidus clinical muscle tests in patients with chronic low back pain. *Manual Therapy* 16:573-577.

41. Hides, J., S. Wilson, W. Stanton, S. McMahon, H, Keto, K. McMahon, M. Bryant, and C. Richardson. 2006. An MRI investigation into the function of the transversus abdominis muscle during "drawing-in" of the abdominal wall. *Spine* 31:E175-E178.

42. Hodges, P.W. 1999. Is there a role for transversus abdominis in lumbo-pelvic stability? *Manual Therapy* 4:74-86.

43. Hodges, P.W., J.E. Butler, D.K. McKenzie, and S.C. Gandevia. 1997. Contraction of the human diaphragm during rapid postural adjustments. *Journal of Physiology* 505(Pt. 2):539-548.

44. Huang, Z.-G., Y.-H. Feng, Y.-H. Li, and C.-S. Lv. 2016. Systematic review and meta-analysis: Tai Chi for preventing falls in older adults. *BMJ Open* 7:e013661. https://doi.org/10.1136/bmjopen-2016-013661.

45. Hui, S.S., and P.Y. Yuen. 2000. Validity of the modified back-saver sit-and-reach test: A comparison with other protocols. *Medicine & Science in Sports & Exercise* 32:1655-1659.

46. International Association for the Study of Pain. 2021. The global burden of low back pain. www.iasp-pain.org/resources/fact-sheets/the-global-burden-of-low-back-pain/

47. International Osteoporosis Foundation (IOF). 2022. What is osteoporosis? Accessed October 2022. https://www.osteoporosis.foundation/patients/about-osteoporosis

48. Intolo, P., S. Milosavljevic, D.G. Baxter, A.B. Carman, P. Pal, and J. Munn. 2009. The effect of age on lumbar range of motion: A systematic review. *Manual Therapy* 14:596-604.

49. Jahnke, R., L. Larkey, C. Rogers, J. Etnier, and F. Lin. 2010. A comprehensive review of health benefits of qigong and tai chi. *American Journal of Health Promotion* 41:e1-e25.

50. Jeong, H.S., S.-C. Lee, J. Hyunseok, J.B. Song, H.S. Chang, and S.Y. Lee. 2019. Proprioceptive training and outcomes of patients with knee osteoarthritis: A meta-analysis of randomized controlled trials. *Journal of Athletic Training* 54:148-428.

51. Jones, C.J., and R.E. Rikli. 2002. Measuring functional fitness of older adults. *Journal on Active Aging* 3(5):24-30.

52. Kang, M.-H., D.-H. Jung, D.-H. An, W.-G. Yoo, and J.-S. Oh. 2013. Acute effects of hamstring-stretching exercises on the kinematics of the lumbar spine and hip during stoop lifting. *Journal of Back and Musculoskeletal Rehabilitation* 26:329-336.

53. Kendall, F.P., E.K. McCreary, and P.G. Provance. 1993. *Muscles: Testing and function.* Philadelphia: Lippincott Williams & Wilkins.

54. Kippers, V., and A.W. Parker. 1987. Toe-touch test: A measure of its validity. *Physical Therapy* 67:1680-1684.

55. Koushyar, H., K.A. Bieryla, M.A. Mussbaum, and M.L. Madigan. 2019. Age-related strength loss affects non-stepping balance recovery. *PLoS ONE* 14(1):e0210049. https://doi.org/10.1371/journal.pone.0210049.

56. Kweon, M., S. Hong, G.U. Jang, Y.M. Ko, and J.W. Park. 2013. The neural control of spinal stability muscles during different respiratory patterns. *Journal of Physical Therapy Science* 25:1421-1424.

57. Lesinski, M., T. Hortobagyi, T. Muehlbauer, and A. Gollhoffer. 2015. Effects of balance training on balance performance in healthy older adults: A systematic review and meta-analysis. *Sports Medicine* 45:1721-1738.

58. Li, W.S., S.B. Wang, Q. Xia, P. Passias, M. Kozanek, K. Wood, and G.A. Li. 2011. Lumbar facet joint motion in patients with degenerative disc disease at affected and adjacent levels: An in vivo biomechanical study. *Spine* 36:E629-E637.

59. Liemohn, W., S.B. Martin, and G.L. Pariser. 1997. The effect of ankle posture on sit-and-reach test performance. *Journal of Strength and Conditioning Research* 11:239-241.

60. Martin, S.B., A. Jackson, J.R. Morrow, and W. Liemohn. 1998. The rationale for the sit-and-reach test revisited. *Measurement in Physical Education and Exercise Science* 2:85-92.

61. Mayer, T.G., A.F. Tencer, S. Kristoferson, and V. Mooney. 1984. Use of noninvasive techniques for quantification of spinal range-of-motion in normal subjects and chronic low-back dysfunction patients. *Spine* 9:588-595.

62. Mayorga-Vega, D., R. Merino-Marban, and J. Viciana. 2014. Criterion-related validity of sit-and-reach tests for estimating hamstring and lumbar extensibility: A meta-analysis. *Journal of Sports Science and Medicine* 13:1-14.

63. McGill, S. 2004. *Ultimate back fitness and performance.* Waterloo, ON: Wabuno.

64. McGill, S.M., V.R. Yingling, and J.P. Peach. 1999. Three-dimensional kinematics and trunk muscle myoelectric activity in the elderly spine—A database compared to young people. *Clinical Biomechanics* 14:389-395.

65. Medeiros, H.B.D., D. de Araujo, and C.G.S. de Araujo. 2013. Age-related mobility loss is joint-specific: An analysis from 6,000 Flexitest results. *Age* 35:2399-2407.

66. Mookerjee, S., and M.J. McMahon. 2014. Electromyographic analysis of muscle activation during sit-and-reach flexibility tests. *Journal of Strength and Conditioning Research* 28:3496-3501.

67. Nachemson, A. 1975. Towards a better understanding of low back pain: A review of the mechanics of the lumbar spine. *Rheumatology and Rehabilitation* 14:129-143.

68. Nadler, S.F., G.A. Malanga, M. DePrince, T.P. Stitik, and J.H. Feinberg. 2000. The relationship between lower extremity injury, low back pain, and hip muscle strength in male and female collegiate athletes. *Clinical Journal of Sport Medicine* 10:89-97.

69. Nadler, S.F., G.A. Malanga, J.H. Feinberg, M. Prybicien, T.P. Stitik, and M. DePrince. 2001. Relationship between hip muscle imbalance and occurrence of low back pain in collegiate athletes: A prospective study. *American Journal of Physical Medicine and Rehabilitation* 80:572-577.

70. Nordin, M.F.V. 2001. *Basic biomechanics of the musculoskeletal system*. Philadelphia: Lippincott Williams & Wilkins.

71. Osteoarthritis Action Alliance. 2022. OA prevalence and burden. https://oaaction.unc.edu/oa-module/oa-prevalence-and-burden/.

72. Richardson, C.A., C.J. Snijders, J.A. Hides, L. Damen, M.S. Pas, and J. Storm. 2002. The relation between the transversus abdominis muscles, sacroiliac joint mechanics, and low back pain. *Spine* 27:399-405.

73. Rikli, R.E., and C.J. Jones. 2013. *Senior Fitness Test manual*. 2nd ed. Champaign IL: Human Kinetics.

74. Rozanska-Kirschke, A., P. Kocur, M. Wilk, and P. Dylewicz. 2006. The Fuller Fitness Test as an index of fitness in the elderly. *Medical Rehabilitation* 10:9-16.

75. Saal, J., and J. Saal. 1991. Strength training and flexibility. In *The conservative care of low back pain*, ed. A.H. White and R. Anderson, 65-77. Baltimore: Williams & Wilkins.

76. Sahrmann, S. 2001. *Diagnosis and treatment of movement impairment syndromes*. Maryland Heights, MD: Mosby.

77. Springer, B.A., R. Marin, T. Cyhan, H. Roberts, and N.W. Gill. 2007. Normative values for the unipedal stance test with eyes open and closed. *Journal of Geriatric Physical Therapy* 30(1):8-15.

78. Tidstrand, J., and E. Horneij. 2009. Inter-rater reliability of three standardized functional tests in patients with low back pain. *BMC Musculoskeletal Disorders* 10(58). https://doi.org/10.1186/1471-2474-10-58.

79. Troke, M., A.P. Moore, F.J. Maillardet, and E. Cheek. 2005. A normative database of lumbar spine ranges of motion. *Manual Therapy* 10:198-206.

80. Urquhart, D.M., P.W. Hodges, T.J. Allen, and I.H. Story. 2005. Abdominal muscle recruitment during a range of voluntary exercises. *Manual Therapy* 10:144-153.

81. Wagner, A.R., O. Akinsola, A.M.W. Chaudhari, K.E. Bigelow, and D.M. Merfeld. 2021. Measuring vestibular contributions to age-related balance impairment: A review. *Frontiers in Neurology* 12:635305. https://doi.org/10.3389/fneur.2021.635305.

Chapter 11

1. Ackland, T.R., T.G. Lohman, J. Sundgot-Borgen, R.J. Maughan, N.L. Meer, A.D. Stewart, and W. Müller. 2012. Current status of body composition in sports: Review and position statement on behalf of the Ad Hoc Research Working Group on Body Composition Health and Performance, under the auspices of the I.O.C. Medical Commission. *Sports Medicine* 42(3):227-249.

2. American College of Sports Medicine (ACSM). 2022. *ACSM's guidelines for exercise testing and prescription*. 11th ed. Philadelphia: Wolters Kluwer.

3. American College of Sports Medicine (ACSM), T.G. Lohman, and L.A. Milliken. 2020. *ACSM's body composition assessment*. Champaign IL: Human Kinetics.

4. Caleyachetty, R., T.M. Barber, N.I. Mohammad, F.P. Cappuccio, R. Hardy, R. Mathur, A. Banerjee, and P. Gill. 2021. Ethnicity-specific BMI cutoffs for obesity based on type 2 diabetes risk in England: A population-based cohort study. *The Lancet: Diabetes & Endocrinology* 9(7):P419-426.

5. Cataldo, D., and V.H. Heyward. 2000. Pinch an inch: A comparison of several high-quality and plastic skinfold calipers. *ACSM's Health and Fitness Journal* 4:12-16.

6. Centers for Disease Control and Prevention. 2017. Clinical growth charts. www.cdc.gov/growthcharts/clinical_charts.htm#Set1.

7. Centers for Disease Control and Prevention. 2022. About adult BMI. www.cdc.gov/healthyweight/assessing/bmi/adult_bmi/index.html.

8. Centers for Disease Control and Prevention. 2022. Adult obesity facts. www.cdc.gov/obesity/data/adult.html.

9. Centers for Disease Control and Prevention. 2022. BMI percentile calculator for child and teen. www.cdc.gov/healthyweight/bmi/calculator.html.

10. Centers for Disease Control and Prevention. 2022. Childhood obesity facts. www.cdc.gov/obesity/data/childhood.html.

11. Cornier, M.-A., J.-P. Despres, N. Davis, D.A. Grossniklaus, S. Klein, B. Lamarche, F. Lopez-Jimenez, G. Rao, M.-P. St.-Onge, A. Towfighi, and P. Poirier. 2011. Assessing adiposity: A scientific statement from the American Heart Association. *Circulation* 124:1996-2019.

12. Flegal, K.M., B.K. Kit, H. Orpana, and B.I. Graubard. 2013. Association of all-cause mortality with overweight and obesity using standard body mass index categories: A systematic review and meta-analysis. *Journal of the American Medical Association* 309(1):71-82.

13. Goldman, H.I., and M.R. Becklake. 1959. Respiratory function tests. *American Review of Tuberculosis and Pulmonary Disease* 79:457-467.

14. Heyward, V.H., and D.R. Wagner. 2004. *Applied body composition assessment*. 2nd ed. Champaign, IL: Human Kinetics.

15. Jackson, A.S., and M.L. Pollock. 1978. Generalized equations for predicting body density of men. *British Journal of Nutrition* 40:497-504.

16. Jackson, A.S., and M.L. Pollock. 1985. Practical assessment of body composition. *Physician and Sportsmedicine* 13:76-90.

17. Jackson, A.S., M.L. Pollock, and A. Ward. 1980. Generalized equations for predicting body density of women. *Medicine & Science in Sports & Exercise* 12:175-182.

18. National Institute for Health and Care Excellence. 2022. Obesity: Identification, assessment and management: Clinical guideline 189. www.nice.org.uk/guidance/cg189/chapter/Recommendations#identifying-and-assessing-overweight-obesity-and-central-adiposity.

19. Noel, S.E., M.P. Santos, and N.C. Wright, N.C. 2021. Racial and ethnic disparities in bone health and outcomes in the United States. *Journal of Bone and Mineral Research* 36:1881-1905.

20. Ogden, C.L., and K.M. Flegal. 2010. Changes in terminology for childhood overweight and obesity. *National Health Statistics Reports* 25:1-5.

21. Powell-Whiley, T.M., P. Poirier, L.E. Burke, J.-P. Despres, P. Gordon-Larsen, C.J. Lavie, S.A. Lear, et al. 2021. Obesity and cardiovascular disease: A scientific statement from the American Heart Association. *Circulation* 143(21):e984-1010.

22. Ratamess, N. 2014. Body composition status and assessment. In *ACSM's resource manual for guidelines for exercise testing and prescription*, ed. D.P. Swain, 287-308. 7th ed. Baltimore: Lippincott Williams & Wilkins.

23. Serviente, C., and G.A. Sforzo. 2013. A simple yet complicated tool: Measuring waist circumference to determine cardiometabolic risk. *ACSM's Health & Fitness Journal* 17(6):29-34.

24. Siri, W.E. 1961. Body composition from fluid spaces and density: Analysis of methods. In *Techniques for measuring body composition*, ed. J. Brozek and A. Henschel, 223-244. Washington, DC: National Academy of Sciences.

25. Williams, M.H. 2007. *Nutrition for health, fitness, and sport*. 8th ed. New York: McGraw-Hill.

26. Wilmore, J. 1969. A simplified method for determination of residual volume. *Journal of Applied Physiology* 27:96-100.

27. World Health Organization. 2021. Obesity and overweight. www.who.int/news-room/fact-sheets/detail/obesity-and-overweight.

Chapter 12

1. American College of Sports Medicine (ACSM). 2022. *ACSM's guidelines for exercise testing and prescription*. 11th ed. Philadelphia: Wolters Kluwer.

2. American College of Sports Medicine (ACSM) and American Heart Association (AHA). 2002. Joint position statement: Automated external defibrillators in health/fitness facilities. *Medicine & Science in Sports & Exercise* 34(3):561-564.

2a. American Heart Association. 2015. Heart attack symptoms in women. www.heart.org/en/health-topics/heart-attack/warning-signs-of-a-heart-attack/heart-attack-symptoms-in-women.

3. American Hospital Formulary Service. 2015. *Drug information 2015*. Bethesda, MD: American Society of Hospital Pharmacists.

4. Berne, R.M., and M.N. Levy. 2001. *Cardiovascular physiology*. 8th ed. St. Louis: Mosby.

5. Chang, K., and K.F. Hossack. 1982. Effect of diltiazem on heart rate responses and respiratory variables during exercise: Implications for exercise prescription and cardiac rehabilitation. *Journal of Cardiac Rehabilitation* 2:326-332.

6. Conover, M.B. 1996. *Understanding electrocardiography*. 7th ed. St. Louis: Mosby.

7. Donnelly, J.E. 1990. *Living anatomy*. 2nd ed. Champaign, IL: Human Kinetics.

8. Dubin, D. 2000. *Rapid interpretation of EKGs*. 6th ed. Tampa: Cover.

9. Ellestad, M.H. 2003 *Stress testing: Principles and practice*. 5th ed. New York: Oxford University Press.

9a. Huff, J. 2022. *ECG workout: Exercises in arrhythmia interpretation*. 8th ed. Philadelphia: Wolters Kluwer Health.

10. Hurst, J.W. 1994. *Diagnostic atlas of the heart*. Philadelphia: Lippincott-Raven.

11. Kannel, W.B., and R.D. Abbot. 1984. Incidence and prognosis of unrecognized myocardial infarction. *New England Journal of Medicine* 311:1144-1147.

12. Stein, E. 2000. *Rapid analysis of electrocardiograms: A self-study program*. 3rd ed. Philadelphia: Lea & Febiger.

Chapter 13

1. American College of Sports Medicine (ACSM). 2006. Prevention of cold injuries during exercise. *Medicine & Science in Sports & Exercise* 38:2012-2029.

2. American College of Sports Medicine (ACSM). 2007. Exertional heat illness during training and competition. *Medicine & Science in Sports & Exercise* 39:556-572.

3. American College of Sports Medicine (ACSM). 2011. The recommended quantity and quality of exercise for developing and maintaining cardiorespiratory, musculoskeletal, and neuromotor fitness in apparently healthy adults: Guidance for prescribing exercise. *Medicine & Science of Sports & Exercise* 43(7):1334-1359.

4. American College of Sports Medicine (ACSM). 2018. *ACSM's guidelines for exercise testing and prescription*. 10th ed. Philadelphia: Lippincott Williams & Wilkins.

5. American College of Sports Medicine (ACSM). 2022. *ACSM's guidelines for exercise testing and prescription*. 11th ed. Philadelphia: Wolters Kluwer.

6. American College of Sports Medicine, American Dietetic Association, Dietitians of Canada. 2009. Joint position stand. Nutrition and athletic performance. *Medicine & Science in Sports & Exercise* 41(3):709-31.

7. Blair, S.N., H.W. Kohl III, R.S. Paffenbarger Jr., D.G. Clark, K.H. Cooper, and L.W. Gibbons. 1989. Physical fitness and all-cause mortality. *Journal of the American Medical Association* 262:2395-2401.

8. Borg, G. 1998. *Borg's perceived exertion and pain scales*. Champaign, IL: Human Kinetics.

9. Burton, A.C., and O.G. Edholm. 1955. *Man in a cold environment*. London: Edward Arnold.

10. Buskirk, E.R., and D.E. Bass. 1974. Climate and exercise. In *Science and medicine of exercise and sport*, ed. W.R. Johnson and E.R. Buskirk, 190-205. New York: Harper & Row.

11. Campbell, M.E., Q. Li, S.E. Gingrich, R.G. Macfarlane, and S. Cheng. 2005. Should people be physically active outdoors on smog alert days? *Canadian Journal of Public Health* 96:24-28.

12. Campbell, W.W., W.E. Kraus, and K.E. Powell, et al. for the 2018 Physical Activity Guidelines Advisory Committee. 2019. High-intensity interval training for cardiometabolic disease prevention. *Medicine & Science in Sports & Exercise* 51(6):1220-1226.

13. Dehn, M.M., and C.B. Mullins. 1977. Physiologic effects and importance of exercise in patients with coronary artery disease. *Cardiovascular Medicine* 2:365.

14. Derby, R., and K. deWeber. 2010. The athlete and high altitude. *Current Sports Medicine Reports* 9(2):79-85.

15. Dionne, F.T., L. Turcotte, M.-C. Thibault, M.R. Boulay, J.S. Skinner, and C. Bouchard. 1991. Mitochondrial DNA sequence polymorphism, $\dot{V}O_2$max, and response to endurance training. *Medicine & Science in Sports & Exercise* 23:177-185.

16. Drinkwater, B.L., J.E. Denton, I.C. Kupprat, T.S. Talag, and S.M. Horvath. 1976. Aerobic power as a factor in women's response to work within hot environments. *Journal of Applied Physiology* 41:815-821.

17. Exercise is Medicine. 2021. Exercise is Medicine: A global health initiative. www.exerciseismedicine.org.

18. Exercise is Medicine. 2021. Exercise professionals: Expanding the reach of health care. www.exerciseismedicine.org/eim-in-action/exercise-professionals/.

19. Folinsbee, L.J. 1990. Discussion: Exercise and the environment. In *Exercise, fitness, and health*, ed. C. Bouchard, R.J. Shephard, T. Stephens, J.R. Sutton, and B.D. McPherson, 179-183. Champaign, IL: Human Kinetics.

20. Fountaine, C.J. 2021. Introduction to high-intensity interval training and chronic diseases. *ACSM's Health & Fitness Journal* 25(5):11-12.

21. Frampton, M.W., M.J. Utell, W. Zareba, G. Oberdorster, C. Cox, L.S. Huang, P.E. Morrow, F.E. Lee, D. Chalupa, L.M. Frasier, D.M. Speers, and J. Stewart. 2004. Effects of exposure to ultrafine carbon particles in healthy subjects and subjects with asthma. *Research Report—Health Effects Institute* 126:1-63.

22. Garber, C.E., B. Blissmer, M.R. Deschenes, B.A. Franklin, M.J. Lamonte, I.-M. Lee, D.C. Nieman, and D.P. Swain. 2011. Quantity and quality of exercise for developing and maintaining cardiorespiratory, musculoskeletal, and neuromotor fitness in apparently healthy adults: Guidance for prescribing exercise. *Medicine & Science in Sports & Exercise* 43(7):1334-1359.

23. Gellish, R.L., B.R. Golsin, R.E. Olson, A. McDonald, G.D. Russi, and V.K. Moudgil. 2007. Longitudinal modeling of the relationship between age and maximal heart rate. *Medicine & Science in Sports & Exercise* 39(5):822-829.

24. Gisolfi, G.V., and J. Cohen. 1979. Relationships among training, heat acclimation, and heat tolerance in men and women: The controversy revisited. *Medicine & Science in Sports & Exercise* 11:56-59.

25. Goodman, L.S., and A. Gilman, eds. 1975. *The pharmacological basis of therapeutics*. New York: Macmillan.

26. Grover, R., J. Reeves, E. Grover, and J. Leathers. 1967. Muscular exercise in young men native to 3,100 m altitude. *Journal of Applied Physiology* 22:555-564.

27. Hardy, J.D., and P. Bard. 1974. Body temperature regulation. In vol. 2 of *Medical physiology*, 13th ed., ed. V.B. Mountcastle, 1305-1342. St. Louis: Mosby.

28. Haskell, W.L. 1978. Design and implementation of cardiac conditioning programs. In *Rehabilitation of the coronary patient*, ed. N.K. Wenger and H.K. Hellerstein, 203-241. New York: Wiley.

29. Haskell, W.L. 1984. The influence of exercise on the concentrations of triglyceride and cholesterol in human plasma. *Exercise and Sport Sciences Reviews* 12:205-244.

30. Haskell, W.L. 2001. What to look for in assessing responsiveness to exercise in a health context. *Medicine & Science in Sports & Exercise* 33:S454-S458.

31. Haskell, W.L., I.-M. Lee, R.R. Pate, K.E. Powell, S.N. Blair, B.A. Franklin, C.A. Macera, G.W. Heath, P.D. Thompson, and A. Bauman. 2007. Physical activity and public health: Updated recommendations for adults from the American College of Sports Medicine and the American Heart Association. *Medicine & Science in Sports & Exercise* 39:1423-1434.

32. Hayward, M.G., and W.R. Keatinge. 1981. Roles of subcutaneous fat and thermoregulatory reflexes in determining ability to stabilize body temperature in water. *Journal of Physiology* 320:229-251.

33. Hellerstein, H.K., and B.A. Franklin. 1984. Exercise testing and prescription. In *Rehabilitation of the coronary patient*, 2nd ed., ed. N.K. Wenger and H.K. Hellerstein, 197-284. New York: Wiley.

34. Holmer, I. 1979. Physiology of swimming man. *Exercise and Sport Sciences Reviews* 7:87-123.

35. Horvath, S.M. 1981. Exercise in a cold environment. *Exercise and Sport Sciences Reviews* 9:221-263.

36. Horvath, S.M., P.R. Raven, T.E. Dahms, and D.J. Gray. 1975. Maximal aerobic capacity of different levels of carboxyhemoglobin. *Journal of Applied Physiology* 38:300-303.

37. Howley, E.T. 1980. Effect of altitude on physical performance. In *Encyclopedia of physical education, fitness, and sports: Training, environment, nutrition, and fitness*, ed. G.A. Stull and T.K. Cureton, 177-187. Salt Lake City: Brighton.

38. Howley, E.T. 2001. Type of activity: Resistance, aerobic and leisure versus occupational physical activity. *Medicine & Science in Sports & Exercise* 33:S364-S369.

39. Jennings, G.L., G. Deakin, P. Korner, I. Meredith, B. Kingwell, and L. Nelson. 1991. What is the dose–response relationship between exercise training and blood pressure? *Annals of Medicine* 23:313-318.

40. Karlsen, T., I.-L. Aamot, M. Haykowsky, and Ø. Rognmo. 2017. High intensity interval training for maximizing health outcomes. *Progress in Cardiovascular Diseases* 60:67-77.

41. Karstoft, K., K. Winding, S.H. Knudsen, J.S. Nielsen, C. Thomsen, B.K. Pedersen, and T.P.J. Solomon. 2013. The effects of free-living interval-walking training on glycemic control, body composition, and physical fitness in type 2 diabetic patients. *Diabetes Care* 36(2):228-236.

42. Karvonen, M.J., E. Kentala, and O. Mustala. 1957. The effects of training heart rate: A longitudinal study. *Annales Medicinae Experimentalis et Biologiae Fenniae* 35:307-315.

43. Kesaniemi, Y.K., E. Danforth Jr., M.D. Jensen, P.G. Kopelman, P. Lefèbvre, and B.A. Reeder. Dose–response issues concerning physical activity and health: An evidence-based symposium. 2001. *Medicine & Science in Sports & Exercise* 33(6 Suppl.):S351-358.

44. Londeree, B.R., and S.A. Ames. 1976. Trend analysis of the %$\dot{V}O_2$max-HRregression. *Medicine and Science in Sports* 8:122-125.

45. Londeree, B.R., and M.L. Moeschberger. 1982. Effect of age and other factors on maximal heart rate. *Research Quarterly for Exercise and Sport* 53:297-304.

46. Mann, T., R.P. Lamberts, and M.I. Lambert. 2013. Methods of prescribing relative exercise intensity: Physiological and practical considerations. *Sports Medicine* 43:613-625.

47. McArdle, W.D., J.R. Magel, T.J. Gergley, R.J. Spina, and M.M. Toner. 1984. Thermal adjustment to cold-water exposure in resting men and women. *Journal of Physiology: Respiratory, Environmental and Exercise Physiology* 56:1565-1571.

48. McArdle, W.D., J.R. Magel, R.J. Spina, T.J. Gergley, and M.M. Toner. 1984. Thermal adjustments to cold-water exposure in exercising men and women. *Journal of Applied Physiology* 56:1572-1577.

49. Mezzani, A., L.F. Hamm, A.M. Jones, P.E. McBride, T. Moholdt, J.A. Stone, A. Urhausen, and M.A. Williams. 2013. Aerobic exercise intensity assessment and prescription in cardiac rehabilitation: A joint position statement of the European Association for Cardiovascular Prevention and Rehabilitation, the American Association of Cardiovascular and Pulmonary Rehabilitation and the Canadian Association of Cardiac Rehabilitation. *European Journal of Preventive Cardiology* 20(3):422-467.

50. Myers, J., M. Prakash, V. Froelicher, D. Do, S. Partington, and J.E. Atwood. 2002. Exercise capacity and mortality among men referred for exercise testing. *New England Journal of Medicine* 346:793-801.

51. National Weather Service. Wet bulb globe temperature: How and when to use it. www.weather.gov/news/211009-WBGT

52. Paffenbarger, R.S., R.T. Hyde, and A.L. Wing. 1986. Physical activity, all-cause mortality, and longevity of college alumni. *New England Journal of Medicine* 314:605-613.

53. Pollock, M.L., L.R. Gettman, C.A. Mileses, M.D. Bah, J.L. Durstine, and R.B. Johnson. 1977. Effects of frequency and duration of training on attrition and incidence of injury. *Medicine and Science in Sports* 9:31-36.

54. Pollock, M.L., and J.H. Wilmore. 1990. *Exercise in health and disease.* 2nd ed. Philadelphia: Saunders.

55. Powers, S.K., and E.T. Howley. 2015. *Exercise physiology.* New York: McGraw-Hill.

56. Pugh, L.G.C. 1964. Deaths from exposure in Four Inns Walking Competition, March 14-15, 1964. *Lancet* 1:1210-1212.

57. Pugh, L.G.C., and O.G. Edholm. 1955. The physiology of Channel swimmers. *Lancet* 2:761-768.

58. Raven, P.B. 1980. Effects of air pollution on physical performance. In vol. 2 of *Encyclopedia of physical education: Physical fitness, training, environment and nutrition related to performance*, ed. G.A. Stull and T.K. Cureton, 201-216. Salt Lake City: Brighton.

59. Raven, P.B., B.L. Drinkwater, R.O. Ruhling, N. Bolduan, S. Taguchi, J. Gliner, and S.M. Horvath. 1974. Effect of carbon monoxide and peroxyacetylnitrate on man's maximal aerobic capacity. *Journal of Applied Physiology* 36:288-293.

60. Sawka M.N., L.M. Burke, E.R. Eichner, R.J. Maughan, S.J. Montain, and N.S. Stachenfeld. 2007. American College of Sports Medicine position stand. Exercise and fluid replacement. *Medicine & Science in Sports & Exercise* 39(2):377-90

61. Sawka, M.N., R.P. Francesconi, A.J. Young, and K.B. Pandolf. 1984. Influence of hydration level and body fluids on exercise performance in the heat. *Journal of the American Medical Association* 252(9):1165-1169.

62. Sawka, M.N., A.J. Young, R.P. Francesconi, S.R. Muza, and K.B. Pandolf. 1985. Thermoregulatory and blood responses during exercise at graded hypohydration levels. *Journal of Applied Physiology* 59:1394-1401.

63. Sharman, J.E., J.R. Cockcroft, and J.S. Coombes. 2004. Cardiovascular implications of exposure to traffic air pollution during exercise. *QJM* 97:637-643.

64. Swain, D.P., K.S. Abernathy, C.S. Smith, S.J. Lee, and S.A. Bunn. 1994. Target heart rates for the development of cardiorespiratory fitness. *Medicine & Science in Sports & Exercise* 26:112-116.

65. Swain, D.P., and B.A. Franklin. 2002. $\dot{V}O_2$ reserve and the minimal intensity for improving cardiorespiratory fitness. *Medicine & Science in Sports & Exercise* 34:152-157.

66. Swain, D.P., and B.C. Leutholtz. 1997. Heart rate reserve is equivalent to %$\dot{V}O_2$ reserve, not to %$\dot{V}O_2$max. *Medicine & Science in Sports & Exercise* 29:410-414.

67. Swain, D.P., B.C. Leutholtz, M.E. King, L.A. Haas, and J.D. Branch. 1998. Relationship between % heart rate reserve and % $\dot{V}O_2$ reserve in treadmill exercise. *Medicine & Science in Sports & Exercise* 30:318-321.

68. Tanaka, H., K.D. Monahan, and D.R. Seals. 2001. Age-predicted maximal heart rate revisited. *Journal of the American College of Cardiology* 37:153-156.

69. Taylor, J.L., D.J. Holland, J.G. Spathis, K.S. Beetham, U. Wisløff, S.E. Keating, and J.S. Coombes. 2019. Guidelines for the delivery and monitoring of high intensity interval training in clinical populations. *Progress in Cardiovascular Diseases* 62(2):140-146.

70. U.S. Department of Health and Human Services (HHS). 1996. *Surgeon General's report on physical activity and health.* Washington, DC: Author.

71. U.S. Department of Health and Human Services (HHS). 2008. Physical Activity Guidelines Advisory Committee report 2008. www.health.gov/paguidelines/committeereport.aspx.

72. U.S. Department of Health and Human Services (HHS). 2008. *2008 Physical Activity Guidelines for Americans.* https://health.gov/paguidelines/guidelines/default.aspx.

73. U.S. Department of Health and Human Services (HHS). 2018. Physical Activity Guidelines Advisory Committee scientific report. https://health.gov/paguidelines/second-edition/report/.

74. U.S. Department of Health and Human Services (HHS). 2018. *Physical Activity Guidelines for Americans.* 2nd ed. https://health.gov/our-work/nutrition-physical-activity/physical-activity-guidelines/current-guidelines.

75. U.S. Department of Health and Human Services (HHS). 2020. *Healthy people 2030.* https://health.gov/healthypeople/objectives-and-data/leading-health-indicators.

76. U.S. Environmental Protection Agency. 2014. Air quality index: A guide to air quality and your health. EPA-456/F-14-002. www.airnow.gov/publications/air-quality-index/air-quality-index-a-guide-to-air-quality-and-your-health/.

77. Zanobetti, A., M.J. Canner, P.H. Stone, J. Schwartz, D. Sher, E. Eagan-Bengston, K.A. Gates, L.H. Hartley, H. Suh, and D.R. Gold. 2004. Ambient pollution and blood pressure in cardiac rehabilitation patients. *Circulation* 110:2184-2189.

Chapter 14

1. American Association for Cardiovascular and Pulmonary Rehabilitation (AACVPR). 2021. *Guidelines for cardiac rehabilitation programs.* 6th ed. Champaign, IL: Human Kinetics.

2. American College of Obstetricians and Gynecologists (ACOG). 2020. Physical activity and exercise during pregnancy and the postpartum period. *Obstetrics and Gynecology* 135:e178-e188.

3. American College of Sports Medicine (ACSM). 2009. Exercise and physical activity for older adults. *Medicine & Science in Sports & Exercise* 41:1510-1530.

4. American College of Sports Medicine (ACSM). 2009. Progression models in resistance training for healthy adults. *Medicine & Science in Sports & Exercise* 41:687-708.

5. American College of Sports Medicine (ACSM). 2022. *ACSM's guidelines for exercise testing and prescription.* 11th ed. Philadelphia: Wolters Kluwer.

6. Androulakis-Korakakis, P., J.P. Fisher, and J. Steele. 2020. The minimum effective training dose required to increase 1RM strength in resistance-trained men: A systematic review and meta-analysis. *Sports Medicine* 50:751-765.

7. Ashton, R., G. Tew, J. Aning, S. Gilbert, L. Lewis, and J. Saxton. 2020. Effects of short-term, medium-term and long-term resistance exercise training on cardiometabolic health outcomes in adults: Systematic review with meta-analysis. *British Journal of Sports Medicine* 54:341-348.

8. Balachandran, A., J. Steele, D. Angielczyk, M. Belio, B. Schoenfeld, N. Quiles, N. Askin, and A. Abou-Setta. 2022. Comparison of power training vs traditional strength training on physical function in older adults: A systematic review and meta-analysis. *JAMA Network Open* 5:e2211623.

9. Barakat, R., and M. Perales. 2016. Resistance exercise in pregnancy and outcome. *Clinical Obstetrics and Gynecology* 59:591-599.

10. Behm, D., A. Blazevich, A. Kay, and M. McHugh. 2016. Acute effects of muscle stretching on physical performance, range of motion, and injury incidence in healthy active individuals: A systematic review. *Applied Physiology, Nutrition and Metabolism* 41:1-11.

11. Behm, D., and J. Colado Sanchez. 2013. Instability resistance training across the exercise continuum. *Sports Health* 5:500-503.

12. Behm, D., A. Faigenbaum, B. Falk, and P. Klentrou. 2008. Canadian Society for Exercise Physiology position paper: Resistance training for children and adolescents. *Applied Physiology Nutrition and Metabolism* 33:547-561.

13. Behringer, M., A. Vom Heede, Z. Yue, and J. Mester. 2010. Effects of resistance training in children and adolescents: A meta-analysis. *Pediatrics* 126:e1199-210.

14. Bennie, J., K. De Cocker, J. Smith, and G. Wiesner. 2020. The epidemiology of muscle-strengthening exercise in Europe: A 28-country comparison including 280,605 adults. *PLoS One* 15:e0242220.

15. Bernárdez-Vázquez, R., J. Raya-González, D. Castillo, and M. Beato. 2022. Resistance training variables for optimization of muscle hypertrophy: An umbrella review. *Frontiers in Sports and Active Living* 4:949021.

16. Blazevich, A., and N. Babault. 2019. Post-activation potentiation versus post-activation performance enhancement in humans: Historical perspective, underlying mechanisms, and current issues. *Frontiers in Physiology* 1(10):1359.

17. Bø, K., R. Artal, R. Barakat, W. Brown, G. Davies, M. Dooley, K. Evenson, et al. 2017. Exercise and pregnancy in recreational and elite athletes: 2016/17 evidence summary from the IOC Expert Group Meeting, Lausanne. Part 3-exercise in the postpartum period. *British Journal of Sports Medicine* 51:1516-1525.

18. Bompa, T., and G. Haff. 2009. *Periodization*. 5th ed. Champaign, IL: Human Kinetics.

19. Borde, R., T. Hortobágyi, and U. Granacher. 2015. Dose-response relationships of resistance training in healthy old adults: A systematic review and meta-analysis. *Sports Medicine* 45:1693-720.

20. Chaabene, H., D. Behm, Y. Negra, and U. Granacher. 2019. Acute effects of static stretching on muscle strength and power: An attempt to clarify previous caveats. *Frontiers in Physiology* 10:1468.

21. Chang, Y.K., C.Y. Pan, F.T. Chen, C.L. Tsai, and C.C. Huang. 2012. Effect of resistance-exercise training on cognitive function in healthy older adults: A review. *Journal of Aging and Physical Activity* 20:497-517.

22. Chu, D., and G. Myer. 2013. *Plyometrics*. Champaign, IL: Human Kinetics.

23. Clark, B., and T. Manini. 2010. Functional consequences of sarcopenia and dynapenia in the elderly. *Current Opinion in Clinical Nutrition and Metabolic Care* 13:271-276.

24. Coelho-Júnior, H., I. Gonçalves, R. Sampaio, P. Sampaio, E. Lusa Cadore, R. Calvani, A. Picca, M. Izquierdo, E. Marzetti, and M. Uchida. 2020. Effects of combined resistance and power training on cognitive function in older women: A randomized controlled trial. *International Journal of Environmental Research and Public Health* 17:3435.

25. Coetsee, C., and E. Terblanche. 2015. The time course of changes induced by resistance training and detraining on muscular and physical function in older adults. *European Review of Aging and Physical Activity* 12:7.

26. Collins, H., J. Booth, A. Duncan, and S. Fawkner. 2019. The effect of resistance training interventions on fundamental movement skills in youth: A meta-analysis. *Sports Medicine Open* 5:17.

27. Collins, H., J. Booth, A. Duncan, S. Fawkner, and A. Niven. 2019. The effect of resistance training interventions on "The Self" in youth: A systematic review and meta-analysis. *Sports Medicine Open* 5:29.

28. Conlon, J., G. Haff, J. Tufan, and R. Newton. 2018. Training load indices, perceived tolerance, and enjoyment among different models of resistance training in older adults. *Journal of Strength and Conditioning Research* 32:867-875.

29. Consitt, L., C. Dudley, and G. Saxena. 2019. Impact of endurance and resistance training on skeletal muscle glucose metabolism in older adults. *Nutrients* 11:2636.

30. Coulombe, B., K. Games, E. Neil, and L. Eberman. 2017. Core stability exercise versus general exercise for chronic low back pain. *Journal of Athletic Training* 52:71-72.

31. Davenport, M., A. Marchand, M. Mottola, V. Poitras, C. Gray, A. Jaramillo, N. Garcia, et al. 2019. Exercise for the prevention and treatment of low back, pelvic girdle and lumbopelvic pain during pregnancy: A systematic review and meta-analysis. *British Journal of Sports Medicine* 53:90-98.

32. Davies, T., K. Kuang, R. Orr, M. Halaki, and D. Hackett. 2017. Effect of movement velocity during resistance training on dynamic muscular strength: A systematic review and meta-analysis. *Sports Medicine* 47:1603-1617.

33. DeLorme, T., and A. Watkins. 1948. Techniques of progressive resistance exercise. *Archives of Physical Medicine and Rehabilitation* 29:263-273.

34. Días, I., P. Farinatti, M. De Souza, D. Manhanini, E. Balthazar, D. Dantas, E. De Andrade Pinto, E. Bouskela, and L. Kraemer-Aguiar. 2015. Effects of resistance training on obese adolescents. *Medicine & Science in Sports & Exercise* 47:2636-2344.

35. Dias, M., R. Simão, F. Saavedra, and N. Ratamess. 2017. Influence of a personal trainer on self-selected loading during resistance exercise. *Journal of Strength and Conditioning Research* 31:1925-1930.

36. Dibben, G., J. Faulkner, N. Oldridge, K. Rees, D. Thompson, A. Zwisler, and R. Taylor. 2021. Exercise-based cardiac rehabilitation for coronary heart disease. *Cochrane Database of Systematic Reviews* 11:CD001800.

37. Dipietro, L., K. Evenson, B. Bloodgood, K. Sprow, R. Troiano, K. Piercy, A. Vaux-Bjerke, and K. Powell. 2019. Benefits of physical activity during pregnancy and postpartum: An umbrella review. *Medicine & Science in Sports & Exercise* 51:1292-1302.

38. El Hadouchi, M., H. Kiers, R. de Vries, C. Veenhof, and J. van Dieën. 2022. Effectiveness of power training compared to strength training in older adults: A systematic review and meta-analysis. *European Review of Aging and Physical Activity* 19:18.

39. Faigenbaum, A., W. Kraemer, C. Blimkie, I. Jeffreys, L. Micheli, M. Nitka, and T. Rowland. 2009. Youth resistance training: Updated position statement paper from the National Strength and Conditioning Association. *Journal of Strength and Conditioning Research* 23(Suppl. 5):S60-S79.

40. Faigenbaum, A., R. Lloyd, J. MacDonald, and G. Myer. 2016. Citius, altius, fortius. Beneficial effects of resistance training for young athletes. *British Journal of Sports Medicine* 50:3-7.

41. Faigenbaum, A., R. Lloyd, and J. Oliver. 2020. *Essentials of youth fitness.* Champaign, IL: Human Kinetics.

42. Faigenbaum, A., J. MacDonald, A. Stracciolini, and T. Rebullido. 2020. Making a strong case for prioritizing muscular fitness in youth physical activity guidelines. *Current Sports Medicine Reports* 19:530-536.

43. Faigenbaum, A., and J. McFarland. 2023. Developing resistance training skill literacy in youth. *Journal of Physical Education, Recreation and Dance* 94(2):5-10.

44. Faigenbaum, A., and G. Myer. 2010. Resistance training among young athletes: Safety, efficacy and injury prevention effects. *British Journal of Sports Medicine* 44:56-63.

45. Faigenbaum, A., T. Rebullido, and L. Zaichkowsky. 2022. Heads-up. Effective strategies for promoting mental health literacy in youth fitness programs. *ACSM Health and Fitness Journal* 26:12-19.

46. Fan, Y., M. Yu, J. Li, H. Zhang, Q. Liu, L. Zhao, T. Wang, and H. Xu. 2021. Efficacy and safety of resistance training for coronary heart disease rehabilitation: A systematic review of randomized controlled trials. *Frontiers in Cardiovascular Medicine* 8:754794.

47. Fassett, Z., A. Jagodinsky, D. Thomas, and S. Williams. 2022. Peak loads associated with high-impact physical activities in children. *Pediatric Exercise Science* 14:1-4.

48. Fiatarone, M.A., E.C. Marks, N.D. Ryan, C.N. Meredith, L.A. Lipsitz, and W. Evans. 1990. High-intensity strength training in nonagenarians: Effects on skeletal muscle. *Journal of the American Medical Association* 263:3029-3034.

49. Fleck, S., and W. Kraemer. 2014. *Designing resistance training programs.* 4th ed. Champaign, IL: Human Kinetics.

50. Fleg, J., D. Forman, K. Berra, V. Bittner, J. Blumenthal, M. Chen, S. Cheng, D. Kitzman, M. Maurer, M. Rich, W. Shen, M. Williams, S. Zieman, and American Heart Association Committees on Older Populations and Exercise Cardiac Rehabilitation and Prevention of the Council on Clinical Cardiology, Council on Cardiovascular and Stroke Nursing, and Council on Lifestyle and Cardiometabolic Health. 2013. Secondary prevention of atherosclerotic cardiovascular disease in older adults: A scientific statement from the American Heart Association. *Circulation* 128:2422-2446.

51. Fletcher, G.F., P.A. Ades, P. Kligfield, R. Arena, G.J. Balady, V.A. Bittner, L.A. Coke, J.L. Fleg, D.E. Forman, T.C. Gerber, M. Gulati, K. Madan, J. Rhodes, P.D. Thompson, M.A. Williams, and American Heart Association Exercise, Cardiac Rehabilitation, and Prevention Committee of the Council on Clinical Cardiology, Council on Nutrition, Physical Activity and Metabolism, Council on Cardiovascular and Stroke Nursing, and Council on Epidemiology and Prevention. 2013. Exercise standards for testing and training: A scientific statement from the American Heart Association. *Circulation* 128:873-934.

52. Flint, K., J. Stevens-Lapsley, and D. Forman. 2020. Cardiac rehabilitation in frail older adults with cardiovascular disease: A new diagnostic and treatment paradigm. *Journal of Cardiopulmonary Rehabilitation and Prevention* 40:72-78.

53. Fragala, M., E. Cadore, S. Dorgo, M. Izquierdo, W. Kraemer, M. Peterson, and E. Ryan. 2019. Resistance training for older adults: Position statement from the National Strength and Conditioning Association. *Journal of Strength and Conditioning Research* 33:2019-2052.

54. French, D., and L. Torres Ronda. 2022. *NSCA's essentials of sport science.* Champaign, IL: Human Kinetics.

55. Garber, C., B. Blissmer, M.R. Deschenes, B.A. Franklin, M.J. Lamonte, I. Lee, D.C. Nieman, and D.P. Swain. 2011. American College of Sports Medicine position stand. Quantity and quality of exercise for developing and maintaining cardiorespiratory, musculoskeletal, and neuromotor fitness in apparently healthy adults: Guidance for prescribing exercise. *Medicine & Science in Sports & Exercise* 43:1334-1359.

56. García-Hermoso, A, R. Ramírez-Campillo, and M. Izquierdo. 2019. Is muscular fitness associated with future health benefits in children and adolescents? A systematic review and meta-analysis of longitudinal studies. *Sports Medicine* 49:1079-1094.

57. García-Hermoso, A., R. Ramírez-Vélez, R. Ramírez-Campillo, M. Peterson, and V. Martínez-Vizcaíno. 2018. Concurrent aerobic plus resistance exercise versus aerobic exercise alone to improve health outcomes in paediatric obesity: A systematic review and meta-analysis. *British Journal of Sports Medicine* 52:161.

58. Gentil, P., J. Fisher, and J. Steele. 2017. A review of the acute effects and long-term adaptations of single- and multi-joint exercises during resistance training. *Sports Medicine* 47:843-855.

59. Goldberg, L., and P. Twist. 2007. *Strength ball training.* Champaign, IL: Human Kinetics.

60. Gómez-Bruton, A., A. Matute-Llorente, A. González-Agüero, J. Casajús, and G. Vicente-Rodríguez. 2017. Plyometric exercise and bone health in children and adolescents: A systematic review. *World Journal of Pediatrics* 13:112-121.

61. Gordon, B., C. McDowell, M. Hallgren, J. Meyer, M. Lyons, and M. Herring. 2018. Association of efficacy of resistance exercise training with depressive symptoms: Meta-analysis and meta-regression analysis of randomized clinical trials. *JAMA Psychiatry* 75:566-576.

62. Gordon, B., C. McDowell, M. Lyons, and M. Herring. 2017. The effects of resistance exercise training on anxiety: A meta-analysis and meta-regression analysis of randomized controlled trials. *Sports Medicine* 47:2521-2532.

63. Granacher, U., A. Gollhofer, T., Hortobágyi, R. Kressig, and T. Muehlbauer. 2013. The importance of trunk muscle strength for balance, functional performance, and fall prevention in seniors: A systematic review. *Sports Medicine* 43:627-641.

64. Grandou, C., L. Wallace, F. Impellizzeri, N. Allen, and C. Coutts. 2020. Overtraining in resistance exercise: An exploratory systematic review and methodological appraisal of the literature. *Sports Medicine* 50:815-828.

65. Grgic, J., B. Lazinica, P. Mikulic, J. Krieger, and B. Schoenfeld. 2017. The effects of short versus long inter-set rest

intervals in resistance training on measures of muscle hypertrophy: A systematic review. *European Journal of Sport Science* 17:983-993.

66. Grgic, J., B. Schoenfeld, T. Davies, B. Lazinica, J. Krieger, and Z. Pedisic. 2018. Effect of resistance training frequency on gains in muscular strength: A systematic review and meta-analysis. *Sports Medicine* 48:1207-1220.

67. Grgic, J., B. Schoenfeld, J. Orazem, and F. Sabol. 2022. Effects of resistance training performed to repetition failure or non-failure on muscular strength and hypertrophy: A systematic review and meta-analysis. *Journal of Sport and Health Science* 11:202-211.

68. Grgic, J., B. Schoenfeld, M. Skrepnik, T. Davies, and P. Mikulic. 2018. Effects of rest interval duration in resistance training on measures of muscular strength: A systematic review. *Sports Medicine* 48:137-151

69. Haff, G., and T. Triplett. 2016. *Essentials of strength training and conditioning.* 4th ed. Champaign, IL: Human Kinetics.

70. Harris, C., M. DeBeliso, K.J. Adams, B. Irmischer, and T. Spitzer Gibson. 2007. Detraining in the older adult: Effects of prior training intensity on strength retention. *Journal of Strength and Conditioning Research* 21:813-818.

71. Hartvigsen, J., M. Hancock, A. Kongsted, Q. Louw, M. Ferreira, S. Genevay, D. Hoy, et al. 2018. What low back pain is and why we need to pay attention. *Lancet* 391:2356-2367.

72. Hatfield, D., W.J. Kraemer, B. Spiering, K. Häkkinen, J.S. Volek, T. Shimano, L. Spreuwenberg, R. Silvestre, J. Vingren, M. Fragala, A. Gómez, S. Fleck, R. Newton, and C. Maresh. 2006. The impact of velocity of movement on performance factors in resistance exercise. *Journal of Strength and Conditioning Research* 20:760-766.

73. Hettinger, R., and E. Muller. 1953. Muskelleistung und muskeltraining (Muscle achievement and muscle training). *ArbeitsPhysiologie* 15:111-126.

74. Hollings, M., Y. Mavros, J. Freeston, and M. Fiatarone Singh. 2017. The effect of progressive resistance training on aerobic fitness and strength in adults with coronary heart disease: A systematic review and meta-analysis of randomised controlled trials. *European Journal of Preventive Cardiology* 24:1242-1259.

75. Hu, K., and A. Staiano. 2022. Trends in obesity prevalence among children and adolescents aged 2 to 19 years in the US from 2011 to 2022. *JAMA Pediatrics* 176:1037-1039.

76. Hyde, E., G. Whitfield, J. Omura, J. Fulton, and S. Carlson. 2021. Trends in meeting the physical activity guidelines: Muscle-strengthening alone and combined with aerobic activity, United States, 1998-2018. *Journal of Physical Activity and Health* 18:S37-S44.

77. Iversen, V., M. Norum, B. Schoenfeld, and M. Fimland. No time to lift? Designing time-efficient training programs for strength and hypertrophy: A narrative review. 2021. *Sports Medicine* 51:2079-2095.

78. Joyce, D., and D. Lewindon. 2022. *High-performance training for sports.* Champaign, IL: Human Kinetics.

79. Karandikar, N., and O. Vargas. 2011. Kinetic chains: A review of the concept and its clinical applications. *Physical Medicine and Rehabilitation* 3:739-745.

80. Kerr, Z., C. Collins, and R. Comstock. 2010. Epidemiology of weight training related injuries presenting to United States emergency room departments, 1990-2007. *American Journal of Sports Medicine* 38:765-771.

81. Khodadad Kashi, S., Z. Mirzazadeh, and V. Saatchian. 2023. A systematic review and meta-analysis of resistance training on quality of life, depression, muscle strength, and functional exercise capacity in older adults aged 60 years or more. *Biological Research for Nursing.* 25(1):88-106.

82. Kirkman, D., D. Lee, and S. Carbone. 2022. Resistance exercise for cardiac rehabilitation. *Progress in Cardiovascular Disease* 70:66-72.

83. Lacroix, A., T. Hortobágyi, R. Beurskens, and U. Granacher. 2017. Effects of supervised vs. unsupervised training programs on balance and muscle strength in older adults: A systematic review and meta-analysis. *Sports Medicine* 47:2341-2361.

84. Lee, J., and A. Stone. 2020. Combined aerobic and resistance training for cardiorespiratory fitness, muscle strength, and walking capacity after stroke: A systematic review and meta-analysis. *Journal of Stroke and Cerebrovascular Disease* 29:104498.

85. Lesinski, M., M. Herz, A. Schmelcher, and U. Granacher. 2020. Effects of resistance training on physical fitness in healthy children and adolescents: An umbrella review. *Sports Medicine* 50:1901-1928.

86. Lloyd, R., A. Faigenbaum, M. Stone, J. Oliver, I. Jeffreys, J.A. Moody, C. Brewer, K. Pierce, T. McCambridge, R. Howard, L. Herrington, B. Hainline, L. Micheli, R. Jaques, W. Kraemer, M. McBride, T. Best, D. Chu, B. Alvar, and G. Myer. 2014. Position statement on youth resistance training: The 2014 International Consensus. *British Journal of Sports Medicine* 48:498-505.

87. Lobstein, T., and R. Jackson-Leach. 2016. Planning for the worst: Estimates of obesity and comorbidities in school-age children in 2025. *Pediatric Obesity* 11:321-325.

88. Lopez, P., R. Pinto, R. Radaelli, A. Rech, R. Grazioli, M. Izquierdo, and E. Cadore. 2018. Benefits of resistance training in physically frail elderly: A systematic review. *Aging Clinical Experimental Research* 30:889-899.

89. Lopez, P., R. Radaelli, D. Taaffe, D. Galvão, R. Newton, E. Nonemacher, V. Wendt, R. Bassanesi, D. Turella, and A. Rech. 2022. Moderators of resistance training effects in overweight and obese adults: A systematic review and meta-analysis. *Medicine & Science in Sports & Exercise* 54(11):1804-1816.

90. Lopez, P., R. Radaelli, D. Taaffe, R. Newton, D. Galvão, G. Trajano, J. Teodoro, W. Kraemer, K. Häkkinen, and R. Pinto. 2021. Resistance training load effects on muscle hypertrophy and strength gain: Systematic review and network meta-analysis. *Medicine & Science in Sports & Exercise* 53:1206-1216.

91. Maestroni, L., P. Read, C. Bishop, K. Papadopoulos, T. Suchomel, P. Comfort, and A. Turner. 2020. The benefits of strength training on musculoskeletal system health: Practical applications for interdisciplinary care. *Sports Medicine* 50:1431-1450.

92. Magro-Malosso, E., G. Saccone, M. Di Tommaso, A. Roman, and V. Berghella. 2017. Exercise during pregnancy and risk of gestational hypertensive disorders: A systematic review and meta-analysis. *Acta Obstetricia el Gynecologica Scandinavica* 96:921-931.

93. Malina, R. 2006. Weight training in youth—growth, maturation and safety: An evidenced-based review. *Clinical Journal of Sports Medicine* 16:478-487.

94. Mazzetti, S., W. Kraemer, J. Volek, N. Duncan, N. Ratamess, A. Gomez, R. Newton, K. Hakkinen, and S. Fleck. 2000. The influence of direct supervision of resistance training on strength performance. *Medicine & Science in Sports & Exercise* 32:1175-1184.

95. McGowan, C., D. Pyne, K. Thompson, and B. Rattray. 2015. Warm-up strategies for sport and exercise: Mechanisms and applications. *Sports Medicine* 45:1523-1546.

96. McLeod, K., M. Jones, J. Thom, and B. Parmenter. 2022. Resistance training and high-intensity interval training improve cardiometabolic health in high risk older adults: A systematic review and meta-analysis. *International Journal of Sports Medicine* 43:206-218.

97. Mcleod, J., T. Stokes, and S. Phillips. 2019. Resistance exercise training as a primary countermeasure to age-related chronic disease. *Frontiers in Physiology* 10:645.

98. McMichan, L., M. Dick, D. Skelton, S. Chastin, N. Owen, D. Dunstan, W. Fraser, J. Tang, C. Greig, S. Agyapong-Badu, and A. Mavroeidi. 2021. Sedentary behaviour and bone health in older adults: A systematic review. *Osteoporosis International* 32:1487-1497.

99. Mediate, P., and A. Faigenbaum. 2007. *Medicine ball training for all kids*. Monterey Bay, CA: Healthy Learning.

100. Meeusen, R., M. Duclos, C. Foster, A. Fry, M. Gleeson, D. Nieman, J. Raglin, G. Rietjens, J. Steinacker, A. Urhausen, European College of Sport Science, and American College of Sports Medicine. 2013. Prevention, diagnosis, and treatment of the overtraining syndrome: Joint consensus statement of the European College of Sport Science and the American College of Sports Medicine. *Medicine & Science in Sports & Exercise* 45:186-205.

101. Méndez-Hernández, L., E. Ramírez-Moreno, R. Barrera-Gálvez, M. Cabrera-Morales, J. Reynoso-Vázquez, O. Flores-Chávez, L. Morales-Castillejos, N. Cruz-Cansino, R. Jiménez-Sánchez, and J. Arias-Rico. 2022. Effects of strength training on body fat in children and adolescents with overweight and obesity: A systematic review with meta-analysis. *Children (Basel)* 9:995.

102. Moesgaard, L., M. Beck, L. Christiansen, P. Aagaard, and J. Lundbye-Jensen. 2022. Effects of periodization on strength and muscle hypertrophy in volume-equated resistance training programs: A systematic review and meta-analysis. *Sports Medicine* 52:1647-1666.

103. Momma, H., R. Kawakami, T. Honda, and S. Sawada. 2022. Muscle-strengthening activities are associated with lower risk and mortality in major non-communicable diseases: A systematic review and meta-analysis of cohort studies. *British Journal of Sports Medicine* 56:755-763.

104. Moraes, H., H. Silveira, N. Oliveira, E. Matta Mello Portugal, N. Araújo, P. Vasques, A. Bergland, et al. 2020. Is strength training as effective as aerobic training for depression in older adults? A randomized controlled trial. *Neuropsychobiology* 79:141-149.

105. Moran, J., R. Ramirez-Campillo, and U. Granacher. 2018. Effects of jumping exercise on muscular power in older adults: A meta-analysis. *Sports Medicine* 48:2843-2857.

106. Morris, S., J. Oliver, J. Pedley, G. Haff, and R. Lloyd. 2022. Comparison of weightlifting, traditional resistance training and plyometrics on strength, power and speed: A systematic review with meta-analysis. *Sports Medicine* 52:1533-1554.

107. Mottola, M., M. Davenport, S. Ruchat, G. Davies, V. Poitras, C. Gray, A. Jaramillo Garcia, et al. 2019. Canadian guideline for physical activity throughout pregnancy. *British Journal of Sports Medicine* 52:1339-1346.

108. Myer, G., A.D. Faigenbaum, K. Ford, T. Best, M. Bergeron, and T. Hewett. 2011. When to initiate integrative neuromuscular training to reduce sports-related injuries and enhance health in youth? *Current Sports Medicine Reports* 10:155-166.

109. Myer, G., C. Quatman, J. Khoury, E. Wall, and T. Hewett. 2009. Youth vs. adult "weightlifting" injuries presented to United States emergency rooms: Accidental vs. non-accidental injury mechanisms. *Journal of Strength and Conditioning Research* 23:2054-2060.

110. Northey, J., N. Cherbuin, K. Pumpa, D. Smee, and B. Rattray. 2018. Exercise interventions for cognitive function in adults older than 50: A systematic review with meta-analysis. *British Journal Sports Medicine* 52:154-160.

111. Nunes J., J. Grgic, P. Cunha, A. Ribeiro, B. Schoenfeld, B. de Salles, and E. Cyrino. 2021. What influence does resistance exercise order have on muscular strength gains and muscle hypertrophy? A systematic review and meta-analysis. *European Journal of Sports Science* 2:149-157.

112. Nunes, E., T. Stokes, J. McKendry, B. Currier, and S. Phillips. 2022. Disuse-induced skeletal muscle atrophy in disease and nondisease states in humans: Mechanisms, prevention, and recovery strategies. *American Journal of Physiology and Cell Physiology* 322:C1068-C1084.

113. Oliva-Lozano, J., and J. Muyor. 2020. Core muscle activity during physical fitness exercises: A systematic review. *International Journal of Environmental Research and Public Health* 17:4306.

114. Ortega, F., J. Mora-Gonzalez, C. Cadenas-Sanchez, I. Esteban-Cornejo, J. Migueles, P. Solis-Urra, J. Verdejo-Román, et al. 2022. Effects of an exercise program on brain health outcomes for children with overweight or obesity: The ActiveBrains randomized clinical trial. *JAMA Network Open* 5:e2227893.

115. Petrov Fieril, K., M. Fagevik Olsén, A. Glantz, and M. Larsson. 2014. Experiences of exercise during pregnancy among women who perform regular resistance training: A qualitative study. *Physical Therapy* 94:1135-1143.

116. Petrov Fieril, K., A. Glantz, and M. Fagevik Olsen. 2015. The efficacy of moderate-to-vigorous resistance exercise during pregnancy: A randomized controlled trial. *Acta Obstetricia Gynecologica Scandinavica* 94:35-42.

117. Petushek, E., D. Sugimoto, M. Stoolmiller, G. Smith, and G. Myer. 2019. Evidence-based best-practice guidelines for preventing anterior cruciate ligament injuries in young female athletes: A systematic review and meta-analysis. *American Journal of Sports Medicine* 47:1744-1753.

118. Quatman, C., G. Myer, J. Khoury, E. Wall, and T. Hewett. 2009. Sex differences in "weightlifting" injuries presenting to United States emergency rooms. *Journal of Strength and Conditioning Research* 23:2061-2067.

119. Radaelli, R., S. Fleck, T. Leite, R. Leite, R. Pinto, L. Fernandes, and R. Simão. 2015. Dose-response of 1, 3, and 5 sets of resistance exercise on strength, local muscular endurance, and hypertrophy. *Journal of Strength and Conditioning Research* 29:1349-58.

120. Radaelli, R., G. Trajano, S. Freitas, M. Izquierdo, E. Cadore, and R. Pinto. 2023. Power training prescription in older individuals: Is it safe and effective to promote neuromuscular functional improvements? *Sports Medicine.* 53(3):569-576.

121. Ralston, G., L. Kilgore, F. Wyatt, and J. Baker. 2017. The effect of weekly set volume on strength gain: A meta-analysis. *Sports Medicine* 47:2585-2601.

122. Ramos-Campo, D., L. Andreu-Caravaca, M. Carrasco-Poyatos, P. Benito, and J. Rubio-Arias. 2021. Effects of circuit resistance training on body composition, strength, and cardiorespiratory fitness in middle-aged and older women: A systematic review and meta-analysis. *Journal of Aging and Physical Activity* 9:1-14.

123. Ratamess, N. 2022. *ACSM's foundations of strength training and conditioning*. 2nd ed. Philadelphia: Wolters Kluwer.

124. Ratamess, N., A. Faigenbaum, J. Hoffman, and J. Kang. 2008. Self-selected resistance training intensity in healthy women: The influence of a personal trainer. *Journal of Strength and Conditioning Research* 22:103-111.

125. Ratamess, N., M. Falvo, G. Mangine, J. Hoffman, A. Faigenbaum, and J. Kang. 2007. The effect of rest interval length on metabolic responses to the bench press exercise. *European Journal of Applied Physiology* 100:1-17.

126. Rhodes, R., D. Lubans, N. Karunamuni, S. Kennedy, and R. Plotnikoff. 2017. Factors associated with participation in resistance training: A systematic review. *British Journal of Sports Medicine* 51:1466-1472.

127. Robbins, D., W. Young, D. Behm, and W. Payne. 2010. Agonist-antagonist paired set resistance training: A brief review. *Journal of Strength and Conditioning Research* 24:2873-82.

128. Russo, L., C. Nobles, K. Ertel, L. Chasan-Taber, and B. Whitcomb. 2015. Physical activity interventions in pregnancy and risk of gestational diabetes mellitus: A systematic review and meta-analysis. *Obstetrics and Gynecology* 125:576-582.

129. Sasaki, S., E. Tsuda, Y. Yamamoto, S. Maeda, Y. Kimura, Y. Fujita, and Y. Ishibashi. 2019. Core-muscle training and neuromuscular control of the lower limb and trunk. *Journal of Athletic Training* 54:959-969.

130. Schoenfeld, B., J. Grgic, D. Ogborn, and J. Krieger. 2017. Strength and hypertrophy adaptations between low- vs. high-load resistance training: A systematic review and meta-analysis. *Journal of Strength and Conditioning Research* 31:3508-3523.

131. Schranz, N., G. Tomkinson, and T. Olds. 2013. What is the effect of resistance training on the strength, body composition and psychosocial status of overweight and obese children and adolescents? A systematic review and meta-analysis. *Sports Medicine* 43:893-907.

132. Shaibi, G., M. Cruz, G. Ball, M. Weigensberg, G. Salem, N. Crespo, and M. Goran. 2006. Effects of resistance training on insulin sensitivity in overweight Latino adolescent males. *Medicine & Science in Sports & Exercise* 38:1208-1215.

133. Shailendra, P., K. Baldock, L. Li, J. Bennie, and T. Boyle. 2022. Resistance training and mortality risk: A systematic review and meta-analysis. *American Journal Preventive Medicine* 63:277-285.

134. Sherrington, C., N. Fairhall, G. Wallbank, A. Tiedemann, Z. Michaleff, K. Howard, L. Clemson, S. Hopewell, and S. Lamb. 2019. Exercise for preventing falls in older people living in the community. *Cochrane Database of Systematic Reviews* 1:CD012424.

135. Shimano, T., W. Kraemer, B. Sppiering, J. Volek, D. Hatfield, R. Silvestre, J. Vingren, M. Fragala, C. Maresh, S. Fleck, R. Newton, L. Spreuwenberg, and K. Hakkinen. 2008. Relationship between the number of repetitions and selected percentages of one repetition maximum in free weight exercises in trained and untrained men. *Journal of Strength and Conditioning Research* 20:819-823.

136. Shoepe, T., D. Ramirez, and H. Almstedt. 2010. Elastic band prediction equations for combined free-weight and elastic band bench presses and squats. *Journal of Strength and Conditioning Research* 24:195-200.

137. Sigal, R., A. Alberga, G. Goldfield, D. Prud'homme, S. Hadjiyannakis, R. Gougeon, P. Phillips, H. Tulloch, J. Malcolm, S. Doucette, G. Wells, J. Ma, and G. Kenny. 2014. Effects of aerobic training, resistance training, or both on percentage body fat and cardiometabolic risk markers in obese adolescents: The healthy eating aerobic and resistance training in youth randomized clinical trial. *Journal of the American Medical Association Pediatrics* 168:1006-1014.

138. Smith, J., N. Eather, R. Weaver, N. Riley, M. Beets, and D. Lubans. 2019. Behavioral correlates of muscular fitness in children and adolescents: A systematic review. *Sports Medicine* 49:887-904.

139. Spaulding, A., and L. Kelly. 2010. *Fitness on the ball*. Champaign, IL: Human Kinetics.

140. Squires, R., L. Kaminsky, J. Porcari, J. Ruff, P. Savage, and M. Williams. 2018. Progression of exercise training in early outpatient cardiac rehabilitation: An official statement for the American Association of Cardiovascular and Pulmonary Rehabilitation. *Journal of Cardiopulmonary Rehabilitation and Prevention* 38:139-146.

141. Steele, J., T. Malleron, I. Har-Nir, P. Androulakis-Korakakis, M. Wolf, J. Fisher, and I. Halperin. 2022. Are trainees lifting heavy enough? Self-selected loads in resistance exercise: A scoping review and exploratory meta-analysis. *Sports Medicine* 52(12):2909-2923.

142. Stone, M., W. Hornsby, G. Haff, A. Fry, D. Suarez, J. Liu, J. Gonzalez-Rave, and K. Pierce. 2021. Periodization and block periodization in sports: Emphasis on strength-power training: A provocative and challenging narrative. *Journal of Strength and Conditioning Research* 35:2351-2371.

143. Stricker, P., A. Faigenbaum, T. McCambridge, and the Council on Sports Medicine and Fitness. 2020. Resistance training for children and adolescents. *Pediatrics* 145:e20201011.

144. Suchomel, T., S. Nimphius, C. Bellon, and M. Stone. 2018. The importance of muscular strength: Training considerations. *Sports Medicine* 48:765-785.

145. Tessier, A., S. Wing, E. Rahme, J., Morais, and S. Chevalier. 2019. Physical function-derived cut-points for the diagnosis of sarcopenia and dynapenia from the Canadian longitudinal study on aging. *Journal of Cachexia Sarcopenia and Muscle* 10:985-999.

146. Thompson, W. 2019. *ACSM's clinical exercise physiology*. Philadelphia: Wolters Kluwer.

147. Thompson, W. 2022. Worldwide survey of fitness trends for 2022. *ACSM's Health and Fitness Journal* 26:11-20.

148. Torres-Costoso, A., P. López-Muñoz, V. Martínez-Vizcaíno, C. Álvarez-Bueno, and I. Cavero-Redondo. 2020. Association between muscular strength and bone health from children to young adults: A systematic review and meta-analysis. *Sports Medicine* 50:1163-1190.

149. United States Department of Health and Human Services (HHS). *2018 Physical Activity Guidelines for Americans*. 2nd ed. www.health.gov/paguidelines.

150. Van der Heijden, G., Z. Wang, Z. Chu, G. Toffolo, E. Manesso, P. Sauer, and A. Sunehag. 2010. Strength exercise improves muscle mass and hepatic insulin sensitivity in obese youth. *Medicine & Science in Sports & Exercise* 42:1973-1980.

151. Vetrovsky, T., M. Steffl, P. Stastny, and J. Tufano. 2019. The efficacy and safety of lower-limb plyometric training in older adults: A systematic review. *Sports Medicine* 49:113-131.

152. Wang, D., J. Yao, Y. Zirek, E. Reijnierse, and A. Maier. 2020. Muscle mass, strength, and physical performance predicting activities of daily living: A meta-analysis. *Journal of Cachexia Sarcopenia and Muscle* 11:3-25.

153. Watson, S., B. Weeks, L. Weis, A. Harding, S. Horan, and B. Beck. 2018. High-intensity resistance and impact training improves bone mineral density and physical function in postmenopausal women with osteopenia and osteoporosis: The LIFTMOR randomized controlled trial. *Journal of Bone and Mineral Research* 33:211-220.

154. Westcott, W.L. 2012. Resistance training is medicine: Effects of strength training on health. *Current Sports Medicine Reports* 11:209-216.

155. White, E., J. Pivarnik, and K. Pfeiffer. 2014. Resistance training during pregnancy and perinatal outcomes. *Journal of Physical Activity and Health* 11:1141-1148.

156. Williams, M., W. Haskell, P. Ades, E. Amsterdam, V. Bittner, B. Franklin, M. Gulanick, S. Laing, and K. Stewart. 2007. Resistance exercise in individuals with and without cardiovascular disease: 2007 update. *Circulation* 116:572-584.

157. Williams, T., D. Tolusso, M. Fedewa, and M. Esco. 2017. Comparison of periodized and non-periodized resistance training on maximal strength: A meta-analysis. *Sports Medicine* 47:2083-2100.

158. World Health Organization (WHO). 2020. *WHO guidelines on physical activity and sedentary behaviour.* Geneva: Author.

159. Yamamoto, S., K. Hotta, E. Ota, R. Mori, and A. Matsunaga. 2016. Effects of resistance training on muscle strength, exercise capacity, and mobility in middle-aged and elderly patients with coronary artery disease: A meta-analysis. *Journal of Cardiology* 68:125-34.

160. Yang, Y., S. Chen, C. Chen, C. Hsu, W. Zhou, and K. Chien. 2022. Training session and detraining duration affect lower limb muscle strength in middle-aged and older adults: A systematic review and meta-analysis. *Journal of Aging and Physical Activity* 30:552-566.

Chapter 15

1. Ahmed, R., S. Shakil-ur-Rehman, and F. Sibtain. 2014. Comparison between specific lumber mobilization and core-stability exercises with core-stability exercises alone in mechanical low back pain. *Pakistan Journal of Medical Sciences* 30:157-160.

2. Akuthota, V., A. Ferreiro, T. Moore, and M. Fredericson. 2008. Core stability exercise principles. *Current Sports Medicine Reports* 7:39-44.

3. American College of Sports Medicine (ACSM). 2017. *ACSM's complete guide to fitness and health.* Champaign, IL: Human Kinetics.

4. American College of Sports Medicine (ACSM). 2022. *ACSM's guidelines for exercise testing and prescription.* 11th ed. Philadelphia: Wolters Kluwer.

5. Axler, C.T., and S.M. McGill. 1997. Low back loads over a variety of abdominal exercises: Searching for the safest abdominal challenge. *Medicine & Science in Sports & Exercise* 29:804-811.

6. Ayala, F., P.S. de Baranda, M. De Ste. Croix, and F. Santonja. 2013. Comparison of active stretching technique in males with normal and limited hamstring flexibility. *Physical Therapy in Sport* 14:98-104.

7. Bandy, W.D., J.M. Irion, and M. Briggler. 1998. The effect of static stretch and dynamic range of motion training on the flexibility of the hamstring muscles. *Journal of Orthopaedic & Sports Physical Therapy* 27:295-300.

8. Barker, K.L., D.R. Shamley, and D. Jackson. 2004. Changes in the cross-sectional area of multifidus and psoas in patients with unilateral back pain—the relationship to pain and disability. *Spine* 29:E515-E519.

9. Bergmark, A. 1989. Stability of the lumbar spine: A study in mechanical engineering. *Acta Orthopaedica Scandinavica Supplementum* 230:1-54.

10. Biering-Sorensen, F. 1984. Physical measurements as risk indicators for low-back trouble over a one-year period. *Spine (Phila Pa 1976)* 9:106-119.

11. Bogduk, N. 1998. *Clinical anatomy of the lumbar spine and sacrum.* London: Churchill Livingstone.

12. Borghuis, J., A.L. Hof, and K. Lemmink. 2008. The importance of sensory-motor control in providing core stability implications for measurement and training. *Sports Medicine* 38:893-916.

13. Bressel, E., D.G. Dolny, C. Vandenberg, and J.B. Cronin. 2012. Trunk muscle activity during spine stabilization exercises performed in a pool. *Physical Therapy in Sport* 13:67-72.

14. Chodzko-Zajko, W.J., D.N. Proctor, M.A. Fiatarone Singh, C.T. Minson, C.R. Nigg, G.J. Salem, J.S. Skinner. 2009. Exercise and physical activity for older adults. *Medicine & Science in Sports & Exercise* 41:1510-1530.

15. Cipriani, D., B. Abel, and D. Pirrwitz. 2003. A comparison of two stretching protocols on hip range of motion: Implications for total daily stretch duration. *Journal of Strength and Conditioning Research* 17:274-278.

16. Cramer, H., R. Lauche, H. Haller, and G. Dobos. 2013. A systematic review and meta-analysis of yoga for low back pain. *Clinical Journal of Pain* 29:450-460.

17. De Baranda, P.S., and F. Ayala. 2010. Chronic flexibility improvement after 12 week of stretching program utilizing the ACSM recommendations: Hamstring flexibility. *International Journal of Sports Medicine* 31:389-396.

18. Ellison, J.B., S.J. Rose, and S.A. Sahrmann. 1990. Patterns of hip rotation range of motion: A comparison between healthy subjects and patients with low-back-pain. *Physical Therapy* 70:537-541.

19. Faries, M.D., and M. Greenwood. 2007. Core training: Stabilizing the confusion. *Strength and Conditioning Journal* 29:10-25.

20. Feland, J.B., J.W. Myrer, S.S. Schulthies, G.W. Fellingham, and G.W. Measom. 2001. The effect of duration of stretching of the hamstring muscle group for increasing range of motion in people aged 65 years or older. *Physical Therapy* 81:1110-1117.

21. Garber, C.E., B. Blissmer, M.R. Deschenes, B.A. Franklin, M.J. Lamonte, I.M. Lee, D.C. Nieman, D.P. Swain, and American College of Sports Medicine (ACSM). 2011. American College of Sports Medicine position stand. Quantity and quality of exercise for developing and maintaining

cardiorespiratory, musculoskeletal, and neuromotor fitness in apparently healthy adults: Guidance for prescribing exercise. *Medicine & Science in Sports & Exercise* 43:1334-1359.

22. Garcia-Vaquero, M.P., J.M. Moreside, E. Brontons-Gil, N. Peco-Gonzalez, and F.J. Vera-Garcia. 2012. Trunk muscle activation during stabilization exercises with single and double leg support. *Journal of Electromyography and Kinesiology* 22:398-406.

23. Gulick, D. 2009. *Ortho notes: Clinical examination pocket guide.* Philadelphia: F.A. Davis.

24. Hadala, M., and S. Gryckiewicz. 2014. The effectiveness of lumbar extensor training: Local stabilization or dynamic strengthening exercises: A review of literature. *Ortopedia, Traumatologia, Rehabilitacja* 16:561-572.

25. Hall, A.M., C.G. Maher, P. Lam, M. Ferreira, and J. Latimer. 2011. Tai chi exercise for treatment of pain and disability in people with persistent low back pain: A randomized controlled trial. *Arthritis Care & Research* 63:1576-1583.

26. Hasebe, K., K. Sairyo, Y. Hada, A. Dezawa, Y. Okubo, K. Kaneoka, and Y. Nakamura. 2014. Spino-pelvic rhythm with forward trunk bending in normal subjects without low back pain. *European Journal of Orthopaedic Surgery & Traumatology* 24(Suppl. 1):S193-S199.

27. Hides, J., C. Gilmore, W. Stanton, and E. Bohlscheid. 2008. Multifidus size and symmetry among chronic LBP and healthy asymptomatic subjects. *Manual Therapy* 13:43-49.

28. Hides, J.A., G.A. Jull, and C.A. Richardson. Long-term effects of specific stabilizing exercises for first-episode low back pain. 2001. *Spine* 26:E243-248.

29. Hides, J.A., C.A. Richardson, and G.A. Jull. 1996. Multifidus muscle recovery is not automatic after resolution of acute, first-episode low back pain. *Spine* 21:2763-2769.

30. Hides, J., W. Stanton, M.D. Mendis, and M. Sexton. 2011. The relationship of transversus abdominis and lumbar multifidus clinical muscle tests in patients with chronic low back pain. *Manual Therapy* 16:573-577.

31. Hodges, P.W. 1999. Is there a role for transversus abdominis in lumbo-pelvic stability? *Manual Therapy* 4:74-86.

32. Hodges, P.W., and C.A. Richardson. 1996. Inefficient muscular stabilization of the lumbar spine associated with low back pain: A motor control evaluation of transversus abdominis. *Spine* 21:2640-2650.

33. Hodges, P.W., and C.A. Richardson. 1997. Contraction of the abdominal muscles associated with movement of the lower limb. *Physical Therapy* 77:132-142; discussion 142-144.

34. Hodges, P.W., and C.A. Richardson. 1997. Feedforward contraction of transversus abdominis is not influenced by the direction of arm movement. *Experimental Brain Research* 114:362-370.

35. Hodges, P.W., and C.A. Richardson. 1999. Altered trunk muscle recruitment in people with low back pain with upper limb movement at different speeds. *Archives of Physical Medicine and Rehabilitation* 80:1005-1012.

36. Huang, Z.-G., Y.-H. Feng, Y.-H. Li, and C.-S Lv. 2016. Systematic review and meta-analysis: Tai Chi for preventing falls in older adults. *BMJ Open* 7:e013661. https://doi.org/10.1136/bmjopen-2016-013661.

37. Imai, A., K. Kaneoka, Y. Okubo, I. Shiina, M. Tatsumura, S. Izumi, and H. Shiraki. 2010. Trunk muscle activity during lumbar stabilization exercises on both a stable and unstable surface. *Journal of Orthopaedic & Sports Physical Therapy* 40:369-375.

38. Jahnke, R., L. Larkey, C. Rogers, J. Etnier, and F. Lin. 2010. A comprehensive review of health benefits of qigong and tai chi. *American Journal of Health Promotion* 41:e1-e25.

39. Juker, D., S. McGill, P. Kropf, and T. Steffen. 1998. Quantitative intramuscular myoelectric activity of lumbar portions of psoas and the abdominal wall during a wide variety of tasks. *Medicine & Science in Sports & Exercise* 30:301-310.

40. Kim, M.J., D.W. Oh, and H.J. Park. 2013. Integrating arm movement into bridge exercise: Effect on EMG activity of selected trunk muscles. *Journal of Electromyography and Kinesiology* 23:1119-1123.

41. Kim, S.J., O.Y. Kwon, C.H. Yi, H.S. Jeon, J.S. Oh, H.S. Cynn, and J.H. Weon. 2011. Comparison of abdominal muscle activity during a single-legged hold in the hook-lying position on the floor and on a round foam roll. *Journal of Athletic Training* 46:403-408.

42. Kim, T.H.M., S. Dogra, B. Al-Sahab, and H. Tamim. 2014. Comparison of functional fitness outcomes in experienced and inexperienced older adults after 16-week tai chi program. *Alternative Therapies in Health and Medicine* 20:20-25.

43. Kolber, M.J., and J. Zepeda. 2004. Addressing hamstring flexibility in athletes with lower back pain: A discussion of commonly prescribed stretching exercises. *Strength and Conditioning Journal* 26:18-23.

44. Li, G.C., H. Yuan, and W. Zhang. 2014. Effects of tai chi on health-related quality of life in patients with chronic conditions: A systematic review of randomized controlled trials. *Complementary Therapies in Medicine* 22:743-755.

45. Majewski-Schrage, T., T.A. Evans, and B. Ragan. 2014. Development of a core-stability model: A Delphi approach. *Journal of Sport Rehabilitation* 23:95-106.

46. McGill, S.M. 2001. Low back stability: From formal description to issues for performance and rehabilitation. *Exercise and Sport Sciences Reviews* 29:26-31.

47. McGill, S. 2004. Mechanics and pathomechanics of muscles acting on the lumbar spine. In *Kinesiology: The mechanics and pathomechanics of human movement*, ed. C.A. Oatis. Philadelphia: Lippincott Williams & Wilkins.

48. McGill, S. 2004. *Ultimate back fitness and performance.* Waterloo, ON: Wabuno.

49. McGill, S., D. Juker, and P. Kropf. 1996. Quantitative intramuscular myoelectric activity of quadratus lumborum during a wide variety of tasks. *Clinical Biomechanics* 11:170-172.

50. McGill, S.M., and A. Karpowicz. 2009. Exercises for spine stabilization: Motion/motor patterns, stability progressions, and clinical technique. *Archives of Physical Medicine and Rehabilitation* 90:118-126.

51. Mok, N.W., E.W. Yeung, J.C. Cho, S.C. Hui, K.C. Liu, and C.H. Pang. 2014. Core muscle activity during suspension exercises. *Journal of Science and Medicine in Sport* 18(2): 189-194.

52. Nitz, A.J., and D. Peck. 1986. Comparison of muscle-spindle concentrations in large and small human epaxial muscles acting in parallel combinations. *American Surgeon* 52:273-277.

53. Nordin, M.F.V. 2001. *Basic biomechanics of the musculoskeletal system.* Philadelphia: Lippincott Williams & Wilkins.

54. Okubo, Y., K. Kaneoka, A. Imai, I. Shiina, M. Tatsumura, S. Izumi, and S. Miyakawa. 2010. Electromyographic analysis

of transversus abdominis and lumbar multifidus using wire electrodes during lumbar stabilization exercises. *Journal of Orthopaedic & Sports Physical Therapy* 40:743-750.

55. Panjabi, M.M. 1992. The stabilizing system of the spine, part 1: Function, dysfunction, adaptation, and enhancement. *Journal of Spinal Disorders* 5:383-389.

56. Panjabi, M.M. 1992. The stabilizing system of the spine, part 2: Neutral zone and instability hypothesis. *Journal of Spinal Disorders* 5:390-397.

57. Panjabi, M.M. 2003. Clinical spinal instability and low back pain. *Journal of Electromyography and Kinesiology* 13:371-379.

58. Panjabi, M., K. Abumi, J. Duranceau, and T. Oxland. 1989. Spinal stability and intersegmental muscle forces. A biomechanical model. *Spine (Phila Pa 1976)* 14:194-200.

59. Panjabi, M.M., C. Lydon, A. Vasavada, D. Grob, J.J. Crisco, and J. Dvorak. 1994. On the understanding of clinical instability. *Spine* 19:2642-2650.

60. Sahrmann, S. 2001. *Diagnosis and treatment of movement impairment syndromes.* Maryland Heights, MO: Mosby.

61. Saliba, S.A., T. Croy, R. Guthrie, D. Grooms, A. Weltman, and T.L. Grindstaff. 2010. Differences in transverse abdominis activation with stable and unstable bridging exercises in individuals with low back pain. *North American Journal of Sports Physical Therapy* 5:63-73.

62. Sengupta, D.K., and H.B. Fan. 2014. The basis of mechanical instability in degenerative disc disease: A cadaveric study of abnormal motion versus load distribution. *Spine* 39:1032-1043.

63. Sorosky, S., S. Stilp, and V. Akuthota. 2008. Yoga and Pilates in the management of low back pain. *Current Reviews in Musculoskeletal Medicine* 1:39-47.

64. Stanton, R., P.R. Reaburn, and B. Humphries. 2004. The effect of short-term Swiss ball training on core stability and running economy. *Journal of Strength and Conditioning Research* 18:522-528.

65. Steele, J., S. Bruce-Low, and D. Smith. 2014. A reappraisal of the deconditioning hypothesis in low back pain: Review of evidence from a triumvirate of research methods on specific lumbar extensor deconditioning. *Current Medical Research and Opinion* 30:865-911.

66. Stevens, V.K., P.L. Coorevits, K.G. Bouche, N.N. Mahieu, G.G. Vanderstraeten, and L.A. Danneels. 2007. The influence of specific training on trunk muscle recruitment patterns in healthy subjects during stabilization exercises. *Manual Therapy* 12:271-279.

67. Vera-Garcia, F.J., S.G. Grenier, and S.M. McGill. 2000. Abdominal muscle response during curl-ups on both stable and labile surfaces. *Physical Therapy* 80:564-569.

68. Wilke, H.J., P. Neef, M. Caimi, T. Hoogland, and L.E. Claes. 1999. New in vivo measurements of pressures in the intervertebral disc in daily life. *Spine* 24:755-762.

69. Yue, J.J., J.P. Timm, M.M. Panjabi, and J. Jaramillo-de la Torre. 2007. Clinical application of the Panjabi neutral zone hypothesis: The Stabilimax NZ posterior lumbar dynamic stabilization system. *Neurosurgical Focus* 22:E12.

Chapter 16

1. American College of Sports Medicine. 2014. *ACSM's resource manual for guidelines for exercise testing and prescription.* 7th ed. Philadelphia: Wolters Kluwer, Lippincott Williams & Wilkins.

2. American College of Sports Medicine. 2017. *ACSM's complete guide to fitness & health.* 2nd ed. Champaign, IL: Human Kinetics.

3. American College of Sports Medicine. 2022. *ACSM's guidelines for exercise testing and prescription.* 11th ed. Philadelphia: Wolters Kluwer.

4. Anderson, M. 2018. What is disordered eating? Accessed November 2022. www.eatright.org/health/diseases-and-conditions/eating-disorders/what-is-disordered-eating.

5. Bell, L., A. Ruddock, T. Maden-Wilkinson, and D. Rogerson. 2020. Overreaching and overtraining in strength sports and resistance training: A scoping review. *Journal of Sports Sciences* 38(16):1897-1912.

6. Bompa, T., and C.A. Buzzichelli. 2019. *Periodization.* 6th ed. Champaign, IL: Human Kinetics.

7. Bushman, B.A. 2016. Finding the balance between overload and recovery. *ACSM's Health & Fitness Journal* 20(1):5-8.

8. Cabre, H.E., S.R. Moore, A.E. Smith-Ryan, and A.C. Hackney. 2022. Relative energy deficient in sport (RED-S): Scientific, clinical, and practical implications for the female athlete. *German Journal of Sports Medicine* 73:225-234.

9. Cadegiani, F., and C.E. Kater. 2019. Novel insights of overtraining syndrome discovered from the EROS study. *BMJ Open Sport & Exercise Medicine* 5:e000542.

10. Carrard, J., A.-C. Rigort, C. Appenzeller-Herzog, F. College, K. Königstein, T. Hinrichs, and A. Schmidt-Trucksäss. 2022. Diagnosing overtraining syndrome: A scoping review. *Sports Health* 14(5):665-673.

11. DeSouza, M.J., R.J. Mallinson, N.C.A. Strock, K.J. Koltun, M.P Olmsted, E.A Ricker, J.L. Scheid, et al. 2021. Randomised controlled trial of the effects of increased energy intake on menstrual recovery in exercising women with menstrual disturbance: The "REFUEL" study. *Human Reproduction* 36(8):2285-2297.

12. DeSouza, M.J., A. Nattiv, E. Joy, M. Misra, N.I. Williams, R.J. Mallinson, J.C. Gibbs, M. Olmsted, M. Goolsby, G. Matheson, and Expert Panel. 2014. 2014 Female Athlete Triad Coalition consensus statement on treatment and return to play of the Female Athlete Triad. *British Journal of Sports Medicine* 48:289.

13. DeSouza, M.J., E.A. Ricker, R.J. Mallinson, H.C.M. Allaway, K.J. Kolton, N.C.A. Strock, J.C. Gibbs, P.K. Don, and N.I. Williams. 2022. Bone mineral density in response to increased energy intake in exercising women with oligomenorrhea/amenorrhea: The REFUEL randomized controlled trial. *American Journal of Clinical Nutrition* 115:1457-1472.

14. Female and Male Athlete Triad Coalition. n.d. Accessed November 2022. https://femaleandmaleathletetriad.org/.

15. Fredericson, M., A. Kussman, M. Misra, M.T. Barrack, M.J. De Souza, E. Kraus, K.J. Koltun, N.I. Williams, E. Joy, and A. Nattiv. 2021. The Male Athlete Triad—A consensus statement from the Female and Male Athlete Triad Coalition Part II: Diagnosis, treatment, and return-to-play. *Clinical Journal of Sports Medicine* 31:349-366.

16. Gabbett, T.J. 2020. How much? How fast? How soon? Three simple concepts for progressing training loads to minimize injury risk and enhance performance. *Journal of Orthopaedic & Sports Physical Therapy* 50(10):570-573.

17. Grandou, C., L. Wallace, F. Impellizzeri, N. Allen, and A. Coutts. 2020. Overtraining in resistance exercise: An exploratory systematic review and methodological appraisal of the literature. *Sports Medicine* 50:815-828.

18. Haff, G.G., and N.T. Triplett. 2016. *Essentials of strength training and conditioning.* 4th ed. Champaign, IL: Human Kinetics.

19. Kellman, M., M. Bertollo, L. Bosquet, M. Brink, A.J. Coutts, R. Duffield, and D. Erlacher. 2018. Recovery and performance in sport: Consensus statement. *International Journal of Sports Physiology and Performance* 13:240-245.

20. Koltun, K.J., N.C.A. Strock, E.A. Southmayd, A.P. Oneglia, N.I. Williams, and M.J. DeSouza. 2019. Comparison of Female Athlete Triad Coalition and RED-S risk assessment tools. *Journal of Sports Sciences* 37(21):2433-2442.

21. Kreher, J.B. 2016. Diagnosis and prevention of overtraining syndrome: An opinion on education strategies. *Open Access Journal of Sports Medicine* 7:115-122.

22. Meeusen, R., M. Duclos, C. Foster, A. Fry, M. Gleeson, D. Nieman, J. Raglin, G. Rietjens, J. Steinacker, A. Urhausen, European College of Sport Science, and American College of Sports Medicine. 2013. Prevention, diagnosis, and treatment of the overtraining syndrome: Joint consensus statement of the European College of Sport Science and the American College of Sports Medicine. *Medicine & Science in Sports & Exercise* 45(1):186-205.

23. Moesgaard, L., M.M. Beck, L. Christiansen, P. Aagaard, and J. Lundbye-Jensen. 2022. Effects of periodization on strength and muscle hypertrophy in volume-equated resistance training programs: A systematic review and meta-analysis. *Sports Medicine* 52:1647-1666.

24. Mountjoy, M., J. Sundgot-Borgen, L. Burke, S. Carter, N. Constantini, C. Lebrun, N. Meyer, et al. 2014. The IOC consensus statement: Beyond the Female Athlete Triad—Relative Energy Deficiency in Sport (RED-S). *British Journal of Sports Medicine* 48:491-497.

25. National Eating Disorders Association. n.d. Information by eating disorder. Accessed November 2022. www.nationaleatingdisorders.org/information-eating-disorder.

26. National Institutes of Health. 2021. Eating disorders: About more than food. NIH Publication No. 21-MH-4901. www.nimh.nih.gov/health/publications/eating-disorders.

27. Nattiv, A., M.J. De Souza, K.J. Kotun, M. Misra, A. Kussman, N.I. Williams, M.T. Barrack, E. Kraus, E. Joy, and M. Fredericson. 2021. The Male Athlete Triad—A consensus statement from the Female and Male Athlete Triad Coalition Part 1: Definition and Scientific Basis. *Clinical Journal of Sports Medicine* 31:335-348.

28. Nattiv, A., A.B. Loucks, M.M. Manore, C.F. Sanborn, J. Sungot-Borgen, and M.P. Warren. 2007. The female athlete triad. *Medicine & Science in Sports & Exercise* 39(10):1867-1882.

29. Otis, C.L., B. Drinkwater, M. Johnson, A. Loucks, and J. Wilmore. 1997. ACSM position stand: The female athlete triad. *Medicine & Science in Sports & Exercise* 29(5):i-ix.

30. Ratamess, N., and the American College of Sports Medicine. 2021. *ACSM's foundations of strength and conditioning.* 2nd ed. Philadelphia: Wolters Kluwer.

31. U.S. Department of Health and Human Services. 2018. *Physical activity guidelines for Americans.* 2nd ed. https://health.gov/our-work/nutrition-physical-activity/physical-activity-guidelines/current-guidelines.

32. Weakley, J., S.L. Halson, and I. Mujika. 2022. Overtraining syndrome symptoms and diagnosis in athletes: Where it the research? A systematic review. *International Journal of Sports Physiology and Performance* 17:675-681.

33. Yeager, K.K., R. Agostini, A. Nattiv, and B. Drinkwater. 1993. The female athlete triad: Disordered eating, amenorrhea, osteoporosis. *Medicine & Science in Sports & Exercise* 25(7):775-777.

Chapter 17

1. Álvarez-Bueno, C., C. Pesce, I. Cavero-Redondo, M. Sánchez-López, M. Garrido-Miguel, and V. Martínez-Vizcaíno. 2017. Academic achievement and physical activity: A meta-analysis. *Pediatrics* 140:e20171498.

2. American College of Sports Medicine. 2022. *ACSM's guidelines for exercise testing and prescription.* Baltimore, MD: Wolters Kluwer.

3. Aubert, S., J. Barnes, C. Abdeta, P. Abi Nader, A. Adeniyi, N. Aguilar-Farias, D. Tenesaca, et al. 2018. Global matrix 3.0 physical activity report card grades for children and youth: Results and analysis from 49 countries. *Journal of Physical Activity and Health* 15:S251-S273.

4. Bai, Y., K. Allums-Featherston, P. Saint-Maurice, G. Welk, and N. 2018. Candelaria. Evaluation of youth enjoyment toward physical activity and sedentary behavior. *Pediatric Exercise Science* 30:273-280.

5. Barnett, L., D. Stodden, K. Cohen, J. Smith, D. Lubans, M. Lenoir, S. Iivonen, A. Miller, A. Laukkanen, D. Dudley, N. Lander, H. Brown, and P. Morgan. 2016. Fundamental movement skills: An important focus. *Journal of Teaching in Physical Education* 35:219-225.

6. Belcher, B., J. Zink, A. Azad, C. Campbell, S. Chakravartti, and M. Herting M. 2021. The roles of physical activity, exercise, and fitness in promoting resilience during adolescence: Effects on mental well-being and brain development. *Biological Psychiatry Cognitive Neuroscience and Neuroimaging* 6(2):225-237.

7. Biddle, S., C. Ciaccioni, G. Thomas, and I. Vergeer. 2019. Physical activity and mental health in children and adolescents: An updated review of reviews and analysis of causality. *Psychology of Sports and Exercise* 42:146-155.

8. Bloemers, F., D. Collard, M. Paw, W. Van Mechelen, J. Twisk, and E. Verhagen. 2012. Physical inactivity is a risk factor for physical activity-related injuries in children. *British Journal of Sports Medicine* 46:669-674.

9. Boisseau, N., and P. Delamarche. 2000. Metabolic and hormonal responses to exercise in children and adolescents. *Sports Medicine* 30:405-422.

10. Bolger, L., L. Bolger, C. O'Neill, E. Coughlan, W. O'Brien, S. Lacey, C. Burns, and F. Bardid. 2021. Global levels of fundamental motor skills in children: A systematic review. *Journal of Sports Sciences* 39:717-753.

11. Bruno, L., and A. Farrell. 2017. PE Ninja Warrior. *Strategies* 30:20-32.

12. Budzynski-Seymour, E., M. Jones, and J. Steele. 2022. A physically active experience: Setting the stage for a new approach to engage children in physical activity using themed entertainment experiences. *Sports Medicine* 52(11):2579-2591.

13. Bukowsky, M., A. Faigenbaum, and G. Myer. 2014. FUNdamental Integrative Training (FIT) for physical education. *Journal of Physical Education Recreation and Dance* 85:23-30.

14. Cao, M., M. Quan, and J. Zhuang. 2019. Effect of high-intensity interval training versus moderate-intensity continuous training on cardiorespiratory fitness in children and adolescents: A meta-analysis. *International Journal of Environmental Research and Public Health* 16:E1533.

15. Cao, M., Y. Tang, S. Li, and Y. Zou. 2021. Effects of high-intensity interval training and moderate-intensity continuous training on cardiometabolic risk factors in overweight and obesity children and adolescents: A meta-analysis of randomized controlled trials. *International Journal of Environmental Research and Public Health* 18:11905.

16. Chen, M., J. Liu, Y. Ma, Y. Li, D. Gao, L. Chen, T. Ma, Y. Dong, and J. Ma. 2021. Association between body fat and elevated blood pressure among children and adolescents aged 7-17 years: Using dual-energy X-ray absorptiometry (DEXA) and bioelectrical impedance analysis (BIA) from a cross-sectional study in China. *International Journal of Environmental Research and Public Health* 18:9254.

17. Chen, T., K. Watson, S. Michael, and S. Carlson. 2021. Sex-stratified trends in meeting physical activity guidelines, participating in sports, and attending physical education among US adolescents, Youth Risk Behavior Survey 2009-2019. *Journal of Physical Activity and Health* 18:S102-S113.

18. Cicone, Z., C. Holmes, M. Fedewa, H. MacDonald, and M. Esco. 2019. Age-based prediction of maximal heart rate in children and adolescents: A systematic review and meta-analysis. *Research Quarterly in Exercise and Sport* 90:417-428.

19. Clark, B., and T. Manini. 2012. What is dynapenia? *Nutrition* 28:495-503.

20. Collins, H., J. Booth, A. Duncan, and S. Fawkner. 2019. The effect of resistance training interventions on fundamental movement skills in youth: A meta-analysis. *Sports Medicine Open* 5:17.

21. Collins, H., J. Booth, A. Duncan, S. Fawkner, and A. Niven. 2019. The effect of resistance training Interventions on "the self" in youth: A systematic review and meta-analysis. *Sports Medicine Open* 5:29.

22. Council on Sports Medicine and Fitness and Council on School Health, M. Bergeron, C. Devore, and S. Rice. 2011. Policy statement—Climatic heat stress and exercising children and adolescents. *Pediatrics* 128:e741-e747.

23. De Meester, A., D. Stodden, J. Goodway, L. True, A. Brian, R. Ferkel, and L. Haerens. 2018. Identifying a motor proficiency barrier for meeting physical activity guidelines in children. *Journal of Science and Medicine in Sport* 21:58-62.

24. Dishman, R., R. Motl, R. Saunders, G. Felton, D. Ward, M. Dowda, and R. Pate. 2005. Enjoyment mediates effects of a school-based physical activity intervention. *Medicine & Science in Sports & Exercise* 37:478-487.

25. Donnelly, J., C. Hillman, D. Castelli, J. Etnier, S. Lee, P. Tomporowski, K. Lambourne, and A. Szabo-Reed. 2016. Physical activity, fitness, cognitive function, and academic achievement in children: A systematic review. *Medicine & Science in Sports & Exercise* 48:1197-1222.

26. Eime, R., J. Young, J. Harvey, M. Charity, and W. Payne. 2013. A systematic review of the psychological and social benefits of participation in sport for children and adolescents: Informing development of a conceptual model of health through sport. *International Journal of Behavioral Nutrition and Physical Activity* 10:98.

27. Faigenbaum, A., and L. Bruno. 2017. A fundamental approach for treating pediatric dynapenia in kids. *ACSM's Health and Fitness Journal* 21:18-24.

28. Faigenbaum, A., J. Kang, N. Ratamess, A. Farrell, M. Belfert, S. Duffy, C. Jenson, and J. Bush. 2019. Acute cardiometabolic responses to multi-modal integrative neuromuscular training in children. *Journal of Functional Morphology and Kinesiology* 4:39.

29. Faigenbaum, A., R. Lloyd, J. MacDonald, and G. Myer. 2016. Citius, Altius, Fortius: Beneficial effects of resistance training for young athletes: Narrative review. *British Journal of Sports Medicine* 50:3-7.

30. Faigenbaum, A., R. Lloyd, and G. Myer. 2013. Youth resistance training: Past practices, new perspectives and future directions. *Pediatric Exercise Science* 25:591-604.

31. Faigenbaum, A., R. Lloyd, J. Oliver, and American College of Sports Medicine. 2020. *Essentials of youth fitness.* Champaign, IL: Human Kinetics.

32. Faigenbaum, A., J. MacDonald, A. Straccioloni, and T. Rial Rebullido. 2020. Making a strong case for prioritizing muscular fitness in youth physical activity guidelines. *Current Sports Medicine Reports* 19:530-536.

33. Faigenbaum, A., and T. Rial Rebullido. 2018. Understanding physical literacy in youth. *Strength and Conditioning Journal* 40:90-94.

34. Faigenbaum, A., T. Rial Rebullido, J. Pena, and I. Chulvi-Medrano. 2019. Resistance exercise for the prevention and treatment of pediatric dynapenia. *Journal of Science in Sport and Exercise* 1:208-216.

35. Faigenbaum, A., T. Rial Rebullido, and L. Zaichkowsky. 2022. Heads up: Effective strategies for promoting mental health literacy in youth fitness programs. *ACSM's Health and Fitness Journal* 26:12-19.

36. Falk, B., and R. Dotan. 2006. Child-adult differences in the recovery from high-intensity exercise. *Exercise and Sport Science Reviews* 34:107-112.

37. Falk, B., and R. Dotan. 2019. Measurement and interpretation of maximal aerobic power in children. *Pediatric Exercise Science* 31:144-151.

38. Fraser, B., L. Blizzard, M. Buscot, M. Schmidt, T. Dwyer, A. Venn, and C. Magnussen. 2021. The association between grip strength measured in childhood, young- and mid-adulthood and prediabetes or type 2 diabetes in mid-adulthood. *Sports Medicine* 51:175-183.

39. Fraser, B., L. Blizzard, M. Buscot, M. Schmidt, T. Dwyer, A. Venn, and C. Magnussen. 2021. Muscular strength across the life course: The tracking and trajectory patterns of muscular strength between childhood and mid-adulthood in an Australian cohort. *Journal of Science and Medicine in Sport* 24:696-701.

40. García-Hermoso, A., Y. Ezzatvar, R. Ramírez-Vélez, J. Olloquequi, and M. Izquierdo. 2021. Is device-measured vigorous physical activity associated with health-related outcomes in children and adolescents? A systematic review and meta-analysis. *Journal of Sport and Health Science* 10:296-307.

41. García-Hermoso, A., M. Izquierdo, and R. Ramírez-Vélez. 2022. Tracking of physical fitness levels from childhood and adolescence to adulthood: A systematic review and meta-analysis. *Translational Pediatrics* 11:474-486.

42. García-Hermoso, A., R. Ramírez-Campillo, and M. Izquierdo. 2019. Is muscular fitness associated with future health benefits in children and adolescents? A systematic review and meta-analysis of longitudinal studies. *Sports Medicine* 49:1079-1094.

43. Guthold, R., G. Stevens, L. Riley, and F. Bull. 2020. Global trends in insufficient physical activity among adolescents: A pooled analysis of 298 population-based surveys with

1.6 million participants. *Lancet Child and Adolescent Health* 4:23-35.

44. Han, A., A. Fu, S. Cobley, and R. Sanders. 2017. Effectiveness of exercise intervention on improving fundamental movement skills and motor coordination in overweight/obese children and adolescents: A systematic review. *Journal of Science and Medicine in Sport* 21:89-102.

45. Hardy, L., D. Merom, M. Thomas, and L. Peralta. 2018. 30-year changes in Australian children's standing broad jump: 1985-2015. *Journal of Science and Medicine in Sport* 21:1057-1061.

46. Harrington, D., F. Gillison, S. Broyles, J. Chaput, M. Fogelholm M, G. Hu, R. Kuriyan, et al. 2016. Household-level correlates of children's physical activity levels in and across 12 countries. *Obesity (Silver Spring)* 24: 2150-2157.

47. Henriksson, H., P. Henriksson, P. Tynelius, and F. Ortega. 2019. Muscular weakness in adolescence is associated with disability 30 years later: A population-based cohort study of 1.2 million men *British Journal of Sports Medicine* 53:1221-1230.

48. Hillman, C., K. McDonald, and N. Logan. 2020. A review of the effects of physical activity on cognition and brain health across children and adolescence. *Nestlé Nutrition Institute Workshop Series* 95:116-126.

49. Hulteen, R., P. Morgan, L. Barnett, D. Stodden, and D. Lubans. 2018. Development of foundational movement skills: A conceptual model for physical activity across the lifespan. *Sports Medicine* 48:1533-1540.

50. Institute of Medicine. 2013. *Educating the student body: Taking physical activity and physical education to school.* Washington, DC: The National Academies Press.

51. Janssen, I., and A. LeBlance. 2010. Systematic review of the health benefits of physical activity and fitness in school-aged children and youth. *International Journal of Behavior, Nutrition and Physical Activity* 7:40.

52. Kaster, T., F. Dooley, J. Fitzgerald, T. Walch, M. Annandale, K. Ferrar, J. Lang, J. Smith, and G. Tomkinson. 2020. Temporal trends in the sit-ups performance of 9,939,289 children and adolescents between 1964 and 2017. *Journal of Sport Sciences* 38:1913-1923.

53. Katzmarzyk, P., K. Denstel, K. Beals, J. Carlson, S. Crouter, T. McKenzie, R. Pate, et al. 2018. Results from the United States 2018 report card on physical activity for children and youth. *Journal of Physical Activity and Health* 15:S422-S424.

54. Kavouras, S., G. Arnaoutis, M. Makrillos, C. Garagouni, E. Nikolaou, O. Chira, E. Ellinikaki, and L. Sidossis. 2012. Educational intervention on water intake improves hydration status and enhances exercise performance in athletic youth. *Scandinavian Journal of Medicine and Science in Sports* 22:684-689.

55. Khan, A., E. Lee, S. Rosenbaum, S. Khan, and M. Tremblay. 2021. Dose-dependent and joint associations between screen time, physical activity, and mental wellbeing in adolescents: An international observational study. *Lancet Child and Adolescent Health* 5:729-738.

56. Korczak, D., S. Madigan, and M. Colasanto. 2017. Children's physical activity and depression: A meta-analysis. *Pediatrics* 139:e20162266.

57. Lai, S., S. Costigan, P. Morgan, D. Lubans, D. Stodden, J. Salmon, and L. Barnett. 2014. Do school-based interventions focusing on physical activity, fitness, or fundamental

movement skill competency produce a sustained impact in these outcomes in children and adolescents? A systematic review of follow-up studies. *Sports Medicine* 44:67-79.

58. Lee, B., A. Adam, E. Zenkov, D. Hertenstein, M. Ferguson, P. Wang, M. Wong, et al. 2017. Modeling the economic and health impact of increasing children's physical activity in the United States. *Health Affairs (Millford)* 36:902-908.

59. Lesinski, M., O. Prieske, and U. Granacher. 2016. Effects and dose–response relationships of resistance training on physical performance in youth athletes: A systematic review and meta-analysis. *British Journal of Sports Medicine* 50:781-795.

60. Lloyd, R., J. Cronin, A. Faigenbaum, G. Haff, R. Howard, W. Kraemer, L. Micheli, G. Myer, and J. Oliver. 2016. The National Strength and Conditioning Association position statement on long-term athletic development. *Journal of Strength and Conditioning Research* 30:1491-1509.

61. Lloyd, R., A. Faigenbaum, M. Stone, J. Oliver, I. Jeffreys, J. Moody, C. Brewer, et al. 2014. Position statement on youth resistance training: The 2014 International Consensus. *British Journal of Sports Medicine* 48:498-505.

62. Malina, R., C. Bouchard, and O. Bar-Or. 2004. *Growth, maturation and physical activity.* Champaign, IL: Human Kinetics.

63. Marques, A., D. Santos, C. Hillman, and L. Sardinha. 2018. How does academic achievement relate to cardiorespiratory fitness, self-reported physical activity and objectively reported physical activity: A systematic review in children and adolescents aged 6-18 years. *British Journal of Sports Medicine* 52:1039.

64. Momma, H., R. Kawakami, T. Honda, and S. Sawada. 2022. Muscle-strengthening activities are associated with lower risk and mortality in major non-communicable diseases: A systematic review and meta-analysis of cohort studies. *British Journal of Sports Medicine* 56:755-763.

65. Morgan, P., L. Barnett, D. Cliff, A. Okely, H. Scott, K. Cohen, and D. Lubans. 2013. Fundamental movement skill interventions in youth: A systematic review and meta-analysis. *Pediatrics* 132:e1361-1683.

66. Myer, G., A. Faigenbaum, D. Chu, J. Falkel, K. Ford, T. Best, and T. Hewett. 2011. Integrative training for children and adolescents: Techniques and practices for reducing sports-related injuries and enhancing athletic performance. *Physician and Sports Medicine* 39:74-84.

67. Myer, G., A. Faigenbaum, E. Edwards, J. Clark, T. Best, and R. Sallis. 2015. 60 minutes of what? A developing brain perspective for activation children with an integrative approach. *British Journal of Sports Medicine* 49:1510-1516.

68. National Association for Sport and Physical Education and American Heart Association. 2016. 2016 Shape of the Nation report: Status of physical education in the USA. Reston, VA: American Alliance for Health, Physical Education, Recreation and Dance.

69. Neville, R., K. Lakes, W. Hopkins, G. Tarantino, C. Draper, R. Beck, and S. Madigan. 2022. Global changes in child and adolescent physical activity during the COVID-19 pandemic: A systematic review and meta-analysis. *JAMA Pediatrics* 176:886-894.

70. Notley, S., A. Akerman, R. Meade, G. McGarr, and G. Kenny. 2020. Exercise thermoregulation in prepubertal children: A brief methodological review. *Medicine & Science in Sports & Exercise* 52:2412-2422.

71. Orsso, C., J. Tibaes, C. Oliveira, D. Rubin, C. Field, S. Heymsfield, C. Prado, and A. Haqq. 2019. Low muscle mass and strength in pediatrics patients: Why should we care? *Clinical Nutrition* 38:2002-2015.

72. Ortega, F., J. Ruiz, M. Castillo, and M. Sjostrom. 2008. Physical fitness in children and adolescence: A powerful marker of health. *International Journal of Obesity* 32:1-11.

73. Pacheco, M., F. Dos Santos, M. Marques, J. Maia, and G. Tani. 2021. Transitional movement skill dependence on fundamental movement skills: Testing Seefeldt's proficiency barrier. *Research Quarterly for Exercise and Sport* 11:1-10.

74. Pandya, N. 2021. Disparities in youth sports and barriers to participation. *Current Review Musculoskeletal Medicine* 14:441-446.

75. Pesce, C. 2012. Shifting the focus from quantitative to qualitative exercise characteristics in exercise and cognition research. *Journal of Sport and Exercise Psychology* 34:766-786.

76. Petushek, E., D. Sugimoto, M. Stoolmiller, G. Smith, and G. Myer. 2019. Evidence-based best-practice guidelines for preventing anterior cruciate ligament injuries in young female athletes: A systematic review and meta-analysis. *American Journal of Sports Medicine* 47:1744-1753.

77. Pilli, N., T. Kybartas, K. Lagally, and K. Laurson. 2021. Low muscular strength, weight status, and metabolic syndrome in adolescents: National Health and Nutrition Examination Survey 2011-2014. *Pediatric Exercise Science* 33:90-94.

78. Poitras, V., C. Gray, M. Borghese, V. Carson, J. Chaput, I. Janssen, P. Katzmarzyk, et al. 2016. Systematic review of the relationships between objectively measured physical activity and health indicators in school-aged children and youth. *Applied Physiology Nutrition and Metabolism* 41:S197-S239.

79. Robinson, L., D. Stodden, L. Barnett, V. Lopes, S. Logan, L. Rodrigues, and E. D'Hondt. 2015. Motor competence and its effect on positive developmental trajectories of health. *Sports Medicine* 45:1273-1284.

80. Rowland, T. 2007. *Children's exercise physiology.* Champaign, IL: Human Kinetics.

81. Ruiz, R., E. Sommer, D. Tracy, J. Banda, C. Economos, M. JaKa, K. Evenson, M. Buchowski, and S. Barkin. 2018. Novel patterns of physical activity in a large sample of preschool-aged children. *BMC Public Health* 18:242.

82. Sandercock, G., and D. Cohen. 2019. Temporal trends in muscular fitness of English 10-year-olds 1998-2014: An allometric approach. *Journal of Science and Medicine in Sport* 22:201-205.

83. Schwarzfischer, P., D. Gruszfeld, P. Socha, V. Luque, R. Closa-Monasterolo, D. Rousseaux, M. Moretti, B. Mariani, E. Verduci, B. Koletzko, and V. Grote. 2018. Longitudinal analysis of physical activity, sedentary behaviour and anthropometric measures from ages 6 to 11 years. *International Journal of Behavior, Nutrition and Physical Activity* 15:126.

84. Smith, J., N. Eather, R. Weaver, N. Riley, M. Beets, and D. Lubans. Behavioral correlates of muscular fitness in children and adolescents: A systematic review. *Sports Medicine* 49:887-904.

85. Soomro, N., R. Sanders, D. Hackett, T. Hubka, S. Ebrahimi, J. Freeston, and S. Cobley. 2016. The efficacy of injury prevention programs in adolescent team sports: A meta-analysis. *American Journal of Sports Medicine* 44:2415-2424

86. Stodden, D., L. True, S. Langendorfer, and Z. Gao. 2013. Associations among selected motor skills and health-related fitness: Indirect evidence for Seefeldt's proficiency barrier theory in young adults? *Research Quarterly in Exercise and Sport* 84:397-403.

87. Stricker, P., A. Faigenbaum, T. McCambridge, and Council on Sports Medicine and Fitness. 2020. Resistance training for children and adolescents. *Pediatrics* 145:e20201011.

88. Sugimoto, D., G. Myer, K. Barber Foss, M. Pepin, L. Micheli, and T. Hewett. 2016. Critical components of neuromuscular training to reduce ACL injury risk in female athletes: Meta-regression analysis. *British Journal of Sports Medicine* 50:1259-1266.

89. Telama, R. 2009. Tracking of physical activity from childhood to adulthood: A review. *Obesity Facts* 2:187-195.

90. Telama, R., X. Yang, E. Leskinen, A. Kankaanpää, M. Hirvensalo, T. Tammelin, J. Viikari, and O. Raitakari. 2014. Tracking of physical activity from early childhood through youth into adulthood. *Medicine & Science in Sports & Exercise* 46:955-962.

91. Tudor-Locke, C., W. Johnson, and P. Katzmarzyk. 2010. Accelerometer-determined steps per day in US children and adolescents. *Medicine & Science in Sports & Exercise* 42:2244-2250.

92. United States Department of Health and Human Services. 2018. *Physical activity guidelines for Americans.* Washington, DC: Author.

93. van Ekris, E., K. Wijndaele, T. Altenburg, A. Atkin, J. Twisk, L. Andersen, K. Janz, et al. 2020. Tracking of total sedentary time and sedentary patterns in youth: A pooled analysis using the International Children's Accelerometry Database (ICAD). *International Journal of Behavior, Nutrition and Physical Activity* 17:65.

94. Vancampfort, D., G. Ashdown-Franks, L. Smith, J. Firth, T. Van Damme, L. Christiaansen, B. Stubbs, and A. Koyanagi. 2019. Leisure-time sedentary behavior and loneliness among 148,045 adolescents aged 12-15 years from 52 low- and middle-income countries. *Journal of Affective Disorders* 251:149-155.

95. Visek, A., S. Achrati, H. Manning, K. McDonnell, B. Harris, and L. Dipietro. 2015. The Fun Integration Theory: Towards sustaining children and adolescents sport participation. *Journal of Physical Activity and Health* 12:424-433.

96. Walker, G., A. Stracciolini, A. Faigenbaum, and G. Myer. 2018. Physical inactivity in youth. Can exercise deficit disorder alter the way we view preventive care? *ACSM's Health and Fitness Journal* 22:42-46.

97. Webster, K., and T. Hewett. 2018. Meta-analysis of meta-analyses of anterior cruciate ligament injury reduction training programs. *Journal of Orthopaedic Research* 36:2696-2708.

98. Whitehead, M. 2010. *Physical literacy throughout the lifecourse.* London: Routledge, Taylor & Francis Group.

99. Wilk, B., F. Meyer, O. Bar-Or, and B. Timmons. 2014. Mild to moderate hypohydration reduces boys' high-intensity cycling performance in the heat. *European Journal of Applied Physiology* 114:707-713.

100. World Health Organization. 2020. *WHO guidelines on physical activity and sedentary behaviour.* Geneva: Author.

Chapter 18

1. Abe, T., D.V. DeHoyos, M.L. Pollock, and L. Garzarella L. 2000. Time course for strength and muscle thickness changes following upper and lower body resistance

training in men and women. *European Journal of Applied Physiology* 81(3):174-80.

2. American College of Sports Medicine (ACSM). 2011. The recommended quantity and quality of exercise for developing and maintaining cardiorespiratory, musculoskeletal, and neuromotor fitness in apparently healthy adults: Guidance for prescribing exercise. *Medicine & Science in Sports & Exercise* 43(7):1334-1359.

3. American College of Sports Medicine (ACSM). 2022. *ACSM's guidelines for exercise testing and prescription*. 11th ed. Philadelphia: Wolters Kluwer.

4. American Council on Exercise. 1998. *Exercise for the older adult*. Champaign, IL: Human Kinetics.

5. American Geriatrics Society Panel on Exercise and Osteoarthritis. 2001. Exercise prescription for older adults with osteoarthritis pain: Consensus practice recommendations. A supplement to the AGS Clinical Practice Guidelines on the management of chronic pain in older adults. *Journal of the American Geriatrics Society* 49:808-823.

6. Bloomfield, S.A., and S.S. Smith. 2003. Osteoporosis. In *ACSM's exercise management for persons with chronic diseases and disabilities*, 2nd ed., ed. J.L. Durstine and G.E. Moore, 222-229. Champaign, IL: Human Kinetics.

7. Chang, Y.K., J.D. Labban, J.I. Gapin, and J.L. Etnier. 2012. The effects of acute exercise on cognitive performance: A meta-analysis. *Brain Research* 1453:87-101.

8. Chodzko-Zajko, W.J. 1998. Physical activity and aging: Implications for health and quality of life in older persons. *PCPFS Research Digest* 3(4).

9. Chodzko-Zajko, W., and American College of Sports Medicine. 2013. *ACSM's exercise for older adults*. Philadelphia: Lippincott Williams & Wilkins.

10. Chodzko-Zajko, W.J., D.N. Proctor, F. Singh, C.T. Minson, C.R. Nigg, G.J. Salem, and J. Skinner. 2009. Exercise and physical activity for older adults. *Medicine & Science in Sports & Exercise* 41(7):1510-1530.

11. Coe, D.P., and M. Fiatarone Singh. 2014. Exercise prescription in special populations: Women, pregnancy, children, and older adults. In *ACSM's resource manual for guidelines for exercise testing and prescription*, ed. D.P. Swain, 565-595. Baltimore: Wolters Kluwer/Lippincott Williams & Wilkins.

12. Criswell, D.S. 2001. Human development and aging. In *ACSM's health and fitness certification review*, ed. J.L. Roitman and K.W. Bibi, 31-47. Baltimore: Lippincott Williams & Wilkins.

13. Epel, E.S. 2020. The geroscience agenda: Toxic stress, hormetic stress, and the rate of aging. *Ageing Research Reviews* 63:101167.

14. Fiatarone, M.A., E.C. Marks, N.D. Ryan, C.N. Meredith, L.A. Lipsitz, and W.J. Evans. 1990. High-intensity strength training in nonagenarians. *Journal of the American Medical Association* 263:3029-3034.

15. Fitzgerald, M.D., H. Tanaka, Z.V. Tran, and D.R. Seals. 1997. Age-related declines in maximal aerobic capacity in regularly exercising vs. sedentary women: A meta-analysis. *Journal of Applied Physiology* 83:160-165.

16. Frontera, W.R., C.N. Meredith, K.P. O'Reilly, and W.J. Evans. 1990. Strength training and determinants of $\dot{V}O_2$max in older men. *Journal of Applied Physiology* 68:329-333.

17. Frontera, W.R., C.N. Meredith, K.P. O'Reilly, H.G. Knuttgen, and W.J. Evans. 1988. Strength conditioning in older men: Skeletal muscle hypertrophy and improved function. *Journal of Applied Physiology* 64:1038-1044.

18. Holloszy, J.O., and W.M. Kohrt. 1995. Exercise. In *Handbook of physiology, section 11: Aging*, ed. E.J. Masoro, 633-666. New York: Oxford Press.

19. Hostler, D., M.T. Crill, F.C. Hagerman, and R. S. Staron. 2001. The effectiveness of 0.5-lb increments in progressive resistance exercise. *Journal of Strength and Conditioning Research* 15(1):86-91.

20. Howley, E.T. 2001. Type of activity: Resistance, aerobic and leisure versus occupational physical activity. *Medicine & Science in Sports & Exercise* 33:S364-S369.

21. Hubal, M.J., H. Gordish-Dressman, P.D. Thompson, T.B. Price, E.P. Hoffman, T.J. Angelopoulos, P.M. Gordon, et al. 2005. Variability in muscle size and strength gain after unilateral resistance training. *Medicine & Science in Sport & Exercise* 37(6):964-72.

22. Knudson, D.V., P. Magnusson, and M. McHugh. 2000. Current issues in flexibility fitness. *President's Council on Physical Fitness and Sports Research Digest* 3(10):1-8.

23. Konopack, J.F., D.X. Marquez, L. Hu, S. Elavsky, E. McAuley, and A.F. Kramer. 2008. Correlates of functional fitness in older adults. *International Journal of Behavioral Medicine* 15(4):311-318.

24. Kraemer, W.J., S.J. Fleck, and W.J. Evans. 1996. Strength and power training: Physiological mechanisms of adaptations. *Exercise and Sport Sciences Reviews* 24:363-397.

25. Lin, J., L. Chen, S. Ni, Y. Ru, S. Ye, X. Fu, D. Gan, J. Li, S. Han, and S. Zhu. 2019. Association between sleep quality and bone mineral density in Chinese women vary by age and menopausal status. *Sleep Medicine* 53:75-80.

26. Nybo, L., J.F. Schmidt, S. Fritzdorf, and N.B. Nordsborg. 2014. Physiological characteristics of an aging Olympic athlete. *Medicine & Science in Sports & Exercise* 46:2132-2138.

27. Pate, R.R., M. Pratt, S.N. Blair, W.L. Haskell, C.A. Marcera, and C. Bouchard. 1995. Physical activity and public health: A recommendation from the Centers for Disease Control and Prevention and the American College of Sports Medicine. *Journal of the American Medical Association* 273:402-407.

28. Petit, M.A., J.M. Hughes, and J.M. Warpeha. 2007. Exercise prescription for people with osteoporosis. In *ACSM's resource manual for guidelines for exercise testing and prescription*, 6th ed., ed. J.K. Ehrman, 635-650. Baltimore: Lippincott Williams & Wilkins.

29. Ponti, F., A. Santoro, D. Mercatelli, C. Gasperini, M. Conte, M. Martucci, L. Sangiorgi, C. Franceschi, and A. Bazzocchi, 2020. Aging and imaging assessment of body composition: From fat to facts. *Frontiers in Endocrinology* 10:861.

30. Rickson, K.I., C. Hillman, C.M. Stillman, R.M. Ballard, B. Bloodgood, D.E. Conroy, R. Macko, D.X. Marquez, S.J. Petruzzello, and K.E. Powell. 2019. Physical activity, cognition, and brain outcomes: A review of the 2018 Physical Activity Guidelines. *Medicine & Science in Sports & Exercise* 51(6):1242-1251.

31. Rikli, R.E., and C.J. Jones. 2013. *Senior fitness test manual*. 2nd ed. Champaign, IL: Human Kinetics.

32. Roberts, B.M., G. Nuckols, and J.W. Krieger. Sex differences in resistance training: A systematic review and meta-analysis. *Journal of Strength and Conditioning Research* 34(5):1448-1460.

33. Rogers, M.A., and W.J. Evans. 1993. Changes in skeletal muscle with aging: Effects of exercise training. *Exercise and Sport Sciences Reviews* 21:65-102.

34. Salvador, E.P., R.M.R. Dias, A.L.D. Gurjão, A. Avelar, L.G. Pinto, and E.S. Cyrino. 2009. Effect of eight weeks of strength training on fatigue resistance in men and women. *Isokinetics and Exercise Science* 17(2):101-106.

35. Santoro, A., G. Guidarelli, R. Ostan, E. Giampieri, C. Fabbri, C. Bertarelli, C. Nicoletti, et al. 2019. Gender-specific association of body composition with inflammatory and adipose-related markers in healthy elderly Europeans from the NU-AGE study. *European Radiology* 29(9):4968-4979.

36. Scott, D., J. Johansson, L.B. McMillan, P.R. Ebeling, A. Nordstrom, and P. Nordstrom. 2019. Mid-calf skeletal muscle density and its associations with physical activity, bone health and incident 12-month falls in older adults: The Healthy Ageing Initiative. *Bone* 120:446-451.

37. Shephard, R.J. 1997. *Aging, physical activity, and health.* Champaign, IL: Human Kinetics.

38. Skinner, J.S. 2005. Aging for exercise testing and exercise prescription. In *Exercise testing and exercise prescription for special cases*, 3rd ed., ed. J.S. Skinner, 85-99. Baltimore: Lippincott Williams & Wilkins.

39. Spirduso, W.W., and D.L. Cronin. 2001. Exercise dose–response effects on quality of life and independent living in older adults. *Medicine & Science in Sports & Exercise* 33:S598-S608.

40. Spirduso, W.W., K.L. Francis, and P.G. MacRae. 2005. *Physical dimensions of aging.* 2nd ed. Champaign, IL: Human Kinetics.

41. Trappe, S., E. Hayes, A. Galpin, L. Kaminsky, B. Jemiolo, W. Fink, T. Trappe, A. Jansson, T. Gustafsson, and P. Tesch. 2013. New records in aerobic power among octogenarian lifelong endurance athletes. *Journal of Applied Physiology* 114:3-10.

42. U.S. Department of Health and Human Services (HHS). n.d. Healthy People 2030: Data PA-05. Accessed December 2022. https://health.gov/healthypeople/objectives-and-data/browse-objectives/physical-activity/increase-proportion-adults-who-do-enough-aerobic-and-muscle-strengthening-activity-pa-05/data.

43. U.S. Department of Health and Human Services (HHS). 2008. Physical Activity Guidelines Advisory Committee report 2008. http://health.gov/paguidelines/report/pdf/committeereport.pdf.

44. U.S. Department of Health and Human Services (HHS). 2008. *2008 physical activity guidelines for Americans.* www.health.gov/paguidelines/guidelines/default.aspx.

45. U.S. Department of Health and Human Services (HHS). 2018. Physical Activity Guidelines Advisory Committee scientific report. https://health.gov/paguidelines/second-edition/report/.

46. U.S. Department of Health and Human Services (HHS). 2018. *Physical activity guidelines for Americans.* 2nd ed. https://health.gov/our-work/nutrition-physical-activity/physical-activity-guidelines/current-guidelines.

47. U.S. Department of Health and Human Services (HHS). 2021. 2020 Profile of older Americans. https://acl.gov/sites/default/files/aging%20and%20Disability%20In%20America/2020Profileolderamericans.final_.pdf.

48. Valenzuela, P.L., N.A. Maffiuletti, M.J. Joyner, A. Lucia, and R. Lepers. 2020. Lifelong endurance exercise as a counter-measure against age-related $\dot{V}O_2$max decline: Physiological overview and insights from masters athletes. *Sports Medicine* 50(4):703-716.

49. Weiss, L.W., F.C. Clark, and D.G. Howard. 1988. Effects of heavy-resistance triceps surae muscle training on strength and muscularity of men and women. *Physical Therapy* 68(2):208-213.

50. World Health Organization (WHO). 1997. *A summary of the physiological benefits of physical activity for older persons.* Geneva: Author.

51. Wroblewski, A.P., F. Amati, M.A. Smiley, B. Goodpaster, and V. Wright. 2011. Chronic exercise preserves lean muscle mass in masters athletes. *Physician and Sportsmedicine* 39:172-178.

Chapter 19

1. American College of Obstetricians and Gynecologists (ACOG). 2020. Physical activity and exercise during pregnancy and the postpartum period. Committee Opinion No. 804. *Obstetrics and Gynecology* 135:e178-188.

1a. American College of Obstetricians and Gynecologists (ACOG). 1985. Exercise during pregnancy and the postnatal period. ACOG home exercise programs, pages 1-6.

2. American College of Sports Medicine (ACSM). 2022. *ACSM's guidelines for exercise testing and prescription.* 11th ed. Philadelphia: Wolters Kluwer.

3. American Diabetes Association Professional Practice Committee. 2022. 15. Management of diabetes in pregnancy: Standards of Medical Care in Diabetes-2022. *Diabetes Care* 45(Suppl. 1):S232-S2432.

4. Ben Ami, N., and G. Dar. 2018. What is the most effective verbal instruction for correctly contracting the pelvic floor muscles? *Neurourology Urodynamics* 37(8):2904-2910.

5. Bo, K., R. Artal, R. Barakat, W. Brown, G.A.L. Davies, M. Dooley, K.R. Evenson, et al. 2016. Exercise and pregnancy in recreational and elite athletes: 2016 evidence summary from the IOC expert group meeting, Lausanne. *British Journal of Sports Medicine* 50:571-589.

6. Canadian Society for Exercise Physiology. n.d. Pre-screen for physical activity in pregnancy: Get Active Questionnaire for Pregnancy. Accessed October 2022. https://csep.ca/2021/05/27/get-active-questionnaire-for-pregnancy/.

7. Centers for Disease Control and Prevention. 2021. Gestational diabetes. Accessed November 2022. www.cdc.gov/diabetes/basics/gestational.html.

8. Centers for Disease Control and Prevention. 2022. Weight gain during pregnancy. Accessed November 2022. www.cdc.gov/reproductivehealth/maternalinfanthealth/pregnancy-weight-gain.htm.

9. Chen, Y., G. Ma, Y. Hu, Q. Yang, J.M. Deavila, M.-J. Zhu, and M. Du. 2021. Effects of maternal exercise during pregnancy on perinatal growth and childhood obesity outcomes: A meta-analysis and meta-regression. *Sports Medicine* 51:2329-2347.

10. Davenport, M.H., and M. Hayman. 2022. Physical activity during pregnancy: Essential steps for maternal and fetal health. *Obstetric Medicine OnlineFirst* https://journals.sagepub.com/doi/epub/10.1177/1753495X221122540.

11. Davenport, M.H., V.L. Meah, S.-M. Ruchat, G.A. Davies, R.J. Skow, N. Barrowman, K.B. Adamo, et al. 2018. Impact of prenatal exercise on neonatal and childhood outcomes: A systematic review and meta-analysis. *British Journal of Sports Medicine* 52:1386-1396.

12. Davenport, M.H., T.S. Nagpal, M. Mottola, R.J. Skow, L. Riske, V.J. Poitras, M. Jaramillo, et al. 2018. Prenatal exercise (including but not limited to pelvic floor muscle training) and urinary incontinence during and following pregnancy: A systematic review and meta-analysis. *British Journal Sports Medicine* 52:1397-1404.

13. Davenport, M.H., S. Neil-Sztramko, B. Lett, M. Duggan, M.F. Mottola, S.-M. Ruchat, K.B. Adamo, et al. 2022. Development of the Get Active Questionnaire for Pregnancy: Breaking down barriers to prenatal exercise. *Applied Physiology, Nutrition, and Metabolism* 47:787-803.

14. Davenport, M.H., S.-M. Ruchat, V.J. Poitras, A.J. Garcia, C.E. Gray, N. Barrowman, R.J. Skow, et al. 2018. Prenatal exercise for the prevention of gestational diabetes mellitus and hypertensive disorders of pregnancy: A systematic review and meta-analysis. *British Journal of Sports Medicine* 52:1367-1375.

15. Davenport, M.H., R.J. Skow, and C.D. Steinback. 2016. Maternal response to aerobic exercise in pregnancy. *Clinical Obstetrics and Gynecology* 59(3):541-551.

16. Davenport, M.H, C. Yoo, M.F. Mottola, V.J. Poitras, A.J. Garcia C.E. Gray, N. Barrowman, et al. 2018. Effects of prenatal exercise on incidence of congenital anomalies and hyperthermia: A systematic review and meta-analysis. *British Journal of Sports Medicine* 53:116-123.

17. Díaz-Álvarez, L., L. Lorenzo-Gallego, H. Romay-Barrero, V. Prieto-Gómez, M. Torres-Lacomba, and B. Navarro-Brazález. 2022. Does the contractile capability of pelvic floor muscles improve with knowledge acquisition and verbal instructions in healthy women? A systematic review. *International Journal of Environmental Research and Public Health* 19(15):9308.

18. Dipietro, L., K.R. Evenson, B. Bloodgood, K. Sprow, R.P. Troiano, K.L. Piercy, A. Vaux-Bjerke, and K.E. Powell for the 2018 Physical Activity Guidelines Advisory Committee. 2019. Benefits of physical activity during pregnancy and postpartum: An umbrella review. *Medicine & Science in Sports & Exercise* 51(6):1292-1302.

19. Downs, D.S., L. Chasan-Taber, K.R. Evenson, J. Leiferman, and S. Yeo. 2012. Physical activity and pregnancy: Past and present evidence and future recommendations. *Research Quarterly in Exercise and Sport* 83(4):485-502.

20. García-Sánchez, E., V. Ávila-Gandía, J. López-Román, A. Martínez-Rodríguez, and J.Á. Rubio-Arias. 2019. What pelvic floor muscle training load is optimal in minimizing urine loss in women with stress urinary incontinence? A Systematic Review and Meta-Analysis. *International Journal of Environmental Research and Public Health* 16(22):4358.

21. Greg, V.H., and J.E. Ferguson II. 2017. Exercise in pregnancy. *Clinics in Sports Medicine* 36:741-752.

22. Hage-Fransen, M., M. Wiezer, A. Otto, M.S. Wieffer-Platvoet, M.H. Slotman, M. Nijhuis-van der Sanden, and A.L. Pool-Goudzwaard. 2021. Pregnancy- and obstetric-related risk factors for urinary incontinence, fecal incontinence, or pelvic organ prolapse later in life: A systematic review and meta-analysis. *Acta Obstetricia Et Gynecologica Scandinavica* 100(3):373-382.

23. Hod, M., A. Kapur, D.A. Sacks, E. Hadar, M. Agarwal, G.C. Di Renzo, L.C. Roura, H.D. McIntyre, J.L. Morris, and H. Divakar. 2015. The International Federation of Gynecology and Obstetrics (FIGO) Initiative on gestational diabetes mellitus: A pragmatic guide for diagnosis, management, and care. *International Journal of Gynecology and Obstetrics* 131(S3):S173-S211.

24. Moossdorff-Steinhauser, H., B. Berghmans, M. Spaanderman, and E. Bols. 2021. Prevalence, incidence and bothersomeness of urinary incontinence between 6 weeks and 1 year post-partum: A systematic review and meta-analysis. *International Urogynecology Journal* 32(7):1675-1693.

25. Moossdorff-Steinhauser, H., B. Berghmans, M. Spaanderman, and E. Bols. 2021. Prevalence, incidence and bothersomeness of urinary incontinence in pregnancy: A systematic review and meta-analysis. *International Urogynecology Journal* 32(7):1633-1652.

26. Mottola, M.F., M.H. Davenport, S.-M. Ruchat, G.A. Davies, V.J. Poitras, C.E. Gray, and A.J. Garcia. 2018. 2019 Canadian guideline for physical activity throughout pregnancy. *British Journal of Sports Medicine* 52:1339-1346.

27. National Institutes of Health, National Institute of Diabetes and Digestive and Kidney Disease. 2015. Symptoms and causes of diabetes. Accessed October 2022. www.niddk.nih.gov/health-information/diabetes/overview/symptoms-causes.

28. Neels, H., S. De Wachter, J.J. Wyndaele, T. Van Aggelpoel, and A. Vermandel. 2018. Common errors made in attempt to contract the pelvic floor muscles in women early after delivery: A prospective observational study. *European Journal Obstetrics Gynecology Reproductive Biology* 220:113-117.

29. Perales, M., R. Artal, and A. Lucia. 2017. Exercise during pregnancy. *JAMA* 317(11):1113-1114.

30. Plows, J.F., J.L. Stanley, P.N. Baker, C.M. Reynolds, and M.H. Vickers. 2018. *International Journal of Molecular Sciences* 19(11):3342.

31. Prevett, C., M.L. Kimber, L. Forner, M. de Vivo, and M.H. Davenport. 2022. Impact of heavy resistance training on pregnancy and postpartum health outcomes. *International Urogynecology Journal* 34:405-411. https://doi.org/10.1007/s00192-022-05393-1.

32. Romero-Gallard, L., O. Roldan-Reoyo, J. Castro-Piñero, O. Ocon-Hernandez, V.A. Aparicio, A. Soriano-Maldonado, M.F. Mottola, and L.E. May. 2022. Physical fitness assessment during pregnancy. *ACSM's Health & Fitness Journal* 26(5):84-90.

33. Schreiner, L., I. Crivelatti, J.M. de Oliveira, C.C. Nygaard, and T.G. Dos Santos. 2018. Systematic review of pelvic floor interventions during pregnancy. *International Journal of Gynaecology and Obstetrics: The Official Organ of the International Federation of Gynaecology and Obstetrics* 143(1):10-18.

34. Skow, R.J., M.H. Davenport, M.F. Mottola, G.A. Davies, V.J. Poitras, C.E. Gray, and A.J. Garcia. 2018. Effects of prenatal exercise on fetal heart rate, umbilical uterine blood flow: A systematic review and meta-analysis. *British Journal of Sports Medicine* 53:124-133.

35. Talasz, H., G. Himmer-Perschak, E. Marth, J. Fischer-Colbrie, E. Hoefner, and M. Lechleitner. 2008. Evaluation of pelvic floor muscle function in a random group of adult women in Austria. *International Urogynecology Journal Pelvic Floor Dysfunction* 19(1):131-135.

36. Tibaek, S., and C. Dehlendorff. 2014. Pelvic floor muscle function in women with pelvic floor dysfunction: A retrospective chart review, 1992-2008. *International Urogynecology Journal* 25(5):663-669.

37. Tsakiridis, I., S. Giouleka, A. Mamopoulos, A. Kourtis, A. Athanasiadis, D. Filopoulou, and T. Dagklis. 2021. Diagnosis and management of gestational diabetes mellitus: An overview of national and international guidelines. *Obstetrical and Gynecological Survey* 76(6):367-381.

38. Tsakiridis, I., E. Kasapidou, T. Dagklis, I. Leonida, C. Leonida, D.R. Bakaloudi, and M. Chourdakis. 2020. Nutrition in pregnancy: A comparative review of major guidelines. *Obstetrical and Gynecological Survey* 75(11):692-702.

39. U.S. Department of Health and Human Services. 2018. *Physical activity guidelines for Americans*. 2nd ed. https://health.gov/our-work/nutrition-physical-activity/physical-activity-guidelines/current-guidelines.

40. U.S. Department of Health and Human Services. 2018. 2018 Physical Activity Guidelines Advisory Committee scientific report. https://health.gov/our-work/nutrition-physical-activity/physical-activity-guidelines/current-guidelines/scientific-report#.

41. U.S. Department of Health and Human Services (HHS) and U.S. Department of Agriculture (USDA). 2020. Dietary guidelines for Americans, 2020-2025. www.dietaryguidelines.gov/.

42. Vermandel, A., S. De Wachter, T. Beyltjens, D. D'Hondt, Y. Jacquemyn, and J.J. Wyndaele. 2015. Pelvic floor awareness and the positive effect of verbal instructions in 958 women early postdelivery. *International Urogynecology Journal* 26(2):223-228.

43. Woodley, S.J., P. Lawrenson, R. Boyle, J.D. Cody, S. Mørkved, A. Kernohan, and E. Hay-Smith. 2020. Pelvic floor muscle training for preventing and treating urinary and faecal incontinence in antenatal and postnatal women. *The Cochrane Database of Systematic Reviews* 5(5):CD007471.

44. Wowdzia, J.B., and M.H. Davenport. 2021. Cardiopulmonary exercise testing during pregnancy. *Birth Defects Research* 113:248-264.

Chapter 20

1. American Diabetes Association. 2020. Obesity management for the treatment of type 2 diabetes: Standards of medical care in diabetes—2021. *Diabetes Care* 44 (Suppl. 1):S100-S110.

2. American Medical Association. 2013. Recognition of obesity as a disease. https://media.npr.org/documents/2013/jun/ama-resolution-obesity.pdf.

3. American Psychiatric Association. 2013. *Diagnostic and statistical manual of mental disorders: DSM-5*. 5th ed. Washington, DC: American Psychiatric Publishing.

4. Bassett, D.R., P.L. Schneider, and G.E. Huntington. 2004. Physical activity in an old order Amish community. *Medicine & Science in Sports & Exercise* 36(1):79-85.

5. Becker, A.E., D.L. Franko, A. Speck, and D.B. Herzog. 2003. Ethnicity and differential access to care for eating disorder symptoms. *International Journal of Eating Disorders* 33(2):205-212.

6. Bouchard, C., L. Pérusse, C. Leblanc, A. Tremblay, and G. Thériault. 1988. Inheritance of the amount and distribution of human body fat. *International Journal of Obesity* 12(3):205-215.

7. Brown, W.J., E. Kabir, B.K. Clark, and S.R. Gomersall. 2016. Maintaining a healthy BMI: Data from a 16-year study of young Australian women. *American Journal of Preventive Medicine* 51(6):e165-e178.

8. Catenacci, V.A., L.G. Ogden, J. Stuht, S. Phelan, R.R. Wing, J.O. Hill, and H.R. Wyatt. 2008. Physical activity patterns in the National Weight Control Registry. *Obesity (Silver Spring)* 16(1):153-161.

9. Cawley, J., and C. Meyerhoefer. 2012. The medical care costs of obesity: An instrumental variables approach. *Journal of Health Economics* 31(1):219-230.

10. Church, T.S., D.M. Thomas, C. Tudor-Locke, P.T. Katzmarzyk, C.P. Earnest, R.Q. Rodarte, C.K. Martin, S.N. Blair, and C. Bouchard. 2011. Trends over 5 decades in U.S. occupation-related physical activity and their associations with obesity. *PLoS One* 6(5):e19657.

11. Cunningham, J.J. 1991. Body composition as a determinant of energy expenditure: A synthetic review and a proposed general prediction equation. *American Journal of Clinical Nutrition* 54(6):963-969.

12. de Munter, J.S., P. Tynelius, C. Magnusson, and F. Rasmussen. 2015. Longitudinal analysis of lifestyle habits in relation to body mass index, onset of overweight and obesity: Results from a large population-based cohort in Sweden. *Scandinavian Journal of Public Health* 43(3):236-245.

13. de Zwaan, M. 2001. Binge eating disorder and obesity. *International Journal of Obesity and Related Metabolic Disorders* 25(Suppl 1):S51-55.

14. Deloitte Access Economics. 2020. The social and economic cost of eating disorders in the United States of America: A report for the Strategic Training Initiative for the Prevention of Eating Disorders and the Academy for Eating Disorders. www.hsph.harvard.edu/striped/report-economic-costs-of-eating-disorders.

15. Desilver, D. 2016. What's on your table? How America's diet has changed over the decades. www.pewresearch.org/fact-tank/2016/12/13/whats-on-your-table-how-americas-diet-has-changed-over-the-decades.

16. Donnelly, J.E., S.N. Blair, J.M. Jakicic, M.M. Manore, J.W. Rankin, and B.K. Smith. 2009. American College of Sports Medicine position stand. Appropriate physical activity intervention strategies for weight loss and prevention of weight regain for adults. *Medicine & Science in Sports & Exercise* 41(2):459-471.

17. Fontaine, K.R., and I. Barofsky. 2001. Obesity and health-related quality of life. *Obesity Reviews* 2(3):173-182.

18. Fryar, C.D., M.D. Carroll, and C. Ogden. 2012. Prevalence of overweight, obesity, and extreme obesity among adults: United States, trends 1960-1962 through 2009-2010. www.cdc.gov/nchs/data/hestat/obesity_adult_09_10/obesity_adult_09_10.pdf.

19. Garrow, J.S., and J. Webster. 1985. Quetelet's index (W/H2) as a measure of fatness. *International Journal of Obesity* 9(2):147-153.

20. Hall, K.D., G. Sacks, D. Chandramohan, C.C. Chow, Y.C. Wang, S.L. Gortmaker, and B.A. Swinburn. 2011. Quantification of the effect of energy imbalance on bodyweight. *Lancet* 378(9793):826-837.

21. Hamer, M., E.J. Brunner, J. Bell, G.D. Batty, M. Shipley, T. Akbaraly, A. Singh-Manoux, and M. Kivimaki. 2013. Physical activity patterns over 10 years in relation to body mass index and waist circumference: The Whitehall II cohort study. *Obesity (Silver Spring)* 21(12):E755-761.

22. Hankinson, A.L., M.L. Daviglus, C. Bouchard, M. Carnethon, C.E. Lewis, P.J. Schreiner, K. Liu, and S. Sidney. 2010.

Maintaining a high physical activity level over 20 years and weight gain. *JAMA* 304(23):2603-2610.

23. Heymsfield, S.B., D. Thomas, C.K. Martin, L.M. Redman, B. Strauss, A. Bosy-Westphal, M.J. Müller, W. Shen, and A. Martin Nguyen. 2012. Energy content of weight loss: Kinetic features during voluntary caloric restriction. *Metabolism* 61(7):937-943.

24. Hornbuckle, L.M., D.R. Bassett Jr., and D.L. Thompson. 2005. Pedometer-determined walking and body composition variables in African-American women. *Medicine & Science in Sports & Exercise* 37(6):1069-1074.

25. Krumm, E.M., O.L. Dessieux, P. Andrews, and D.L. Thompson. 2006. The relationship between daily steps and body composition in postmenopausal women. *Journal of Women's Health (Larchmont)* 15(2):202-210.

26. Kujala, U.M., T. Leskinen, M. Rottensteiner, S. Aaltonen, M. Ala-Korpela, K. Waller, and J. Kaprio. 2022. Physical activity and health: Findings from Finnish monozygotic twin pairs discordant for physical activity. *Scandinavian Journal of Medicine & Science in Sports* 32(9):1316-1323.

27. Ligibel, J.A., C.M. Alfano, K.S. Courneya, W. Demark-Wahnefried, R.A. Burger, R.T. Chlebowski, C.J. Fabian, et al. 2014. American Society of Clinical Oncology position statement on obesity and cancer. *Journal of Clinical Oncology* 32(31):3568-3574.

28. Liguori, G., ed. *ACSM's guidelines for exercise testing and prescription.* 11th ed. Philadelphia: Wolters Kluwer Health.

29. Locke, A.E., B. Kahali, S.I. Berndt, A.E. Justice, T.H. Pers, F.R. Day, C. Powell, et al. 2015. Genetic studies of body mass index yield new insights for obesity biology. *Nature* 518(7538):197-206.

30. Loos, R.J., and C. Bouchard. 2003. Obesity—is it a genetic disorder? *Journal of Internal Medicine* 254(5):401-425.

31. Loos, R.J.F., and G.S.H. Yeo. 2022. The genetics of obesity: From discovery to biology. *Nature Reviews Genetics* 23(2):120-133.

32. Maciejewski, M.L., D.E. Arterburn, L. Van Scoyoc, V.A. Smith, W.S. Yancy Jr., H.J. Weidenbacher, E.H. Livingston, and M.K. Olsen. 2016. Bariatric surgery and long-term durability of weight loss. *JAMA Surgery* 151(11):1046-1055.

33. Malik, I.-h.O., M.C. Petersen, and S. Klein. 2022. Glucagon-like peptide-1, glucose-dependent insulinotropic polypeptide, and glucagon receptor poly-agonists: A new era in obesity pharmacotherapy. *Obesity* 30(9):1718-1721.

34. Manore, M.M. 2015. Rethinking energy balance: Facts you need to know about weight loss and management. *ACSM's Health & Fitness Journal* 19(5):9-15.

35. Molé, P.A. 1990. Impact of energy intake and exercise on resting metabolic rate. *Sports Medicine* 10(2):72-87.

36. Montoye, H.J., H.C.G. Kemper, W.H.M. Saris, and R.A. Washburn. 1996. *Measuring physical activity and energy expenditure.* Champaign, IL: Human Kinetics.

37. Morgan-Bathke, M., S.D. Baxter, T.M. Halliday, A. Lynch, N. Malik, H.A. Raynor, J.L. Garay, and M. Rozga. 2022. Weight management interventions provided by a dietitian for adults with overweight or obesity: An evidence analysis center systematic review and meta-analysis. *Journal of the Academy of Nutrition and Dietetics* S2212-2672(22):00170-8.

38. National Center for Health Statistics. 2021. National Health and Nutrition Examination Survey 2017–March 2020 prepandemic data files development of files and prevalence estimates for selected health outcomes. *National Health Statistics Reports.* http://dx.doi.org/10.15620/cdc:106273.

39. Nielsen, S.J., and B.M. Popkin. 2003. Patterns and trends in food portion sizes, 1977-1998. *JAMA* 289(4):450-453.

40. Nielsen, S.J., A.M. Siega-Riz, and B.M. Popkin. 2002. Trends in energy intake in U.S. between 1977 and 1996: Similar shifts seen across age groups. *Obesity Research* 10(5):370-378.

41. Poslusna, K., J. Ruprich, J.H. de Vries, M. Jakubikova, and P. van't Veer. 2009. Misreporting of energy and micronutrient intake estimated by food records and 24 hour recalls, control and adjustment methods in practice. *British Journal of Nutrition* 101(Suppl. 2):S73-85.

42. Powell-Wiley, T.M., P. Poirier, L.E. Burke, J.-P. Després, P. Gordon-Larsen, C.J. Lavie, S.A. Lear, et al. 2021. Obesity and cardiovascular disease: A scientific statement from the American Heart Association. *Circulation* 143(21):e984-e1010.

43. Snow, V., P. Barry, N. Fitterman, A. Qaseem, and K. Weiss. 2005. Pharmacologic and surgical management of obesity in primary care: A clinical practice guideline from the American College of Physicians. *Annals of Internal Medicine* 142(7):525-531.

44. Stunkard, A.J., T.I. Sørensen, C. Hanis, T.W. Teasdale, R. Chakraborty, W.J. Schull, and F. Schulsinger. 1986. An adoption study of human obesity. *New England Journal of Medicine* 314(4):193-198.

45. Sundgot-Borgen, J. 1993. Prevalence of eating disorders in elite female athletes. *International Journal of Sport Nutrition and Exercise Metabolish* 3(1):29-40.

46. Thompson, D.L., J. Rakow, and S.M. Perdue. 2004. Relationship between accumulated walking and body composition in middle-aged women. *Medicine & Science in Sports & Exercise* 36(5):911-914.

47. Tremmel, M., U.G. Gerdtham, P.M. Nilsson, and S. Saha. 2017. Economic burden of obesity: A systematic literature review. *International Journal of Environmental Research and Public Health* 14(4):435.

48. Trumbo, P., S. Schlicker, A.A. Yates, and M. Poos. 2002. Dietary reference intakes for energy, carbohydrate, fiber, fat, fatty acids, cholesterol, protein and amino acids. *Journal of the American Dietetic Association* 102(11):1621-1630.

49. U.S. Department of Health and Human Services. 2018. *Physical Activity Guidelines for Americans.* https://health.gov/our-work/nutrition-physical-activity/physical-activity-guidelines/current-guidelines.

50. U.S. Department of Health and Human Services. 2020. *2020-2025 Dietary Guidelines for Americans.* www.dietaryguidelines.gov/resources/2020-2025-dietary-guidelines-online-materials.

51. Vimaleswaran, K.S., and R.J. Loos. 2010. Progress in the genetics of common obesity and type 2 diabetes. *Expert Reviews in Molecular Medicine* 12:e7.

52. Wing, R.R., and J.O. Hill. 2001. Successful weight loss maintenance. *Annual Review of Nutrition* 21:323-341.

53. Wing, R.R., and S. Phelan. 2005. Long-term weight loss maintenance. *American Journal of Clinical Nutrition* 82(1 Suppl.):222s-225s.

54. Wright, J., J. Kennedy-Stephenson, C. Yang, and C. Johnson. 2004. Trends in intake of energy and macronutrients—

United States, 1971-2000. *Morbidity and Mortality Weekly Report* 53(4):80-82.

Chapter 21

1. Alswat, K.A. 2017. Gender disparities in osteoporosis. *Journal of Clinical Medicine Research* 9(5):382-387.

2. American Association for Cancer Research. 2022. AACR Cancer Progress Report 2022: Supporting cancer patients and survivors. https://cancerprogressreport.aacr.org/progress/cpr22-contents/cpr22-supporting-cancer-patients-and-survivors/.

3. American Association for Cardiovascular and Pulmonary Rehabilitation (AACVPR). 2020. *Guidelines for pulmonary rehabilitation programs.* 5th ed. Champaign, IL: Human Kinetics.

4. American Association for Cardiovascular and Pulmonary Rehabilitation (AACVPR). 2021. *Guidelines for cardiac rehabilitation programs.* 6th ed. Champaign, IL: Human Kinetics.

5. American Cancer Society. 2022. Cancer facts & figures 2022. www.cancer.org/research/cancer-facts-statistics/all-cancer-facts-figures/cancer-facts-figures-2022.html

6. American College of Sports Medicine (ACSM). 2022. *ACSM's guidelines for exercise testing and prescription.* 11th ed. Philadelphia: Wolters Kluwer.

7. American College of Sports Medicine (ACSM). 2024. *ACSM's clinical exercise physiology*, 2nd ed., ed. W.R. Thompson and C. Ozemek. Philadelphia: Wolters Kluwer.

8. American Diabetes Association. 2018. Economic costs of diabetes in the U.S. in 2017. *Diabetes Care* 41(5):917-928.

9. American Diabetes Association. 2023. Standards of care in diabetes—2023. *Diabetes Care* 46(1):S1-S291.

10. American Heart Association. 2020. What is atherosclerosis? www.heart.org/en/health-topics/cholesterol/about-cholesterol/atherosclerosis.

11. American Lung Association. n.d. COPD trends brief. Accessed November 2022. www.lung.org/research/trends-in-lung-disease/copd-trends-brief.

12. American Lung Association. n.d. Lung disease lookup. Accessed November 2022. www.lung.org/lung-health-diseases/lung-disease-lookup.

13. American Lung Association. 2020. The basics of pulmonary rehabilitation. www.lung.org/lung-health-diseases/lung-procedures-and-tests/pulmonary-rehab.

14. Asthma and Allergy Foundation of America. 2015. Exercise-induced bronchoconstriction (asthma). www.aafa.org/exercise-induced-asthma/.

15. Asthma and Allergy Foundation of America. 2021. Asthma medications and treatment. www.aafa.org/asthma-treatment/.

16. Berman, L.B., and J.R. Sutton. 1986. Exercise and the pulmonary patient. *Journal of Cardiopulmonary Rehabilitation* 6:52-61.

17. Campbell, K.L., K.M. Winters-Stone, J. Wiskemann, A.M. May, A.L. Schwartz, K.S. Courneya, D.S. Zucker, C.E. Matthews, J.A. Ligibel, L.H. Gerber, et al. 2019. Exercise guidelines for cancer survivors: Consensus statement from International Multidisciplinary Roundtable. *Medicine & Science in Sports & Exercise* 51(11):2375-2390.

18. Centers for Disease Control and Prevention. 2020. 2019 National Health Interview Survey (NHIS) data. www.cdc.gov/asthma/nhis/2019/data.htm.

19. Centers for Disease Control and Prevention. 2022. About chronic diseases. www.cdc.gov/chronicdisease/about/index.htm.

20. Centers for Disease Control and Prevention. 2022. Cystic fibrosis. www.cdc.gov/genomics/disease/cystic_fibrosis.htm.

21. Centers for Disease Control and Prevention. 2022. National Diabetes Statistics Report. www.cdc.gov/diabetes/data/statistics-report/index.html.

22. Chobanian, A.V., G.L. Bakris, H.R. Black, et al., and National High Blood Pressure Education Program Coordinating Committee. 2003. Seventh report of the Joint National Committee on Prevention, Detection, Evaluation, and Treatment of High Blood Pressure. *Hypertension* 42(6):1206-1252.

23. Colberg, S.R., R.J. Sigal, J.E. Yardley, M.C. Riddell, D.W. Dunstan, P.C. Dempsey, E.S. Horton, K. Castorino, and D.F. Tate. 2016. Physical activity/exercise and diabetes: A position statement of the American Diabetes Association. *Diabetes Care* 39(11):2065-2079.

24. Eckel, R.H., J.M. Jakicic, J.D. Ard, J.M. de Jesus, N.H. Miller, V.S. Hubbard, I.-M. Lee, et al. 2014. 2103 AHA/ACC guideline on lifestyle management to reduce cardiovascular risk. *Circulation* 129(25):S76-S99.

25. Fletcher, G.F., P. Ades, P. Kligfield, R. Arena, et al. 2013. Exercise standards for testing and training: A scientific statement from the American Heart Association. *Circulation* 128:873-934.

26. Gerow, M. and P.J. Bruner. 2021 Exercise-induced asthma. www.ncbi.nlm.nih.gov/books/NBK557554/.

27. Global Initiative for Chronic Obstructive Lung Disease. 2022. Pocket guide to COPD diagnosis, management, and prevention: A guide for health care professionals. 2023 ed. https://goldcopd.org/2023-gold-report-2/.

28. 2Grundy, S.M., J.L. Cleeman, S.R. Daniels, K.A. Donato, R.H. Eckel, B.A. Franklin, D.J. Gordon, et al. 2005. Diagnosis and management of the metabolic syndrome: An American Heart Association/National Heart, Lung, and Blood Institute scientific statement (executive summary). *Circulation* 112:285-290.

29. Hirode, G., and R.J. Wong. 2020. Trends in the prevalence of metabolic syndrome in the United States, 2011-2016. *JAMA* 323(24):2526-2528.

30. Irwin, M.L., ed. *ACSM's guide to exercise and cancer survivorship.* 2012. Champaign, IL: Human Kinetics.

31. James, P.A., S. Oparil, B.L. Carter, W.C. Cushman, C. Dennison-Himmelfarb, J. Handler, D.T. Lackland, et al. 2014. 2014 evidence-based guidelines for the management of high blood pressure in adults: Report from the panel members appointed to the eighth Joint National Committee (JNC 8). *JAMA* 311(5):507-520.

32. Kohrt, W.M., S.A. Bloomfield, K.D. Little, M.E. Nelson, and V.R. Yingling. 2004 Physical activity and bone health. *Medicine & Science in Sports & Exercise* 36(11):1985-1996.

33. LeBoff, M.S., S.L. Greenspan, K.L. Insogna, E.M. Lewiecki, K.G. Saag, A.J. Slinger, and E.S. Siris. 2022. Consensus statement: The clinician's guide to prevention and treatment of osteoporosis. www.bonesource.org/clinical-guidelines.

34. Lloyd-Jones, D., N.B. Allen, C.A.M. Anderson, T. Black, L.C. Brewer, R.E. Foraker, M.A. Grandner, et al. 2022. Life's Essential 8: Updating and enhancing the American Heart Association's construct of cardiovascular health: A

presidential advisory from the American Heart Association. *Circulation* 146:e18-e43.

35. Lloyd-Jones, D., H. Ning, D. Labarthe, L. Brewer, G. Sharma, W. Rosamond, and R.E. Foraker. 2022. Status of cardiovascular health in US adults and children using the American Heart Association's new "Life's Essential 8" metrics: Prevalence estimates from the National Health and Nutrition Examination Survey (NHANES), 2013 through 2018. *Circulation* 146(11):822-835.

36. Martinez-Pitre, P.J., B.R. Sabbula, and M. Cascella. 2022. Restrictive lung disease. www.ncbi.nlm.nih.gov/books/NBK560880/.

37. Million Hearts. 2021. Estimated hypertension prevalence, treatment, and control among U.S. adults. https://millionhearts.hhs.gov/data-reports/hypertension-prevalence.html.

38. Moore, G.E., J.L. Durstine, and P.L. Painter, eds. *ACSM's exercise management for persons with chronic diseases and disabilities*. 2016. Champaign, IL: Human Kinetics.

39. National Center for Health Statistics. 2022. Leading causes of death. www.cdc.gov/nchs/fastats/leading-causes-of-death.htm.

40. National Center on Health, Physical Activity and Disability. n.d. Cancer. Accessed November 2022. www.nchpad.org/32/5699/Cancer.

41. National Heart, Lung, and Blood Institute. 2022. What are stents? www.nhlbi.nih.gov/health/stents.

42. National Institutes of Health: Consensus Development Panel on Osteoporosis Prevention, Diagnosis, and Therapy. 2001. Osteoporosis prevention, diagnosis, and therapy. *JAMA* 285(6):785-795.

43. National Institutes of Health: National Heart, Lung, and Blood Institute. 2022. Atherosclerosis: What Is Atherosclerosis? www.nhlbi.nih.gov/health/atherosclerosis/.

44. National Institutes of Health: National Heart, Lung, and Blood Institute. 2022. Cystic fibrosis. www.nhlbi.nih.gov/health/cystic-fibrosis.

45. National Institutes of Health: National Institute of Arthritis and Musculoskeletal and Skin Diseases. 2022. Osteoporosis. www.niams.nih.gov/health-topics/osteoporosis.

46. National Institutes of Health: National Institute on Aging. 2022. Osteoporosis. www.nia.nih.gov/health/osteoporosis.

47. National Library of Medicine. 2021. Chronic bronchitis. https://medlineplus.gov/chronicbronchitis.html.

48. Patel, A.V., C.M. Friedenreich, S.C. Moore, et al. 2019. American College of Sports Medicine roundtable report on physical activity, sedentary behavior, and cancer prevention and control. *Medicine & Science in Sports & Exercise* 51(11):2391-2402.

49. Pescatello, L.S., B.A. Franklin, R. Fagard, W.B. Farquhar, G.A Kelley, and C.A. Ray for ACSM. 2004. American College of Sports Medicine position stand: Exercise and hypertension. *Medicine & Science in Sports & Exercise* 36(3):533-553.

50. Petit, M.A., J.M. Hughes, and L. Scibora. 2014. Exercise prescription for people with osteoporosis. In *ACSM's resource manual for guidelines for exercise testing and prescription*, 7th ed., ed. D.P. Swain, 699-712. Baltimore: Lippincott Williams & Wilkins.

51. Ravn, P., M.L. Hetland, K. Overgaard, and C. Christiansen. 1994. Premenopausal and postmenopausal changes in bone mineral density of the proximal femur measured by dual-energy X-ray absorptiometry. *Journal of Bone and Mineral Research* 9(12):1975-1980.

52. Rock, C.L., C.A. Thomson, T. Gansler, et al. 2020. American Cancer Society guideline for diet and physical activity for cancer prevention. *CA: A Cancer Journal for Clinicians* 70(4):245-271.

53. Rock, C.L., C.A Thomson, K.R. Sullivan, et al. 2022 American Cancer Society nutrition and physical activity guideline for cancer survivors. *CA: A Cancer Journal for Clinicians* 72(3):230-262.

54. Sarafrazi, N., E.A. Wambogo, and J.A. Shepherd. 2021. Osteoporosis or low bone mass in older adults: United States, 2017-2018. NCHS Data Brief, no 405. Hyattsville, MD: National Center for Health Statistics.

55. Schmitz, K.H., ed. 2020. *Exercise oncology: Prescribing physical activity before and after a cancer diagnosis*. Cham, Switzerland: Springer.

56. Sin, D.D., N.R. Anthonisen, J.B. Soriano, and A.G. Agusti. 2006. Mortality in COPD: Role of comorbidities. *European Respiratory Journal* 28:1245-1257.

57. Thanassoulis G., and H. Aziz. 2022. Atherosclerosis. www.merckmanuals.com/home/heart-and-blood-vessel-disorders/atherosclerosis/atherosclerosis.

58. Thomas, R.J., A.L. Beatty, T.M. Beckie, et al. 2019. Home-based cardiac rehabilitation: A scientific statement from the American Association of Cardiovascular and Pulmonary Rehabilitation, the American Heart Association, and the American College of Cardiology. *Circulation* 140:e69-e89.

59. Tsao, C.W., A.W. Aday, Z.I. Almarzooq, A. Alonso, A.Z. Beaton, M.S. Bittencourt, A.K. Boehme, et al. on behalf of the American Heart Association Council on Epidemiology and Prevention Statistics Committee and Stroke Statistics Subcommittee. 2022. Heart disease and stroke statistics—2022 update: A report from the American Heart Association. *Circulation* 145:e153-639.

60. U.S. Department of Health and Human Services. 2018. *Physical activity guidelines for Americans*. 2nd ed. https://health.gov/our-work/nutrition-physical-activity/physical-activity-guidelines/current-guidelines.

61. Whelton, P.K., R.M. Carey, W.S. Aronow, D.E. Casey Jr., K.J. Collins, C. Dennison Himmelfarb, and S.M. DePalma. 2018. 2017 ACC/AHA/AAPA/ABC/ACPM/AGS/APhA/ASH/ASPC/NMA/PCNA guideline for the prevention, detection, evaluation, and management of high blood pressure in adults: A report of the American College of Cardiology/American Heart Association Task Force on Clinical Practice Guidelines. *Hypertension* 71:e13-e115.

62. Winnige P., R. Vysoky, F. Dosbaba, and L. Batalik. 2021. Cardiac rehabilitation and its essential role in the secondary prevention of cardiovascular diseases. *World Journal of Clinical Cases* 9(8):1761-1784.

63. World Health Organization. 2021. Cardiovascular diseases (CVDs). www.who.int/news-room/fact-sheets/detail/cardiovascular-diseases-(cvds)

64. Zhao, G., E.S. Ford, C. Li, and A.H. Mokdad. 2008. Compliance with physical activity recommendations in U.S. adults with diabetes. *Diabetic Medicine* 25:221-227.

Chapter 22

1. Buckworth, J., R.K. Dishman, P. O'Connor, and P. Tomporowski. 2013. *Exercise psychology*. 2nd ed. Champaign, IL: Human Kinetics.

2. Deci, E., and N.D. Ryan. 2008. Self-determination theory: A macrotheory of human motivation, development and health. *Canadian Psychology* 49(3):182-185. https://doi.org/10.1037/a0012801.

3. Dishman, R.K., and J. Buckworth. 1996. Adherence to physical activity. In *Physical activity and mental health*, ed. W.P. Morgan, 63-80. Washington, DC: Taylor & Francis.

4. Hagger, M.S., N.L.D. Chatzisarantis, and S.J.H. Biddle. 2002. A meta-analytic review of the theories of reasoned action and planned behavior in physical activity: Predictive validity and the contribution of additional variables. *Journal of Sport and Exercise Psychology* 24:3-32.

5. Joseph, R.P., C.L. Daniel, H. Thind, T.J. Benitez, and D. Pekmezi. 2016. Applying psychological theories to promote long-term maintenance of health behaviors. *American Journal of Lifestyle Medicine* 10(6):356-368. https://doi.org/10.1177/1559827614554594.

6. Keeley, R., M. Engel, A. Reed, D. Brody, and B.L. Burke. 2018. Toward an emerging role for motivational interviewing in primary care. *Current Psychiatry Reports* 20(6):41. https://doi.org/10.1007/s11920-018-0901-3.

7. Keller, C., B. Ainsworth, K. Records, M. Todd, M. Belyea, S. Vega-López, et al. 2014. A comparison of a social support physical activity intervention in weight management among post-partum Latinas. *Biomedical Central Public Health* 14(1):1-15.

8. King, A.C., J.E. Martin, and C. Castro. 2006. Behavioral strategies to enhance physical activity participation. In *ACSM's resource manual for guidelines for exercise testing and prescription*, ed. L.A. Kaminsky and K.A. Bonzheim, 572-580. Philadelphia: Lippincott Williams & Wilkins.

9. King, A.C., D. Stokols, E. Talen, G.S. Brassington, and R. Killingsworth. 2002. Theoretical approaches to the promotion of physical activity: Forging a transdisciplinary paradigm. *American Journal of Preventive Medicine* 23:15-25.

10. Kleis, R.R., M.C. Hoch, R. Hogg-Graham, and J.M. Hoch. 2021. The effectiveness of the transtheoretical model to improve physical activity in healthy adults: A systematic review. *Journal of Physical Activity and Health* 18(1):94-108. https://doi.org/10.1123/jpah.2020-0334.

11. Knapp, D.N. 1988. Behavioral management techniques and exercise promotion. In *Exercise adherence*, ed. R.K. Dishman, 203-236. Champaign, IL: Human Kinetics.

12. Kyllo, L.B., and D.M. Landers. 1995. Goal setting in sport and exercise: A research synthesis to resolve the controversy. *Journal of Sport and Exercise Psychology* 17:117-137.

13. Marcus, B.H., P.M. Dubbert, L.H. Forsyth, T.L. McKenzie, E.J. Stone, A.L. Dunn, and S.N. Blair. 2000. Physical activity behavior change: Issues in adoption and maintenance. *Health Psychology* 19:32-41.

14. Marcus, B.H., and L. Forsyth. 2009. *Motivating people to be physically active.* 2nd ed. Champaign, IL: Human Kinetics.

15. Markland, D., and L. Hardy. 1993. The exercise motivation inventory: Preliminary development and validity of a measure of individuals' reasons for participation in regular physical exercise. *Personality and Individual Differences* 15:289-296.

16. Marlatt, G.A., and J.R. Gordon. 1985. *Relapse prevention: Maintenance strategies in the treatment of addictive behaviors.* New York: Guilford Press.

17. Nigg, C., ed. 2014. *ACSM's behavioral aspects of physical activity and exercise.* Philadelphia: Lippincott Williams & Wilkins.

18. Orstad, S.L., K. Szuhany, K. Tamura, L.E. Thorpe, and M. Jay. 2020. Park proximity and use for physical activity among urban residents: Associations with mental health. *International Journal of Environmental Research and Public Health* 17(13). https://doi.org/10.3390/ijerph17134885.

19. Osuka, Y., S. Jung, T. Kim, Y. Okubo, E. Kim, and K. Tanaka. 2017. Does attending an exercise class with a spouse improve long-term exercise adherence among people aged 65 years and older: A 6-month prospective follow-up study. *BMC Geriatrics* 17(1):170. https://doi.org/10.1186/s12877-017-0554-9.

20. Prochaska, J.O., and B.H. Marcus. 1994. The transtheoretical model: Applications to exercise. In *Advances in exercise adherence*, ed. R.K. Dishman, 161-180. Champaign, IL: Human Kinetics.

21. Prochaska, J.O., and W.F. Velicer. 1997. The transtheoretical model of behavior change. *American Journal of Health Promotion* 12:38-48.

22. Rollnick, S., W.R. Miller, and C.C. Butler. 2007. *Motivational interviewing in health care: Helping patients change behavior.* New York: Guilford Press.

23. Ryan, R., C. Frederick, D. Lepes, N. Rubio, and K. Sheldon. 1997. Intrinsic motivation and exercise adherence. *International Journal of Sport Psychology* 28:335-354.

24. Sonstroem, R.J. 1988. Psychological models. In *Exercise adherence: Its impact on public health*, ed. R.K. Dishman, 125-153. Champaign, IL: Human Kinetics.

25. Stetson, B.A., A.O. Beacham, S.J. Frommelt, K.N. Boutelle, J.D. Cole, C.H. Ziegler, et al. 2005. Exercise slips in high-risk situations and activity patterns in long-term exercisers: An application of the relapse prevention model. *Annals of Behavioral Medicine* 30(1):25-35.

26. Teixeira, P.J., E.V. Carraca, D. Markland, M.N. Silva, and R.M. Ryan. 2012. Exercise, physical activity, and self-determination theory: A systematic review. *International Journal of Behavioral Nutrition and Physical Activity* 9:78.

27. Teixeira, P.J., E.V. Carraca, M.M. Marques, H. Rutter, J.M. Oppert, I. De Bourdeaudhuij, J. Lakerveld, and J. Brug. 2015. Successful behavior change in obesity interventions in adults: A systematic review of self-regulation mediators. *BMC Medicine* 13:84. https://doi.org/10.1186/s12916-015-0323-6.

28. Trost, S.G., N. Owen, A. Bauman, J.F. Sallis, and W.J. Brown. 2002. Correlates of adults' participation in physical activity: Review and update. *Medicine & Science in Sports & Exercise* 34:1996-2001.

29. U.S. Department of Health and Human Services. 2018. *Physical activity guidelines for Americans.* 2nd ed. https://health.gov/our-work/nutrition-physical-activity/physical-activity-guidelines/current-guidelines.

30. Whiteley, J.A., B.A. Lewis, M.A. Napolitano, and B.H. Marcus. 2009. Health behavior counseling. In *ACSM's resource manual for guidelines for exercise testing and prescription*, ed. J.K. Ehrman, 723-733. Baltimore: Williams & Wilkins.

31. Wilson, K., and D. Brookfield. 2009. Effect of goal setting on motivation and adherence in a six-week exercise program. *International Journal of Sport and Exercise Psychology* 7:89-100.

Chapter 23

1. American Diabetes Association (ADA). 2018. Low blood glucose (hypoglycemia). https://professional.diabetes.org/sites/professional.diabetes.org/files/pel/source/sci-advisor_2018_low_blood_glucose_hypoglycemia-newb-final.pdf.

2. American Heart Association (AHA). 2020. Highlights of the 2020 American Heart Association guidelines update for CPR and ECC. https://cpr.heart.org/-/media/CPR-Files/CPR-Guidelines-Files/Highlights/Hghlghts_2020_ECC_Guidelines_English.pdf.

3. American Red Cross (ARC). 2016. CPR/AED for professional rescuers: Participant's handbook. www.redcross.org/content/dam/redcross/uncategorized/6/CPro_PM_digital.pdf.

4. Anderson, J.C., R.W. Courson, D.M. Kleiner, and T.A. McLoda. 2002. National Athletic Trainers' Association position statement: Emergency planning in athletics. *Journal of Athletic Training* 37(1):99-104.

5. Anderson, M.K., and M.G. Barnum. 2022. *Foundations of athletic training: Prevention, assessment, and management.* 7th ed. Philadelphia: Wolters Kluwer.

6. Anzalone, M.L., V.S. Green, M. Buja, R.I. Harrykissoon, and E.R. Eichner. 2010. Sickle cell trait and fatal rhabdomyolysis in football training: A case study. *Medicine & Science in Sports & Exercise* 42(1):3-7.

7. Armstrong, A.B. 1984. Mechanisms of exercise-induced delayed onset muscular soreness: A brief review. *Medicine & Science in Sports & Exercise* 16(6):529-538.

8. Boden, B.P., K.M. Fine, T.A. Spencer, I. Breit, and S.A. Anderson. 2020. Nontraumatic exertional fatalities in football players, part 2: Excess conditioning kills. *The Orthopaedic Journal of Sports Medicine* 8(8):1-10.

9. Bosh, X., P. Esteban, and J. Grau. 2009. Rhabdomyolysis and acute kidney injury. *New England Journal of Medicine* 361:62-72.

10. Byrnes, W.C., P.M. Clarkson, J.S. White, S.S. Hsieh, P.N. Frykman, and R.J. Maughan. 1985. Delayed onset muscle soreness following repeated bouts of downhill running. *Journal of Applied Physiology* 59(3):710-715.

11. Cappaert, T.A., J.A. Stone, J.W. Castellani, B.A. Krause, D. Smith, and B.A. Stephens. 2008. National Athletic Trainers' Association position statement: Environmental cold injuries. *Journal of Athletic Training* 43(6):640-658.

12. Casa, D.J., S.A. Anderson, L. Baker, S. Bennett, M.F. Bergeron, D. Connolly, R. Courson, J.A. Drezner, E.R. Eichner, B. Epley, S. Fleck, R. Franks, K.M. Guskiewicz, K.G. Harmon, J. Hoffman, J.C. Holschen, J. Jost, A. Kinniburgh, D. Klossner, R.M. Lopez, G. Martin, B.P. McDermott, J.P. Mihalik, T. Myslinski, K. Pagnotta, S. Poddar, G. Rodgers, A. Russell, L. Sales, D. Sandler, R.L. Stearns, C. Stiggins, and C. Thompson. 2012. The inter-association task force for preventing sudden death in collegiate conditioning sessions: Best practices recommendations. *Journal of Athletic Training* 47(4):477-480.

13. Casa, D.J., and D. Csillan. 2009. Preseason heat-acclimatization guidelines for secondary school athletics. *Journal of Athletic Training* 44(3):332-333.

14. Casa, D.J., J.K. DeMartini, M.F. Bergeron, D. Csillan, E.R. Eichner, R.M. Lopez, M.S. Ferrara, K.C. Miller, F. O'Connor, M.N. Sawka, and S.W. Yeargin. 2015. National Athletic Trainers' Association position statement: Exertional heat illness. *Journal of Athletic Training* 50(9):986-1000.

15. Casa, D.J., K.M. Guskiewicz, S.A. Anderson, R.W. Courson, J.F. Heck, C.C. Jimenez, B.P. McDermott, M.G. Miller, R.L. Stearns, E.E. Swartz, and K.M. Walsh. 2012. National Athletic Trainers' Association position statement: Preventing sudden death in sports. *Journal of Athletic Training* 47(1):96-118.

16. Casa, D.J., and R.L. Stearns. 2015. *Emergency management for sport and physical activity.* Burlington, MA: Jones & Bartlett Learning.

17. Caterisano, A., D. Decker, B. Snyder, M. Feigenbaum, R. Glass, P. House, C. Sharp, M. Waller, and Z. Witherspoon. 2019. CSCCa and NSCA joint consensus guidelines for transition periods: Safe return to training following inactivity. *Strength and Conditioning Journal* 41(3):1-23.

18. Centers for Disease Control and Prevention (CDC). 2022. General information about MRSA in healthcare settings. www.cdc.gov/mrsa/healthcare/index.html.

19. Centers for Disease Control and Prevention (CDC). 2022. Handwashing in community settings. www.cdc.gov/handwashing/when-how-handwashing.html.

20. Centers for Disease Control and Prevention (CDC). n.d. Personal protective equipment (PPE) sequence. Accessed July 2023. www.cdc.gov/hai/pdfs/ppe/ppe-sequence.pdf.

21. Cheung, K., P.A. Hume, and L. Maxwell. 2003. Delayed-onset muscle soreness: Treatment strategies and performance factors. *Sports Medicine* 33(2):145-164.

22. Connolly, D.A., S.E. Sayers, and M.P. Mchugh. 2003. Treatment and prevention of delayed onset muscle soreness. *Journal of Strength and Conditioning Research* 17(1):197-208.

23. Covassin, T., and R.J. Elbin. 2010. The cognitive effects and decrements following concussion. *Journal of Sports Medicine* 1:55-61.

24. Eckner, J.T., and J.S. Kutcher. 2010. Concussion symptom scales and sideline assessment tools: A critical literature update. *Current Sports Medicine Reports ACSM* 9(1):8-15.

25. Faul, M., L. Xu, M.M. Wald, and V.G. Coronado. 2010. *Traumatic brain injury in the United States: Emergency department visits, hospitalizations and deaths 2002-2006.* Atlanta: Centers for Disease Control and Prevention, National Center for Injury Prevention and Control.

26. Gardner, J.W., and J.A. Kark. 1994. Fatal rhabdomyolysis presenting as mild heat illness in military training. *Military Medicine* 159:160-163.

27. Glover, J. 2016. *Sports medicine essentials: Core concepts in athletic training and fitness instruction.* 3rd ed. Clifton Park, NY: Thompson Delmar Learning.

28. Guskiewicz, K.M., S.L. Bruce, R.C. Cantu, M.S. Ferrara, J.P. Kelly, M. McCrea, M. Putukian, and T.C. Valovich McLeod. 2004. National Athletic Trainers' Association position statement: Management of sport-related concussion. *Journal of Athletic Training* 39(3):280-297.

29. Hainline, B., J. Drezner, A. Baggish, K.G. Harmon, M.S. Emery, R.J. Myerburg, E. Sanchez, S. Molossi, J.T. Parsons, and P.D. Thompson. 2017. Interassociation consensus statement on cardiovascular care of college student-athletes. *British Journal of Sports Medicine* 51(2):74-85.

30. Harmon, K.G., et al. 2013. American Medical Society for Sports Medicine position statement: Concussion in sport. *Clinical Journal of Sports Medicine* 23:1-18.

31. Harrelson, G.L., A.L. Fincher, and J.B. Robinson. 1995. Acute exertional rhabdomyolysis and its relationship to sickle cell trait. *Journal of Athletic Training* 30(4):309-312.

32. Jimenez, C.C, M.H. Corcoran, J.T. Crawley, W.G. Hornsby, K.S. Peer, R.D. Philbin, and M.C. Riddell. 2007. National Athletic Trainers' Association position statement: Management of the athlete with type 1 diabetes mellitus. *Journal of Athletic Training* 42(4):536-545.

33. McCrory, P., et al. 2013. Consensus statement on concussion in sport: The 4th International Conference on Concussion in Sport, Zurich, November 2012. *British Journal of Sports Medicine* 47:250-258.

34. McDermott, B.P., S.A. Anderson, L.E. Armstrong, D.J. Casa, S.N. Cheuvront, L. Cooper, L. Kenney, F.G. O'Conner, and W.O. Roberts. 2017. National Athletic Trainers' Association position statement: Fluid replacement for the physically active. *Journal of Athletic Training* 52(9):877-895.

35. National Athletic Trainers' Association (NATA). 2005. Official statement from the National Athletic Trainers' Association on community-acquired MRSA infections (CA-MRSA). www.nata.org/sites/default/files/MRSA.pdf.

36. National Collegiate Athletic Association (NCAA). *2014-2015 NCAA sports medicine handbook*, 25th ed., ed. J.T. Parsons. Indianapolis: Author.

37. Patricios, J.S., K.J. Schneider, J. Dvorak, et al. 2023. Consensus statement on concussion in sport: The 6th International Conference on Concussion in Sport, Amsterdam, October 2022. *British Journal of Sports Medicine* 57:695-711.

38. Prentice, W.E. 2014. *Principles of athletic training: A competency-based approach.* 15th ed. New York: McGraw-Hill Higher Education.

39. Prentice, W.E. 2020. *Essentials of athletic injury management.* 11th ed. New York: McGraw-Hill.

40. Roberts, O.W., L.E. Armstrong, M.N. Swaka, S.W. Yeargin, Y. Heled, and F.G. O'Connor. 2021. ACSM expert consensus statement on exertional heat illness: Recognition, management, and return to activity. *Current Sports Medicine Report* 20(9):470-484.

41. Sanders, M.E., ed. 2018. *ACSM's health/fitness facility standards and guidelines.* 5th ed. Champaign, IL: Human Kinetics.

42. Sayers, S.P., P.M. Clarkson, P.A. Pierre, and G. Kamen. 1999. Adverse events associated with eccentric exercise protocols: Six case studies. *Medicine & Science in Sports & Exercise* 31(12):1697.

43. Siegel, J.D., E. Rhinehart, M. Jackson, L. Chiarello, and the Healthcare Infection Control Practices Advisory Committee. 2019. 2007 guideline for isolation precautions: Preventing transmission of infectious agents in healthcare settings. www.cdc.gov/infectioncontrol/guidelines/isolation/index.html.

44. U.S. Preventive Services Task Force (USPSTF). 2016. Sickle cell disease (hemoglobinopathies) in newborns: Screening. www.uspreventiveservicestaskforce.org/uspstf07/sicklecell/sicklers.htm.

45. Walsh, K.M., B. Bennett, M.A. Cooper, R. Holle, V.A. Rakov, W.P. Roederll, and M. Ryan. 2013. National Athletic Trainers' Association position statement: Lightning safety for athletics and recreation. *Journal of Athletic Training* 48(2):258-270.

46. Ward, M.M. 1988. Factors predictive of acute renal failure in rhabdomyolysis. *Archives of Internal Medicine* 148(7):1553-1557.

Chapter 24

1. Abbott, A.A. 2013. Cardiac arrest litigations. *ACSM's Health & Fitness Journal* 17(1):31-34.

2. American College of Sports Medicine (ACSM). n.d. ACSM exercise professional licensure statement. Accessed November 20, 2018. www.acsm.org/get-stay-certified/policies-procedures/professional-licensure-statement.

3. American College of Sports Medicine (ACSM). 2009. Position stand. Progression models in resistance training for healthy adults. *Medicine & Science in Sports & Exercise* 41(3):687-708.

4. American Law Institute. *A concise restatement of torts.* 3rd ed. 2013. Compiled by E.M. Bublick and J.E. Rogers. St. Paul, MN: Author.

5. Americans with Disabilities Act. 2010. 2010 ADA standards for accessible design. www.ada.gov/2010ADAstandards_index.htm.

6. Americans with Disabilities Act of 1990 (original text). n.d. Accessed November 6, 2022. www.eeoc.gov/americans-disabilities-act-1990-original-text.

7. ASTM International. ASTM F1749. 2015. Standard specification for fitness equipment and fitness facility safety signage and labels. West Conshohocken, PA: ASTM International.

8. ASTM International. ASTM F2115. 2018. Standard specification for motorized treadmills. West Conshohocken, PA: ASTM International.

9. ASTM International. ASTM F3021. 2017. Standard specification for universal design of fitness equipment for inclusive use by persons with functional limitations and impairments. West Conshohocken, PA: ASTM International.

10. *Baldi-Perry v. Glenn Kaifas and 360 Fitness Center, Inc.* Complaint. Index No. 2010-1927, Supreme Court, Erie County, New York. February 19, 2010.

11. *Bartlett v. Push to Walk*, No. 2:15-cv-7167-KM-JBC, 2018 WL 1726262 (D. N.J., 2018).

12. Bergeron M.F., B.C. Nindl, P.A. Deuster, et al. 2011. Consortium for health and military performance and American College of Sports Medicine consensus paper on extreme conditioning programs in military personnel. *Current Sports Medicine Reports* 10(6):383-389.

13. *Bloodborne pathogens.* Occupational safety and health standards. March 6, 1992. 29 C.F.R. § 1910.1030. Accessed November 6, 2022. www.osha.gov/laws-regs/regulations/standardnumber/1910/1910.1030. OSHA Fact Sheet: www.osha.gov/sites/default/files/publications/bbfact01.pdf.

14. *Boggus obo Casey v. Texas Racquet & Spa, Inc.*, 2018 WL 3911090 (Tex. App., 2018).

15. Brathwaite, A., D. Davidson, and J.M. Eickhoff-Shemek. 2006. Recruiting, training, and retaining qualified group exercise leaders: Part I. *ACSM's Health & Fitness Journal* 10(2):14-18.

16. Brathwaite, A., and J.M. Eickhoff-Shemek. 2007. Preparing quality personal trainers: A successful pilot program. *Exercise Standards and Malpractice Reporter* 21(2):25-31.

17. Breach notification rule. Office of Civil Rights. 2013. Accessed November 7, 2022. www.hhs.gov/hipaa/for-professionals/breach-notification/index.html.

18. Bushman, B.A. 2014. Determining the i (intensity) for the FITT-VP aerobic exercise prescription. *ACSM's Health & Fitness Journal* 18(3):4-7.

19. Carper, D.L., and J.A. McKinsey. 2012. *Understanding the law.* 6th ed. Mason, OH: South-Western, Cengage Learning.

20. Casa, D.J., J.K. DeMartini, M.F. Bergeron, et al. 2015. National Athletic Trainers' Association position statement: Exertional heat illnesses. *Journal of Athletic Training* 50(9):986-1000.

21. *CDC injury research agenda 2009-2018.* 2009. National Center for Injury Prevention and Control. Accessed November 9, 2022. https://stacks.cdc.gov/view/cdc/21769.

22. *Chavez v. 24 Hour Fitness,* 189 Cal. Rptr. 3d. 449 (Cal. Ct. App., 2016).

23. Civil monetary penalties inflation adjustment under Title III. 2014. Accessed November 6, 2022. www.ada.gov/civil_penalties_2014.htm.

24. Clarkson, K.W., R.L. Miller, G.A. Jentz, and F.B. Cross. 2001. *West's business law.* 8th ed. St. Paul, MN: West.

25. *Corrigan v. Musclemakers, Inc.,* 258 A.D.2d 861 (N.Y. App. Div., 1999).

26. Cotten, D.J., and M.B. Cotten. 2019. *Waivers and releases of liability.* 10th ed. Statesboro, GA: Sport Risk Consulting.

27. *Covenant Health System v. Barnett,* 342 S.W.3d 226 (Tex. App. LEXIS 3665, 2011).

28. Craig, A., and J.M. Eickhoff-Shemek. 2009. Educating and training the personal fitness trainer: A pedagogical approach. *ACSM's Health & Fitness Journal* 13(2):8-15.

29. *Crossing-Lyons v. Town Sports International, Inc.,* No. L-2024-14, 2017 WL 2953388 (N.J. Super. Ct. App. Div., 2017).

30. Davidson, D., A. Brathwaite, and J.M. Eickhoff-Shemek. 2006. Recruiting, training, and retaining qualified group exercise leaders: Part II. *ACSM's Health & Fitness Journal* 10(3):22-26.

31. *Del Castillo v. Secretary, Florida Department of State,* 26 F. 4th 1214 (11th Cir., 2022).

32. *Diniro v. Aspen Athletic Club, LLC,* 173 A.D.3d 1789 (N.Y. App. 4th, 2019).

33. Dobbs, D.B. 2000. *The law of torts.* St. Paul, MN: West.

34. Dougherty, N.J., A.S. Goldberger, and L.J. Carpenter. 2007. *Sport, physical activity, and the law.* 3rd ed. Champaign, IL: Sagamore Publishing.

35. *Duncan v. World Wide Health Studios,* 232 S.2d 835 (La. Ct. App., 1970).

36. Eickhoff-Shemek, J. 2010. Treadmill injuries: An analysis of case law. *ACSM's Health & Fitness Journal* 14(1):39-41.

37. Eickhoff-Shemek, J.M. 2021. HIIT for clinical populations: Safety and legal liability issues for community fitness facilities. *ACSM's Health & Fitness Journal* 25(5):65-67.

38. Eickhoff-Shemek, J.M. 2022. Establishing safety policies and procedures for fitness assessments. *ACSM's Health & Fitness Journal* 26(5):100-102.

39. Eickhoff-Shemek, J.M., and A.C. Craig. 2017. Putting the new ACSM's pre-activity health screening guidelines into practice. *ACSM's Health & Fitness Journal* 21(3):11-21.

40. Eickhoff-Shemek, J.M., and D.L. Herbert. 2007. Is licensure in your future? Issues to consider—part 1. *ACSM's Health & Fitness Journal* 11(5):35-37.

41. Eickhoff-Shemek, J.M., and D.L Herbert. 2008. Is licensure in your future? Issues to consider—part 2. *ACSM's Health & Fitness Journal* 12(1):36-38.

42. Eickhoff-Shemek, J.M., and D.L. Herbert. 2008. Is licensure in your future? Issues to consider—part 3. *ACSM's Health & Fitness Journal* 12(3):36-38.

43. Eickhoff-Shemek, J.M., and H. Kim. 2022. Virtual fitness programs: Safety and legal liability issues to consider: Part 2. *ACSM's Health & Fitness Journal* 26(3):45-48.

44. Eickhoff-Shemek, J.M., and T. Topalian. 2022. Virtual fitness programs: Safety and legal liability issues to consider: Part 1. *ACSM's Health & Fitness Journal* 26(1):48-51.

45. Eickhoff-Shemek, J.M., B.J. Zabawa, and P.R. Fenaroli. 2020. *Law for fitness managers and exercise professionals.* Parrish, FL: Fitness Law Academy, LLC.

46. *Elledge v. Richland/Lexington School District Five,* LEXIS 108 (S.C. Ct. App. 2000).

47. Federation of State Medical Boards. Assessing scope of practice in health care delivery: Critical questions in assuring public access and safety. 2005. Accessed November 7, 2022. www.fsmb.org/siteassets/advocacy/policies/assessing-scope-of-practice-in-health-care-delivery.pdf.

48. Feeling the burn: At-home exercise injuries surge during the pandemic. 2021. Accessed November 7, 2022. www.medicareadvantage.com/news/covid-at-home-exercise-injuries-report.

49. First aid and CPR training for employees of fitness centers, Wis. DHS § 174.04 (1999).

50. *Goynias v. Spa Health Clubs, Inc.,* 148 N.C. App. 554 (N.C. Ct. App., 2002).

51. *Grebing v. 24 Hour Fitness,* 184 Cal. Rptr. 3d. 155 (Cal. Ct. App., 2015).

52. Head, G.L., and S. Horn. 1997. *Essentials of risk management: Vol. I.* 3rd ed. Malvern, PA: Insurance Institute of America.

53. Health studios; acquisition, maintenance, training, and use of automated external defibrillators; civil liability for emergency care or treatment; public safety requirements; waiver. Cal. Health & Safety Code § 104113 (2020).

54. Herbert, D.L. n.d. Recent verdict against personal trainer—lessons to be learned. CPH & Associates. Accessed November 4, 2022. www.cphins.com/recent-verdict-against-personal-trainer-lessons-to-be-learned/.

55. Herbert, D.L., and W.G. Herbert. 2002. *Legal aspects of preventive, rehabilitative and recreational exercise programs.* 4th ed. Canton, OH: PRC.

56. *Howard v. Missouri Bone and Joint Center,* 615 F.3d 991 (8th Cir., 2010).

57. *Jimenez v. 24 Hour Fitness,* 188 Cal. Rptr. 3d. 228 (Cal. Ct. App., 2015).

58. Kerr, Z.Y., C.L. Collins, and R.D. Comstock. 2010. Epidemiology of weight-training-related injuries presenting to the United States emergency departments, 1990 to 2007. *American Journal of Sports Medicine* 38(4):765-771.

59. Kruskall, L.J., M.M. Manore, J.M. Eickhoff-Shemek, et al. 2017. Drawing the line: Understanding the scope of practice among registered dietitian nutritionists and exercise professionals. *ACSM's Health & Fitness Journal* 21(1):23-32.

60. Kufahl, P. 2015. Woman's undiscovered death in steam room shows how routines should never become routine. *Club Industry.* Accessed November 7, 2022. www.clubindustry.com/blog/womans-undiscovered-death-steam-room-shows-how-routines-should-never-become-routine.

61. *Levy v. Town Sports International, Inc.*, 101 A.D.3d 519, 2012 LEXIS 8543 (N.Y. App. Div., 2012).

62. Ligouri, G., ed. 2021. *ACSM's guidelines for exercise testing and prescription.* 11th ed. Philadelphia: Wolters Kluwer.

63. *Lotz v. Claremont Club*, No. B242399, 2013 LEXIS 5748 (Cal. Ct. App., 2013).

64. *Miglino v. Bally Total Fitness of Greater N.Y., Inc.*, 20 N.Y.3d 342 (N.Y. App., 2013).

65. *Mimms v. Ruthless Training Concepts, LLC*, Case No. 78584 (Cir. Ct. of Prince William County, VA, 2008).

66. Moorman, A.M., and J.M. Eickhoff-Shemek. 2007. Risk management strategies for avoiding and responding to sexual assault complaints. *ACSM's Health & Fitness Journal* 11(3):35-37.

67. NSCA strength and conditioning professional standards and guidelines. 2017. *Strength and Conditioning Journal* 39(6):1-24.

68. *Ohio Board of Dietetics v. Brown*, 83 Ohio App. 3rd 242 (Ohio App. LEXIS 88, 1993).

69. Panish Shea & Boyle LLP announces record $39.5 million settlement for college student who suffered heat stroke during outdoor jogging class. 2021. Accessed November 6, 2022. www.businesswire.com/news/home/20210222005958/en/Panish-Shea-Boyle-LLP-Announces-Record-39.5-Million-Settlement-for-College-Student-Who-Suffered-Heat-Stroke-During-Outdoor-Jogging-Class.

70. *Pellham v. Let's Go Tubing, Inc.* 398 P.3d 1205 (Wash. Ct. App. 2017).

71. Perkins, J. September 19, 2019. Your fitness business suffered a data breach. Now what? IHRSA. Accessed November 7, 2022. www.ihrsa.org/improve-your-club/your-fitness-business-suffered-a-data-breach-now-what/.

72. *Proffitt v. Global Fitness Holdings, LLC, et al.* In: Herbert D.L. 2013. New lawsuit against personal trainer and facility in Kentucky—rhabdomyolysis alleged. *Exercise, Sports and Sports Medicine Standards and Malpractice Reporter* 2(1):1, 3-10.

73. Rhabdomyolysis lawsuit in Kentucky settled. 2013. *Exercise, Sports and Sports Medicine Standards and Malpractice Reporter* 2(4):58.

74. Riebe. D., B.A. Franklin, P.D. Thompson, et al. 2015. Updating the American College of Sports Medicine's recommendations for the exercise pre-participation health screening process. *Medicine & Science in Sports & Exercise* 47(11):2473-2479.

75. Rule 4759-2-01. Definitions. Ohio administrative code. Chapter 4759-2. November 30, 2019. Accessed November 7, 2022. https://codes.ohio.gov/ohio-administrative-code/rule-4759-2-01.

76. *Rutnik v. Colonie Center Court Club, Inc.*, 672 N.Y.S 2d 451 (1998 N.Y. App. Div. LEXIS 4845).

77. Sanders, M.E., ed. 2019. *ACSM's health/fitness facility standards and guidelines.* 5th ed. Champaign, IL: Human Kinetics.

78. *Santana v. Women's Workout and Weight Loss Centers, Inc.* (2001 Cal. App. LEXIS 1186).

79. *Scheck v. Soul Cycle*, No. 104046/10, 2012 LEXIS 3719 (N.Y. Misc., 2012).

80. Security of confidential personal information, FL Stat § 501.171, 2019. Accessed November 7, 2022. www.flsenate.gov/Laws/Statutes/2019/501.171.

81. Sitzler, B. NCAA addresses exertional rhabdomyolysis. February 1, 2018. Accessed November 7, 2022. www.nata.org/blog/beth-sitzler/ncaa-addresses-exertional-rhabdomyolysis.

82. *Stelluti v. Casapenn Enterprises, LLC*, 203 N.J. 286 (N.J. LEXIS 750, 2010). Accessed November 7, 2022. https://casetext.com/case/stelluti-v-casapenn-enterprises.

83. Summary of the HIPAA privacy rule. Office of Civil Rights. October 19, 2022. Accessed November 7, 2022. www.hhs.gov/hipaa/for-professionals/privacy/laws-regulations/index.html.

84. Summary of the HIPAA security rule. Office for Civil Rights. October 19, 2022. Accessed November 6, 2022. www.hhs.gov/hipaa/for-professionals/security/laws-regulations/index.html.

85. Taylor, J.L., D.J. Holland, J.G. Spathis, et al. 2019. Guidelines for the delivery and monitoring of high intensity interval training in clinical populations. *Progress in Cardiovascular Diseases* 62(2):140146.

86. *Thomas v. Sport City, Inc.* 738 So. 2d 1153 (La. Ct. App. 2 Cir., 1999).

87. Thompson, W.R., ed. 2010. *ACSM's guidelines for exercise testing and prescription.* 8th ed. Philadelphia: Lippincott Williams & Wilkins.

88. Thompson, W.R. 2023. Worldwide survey of fitness trends for 2023. *ACSM's Health & Fitness Journal* 27(1):9-18. .

89. *Vaid v. Equinox*, CV136019426, 2016, LEXIS 828 (Conn. Super. Ct. 2016).

90. van der Smissen B. 1990. *Legal liability and risk management for public and private entities. Vol. one*, § 2.111 inherent in the situation. Cincinnati, OH: Anderson Publishing.

91. van der Smissen, B. 1990. *Legal liability and risk management for public and private entities: Vol. two*, chapter 18. Cincinnati, OH: Anderson Publishing.

92. van der Smissen, B. 2007. Elements of negligence. In *Law for recreation and sport managers*, 4th ed., ed. D.J. Cotton and J.T. Wolohan, 36-45. Dubuque, IA: Kendall/Hunt.

93. Voris, H.C., and M. Rabinoff. 2011. When is a standard of care not a standard of care? *Exercise Standards and Malpractice Reporter* 25(2):20-21.

94. Warburton, D.E.R., S.S.D. Bredin, S.A. Charlesworth, et al. 2011. Evidence-based risk recommendations for best practices in the training of qualified exercise professionals working with clinical populations. *Applied Physiology Nutrition and Metabolism* 36:S232-S265.

95. What percentage of lawsuits settle before trial? What are some statistics on personal injury settlements? n.d. *The law dictionary. Your free online legal dictionary featuring Black's Law Dictionary.* 2nd ed. Accessed November 4, 2022. https://thelawdictionary.org/article/what-percentage-of-lawsuits-settle-before-trial-what-are-some-statistics-on-personal-injury-settlements/.

96. *York Insurance Company v. Houston Wellness Center, Inc.*, 261 Ga. App. 854 (Ga. Ct. App., 2003).

97. Zabawa, B.J., and J.M. Eickhoff-Shemek. 2021. *Rule the rules of workplace wellness programs.* 2nd ed. Chicago: American Bar Association.

INDEX

Note: The italicized *f* and *t* following page numbers refer to figure and tables, respectively.

ABOUT THE EDITOR

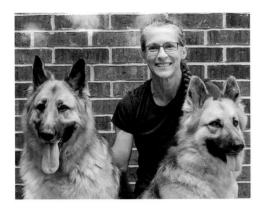

Barbara A. Bushman, PhD, FACSM, earned her bachelor's degree from Grand Valley State University and her doctorate from the University of Toledo. In 1995, she joined the faculty at Southwest Missouri State University in Springfield; the university name changed to Missouri State University in 2005. During her 27 years at Missouri State, she taught a wide variety of courses, both undergraduate and graduate, including anatomy, physiology, exercise physiology, sports conditioning, research methods, and health appraisal and exercise testing. She retired as a full professor in 2022 and is currently a faculty emeritus.

Dr. Bushman is a fellow of the American College of Sports Medicine (ACSM) and holds four ACSM certifications (Personal Trainer, Exercise Physiologist, Clinical Exercise Physiologist, and Program Director) in addition to the Exercise is Medicine Level 3 credential. She has been very active within ACSM, serving on the Membership Committee; Certification and Registry Committee; Women, Sport and Physical Activity Strategic Health Initiative; and Media Referral Network, among others. Within the Central States Chapter of ACSM she has served as president and secretary-treasurer and has served on several committees.

Dr. Bushman has been involved in numerous book projects, including being the lead author of ACSM's *Action Plan for Menopause*; associate editor of *ACSM's Resources for the Personal Trainer, Third Edition*; senior editor of *ACSM's Resources for the Personal Trainer, Fourth Edition*; and editor of *ACSM's Complete Guide to Fitness & Health, First Edition*, and *ACSM's Complete Guide to Fitness & Health, Second Edition*. She has been an associate editor of *ACSM's Health & Fitness Journal* since 2011 and writes the "Wouldn't You Like to Know" column, which covers a wide range of topics of interest to fitness professionals.

Over her lifetime, Dr. Bushman has maintained a regular exercise program; she enjoys running, cycling, and resistance training. Leisure pursuits include hiking, open-water kayaking, and, more recently, woodworking. She and her husband enjoy walks with their two German shepherds, who have been her faithful office companions during the work on this textbook.

ABOUT THE CONTRIBUTORS

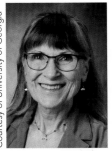
Courtesy of University of Georgia

Janet Buckworth, PhD, has several notable publications in exercise psychology, and is the lead author on the textbook, *Exercise Psychology*. She has been invited as a keynote presenter for several conferences on the subject. Dr. Buckworth completed her PhD in exercise psychology at the University of Georgia (UGA), an extension of her academic and professional backgrounds that include master's degrees in clinical social work and health education and work experiences in medical and college settings. Dr. Buckworth was a faculty member in exercise science at The Ohio State University and served in several leadership roles during her 18 years on the faculty. She was department head of kinesiology in the Mary Frances Early College of Education at UGA from 2014 to 2023. She is a fellow of the American College of Sports Medicine (ACSM) and served on the Behavioral Strategies Special Interest Group from 2002 to 2022.

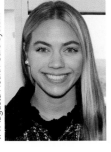
VA Augusta Health Care System

Lauren R. Chaney, PharmD, graduated from Ohio Northern University Raabe College of Pharmacy in 2021. After this, she completed 2 years of pharmacy residency at the Chillicothe VA Medical Center, where she specialized in psychiatric pharmacy. She now practices as a mental health clinical pharmacy specialist at Charlie Norwood VA Medical Center in Augusta, Georgia. Throughout her practice, she has conducted research and published articles focused on the topics of mental health and substance use disorders. Chaney's contributions to this text were done outside of her current employment and do not represent the views of the U.S. Department of Veteran's Affairs or the United States Government.

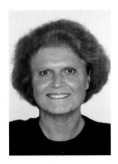

JoAnn M. Eickhoff-Shemek, PhD, FACSM, FAWHP, professor emeritus of exercise science at the University of South Florida and president of the Fitness Law Academy, LLC, is an internationally known author and speaker. For more than 35 years, her teaching and research have focused on fit-

ness safety, legal liability, and risk management issues. Dr. Eickhoff-Shemek is the lead author of a groundbreaking textbook, *Law for Fitness Managers and Exercise Professionals*, and coauthor of another textbook, *Rule the Rules of Workplace Wellness Programs*, published in 2020 and 2021, respectively. She was invited to be a contributing author for a resource widely used in Australia, *The Australian Fitness Industry Risk Management Manual*, published in 2014. Dr. Eickhoff-Shemek has authored several book chapters and authored or coauthored over 95 articles in refereed journals. She served as the legal columnist for *ACSM's Health & Fitness Journal* for 10 years (2001-2010) and currently serves as the fitness safety columnist for the same journal.

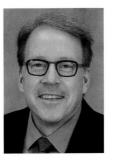

Avery D. Faigenbaum, EdD, FACSM, FNSCA, FNAK, is a full professor in the department of kinesiology and health sciences at The College of New Jersey. His research interests focus on resistance exercise, youth fitness, and long-term athletic development. He has coauthored over 250 scientific publications, 50 book chapters, and 10 books, including *Essentials of Youth Fitness*. He holds the Clinical Exercise Physiologist certification from the American College of Sports Medicine (ACSM) and Certified Strength and Conditioning Specialist credential from the National Strength and Conditioning Association (NSCA). Dr. Faigenbaum is a fellow of the ACSM, the NSCA, and the National Academy of Kinesiology. He was awarded the Lifetime Achievement Award from the National Strength and Conditioning Association in 2017.

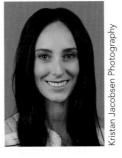
Kristan Jacobsen Photography

Tanya M. Halliday, PhD, RD, is an assistant professor in the department of health and kinesiology at the University of Utah. Her research program is focused on diet and exercise interventions for weight management and diabetes prevention with an emphasis on enhancing our understanding of appetite regulation. Before starting her faculty career at the University of Utah, Dr. Halliday completed postdoctoral research training at the University of Colorado's Anschutz Medical Center, her PhD at Virginia

Tech, her dietetic internship at the University of Houston, and her bachelor's degree at the University of Wyoming. Originally from Boston, Dr. Halliday has come to appreciate the Rocky Mountain region and enjoys hiking, trail running, skiing, and horseback riding in Salt Lake City and the surrounding Wasatch mountain range.

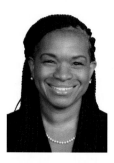

NiCole R. Keith, PhD, FACSM, FNAK, is a research scientist at Indiana University Center for Aging Research and Regenstrief Institute and a professor of kinesiology and executive associate dean at Indiana University School of Public Health Bloomington. She is a fellow of the ACSM and the National Academy of Kinesiology. She was the 2020-2021 president of ACSM and serves on several other ACSM national committees. In 2022 Dr. Keith served on the President's Council on Sports, Fitness & Nutrition Science Board, Physical Activity Midcourse Report focused on physical activity recommendations for older adults. She is a member of the National Physical Activity Plan Executive Committee. Dr. Keith examines ways to improve physical fitness and health as individuals age. She is dedicated to research that increases physical activity participation, improves fitness, and positively influences health outcomes for socioeconomically challenged community residents.

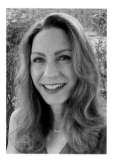

Laura J. Kruskall, PhD, received her master's degree in human nutrition from Columbia University, her PhD in nutrition from Pennsylvania State University, and is a fellow of both the ACSM and Academy of Nutrition and Dietetics (AND). In addition, she is a Registered Dietitian Nutritionist and holds the Certified Specialist in Sports Dietetics credential. She is an associate professor at University of Nevada, Las Vegas (UNLV), the founding director of the UNLV Nutrition Center, the founding director of the dietetic internship, and creator and graduate coordinator of the master's program in nutrition sciences. Dr. Kruskall created the existing nutrition sciences educational programs at UNLV and made it her mission over the last 23 years to be the driving force that makes UNLV Nutrition Sciences the primary source of newly credentialed nutrition and dietetic professionals in southern Nevada. Her areas of expertise are sport nutrition, weight management, and medical nutrition therapy.

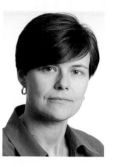

Clare E. Milner, PhD, FACSM, is an associate professor in the department of physical therapy and rehabilitation sciences at Drexel University in Philadelphia. Her research interests are in the biomechanics of lower-extremity injury, injury prevention, and rehabilitation. She focuses on overuse injuries in runners and the quality of walking and other activities of daily living in people with functional limitations. Dr. Milner teaches graduate courses in research methods and biomechanics. She is a fellow of the ACSM.

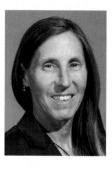

Jenny Moshak, MS, ATC, CSCS, is currently serving as the treasurer and board member of the College Athletic Trainers' Society. From 2014 to 2019 she provided rehabilitation and strength and conditioning services to the UMMC Basketball Club, a women's professional team in Yekaterinburg, Russia. She retired from the University of Tennessee in 2013 after a 24-year career leading the women's athletics sports medicine department, primarily working with Lady Vol basketball. Her vision led to the creation of Team ENHANCE, a nutritional, mental, and emotional wellness program that creates a healthy culture for Lady Vol student-athletes so they can succeed in their sports and in their lives. Moshak's book, *Ice 'n' Go: Score in Sports and Life*, released in 2013, presents a model for healthy living that focuses on physical, mental, and emotional development and tells her story of achieving her national championship as she discovers the thrills of the journey. She is an avid cyclist.

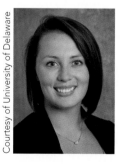

Courtesy of University of Delaware

Brittany Overstreet, PhD, ACSM-CEP, FACSM, is an assistant professor in the department of kinesiology and applied physiology at the University of Delaware. She holds the ACSM Clinical Exercise Physiologist certification. She earned her BS at Salisbury University (2011), MS at Ball State University (2013), and PhD at the University of Tennessee (2016). At the University of Delaware, she is the program director for the clinical exercise physiology graduate program, which was nationally accredited in 2022 through the Commission on Accreditation of Allied Health Education Programs. Dr. Overstreet has held several roles within ACSM, including being the secretary for MARC ACSM, member of the ACSM CCRB CEP committee, and member of the CEP/CPT Task Force. She is the current secretary and chair of the Clinical Exercise Physiology Association's (CEPA) Legislative Committee. Recently, Dr. Overstreet became a member of the American Heart Association's Executive Leadership Team for the Wilmington, Delaware, Heart Walk.

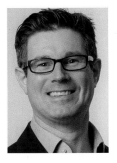

Brian Parr, PhD, FACSM, is a professor in the department of exercise and sports science at the University of South Carolina Aiken, where he teaches courses in exercise physiology, electrocardiography, clinical exercise physiology, and research methods. He also mentors undergraduate students in exercise science research. His current research interests include obesity, exercise, and functional limitations. Dr. Parr is a fellow of the ACSM and holds their Certified Clinical Exercise Physiologist credential.

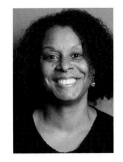

Erica M. Taylor, PhD, is the associate dean for health professions at Columbus State University in Columbus, Georgia. She holds a PhD in exercise science specializing in exercise psychology. Her research focused on physical activity and stress in Black women at increased risk for hypertension. Additional interests include promoting physical activity to address health disparities in women and racial minority populations. In addition to exercise psychology, Dr. Taylor has taught physical activity epidemiology, research methods, exercise for special populations, and exercise testing and prescription. She was a coauthor or contributing author for three editions of *Total Fitness and Wellness*, and she has contributed to revisions for other wellness texts and *ACSM's Clinical Exercise Physiology, Second Edition*. Dr. Taylor is active in ACSM, has been a fellow since 2009, and has served on the Board of Trustees. She enjoys spending time with her family and competing in road races and duathlons.

ABOUT
THE CASE STUDY CONTRIBUTORS

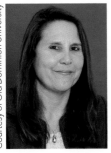

Sheri R. Colberg, PhD, FACSM, is a professor emerita of exercise science of Old Dominion University and an internationally recognized authority on diabetes and exercise. She is the author of 13 books, including *Exercise and Diabetes: A Clinician's Guide to Prescribing Physical Activity*, published by the American Diabetes Association (ADA) in 2013; *Diabetes & Keeping Fit for Dummies*, copublished by ADA and Wiley in 2018; and *The Athlete's Guide to Diabetes* in 2019. In addition, she has published 36 book chapters and over 400 articles, such as the latest ADA and American College of Sports Medicine (ACSM) position statements on physical activity and diabetes and Association of Diabetes Care and Education Specialists (ADCES) chapters and curriculum materials related to being active. She was honored with the 2016 ADA Outstanding Educator in Diabetes Award.

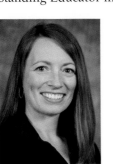

Margie Davenport, PhD, is an exercise physiologist and professor in the faculty of kinesiology, sport, and recreation at the University of Alberta. She holds the Christenson Professorship in Active Healthy Living and is director of the Program for Pregnancy and Postpartum Health (www.exerciseandpregnancy.ca). Dr. Davenport was the chair of the SOGC/CSEP 2019 Canadian Guideline for Physical Activity Throughout Pregnancy, the Get Active Questionnaire for Pregnancy, and the CSEP Pre & Postnatal Exercise Specialization.

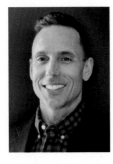

Nicholas H. Evans, PhD, received a BEd degree in exercise and sports science from the University of Georgia, an MHS in human movement studies from the Queensland University of Technology, and a PhD in applied physiology from the Georgia Institute of Technology. He currently holds dual positions at Shepherd Center in Atlanta in an outpatient neurorehabilitation program (Beyond Therapy) and in the Hulse Spinal Cord Injury Laboratory, where he serves as an exercise physiologist and research associate. In his clinical role, Dr. Evans has been involved in the programming and development of exercise and motor training interventions aimed at facilitating functional recovery and improving the health status of persons living with neurological injuries, including spinal cord injury and acquired brain injury. In his research role, he provides support for grant-funded studies investigating the effects of intensive exercise combined with neuromodulation technologies (e.g., transcranial direct current stimulation and transcutaneous spinal cord stimulation) with the goal of improving lower-extremity motor function and functional independence for persons with spinal cord injury.

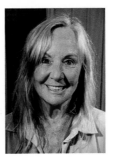

Carol L. Otis, MD, FACSM, is an internationally recognized primary care sports medicine physician, consultant, and advocate for women's issues. Dr. Otis worked as team physician and internist at UCLA (1982-2000) and as director of women's sports medicine at the Kerlan-Jobe Clinic (Los Angeles, 2000-2003), and is chairperson of the WTA Tennis Professional Development Panel (1994-present). She is the lead author of ACSM's Position Stand on the Female Athlete Triad (1997) and two articles on the WTA age eligibility and professional development programs (*British Journal of Sports Medicine*, 2006, 2022). Highlights of her international sports medicine experience include serving as physician for the 1984 Olympic Games (gymnastics), 2000 Olympic Games (U.S. tennis), U.S. Fed Cup teams, and WTA Championships (2002). She has been a physician for WTA (1998-2000), U.S. track and field, U.S. figure skating, UCLA athletic teams, NCAA Women's Volleyball Final Four, and a consultant to the LPGA and WTA on professional player development.

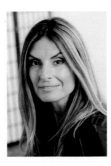

Tamara Rial, PhD, C-EP, CSPS, is a specialist professor in the department of health and physical education at Monmouth University, New Jersey. Her research interests focus on women's health, pelvic floor fitness, and hypopressive exercise. She holds the Certified Exercise Physiologist credential from the ACSM and the Certified

Special Population Specialist credential from the NSCA, and she is a certified yoga teacher. She is the author of several scientific publications and books. She is an internationally recognized speaker and has presented at conferences in Argentina, Canada, Mexico, Portugal, Spain, Brazil, the United Kingdom, and the United States.

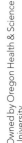

Kerri Winters-Stone, PhD, FACSM, is an exercise scientist and professor and section head of cancer population sciences in the division of oncological sciences at Oregon Health & Science University. She also is codirector of the Knight Community Partnership Program and coprogram leader of the Cancer Prevention and Control Program for the OHSU Knight Cancer Institute, an NCI-designated comprehensive cancer center. As a scientist, Dr. Winters-Stone's research focuses on the effects of cancer treatment on musculoskeletal health and cancer recurrence risk and on the ability of exercise to improve health and longevity in cancer survivors. Dr. Winters-Stone has been funded by the National Cancer Institute; National Heart, Blood, and Lung Institute; the American Cancer Society; and the Susan G. Komen for the Cure, Livestrong, and Movember foundations. She has conducted 14 controlled clinical exercise trials that have trained over 2,500 cancer survivors in different exercise modalities that are used as specific countermeasures to treatment-related toxicities. She has also co-led the update of the ACSM Exercise Guidelines for Cancer Survivors, released in October 2019.